PHARMACOLOGY
for Pharmacy Technicians

Kathy Moscou, RPh, MPH
Research Officer
Faculty of Health
York University
Toronto, Ontario, Canada
Former Director, Pharmacy Technician Program (1989-2006)
North Seattle Community College
Seattle, Washington

Karen R. Shipe, CPhT, MEd
Pharmacy Technician Program Coordinator
Department Head, Diagnostic and Imaging Services
Trident Technical College
Charleston, South Carolina

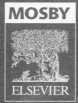

MOSBY

ELSEVIER

11830 Westline Industrial Drive
St. Louis, Missouri 63146

PHARMACOLOGY FOR PHARMACY TECHNICIANS

ISBN: 978-0-323-04720-3

Notice

Knowledge and best practice in this field are constantly changing. As new research and experience broaden our knowledge, changes in practice, treatment and drug therapy may become necessary or appropriate. Readers are advised to check the most current information provided (i) on procedures featured or (ii) by the manufacturer of each product to be administered, to verify the recommended dose or formula, the method and duration of administration, and contraindications. It is the responsibility of the practitioner, relying on their own experience and knowledge of the patient, to make diagnoses, to determine dosages and the best treatment for each individual patient, and to take all appropriate safety precautions. To the fullest extent of the law, neither the Publisher nor the Authors assumes any liability for any injury and/or damage to persons or property arising out of or related to any use of the material contained in this book.

The Publisher

Library of Congress Control Number 2008925496

Publishing Director: Andrew Allen
Acquisitions Editor: Jennifer Allen
Senior Developmental Editor: Ellen Wurm-Cutter
Associate Developmental Editor: Kelly Brinkman
Publishing Services Manager: Julie Eddy
Project Manager: Marquita Parker
Designer: Andrea Lutes

Printed in Canada

Last digit is the print number: 9 8 7 6 5 4 3 2 1

Reviewers

Terri L. Levien, PharmD
Clinical Associate Professor
Pharmacotherapy Department
College of Pharmacy
Washington State University Spokane
Spokane, Washington

Helene E. Benaim Hachuel, CPhT
New York, New York

Elizabeth E. Leavy, BA, BS, CPhT
PPMC Pharmaceutical Services
San Francisco, California

Marcy May, MAEd, CPhT, PhRT
Adjunct Faculty
Virginia College at Austin
Austin, Texas

Kelly Meyer, BS, CPhT
Cisco Junior College
Abilene, Texas

Teresa Lanette Moore, BS, PharmD
Albany Technical College
Albany State University
Albany, Georgia

Richard R. Nunez, BS, CPhT
California Board of Pharmacy
Certified Pharmacy Technician
Everest College
San Francisco, California

Kathleen M. O'Malley, CPhT
American Medical Careers
Flint, Michigan

Sherry Rodriquez, CMA
Kaiser Permanente
Oakland, California

Rebecca Schonsheck, BS, CPhT
High-Tech Institute
Phoenix, Arizona

John J. Smith, EdD
Corinthian College, Inc
Santa Ana, California

Sandra J. Tschritter, BA, CPhT
Spokane Community College
Spokane, Washington

Preface

The pharmacy technician profession is growing by leaps and bounds due to the increase in the number of prescriptions written, the aging of the population, and the increasing number of new pharmacies. The role of the pharmacy technician has expanded to address the growing need for pharmaceutical services coupled with increasing requirements for pharmacists to provide cognitive services and direct patient care. It does not matter what type of pharmacy setting one is employed, a basic understanding of pharmacology is needed to effectively assist the pharmacist in the dispensing of medications and education of the clients of the pharmacy. To this end, *Pharmacology for Pharmacy Technicians* seeks to provide the body of knowledge that would enable the pharmacy technician to understand the principles of pharmacology and apply them to the daily activities and challenges presented in all pharmacy practice settings.

BACKGROUND

This book was conceived by both a pharmacist and a pharmacy technician involved in the training of pharmacy technicians who saw the need for a comprehensive pharmacology text that would provide both knowledge and application to students in the field of pharmacy practice.

WHO WILL BENEFIT FROM THIS BOOK?

Pharmacology for Pharmacy Technicians will provide students with comprehensive coverage of pharmacology and also give the instructor the tools necessary to present this information in an effective manner. Today's pharmacy technicians are increasingly called upon to perform highly technical tasks that were previously the responsibility of the pharmacist. In all practice settings pharmacy technicians are required to perform their duties maintaining accuracy and professionalism. Given the volume of medication doses currently dispensed, pharmacy technicians need to understand the general principles of pharmacology to be able to assist the pharmacist in spotting medication errors, drug interactions, and therapeutic duplication. Knowledge of pharmacology will increase the pharmacy technician's brand/generic name recognition. Moreover, study of pharmacology will help pharmacy technicians identify appropriate warning labels to affix to prescription vials and can speed the process of identifying the drug requested for refill when the patient can't remember the drug name.

WHY IS THIS BOOK IMPORTANT TO THE PROFESSION?

Although there are many pharmacology texts on the market geared toward pharmacy technicians, this textbook seeks to go beyond the basic required knowledge to provide up-to-date drug information, tools to enhance learning, and tech alerts and tech notes that are key to preventing medication errors in a way that is easily understood and grasped by the reader.

ORGANIZATION

Pharmacology for Pharmacy Technicians is organized to support teaching of a 2-term (semester or quarter) pharmacology course. The pharmacology text is organized to provide an integrated approach to the understanding of pharmacology and pharmacotherapy. Unit 1 provides the basic foundation for understanding pharmacology. Unit 1 includes content on pharmaceutics, pharmacokinetics, and pharmacodynamics. Unit 2 through Unit 11 are organized according to body systems: Nervous System, Musculoskeletal System, Otic and Ophthalmic

System, Cardiovascular System, Endocrine System, Genitourinary System, Respiratory System, and Integumentary System. An overview of common disorders of each body system is described, including symptoms. This will help students understand why a given medication is useful for treatment of the condition. The mechanism of action for drugs is also presented. It builds on foundation knowledge presented in Unit 1 and aids in understanding pharmacotherapeutics. Duplicate entries of some drugs are found throughout the text for those that are prescribed for the treatment of more than one medical condition. The rationale for usage may differ according to the medical condition being treated. Each chapter contains a list of basic terminology, a chapter summary, review questions, and critical thinking exercises. Common endings of drugs classifications are provided to aid in memorizing drugs and their use.

DISTINCTIVE FEATURES

Pharmacology for Pharmacy Technicians makes extensive use of tables and figures to enhance learning. U.S. and Canadian brand names are provided for each generic name product. Available strengths and dosage forms are placed in tables along with photographs of many of the top 200 selling drugs to aid in product identification.

Additional unique features include common endings of drugs classifications, warning labels for every drug, Tech Alerts for drug look-alike and sound-alike issues, and Tech Notes for important need-to-know information. As compared to existing pharmacology books, *Pharmacology for Pharmacy Technicians* is comprehensive and contains hundreds of pharmaceuticals.

LEARNING AIDS

A variety of pedagogical features are included in the book to aid in learning:

- **Learning Objectives** listed at the beginning of each chapter clearly outline what students are expected to learn from the chapter materials.
- A list of **Key Terms** follows the Learning Objectives and identifies new terminology and makes it easier for students to learn this new vocabulary; learning this new terminology is vital to success on the job.
- **Tech Alerts** are found in the margins of the text and alert the student to drug look-alike and sound-alike issues.

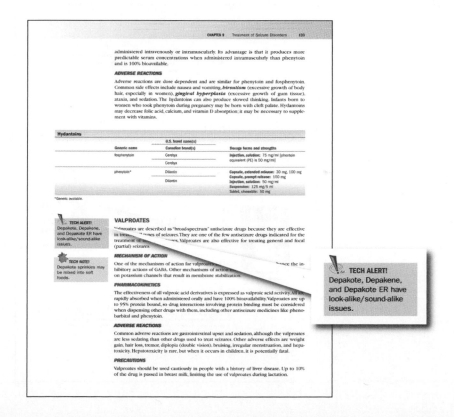

- Helpful **Tech Notes** are dispersed throughout the chapters and provide critical, need-to-know information regarding dispensing concerns and interesting points about pharmacology.

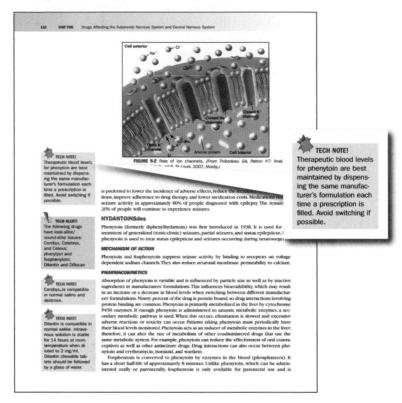

- **Mini drug monographs** with pill photos are provided in every body systems and drug classification chapter. These include generic and trade names, strength of medication, route of administration, dosage, and warning label.

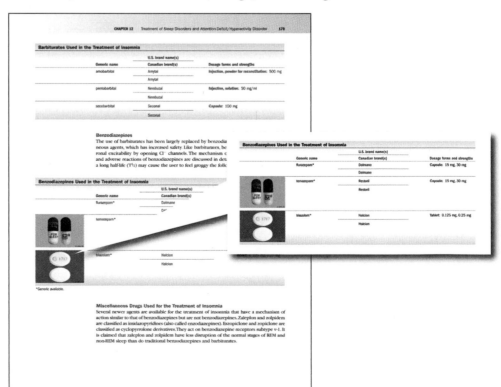

- A **Chapter Summary** is found at the end of each chapter and summarizes the key concepts of the chapter.
- **Review Questions** further enhance student review and retention of chapter content by testing them on the key content within the chapter.
- The Technician's Corner provides critical thinking exercises that help students prepare for on-the-job experiences by challenging them to pull together a collection of facts and information to reach a conclusion.

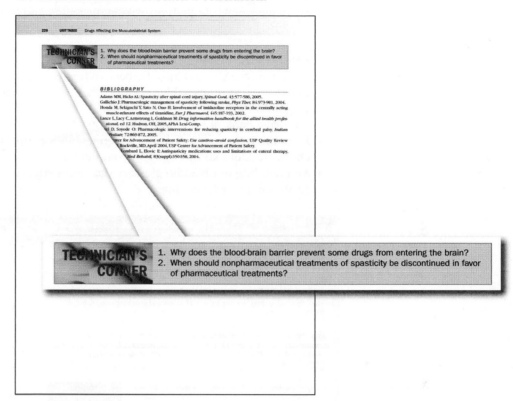

- The Bibliography provides a list of sources that students and instructors can use for additional information on the chapter's topic.

ANCILLARIES

For the Instructor
Evolve

We are offering several assets on Evolve to aid instructors:

- Test bank: an ExamView test bank of 700 multiple-choice questions that feature rationales, cognitive levels, and page number references to the text. This can be used as review in class or for test development.
- PowerPoint presentations: one PowerPoint presentation per chapter, these can be used "as is" or as a template to prepare lectures.
- Image Collection: all of the images from the book are available as JPGs and can be downloaded into PowerPoint presentations. These can be used during lecture to illustrate important concepts.
- Text Answer Key: All of the answers to the Review Questions and Technician's Corner questions from the text.
- Workbook Answer Key: All of the answers to the Workbook exercises.
- TEACH Online Pharmacy Technician Program Guide: assists instructors seeking to start or expand a pharmacy technician program.

- **TEACH:** including a lesson plans, lecture outlines, and PowerPoint slides, all available via Evolve. The TEACH Lesson Plan Manual provides instructors with customizable lesson plans and lecture outlines based on learning objectives. With these valuable resources, instructors will save valuable preparation time and create a learning environment that fully engages students in classroom preparation. The lesson plans are keyed chapter-by-chapter and are divided into 50-minute units in a 3-column format. In addition to the lesson plans, instructors will have unique lecture outlines in PowerPoint with talking points, thought-provoking questions, and unique ideas for lectures.

FOR THE STUDENT

COMPANION CD

The Companion CD, bound into the back of textbook, provides students with:

- Interactive exercises, which include drag and drop exercises and fill in the blank questions.
- An image bank of pill photos that shows the top 200 selling drugs.
- A comprehensive mock exam, which includes approximately 700 questions to check students' knowledge and comprehension.
- An English/Spanish audio glossary that helps students master key terms, while also reinforcing word meanings.

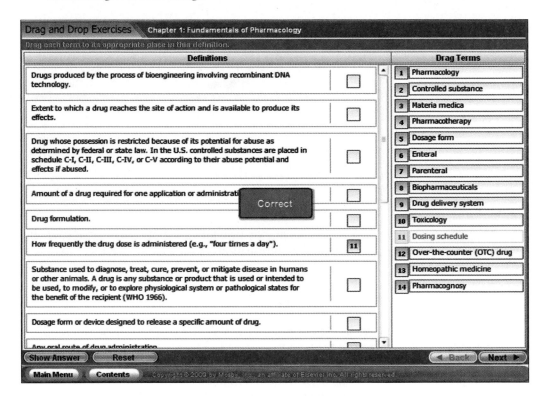

STUDENT WORKBOOK

The student workbook includes:

- Fill in the Blank Exercises, Multiple-Choice Questions, Matching Questions, and True/False Questions reinforce the concepts presented in the textbook.
- Internet Research Activities teach students how to keep current with an ever-changing industry.
- Critical Thinking Exercises help students apply the knowledge they learn in class to real-life scenarios, including testing knowledge of pharmacy calculations.

EVOLVE

The student resources on Evolve include:

- A comprehensive mock exam, which includes approximately 700 questions to check students' knowledge and comprehension.
- An English/Spanish audio glossary that helps students master key terms, while also reinforcing word meanings.
- Several appendices, which feature additional information relevant to pharmacology, including the top 200 selling drugs, the top 30 selling herbals, abbreviations commonly used in the pharmacy, and abbreviations that shouldn't be used.
- Weblinks, which link to places of interest on the web specifically for pharmacy technicians.
- Mosby's Essential Drugs for Pharmacy Technicians: detailed drug monographs, including full-color pill photos, for the top 200 dispensed drugs in the United States.

Note to the Student

Pharmacology for Pharmacy Technicians was created to provide pharmacy technicians with a strong foundation in pharmacology. As you proceed through this text you will notice that key concepts are repeated to reinforce learning. Review the Key Terms before you begin to read the chapter as this will help you better understand the chapter. The Chapter Summary provides a synopsis of key concepts in each chapter. You will want to refer often to the tables of brand and generic names. Knowledge of brand and generic names is critical for your profession. The drug photos of the top 200 selling drugs will help you learn to identify commonly prescribed medicines; familiarity with product appearance helps to reduce medication errors. You may also find this text useful in other pharmacy technician courses.

Acknowledgments and Dedication

The education of pharmacy technicians to assume ever expanding professional responsibilities has been the focus of most of my professional career. This book is dedicated to all of my former students at North Seattle Community College, whom I have challenged and hopefully inspired to achieve their best, for themselves and the profession. I dedicate this book to my husband, Gervan Fearon, who has supported me throughout the arduous process of writing this textbook, and my children, Gyasi and Chi Moscou-Jackson, who are on the cusp of starting their own professional careers. Finally, I would like to thank my co-author, Karen Snipe, for her enthusiasm and motivation throughout the writing of this book and the Pharmacy Technician Educators Council, and other organizations, for encouraging the development of instructional materials for pharmacy technicians.

— KATHY MOSCOU

I would like to thank my family, for without their continuous support, I would not have pursued this project. Thank you to my writing partner, Kathy, whose encouragement was priceless throughout this project. I dedicate this text to my pharmacy technician students for inspiring me to write teaching materials that are relevant and pertinent to their training.

— KAREN SNIPE

Contents

UNIT 1:   **Introduction to Pharmacology**

Chapter 1:   Fundamentals of Pharmacology, *2*
Chapter 2:   Principles of Pharmacology, *21*
Chapter 3:   Pharmacodynamics, *40*
Chapter 4:   Drug Interactions and Medication Errors, *53*

UNIT 2:   **Drugs Affecting the Autonomic Nervous System and Central Nervous System**

Chapter 5:   Treatment of Anxiety, *74*
Chapter 6:   Treatment of Depression, *86*
Chapter 7:   Treatment of Schizophrenia and Other Psychoses, *103*
Chapter 8:   Treatment of Parkinson's Disease and Huntington's Disease, *116*
Chapter 9:   Treatment of Seizure Disorders, *129*
Chapter 10:   Treatment of Pain, *144*
Chapter 11:   Treatment of Migraine Headache and Alzheimer's Disease, *163*
Chapter 12:   Treatment of Sleep Disorders and Attention-Deficit Hyperactivity Disorder, *175*

UNIT 3:   **Drugs Affecting the Musculoskeletal System**

Chapter 13:   Neuromuscular Blockade, *196*
Chapter 14:   Treatment of Muscle Spasms, *209*
Chapter 15:   Treatment of Autoimmune Diseases That Affect the Musculoskeletal System, *221*
Chapter 16:   Treatment of Osteoporosis and Paget's Disease of the Bone, *242*
Chapter 17:   Treatment of Hyperuricemia and Gout, *256*

UNIT 4:   **Treatment of Diseases of the Ophthalmic and Otic Systems**

Chapter 18:   Treatment of Glaucoma, *270*
Chapter 19:   Treatment of Vertigo and Other Disorders of the Ear, *281*
Chapter 20:   Treatment of Ophthalmic and Otic Infections, *292*

UNIT 5:   **Drugs Affecting the Cardiovascular System**

Chapter 21:   Treatment of Angina, *317*
Chapter 22:   Treatment of Hypertension, *332*
Chapter 23:   Treatment of Heart Failure, *360*
Chapter 24:   Treatment of Myocardial Infarction and Stroke, *371*
Chapter 25:   Treatment of Arrhythmia, *391*

UNIT 6:   Drugs Affecting the Gastrointestinal System

Chapter 26:   Treatment of Gastroesophageal Reflux Disease, Laryngopharyngeal
               Reflux and Peptic Ulcer Disease, *407*
Chapter 27:   Treatment of Irritable Bowel Syndrome, Ulcerative Colitis, and Crohn's
               Disease, *423*

UNIT 7:   Drugs Affecting the Respiratory System

Chapter 28:   Treatment of Asthma and Chronic Obstructive Pulmonary Disease, *443*
Chapter 29:   Treatment of Allergies, *461*

UNIT 8:   Drugs Affecting the Urinary System

Chapter 30:   Treatment of Prostate Disease and Erectile Dysfunction, *477*
Chapter 31:   Treatment of Fluid and Electrolyte Disorders, *490*

UNIT 9:   Drugs Affecting the Endocrine System

Chapter 32:   Treatment of Thyroid Disorders, *514*
Chapter 33:   Treatment of Diabetes Mellitus, *525*
Chapter 34:   Drugs That Affect the Reproductive System, *545*

UNIT 10:   Drugs Affecting the Immunological System

Chapter 35:   Treatment of Bacterial Infection, *578*
Chapter 36:   Treatment of Viral Infections, *601*
Chapter 37:   Treatment of Cancers, *624*
Chapter 38:   Vaccines, Immunomodulators, and Immunosuppresants, *649*

UNIT 11:   Drugs Affecting the Integumentary System

Chapter 39:   Treatment of Fungal Infections, *672*
Chapter 40:   Treatment of Decubitus Ulcers and Burns, *687*
Chapter 41:   Treatment of Acne, *700*
Chapter 42:   Treatment of Eczema and Psoriasis, *715*
Chapter 43:   Treatment of Lice and Scabies, *730*

Introduction to Pharmacology

CHAPTER

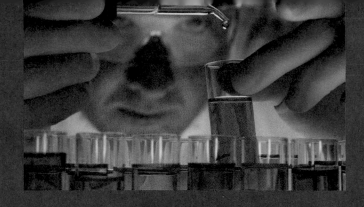

Fundamentals of Pharmacology

- Explain why the study of pharmacology is necessary for pharmacy technicians.
- Illustrate the global contribution to the knowledge of pharmaceuticals.
- Identify key legislation responsible for protecting public health and regulating drug distribution.
- Describe the drug approval process.
- Describe commonly dispensed dosage forms.
- Compare and contrast routes of drug administration.
- Learn the terminology associated with the fundamentals of pharmacology.

KEY TERMS

Bioavailability: Extent to which a drug reaches the site of action and is available to produce its effects.

Biopharmaceuticals: Drugs produced by the process of bioengineering involving recombinant DNA technology.

Controlled substance: Drug whose possession is restricted because of its potential for abuse as determined by federal or state law. Controlled substances are placed in schedule C-I, C-II, C-III, C-IV, or C-V according to their abuse potential and effects if abused.

Dosage form: Drug formulation.

Dose: Amount of a drug required for one application or administration.

Dosing schedule: How frequently the drug dose is administered (e.g., "four times a day")

Drug: Substance used to diagnose, treat, cure, prevent, or mitigate disease in humans or other animals. A drug is any substance or product that is used or intended to be used, to modify, or to explore physiological system or pathological states for the benefit of the recipient (WHO, 1966).

Drug delivery system: Dosage form or device designed to release a specific amount of drug.

Enteral: Any oral route of drug administration.

Homeopathic medicine: Drugs that are administered in minute quantities and stimulate natural body healing systems.

Legend drug: Drug that is required by state or federal law to be dispensed by a prescription only. Prescriptions must be written for a legitimate medical condition and issued by a practitioner authorized to prescribe.

Materia medica: Medicinal materials.

Over-the-counter (OTC) drug: Drug that may be obtained without a prescription.

Parenteral: Drug dosage form that is administered by injection or infusion.

Pharmacognosy: Science dealing with the biologic, biochemical features of natural drugs and their constituents. It is the study of drugs of plant and animal origins.

Pharmacology: Study of drugs and their interactions with living systems including chemical and physical properties, toxicology, and therapeutics.

Pharmacotherapy: Use of drugs in the treatment of disease.

Toxicology: Science dealing with the study of poisons.

Pharmacology is the study of drugs and their interactions with living systems including chemical and physical properties, toxicology, and therapeutics. Knowledge of *pharmacology* is essential to the accurate, effective, and efficient performance of the responsibilities of pharmacy technicians. Pharmacy technicians educated in pharmacology have the skills to properly identify the drug from a patient's profile when refills are requested and the patient does not remember the drug name. Less time is spent searching for drugs when pharmacy technicians have good brand/generic name recognition. Pharmacy technicians possessing a substantial knowledge of pharmacology may be able to reduce dispensing errors associated with look-alike or sound-alike drugs, incorrect drug or strength, incorrect dosage form, and improper dosing schedule. Knowledge of pharmacology facilitates selection of warning labels for drugs dispensed. Pharmacy technicians who possess a good knowledge of pharmacology understand the importance of recognizing drug interactions, therapeutic duplication, and excessive dose alerts screened by the computer. Overall, pharmacy technicians who have a working knowledge of pharmacology can perform duties, within their scope of practice, with greater independence.

History of Medicines and Their Use

Plants have been collected, cultivated, and harvested for their healing properties and used in the treatment of illness for centuries. Contributors to the current knowledge about drugs span the globe. Records dating as early as 3000 BC document the pharmacological knowledge by the people of ancient Egypt, Mesopotamia, India, and China. *Papyrus Ebers* (1550 BC), which was found in Egypt and describes more than 700 medical compounds and lists more than 811 prescriptions, is thought to be a copy of an ancient manuscript that dates to 3000 BC. More than 800 clay tablets have been unearthed describing more than 500 remedies in Mesopotamia (Persian Gulf 2500 BC), and Emperor Shen Nung is credited with writing *Pen T'sao Ching* (2750 BC), in which more than 1000 medicinal compounds are described and 11,000 prescription remedies are listed. The *Dravyaguna* (2500 BC) is an ancient Aryuvedic manuscript (India) of *materia medica* (medicinal materials) and includes sources, descriptions, criteria for identification, properties, methods for preparation, and therapeutic uses of hundreds of medicinal herbs. Some of the medicinal compounds described in these ancient manuscripts are still used today for essentially the same purposes. For example, castor oil and tincture opii were described in *Papyrus Ebers.*

Theophratus (300 BC), the "father of pharmacology," was a Greek physician known for his accurate observation of medicinal plants. By the first century, Discorides, another Greek physician, described approximately 600 medicinal plants in *De Materia Medica.* Aloe, belladonna, ergot, and opium are a few of the medicines described in the manuscript that are still in use today.

Since the 20th century, research into medicines and the introduction of new drugs and vaccines have grown exponentially. Antiinfective agents; the discovery of insulin and its use for the treatment of diabetes; and antiretroviral drugs for the treatment of HIV/AIDS were all discovered between the 1930s and present time. The Human Genome Project, a study of human genes, has provided data useful in understanding diseases that are caused by genetic defects or are linked to heredity. The study of genes has also enabled scientists to develop new genetically modified drugs, such as human insulin. Bioengineering is the process used to produce *biopharmaceuticals*. Erythropoietin and human insulin are examples of biopharmaceuticals.

Pharmacology Timeline

3000 BC   Imhoptep, Egyptian god of medicine

2750 BC   Emperor Shen Nung (China) is credited with writing *Pen T'sao Ching*. More than 1000 medicinal compounds are described and 11,000 prescription remedies are listed.

2500 BC   More than 800 clay tablets have been unearthed in Mesopotamia, describing greater than 500 remedies.

2500 BC   The *Dravyaguna*, an ancient Aryuvedic manuscript of medicinal materials, sources, descriptions, criteria for identification, properties, methods for preparation and therapeutic uses of hundreds of medicinal herbs is written in India.

1550 BC   *Papyrus Ebers*, thought to be a copy of an ancient Egyptian manuscript that dates back to 3000 BC, describes more than 700 medical compounds and lists greater than 811 prescriptions.

1000 BC   Charaka described more than 2000 medicinal substances (including mercury compound,e.g., merthiolate), methods to improve palatability and metrology (measurements and dosages).

400 BC   Hippocrates ("Father of Medicine")

300 BC   Theophratus, the "father of pharmacology," was a Greek physician known for his accurate observation of medicinal plants.

AD 100   Dioscorides, the "Father of Pharmacology," botanist and pharmacologist, authored *"Dioscorides Herbal"*.

AD 120 to 200   Galen, the "Father of Pharmacotherapy," promoted Humoral theory, the dominant theory of disease and treatment for 1500+ years. Illness is caused by an imbalance of 'humors' and is treated with Simples, Compostites, and Entities.

AD 1000   Avicenna Ibn Sina, known as the "Persian Galen," whose writings unified pharmaceutical and medicinal knowledge of his time and teachings were accepted in West until the 17th Century.

AD 1500s   Paracelsus, "Father of the Pharmaceutical Revolution," promoted the concept that disease is a chemical abnormality to be treated with chemicals. Introduced laudanum, a drug derived from opium that deadens pain.

AD 1500s   Indians of the Americas had pharmacological knowledge of up to 1200 plants including:
- W Indies: guaiacum (evergreen tree)
- S America: cocaine (coca leaves), curare
- Mexico: jalap (laxative)
- Peru: quinine (chinchona)
- Brazil: balsam Tolu (expectorant)

AD 1700s   William Withering (United Kingdom) isolated digitalis from foxglove.
Edward Jenner (United Kingdom) vaccine against cowpox. His research led to the development of the smallpox vaccine.
Bernard Courtois (France) discovered iodine, used to treat goiter and to decrease mucus (mucolytic).
Joseph Caventou and Pierre Pelletier (France) discovered quinine, which is used to treat malaria.
Johannes Buchner (Germany) identified salicin from willow bark (ASA) and nicotine in tobacco (niacin).
Emil von Behring (Germany) worked with antitoxins resulted in diphtheria and tetanus vaccine.
Gregor Mendel (Austria), a famous scientist and monk, discovered the basis of genetics and how genes are woven into heredity.

1800s   Frederich Serturner (Germany) extracted morphone from opium.
Louis Pasteur's experiments showing that microorganisms can cause disease and heat can kill them became the basis of "germ theory."

1900s   Frederick Banting and Charles Best (Canada) discovered that insulin lowers blood sugar levels and can be used to treat diabetes.
Gerhardt Domagk (Germany) introduced the sulfonamide prontosil, the first antiinfective agent.
Alexander Fleming (United Kingdom) discovers penicillin, a chemical produced by a fungus.
Beyer (United States), instrumental in the development of thiazide diuretics, derivatives of sulfonamides and other drugs.

Pharmacology timeline.

Origin of Drugs

Pharmacognosy, a term derived from the Greek words *pharmakon* ("drug") and *gnosis* ("knowledge"), is the branch of science dealing with the study of the natural origin of drugs. Pharmacognosy is the study of the constituents of natural drugs that are responsible for their effects. A *drug* is a substance that affects the normal function or structure of humans or animals and may be used to diagnose, treat, mitigate, cure, or prevent disease. Drugs may come from natural or synthetic origins. Natural drugs may be derived from plants (e.g., digitalis, quinine), animals (e.g., thyroid USP, pepsin), or minerals (e.g., silver nitrate). Some natural drugs are administered in their crude form; however, most frequently, the chief active ingredient(s) are extracted from the crude source.

Synthetic drugs may be a chemical modification of a natural drug or manufactured entirely from chemical ingredients unrelated to the natural drug. The synthetic drug may be equally potent or more potent to the natural drug. Fentanyl is a synthetically manufactured analgesic that is more potent than the natural drug, morphine (a naturally derived analgesic from the opium poppy). Drugs may also be produced via the process of bioengineering. Drugs produced via bioengineering are called *biopharmaceuticals*. Erythropoietin and human insulin are examples of biopharmaceuticals.

What Is Pharmacology?

Pharmacognosy and pharmacology are both sciences that involve the study of medicinal substances, however, the science of *pharmacology* involves the action of drugs on humans and animals. The aim of drug therapy is to diagnose, treat, cure, or lessen the symptoms of disease. The study of pharmacology applies knowledge of properties of drugs, mechanism of drug action, anatomy and physiology, and pathology. Selection of the appropriate drug for a patient in the proper *dose* and dosage form, administered at an appropriate *dosing schedule,* requires knowledge of pharmacology. The drug dose is the amount of drug units given for a single administration (e.g., two tablets). The dosing schedule is the number of times the drug dose is administered per day.

RESEARCH AND DEVELOPMENT

In 1906, the Pure Food and Drug Act was passed to protect the public from ineffective and harmful drugs. This act was expanded in 1938 and standards for allowing new drugs onto the market were set. Today, it can take several years to move a new drug from the idea phase to making it available to the public. Thousands of chemical compounds may be tested before one is discovered that can produce the desired effects with an acceptable level of adverse effects.

There are many steps in the drug development process (Figure 1-1). The steps from the test tube to production and distribution of a new drug involve preclinical research, clinical studies, new drug application process, and review. Manufacturers of new drugs must submit data showing that their drug is reasonably safe before preliminary small-scale clinical

TECH NOTE!
Some common beverages and foods are natural drugs. Coffee and tea contain the drug caffeine. Ginger and peppermint contain ingredients that can reduce nausea.

Drugs and Their Sources

Classification	Source	Generic name	Use
Plant	Foxglove	Digitalis	Heart failure (CHF)
	Chinchona	Quinine	Malaria
	Opium poppy	Morphine	Pain
Animal	Thyroid gland	Thyroid, USP	Hypothyroidism
	Pancreas	Pancreatin	Digestive aid
Mineral	Silver	Silver sulfidiazine	Burns (antiinfective)
	Gold	Auranofin	Arthritis
Synthetic	Synthetic opioid	Fentanyl	Pain
	Red azo dye	Sulfonamides	Infection
Bioengineering (recombinant DNA technology)	Isolated DNA + *Escherichia coli* bacteria	Hepatitis B vaccine	Hepatitis B prevention
		Human insulin	Diabetes mellitus

Source of Hepatitis B vaccine is viral DNA copied into a yeast cell.
Source of Human insulin is isolated DNA + *Escherichia coli* bacteria.

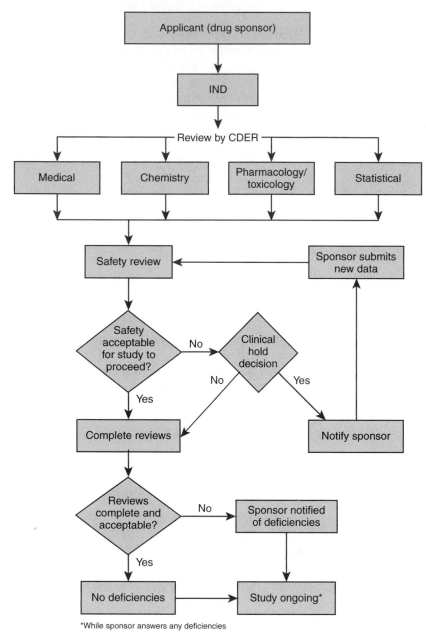

FIGURE 1-1 Investigational new drug process.

study is approved. Preclinical research is conducted to determine a pharmacological profile for the drug and acute toxicity of the drug in at least two species of animals. Upon completion of the preclinical phase, drug manufacturers file an Investigational New Drug (IND) application. Only approved investigational new drugs move to the clinical study phase.

There are three clinical study phases (Figure 1-2). In Phase 1 clinical trials, the drug is administered to a small number of healthy volunteers who are enrolled in the clinical study. Preliminary information about the drug's pharmacology, mechanism of action, and effectiveness in humans is gathered in Phase 1. If appropriate, the drug enters Phase 2 clinical studies. Phase 2 studies are controlled trials with a limited number of patients with the condition to be treated. During this phase, data are collected to determine the drug's effectiveness and the drug's side effects in patients with the disease. Phase 3 clinical studies involve many more patients. Drug safety is evaluated and the benefit of taking the drug is compared with the risks associated with taking the drug. If safety and effectiveness are

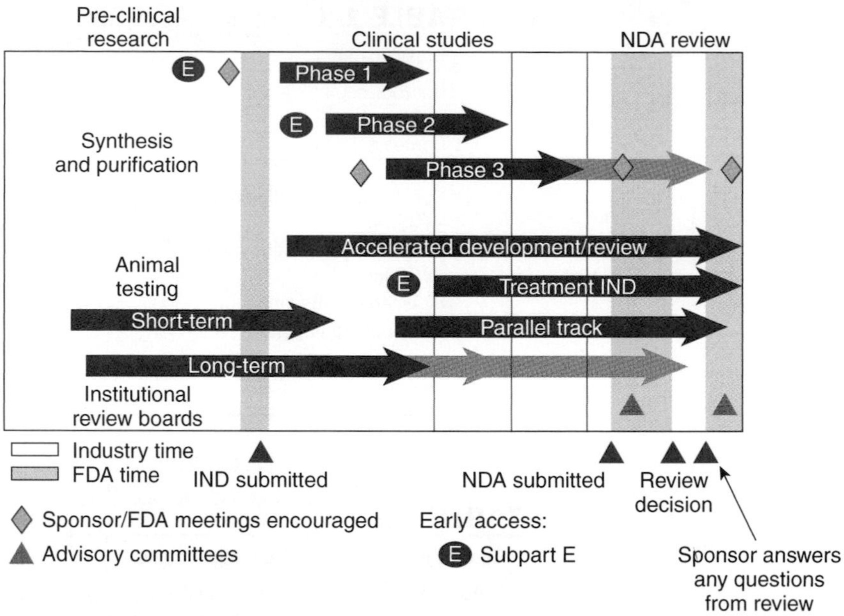

FIGURE 1-2 Phase I through Phase IV development process. *(From The New Drug Development Process, Food and Drug Administration:* The new drug development process. *Retrieved from http://www.fda.gov/cder/handbook/. Accessed May 9, 2006.)*

proved, the drug begins the new drug application process and then moves on to review. An accelerated process exists to speed drug development and review when the drug provides significant benefit over existing therapies or a life-threatening illness is present. Additional safety information is collected in the postmarketing phase. Phase 4 trials are drug safety studies that are conducted after the drug is marketed to the public.

In 1992, the Prescription Drug User Fees Act passed to allow companies to pay a fee to the U.S. Food and Drug Administration (FDA) in return for a faster review period. The Prescription Drug User Fees Act was renewed in 1997 and 2002.

Drug approval and marketing of new drugs are also regulated in Canada. The Health Products and Food Branch of Health Canada regulates the use of therapeutic drugs in Canada. Preclinical and Phase I–IV clinical studies are also required in Canada. A Notice of Compliance (NOC) and Drug Identification Number (DIN) are issued before a new drug is marketed in Canada.

DRUG NOMENCLATURE

All drugs are identified by a generic name, a chemical name, and a proprietary name. The name of a new drug is made according to standards set by the Center for Drug Evaluation and Research (CDER). The standards published in the CDER *Data Standards Manual* (DSM) are used by the Drug Product Reference File (DPRF) and the Drug Registration and Listing System (DRLS) (CDER Data Standards Manual is available at http://www.fda.gov/cder/dsm/index.htm).

The official name of the drug is the ***generic name***. Only the official name of the drug is published in an official compendium like the *United States Pharmacopoeia.* Official names are selected by the U.S. Adopted Name Council and must be approved by the FDA. If a drug contains more than one active ingredient, all official drug names must be listed. The ending of the official name of many drugs indicates the pharmacological class to which the drug belongs (Table 1-1). For example, many local anesthetics have the common ending *"-caine."*

The ***chemical name*** describes the molecular structure of the drug. The chemical structure of the drug determines its activity and side effects.

TABLE 1-1   Examples of Common Endings to Official Drug Names

Classification	Common ending	Prototypical drug
Benzodiazepine	-zepam	diazepam
	-zolam	triazolam
Corticosteroid	-sone	prednisone
	-lone	prednisolone
Nonsteroidal antiinflammatory drug (NSAID)	-profen	ibuprofen
	-olac	ketorolac
β-Adrenergic blocking drug (β-blocker)	-olol	propranolol
H$_2$ receptor antagonist	-tidine	cimetidine
Proton pump inhibitor	-prazole	omeprazole
Calcium channel blocker	-dipine	nifedipine
Macrolide antiinfective	-thromycin	erythromycin

TABLE 1-2   Examples of Chemical, Generic, and Proprietary Names

Generic name	Chemical name	Brand name
fluoxetine HCl	(±)-N-Methyl-3-phenyl-[(α,α,α-trifluoro-p-tolyl)oxy]propylamine	Prozac
acetaminophen	4′-Hydroxyacetanilide	Tylenol
ibuprofen	(±)-2-(p-Isobutylphenyl)propionic acid	Motrin

The ***proprietary name,*** or ***brand name,*** is assigned by the drug manufacture according to recommendations made by the CDER Labeling and Nomenclature Committee. Factors considered when selecting a suitable proprietary name are existing "look-alike" and "sound-alike" names and ease of association with the generic name and/or active ingredient name (Table 1-2).

COMPARISONS BETWEEN BRAND NAME DRUGS AND GENERIC DRUGS

The innovator of a new drug may apply for patent protection. If awarded, the manufacturer is given up to 20 years' exclusive right to manufacture and distribute the new drug. The manufacturer selects a brand name for the drug according to CDER recommendations. Once the drug is off patent, other drug companies may manufacturer a generic equivalent. Generic drugs contain the same active ingredient as the original manufacturer's drug, in the same strength and in the same dosage form. Generic drugs may contain different inactive ingredients. Occasionally, these inactive ingredients result in slight differences between brand name and generic products that affect how much of the drug is available to produce drug action or how quickly drug effect is produced. Generic drugs that are not significantly different from the innovator's product receive an "A" rating from the FDA and may be substituted for the brand name product according to state and federal product substitution laws.

Generic drugs are always less expensive than brand name drugs. In many states, pharmacists routinely dispense generic drugs. Most prescription drug insurance plans require that generic drugs be dispensed and brand name drugs are only dispensed when the prescriber insists that a brand name drug is necessary.

Drug Legislation

The Pure Food and Drug Act (1906) was the first significant legislation passed to protect the public from harmful and ineffective drugs. Over the years, many more laws have been passed that regulate drug manufacture and distribution. The Durham-Humphrey Amendment (1951) established the distinction between ***legend drugs*** and drugs that could safely be used by the public without supervision by a health care provider. Legend drugs can only be obtained by prescription, whereas ***over-the-counter (OTC)*** drugs do not require a prescription. "Rx only" must be printed on the label of all legend drugs. The Kefauver-Harris Amendment (1962) requires that all drugs be safe and effective before they are made

TECH NOTE!
Every drug has a generic name; however, the drug cannot be manufactured by a generic manufacturer until the patent expires.

TECH NOTE!
Technicians must concentrate on memorizing the generic name and the brand name. Medication errors can also be avoided by arranging drugs on the pharmacy shelves according to the generic names.

available to the public. Investigational new drugs are limited to drug study participants until clinical studies have shown them to be safe and effective. The Drug Price Competition Act and Patent Restoration Act (1984) encouraged the creation of generic drugs by streamlining the drug approval process for drugs no longer patented. A patent permits manufacturers of proprietary drugs up to 20 years' exclusive production rights. Once a patent has expired, manufacturers of generic drugs are no longer required to conduct additional studies to prove safety and effectiveness but instead are permitted to rely on safety data submitted by the manufacturer of the proprietary drug. The Combat Methamphetamine Epidemic Act of 2005 (CMEA) was passed to curb the illegal manufacture and use of "crystal meth." The CMEA was signed into law on March 6, 2006, to regulate, among other things, retail over-the-counter sales of ephedrine, pseudoephedrine, and phenylpropanolamine products used to manufacture crystal meth. Purchase limits, placement of product out of direct customer access, sales logbooks, customer ID verification, employee training, and self-certification of regulated sellers are required provisions of the CMEA.

The Comprehensive Drug Abuse Prevention and Control Act, also known as the Controlled Substance Act (CSA), was passed by Congress in 1970. It regulates drugs that have a history for abuse (Table 1-3). Access to *controlled substances* is more restrictive than access to legend drugs. Controlled substances are placed in schedule C-I, C-II, C-III, C-IV, or C-V category according to their abuse potential and effects if abused. Controlled substance schedules are determined by federal and state laws.

TABLE 1-3 Controlled Substances: Schedules, Classification, Dispensing Rules, and Examples

Schedule	Classification	Dispensing rules	Examples
C-I	The drug has a high potential for abuse. The drug has no currently accepted medical use in treatment in the United States.	Only with approved protocol or investigational use	Ecstasy, heroin, LSD, marijuana, PCP
C-II	The drug has a high potential for abuse. Abuse of the drug may lead to severe psychological or physical dependence The drug has an accepted medical use In treatment In the United States.	Written prescription (if called in or faxed in, a written prescription must follow within 72 hours) No refills allowed	Methylphenidate, codeine, meperidine, oxycodone, secobarbital
C-III	The drug has a potential for abuse less than that of C-II drugs. Abuse may lead to moderate or low physical dependence or high psychological dependence. The drug has an accepted medical use in treatment in the United States.	Written, oral, or faxed prescription Prescription expires within 6 months Refillable (no more than five refills within 6 months)	Codeine + acetaminophen, hydrocodone + acetaminophen, methyltestosterone, phendimetrazine
C-IV	The drug has a potential for abuse less than that of C-III drugs. Abuse may lead to limited physical dependence or psychological dependence relative to the C-III drugs. The drug has an accepted medical use in treatment in the United States.	Written, oral, or faxed prescription Prescription expires within 6 months Refillable (no more than five refills within 6 months)	Alprazolam, buprenorphine butorphanol, diazepam, diethylpropion, pentozocine + naloxone, phentermine, propoxyphene, triazolam
C-V	The drug has a potential for abuse less than that of C-IV drugs. Abuse may lead to limited physical dependence or psychological dependence relative to C-IV drugs. The drug has an accepted medical use in treatment in the United States.	*Prescription:* Written, oral, or faxed prescription Prescription expires within 6 months Refillable (no more than five refills within 6 months) *Over-the counter (OTC):* Rules vary for each state	Diphenoxylate + atropine,

Canada, like the United States, has passed legislation to limit the access to drugs with a potential for abuse. Controlled substance schedules are outlined in the Canadian Food and Drugs Act. Narcotics are classified Schedule N and include codeine, morphine, oxycodone, and related drugs. They are identified by a (N) symbol on the product label. Schedule G controlled substances are identified by a ⟨C⟩ symbol on the product label. Schedule G controlled substances include amphetamines, methylphenidate, and barbiturates such as secobarbital.

Drug Dosage Forms and Delivery Systems

Drugs are formulated for delivery by mouth (oral), injection (parenteral), inhalation, or topical application to skin or a mucous membrane. Factors influencing the choice for drug formulation are chemical properties of the drug and human physiology. Chemical properties of the drug influence absorption, distribution, metabolism, and elimination of the drug in the body. Normal physiological processes can influence effectiveness of the drug. For example, drugs formulated for transdermal administration must have sufficient lipid solubility to enable the drug to pass through the cell membranes of skin and get to the site of action. Insulin is formulated for subcutaneous injection because it is composed of two amino acid strands and, if it is formulated for oral delivery, would be destroyed by the digestive enzymes that break down protein foods.

DOSAGE FORMS FOR ORAL (ENTERAL) ADMINISTRATION

Oral administration is safe, easy, and generally more economical than parenteral administration. Common oral formulations include tablets, capsules, solutions, emulsions, syrups, suspensions, and elixirs.

Tablets. Tablets are solid dosage forms containing one or more active ingredient plus binders and fillers. Binders are added to aid in compressing drug into a tablet shape. Fillers make up the required bulk and help bind the tablet. Binders and fillers are inactive ingredients but may influence rate of drug absorption. Tablets are formulated to deliver their contents immediately or over time.

Repeat-action tablets are layered. The outer layer rapidly disintegrates in the stomach, and the inner layer dissolves in the small intestine.

Delayed-action tablets slow the release of drug to avoid stomach upset, improve absorption, or prevent drug destruction in the stomach.

Enteric-coated tablets are a type of delayed-action tablet (Figure 1-3). Enteric-coated tablets do not dissolve in the stomach. They release their contents in the small intestine.

TECH NOTE!

The Latin abbreviation for by mouth is P. O. (per OS). It can be easily remembered as per oral.

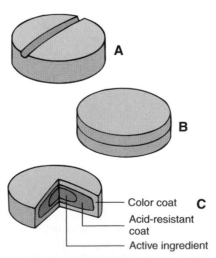

Color coat
Acid-resistant coat
Active ingredient

FIGURE 1-3 Enteric-coated tablets. *A,* Scored side. *B,* Unscored side. *C,* Interior of tablet. *(From Clayton BD, Stock YN, Harroun RD:* Basic pharmacology for nurses, *ed 14, St Louis, 2007, Mosby.)*

Sustained-release and *time-release tablets* deliver their contents over time. Some drugs are formulated to deliver their contents over 24 hours and only need to be taken once a day. Sustained-release drugs should be swallowed whole; crushing may cause the contents to be released immediately. Sustained release and time release are patented processes.

Film coating and *sugar coating* tablets make them easier to swallow and improves taste.

Chewable tablets are formulated for people who have difficulty swallowing pills. Many children's medicines are available in a chewable dosage form.

Sublingual tablets and *buccal tablets* dissolve in the mouth. Sublingual tablets are dissolved under the tongue, and buccal tablets are dissolved in the cheek pouch. Many blood vessels are located in the mouth. Drugs that are destroyed by stomach acids or need to get into the bloodstream rapidly (e.g., nitroglycerin) may be formulated for sublingual or buccal administration.

Troches and *lozenges* are dissolved in the mouth.

CAPSULES

TECH NOTE!
Pharmacy technicians must carefully read the labels of medications available for immediate release, sustained release, and delayed release to avoid errors. Many are available in the same strength.

Capsules are solid dosage forms containing one or more active ingredient plus binders and fillers (Figure 1-4). Capsules are formulated to deliver their contents immediately or over time.

ORAL LIQUIDS

Oral liquids include suspensions, solutions, syrups, elixirs, tinctures, and emulsions. Typically, they are water based. Drugs formulated in liquids are easy to swallow. Liquid medicines work more rapidly than tablets or capsules.

Suspensions contain small drug particles (solute) suspended in a solvent (Figure 1-5). Drug particles settle to the bottom of the bottle when suspensions are left standing. Solutions are dosage forms where drug particles completely dissolve in the liquid. Solutions remain clear. Suspensions may be administered orally, topically, or rectally.

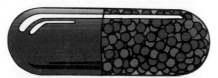

FIGURE 1-4 Capsules. *(From Clayton BD, Stock YN, Harroun RD: Basic pharmacology for nurses, ed 14, St Louis, 2007, Mosby.)*

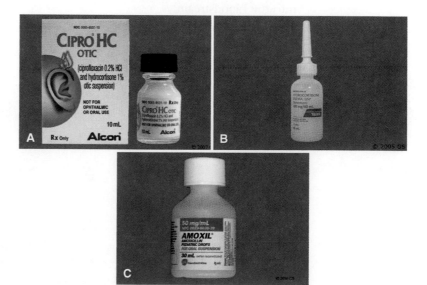

FIGURE 1-5 Suspensions. *A,* Otic suspensions. *B,* Rectal suspension. *C,* Oral suspension. *(Copyright © Gold Standard, Inc., 2007)*

Syrups contain a high concentration of sucrose or other sugar.

Elixirs contain between 5% and 40% alcohol.

Tinctures may contain as little 17% alcohol or as much as 80% alcohol.

Emulsions are similar to suspensions. Drugs suspended in oil may be dispersed in water (O/W) or drugs suspended in water may be dispersed in oil (W/O).

DOSAGE FORMS FOR TOPICAL ADMINISTRATION

Solutions, suspensions, and emulsions are also formulated for topical application to the skin, eye, ear, and mucous membranes of the rectum and vagina. Topical dosage forms not previously described include ointments, creams, and suppositories.

OINTMENTS

Ointments are semisolid preparations containing petrolatum or another oily base (lanolin, wool fat). They soften dry, scaly skin and protect the skin by forming a barrier between the skin and harmful substances.

Creams. Creams are semisolid emulsions. Vanishing creams have high water content (O/W), and cold cream is an oil-in-water emulsion (W/O).

Suppositories. Suppositories are solid or semisolid dosage forms intended to be inserted into a body orifice. They are shaped for vaginal, urethral, or rectal insertion. Suppositories melt at body temperature, dispersing the medicine (Figure 1-6).

TRANSDERMAL DRUG DELIVERY SYSTEMS (PATCHES)

Transdermal patches are controlled-release devices that deliver medication across skin membranes into the general circulation (Figure 1-7). They produce systemic effects (throughout the body) in addition to local effects. Medicines formulated for transdermal application are used to treat angina (e.g., nitroglycerin), male hypogonadism (e.g., testosterone), menopause (e.g., estrogen), and pain (e.g., fentanyl).

DOSAGE FORMS FOR PARENTERAL ADMINISTRATION

Parenteral drugs are injected or infused (slowly injected) directly into a blood vessel, muscle, skin, or joint (Figure 1-8). Parenterally administered drugs enter the bloodstream, often producing rapid action. Once in the bloodstream, the side effects cannot be easily stopped. Parenterally administered drugs must be prepared using aseptic technique in a sterile environment to avoid introducing contaminants that are harmful if injected into a patient.

Intravenous (IV) solutions are injected or infused directly into a vein and go immediately into the bloodstream.

Intramuscular (IM) solutions and suspensions are injected deep into a skeletal muscle.

TECH NOTE!
When suspensions are dispensed, a SHAKE WELL auxiliary label should be placed on the prescription bottle.

TECH NOTE!
Patients should be advised to remove the foil or outer wrapper from the suppository before inserting it into the rectum or vagina.

TECH NOTE!
Please make sure to double-check your calculations for parenteral medications. Once administered, drug action cannot be stopped.

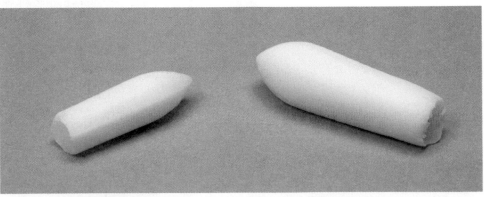

FIGURE 1-6 Typical shapes of suppositories. *(Courtesy Rick Brady Riva, MD. From Lilley LL, Harrington S, Snyder JS: Pharmacology and the nursing process, ed 5, St Louis, 2007, Mosby.)*

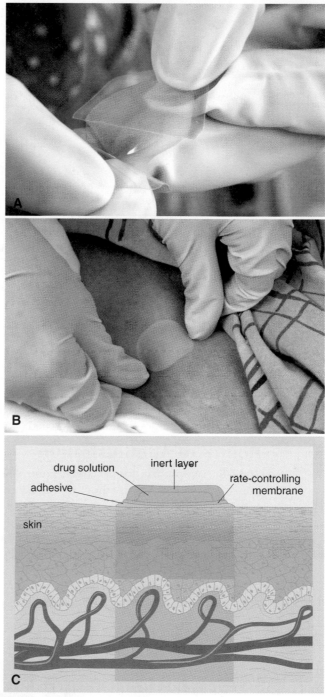

FIGURE 1-7 Transdermal patches. *(A and B, Courtesy Rick Brady Riva, MD. From Lilley LL, Harrington S, Snyder JS:* Pharmacology and the nursing process, *ed 5, St Louis, 2007, Mosby. C, From Page C, et al.:* Integrated pharmacology, *ed 3, Philadelphia, 2006, Mosby.)*

Subcutaneous (SC) solutions and suspensions are injected just beneath the skin.

Intraarticular solutions are injected directly into a joint.

Intradermal solutions are injected into the dermal layer (allergy tests or tuberculosis vaccinations).

Intrathecal solutions are injected directly into the cerebrospinal fluid.

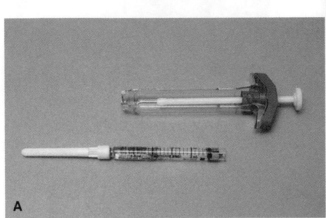
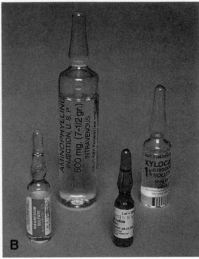

FIGURE 1-8 Typical containers for parenteral medications. *(A, From Potter PA, Perry AG: Basic nursing: theory and practice, ed 3, St Louis, 1995, Mosby. From Potter PA, Perry AG: Fundamentals of nursing, ed 5, St Louis, 2001, Mosby.)*

DOSAGE FORMS FOR RESPIRATORY TRACT ADMINISTRATION

Solutions and suspensions are applied to mucous membranes of the nose as sprays or drops. Micro-fine powders, solutions, and gaseous drugs are inhaled into the lungs using a metered dose aerosol inhaler (Figure 1-9) or a nebulizer. A nebulizer is a device that turns solutions into vapors that can be inhaled.

Routes of Administration

The formulation of a drug is largely controlled by the chemical properties of the drug and human physiology. The method of drug administration is determined by drug dosage form. When a drug is available for administration via more than one route, the selection of one route of administration over another is made according to the properties of the drug (e.g., lipid solubility, ionization, etc.), ease of administration, *pathophysiology* (kidney or liver disease, etc.), and therapeutic objectives (e.g., the need for rapid onset or long duration of action).

The major routes of drug administration are enteral (oral), parenteral (IV, IM, SC), inhalation, and topical. Enteral, parenteral, and inhalation routes typically produce *systemic*

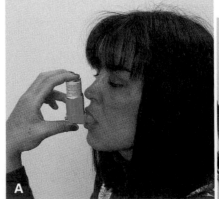
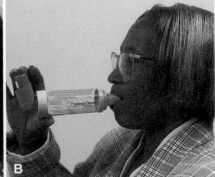

FIGURE 1-9 *A,* Proper use of an inhaler. *B,* Inhaler with spacer *(also known as: aerochamber). (From Hopper T:* Mosby's pharmacy technician, *ed 2, St Louis, 2007, WB Saunders.)*

effects. Systemic effects extend beyond the area of drug application or administration, whereas local effects occur predominantly at or near the site of application. Drugs that are applied topically usually produce a local effect. These are general rules. Some drugs that are administered orally produce a local effect (e.g., antacids, neomycin), and some drugs administered by injection produce a local effect (e.g., local anesthetics). Transdermal patches produce systemic effects.

ENTERAL

Oral administration is safe and easy compared with parenteral administration. No special techniques are required for administration and, if needed, the drug can be removed from the body via vomiting (emesis) or binding with activated charcoal. Drugs available for oral administration are generally less expensive than their parenteral dosage form. All orally administered drugs must disintegrate and dissolve into solution before they can be absorbed and distributed. This process is called the ***pharmaceutical phase*** of drug disposition. Tablets and capsules contain binders and fillers that can influence the rate and extent of disintegration and dissolution.

Disadvantages to oral administration are variable absorption and decreased ***bioavailability*** (Table 1-4). Bioavailability is the extent to which a drug is absorbed and distributed to the site of action. The presence of food in the stomach can delay the absorption of some drugs.

There are other disadvantages to oral administration. Drugs that are swallowed must pass through the gastrointestinal (GI) tract. Stomach contents contain powerful acids and digestive enzymes. These acids and enzymes can significantly decrease the amount of drug to be absorbed or inactivate some drugs (e.g., penicillin G, insulin).

PARENTERAL

Parenteral administration is preferred when the patient is unable to swallow (e.g., unconscious) or is experiencing nausea and vomiting or the drug is poorly absorbed via an oral route. Medicines that are administered parenterally bypass the GI tract. Drugs administered parenterally directly enter the general circulation and therefore are not subject to degradation by GI and liver enzymes. The bioavailability of parenterally administered drugs is greater than that of orally administered drugs. ***Bioavailability*** is defined as the extent to which a drug reaches the site of action and is available to produce its effects. An advantage to parenteral administration is rapid onset of action. The amount of drug delivered parenterally can be carefully controlled by managing flow rates. The exact amount of drug circulating throughout the body cannot be controlled when drugs are administered orally. There are disadvantages to parenteral administration of drugs. Aseptic technique must be used when preparing drugs for parenteral administration in order to avoid introducing life-threatening contaminants into the patient's bloodstream. Once a drug has been administered parentally, it cannot be recalled through vomiting.

Parenteral drugs must be administered using specialized techniques. Proper injection procedures must be followed to avoid harm to the patient (Figure 1-10). High doses of drugs administered intravenously (injected into a vein) must be injected slowly to avoid

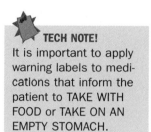

TECH NOTE!
It is important to apply warning labels to medications that inform the patient to TAKE WITH FOOD or TAKE ON AN EMPTY STOMACH.

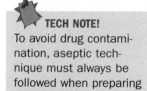

TECH NOTE!
To avoid drug contamination, aseptic technique must always be followed when preparing drugs for parenteral administration.

TABLE 1-4   Summary of Potential Advantages and Disadvantages of Oral Versus Intravascular Administration

Oral	Intravascular
Self-administration: easy	Self-administration: hard
Safe	Dangerous; no recall
Absorption slower	Absorption faster
Less expensive	Expensive
Bioavailability lower	Bioavailability higher
Degraded by gastrointestinal enzymes	Not degraded by gastrointestinal enzymes
Subject to the "first pass effect"	Not subject to the "first-pass effect"
Sterile preparation not critical	Sterile product preparation critical

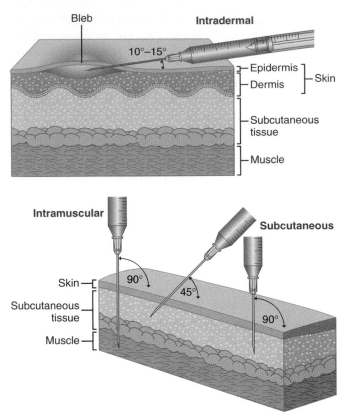

FIGURE 1-10 Forms of injection: intradermal injection, subcutaneous injection, and intramuscular injection. *(From Kee JL, Hayes ER, McCuistion LE: Pharmacology: a nursing process approach, ed 5, St Louis, 2006, WB Saunders.)*

the destruction of red blood cells (hemolysis). Drugs formulated for intramuscular administration (injected into a muscle) may produce a rapid onset or a slow onset of action. Rapid-onset formulations are typically prepared in water-soluble solutions. Slow-onset, prolonged-duration-of-action formulations are suspended in oil or other nonaqueous vehicles (solvent). As the vehicle diffuses out of the muscle into which it has been injected, the drug is slowly deposited. The drug is slowly released from the muscle depot.

Drugs intended for subcutaneous injection pose fewer risks than intravascular administration; however, aseptic technique must still be followed, and the site of injection must be rotated to avoid complications.

INHALATION

Inhalation is one of the most effective ways to rapidly deliver drug locally to cells of the respiratory tract and into the general circulation. Absorption problems that are encountered with oral administration are avoided. Some of the side effects associated with oral or parenteral administration are minimized. Inhalation is an effective method for delivery of medications used to treat asthma and other respiratory disorders. Some medicines used to produce general anesthesia are administered by inhalation.

TRANSDERMAL

Drugs that are formulated for transdermal administration are applied to the skin to produce systemic effects. Drugs like nitroglycerin, estrogen, and testosterone are available for transdermal administration. Patients may experience systemic side effects and local side effects from drugs applied as transdermal patches. Local side effects such as skin irritation are often associated with the adhesives used to enable the patch to stay affixed to the skin and can be minimized by rotating the site where the patch is applied.

TOPICAL

Topical administration produces a local effect unless the drug is applied to a large percentage of body surface area. Side effects associated with topical administration are typically localized to the site of application. For example, hydrocortisone cream applied to the skin will reduce itchiness and redness associated with rashes without the serious systemic side effects associated with oral administration of the drug.

TECH NOTE!

Pharmacy technicians must carefully read the label of medications to avoid dispensing errors. Many drugs are available for immediate release and slow depot release. Many are available in the same strength.

CHAPTER SUMMARY

- Knowledge of pharmacology is essential to the accurate, effective, and efficient performance of pharmacy technician responsibilities.
- Pharmacy technicians possessing a substantial knowledge of pharmacology may be able to reduce dispensing errors.
- Less time is spent searching for drugs when pharmacy technicians have good brand/generic name recognition and can perform the duties with greater independence.
- Knowledge of pharmacology facilitates selection of warning labels for drugs dispensed.
- Pharmacy technicians who possess a good understanding of pharmacology understand the importance of recognizing drug interactions, therapeutic duplication, and excessive dose alerts screened by the computer.
- People from around the globe have contributed to the knowledge of drugs.
- Drugs may come from natural or synthetic origins.
- Plants have been collected, cultivated, and harvested for their healing properties and used in the treatment of illness for centuries.
- Pharmacognosy is the study of the constituents of natural drugs that are responsible for their effects.
- Natural drugs may be derived from plants, animals, or minerals.
- Synthetic drugs may be a chemical modification of a natural drug or manufactured entirely from chemical ingredients unrelated to the natural drug.
- Drugs may also be produced by the process of bioengineering. Drugs produced by bioengineering are called biopharmaceuticals.
- Pharmacology is the study of the action of drugs on humans and animals.
- The new drug application process takes years to complete and includes preclinical research; clinical studies; Phase 1, Phase 2, and Phase 3 drug trials; and review.
- The Food and Drug Administration regulates the new drug and investigational new drug process in the United States. Health Products and Food Branch of Health Canada regulates the use of therapeutic drugs in Canada.
- The name of a new drug is made according to standards set by the Center for Drug Evaluation and Research.
- The official name of the drug is the generic name.
- The chemical name describes the molecular structure of the drug.
- The proprietary name, or brand name, is assigned by the drug manufacturer. Factors considered when selecting a suitable proprietary name are existing "look-alike" and "sound-alike" names and ease of association with the generic name and/or active ingredient name.
- Patent holders for new drugs are given up to 20 years exclusive right to manufacture and distribute the new drug.
- Generic drugs contain the same active ingredient as the original manufacturer's drug, in the same strength and in the same dosage form.
- Generic drugs may contain different inactive ingredients.
- Generic drugs are less expensive than brand name drugs.
- The Durham-Humphrey Amendment established the distinction between legend drugs and over-the-counter drugs.
- The Kefauver-Harris Amendment requires all drugs be safe and effective before they are made available to the public.
- The Drug Price Competition Act and Patent Restoration Act (1984) encouraged the creation of generic drugs.

- Access to controlled substances is more restrictive than access to legend drugs because controlled substances may cause physical or psychological dependence.
- Drugs are formulated for delivery by mouth, injection, inhalation, or topical application to skin or a mucous membrane. Factors influencing the choice for drug formulation are chemical properties of the drug and human physiology.
- The formulation of a drug is largely controlled by the chemical properties of the drug and human physiology.
- When a drug is available for administration by more than one route, the selection of one route of administration over another is made according to the properties of the drug, ease of administration, therapeutic objectives, and whether the patient has a preexisting disease.
- The major routes of drug administration are enteral (oral), parenteral (IV, IM, SC), inhalation, and topical.
- Enteral, parenteral, and inhalation routes typically produce systemic effects.
- Topical administration typically produces local effects.
- Orally administered drugs must disintegrate and dissolve into solution before they can be absorbed and distributed. This process is called the pharmaceutical phase.
- Drugs that are swallowed must pass through the gastrointestinal tract. Acids in the stomach and digestive enzymes can inactivate some drugs (e.g., penicillin G).
- Medicines that are administered parenterally bypass the gastrointestinal tract. Drugs administered parenterally directly enter the general circulation and therefore are not subject to the degradation by gastrointestinal and liver enzymes.
- An advantage to parenteral administration is rapid onset of action.
- Aseptic technique must be used when preparing drugs for parenteral administration in order to avoid introducing life-threatening contaminants into the patient's bloodstream.
- High doses of drugs administered intravenously (injected into a vein) must be injected slowly to avoid destruction of red blood cells (hemolysis).
- Drugs formulated for intramuscular administration (injected into a muscle) may produce a rapid onset or a slow onset of action. Rapid onset formulations are typically prepared in water-soluble solutions and slow onset, prolonged duration of action formulations are suspended in oil or other nonaqueous vehicles (solvent).
- Inhalation is one of the most effective ways to rapidly deliver drug locally to cells of the respiratory tract and into the general circulation. Inhalation is an effective method for delivery of medications used to treat asthma, other respiratory disorders, and general anesthetics.
- Drugs like nitroglycerin, estrogen, and testosterone are formulated for transdermal administration (applied to the skin) but produce systemic effects.
- Transdermal patches may cause skin irritation, which is associated with the adhesive. Rotating the site of patch application can reduce risk of skin irritation.

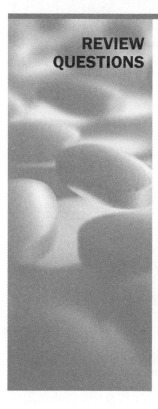

REVIEW QUESTIONS

Multiple Choice

1. Who was called the "father of pharmacology" and was a Greek physician known for his accurate observation of medicinal plants?
    a. Discorides
    b. Theophrastus
    c. Hippocrates
    d. Shen Nung

2. What is the study of the constituents of natural drugs that are responsible for their effects?
    a. pharmacology
    b. pharacogenomics
    c. pharmacognosy
    d. pharmacokinetics

3. In 1906, what law was passed to protect the public from ineffective and harmful drugs?
    a. Pure Food and Drug Act
    b. Harrison Narcotic Act
    c. Pure Food Drug and Cosmetic Act
    d. none of the above

4. Which of the following drugs was *not* made from a plant?
    a. morphine
    b. fentanyl
    c. quinine
    d. digitalis

5. The study of pharmacology applies knowledge of
    a. properties of drugs
    b. mechanism of drug action
    c. anatomy, physiology, and pathology
    d. all of the above

6. Which of the following is *not* a step in developing and receiving approval for a new drug?
    a. preclinical research
    b. clinical studies
    c. marketing
    d. new drug application process and review

7. The official name of the drug is the
    a. generic name
    b. proprietary name
    c. brand name
    d. chemical name

8. Which drugs can be obtained *only* by prescription?
    a. herbal remedies
    b. legend
    c. compounded
    d. all of the above

9. Which of the following is *not* an oral formulation?
    a. tablet
    b. capsule
    c. suspension
    d. suppository

10. Parenterally administered drugs must be prepared using
    a. aseptic technique in sterile environment
    b. countertops cleaned with alcohol
    c. patient carts in nursing units
    d. none of the above

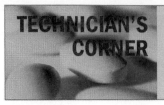

TECHNICIAN'S CORNER

1. The Kefauver-Harris Amendment (1962) requires all drugs be safe and effective before they are made available to the public. Exactly what is involved in making a drug "safe and effective" for public use?
2. How would you explain to a client that a generic drug works just as well as a brand drug?

BIBLIOGRAPHY

Basch E, Ulbricht C: *Natural standard herb & supplement handbook: the clinical bottom line,* St Louis, 2005, Mosby.

Food and Drug Administration: *CDER data standards manual.* Retrieved from http://www.fda.gov/cder/dsm/index.htm. Accessed May 9, 2006.

Food and Drug Administration: *The new drug development process.* Retrieved from http://www.fda.gov/cder/handbook/. Accessed May 9, 2006.

Goodman L, Gilman A: *The pharmacological basis of therapeutics* (pp 1-8), ed 5, New York, 1975, MacMillan.

Haas LF: Neurological stamp: Papyrus of Ebers and Smith, *J Neurol Neurosurg Psychiatry* 67:578, 1999.

Merck manual home edition: *Introduction: overview of drugs.* Retrieved from http://www.merck.com/mmhe/sec02/ch010/ch010a.html. Accessed October 30, 2007.

National Library of Medicine, History of Medicine Division: *Classics of traditional Chinese medicine.* Retrieved from http://www.nlm.nih.gov/hmd/chinese/emperors.html. Accessed May 6, 2006.

Shargel L, Mutnick A, Souney P, Swanson L: *Comprehensive pharmacy review* (pp 28-66), ed 4, Philadelphia, 2001, Lippincott Williams & Wilkins.

Tyler V, Brady L, Robbers J: *Pharmacognosy* (pp 1-6), ed 9, Philadelphia, 1988, Lea & Febiger.

United States Drug Enforcement Administration: *Title 21: food and drugs, chapter 13: drug abuse prevention and control.* Retrieved from http://www.dea.gov/pubs/csa.html. Accessed May 9, 2006.

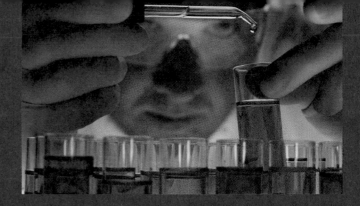

Principles of Pharmacology

LEARNING OBJECTIVES

- Give a definition for each pharmacokinetic phase.
- Describe factors influencing each pharmacokinetic phase.
- Explain the importance of the first-pass effect.
- Describe the function of the blood-brain barrier.
- List major routes of drug elimination.
- Describe elimination half-life.
- Explain the importance of bioavailability to generic drug substitution.
- Learn the terminology associated with the principles of pharmacology.

KEY TERMS

Absorption: Process involving the movement of drug molecules from the site of administration into the circulatory system.

Bioavailability: Extent to which a drug reaches the site of action and is available to produce its effects.

Bioequivalent drug: Drug that shows no statistical differences in the rate and extent of absorption when it is administered in the same strength, dosage form, and route of administration as the brand name product.

Biotransformation: Process of drug metabolism in the body that transforms a drug to a more active, equally active, or inactive metabolite.

Diffusion: Passive movement of molecules across cell membranes from an area of high drug concentration to lower concentration.

Distribution: Process of movement of the drug from the circulatory system across barrier membranes, to the site of drug action.

Duration of action: Time between the onset of action and discontinuation of drug action.

Elimination: Process that results in removal of drug from the body and discontinuation of drug action.

Enzyme: Protein capable of causing a chemical reaction. Enzymes may increase the metabolism of drugs.

First-pass effect: Process whereby the liver metabolizes nearly all of a drug before it passes into the general circulation.

Half-life (T½): Length of time it takes for the plasma concentration of an administered drug to be reduced by one half.

Hydrophilic: Water loving.

Hydrophobic: Water hating.

Ionization: Chemical process involving the release of a proton (H^+). Ionized drug molecules may have a positive or negative charge.

Lipid: Fat-like substance.

Lipophilic: Lipid loving.

Metabolism: Biochemical process involving transformation of active drugs to a compound that can be easily eliminated or prodrugs to active drugs.

Metabolite: Product of drug metabolism. Metabolites may be an inactivated drugs or active drugs with equal or greater activity than the parent drug.

Onset of action: Time it takes a drug to reach the concentration necessary to produce a therapeutic effect.

Pathophysiology: Study of structural and functional changes that are produced by disease.

Peak effect: Maximum drug effect produced by drug is achieved once the drug has reached its maximum concentration in body.

Pharmaceutical alternative: Contains the same active ingredient as the brand name drug; however, the strength and dosage form may be different.

Pharmaceutical equivalent: Drug that contains identical amount of active ingredient as brand name drug but may have different inactive ingredients, be manufactured in a different dosage form, and exhibit different rates of absorption.

Pharmacokinetics: Science dealing with the dynamic process drug undergoes to produce its therapeutic effect.

Prodrug: Drug administered in an inactive form that is metabolized in the body to an active form.

Therapeutic alternative: Drug that contains different active ingredient(s) than the brand name drug yet produces the same desired therapeutic outcome.

Pharmacokinetics

The word **pharmacokinetics** is derived from the Greek words *pharmaco* ("drug") and *kinesis* ("movement"). Absorption, distribution, metabolism, and elimination are four pharmacokinetic phases. Drugs that are administered must be absorbed into the bloodstream and distributed to their site of action before they can begin to produce their effect. The body metabolizes the drug and then it is eliminated. As a drug moves throughout the body, it undergoes changes that may increase or decrease its absorption, distribution, metabolism, or elimination. These pharmacokinetic phases control the intensity of the drug's effect and the duration of the drug action (Figure 2-1).

The time it takes for a drug to reach the concentration necessary to produce a therapeutic effect is called the ***onset of action***. The onset of action is not achieved until the drug reaches a minimum concentration in the body. The maximum drug effect or ***peak effect*** occurs after the maximum drug concentration is reached in the body. ***Duration of action*** is the time between the onset of action and discontinuation of drug action. Duration of action is the amount of time the drug concentration remains within the therapeutic range (Figure 2-2).

Pharmacokinetic Phases

ABSORPTION

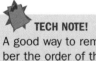

TECH NOTE!
A good way to remember the order of the pharmacokinetic phases is to use the acronym ADME.

Absorption is the first pharmacokinetic phase. **Absorption** is the process that involves the movement of drug molecules from the site of administration, across cell membranes, into the circulatory system of the body (blood or lymphatic system). Absorption may occur across the skin or cells that line blood vessels. How quickly or slowly a drug is absorbed is determined by the characteristics of the drug, the drug dosage form, route of administration, human anatomy, and physiology. The amount of drug absorbed is also influenced by many factors. Drugs that are administered intravenously are completely absorbed into the bloodstream if they are injected directly into the vein. Other routes of drug administration result in partial absorption. Absorption of drugs taken by mouth may be delayed when food is present in the stomach. Absorption of pills that have been swallowed does not begin until after the drug goes into solution, so factors effecting disintegration or dissolution of the drug (pharmaceutical phase) can decrease absorption (see Chapter 1). The ease in

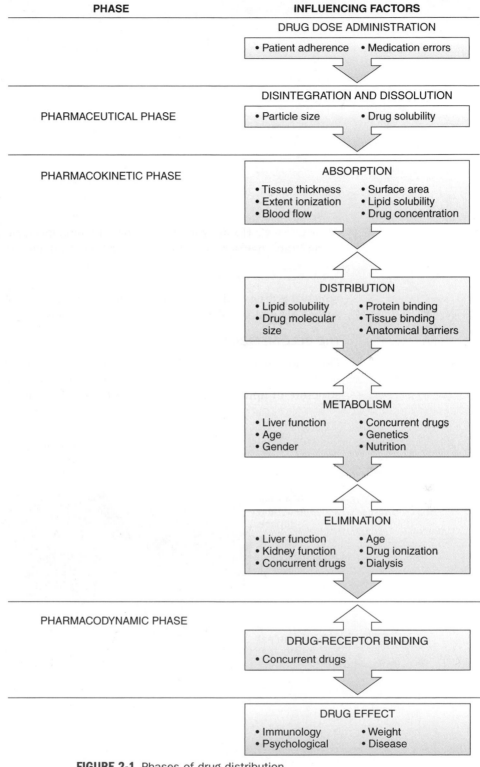

FIGURE 2-1 Phases of drug distribution.

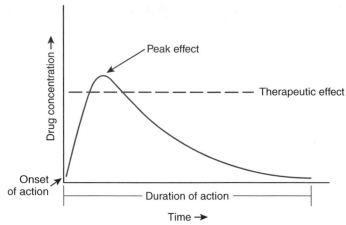

FIGURE 2-2 Onset of action, peak effect, duration of action, and therapeutic effect.

which the drug is able to cross cell membranes is a factor in how readily the drug is absorbed via oral, rectal, vaginal, and other routes of administration.

THE CELL MEMBRANE

Drug movement from the site of administration into the circulatory system is dependent on the ability of the drug to move across cell membranes. The cell membrane is a complex structure of lipids (fats), protein, and water-filled channels (Figure 2-3). Movement across

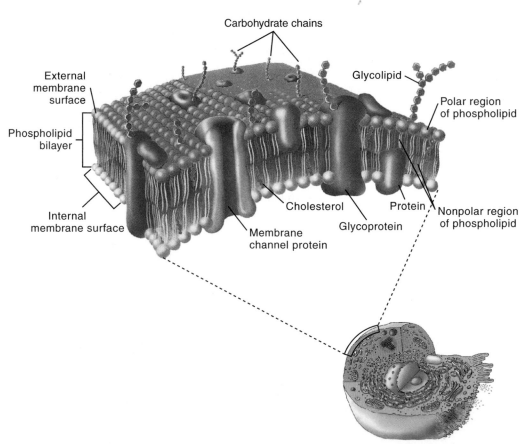

FIGURE 2-3 Plasma membrane. *(From Thibodeau GA, Patton KT:* Anatomy and physiology, *ed 6, St Louis, 2007, Mosby.)*

the cell membrane is restricted unless the drug can pass through the lipid layers of the cell membrane or is small enough to pass through the small water-filled (aqueous) channels. A lipid-soluble drug can move easily across the cell membrane. Drugs that enter the cell through aqueous channels are listed in Box 2-1.

DRUG TRANSPORT MECHANISMS

Passive Transport

Drug absorption across the cell membrane may occur via passive or active transport mechanisms. Drugs that are absorbed by passive *diffusion* move from a region of greater concentration to a region of lesser concentration. When the drug first enters the body, the concentration at the administration site is greater than in the bloodstream. Lipid-soluble drugs will easily diffuse across the cell membrane of the blood vessel into the bloodstream, where the concentration of the drug is small. Lipid-soluble drugs are *lipophilic* (lipid-loving) and *hydrophobic* or water-hating. Water-soluble drugs are *hydrophilic* or water-loving and move through the small water channels in the cell membrane. Most drugs are transported via passive transport.

Active Transport

Active transport mechanisms permit the drug to move across cell membranes without regard to concentration. A drug can move from an area where drug concentration is low to an area where the concentration is high. Active transport takes energy and requires special carrier proteins or pumps to "carry the drug" across the cell membrane. (Figure 2-4)

FACTORS INFLUENCING ABSORPTION

Effect of pH on Drug Absorption

Most drugs are either weak acids or weak bases. In solution, weak acids and weak bases exist between the ionized and the nonionized state. In solution, weak acids (HA) disassociate, releasing a proton (H^+) and negatively charged anion (A^-).

$$HA \rightleftharpoons H^+ + A^-$$

BOX 2-1 DRUGS THAT ENTER THE CELL THROUGH AQUEOUS CHANNELS

- Caffeine
- Ascorbic acid (vitamin C)
- Niacin (vitamin B_3)
- Ephedrine

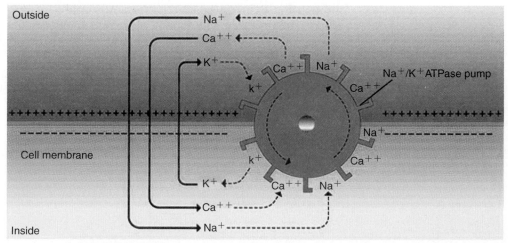

FIGURE 2-4 Active transport: sodium/potassium ATPase pump. *(From Lilley LL, Harrington S, Snyder JS:* Pharmacology and the nursing process, *ed 5, St Louis, 2007, Mosby.)*

Weak bases also release a proton when they are in solution. Loss of a proton results in an uncharged drug molecule.

$$B^+H \rightleftharpoons B+H^+$$

Weakly acidic drugs are more ionized when they are in basic solutions. When the drug is in an acidic solution, it is less ionized. Weakly basic drugs are more ionized when they are in acidic solutions and less ionized in basic solution. This is important because as the drug travels throughout the body, it passes through acidic solutions (e.g., in the stomach) and basic solutions (e.g., in the small intestine). The ability of a drug to diffuse across the cell membrane is dependent on properties of the drug and the pH of the body fluid in which it is dissolved. The *pH* is a measure of how acidic or alkaline (or basic) a solution is. A pH of 1 is very acidic (e.g., stomach acids [HCl]). A pH of 7 is neutral. Plasma has a pH between the range of 7.35 and 7.45. A pH of greater than 7 is alkaline.

Diffusion across the cell membrane is greatest when the drug is lipid soluble and nonionized (uncharged). When a weakly acidic drug like phenobarbital is in the stomach, it is less ionized and can readily cross the cell membranes (Figure 2-5). Absorption is high. When the drug moves into the small intestine, ionization increases and absorption is reduced.

Effect of Blood Flow on Drug Absorption

Absorption is greatest in areas of the body that have a good blood supply. Medications administered sublingually have good absorption because of the many blood vessels located under the tongue. Absorption of orally administered drugs is greatest in the small intestine. The structure of the intestine is designed to perform the specialized job of absorption. Thousands of microvilli line the walls of the small intestine (Figure 2-6). The microvilli are filled with blood vessels. As the drug passes through the cell membrane of the microvilli, it is quickly absorbed into the bloodstream. Absorption of drugs that are injected intramuscularly or subcutaneously is enhanced when the patient applies heat to the muscle, exercises, or does some other activity to stimulate blood flow to the site of administration.

Effect of Surface Area on Drug Absorption

Microvilli also increase the surface area of the small intestine, making it the largest absorbing surface in the body (Figure 2-7). The area for absorption in the small intestine is about 1000 times greater than that in the stomach.

Effect of Contact Time at the Absorption Surface

Drug absorption increases the longer the drug is in contact with the absorbing surface. Drug absorption is decreased if the patient has diarrhea because the rapid passage of contents through the gastrointestinal (GI) tract. Absorption of delayed release drugs is increased when a drug is taken with food because of delayed gastric emptying.

Effect of Tissue Thickness on Absorption

Drug absorption is greater across single cell membranes than multiple cell layers because some drugs may become trapped in cell layers. As tissue thickness increases, the portion of the drug trapped in the cell layers increases.

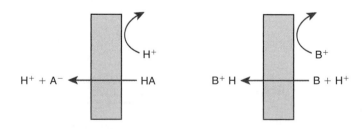

Weak acid drug   Weak base drug

FIGURE 2-5 Weak acid and weak bases crossing cell membranes.

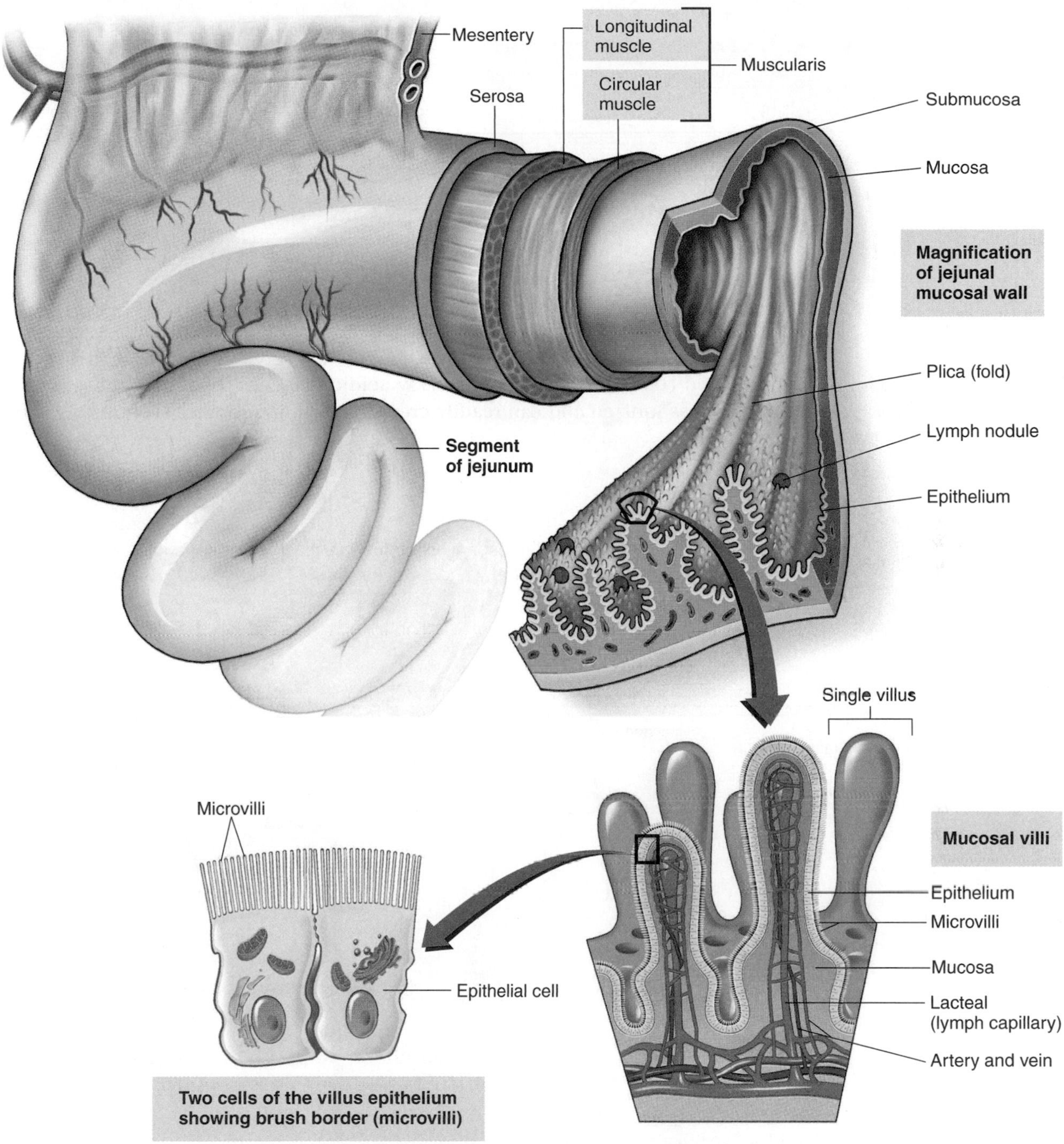

FIGURE 2-6 Wall of intestine with villi. *(From Thibodeau GA, Patton KT:* Anatomy and physiology, *ed 6, St Louis, 2007, Mosby.)*

DISTRIBUTION

Distribution is the process of movement of the drug from the circulatory system, across barrier membranes, to the site of drug action (Figure 2-8). It is the second pharmacokinetic phase. The volume of drug that is distributed is influenced by the properties of the drug, the extent of drug binding to blood proteins or tissue, the blood supply to the region, and the ability of the drug to cross natural body barriers. The drug may be distributed to water compartments of the body or to fat cells or proteins. Water compartments include plasma, extracellular fluid, and total body water.

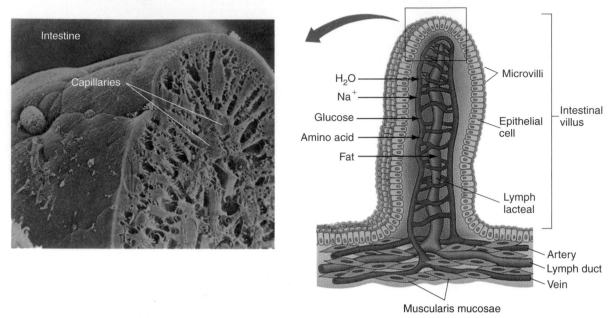

FIGURE 2-7 Intestinal villi showing absorbing surfaces. *(From Thibodeau GA, Patton KT:* Anatomy and physiology, *ed 6, St Louis, 2007, Mosby.)*

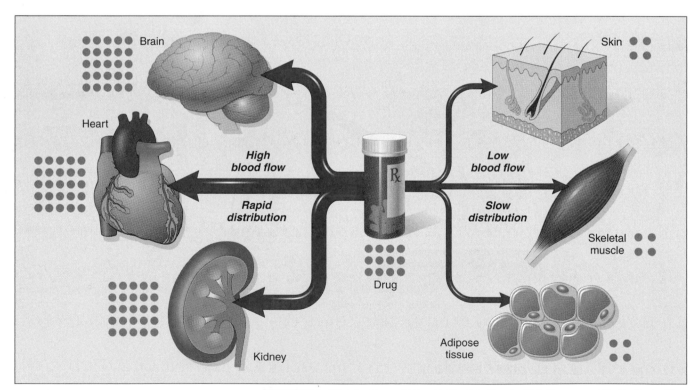

FIGURE 2-8 Distribution. *(From Raffa RB, Rawls SM, Beyzarov EP:* Netter's illustrated pharmacology. *Philadelphia, 2005, WB Saunders.)*

FACTORS INFLUENCING DISTRIBUTION

Effect of Drug Properties on Distribution

Distribution of the drug across the cell membrane of the blood vessel and transport to its site of action is influenced by the chemical nature of the drug. The drug must be hydrophobic, lipid soluble, nonionized, or small enough to pass through slit junctions in the capillary wall. Slit junctions located in the capillaries vary in size. Slit junctions in the capillaries of the brain are so tight that drugs cannot pass through them. On the other hand, slit junctions in the capillaries of the liver and spleen are larger and the size of the drug molecule is less of a limiting factor to drug distribution.

Effect of Protein Binding on Distribution

The blood contains albumin, a plasma protein. Many drugs have an *affinity* for albumin and the result is reversible binding of the drug to the protein. When the drug is bound to plasma proteins, it is unable to diffuse out of the blood vessel to get to the site of drug action. As the concentration of unbound or "free" drug decreases in the bloodstream, the drug that is bound to the plasma protein is released and transported to the site of action.

Plasma proteins act like a drug reservoir for bound drug trapped within the blood vessels. When two drugs are administered that both have an affinity for plasma albumin, the drug with the greatest affinity will competitively bind to the protein. Albumin has the greatest affinity for weak acids and hydrophobic drugs. This competition for albumin binding can result in the release of bound drug enabling it to get to its site of action. (Severe burns can decrease plasma protein levels [hypoalbuminemia] that may alter the level of "free drug".) Competitive protein binding represents a mechanism for drug interactions (Figure 2-9).

Anatomical Barriers to Distribution

Access to the site of drug action may be limited by natural body barriers. Anatomical structures that selectively limit drug access are the blood-brain barrier, blood-placenta barrier, and blood-testicular barrier.

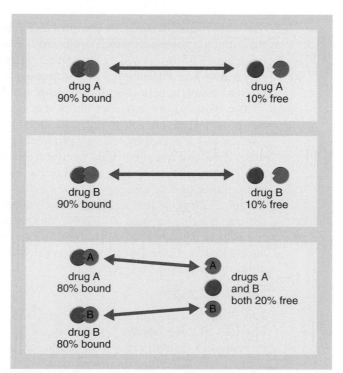

FIGURE 2-9 Protein binding and free fraction of drugs. *(From Page C, et al.: Integrated pharmacology, ed 3. Philadelphia, 2006, Mosby.)*

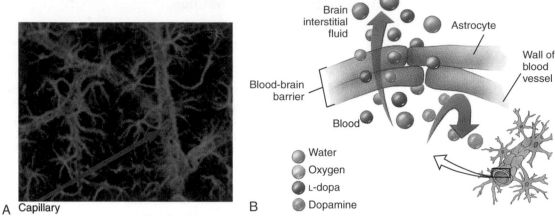

A Capillary   B

FIGURE 2-10 Barriers. (**A,** *From Marie Simar Couldwell, MD and Maiken Neder-gaard.* **B,** *From Thibodeau GA, Patton KT:* Anatomy of Physiology, *6th edition. St Louis, Mosby, 2007.)*

TABLE 2-1   Pregnancy Safety Categories

Category	Description
Category A	Studies indicate no risk to the fetus.
Category B	Studies indicate no risk to animal fetus; information in humans in not available.
Category C	Adverse effects reported in animal fetus; information in humans is not available.
Category D	Possible fetal risk in humans reported; however, considering potential benefit versus risk may, in selected cases, warrant the use of these drugs in pregnant women.
Category X	Fetal abnormalities reported and positive evidence of fetal risk in humans is available from animal and/or human studies. These drugs should not be used in pregnant women.

From Lilley LL, Harrington S, Snyder JS: *Pharmacology and the nursing process,* ed 5, St Louis, 2007, Mosby.

The blood-brain barrier is composed of cells lining the capillaries of the brain that form tight junctions through which drugs are able to pass (Figure 2-10). The blood vessels in the brain are also surrounded by fatty structures called glial feet (also known as astrocyte foot processes). These structures permit passage of lipid-soluble, hydrophobic drugs into the brain and limit access of ionized hydrophilic drugs.

The blood-placenta barrier limits access of drugs taken by a pregnant woman to the fetus. Many drugs are able to cross the blood-placenta barrier, so it is important for pregnant women to ask their physician or pharmacist about potential safety issues before taking a drug. There are five pregnancy safety categories (Table 2-1). Drugs classified in pregnancy safety category A have been shown to be safe when taken during pregnancy. Drugs listed in pregnancy safety category B have been shown to be safe when studied in animals but no information for humans is available. Category C contains a list of drugs with reported adverse effects in animal fetuses. No information for humans is available. Adverse effects in humans are possible for drugs listed in pregnancy safety category D, so use must be balanced against the risks for use. Drugs listed in category X should be avoided because fetal abnormalities have been reported.

METABOLISM

Few drugs that are administered are eliminated unchanged. Most drugs are transformed by enzymes to a *metabolite(s)* that is more active or less active than the original drug. An *enzyme* is a protein capable of causing a chemical reaction. A metabolite is a product of drug metabolism. *Biotransformation* is the process of drug metabolism in the body that transforms a drug to a more active, equally active, or inactive metabolite. The primary site of biotransformation is the liver; however, metabolism may occur in the intestines, lung, kidney, or other cells in the body. Microsomal enzymes in the liver are responsible for transforming lipophilic drugs to compounds that can be more easily eliminated by the kidney. The cytochrome P-450 (CYP450) system is frequently involved in this process. Drugs that interfere with the enzymes of the cytochrome P-450 system can enhance or inhibit the metabolism of other drugs that are taken concurrently (Figure 2-11). Phenobarbital, a drug used in the treatment of epilepsy, increases metabolic enzyme activity of other antiseizure medications (phenytoin, valproic acid), resulting in increased elimination of the drugs. This

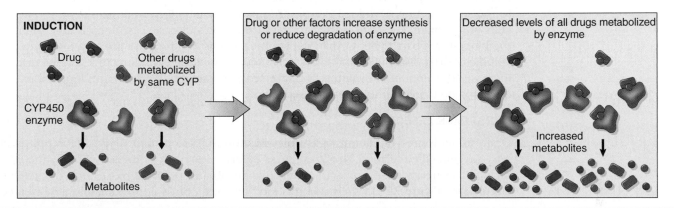

CYP	Inducers	Inhibitors
1A2	Smoking, charbroiled foods, cruciferous vegetables, insulin, modafinil, nafcillin, omeprazole, phenobarbital, primidone, rifampin	Amiodarone, anastrozole, cimetidine, ciprofloxacin, diltiazem, enoxacin, erythromycin, fluoroquinolones, fluvoxamine, grapefruit (juice), mexiletine, norfloxacin, ritonavir, tacrine, ticlopidine
2A6	Dexamethasone, phenobarbital	Methoxsalen, ritonavir, tranylcypromine
2B6	Cyclophosphamide, dexamethasone, phenobarbitol, phenytoin, primidone, rifampin	Efavirenz, nelfinavlr, orphenadrine, ritonavir, thiotepa, ticlopidine
2C8/9	Dexamethasone, primidone, rifampin, secobarbital	Anastrozole, amiodarone, cimetidine, diclofenac, disulfiram, fluconazole, luvoxamine, flurbiprofen, fluvastatin, isoniazid, ketoprofen, lovastatin, metronidazole, omeprazole, paroxetine, phenylbutazone, ritonavir, sertraline, sulfinpyrazone, sulfonamides, sulfamethoxazole, trimethoprim, troglitazone, zafirlukast
2C19	Barbituates, rifampin	Cimetidine, ketoconazole, modafinil, omeprazole, oxcarbazepine, ticlopidine
2D6	Dexamethasone, quinidine, rifampin	Amiodarone, buproprion, celecoxib, chlorpromazine, chlorpheniramine, cimetidine, clomipramine, cocaine, doxorubicin, fluoxetine, fluphenazine, fluvoxamine, haloperidol, lomustine, metoclopramide, methadone, norfluoxetine, paroxetine, perphenazine, propafenone, quinidine, ranitidine, ritonavir, sertindole, sertraine, terbinafine, thioridazine, venlafaxine, vinblastine, vinorelbine
2E1	Acetone, ethanol, isoniazid	Disulfiram, ritonavir
3A4	Barbituates, carbamazepine, dexamethasone, efavirenz, macrolides, glucocorticoids, modafinil, nevirapine, oxcarbazepine, phenobarbital, phenylbutazone, pioglitazone, phenytoin, primidone, rifabutin, rifampin, St John's wort, sulfinpyrazone, troglitazone	Amiodarone, anastrozole, chloramphenicol, cimetidine, ciprofloxacin, clarithromycin, clotrimazole, danazol, delavirdine, diltiazem, erythromycin, fluconazole, fluoxetine, fluvoxamine, grapefruit juice, indinavir, itraconazole, ketoconazole, metronidazole, mibefradil, miconazole, nefazodone, nelfinavir, nevirapine, norfloxacin, norfluoxetine, omeprazole, paroxetine, propoxyphene, quinidine, ranitidine, ritonavir, saquinavir, sertindole, troglitazone, troleandomycin, verapamil, zafirlukast, zileuton

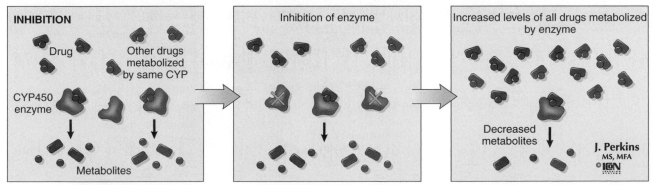

FIGURE 2-11 Metabolic enzyme induction and inhibition. *(From Raffa RB, Rawls SM, Beyzarov EP:* Netter's illustrated pharmacology. *Philadelphia, 2005, WB Saunders.)*

decreases their effectiveness. A high level of CYP450 activity is also found in the mucous membranes of the nose. Metabolic enzymes are found in saliva and are also secreted by bacteria in the intestines.

Not all drugs are metabolized to inactive metabolites. Table 2-2 shows the potential products of metabolism.

Dipivefrin is a drug that is used to treat glaucoma. It is an example of a drug that is metabolized in the eye rather than in the liver. It is also a good example of a prodrug. Prodrugs are drugs that are administered in an inactive form and must be metabolized to their active form. Drugs may be formulated as prodrugs to avoid side effects or to increase distribution to the site of action. Levodopa is a prodrug that is metabolized to dopamine in the nerve cells of the brain. The drug is used to treat Parkinson's disease. Levodopa is able to cross the blood-brain barrier better than dopamine. Administration of the prodrug increases the volume of drug distributed into nerve cells. Adding the drug carbidopa to levodopa further increases the amount of drug that is converted to dopamine because carbidopa interrupts levodopa metabolism in the intestines.

"FIRST-PASS EFFECT"

Orally administered drugs must pass into hepatoportal circulation (liver) before entering into the general circulation. The *"first-pass effect"* describes a process whereby the liver metabolizes nearly all of a drug to an inactive metabolite; before it passes into the general circulation (Figure 2-12). Orally administered nitroglycerin is approximately 90% cleared

TABLE 2-2   Products of Metabolism

Parent drug	Example	Metabolite	Example
Active drug	6-Mercaptopurine	Inactive drug	6-Mercapturic acid
Active drug	Prednisolone	Equally active drug	Prednisone
	Imipramine		Desipramine
Active drug	Diazepam	More active drug	Oxazepam
	Codeine		Morphine
Inactive drug	Dipivefrin	Active drug	Epinephrine
	Levodopa		Dopamine

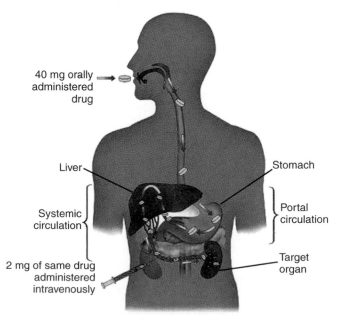

FIGURE 2-12 The first-pass effect. *(From Lilley LL, Aucker RS:* Pharmacology and the nursing process, *ed 3, St Louis, 2001, Mosby.)*

during a single pass through the liver. Sublingual administration avoids the first-pass effect. Many blood vessels are located under the tongue, so drugs administered by this route can pass directly into the general circulation before passing through the liver. Morphine is also subject to the first-pass effect.

FACTORS INFLUENCING METABOLISM

When metabolism is increased, the duration of effect of many drugs is reduced. The effects of drugs that must be metabolized to their active form are prolonged when metabolism is increased.

Effect of Liver Function on Metabolism

The liver is the primary site for metabolism. If the liver is functioning below capacity, metabolism is decreased. Drug doses should often be reduced in the presence of liver dysfunction.

Effect of Disease on Metabolism

Diseases like hepatitis decrease the metabolic capacity of the liver. The liver, however, is not the only site of metabolism. Lung disease and kidney disease can also reduce the ability of the body to metabolize drugs. Congestive heart disease decreases blood flood to the liver, altering the extent of drug metabolism.

Effect of Age on Metabolism

Metabolism in the liver is decreased in the elderly and in infants. Age-related changes in the liver decrease metabolic enzyme function in the elderly. Metabolizing enzyme systems (cytochrome P-450 system) is not fully developed in infants; therefore, their ability to metabolize drugs is decreased. Infants and the elderly require lower doses of drug to produce therapeutic effects.

Effect of Concurrent Administration of Drugs (Interactions)

Administration of two or more drugs that both use the same metabolic pathways can alter the metabolism of each other. Phenytoin is a drug used in the treatment of epilepsy. It is metabolized by the cytochrome P-450 isoform (CYP2C). Phenytoin can stimulate the metabolism of warfarin, a drug used to decrease blood clotting that is also metabolized by CYP2C metabolic enzymes.

Cigarette smoke contains ingredients that can stimulate the activity of metabolic enzymes. These enzymes increase the metabolism and clearance of theophylline, a drug used to treat asthma.

Effect of Genetics on Metabolism

A genetic deficiency of a metabolic enzyme can reduce the body's ability to metabolize drugs that use the enzyme. Nutrasweet (aspartame) is a common sweetener found in diet foods and beverages. It is a derivative of the amino acid phenylalanine. People diagnosed with the disorder phenylketonuria lack the enzyme needed to metabolize the amino acid phenylalanine to tyrosine. If they consume products containing aspartame, then they may build up toxic levels of phenylalanine.

Effect of Nutrition on Metabolism

Metabolism is decreased when nutritional status is severely depressed as in starvation. Low-protein diets and diets deficient in essential fatty acids can reduce the synthesis of drug-metabolizing enzymes and decrease metabolism. Deficiencies of vitamins and minerals can affect metabolism because they catalyze biochemical reactions in the body. For example, vitamin B_2 catalyzes oxidation-reduction reactions. Oxidation and reduction are metabolic processes that result in drug inactivation.

Foods can influence metabolism of drugs. Many drug interactions are linked to consumption of grapefruit juice. Grapefruit juice is a powerful inhibitor of metabolic enzyme CYP3A4. When the anticholesterol drugs (e.g., lovastatin) and antiretroviral drugs

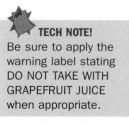

TECH NOTE!
Be sure to apply the warning label stating DO NOT TAKE WITH GRAPEFRUIT JUICE when appropriate.

(e.g., saquinavir) are taken with grapefruit juice, blood levels of the drugs are increased along with drug effects.

Effect of Gender on Metabolism

The rate of metabolism of some drugs varies between men and women, suggesting the sex hormones may influence metabolism. Men metabolize propranolol (a heart drug) faster than do women. Women metabolize acetaminophen (an analgesic) slightly faster than do men.

ELIMINATION

Elimination is the final pharmacokinetic phase. Elimination results in removal of the drug from the body and discontinuation of drug action. The three major routes of drug elimination are the kidney, lung, and bowel (Table 2-3).

The normal function of the kidney is to filter the blood and remove things that are foreign or harmful. This job is done by the **nephrons** of the kidney (Figure 2-13). Free drug (not bound to albumin) is transported to Bowman's capsule, where it is filtered by the **glomerulus**. As the drug moves through the nephron to the distal convoluted tubule, its concentration increases. If the drug is nonionized, it may diffuse out of the nephron back into the systemic circulation and continue to produce drug action.

FACTORS INFLUENCING ELIMINATION

Effect of Kidney Function on Elimination

Kidney dysfunction can have a profound effect on elimination of drugs from the body. Decreased kidney function decreases the extent of drug cleared and the rate of clearance. This can cause a build-up of drug in the body and produce toxic drug effects. When kidney function is critically reduced, dialysis is needed. Dialysis mechanically filters the blood and can increase drug elimination.

Effect of Disease on Elimination

Lung disease decreases the body's capacity to eliminate drugs and their metabolites. Bowel disease may increase of decrease elimination. Crohn's disease causes excessive diarrhea, which speeds the elimination of drugs. When movement of contents of the bowel is slowed, drug elimination is delayed.

Effect of Drug Ionization on Elimination

Changes in the acidity of the urine can influence the rate in which a drug is cleared from the body. Weakly acidic drugs are less ionized in acidic urine. As the pH of the urine becomes more basic, the ionization of acidic drugs increases. Weak bases are more ionized when the urine is acidic and less ionized when the urine is basic. Drugs that are ionized

TABLE 2-3   Routes of Drug Elimination

	Eliminated in
Major Routes	
Kidney	Urine
Lung	Expired air
Bowel	Feces
Minor Routes	
Liver	Bile
Skin	Sweat
Eyes	Tears
Mouth	Saliva
Nose	Mucus
Penis	Semen
Breast	Breast milk

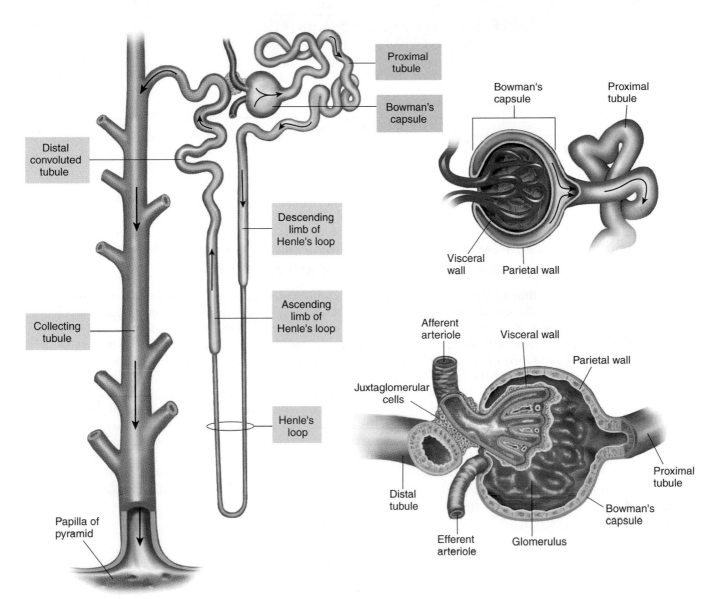

FIGURE 2-13 Nephron. *(From Thibodeau GA, Patton KT: Anatomy and physiology, ed 6, St Louis, 2007, Mosby.)*

are eliminated in the urine. Nonionized drugs are reabsorbed back into the circulatory system to continue their drug action.

Effect of Concurrent Administration of Drugs (Interactions)

Drug interactions can result in increased or decreased elimination of drugs. Pharmacists and health care providers may purposefully recommend coadministration of two drugs to delay elimination and prolong drug action or to speed elimination. Urinary acidifiers (e.g., vitamin C) decrease the elimination of acidic drugs. Urinary alkalinizers (e.g., sodium bicarbonate) decrease the elimination of basic drugs.

ELIMINATION HALF-LIFE (T½)

Elimination half-life (T½) refers to the time it takes for 50% of the drug to be cleared from the bloodstream (Table 2-4). It takes approximately eight half-lives to entirely eliminate a drug from the body. Every drug has a unique half-life that is dependent on characteristics of the drug (e.g., active metabolites). Knowledge of elimination half-life is important; it is

TABLE 2-4   The Concept of Drug Half-Life

Different perspectives			Changing values			
Drug concentration (mg/L)	100	50	25	12.5	6.25	3.125
Hours after peak concentration	0	8	16	24	32	40
Number of half-lives	0	1	2	3	4	5
Percentage of drug removed	0	50	75	88	94	97

From Lilley LL, Harrington S, Snyder JS: *Pharmacology and the nursing process*, ed 5, St Louis, 2007, Mosby.

an indicator of how long a drug will produce effects in the body. The half-life of a drug can be as short as a few minutes (e.g., drugs used to produce general anesthesia) or as long as several days (e.g., levothyroxine, a drug used to treat hypothyroidism). Drugs with a long half-life are dosed less frequently than are drugs with a very short half-life.

BIOAVAILABILITY AND BIOEQUIVALENCE OF DRUGS

Bioavailability describes the extent to which an administered amount of drug reaches the site of action and is available to produce drug effect(s). The bioavailability of a drug is influenced by drug absorption and distribution to the site of action. The bioavailability of generic drugs is compared with the innovators product to determine if the generic is bioequivalent. Tests are conducted to measure maximum concentration (C_{max}) of the drug in the bloodstream after a single dose is administered. The time it takes to reach maximum concentration (T_{max}) is also measured. A graph showing rise and fall of drug blood levels following the administration of a single dose of drug looks like a curve. The area under the curve (AUC) is a measure to the drug bioavailability. Bioavailability tests are conducted to determine if the generic drug achieves the same maximum blood concentration, in the same time as the brand name drug. The generic is *bioequivalent* if no statistical differences are found in the rate and extent of absorption when the drug is administered in the same strength, dosage form, and route of administration as the brand name product (Figure 2-14).

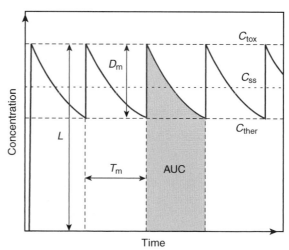

L = loading dose
D_m = maintence dose
T_m = maintence interval
C_{ther} = therapeutic concentration
C_{tox} = toxic concentration
C_{ss} = average steady state concentration
AUC = area under the curve

FIGURE 2-14 Plasma concentrations following repeated dose. *(From: Kalant H, Grant DM, Mitchell J: Principles of medical pharmacology, ed 7, Philadelphia, 2007, WB Saunders.)*

PHARMACEUTICAL EQUIVALENTS AND PHARMACEUTICAL ALTERNATIVES

Pharmaceutical equivalents differ from bioequivalents. Bioequivalent drugs and pharmaceutical equivalent drugs both contain the same active ingredient in the same strength as the innovator's drug (brand name). *Pharmaceutical equivalents* may have different inactive ingredients, be manufactured in a different dosage form, and exhibit different rates of absorption than the brand name. *Pharmaceutical alternatives* contain the same active ingredient as the brand name product; however, the strength and dosage form may be different. A *therapeutic alternative* may contain different active ingredients yet produce the same desired therapeutic outcome.

CHAPTER SUMMARY

- There are four pharmacokinetic phases: absorption, distribution, metabolism, and elimination.
- As a drug moves throughout the body, it undergoes changes that may increase or decrease its absorption, distribution, metabolism, or elimination.
- Pharmacokinetic phases control the intensity of the drug's effect and the duration of the drug action.
- The time it takes for a drug to reach the concentration necessary to produce a therapeutic effect is called the onset of action.
- The peak effect occurs once the maximum concentration of the drug is reached in the body.
- Duration of action is the time between the onset of action and discontinuation of drug action.
- The pharmaceutical phase of drug disposition involves drug disintegration and dissolution.
- Drugs administered parenterally enter directly into the general circulation; therefore, they are not subject to the first-pass effect and are not degraded by gastrointestinal enzymes.
- The bioavailability of parenterally administered drugs is greater than orally administered drugs.
- Absorption is the process that involves the movement of drug molecules from the site of administration, across cell membranes, into the circulatory system of the body (blood or lymphatic system).
- Drugs are absorbed across cell membranes via active and passive transport mechanisms.
- Factors influencing absorption are chemical nature of the drug, pH, blood flow, surface area, and tissue thickness.
- Distribution is the process of movement of the drug from the circulatory system, across barrier membranes, to the site of drug action.
- Factors influencing distribution are the chemical nature of the drug, protein and tissue binding, and ability to move across anatomical barriers.
- Metabolism is a biochemical process involving enzymes that convert the administered drug to metabolites that are or more active or less active than the original drug.
- Drugs that interfere with the enzymes of the cytochrome P-450 system can enhance or inhibit the metabolism of other drugs that are taken concurrently.
- First-pass metabolism describes a process whereby the liver clears nearly all of a drug before it passes into the general circulation.
- Factors influencing metabolism are liver function, disease, age, drug interactions, genetics, nutrition, and gender.
- Elimination results in removal of the drug from the body and discontinuation of drug action.
- Factors influencing elimination are kidney function, diseases, drug ionization, and drug interactions.
- Elimination half-life ($T\frac{1}{2}$) refers to the time it takes for 50% of the drug to be cleared from the bloodstream. It takes approximately eight half-lives to eliminate a drug from the body.

- Bioavailability is the extent to which a drug is absorbed and distributed to the site of action.
- A generic drug is bioequivalent if no statistical differences are found in the rate and extent of absorption when the drug is administered in the same strength, dosage form, and route of administration as the brand name product.
- Pharmaceutical equivalents may have different inactive ingredients, be manufactured in a different dosage form, and exhibit different rates of absorption than the brand name.
- Pharmaceutical alternatives contain the same active ingredient as the brand name drug; however, the strength and dosage form may be different.
- A therapeutic alternative may contain different active ingredients yet produce the same desired therapeutic outcome.

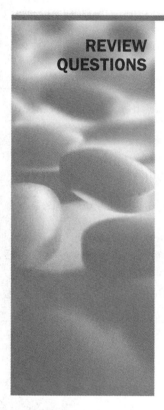

REVIEW QUESTIONS

Multiple Choice

1. **Name the four phases of pharmacokinetics.**
   a. absorption, dissolution, catabolism, elimination
   b. absorption, distribution, metabolism, elimination
   c. assimilation, dissolution, metabolism, excretion
   d. assimilation, distribution, anabolism, excretion

2. **Lipid-soluble drugs are _____.**
   a. hydrophobic
   b. lipophobic
   c. lipophilic
   d. a and c

3. **A process whereby the liver clears nearly all of a drug before it passes into the general circulation is known as the**
   a. first-pass effect
   b. dissolution effect
   c. metabolite effect
   d. liver-pass effect

4. **Drugs that contain different active ingredient(s) than the brand name drug yet produces the same desired therapeutic outcome are called a therapeutic _____.**
   a. equivalent
   b. alternative
   c. substitution
   d. replacement

5. **The process that involves the movement of drug molecules from the site of administration, across cell membranes into the circulatory system of the body is known as**
   a. distribution
   b. metabolism
   c. absorption
   d. elimination

6. **Drugs are assigned to one of five categories according to their safety if taken during pregnancy. Which one of the following is the safest?**
   a. category A
   b. category C
   c. category D
   d. category X

7. The transformation of drugs via biochemical processes involving enzymes to metabolites is termed
   a. bioequivalence
   b. biotransformation
   c. bioavailability
   d. bioeffect

8. Drugs that are administered in an inactive form and must be metabolized to their active form is called a(an)
   a. investigational drug
   b. metabolite
   c. prodrug
   d. none of the above

9. Which body organ serves as the primary site of the metabolism of drugs?
   a. kidney
   b. lungs
   c. stomach
   d. liver

10. The time it takes for 50% of the drug to be cleared from the bloodstream is termed the
   a. distribution half-life ($T\frac{1}{2}$)
   b. elimination half-life ($T\frac{1}{2}$)
   c. metabolism half-life ($T\frac{1}{2}$)
   d. absorption half-life ($T\frac{1}{2}$)

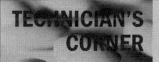 **TECHNICIAN'S CORNER** What is the difference between bioavailability and bioequivalence?

BIBLIOGRAPHY

Fulcher E, Soto C, Fulcher R: *Pharmacology: Principles and applications. A worktext for allied health professionals* (pp 21-22, 60-65, 83), Philadelphia, 2003, WB Saunders.

Lance L, Lacy C, Armstrong L, Goldman M: *Drug information handbook for the allied health professional,* ed 12, Hudson, OH, 2005, APhA Lexi-Comp.

Page C, et al.: *Integrated pharmacology* (pp 57-70), Philadelphia, 2005, Elsevier Mosby.

Raffa RB, Rawls SM, Beyzarov EP: *Netter's illustrated pharmacology* (pp 10-11, 25-27). Philadelphia, 2005, WB Saunders

Shargel L, Mutnick A, Souney P, Swanson L: *Comprehensive pharmacy review* (pp 78-84, 42-65, 131-132), ed 4, Baltimore, 2001, Lippincott Williams & Wilkins.

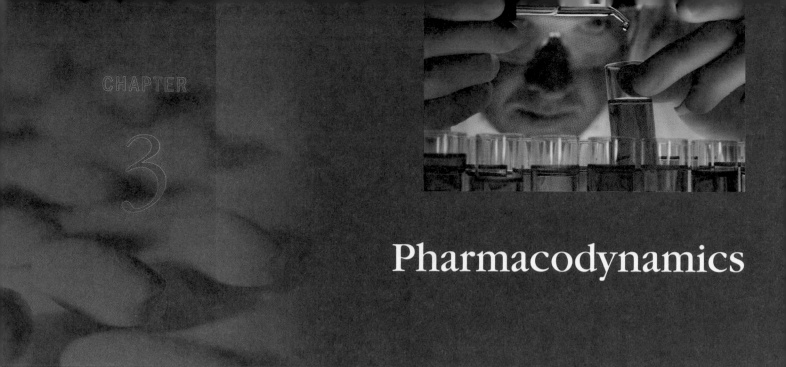

CHAPTER 3

Pharmacodynamics

LEARNING OBJECTIVES

- Explain the drug-receptor theory.
- Compare and contrast agonists, antagonists, and partial agonists.
- Illustrate the relationship between drug effectiveness and potency.
- Discuss the importance of pharmacodynamics to drug action.
- Discuss the factors influencing patient response to drug therapy.
- List ways to improve patient adherence to drug therapy.
- Learn terminology associated with pharmacodynamics and drug action.

KEY TERMS

Affinity: Attraction that the receptor site has for the drug.

Agonist: Drug that binds to its receptor site and stimulates a cellular response.

Antagonist: Drug that binds to the receptor site and does not produce an action. An antagonist prevents another drug or natural body chemical from binding to the receptor site.

Drug-Receptor Theory: Theory that states that a drug must interact or bind with targeted cells in the body if drug action is to be produced.

Efficacy: Measure of the drug's effectiveness.

Hepatoxicity: Serious adverse reaction that occurs in the liver.

Idiosyncratic reaction: Unexpected drug reaction.

Inverse agonist: Drug that has affinity and activity at the receptor site. The drug can turn "off" a receptor that is activated or turn "on" a receptor that is not currently active.

Mechanism of action (MOA): Manner in which a drug produces its effect.

Nephrotoxicity: Serious adverse effect that occurs in the kidney.

Noncompetitive antagonist: Drug that binds to the same receptor site as the antagonist or an alternative receptor site, preventing the agonist from binding to and producing its desired action.

Partial agonist: Drug that behaves like an agonist under some conditions and acts like an antagonist under different conditions.

Pharmacodynamics: Study of drugs and their action on the living organism.

Pharmacotherapeutics: Use of drugs in the treatment of disease. It is the study of factors that influence patient response to drugs.

Potency: Measure of the amount of drug required to produce a response. It is the effective dose concentration.

Receptor site: Location of drug-cell binding.

Therapeutic index (TI): Ratio of the effective dose to the lethal dose.

Pharmacodynamics

In the previous chapter, we looked at how the drug was altered as it traveled throughout the compartments of the body. ***Pharmacodynamics*** is the study of drugs and their action on the living organism. Pharmacodynamics looks at how the body responds to drugs that are administered. The ***mechanism of action (MOA)*** describes how the drug produces its effect. An understanding of pathophysiology and drug mechanism of action will facilitate the selection of the best drug to treat the patient's medical condition. ***Pathophysiology*** is the study of disease in the body.

DRUG-RECEPTOR INTERACTIONS

According to ***drug-receptor theory,*** drugs interact or bind with targeted cells in the body to produce pharmacologic action. Most drugs bind with specific proteins in the body; however, they may also bind to carbohydrates, lipids, or enzymes. The location of drug-cell binding is called the ***receptor site***. Drug-receptor binding is similar to the action of a lock and key (Figure 3-1). The drug is the key and the receptor site is the lock. The more similar the drug is to the shape of the receptor site, the greater is the ***affinity,*** or attraction, that the receptor site has for the drug. When two or more drugs are administered, the receptor site will preferentially bind with the drug for which it has the greatest affinity (the drug that best fits the lock). Drug binding to the receptor is reversible. Drugs spontaneously bind and disassociate with the receptor site.

Some drugs do not produce their actions by directly binding to a receptor site on the cell. They are able to produce a change in cell membrane stability or excitability through nonspecific mechanisms. Some general anesthetics gases produce effect via nonspecific interactions.

SECOND MESSENGERS

Drug response does not always occur on stimulation of the primary drug receptor. In some cases, stimulation of the primary receptor causes a second receptor to be activated, and it is only after the release of the ***second messenger*** that the desired drug effect is produced.

TYPES OF DRUG-RECEPTOR INTERACTIONS

Drugs are described as agonist, partial agonist, antagonist, competitive antagonist, and non-competitive antagonist based on their effect at the receptor site (Table 3-1).

Agonists

An ***agonist*** is a drug that binds to and activates the receptor site eliciting a cellular response (Figure 3-2). Agonist binding may activate a receptor that was resting or turn off a receptor that was activated. ***Inverse agonists*** (Figure 3-2) are drugs that have affinity at the receptor site but produce opposite actions (turn "off" a receptor that is activated or turn "on" a receptor that is not currently active). When two or more agonists are administered together, a competition for drug-receptor binding sites occurs. The drug with the greatest affinity will bind to the receptor site. The result of agonist binding may mimic the effects produced by binding of normal body chemicals to their target receptor. An example

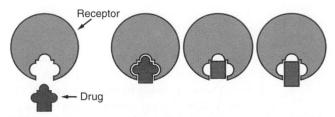

FIGURE 3-1 Drug-receptor interactions. *(From Clayton BD, Stock YN, Harroun RD: Basic pharmacology for nurses, ed 14, St Louis, 2007, Mosby.)*

TABLE 3-1   Summary of Effects of Drug-Receptor Binding

Interaction term	Definition
Agonist	Drug binds to a receptor, and there is a response.
Partial agonist	Drug binds to a receptor, and there is a diminished response compared with that elicited by the agonist.
Antagonist	Drug binds to receptor, but there is no response. Drug prevents binding of agonists.
Competitive antagonist	Drug competes with the agonist for binding to receptor. If it binds, there is no response.
Noncompetitive antagonist	Drug combines with different parts of receptor and inactivates it, so agonist has no effect.

From Lilly LL, Harrington S, Snyder JS: *Pharmacology and the nursing process,* ed 5, St Louis, 2007, Mosby.

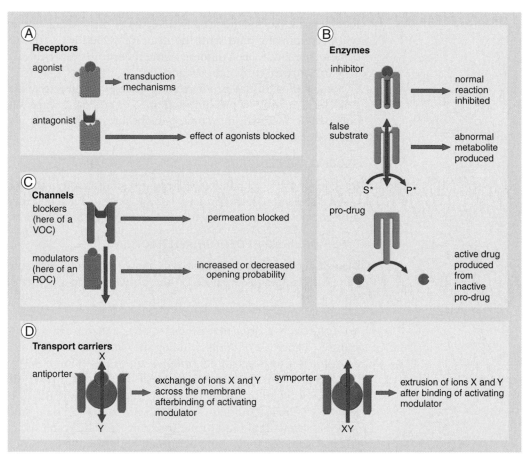

FIGURE 3-2 Effect of agonist and antagonist binding. *(From Page C, et al.: Integrated pharmacology, ed 3. Philadelphia, 2006, Mosby.)*

is the binding of barbiturates to their drug-receptor site. This mimics the effects produced by the neurotransmitter γ-aminobutyric acid GABA (a chemical messenger of the nervous system) when it binds to its receptor site. Drug-receptor binding may stimulate the release of a normal biological chemical and in doing so produce the desired action. When the drug amantadine is administered, it stimulates the release of the neurotransmitter dopamine. An increase in dopamine levels reduces the symptoms associated with Parkinson's disease.

Antagonists

Antagonists bind to the receptor site and do not produce an action. They prevent another drug or natural body chemical from binding by occupying or activating the receptor site. Antagonists block the actions of agonists, inverse agonists, and partial agonists.

Naloxone is an example of a pure antagonist. Administration reverses the effects of opiates (e.g., heroin) by occupying the receptor site and preventing the heroin from binding.

Noncompetitive antagonists bind to an alternative site on the same receptor site as the agonist. Noncompetitive antagonist binding results in inactivation of the receptor site.

Partial Agonists

A *partial agonist* behaves like an agonist under some conditions and acts like an antagonist under different conditions. The drug butorphanol (Stadol) is an example of a partial agonist. Partial agonists behave like antagonists in the presence of a high concentration of a full agonist or when administered after recent exposure to high concentrations of an agonist.

DOSE-RESPONSE RELATIONSHIP

Typically, increasing the drug dose will increase the cellular response and drug effect; however, many other factors may influence the strength of the response to a dose of administered drug. Pharmacokinetic factors (absorption, distribution, metabolism, and elimination) and individual properties of a drug also influence drug response. A dose-response curve shows the relationship between the effectiveness of a drug at the administered dose. The effects produced by a given drug dose can be quantified and graphed. The graph is called a dose-response curve. The ***dose-response*** curve shows the drug's relative efficacy and potency (Figure 3-3). A steep dose-response curve indicates that a small change in drug dose will produce a large change in the drug response. A flatter dose-response curve shows that small changes in drug dose produce little change. A large increase in the dose of the drug administered is needed to produce a greater drug response.

EFFICACY

Efficacy describes the maximum response produced by a drug (Figure 3-4). It is a measure of the drug's effectiveness. Agonists produce the maximum drug response. The drug response produced by partial agonists is less than maximal. The efficacy of antagonists is measured by the extent to which they intefere with the effect of an agonist. Efficacy can be measured for each effect produced by a drug. It is not necessary for all drug receptor sites to be occupied before the maximum drug effect is achieved.

POTENCY

Efficacy and potency are related. Drugs that have a high efficacy at a low dose are very potent. In other words, only a small dose is required to produce the maximum drug effect. Drugs that must be administered in very high doses in order to produce a minimal effect

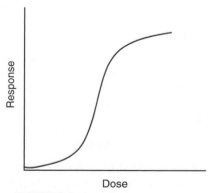

FIGURE 3-3 Dose-response curve.

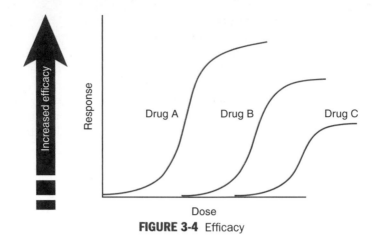

FIGURE 3-4 Efficacy

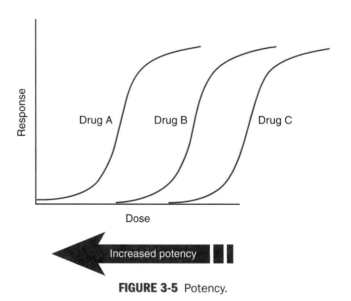

FIGURE 3-5 Potency.

have low efficacy. In Figure 3-5, drug A is more potent than drug B and drug C because a lower dose produces an equal response.

Efficacy is more important than potency when determining usefulness of a drug unless the dose that is required to produce the therapeutic effect is so large it is impractical to administer. When choosing between two equally effective drugs, pharmacokinetic factors, disease, and the ability of the patient to tolerate the side effects of the drug become more important than the dose that is required to produce an effect.

CEILING EFFECT

A graded dose-response curve shows that as the drug dose increases, the drug effect increases. Drug effects increase up to a ceiling. This ceiling effect may be reached when all drug receptors are saturated or when the maximum possible effect that could be produced is reached. For example, the ceiling effect for opioid analgesics is reached at the point when no more pain relief is achieved even if additional opioid is administered.

THERAPEUTIC INDEX

All drugs produce toxic effects that can lead to death. When the lethal dose of a drug is close to the effective dose, the drug is not very safe. The safest drugs have a wide margin between the lethal dose and the effective dose. *Therapeutic index (TI)* is the ratio of the effective dose to the lethal dose; the formula is shown below. ED_{50} represents the effective dose for 50% of a population and LD_{50} is the lethal dose for 50% of a population.

$$\text{Therapeutic Index (TI)} = \frac{\text{Lethal Dose (LD}_{50})}{\text{Effective Dose (ED}_{50})}$$

TECH NOTE!
Product substitution must be considered carefully when the therapeutic index is narrow or bioequivalency problems are present.

Digoxin, a drug used to treat heart disease, has a narrow TI. The drug dose needed to increase the force of heart contractions is similar to the drug dose that can cause the heart to stop beating. Another drug with a small TI is warfarin. The dose required to prolonged blood clotting time is near the dose that causes hemorrhage and death. Patients respond differently to different doses of drug. Variation in patient response to a drug can become critical when the TI is narrow.

FACTORS INFLUENCING PHARMACOTHERAPEUTICS

Pharmacotherapeutics describes the process of using drugs in the treatment of disease. Factors that influence patient response to drugs range from pharmacokinetics to patient-specific factors. Successful drug therapy is also influenced by a variety of factors ranging from the patient's belief that the therapy will be beneficial to drug interactions. Patient-related factors such as the presence of chronic disease, drug allergies, age, obesity, or gender increase or decrease a person's response to an administered drug. Prior exposure to the drug can result in a heightened drug response if the patient has developed an allergy to the drug. Drug response is decreased in situations where the patient has become desensitized to the effects of the drug. The patient's response to a drug is not always predictable; however, drug doses and dosing schedules should be modified to control for known factors that influence patient drug response. Successful drug therapy is strongly influenced by whether the patient takes the medication as prescribed or whether medication is taken at all.

PATIENT PHYSIOLOGICAL FACTORS

Humans are unique and individual variability influences the outcome of drug therapy. Desired therapeutic effects are achieved when optimum drug doses are administered. Doses that are too low result in subtherapeutic effects. Doses that are too high result in toxic effects.

Age

The human body undergoes physiologic and hormonal changes between birth and death. Age-related changes influence how effectively the body is able to handle drugs. Neonates and infants have an underdeveloped capacity to absorb, distribute, metabolize, and eliminate drugs. The ability of the lungs, liver, and kidney to process and eliminate drugs declines as humans age. The elderly and infants require lower drug doses.

Weight

Drug doses for children are often calculated according to the child's weight; however, dose calculations based on body surface area are more accurate than those based on weight. Dose adjustments may need to be considered for obese or severely underweight adults. Drug doses must be increased in obese patients to produce therapeutic effects. Doses are decreased in severely underweight or emaciated adults and children to avoid toxic side effects.

Gender

Gender may influence drug distribution and metabolism. The fat-to-muscle ratio varies between women and men and may influence the volume of drug distribution. Additionally, the rate of metabolism of some drugs varies between men and women, suggesting the sex hormones may influence metabolism.

Genetics

Genetics influence enzyme and protein production in the body. Absence of certain enzymes can produce deadly side effects in people who take drugs that require the enzyme for metabolism and elimination.

Disease

The presence of disease can significantly influence pharmacotherapeutics. More severe drug reactions occur in patients with kidney disease, liver disease, and/or lung disease, because the ability to distribute, metabolize, and eliminate drugs is compromised. The effects of a drug may diminish because the disease itself becomes more debilitating over time. Parkinson's disease is linked to destruction of dopamine releasing nerve cells in the body. The ability of anti–Parkinson's disease drugs to improve patient symptoms decreases as the disease progresses.

Pregnancy

Drug absorption may decrease during pregnancy because of pregnancy-related decreased movement through the gastrointestinal tract. These may decrease drug effects. Pregnancy causes increased urination, thereby increasing the rate of drug elimination. The duration of drug effects may be reduced in pregnancy.

IMMUNOLOGIC FACTORS

Excessive reactions can occur at any dose. Hypersensitivity reactions are extreme allergic reactions and can occur after a single dose of the drug or after multiple exposures to the drug. The reaction occurs because the patient develops antibodies to the drug. The presence of antibodies, causes the release of histamine and other body chemicals that produce allergic symptoms. Symptoms may range from a mild rash to anaphylactic shock.

DESENSITIZATION

Repeated exposures to a drug may result in a decreased drug response. Desensitization is caused by changes to drug receptor (especially proteins) that decrease drug-receptor binding or reduce receptor site activation when binding occurs. When desensitization occurs, the effects can be limited to a single receptor or may influence multiple receptors. When drug-receptor binding involves a second messenger, the result may be desensitization to the effects that would have been produced by binding to multiple receptors (i.e., all of the receptors normally activated by binding of the drug to its primary receptor).

IDIOSYNCRATIC REACTIONS

Sometimes the response to a drug cannot be predicted. Unexpected drug reactions are known as *idiosyncratic reactions.*

PSYCHOLOGICAL FACTORS

Drug therapy is influenced by patient belief that the therapy will be beneficial. Studies have shown that sugar pills can produce the desired effect if the patient believes it will be effective. This is known as the *placebo effect.* Double-blind clinical studies are conducted to control for the placebo effect. In a **double-blind study,** some of the people in the study will receive a drug containing active ingredient and other will receive a drug look-alike that does not contain active ingredients. Neither the people taking the drugs nor their care providers know who is receiving the real drug. This reduces the risk that drug effects reported are caused by placebo effect. This also decreases the likelihood that care providers will treat their patient differently because they know they are receiving the active drug. Increased attention can also improve patient outcomes.

ADVERSE DRUG REACTIONS

Few drugs are so specific that they only produce their desired effect. Drugs produce desired effects (therapeutic effects) and undesired effects. Undesired effects are called *adverse reactions.* Approximately 10% of people who receive health care in industrialized countries will experience a preventable adverse drug reaction (ADR).

ADRs have an impact on patients, family members, employers, pharmacies, health care facilities, and society. The cost of drug-related illness, hospitalization, and death in the

United States is estimated to be more than $100 billion. In Canada, 2% of all hospitalized patients experience a preventable adverse drug event and 700 deaths per year are attributed to medication errors.

Some populations are more at risk for adverse drug reactions than others. The elderly have an increased risk for ADRs, because they are more likely to be on multiple drug therapy and their capacity to metabolize and eliminate drugs is less than that of younger adults. Multiple drug therapy *(polypharmacy)* is a risk factor for hospitalized patients, too. The average patient in the hospital is prescribed up to 10 drugs. The risk for drug side effects and drug interactions increases with the number of medications a person is administered.

ADRs may be localized and only occur at the site where the drug was administered. Other adverse reactions are widespread, occurring at other regions of the body. Adverse effects may cause minor discomfort such as a rash, or they may be life threatening (e.g., coma and death).

Common adverse effects that occur in the central nervous system are drowsiness, dizziness, stimulation, or confusion. Life-threatening central nervous system effects include respiratory depression, coma, and death. ***Hepatoxicity*** is a toxic adverse reaction that occurs in the liver. Some common drugs that can produce hepatoxicity are acetaminophen and isoniazid (a drug used to treat tuberculosis). ***Nephrotoxicity*** is a serious adverse effect that occurs in the kidney. Nonsteroidal antiinflammatory drugs such as ibuprofen and naproxen can produce nephrotoxicity.

ADRs also occur as a result of nonsterile drug preparation. Intravenous fluids and other parenterals must be prepared using aseptic technique. Failure to use aseptic technique can result in the introduction of contaminants, pathogens, and fever-causing agents into the solution. Prolonged illness or death may occur if the solution is injected into a patient.

TECH NOTE!
New clean room standards have been adopted to reduce contamination of sterile products. The new standards are outlined in the USP 797 regulations for sterile product preparation.

Teratogenicity

ADRs that produce harm to a developing fetus are called *teratogenic effects.* To reduce possible harm to the fetus, pregnant women and their health care providers must weigh the risks versus the benefit of taking drugs. To assist in their decision-making, pregnancy safety categories have been created. Drugs with no known teratogenic effects in humans are listed in category A. Drugs known to produce teratogenic effects are listed in category X (see Table 2-1).

Carcinogenicity

Drugs and natural products that stimulate the growth of cancers are classified as carcinogens. Carcinogenic drugs interact with DNA and produce permanent genetic mutations. Many of the drugs used to treat one type of cancer are capable of producing cancers in other areas. Drugs used to treat ovarian cancer increase the risk for acute nonlymphocytic leukemia (ANLL). Melphalan is a drug used to treat breast cancer that can increase the risk for ANLL. The synthetic estrogen diethylstilbesterol (DES) is no longer prescribed to women to prevent miscarriage because it increases the risks for breast and uterine cancer. The drug is still prescribed for the treatment of prostate cancer. Sassafras tea was widely used as a cleansing tea or tonic until it was discovered to be carcinogenic in the 1960s.

Dependence and Tolerance

Dependence and *tolerance* are adverse reactions associated with controlled substances. Drugs are placed in controlled substance schedules according to their likelihood to produce physiological or psychological dependence. Patients who have developed dependence to a drug must continue to take the drug in order to prevent the onset of withdrawal symptoms. Once tolerance to a drug has developed, the patient must take increasing doses of the drug to produce the same effects as was previously produced by a lower dose. Tolerance may occur to the therapeutic effect or side effects. Tolerance develops to the sedation produced by some antiseizure drugs like alprazolam before tolerance develops to the desired antiseizure effects.

Improving Adherence to Drug Therapy

Drug therapy is strongly influenced by whether the patient takes the medication as prescribed or whether medication is taken at all. Adherence to drug therapy is defined as taking the prescribed medication in the correct dose, at the right time, and without missed doses. Today, it is recognized that patients and their caregivers must be actively involved to making decisions about drug therapy. Patients who recognize the importance of the drug therapy and are involved in selecting the medication best suited for their individual needs are more likely to adhere to therapy.

FACTORS INFLUENCING ADHERENCE TO DRUG THERAPY

Lack of adherence to drug therapy is associated with poor health outcomes. Understanding why medications are not taken as prescribed is important for the design of strategies to improve adherence. Strategies for improving adherence must be targeted at patients, caregivers, pharmacists, pharmacy technicians, clinicians, and other health care providers.

BELIEF THAT THERAPY IS BENEFICIAL

Adherence to drug therapy is increased when patients believe therapy is beneficial. This is particularly important when the medication has substantial adverse effects. Hypertension is known as the silent killer because often no symptoms are present. Medications to treat hypertension may cause dizziness, upset stomach, impotence, or even depression, causing many patients to discontinue drug therapy. Adherence to drug therapy to avoid complications associated with untreated hypertension is essential.

ADVERSE DRUG REACTIONS

ADRs are a principal cause for discontinuation of drug therapy. Even fear of potential adverse reactions is a sufficient disincentive for some patients to avoid taking their medication. Many drug formulations have been developed to minimize drug side effects. Enteric-coated formulations reduce the risk of stomach upset. Gastrointestinal side effects are avoided by use of drugs formulated for transdermal application.

Pharmacy technicians can assist the pharmacist in reducing the patient's anxiety about adverse reactions by making certain patients get the information they need to reduce their risk for drug side effects. Warning labels, also called auxiliary labels, are affixed to the prescription vial and provide information to ensure maximum benefits of drug therapy are achieved with minimum side effects. Taking medication with food or a glass of water can decrease the risk for upset stomach. Pharmacy technicians can play a key role in helping patients limit adverse reactions by distributing patient drug information leaflets and alerting the pharmacist when counseling is required.

LACK OF ANY MEDICATION ADMINISTRATION ROUTINE

Adherence is improved when patients develop a regular routine for taking medicine. The pharmacist and pharmacy technician can work with patients to develop a routine for taking medications that fits the patient's lifestyle. Some pharmacies sell devices that prompt the patient to remember to take medicines.

UNDERSTANDABLE DOSING SCHEDULE

Dosing schedules must be convenient and understandable if patients are to avoid missed doses or taking double doses. Adherence to drug therapy increases in difficulty as the number of medications prescribed increases. Selection of drug formulations that are taken once a day may improve adherence.

ABILITY TO AFFORD DRUG THERAPY

The poor are at increased risk for ADRs. Poverty decreases the ability to afford medications and decreases access to health care when adverse events are experienced. When drug therapy is expensive, prescriptions may not be filled. When prescriptions are filled, patients

TECH NOTE!
Many pharmacy computer systems now print auxiliary labels directly onto the prescription label, using a different color for identification purposes.

TECH NOTE!
Extended release medications promote patient adherence. Instead of taking medications 3 or 4 times a day, an extended release (ER), sustained release (SR), or controlled dose (CD) tablet may be taken once daily.

U.S. Department of Health and Human Services

MedWatch

The FDA Safety Information and
Adverse Event Reporting Program

For VOLUNTARY reporting of
adverse events, product problems and
product use errors

Page ____ of ____

Form Approved: OMB No. 0910-0291, Expires: 10/31/08
See OMB statement on reverse.

FDA USE ONLY
Triage unit sequence #

A. PATIENT INFORMATION

1. Patient Identifier	2. Age at Time of Event, or Date of Birth:	3. Sex	4. Weight
In confidence		☐ Female ☐ Male	_____ lb or _____ kg

B. ADVERSE EVENT, PRODUCT PROBLEM OR ERROR

Check all that apply:

1. ☐ Adverse Event   ☐ Product Problem (e.g., defects/malfunctions)
   ☐ Product Use Error   ☐ Problem with Different Manufacturer of Same Medicine

2. Outcomes Attributed to Adverse Event
   (Check all that apply)

☐ Death: _____ (mm/dd/yyyy)   ☐ Disability or Permanent Damage

☐ Life-threatening   ☐ Congenital Anomaly/Birth Defect

☐ Hospitalization - initial or prolonged   ☐ Other Serious (Important Medical Events)

☐ Required Intervention to Prevent Permanent Impairment/Damage (Devices)

3. Date of Event (mm/dd/yyyy)	4. Date of this Report (mm/dd/yyyy)

5. Describe Event, Problem or Product Use Error

6. Relevant Tests/Laboratory Data, Including Dates

7. Other Relevant History, Including Preexisting Medical Conditions (e.g., allergies, race, pregnancy, smoking and alcohol use, liver/kidney problems, etc.)

PLEASE TYPE OR USE BLACK INK

C. PRODUCT AVAILABILITY

Product Available for Evaluation? (Do not send product to FDA)

☐ Yes   ☐ No   ☐ Returned to Manufacturer on: _____ (mm/dd/yyyy)

D. SUSPECT PRODUCT(S)

1. Name, Strength, Manufacturer (from product label)

#1 _____

#2 _____

2.	Dose or Amount	Frequency	Route
#1			
#2			

3. Dates of Use (If unknown, give duration) from/to (or best estimate)	5. Event Abated After Use Stopped or Dose Reduced?
#1	#1 ☐ Yes ☐ No ☐ Doesn't Apply
#2	#2 ☐ Yes ☐ No ☐ Doesn't Apply

4. Diagnosis or Reason for Use (Indication)	8. Event Reappeared After Reintroduction?
#1	#1 ☐ Yes ☐ No ☐ Doesn't Apply
#2	#2 ☐ Yes ☐ No ☐ Doesn't Apply

6. Lot #	7. Expiration Date	9. NDC # or Unique ID
#1	#1	
#2	#2	

E. SUSPECT MEDICAL DEVICE

1. Brand Name

2. Common Device Name

3. Manufacturer Name, City and State

4. Model #	Lot #	5. Operator of Device
Catalog #	Expiration Date (mm/dd/yyyy)	☐ Health Professional
Serial #	Other #	☐ Lay User/Patient ☐ Other: _____

6. If Implanted, Give Date (mm/dd/yyyy)	7. If Explanted, Give Date (mm/dd/yyyy)

8. Is this a Single-use Device that was Reprocessed and Reused on a Patient?
   ☐ Yes   ☐ No

9. If Yes to Item No. 8, Enter Name and Address of Reprocessor

F. OTHER (CONCOMITANT) MEDICAL PRODUCTS

Product names and therapy dates (exclude treatment of event)

G. REPORTER (See confidentiality section on back)

1. Name and Address

Phone #	E-mail

2. Health Professional?	3. Occupation	4. Also Reported to:
☐ Yes ☐ No		☐ Manufacturer
5. If you do NOT want your identity disclosed to the manufacturer, place an "X" in this box: ☐		☐ User Facility ☐ Distributor/Importer

FORM FDA 3500 (10/05)   Submission of a report does not constitute an admission that medical personnel or the product caused or contributed to the event.

FIGURE 3-6 FDA Voluntary Reporting Form 3500. *(Courtesy U.S. Food and Drug Administration, Rockville, MD.)*

may take less than the dose prescribed, to make the prescription last longer. Pharmacy personnel can work with prescribers to ensure effective and affordable drugs are prescribed. Pharmacy technicians can contact insurance companies to obtain approval for nonformulary medicines.

REPORTING ADVERSE DRUG EVENTS

ADRs are reported to the U.S. Food and Drug Administration (FDA) by drug manufacturers, health care professionals, and consumers using FDA Voluntary Reporting Form 3500 (Figure 3-6). These reports of ADRs are compiled into a computerized information database called the Adverse Event Reporting System (AERS). The reports are analyzed and used to update product labeling, send out a "Dear Health Care Professional" letter, or even reevaluate the drug approval decision. If reevaluation results in a decision to withdraw approval of the drug, then a recall will be issued. The AERS also issues safety alerts for drugs, biologics, devices, and dietary supplements. Patient and consumer information sheets are also available from the FDA.

CHAPTER SUMMARY

- Pharmacodynamics looks at how the body responds to drugs that are administered.
- Drugs interact or bind with targeted cells in the body to produce pharmacologic action.
- Drug-receptor binding is similar to a lock and key. The more similar the drug is to the shape of the receptor site, the greater is the affinity the receptor site has for the drug.
- Drug-receptor binding enhances or inhibits normal biological processes. Binding may reverse the action of a currently administered drug.
- An agonist is a drug that binds to its receptor site and stimulates a cellular response. Agonist binding may activate a receptor that was resting or turn off a receptor that was activated.
- Antagonists bind to the receptor site and do not produce an action. They prevent another drug or natural body chemical from binding by occupying or activating the receptor site.
- Partial agonists behave like antagonists in the presence of a high concentration of a full agonist or when administered after recent exposure to high concentrations of an agonist.
- Efficacy is a measure of the drug's effectiveness.
- Drugs that are administered in very low doses yet produce a maximum effect have high efficacy.
- The dose-response curve shows the drug's relative efficacy and potency. A steep dose-response curve indicates that a small change in drug dose will produce a big change in the drug response.
- The therapeutic index (TI) is ratio of the effective dose to the lethal dose. Safe drugs have a wide margin between the lethal dose and the effective dose.
- Successful drug therapy is influenced by a variety of factors. The patient's response to a drug is not always predictable.
- Age, gender, disease, pregnancy, weight, and genetics are patient-related factors that influence drug response.
- Drug allergies cause a heightened response to drugs and can occur after one or more exposures to a drug.
- Patients may become desensitized to the effects of drugs.
- Idiosyncratic reactions are unpredictable.
- Psychological factors can influence drug response. The placebo effect demonstrates that patients can experience drug effects even when no active drug has been administered.
- Drugs produce desired effects (therapeutic effects) and undesired effects. Undesired effects are called adverse reactions.
- Multiple drug therapy increases risks for adverse drug reactions (ADRs). The elderly and poor also have increased risks for ADRs.
- ADRs can be mild or severe. Effects range from rash, upset stomach, and sedation to hepatoxicity, teratogenicity, and anaphylactic shock.
- Dependence and tolerance are adverse reactions associated with controlled substances. When tolerance develops, the patient must take increasing doses of the drug to get the

desired effect. When dependence has developed, patients must continue to take the drug to prevent withdrawal symptoms.

- Patients, caregivers, pharmacists, pharmacy technicians, clinicians, and other health care providers must work as a team to improve adherence to drug therapy.
- Adherence to drug therapy is influenced by patient belief that the therapy will be beneficial.
- Selection of effective, affordable medicines that has few side effects and that are dosed in convenient schedules improves adherence to drug therapy.

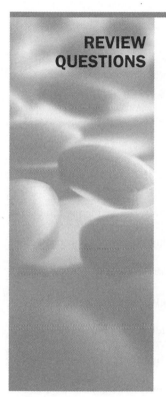

REVIEW QUESTIONS

Multiple Choice

1. An _____ is a drug that binds to a receptor site and elicits cellular response.
   - a. agonist
   - b. antagonist
   - c. alternative
   - d. anti-metabolite

2. All drugs produce toxic effects that can lead to death. The Therapeutic _____ is the ratio of the effective dose to the lethal dose.
   - a. equivalence
   - b. derivative
   - c. index
   - d. window

3. The process of using drugs in the treatment of disease is called
   - a. pharmacodynamics
   - b. pharamacotherapeutics
   - c. pharmacokinetics
   - d. pharmacognosy

4. What is the measure of a drug's effectiveness called?
   - a. availability
   - b. bioequivalence
   - c. efficacy
   - d. potency

5. Humans are unique and individual variability influences the outcome of drug therapy. Name some physiological factors that influence drug therapy.
   - a. age, weight, gender
   - b. genetics, disease, pregnancy
   - c. allergies, hypersensitivities, desensitization
   - d. both a and b

6. Toxic adverse reactions that cause heptotoxicity occur in the _____, and toxic adverse reactions that cause neprotoxicity occur in the _____ .
   - a. liver, lungs
   - b. liver, kidneys
   - c. kidneys, bladder
   - d. kidneys, nephrons

7. Two adverse reactions associated with controlled substances are
   - a. hypersensitivities and dependence
   - b. tolerance and toxicity
   - c. dependence and tolerance
   - d. toxicity and anaphalaxis

8. **To which government agency are adverse reactions reported?**
    a. DEA
    b. TJC
    c. CMS
    d. FDA

9. **An adverse effect produced by drugs on fetuses is called**
    a. carcinogenicity
    b. teratogenicity
    c. pathogenicity
    d. toxicity

10. **One drug that has a narrow therapeutic index is**
    a. acetaminophen
    b. penicillin
    c. digoxin
    d. melphalan

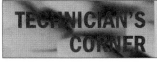

1. How can pharmacy technicians assist patients in reducing anxiety about adverse reactions?
2. Explain how the poor are at an increased risk for adverse reactions.

BIBLIOGRAPHY

Baker GR, Norton PG, Flintolf V, et al.: The Canadian Adverse Events Study. The incidence of adverse events among hospital patients in Canada, *Can Med Assoc J,* 170:1678-1686, 2004.

Edwards IR: The WHO World Alliance for Patient Safety: A new challenge or an old one neglected? *Drug Safety,* 28:379-386, 2005.

Lance L, Lacy C, Armstrong L, Goldman M: *Drug information handbook for the allied health professional,* ed 12, Hudson, OH, 2005, APhA Lexi-Comp.

Page C, Curtis M, Sutter M, Walker M, Hoffman B: *Integrated pharmacology* (pp 57-70, 314), Philadelphia, 2005, Elsevier Mosby, Philadelphia, PA 2005.

Passarelli M, Jacob-Filho W, Figueras A: Adverse drug reactions in an elderly hospitalised population: Inappropriate prescription is a leading cause, *Drugs Aging,* 22:767-777, 2005.

Raffa RB, Rawls SM, Beyzarov EP: *Netter's illustrated pharmacology* (pp 10-11, 21-23), Philadelphia, WB Saunders, 2005.

Ratajczak H: Drug-induced hypersensitivity: Role in drug development, *Toxicol Rev,* 23:265-280, 2004.

Sorensen L, Stokes J, Purdie D, Woodward M, Roberts M: Medication management at home: Medication-related risk factors associated with poor health outcomes, *Age Ageing* 34:626-632, 2005.

Tyler V, Brady L, Robbers J: *Pharmacognosy* (p 486), ed 9, Philadelphia, 1988, Lea & Febiger, 1988.

U.S. Food and Drug Administration: *Adverse Event Reporting System.* Retrieved from http://www.fda.gov/cder/aers/default.htm. Accessed June 2, 2006.

Wu WK, Pantaleo N: Evaluation of outpatient adverse drug reactions leading to hospitalization, *Am J Health Syst Pharm,* 60:253-259, 2003.

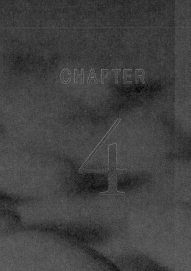

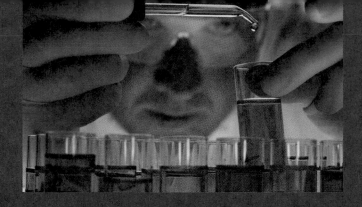

Drug Interactions and Medication Errors

- Give examples of drug-drug interactions, drug-food interactions, and drug-disease contraindications.
- Describe several mechanisms for drug interactions.
- List ways to avoid drug interactions.
- Categorize medication errors.
- Identify medication errors made by pharmacists and pharmacy technicians.
- Describe techniques used to avoid medication errors in the pharmacy.
- Learn the terminology associated with drug interactions and medication errors.

KEY TERMS

Additive effect: Increased drug effect that is produced when a second similar drug is added to therapy that Is greater than the effects produced by either drug alone.

Antagonism: Drug-drug interaction or drug-food interaction that causes decreased effects.

Drug contraindication: Conditions under which a drug is not indicated and should not be administered.

Drug-disease contraindication: Administration of the drug should be avoided because it may worsen the patient's medical condition.

Drug-drug interaction: Reaction that occurs when two or more drugs are administered at the same time.

Drug-food interaction: Altered drug response that occurs when a drug is administered with certain foods.

Medication error: Error made in the process of prescribing, preparing, dispensing, or administering drug therapy.

Potentiation: Process where one drug, acting at a separate site or via a different mechanism of action, increases the effect of another drug, yet produces no effect when administered alone. Food can also potentiate the effects of a drug.

Synergistic effects: Drug-drug or drug-food interaction between two drugs that produces an effect that is greater than would be produced if either drug were administered alone.

Therapeutic duplication: Administration of two drugs that produce similar effects and side effects. These drugs may belong to the same therapeutic class.

Drug Interactions

Drug effects are influenced by joint administration with foods and other drugs. The more drugs that are administered to a patient, the more likely it is that interactions will occur. Drug-drug interactions and drug-food interactions can increase or decrease the intended drug effects. They may also increase or decrease drug side effects. Drug interactions may produce life-threatening or minor undesired effects or they may enhance the desired drug effect. Low doses of antidepressant drugs like amitriptyline are administered along with pain medications such as hydrocodone to enhance pain relief. By administering these two drugs together, less hydrocodone is needed and the patient's risk for development of tolerance and dependence from the hydrocodone is reduced. The study of pharmacology is important because it enables the prediction of the likelihood a drug interaction may occur.

DRUG-DRUG INTERACTIONS

An interaction that occurs between two or more drugs administered at the same time is called a ***drug-drug interaction.*** Drug-drug interactions may increase or decrease the effect or side effects of the drug. Tetracycline and penicillin both treat infections. If the drugs are administered together, the infection-fighting ability of penicillin is reduced by the tetracycline. The action to the antifungal ketoconazole is reduced if it is taken with antacids. Antiulcer drugs such as cimetidine increase the effects of alcohol. Amoxicillin reduces the effectiveness of oral contraceptives.

DRUG-FOOD INTERACTIONS

An interaction between an administered drug and food(s) consumed at the same time is called a *drug-food interaction.* The foods may contain enzymes, vitamins, or minerals that enhance or interfere with drug effects. The interaction may influence side effects, too. A classic example is the interaction between dairy products and the antiinfective tetracycline. Tetracycline binds with the calcium in milk or cheese and its effect is diminished. Another example is levothyroxine, a synthetic thyroid hormone; its effect is decreased when iron supplements are taken.

ADDITIVE EFFECTS

Additive effects may occur when two drugs are administered concurrently. The effects produced by one or both of the drugs may be increased. The increase is equal to the sum of the individual effects produced by each of the drugs alone. Many drug interactions produce additive effects. The sleeping pill triazolam is administered to promote drowsiness. Alcoholic beverages also cause drowsiness. When alcoholic beverages are consumed together with trazolam, additional drowsiness is caused. The sedation caused by triazolam adds to the sedation caused by alcohol.

   Additive effects can be described using the equation

$$1 + 1 = 2$$

SYNERGISTIC EFFECTS

Drug-drug interactions and drug-food interactions may produce synergistic effects. Synergistic effects result when two drugs administered together produce effects that are greater than would be produced if either drug were administered alone. Bleeding is a potential side effect of warfarin and aspirin. When warfarin and aspirin are administered together, excessive bleeding occurs.

   Synergistic effects can be described using the equation

$$1 + 1 = 3$$

POTENTIATION

The process where one drug, or a food, increases the effects of another drug, yet does not produce any effect when administered alone, is called ***potentiation***. Carbidopa is an inactive drug. When added to levodopa, the anti–Parkinson's disease effects of levodopa are

TECH NOTE!

The pharmacist usually counsels a patient who has a prescription for amoxicillin and who is also taking oral contraceptives to use additional contraceptive measures while on the antibiotic, to prevent pregnancy.

increased. Carbidopa is able to decrease the destruction of levodopa in the gastrointestinal tract so more of the levodopa can get to its site of action in the nerve cells of the brain. Grapefruit juice increases the effects of some anticholesterol drugs because it inhibits metabolic enzymes. The action of the antifungal griseofulvin is increased when it is taken with fatty foods because food increases the absorption of the drug.

Potentiation can be described using the equation:

$$1 + 0 = 2$$

ANTAGONISM

Antagonism is a drug-drug interaction or drug-food interaction that causes decreased drug effects. Naloxone is administered to block the respiratory depression produced by morphine and heroin. Vitamin K is an antidote for the drug warfarin. It is administered in warfarin overdose to stop bleeding.

Antagonism can be described using the equation

$$1 + 1 = 0$$

Mechanisms of Drug Interactions

Drug-drug interactions and drug-food interactions occur via many different mechanisms (Figure 4-1). Coadministration of drugs and foods can increase absorption, distribution, metabolism, or elimination and results in increased or decreased drug action or side effects. Epinephrine is added to local anesthetics to constrict blood vessels at the site of injection and thereby augment the local anesthetic effects at the injection site. Absorption of a drug can also be increased by administering a second drug that alters the movement of the gastrointestinal system. Prokinetic drugs like metoclopramide stimulate movement through the stomach and increase the absorption of drugs that are primarily absorbed in the small intestine and decrease absorption of drugs that are absorbed in the stomach. Drugs that decrease the rate of gastric emptying and movement through the intestines, like codeine or loperamide, can increase the absorption and effects of drugs. (Figure 4-1)

Drugs that are weak acids and weak bases are involved in many drug interactions. The absorption of cimetidine (H_2 receptor antagonist) is decreased when taken with antacids because antacids make the pH more alkaline. Absorption of cimetidine is greatest in an

> **TECH NOTE!**
> Grapefruit juice is implicated in many drug-food interactions. When grapefruit juice is known to affect a drug's action, place an auxiliary label on the medication vial and let the patient know to avoid grapefruit juice when taking the medication.

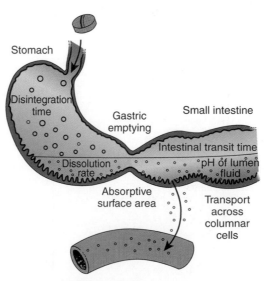

FIGURE 4-1 Factors involved in GI drug interactions. *(From: Kalant H, Grant DM, Mitchell J:* Principles of medical pharmacology, *ed 7, Philadelphia, 2007, WB Saunders.)*

acidic pH. Intravenous solutions of acids and bases are incompatible and, when combined, form solid particles (precipitate). The resulting intravenous solution is not usable.

Displacement from protein binding sites is a mechanism for drug interactions that influences the distribution of a drug. Displacement increases the amount of drug that is free to get to its site of action and produce effects (Figure 2-9). Warfarin is a drug that is highly protein bound. Even a small change in the percent of drug that is free to get to the binding site can increase drug effects and risk of hemorrhage. Sulfonamides are a class of antiinfectives that are also strongly protein bound. When a sulfonamide and warfarin are both administered, displacement occurs.

Interactions that alter the rate of drug metabolism are caused by induction or inhibition of metabolic enzymes. Barbiturates like phenobarbital stimulate metabolic enzymes of other antiseizure medications (phenytoin, valproic acid). Grapefruit juice is a powerful inhibitor of metabolic enzyme CYP3A4 and potentiates the effect of anticholesterol drugs like lovastatin. H_2 receptor antagonists alter the metabolism of alcohol. When drugs like cimetidine or ranitidine are taken with alcohol, the effects of alcohol may be increased and may last longer (Table 4-1).

Some drug interactions influence elimination of drugs. Alteration of the pH of the urine can increase the elimination of a drug or enhance its reabsorption. Elimination of acidic

TABLE 4-1   Selected Substrates, Inhibitors, and Inducers of Specific Cytochromes P450* (CYPs)

CYP isoform	Substrate	Inhibitor	Inducer	CYP isoform	Substrate	Inhibitor	Inducer
1A2	Clozapine	Cimetidine	Tobacco	2E1	Acetaminophen	Disulfiram	Ethanol
	Imipramine	Fluoroquinolones			Chlorzoxazone		
		Fluvoxamine			Ethanol		
		Ticlopidine		3A4/5	Clarithromycin	Indinavir	Carbamazepine
2C19	Diazepam	Fluvoxamine			Erythromycin	Nelfinavir	Phenobarbital
	Phenytoin	Ketoconazole			Quinidine	Ritonavir	Phenytoin
	Amitriptyline	Lansoprazole			Alprazolam	Saquinavir	Rifabutin
	Clomipramine	Omeprazole			Diazepam	Amiodarone	Rifampin
	Cyclophosphamide	Ticlopidine			Midazolam	Cimetidine	St. John's wort
2C9	Tolbutamide	Amiodarone	Rifampin		Triazolam	Clarithromycin	Troglitazone
	Glyburide	Fluconazole			Cyclosporin	Diltiazem	
	Irbesartan	Isoniazid			Tacrolimus	Erythromycin	
	Losartan	Ticlopidine			Indinavir	Fluvoxamine	
	Phenytoin				Ritonavir	Grapefruit juice	
	Tamoxifen				Saquinavir	Itraconazole	
	Tolbutamide				Amlodipine	Ketoconazole	
	Warfarin				Diltiazem	Mibefradil	
2D6	S-Metoprolol	Amiodarone			Felodipine	Nefazodone	
	Propafenone	Chlorpheniramine			Nifedipine	Troleandomycin	
	Timolol	Cimetidine			Nisoldipine	Verapamil	
	Amitriptylline	Clomipramine			Verapamil		
	Clomipramine	Fluoxetine			Atorvastatin		
	Desipramine	Haloperidol			Cerivastatin		
	Imipramine	Methadone			Lovastatin		
	Haloperidol	Paroxetine			Simvastatin		
	Risperidone	Quinidine			Methadone		
	Thioridazine	Ritonavir			Pimozide		
	Codeine				Tamoxifen		
	Dextromethorphan				Trazodone		
	Flecainide				Vincristine		
	Mexiletine						
	Ondansetron						
	Tamoxifen						
	Tramadol						
	Venlafaxine						

*This table can be used to anticipate some potential interactions between drugs that are substrates and those that are inhibitors or inducers.
(From: Kalant H, Grant DM, Mitchell J: *Principles of medical pharmacology*, ed 7, Philadelphia, 2007, WB Saunders.)

drugs is increased when drugs that make the urine alkaline are administered. Elimination of alkaline drugs is increased when drugs that make the urine more acidic are administered.

Drug interactions that involve competition for a common transport system in the kidney can effect the elimination of some drugs. This describes the drug-drug interaction between penicillin and probenecid. When the drugs are administered together, elimination of penicillin is decreased.

Avoiding Undesired Drug Interactions

Studies indicate that between 7% and 22% of adverse drug reactions (ADRs) are caused by drug-drug interactions. Drug interactions that produce undesired effects should be avoided. Undesired drug interactions can result in cancellation of desired drug effect or reduced drug effect. At the opposite extreme, a drug interaction can produce toxic or harmful effects (Table 4-2). Failure to recognize drug interactions can harm the patient or prolong patient illness. It is the responsibility of pharmacists and pharmacy technicians to screen all prescriptions for potential drug interactions before dispensing the medication. Pharmacy technicians play a significant role in the screening process.

Pharmacy technicians play a key role in entering patient data into the pharmacy's prescription filling software. Data entered into the computer must be complete and accurate if the screening for drug interactions is to be effective. Drug-disease contradictions can be avoided by maintaining an up-to-date patient history of chronic and acute medical conditions. Computers prospectively screen for drug interactions so adjustments can be made to the patient drug therapy before the drug is dispensed. When a drug-disease contradiction is identified by computer software, the pharmacy technician must alert the pharmacist so the significance of the computer-screened drug-disease contraindication can be evaluated. Drug-drug interactions can also be avoided by maintenance of an up-to-date patient profile. Pharmacy technicians and pharmacists should query patients about current nonprescription drug use as well as prescription drug usage. Information about prescriptions filled at other pharmacies should be obtained, if possible, and entered into the pharmacy's computer system.

Pharmacy technicians must also be knowledgeable of intravenous drug incompatibilities. Combining acidic intravenous solutions and alkaline solutions causes the precipitation of drug out of the solution. Intravenous solutions that contain precipitates cannot be used and must be destroyed.

Drug-food interactions are avoided by counseling patients to avoid certain foods at the same time as their medication. Spacing the time between food consumption and medication

TECH NOTE!
When taking a patient's medication history, ask the following: "Are you taking any over-the-counter medications? Are you taking any herbal supplements or vitamins? What other prescription drugs are you taking?"

TABLE 4-2 Summary of Selected Drug Interactions

Drug	Effects/side effects increased by:	Effects/side effects decreased by:
Tetracycline		Penicillin
		Antacids
		Dairy products
Ketoconazole		Antacids
Alcoholic beverage	Cimetidine	
Oral contraceptives		Amoxicillin
Levothyroxine		Iron supplements
Triazolam	Alcoholic beverages	
Warfarin	Aspirin	Vitamin K
Levodopa	Carbidopa	
Verapamil	Grapefruit juice	
Griseofulvin	Fatty foods	
Morphine		Naloxone
Lidocaine	Epinephrine	
Cimetidine		Antacids
Phenobarbital		Phenytoin
		Sodium bicarbonate
Penicillin	Probenicid	

administration is often sufficient to avoid an undesired interaction. Pharmacy technicians can play an active role in ensuring that appropriate warning labels are affixed to prescription containers.

Medication Errors

The National Coordinating Council for Medication Error Reporting and Prevention defines a medication error as "any preventable event that may cause or lead to inappropriate medication use or patient harm while the medication is in the control of the health care professional, patient, or consumer. Such events may be related to professional practice, health care products, procedures, and systems, including prescribing; order communication; product labeling, packaging, and nomenclature; compounding; dispensing; distribution; administration; education; monitoring; and use." Preventable medication errors are the cause of nearly 98,000 deaths in the United States annually and exceed deaths due to motor vehicle accidents, breast cancer, and AIDS. Medication errors may also result in hospitalization and account for increased medical cost, income loss, missed school days, and prolonged illness.

Medication errors may be made by physicians, pharmacists, nurses, and pharmacy technicians in the health care setting. Medication errors typically occur in the process of ordering, transcribing, dispensing, and administering medications. Adverse drug events result from prescribing inappropriate medicines for patients, translating prescription orders, improper preparation and selection of drug to dispense, and improper drug administration. Medication errors may also be made by the patient. Patient errors typically involve taking the wrong dose or forgetting to take a dose.

MEDICATION ERRORS MADE BY HEALTH CARE PROVIDERS WHO PRESCRIBE MEDICATION

As many as 57 of 1000 medication orders have an error. Errors made in ordering medications are made by physicians, nurse practitioners, pharmacists, dentists, and other health professionals legally able to prescribe medicines. Medication errors associated with prescribers are often a result of miscommunication or misinformation.

MISCOMMUNICATION

Miscommunication of the drug ordered may involve poor handwriting, confusion between drugs with similar names, misuse of zeroes and decimal points, confusion of metric and other dosing units, or inappropriate abbreviations.

Poor Handwriting

Many jokes have been made about physicians' poor handwriting (often called "chicken scratch"); however, medication errors that are made because the prescription was not decipherable are no laughing matter. When prescriptions are illegible, there may be confusion between drugs with similar names.

Confusion Between Drugs With Similar Names

Although the Center for Disease Evaluation and Research (CDER) tries to avoid assigning names to new drugs that are similar to existing drugs, sometimes this happens. According to the FDA MedWatch, medication errors have recently been made involving Zyrtec and Zantac, Zantac and Xanax, Keppra and Kaletra, Flomax and Volmax, Zyprexa and Celexa, and Serzone and Seroquel. When prescribers fail to write legibly, confusion about the drug to dispense arises.

Misuse of Zeroes and Decimal Points

Orders for medication may be incorrect because the strength is written incorrectly or is illegible. Haloperidol is a drug used to treat schizophrenia. It is available as a 0.5-mg tablet and as a 5-mg tablet. If the decimal point to the left is illegible or the zero is omitted, there may be confusion about which strength to dispense. On the other hand, if the 5-mg tablet was ordered and the prescription was written as 5.0 mg, it could be confused with 50 mg. In both cases, if the error is not caught, the patient receives 10 times the desired dose (Figure 4-2).

FIGURE 4-2 Decimal point error example.

Confusion of Metric and Other Dosing Units or Inappropriate Abbreviations

Prescriptions may be written using metric units or apothecary units. Medication errors have been caused by improper conversion between the two systems of measurement. For example, the apothecary symbol for 1 dram (ℨi) has been interpreted as 3 ml, 4 ml, and 5 ml. Most pharmacists and pharmacy technicians interpret ℨi = 5ml = 1 teaspoonful. Prescribers unfamiliar with apothecary symbols may confuse the symbol for ounce (℥) and dram (ℨ), causing toxic or subtherapeutic effects.

MISINFORMATION

Medication errors made by prescribers occur because of lack of information or misinformation. Limited information about the patient occurs because no medical or drug history was taken or insufficient information was collected from the patient. Studies have shown that greater than 25% of the prescribing errors made in hospitals are associated with incomplete medication histories being obtained at the time of admission. A complete history is needed of patients' allergies, other medicines they are taking, previous diagnoses, and lab results to prevent medication errors.

Errors of Omission

An error of omission occurs when information is not collected or recorded in the patient's medical history. Studies have shown a 67% error rate in obtaining prescription medication histories. Medication histories taken by physicians were less accurate than histories taken by pharmacists. An incomplete drug history may be the reason for prescribing a drug similar to one currently being administered. This is called ***therapeutic duplication.*** Therapeutic duplication may increase or decrease desired effects. If both drugs compete for the same drug receptor binding sites or the same transport systems, the drug with the greatest affinity will bind. If the drug bound to the receptor is less potent, a decreased desired effect results. Therapeutic duplication may cause an increase in adverse reactions. Omission of drug allergy information could result in a prescription written and filled for a medicine that may cause extreme harm to the patient. Errors of omission are the source of prescriptions written for drugs that are contraindicated due to the patient's disease state or allergies. An example of a drug-disease contraindication is the administration of the antidepressant bupropion to patients with a history of seizures.

Errors of Commission

Commission errors result when a previously discontinued drug is accidentally restarted or a nonprescribed drug is accidentally added to the patient's medication history. This can occur when inaccurate drug histories are collected from caregivers (the patient is too ill to provide his or her own drug history) or from patient confusion. When this occurs, non-needed drugs are taken and the patient is at risk for adverse reactions.

Prescriptions written for the wrong strength or wrong dosing schedule are medication errors that are not specifically errors of omission or commission but do involve prescribers. This type of error occurs when the prescriber lacks familiarity with the drug that is being prescribed. The error may occur when drug dose and dosing frequency are determined according to patient weight and inaccurate weight information is given in the medical history.

MEDICATION ERRORS MADE BY HEALTH CARE PROVIDERS WHO DISPENSE MEDICATION

Pharmacists, pharmacy technicians, and pharmacy assistants make preventable medication errors, too! Medication errors made by pharmacy personnel usually involve transcribing errors, incorrect interpretation of prescription contents, improper product preparation, lack of prescription monitoring, product labeling, and inaccurate dispensing. Some dispensing errors are caused by distractions in the pharmacy. The pharmacist or pharmacy technician filling a medication order may become distracted when their workflow is interrupted by the telephone ringing or by questions from a patient at the pharmacy counter.

CONFUSION OF METRIC AND OTHER DOSING UNITS OR INAPPROPRIATE ABBREVIATIONS

Serious medication errors have been caused by confusing abbreviations. This problem is so serious that The Joint Commission (formerly JCAHO) has recommended abolishment of the use of certain abbreviations and has published them in their official "Do Not Use" list (Table 4-3). The National Coordinating Council for Medication Error Reporting and Prevention has also developed a list of dangerous abbreviations (Table 4-4).

> **TECH NOTE!**
> Always check the original prescription against the prescription label and the NDC number on the stock medication chosen to ensure accuracy.

TABLE 4-3 The Joint Commission Official "Do Not Use" List*

Do not use	Potential problem	Use instead
U (unit)	Mistaken for "0" (zero), the number "4" (four) or "cc"	Write "unit"
IU (International Unit)	Mistaken for IV (intravenous) or the number 10 (ten)	Write "International Unit"
Q.D., QD, q.d., qd (daily)	Mistaken for each other	Write "daily"
Q.O.D., QOD, q.o.d, qod (every other day)	Period after the Q mistaken for "I" and the "O" mistaken for "I"	Write "every other day"
Trailing zero (X.0 mg)†	Decimal point is missed	Write X mg
Lack of leading zero (.X mg)	Decimal point is missed	Write 0.X mg
MS	Can mean morphine sulfate or magnesium sulfate	Write "morphine sulfate"
MSO_4 and $MgSO_4$	Confused for one another	Write "magnesium sulfate"

Additional abbreviations, acronyms and symbols (for possible future inclusion in the official "Do Not Use" list)

> (greater than) and < (less than)	Misinterpreted as the number "7" (seven) or the letter "L"; confused for each other	Write "greater than" and "less than"
Abbreviations for drug names	Misinterpreted due to similar abbreviations for multiple drugs	Write drug names in full
Apothecary units	Unfamiliar to many practitioners; confused with metric units	Use metric units
@	Mistaken for the number "2" (two)	Write "at"
cc	Mistaken for U (units) when poorly written	Write "ml" or "milliliters"
Mg	Mistaken for mg (milligrams) resulting in 1000-fold overdose	Write "mcg" or "micrograms"

*Applies to all orders and all medication-related documentation that is handwritten (including free-text computer entry) or on pre-printed forms.
†**Exception:** A "trailing zero" may be used only where required to demonstrate the level of precision of the value being reported, such as for laboratory results, imaging studies that report size of lesions, or catheter/tube sizes. It may not be used in medication orders or other medication-related documentation.
Courtesy of The Joint Commission, May 2005.

TABLE 4-4   National Coordinating Council for Medication Error Reporting and Prevention: Dangerous Errors

Abbreviation	Intended meaning	Common error
U	Units	Mistaken as a zero or a four (4) resulting in overdose. Also mistaken for "cc" (cubic centimeters) when poorly written.
μg	Micrograms	Mistaken for "mg" (milligrams) resulting in an overdose.
Q.D.	Latin abbreviation for every day	The period after the "Q" has sometimes been mistaken for an "I," and the drug has been given "QID" (four times daily) rather than daily.
Q.O.D.	Latin abbreviation for every other day	Misinterpreted as "QD" (daily) or "QID" (four times daily). If the "O" is poorly written, it looks like a period or "I."
SC or SQ	Subcutaneous	Mistaken as "SL" (sublingual) when poorly written.
T I W	Three times a week	Misinterpreted as "three times a day" or "twice a week."
D/C	Discharge; also discontinue	Patient's medications have been prematurely discontinued when D/C, (intended to mean "discharge") was misinterpreted as "discontinue," because it was followed by a list of drugs.
HS	Half strength	Misinterpreted as the Latin abbreviation "HS" (hour of sleep).
cc	Cubic centimeters	Mistaken as "U" (units) when poorly written.
AU, AS, AD	Latin abbreviations for both ears; left ear; right ear	Misinterpreted as the Latin abbreviation "OU" (both eyes); "OS" (left eye); "OD" (right eye).
IU	International Unit	Mistaken as IV (intravenous) or 10 (ten).
MS, MSO$_4$, MgSO$_4$	Confused for one another	Can mean morphine sulfate or magnesium sulfate

TECH NOTE!

When in doubt about what is written on a prescription, always get a second opinion. Never guess at what the medication might be. Ask for help to verify the drug in question.

TECH NOTE!

It is vitally important to adopt an "aseptic attitude" when preparing parenteral medications. Hand-washing, hood cleaning, dose calculating, and proper technique will ensure that the sterile products are not contaminated or inaccurate.

INACCURATE TRANSCRIBING

Poor handwriting is responsible for many transcription errors. Medication orders received by the pharmacy must be translated and entered into the computer. If the order is illegible, the pharmacy must verify the order to prevent incorrect selection of the drug and strength ordered. Medication orders received by telephone or left on a computer messaging system are also subject to transcription errors. Verbal medication orders must be written down accurately or medication errors result.

INSUFFICIENT MONITORING OF DRUG THERAPY

An important role of the pharmacist is to monitor appropriateness of drug therapy. Pharmacy technicians assist the pharmacist with this task. Together they review each prescription to determine whether the medication ordered, dose, and dosing frequency are appropriate for the patient. They also monitor drug therapy for drug interactions and drug allergies. Medication errors occur when the pharmacy fails to carefully monitor drug therapy. Monitoring of drug therapy reduces therapeutic duplication. Pharmacy technicians and pharmacists work together to alert the prescriber when they see that two therapeutically equivalent drugs are ordered for the patient. Monitoring also prevents refills of discontinued medication.

IMPROPER MEDICATION PREPARATION

Another medication error made by pharmacy staff is improper sterile and nonsterile compounding. Medications for parenteral administration must be prepared using aseptic technique. Medication errors associated with incorrect calculations occur, too. Combining incompatible drugs is also a source of medication errors.

IMPROPER LABELING

Several medication errors involve improper labeling of the drug to be dispensed. A labeling error has occurred when the correct drug is selected but the container is labeled with the wrong drug name, dosage form, strength, or quantity. Putting the wrong patient's name on the label is also a labeling error. Incorrect or incomplete directions typed on the label are another preventable label error.

PRODUCT SELECTION ERRORS

Selection of the wrong drug to dispense is a preventable error. This type of error most often occurs when drugs have similar names or similar packaging (Figure 4-3). Other product selection errors include dispensing the wrong strength or wrong dosage form.

BAGGING ERRORS

Placing the correct prescription in the wrong patient's bag is a bagging error. Placing additional prescriptions into a patient's bag or omitting a prescription from the bag are bagging errors, too.

MISCELLANEOUS DISPENSING ERRORS

A properly filled prescription that is dispensed to the wrong patient is a medication error. This may occur when two customers have similar names. The pharmacy staff may incorrectly hear the name of the person who wants to pick up their prescription. The patient may incorrectly hear the name of the person the pharmacy staff has announced. This error is preventable. Always verify the name and identification of the person picking up a prescription.

MEDICATION ERRORS MADE BY HEALTH CARE PROVIDERS WHO ADMINISTER MEDICATION

Medication errors are made by health care providers and caregivers who administer medications. One error associated with drug administration can result in a drug being given to the wrong patient. Sometimes, the correct drug is given to the right patient; however, the drug strength, dosing frequency, and dosage form are incorrect. That is a medication error, too.

MEDICATION ERRORS ARE MADE BY PATIENTS

Medication errors are made by patients, too! Pharmacists, pharmacy technicians, and other health care providers can help patients prevent medication errors. Patients are often confused by generic and trade names. Their medicines may be labeled using the generic name in the hospital. The community pharmacy may label the same drug with the brand name. The patient may not realize the drugs are the same and take a double dose. A similar situation occurs when two similar medicines are prescribed by different physicians. The patient is unaware that taking both medicines is therapeutic duplication. Confusion is also the reason why patients refill medications that have been discontinued by their health care provider.

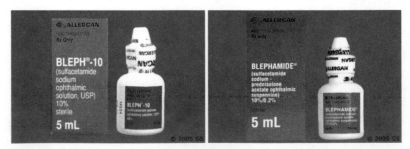

FIGURE 4-3 Example of similar packaging. *(Copyright © Gold Standard, Inc., 2007)*

Two other medication errors are important to note. They are (1) taking too much medicine and (2) taking too little medicine. Some patients believe the saying, "If one pill is good, than two pills is better." Others do not realize the importance of taking medicines without missing doses. They do not realize that a chronic illness becomes worse or drug resistance can develop when doses are skipped. For some patients, the medication is too expensive and they take less than the prescribed dose to try to "stretch" the prescription and make it last longer. Regardless of the reason, taking too little or too much medicine can negatively influence drug therapy outcomes.

Avoiding Medication Errors

Pharmacy technicians can play an important role in preventing medication errors. Some tips for preventing medication errors are listed next.

- Always verify prescriptions with similar drug names. Verify spelling and strength.
- Always verify unfamiliar abbreviation or abbreviations published in the TJC "Do Not Use" list or the National Coordinating Council for Medication Error Reporting and Prevention dangerous abbreviation list.
- Always confirm drug, strength, and dosing schedule when prescriptions are written and the handwriting is illegible. **Never guess**.
- Avoid product selection errors by using the Pull-Dispense-Review (PDR) system. Verify the drug name and NDC No. or DIN No. when selecting (pulling) the drug from the shelf. Check drug name, strength, and dosage form against medication order. Confirm the drug a third time when returning medicine to the shelf.
- Become familiar with brand and generic names of commonly dispensed drugs.
- Become familiar with strength, dosage form, and dosing frequency of commonly dispensed drugs.
- Alert the pharmacist of all drug interactions and therapeutic duplications.
- Develop a routine to avoid errors associated with distractions.
- Check the identification of persons picking up prescriptions.
- Dispense patient information sheets as required.
- Affix warning labels to prescription vials as required.
- Verify all calculations.
- Check all labels for accuracy.

CHAPTER SUMMARY

- Drug-drug interactions and drug-food interactions can increase or decrease intended drug effects.
- The more drugs that are administered to a patient, the more likely it is that interactions will occur.
- Drug-drug interactions may increase or decrease side effects of the drug.
- Foods may contain enzymes, vitamins, or minerals that enhance or interfere with drug effects.
- Additive effects occur when two drugs are administered together and the effects produced by one or both of the drugs are increased.
- Synergistic effects result when two drugs administered together produce effects that are greater than would be produced if either drug were administered alone.
- The process where one drug, or a food, increases the effects of another drug, yet does not produce any effect when administered by alone, is called potentiation.
- Antagonism is a drug-drug interaction or drug-food interaction that causes decreased drug effects.
- Coadministration of drugs and foods can increase absorption, distribution, metabolism, or elimination.
- Intravenous solutions of acids and bases are incompatible and, when combined, form solid particles (precipitate).
- Displacement from binding sites increases the amount of drug that is free to get to its site of action. Even a small change in the percent of drug that is free to get to the binding site can increase drug effects.

- Interactions that alter the rate of drug metabolism are caused by induction or inhibition of metabolic enzymes.
- Interactions that involve competition for a common transport system in the kidney can affect the elimination of some drugs.
- It is the responsibility of pharmacists and pharmacy technicians to screen all prescriptions for potential drug interactions before dispensing the medication.
- Drug-disease contradictions and drug-drug interactions can be avoided by maintaining an up-to-date history of the patients' chronic and acute medical conditions.
- Computers prospectively screen for drug interactions so adjustments can be made to the patient drug therapy before the drug is dispensed.
- Pharmacy technicians must also be knowledgeable of intravenous drug incompatibilities. Combining acidic intravenous solutions to alkaline solutions causes the precipitation of drug out of the solution.
- Medication errors in the health care setting typically occur in the process of ordering, transcribing, dispensing, and administering medications.
- Poor handwriting is responsible for many medication errors. When prescriptions are illegible, there may be confusion between drugs with similar names.
- Medication errors occur because of misplacement of zeros and decimal points.
- Medication errors have been caused by improper conversion between systems of measurement.
- Medication errors occur when pharmacists, pharmacy technicians, physicians, and other health care workers lack familiarity with the drug that is being prescribed.
- Medication errors made by pharmacy personnel usually involve transcribing errors, incorrect interpretation of prescription contents, improper product preparation, lack of prescription monitoring, product labeling, and inaccurate dispensing.
- Some dispensing errors are caused by distractions in the pharmacy.
- Medication errors made by patients can be minimized by proper education.
- Medication errors can be avoided by verifying prescriptions with similar drug names and unfamiliar abbreviations.
- Avoid product selection errors by using the Pull-Dispense-Review (PDR) system and checking all labels for accuracy.
- Prevent medication errors by becoming familiar with brand and generic names, strength, dosage form, and dosing frequency of commonly dispensed drugs.
- Medication errors can be minimized by verifying all calculations.

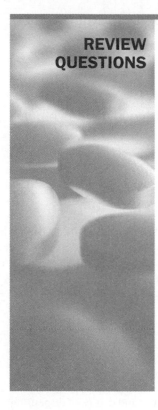

REVIEW QUESTIONS

Multiple Choice

1. State whether the following statement is true or false: Drug-drug interactions may increase or decrease the effect or side effects of the drug.
   a. true
   b. false

2. _____ effects occur when two drugs are administered together and the effects produced by one or both of the drugs are increased.
   a. Antagonistic
   b. Additive
   c. Adverse
   d. Absorption

3. When warfarin and aspirin are administered together, excessive bleeding occurs. This type of effect is _____.
   a. antagonistic
   b. idiosyncratic
   c. both a and b
   d. synergistic

4. Whose responsibility is it to screen all prescriptions for potential drug interactions before dispensing the medication?
   a. pharmacist
   b. technician
   c. pharmacist and technician
   d. pharmacy manager

5. Medication errors in the health care setting typically occur in the process of
   a. ordering medications
   b. transcribing medications
   c. dispensing and administering medications
   d. a, b, and c

6. Orders for medication may be incorrect because the strength is written incorrectly or is illegible. Which of the following is the correct way of writing the dose for digoxin?
   a. digoxin 0.25 mg
   b. digoxin 25 mg
   c. digoxin .25 mg
   d. digoxin 025 mg

7. Selection of the wrong drug to dispense is a preventable error. Which of the following is the correct drug for the following prescription order?
   "i tab bid for joint pain"
   a. Celebrex
   b. Celexa
   c. Cerebyx
   d. Cerebra

8. To which federal agency should medication errors be reported to using the program MedWatch?
   a. DEA
   b. FDA
   c. TJC
   d. CMS

9. **Which agency developed a "Do Not Use" abbreviation list to avoid medication errors?**
    a. FDA
    b. DEA
    c. HIPAA
    d. TJC

10. **Is the following statement true or false? "If one pill is good, than two pills is better."**
    a. true
    b. false

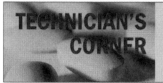

TECHNICIAN'S CORNER

1. What are three "checks" to ensure that the right medication is pulled from the pharmacy shelf when preparing a prescription?
2. What should a pharmacy technician do if unsure about the name of a medication handwritten on a prescription?

BIBLIOGRAPHY

Adubofour K, Keenan C, Daftary A, Mensah-Adubofour J: Strategies to reduce medication errors in ambulatory practice, *J Natl Med Assoc,* 96:1558, 2004.

Ashcroft D, Quinlan P, Blenkins A: Prospective study of the incidence, nature and causes of dispensing errors in community pharmacies, *Pharmacoepidemiol Drug Safety,* 14:327-332, 2005.

Lance L, Lacy C, Armstrong L, Goldman M: *Drug information handbook for the allied health professional,* ed 12, Hudson, OH, 2005, APhA Lexi-Comp.

National Coordinating Council for Medication Error Reporting and Prevention: *Dangerous abbreviations.* Retrieved from http://nccmerp.org. Accessed November 1, 2007.

Page C, Curtis M, Sutter M, Walker M, Hoffman B: *Integrated pharmacology* (pp 57-70), Philadelphia, 2005, Elsevier Mosby.

Passarelli M, Jacob-Filho W, Figueras A: Adverse drug reactions in an elderly hospitalised population: Inappropriate prescription is a leading cause, *Drugs Aging,* 22:767-777, 2005.

Rados C: Drug name confusion: Preventing medication errors, *FDA Consumer,* 39:35, 2005, Health Module.

Shargel L, Mutnick A, Souney P, Swanson L: *Comprehensive pharmacy review* (pp 78-84, 42-65, 131-132), ed 4, Baltimore, 2001, Lippincott Williams & Wilkins.

St Onge E, Dea M, Rose R: Medication errors and strategies to improve patient safety, *Drug Topics,* 150:36, 2006.

Tam V, Knowles S, Cornish P, Fine N, Marchesano R, Etchells E: Frequency, type and clinical importance of medication history errors at admission to hospital: A systematic review, *JAMC* 173(5), 2005.

The Joint Commission: *The official "Do Not Use" list.* Retrieved from http://www.jointcommission.org/PatientSafety/DoNotUseList/. Accessed November 1, 2007.

U.S. Food and Drug Administration: *Medication errors.* Retrieved from http://www.fda.gov/cder/drug/MedErrors/default.htm. Accessed November 1, 2007.

II

Drugs Affecting the Autonomic Nervous System and Central Nervous System

- List the divisions of the nervous system.
- Describe the process of nerve impulse transmission.
- Explain the "all-or-none" law.
- Describe the function of neurotransmitters.
- List neurotransmitters important to the autonomic nervous system.
- Compare and contrast the "fight-or-flight" response with the "rest-and-digest" response.

Overview

The nervous system is a complex communication system that is made up of the brain, spinal cord, and nerves and is organized to detect changes in the internal and external environment, evaluate that information, and possibly respond by initiating changes in muscles or glands. Messages are transmitted throughout the nervous system along nerve cells called neurons. Two main types of cells compose the nervous system: neurons and glia. *Neurons* conduct all the impulses that make the nervous system function. Glia, or glial cells, support the function of the neurons. All neurons consist of a cell body and its extensions, one axon, and many dendrites. At the end of every axon is a *synapse,* or space, that must be bridged for the impulse to continue on to its destination. Proteins called *neurotransmitters* are released as the impulses approach the synapse and provide the means for the impulse to cross the synapse. There are three types of neurons: afferent (sensory) neurons that transmit nerve impulses to the brain or spinal cord, efferent (motor) neurons that transmit nerve impulses away from the brain or spinal cords and toward the muscles and glands, and interneurons that conduct impulses from afferent neurons to efferent neurons. Interneurons are found only in the central nervous system (CNS).

Glial cells form the blood-brain barrier and support the function of the neurons by engulfing and destroying bacteria and cellular debris (phagocytosis), lining the fluid-filled ventricles of the brain, and producing fatty myelin sheaths that insulate nerve fibers.

Mechanism of Communication Between Nerve Cells

NERVE IMPULSES

Neurons initiate and conduct signals called *action potentials* or *nerve impulses.* They exhibit both excitability and conductivity. A nerve impulse can be described as a wave of electrical fluctuation that travels along the plasma membrane. A synapse is the space between the *presynaptic neuron* and the *postsynaptic neuron* or effector site, such as a muscle where a chemical transmitter called a neurotransmitter is released. It is the place where signals are transmitted, sending the "message" from the presynaptic to the postsynaptic cell.

NEUROTRANSMITTERS

Neurotransmitters are the means by which neurons "talk" to each other. Neurotransmitters are commonly classified by their functions (excitatory or inhibitory) or by their chemical structure (small-molecule and large-molecule transmitters). Small-molecule transmitters are single amino acids, and large-molecule transmitters are chains of 20 to 40 amino acids.

SMALL-MOLECULE TRANSMITTERS

Small-molecule transmitters are divided into four main chemical classes: *acetylcholine* (ACh), *amines* (e.g., serotonin and histamine), *catecholamines* (e.g., epinephrine and norepinephrine) and *hormones.* Norepinephrine and epinephrine are also classified as hormones because they are released directly into the bloodstream.

Divisions of the Nervous System

The nervous system is divided into two anatomical divisions: the CNS and the peripheral nervous system (PNS). The PNS is further subdivided into efferent and afferent divisions. The efferent division is subdivided again into the autonomic system and the somatic system. The final subdivisions of the autonomic nervous system (ANS) are the parasympathetic system and the sympathetic system.

CENTRAL NERVOUS SYSTEM

The CNS is composed of both the brain and the spinal cord and is the principal integrator of sensory input and motor output.

THE BRAIN

There are six divisions of the brain—cerebellum, diencephalon, cerebrum, medulla oblongata (lowest part), pons (middle), and midbrain (upper)—collectively known as the brain stem.

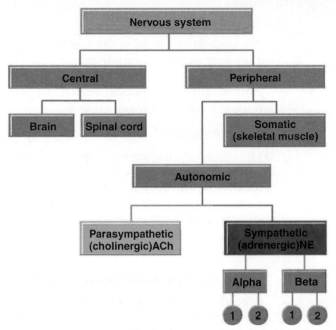

(From Lilley LL, Harrington S, Snyder JS: Pharmacology and the nursing process, *ed 5, St. Louis, 2007, Mosby.)*

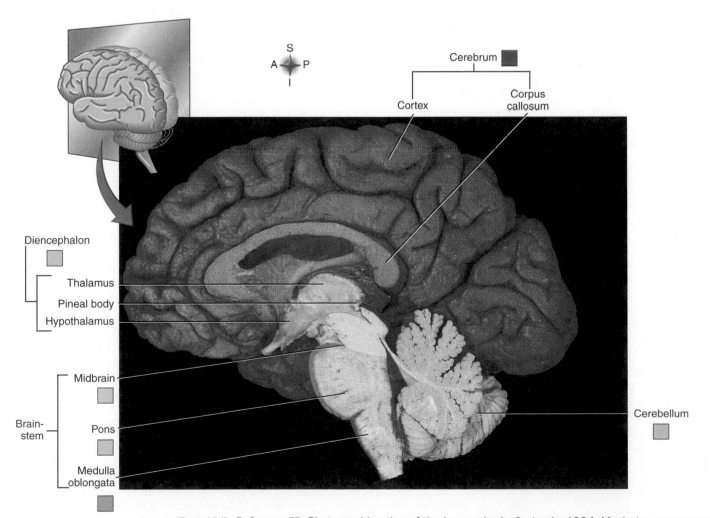

(From Vidic B, Suarez FR: Photographic atlas of the human body, *St. Louis, 1984, Mosby.)*

THE BRAIN STEM

The medulla oblongata is attached to the spinal cord and is composed of white matter and a network of gray and white matter called the reticular formation. The pons and the midbrain contain both white matter and reticular formation. The brain stem, like the spinal cord, performs sensory, motor, and reflex functions and contains control centers for cardiac, respiratory, and vasomotor control.

THE CEREBRUM

The cerebrum, the largest, uppermost division of the brain, consists of two halves: the right and the left cerebral hemisphere. Connecting both hemispheres is a band of neurons called the corpus callosum that integrates the actions of both hemispheres. The surface of the cerebrum—called the cerebral cortex—is made up of gray matter and contains convolutions and deep grooves called fissures. These fissures divide the cerebral hemisphere into five lobes: frontal lobe, parietal lobe, temporal lobe, and occipital lobe and insula.

CEREBRAL TRACTS AND BASAL NUCLEI

Beneath the cerebral cortex are the basal nuclei or basal ganglia, important for regulating voluntary motor functions (see Chapter 8). Normally, the basal nuclei secrete dopamine, an inhibitory neurotransmitter.

SPECIALIZATION OF CEREBRAL HEMISPHERES

The right and left hemispheres specialize in different functions. The left hemisphere specializes in language functions and certain hand movements like skilled and gesturing movements. The right hemisphere specializes in the perception of certain types of auditory stimuli, nonspeech sounds such as melodies, coughing, crying, and laughing. The left hemisphere also functions better at tactile perception and perceiving visual and spatial relationships.

THE CEREBELLUM

The cerebellum is the second largest part of the brain but has more neurons than all of the other parts of the nervous system combined. Its main functions are coordination and balance.

DIENCEPHALON

The diencephalon is the part of the brain located between the cerebrum and the midbrain (mesencephalon). Its main structures are the thalamus and the hypothalamus, the optic chiasma, and the pineal gland. The thalamus serves as a major relay station for sensory impulses on their way to the cerebral cortex and (1) performs the function of conscious recognition of pain, temperature, and touch; (2) plays a part in the mechanisms responsible for emotions by associating sensory impulses with feelings of pleasantness and unpleasantness; (3) plays a part in the arousal or alerting mechanism; and (4) plays a part in mechanisms that produce complex movements. The hypothalamus performs many functions important for both survival and the enjoyment of life. For instance, it functions as a link between the psyche (mind) and the soma (body). It also links the endocrine system to the nervous system. Certain areas of the hypothalamus function as pleasure centers or reward centers for the primary drives such as eating, drinking, and sex.

The functions of the pineal gland are still not completely understood. However, we do know that is an important part of the biological clock mechanism. The body's biological clock depends partly on the pineal gland varying its secretion of the hormone melatonin. Changes in light levels throughout the day and night affect the body's circadian rhythm and trigger changes in the rate of melatonin secretion. When sunlight levels are high, melatonin secretion decreases; when light levels are low, melatonin levels increase proportionally.

THE SPINAL CORD

The spinal cord lies within the spinal cavity. Two bundles of nerve fibers called *nerve roots* project from each side of the spinal cord. Fibers comprising the dorsal (posterior) nerve root carry sensory information into the spinal cord, and fibers of the ventral (anterior) nerve root carry motor information out of the spinal cord. On each side of the spinal cord, the dorsal and ventral nerve roots join together to form a single mixed nerve called a *spinal nerve*. The spinal cord provides conduction routes to and from the brain and serves as a reflex center. Ascending tracts conduct sensory impulses up the cord to the brain and descending tracts conduct motor impulses down the cord from the brain.

The Peripheral Nervous System

The PNS consists of nerve tissue that lies in the periphery, or "outer regions," of the nervous system. The PNS is made up of 31 pairs of spinal nerves that emerge from the spinal cord, the 12 pairs of cranial nerves that emerge from the brain, and all the smaller nerves that branch from the "main" nerves. The PNS includes all the nerve pathways outside the brain and spinal cord and all their individual branches. The PNS is composed of the ANS and the somatic nervous system (SNS). The PNS has two functional divisions: the sensory (efferent) and the motor (afferent) divisions. The SNS comprises of all the voluntary motor pathways outside the CNS, like the peripheral pathways to the skeletal muscles, which are somatic effectors.

Autonomic Nervous System

The ANS is a subdivision of the PNS that regulates involuntary actions. The major function of the ANS is to regulate the heartbeat, smooth muscle contraction, and glandular secretions to maintain homeostasis. The ANS is also divided into two divisions: the sympathetic and parasympathetic divisions. The sympathetic and the parasympathetic divisions produce opposite effects.

THE SYMPATHETIC SYSTEM

The major function of the **sympathetic system** is to serve as an "emergency" system. It is also called the "fight-or-flight" system. Whenever the body is undergoing physical or psychological stress, outgoing sympathetic signals increase greatly. Sympathetic impulses to the adrenal medulla stimulate the secretion of epinephrine and norepinephrine. The "flight-or-fight" reaction is normal in times of stress.

THE PARASYMPATHETIC SYSTEM

The **parasympathetic system** is the dominant controller of most autonomic effectors. Whereas the sympathetic system dominates during times of stress, the parasympathetic system dominates during time of "rest and digest."

NEUROTRANSMITTERS

Axon terminals of autonomic neurons release the neurotransmitters norepinephrine, epinephrine, or ACh. Neurons that release norepinephrine and epinephrine are known as adrenergic neurons and bind to adrenergic receptors. Cholinergic neurons release acetylcholine and bind to cholinergic receptors.

ADRENERGIC RECEPTORS

There are two types of adrenergic receptors: alpha (α)-receptors and beta (β)-receptors. Subtypes of these receptors are α_1, α_2, β_1, and β_2. The binding of norepinephine to α-receptors in the smooth muscle of blood vessels has a stimulating effect on the muscle that causes the muscle to constrict. The binding of norepinephrine to β-receptors in smooth muscle of a different blood vessel produces opposite effects. The binding of norepinephrine to β-receptors in cardiac muscle has a stimulating effect that results in a faster and stronger heartbeat. The actions of norepinephrine and epinephrine are terminated in two ways. Most of the neurotransmitter molecules are taken back up by the synaptic knob of the postganglionic

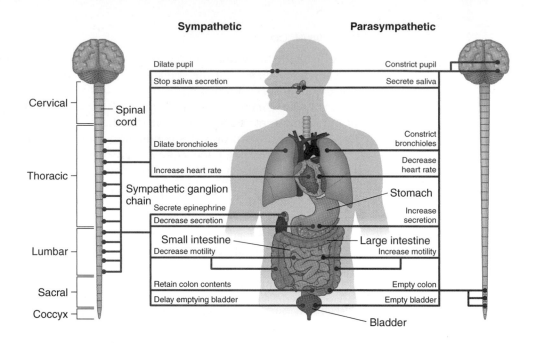

neurons, where they are broken down by the enzyme monoamine oxidase (MAO). The remaining neurotransmitter molecules are eventually broken down by another enzyme, catechol-*O*-methyl transferase (COMT).

CHOLINERGIC RECEPTORS

Acetylcholine binds to cholinergic receptors. The two main types of cholinergic receptors are nicotinic (N) receptors and muscarinic (M) receptors. Like the adrenergic receptors, cholinergic receptors have subtypes such as nicotinic-1 (N1), nicotinic-2 (N2), muscarinic-1 (M1), and muscarinic-2 (M2). The action of ACh is quickly terminated through hydrolysis by the enzyme acetylcholinesterase.

Drugs Used to Affect the Autonomic and Somatic Nervous System

Drug	Primary receptors	Primary use
Selected cholinergics		
bethanechol	Cholinergic	Increase urination
pilocarpine	Cholinergic (eye)	Glaucoma
pyridostigmine	Cholinergic	Myesthenia gravis
tacrine	Cholinergic	Alzhiemer's disease
Selected anticholinergics		
atropine	Cholinergic	Dilate pupils and increase heart rate
benztropine	Cholinergic	Parkinson's disease
ipratropium bromide	Cholinergic	Asthma
oxybutinin	Cholinergic	Incontinence
scopolamine	Cholinergic	Motion sickness
Selected sympathomimetics		
albuterol	β_2	Asthma
clonidine	α_2	Hypertension
dobutamine	β_1	Cardiac stimulant
norepinephrine	α_1 and β_1	Shock
salmeterol	β_2	Asthma
Selected adrenergic antagonists		
atenolol	β_1	Hypertension
carvedilol	α_1, β_1, and β_2	Hypertension
doxazocin	α_1	Hypertension
propranolol	β_1 and β_2	Angina and hypertension
terazocin	α_1	Benign prostatic hypertrophy and hypertension

BIBLIOGRAPHY

Chabner E: *The language of medicine,* ed 8, St. Louis, 2007, WB Saunders.
Patton K: *Survival guide for anatomy and physiology,* St. Louis, 2006, Mosby.
Thibodeau G, Patton K: *Anatomy and physiology,* ed 6, St. Louis, 2007, Mosby.

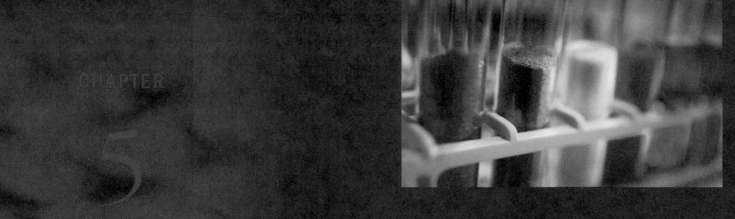

CHAPTER 5

Treatment of Anxiety

LEARNING OBJECTIVES

- List and describe the function of neurotransmitters associated with symptoms of anxiety.
- Classify medications used to treat anxiety.
- Describe the mechanism of action for each class of drugs used to treat anxiety.
- Identify warning labels and precautionary messages associated with medications used to treat anxiety.
- Identify significant drug look-alike/sound-alike issues.

KEY TERMS

Anxiety: Condition associated with tension, apprehension, fear, or panic.

Anxiolytic: Drug used to treat anxiety.

Drug dependence: Person taking the drug must continue to take the drug in order to avoid the onset of physical and/or psychological withdrawal symptoms.

Generalized anxiety disorder: Condition that is associated with excessive worrying and tension that is experienced daily for more than 6 months.

Obsessive-compulsive disorder (OCD): A condition associated with an inability to control or stop repeated unwanted thoughts or behaviors.

Panic disorder: Condition associated with repeated sudden onset of feelings of terror.

Phobia: Irrational fear of things or situations that produce symptoms of intense anxiety.

Post-traumatic stress disorder (PTSD): Stress disorder that develops in persons who have participated in, witnessed, or been a victim of a terrifying event.

Tolerance: Increasing doses of a drug are required in order to achieve the same effects as were achieved previously at lower doses.

Overview

Anxiety disorder is the leading mental health illness and affects more than 40 million U.S. adults, according to Anxiety Disorders Association of America. The prevalence in Canada is 12% of the population. The cause of anxiety disorders may be environmental, biological, developmental, associated with socioeconomic conditions, or a combination of several of these individual factors.

There are four major types of anxiety disorders—generalized anxiety disorder, panic disorder, obsessive-compulsive disorder (OCD), and post-traumatic stress disorder (PTSD). Individuals diagnosed with anxiety disorders experience intense fear, apprehension, tension, or panic out of proportion to the actual threat or danger.

Certain physiological symptoms are diagnostic for individual anxiety disorders; however, some symptoms are common to all anxiety disorders. Common physiological symptoms include increased heart rate, palpitations, shortness of breath, rapid breathing, nausea, sweating, and dry mouth. All of these symptoms are associated with hyperactivity of the autonomic nervous system. More specifically, the physiological symptoms produced by anxiety are related to stimulation of the sympathetic nervous system and the parasympathetic nervous system.

GENERALIZED ANXIETY DISORDER

Although most adults will experience anxiety at one point in their life, excessive worrying and tension that are experienced daily for longer than 6 months is an indication of generalized anxiety disorder. Generalized anxiety disorder affects up to 6.8 million Americans, according to Anxiety Disorders Association of America, and is the most common type of anxiety disorder. Approximately 1.1% of Canadians between the ages of 15 and 64 years are diagnosed with generalized anxiety disorder, and women are twice as likely as men to be diagnosed with generalized anxiety disorder.

PANIC DISORDER

Panic disorder affects approximately 2.7% of the adult population, and it occurs twice as frequently in women than in men. It may be accompanied by major depression. Signs and symptoms of panic disorder include sudden onset of terror, shortness of breath, increased heart rate, trembling, and nausea. The person may feel paralyzed by the fear and unable to perform their routine daily activities. If these symptoms occur at least four times in 4 weeks or if a single panic attack is followed by persistent fear of another attack, lasting for a minimum of 1 month, a diagnosis of panic disorder is made. Most symptoms of panic disorder last for only a few minutes.

Panic attacks may be triggered by a phobia. A *phobia* is an irrational fear of things or situations that produce symptoms of intense anxiety. Phobias cause the person to try to avoid the thing that is feared. Agoraphobia is a condition where a person becomes so fearful of situations that may produce "panicky feelings" that they may isolate themselves or severely restrict their activities. Other more common phobias are claustrophobia (fear of being in confined spaces), aviophobia (fear of flying), and acrophobia (fear of heights). Social phobias cause affected individuals to shy away from social situations where they fear embarrassment or humiliation. Fear of public speaking or asking questions in a public forum setting is often associated with a social phobia. Approximately 8% of the population in the United States and Canada have some type of phobia.

OBSESSIVE-COMPULSIVE DISORDER

Obsessive-compulsive disorder (OCD) is a condition associated with an inability to control or stop repeated unwanted thoughts or behaviors. Individuals create rituals, which they perform repeatedly, to lessen anxieties about the things they fear. A person who fears germs may wash his or her hands excessively. The prevalence of OCD is 1.8% of the Canadian population between the ages of 15 and 64 years according to the Public Health Agency of Canada Report on Mental Illness in Canada (2002). One percent of the American population is affected and the lifetime incidence of OCD worldwide is 1.7-4%.

POST-TRAUMATIC STRESS DISORDER

Post-traumatic stress disorder (PTSD) may develop in persons who have participated in, witnessed, or been a victim of a terrifying event. According to Anxiety Disorders Association of America, nearly 8 million people in the United States have been diagnosed with PTSD. It may occur in soldiers who have committed atrocities or witnessed horrific events during wartime. Women, men, or children who have been raped have developed PTSD. Up to 65% of men and 45.9% of women who have been raped will develop PTSD. PTSD is likely to develop at some point in the lifetime of children who have been sexually abused. Some people have developed PTSD after natural disasters such as earthquakes and floods or human disasters such as airplane crashes.

Neurochemistry of Anxiety

Pharmaceutical treatment of anxiety is achieved by administering drugs that affect the neurotransmitters γ-aminobutyric acid (GABA), serotonin (5-hydroxytryptamine [5-HT]), and norepinephrine (NE).

ROLE OF γ-AMINOBUTYRIC ACID

The mechanism of action for most anxiolytics is to enhance binding of GABA, a neurotransmitter, to $GABA_A$ and $GABA_B$ receptors. In other words, the anxiolytic agent binds to its specific receptor, which in turn increases GABA binding to GABA receptors. Recall that GABA is the major inhibitory neurotransmitter in the nervous system. $GABA_A$ receptor binding causes chloride ion (Cl^-) channels to open, and $GABA_B$ receptor binding are coupled to G proteins. The influx of chloride ions results in hyperpolarization, which inhibits formation of action potentials. Ultimately, neuronal excitability is reduced and nerve impulse transmission is decreased.

ROLE OF SEROTONIN

Serotonin, also known as 5-HT, plays a minor role in treatment of anxiety. Serotonin is a neurotransmitter, too. More than nine serotonin receptors have been identified. Most are located in the pons and midbrain. The serotonin receptor involved in the treatment of anxiety is $5-HT_{1A}$.

ROLE OF NOREPINEPHRINE

NE is an important neurotransmitter for the sympathetic nervous system. It is responsible for mediating some of the adrenergic-related symptoms of anxiety. While NE plays a critical role in affective disorders such as depression, its role in anxiety is minimal.

Drugs Used to Treat Anxiety

Anxiety disorder is treated by the administration of anxiolytics and psychotherapy, including cognitive behavioral therapy. An *anxiolytic* is a drug that reduces symptoms of anxiety.

BENZODIAZEPINES

TECH NOTE!
Two common endings for drugs that are classified as benzodiazepines are "*-epam*" and "*-olam.*"

Benzodiazepines are the principal class of medications used in the treatment of anxiety (Table 5-2). They are indicated for short-term treatment of anxiety. Benzodiazepines are able to reduce anxiety even when taken in low doses. They reduce anxiety by depressing the limbic system and reticular formation. Other indications for benzodiapines are panic attack, insomnia, seizure disorder, and muscle relaxation. These additional indications are listed under the description of individual benzodiazepines.

MECHANISM OF ACTION

Benzodiazepines bind to receptor sites on the $GABA_A$ complex. This increases the affinity of gamma aminobutyric acid to the GABA receptor. GABA receptor binding opens Cl^- ion channels and lowers the neuronal membrane resting potential from −60 mV to −90 mV. This reduces neuronal excitability. (Figure 5-1)

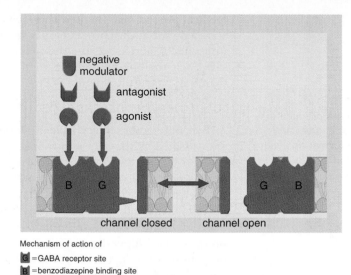

Mechanism of action of

G = GABA receptor site

B = benzodiazepine binding site

FIGURE 5-1 Anxiolytic agents. *(Page C, et al.: Integrated pharmacology, ed 3. Philadelphia, 2006, Mosby.)*

PHARMACOKINETICS

Benzodiazepines have a high degree of lipid solubility, which accounts for their rapid and complete absorption and enables the drugs to readily cross the blood-brain barrier. The duration of action varies from one benzodiazepine to another and may influence the selection of one benzodiazepine over another. A benzodiazepine that has a long duration of action may have long-lasting, unwanted side effects. The effects of some benzodiazepines may persist for up to 3 days (Table 5-1).

The benzodiazepines are fully metabolized, and some agents are metabolized to active metabolites (see Chapter 2). The half-life ($T^{1/2}$) of the active metabolites can be several days and accounts for the long duration of action of some anxiolytics. The long duration of diazepam is associated with the formation of active metabolites.

ADVERSE REACTIONS

Certain side effects are common to all benzodiazepines, while others are drug specific. All benzodiazepines produce some degree of sedation, ataxia, confusion, and reduced motor performance. Benzodiazepines can also interfere with cognitive functions and memory because they produce a type of amnesia. This side effect is sometimes used purposefully such as when benzodiazepines are used to reduce anxiety associated with dental or

TABLE 5-1   Half-life of Benzodizepines

Long Acting	
Chlorazepate	1 to 3 days
Diazepam	1 to 3 days
Chlordiazepoxide	1 to 3 days
Intermediate Acting	
Alprazolam	10 to 20 hours
Lorazepam	8 to 24 hours
Temazepam	Up to 25 hours
Short Acting	
Oxazepam	3 to 8 hours
Triazolam	3 to 8 hours

medical procedures. The person receiving the drug "forgets" the procedure, so anxiety associated with future procedures is reduced. Adverse reactions are dose dependent; therefore, effects increase as the dose increases. As a class of drugs, benzodiazepines are fairly safe. Their therapeutic index is high. The lethal dose is approximately 1000 times greater than the typical therapeutic dose.

TOLERANCE AND DEPENDENCE

All benzodiazepines are capable of producing tolerance and dependence, which is why they are classified as Class IV controlled substances in the United States. Benzodiazepines are categorized as a targeted controlled substance in Canada and listed in Schedule 1 and 2 of the Canadian Controlled Drugs and Substances Act.

Tolerance to a drug is said to have developed when the patient must take increasing doses to achieve the same effects as were achieved previously at lower doses. Tolerance to benzodiazepines can develop in as little as 14 days. Benzodiazepines are also known to produce drug dependence. When drug dependence has developed, the person taking the drug must continue to take the drug in order to avoid the onset of physical and/or psychological withdrawal symptoms. Sudden cessation of benzodiazepines can bring on the onset of withdrawal symptoms such as tremors, anxiety, insomnia, agitation, and confusion. Onset of withdrawal symptoms is drug specific. Withdrawal symptoms develop soon after discontinuation of benzodiazepines with a short half-life ($T\frac{1}{2}$). The onset of withdrawal symptoms is delayed following abrupt discontinuation of benzodiazepines that have a long half-life.

> **TECH NOTE!**
> C-IV drugs produce less risk for physical and psychological addiction than do C-I, C-II, and C-III drugs.

> **TECH ALERT!**
> Xanax, Zantac, and Zyrtec have look-alike/sound-alike issues. Immediate release and extended release have look-alike/sound-alike issues, too!

TABLE 5-2   Benzodiazepines Used in the Treatment of Anxiety

Generic name	U.S. brand name(s) / Canadian brand(s)	Dosage forms and strengths
alprazolam*	Alprazolam Intensol, Niravam, Xanax, Xanax XR	Solution (Alprazolam Intensol): 1 mg/ml Tablets (Xanax): 0.25 mg, 0.5 mg, 1 mg, 2 mg
	Xanax, Xanax TS	Tablets, extended release (Xanax XR, Xanax TS): 0.5 mg, 1 mg, 2 mg, 3 mg Tablet, disintegrating (Niravam): 0.25 mg, 0.5 mg, 1 mg, 2 mg
clonazepam*	Klonopin	Tablet: 0.5 mg, 1 mg, 2mg Tablet, disintegrating: 0.125 mg, 0.25 mg, 0.5 mg, 1 mg, 2 mg
	Clonopam, Klonopin, Rivotril	
clorazepate*	Tranxene, Tranxene SD, Tranxene SD Half Strength	Tablet (Tranxene) 3.75 mg, 7.5 mg, 15 mg Tablet, sustained release (Tranxene SD) 22.5 mg
	generics only	Tablet, sustained release (Tranxene SD Half Strength) 11.25 mg
diazepam*	Diastat, Diazepam Intensol, Valium	Rectal gel (Diastat): 5 mg/ml Injection, solution 5 mg/ml Oral, solution 5 mg/5 ml
	Diastat, Diazemuls, Valium	Oral concentrate (Diazepam Intensol): 5 mg/ml Tablet (Valium): 2 mg, 5 mg, 10 mg
lorazepam*	Ativan, Lorazepam Intensol	Injection, solution (Ativan) 2 mg/ml; 4 mg/ml Solution, oral concentrate (Lorazepam Intensol) 2 mg/ml
	Ativan, Nu-Loraz	Tablet (Ativan) 0.5 mg, 1 mg, 2 mg
midazolam*	generic only	Injection, solution: 1 mg/ml and 5 mg/ml Syrup: 2 mg/ml
	generic only	
oxazepam*	generic	Capsule: 10 mg, 15 mg, 30 mg Tablet (Serax): 10 mg,15 mg, 30 mg
	Serax	

*Generic available.

The risk of developing withdrawal symptoms is minimized when benzodiazepines are discontinued slowly.

PRECAUTIONS

Benzodiazepines potentiate the sedative effects of other central nervous system depressants. They also should be used cautiously in patients who have liver disease. When midazolam is administered, respiratory resuscitation equipment should be readily available. There is a drug interaction between midazolam and cimetidine that results in increased midazolam levels.

AZAPIRONES

Azapirones are effective in management of anxiety disorders (Table 5-3) and have a benefit over benzodiazepines because they do not produce tolerance or dependence.

MECHANISM OF ACTION

The actions produced by azapirones are believed to be caused by binding at dopamine (DA_2) and serotonin ($5\text{-}HT_{1A}$) receptors. Azapirones are partial agonists at the $5\text{-}HT_{1A}$ receptors. Drug-receptor binding at the presynapse is inhibitory and decreases neuronal firing. Azapirones have no effect on GABA receptors and lack central nervous system–depressant activity.

PHARMACOKINETICS

Buspirone is the only drug in this class. The onset of action is slow, and maximum therapeutic effects are achieved 1 to 3 weeks after therapy has been initiated.

Buspirone is metabolized in the liver and eliminated in urine. The elimination half-life is between 2 and 3 hours. Food decreases first-pass metabolism in the liver and increases the drug's bioavailability.

ADVERSE REACTIONS

The most common adverse effects associated with buspirone therapy are dizziness, restlessness, headache, nausea, diarrhea, and insomnia. Buspirone produces only minimal sedation.

PRECAUTIONS

Buspirone should be used with caution in patients with liver or kidney disease.

MISCELLANEOUS ANXIOLYTIC AGENTS

HYDROXYZINE

Hydroxyzine is an antihistamine that is also approved for the treatment of anxiety. It is used in children and adults to reduce anxiety associated with dental and minor medical procedures. It produces a fair bit of sedation but, like buspirone, does not produce tolerance or dependence. Other side effects are dizziness, headache, dry mucous membranes, and urinary retention.

TABLE 5-3   Azapirones Used in the Treatment of Anxiety

Generic name	U.S. brand name(s) / Canadian brand(s)	Dosage forms and strengths
buspirone*	BuSpar	Tablet: 5 mg, 7.5 mg, 10 mg, 15 mg, 30 mg
	BuSpar	

*Generic available

TABLE 5-4   Miscellaneous Drugs Used in the Treatment of Anxiety

Generic name	U.S. brand name(s) Canadian brand(s)	Dosage forms and strengths
hydroxyzine HCl*	Atarax, Antatens	Syrup, as HCl: 10 mg/5 ml
	Atarax	Tablet, as HCl: 10 mg, 25 mg 50 mg Solution, for injection: 50 mg/ml
hydroxyzine pamoate*	generic only	Capsule, as pamoate: 25 mg, 50 mg, 100 mg
	no longer available	Oral suspension, as pamoate: 25 mg/5 ml

*Generic available.

Hydroxyzine HCl and hydroxyzine pamoate are contraindicated in men with prostate disease and lactating women. Sedation is increased when the drug is taken with other central nervous system depressants or alcohol (Table 5-4).

ANTIDEPRESSANTS

Tricyclic antidepressants (TCAs), selective serotonin reuptake inhibitors (SSRIs), and monoamine oxidase inhibitors (MAOIs) are antidepressants with a limited use in the treatment of anxiety (see Chapter 6) (Table 5-5). **Clomipramine**, a TCA, is indicated for the treatment of OCD. **Fluoxetine** and **sertraline** are SSRIs and are indicated for OCD as well. Sertraline is also labeled for use in the treatment of panic disorder, social phobia, and PTSD.

Treatment of OCD with antidepressants requires higher doses than the treatment of depression, and it takes a longer time for maximum benefits to be achieved. TCAs, like clomipramine, may take up to 6 weeks for full effects to be noticed. Maximum benefits of fluoxetine and sertraline are achieved in 1 to 3 weeks.

ADVERSE REACTIONS

Some adverse reactions are common to all the antidepressants used in the treatment of anxiety. Others are drug specific. Clomipramine may produce sedation or decreased alertness; fluoxetine, paroxetine, and sertraline may cause insomnia, decreased appetite, dry mouth, dizziness, and agitation or tremor; and paroxetine may also produce headache, nausea, diarrhea, and sexual dysfunction.

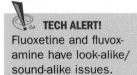

TECH ALERT!
Clomipramine, chlorpromazine, and clomiphene have look-alike/sound-alike issues.

TECH ALERT!
Fluoxetine and fluvoxamine have look-alike/sound-alike issues.

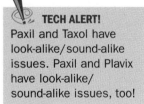

TECH ALERT!
Paxil and Taxol have look-alike/sound-alike issues. Paxil and Plavix have look-alike/sound-alike issues, too!

TABLE 5-5   Antidepressants Used in the Treatment of Anxiety

Generic name	U.S. brand name(s) Canadian brand(s)	Dosage forms and strengths
clomipramine*	Anafranil	Cap sule: 25 mg, 50 mg, 75 mg
	Anafranil	Capsule (Prozac): 10 mg, 20 mg, 40 mg; (Serafem): 10 mg, 20 mg
fluoxetine*	Prozac, Prozac Weekly, Serafem	Oral solution: 20 mg/5 ml
	Prozac	
paroxetine*	Paxil, Paxil CR, Pexeva	Tablet, as HCl (Prozac): 10 mg, 20 mg Suspension, oral: 10 mg/5 ml
	Paxil, Paxil CR	Tablet, as hydrochloride (Paxil): 10 mg, 20 mg,
sertraline*	Zoloft	Solution, oral concentrate: 20 mg/ml
	Zoloft	Tablet: 25 mg, 50 mg, 100 mg

*Generic available.

No tolerance or dependence is associated with any of the antidepressants. However, some serious side effects are possible. Clomipramine may produce seizures. Serotonin syndrome is a serious condition associated with the use of drugs like sertraline and fluoxetine. Serotonin syndrome is potentially fatal and produces symptoms of confusion, agitation, diarrhea, tremors, increased blood pressure, and seizures. A detailed description of specific mechanisms of action and pharmacokinetics of these drugs will be discussed in Chapter 6.

β-ADRENERGIC ANTAGONISTS

Rapid heart rate is a common symptom of anxiety. β-Adrenergic antagonists, also known as β-blockers, are administered to reduce the palpitations. β-Adrenergic antagonists are not U.S. Food and Drug Administration approved for the treatment of anxiety; however, they are prescribed for the management of stage fright.

Summary of Drugs Used in the Treatment of Anxiety Disorders

	Generic name	U.S. brand name	Usual adult oral dose and dosing schedule	Warning labels
	Benzodiazepines			
	alprazolam	Xanax	**Generalized anxiety disorder:** immediate release 0.5 mg to 4 mg daily (in 1 to 3 divided doses) **Panic disorder:** 1.5 mg to 10 mg/day (immediate release); 0.5 mg to 6 mg/day (extended release) **Anxiety associated with depression:** 2.5 mg to 3 mg/day in divided doses)	MAY CAUSE DROWSINESS; MAY IMPAIR ABILITY TO DRIVE AVOID ALCOHOL MAY BE HABIT FORMING
	clonazepam	Klonopin	**Panic disorder:** 0.25 mg to 1 mg twice a day (maximum 4 mg/day)	DO NOT CRUSH, BREAK OR CHEW (extended release)
	clorazepate	Tranxene	**Generalized anxiety disorder:** 7.5 mg to 15 mg 2 to 4 times/day (immediate release); 11.25 mg to 22.5 mg once daily (sustained release) **Ethanol withdrawal:** 30 mg dosed 2 to 4 times per day; increase up to maximum 90 mg/day	
	diazepam	Valium	**Anxiety disorder:** 2 to 10 mg 2 to 4 times /day (oral); 2 to 10 mg every 3 to 4 hours (IM, IV) **Ethanol withdrawal:** 5 to 10 mg IV every 3 to 4 hours as needed	
	lorazepam	Ativan	**Anxiety and sedation:** Oral 1 to 10 mg daily in 2 to 3 divided doses. **Preprocedure sedation:** 0.05 mg/kg IM (maximum 4 mg/dose) or 0.044 mg/kg IV (maximum 2 mg/dose)	

Continued

Summary of Drugs Used in the Treatment of Anxiety Disorders—cont'd

	Generic name	U.S. brand name	Usual adult oral dose and dosing schedule	Warning labels
	midazolam	generic	**Conscious sedation for preoperative procedures:** 0.5 mg to 2 mg slow IV every 2 to 3 minutes (maximum 2.5 mg to 5 mg)	
	oxazepam	generic	**Anxiety:** 10 to 30 mg 3 to 4 times a day **Ethanol withdrawal:** 15 to 30 mg 3 to 4 times a day	
Azapirones				
	buspirone	BuSpar	7.5 mg to 15 mg twice daily (maximum dose 60 mg/day)	MAY CAUSE DROWSINESS; MAY IMPAIR ABILITY TO DRIVE TAKE WITH FOOD
Miscellaneous anxiolytics				
	hydroxyzine hcl hydroxyzine pamoate	Atarax generic	**Anxiety:** 25 to 100 mg 4 times a day (maximum dose 600 mg/day) **Ethanol withdrawal:** 50 mg to 100 mg IM 4 times a day **Preoperative sedation:** 50 to 100 mg as a single dose (oral); 25 mg to 100 mg (IM)	MAY CAUSE DROWSINESS; AVOID ALCOHOL MAY INTENSIFY THIS EFFECT MAY IMPAIR ABILITY TO DRIVE
Antidepressants used in the treatment of anxiety disorders				
	clomipramine	Anafranil	**Obsessive-compulsive disorder:** 25 mg to 100 mg/day in divided doses (maximum 250 mg/day)	MAY CAUSE DROWSINESS; AVOID ALCOHOL MAY INTENSIFY THIS EFFECT MAY IMPAIR ABILITY TO DRIVE
	fluoxetine	Prozac	**Obsessive-compulsive disorder:** 20 mg to 80 mg/day **Panic disorder:** 20 mg/day (maximum 60 mg/day)	MAY CAUSE DIZZINESS AVOID ALCOHOL MAY INTENSIFY THIS EFFECT MAY IMPAIR ABILITY TO DRIVE SWALLOW WHOLE; DON'T CRUSH OR CHEW (delayed release) DO NOT DISCONTINUE WITHOUT MEDICAL SUPERVISION
	paroxetine	Paxil	**Generalized anxiety:** 20 mg to 50 mg/day **Obsessive-compulsive disorder:** 20 mg to 60 mg daily **Panic disorder:** 10 mg to 60 mg daily (Paxil, Pexeva) or 12.75 mg daily (Paxil CR) **Post-traumatic stress disorder:** 12.5 mg to 25 mg daily (Paxil CR) **Social phobias:** 20 mg daily (Paxil) or 12.5 to 27.5 mg daily (Paxil CR)	
	sertraline	Zoloft	**Obsessive-compulsive disorder:** 50 mg/day **Panic disorder, post-traumatic stress disorder, and social phobias:** 50 mg/day (up to 200 mg/day)	

CHAPTER SUMMARY

- Anxiety disorders are the leading mental health illness.
- The cause of anxiety disorders may be environmental, biological, or developmental; associated with socioeconomic conditions; or a combination of several of these individual factors.
- The four major types of anxiety disorders are generalized anxiety disorder, panic disorder, obsessive-compulsive disorder (OCD), and post-traumatic stress disorder (PTSD).
- Common physiological symptoms include increased heart rate, palpitations, shortness of breath, rapid breathing, nausea, sweating, and dry mouth. All of these symptoms are associated with hyperactivity of the autonomic nervous system.
- Generalized anxiety disorder is associated with excessive worry and tension that are experienced daily for longer than 6 months.
- OCD is a condition associated with an inability to control or stop repeated unwanted thoughts or behaviors.
- Panic disorder is a condition associated with repeated sudden onset of feelings of terror.
- A phobia is an irrational fear of things or situations that produce symptoms of intense anxiety.
- Social phobias cause affected individuals to shy away from social situations where they fear embarrassment of humiliation. Fear of public speaking is an example of a social phobia.
- PTSD is a stress disorder that develops in persons who have participated in, witnessed, or been a victim of a terrifying event.
- Anxiety disorder is treated by the administration of anxiolytics and psychotherapy, including cognitive behavioral therapy.
- The mechanism of action for most anxiolytics is to enhance binding of γ-aminobutyric acid (GABA), a neurotransmitter, to $GABA_A$ and $GABA_B$ receptors.
- Benzodiazepines are the principal class of medications used in the treatment of anxiety and bind to receptor sites on the $GABA_A$ complex.
- GABA receptor binding opens Cl^- ion channels, which reduces neuronal excitability.
- The duration of action for benzodiazepines may be long acting, intermediate acting, or short acting.
- Benzodiazepines can produce a type of amnesia that causes the person receiving the drug to "forget," reducing anxiety associated with future dental or medical procedures.
- All benzodiazepines are capable of producing tolerance and dependence.
- Once tolerance develops, increasing doses of a drug are required in order to achieve the same effects as were achieved a previously at lower doses. When drug dependence has developed, the person taking the drug must continue to take the drug in order to avoid the onset of physical and/or psychological withdrawal symptoms.
- All benzodiazepines are scheduled Class IV controlled substances in the United States and are listed in schedule 1 and 2 of the Canadian Controlled Drugs and Substances Act.
- Withdrawal symptoms develop soon after discontinuation of benzodiazepines with a short $T^{1/2}$ and is delayed following abrupt discontinuation of benzodiazepines that have a long half-life.
- Buspirone is an azapirone and is a partial agonist at $5\text{-}HT_{1A}$ receptor. These receptors are inhibitory at the presynapse, so stimulation causes decreased neuronal firing.
- Buspirone does not produce tolerance or dependence. Abrupt discontinuation does not produce withdrawal symptoms.
- Hydroxyzine is an antihistamine that is indicated for the treatment of anxiety. It is used in children and adults to reduce anxiety associated with dental and minor medical procedures.
- Tricyclic antidepressants, selective serotonin reuptake inhibitors, and monoamine oxidase inhibitors are antidepressants with a limited use in the treatment of anxiety.
- Serotonin syndrome is a potentially life threatening adverse drug reaction caused by excessive serotonin that produces symptoms of confusion, agitation, diarrhea, tremors, increased blood pressure, and seizures.
- β-Adrenergic antagonists are administered to reduce the palpitations associated with anxiety and are also useful for the management of stage fright.

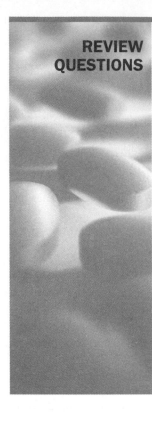

REVIEW QUESTIONS

Multiple Choice

1. Is the following statement true or false? "Women are twice as likely as men to be diagnosed with generalized anxiety disorder."
   a. true
   b. false

2. The _____ treatment of anxiety is associated with increases in drug-receptor binding to the neurotransmitters γ-aminobutyric acid, serotonin, and norepinephrine.
   a. therapeutic
   b. psychological
   c. pharmacological
   d. physiological

3. Anxiety disorder is treated by the administration of _____ and psychotherapy.
   a. antidepressants
   b. anxiolytics
   c. antiinflammatories
   d. antipsychotics

4. Benzodiazepines are indicated for _____ treatment of anxiety.
   a. short-term
   b. long-term

5. _____ to a drug is said to have developed when the patient must take increasing doses to achieve the same effects as were achieved previously at lower doses.
   a. Dependence
   b. Addiction
   c. Tolerance
   d. none of the above

6. Which of the following benzodiazepines is indicated for the treatment of anxiety disorders, ethanol withdrawal, skeletal muscle relaxation, and seizure disorders?
   a. alprazolam
   b. clonazepam
   c. lorazepam
   d. diazepam

7. Buspirone is the only drug in this class.
   a. azapirone
   b. antihistamine
   c. amiodarone
   d. a and c

8. _____ is an antihistamine that is indicated for the treatment of anxiety
   a. promethazine
   b. hydroxyzine
   c. apresoline
   d. none of the above

9. Clomipramine, fluoxetine, and sertraline are antidepressants that are indicated for the treatment of
   a. panic disorders
   b. anxiety
   c. obsessive-compulsive disorder
   d. post-traumatic stress disorder

10. **Rapid heart rate is a common symptom of anxiety. β-Adrenergic antagonists are administered to reduce the palpitations. One example is**

    a. propranolol

    b. Inderal

    c. InnoPran XL

    d. all of the above

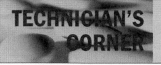

TECHNICIAN'S CORNER

1. What happens if a patient stops using benzodiazepines abruptly?
2. What is the difference between tolerance and dependence on a drug?

BIBLIOGRAPHY

Anxiety Disorders Association of America: *Statistics and facts.* Retrieved from http://www.adaa.org/AboutADAA/PressRoom/StatsandFacts.asp. Accessed Nov. 30, 2007.

Greenberg, W. and Aronson, S., *Obsessive-Compulsive Disorder.* e Medicine 2007. Retrieved from http://www.emedicine.com/med/topic1654.htm. Accessed Feb 15, 2008.

Lance L, Lacy C, Armstrong L, Goldman M: *Drug information handbook for the allied health professional,* ed 12. Hudson, OH, 2005, APhA Lexi-Comp.

National Institute of Mental Health, Department of Health and Human Services, Public Health Service, National Institutes of Health: *Facts about anxiety disorders.* Retrieved from http://www.nlm.nih.gov/medlineplus. Accessed June 15, 2006.

National Mental Health Information Center: *Anxiety disorders.* Retrieved from www.mwntalhealth.samhsa.gov/publications/allpubs/ken98-0045/default.asp

Page C, Curtis M, Sutter M, Walker M, Hoffman B: *Integrated pharmacology* (pp 239-241), Philadelphia, 2005, Elsevier Mosby.

Public Health Agency of Canada: *A report on mental illness in Canada.* Retrieved from http://www.phac-aspc.gc.ca/publicat/miic-mmac/chap_4_. Accessed June 15, 2006.

Raffa R, Rawls S, Beyzarov E: *Netter's illustrated pharmacology* (pp 65-66), Philadelphia, 2005, WB Saunders.

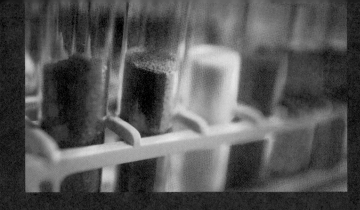

Treatment of Depression

LEARNING OBJECTIVES

- List and describe the function of neurotransmitters associated with symptoms of depression.
- Classify medications used to treat depression.
- Describe mechanism of action for each class of drugs used to treat depression.
- Identify warning labels and precautionary messages associated with medications used to treat depression.
- Identify significant drug look-alike/sound-alike issues.
- Learn the terminology associated with the treatment of depression.

KEY TERMS

Adjunct: Drug that is used to compliment the effects of another drug.

Bipolar disorder: Mental health illness associated with sudden swings in mood between depression and periods of insomnia, racing thoughts, distractibility, and increased goal-directed behavior.

Enuresis: Bedwetting or uncontrollable urination during sleep.

Major depression: Mental health illness associated with persistent feelings of sadness, emptiness, or hopelessness that persists for several weeks.

Monoamine oxidase: Enzyme found in the liver, intestine, and terminal neuron, responsible for degradation of monoamine neurotransmitters and dietary amines.

Mood disorder: Affective disorder involving a change in emotional behavior.

Serotonin syndrome: Potentially life threatening adverse drug reaction caused by excessive serotonin that produces symptoms of confusion, agitation, diarrhea, tremors, increased blood pressure, and seizures.

Overview

Depressive illness affects nearly 20 million Americans and 1.2 million Canadians each year (2007). Depression affects men, women, and children. Depressive disorder may be precipitated by hormonal changes (premenstrual syndrome, pregnancy, postpartum), substance abuse (alcohol and other drugs), or illnesses such as Parkinson's disease, heart attack, or thyroid dysfunction. Heredity plays a role as well, particularly in bipolar disorder, where children born to a parent with bipolar disorder are at increased risk for the illness.

Depressive illness influences most aspects of a person's life and lifestyle. It affects self-esteem, mood, thoughts, eating, and sleeping. Depression reduces the ability to think and concentrate. Feelings of worthlessness or guilt often accompany depressive episodes. As many as 12% of depressed patients contemplate or attempt suicide. Without treatment, symptoms of depression can persist for a few weeks to years.

There are three primary types of depressive disorders: major depression, bipolar disorder, and dysthymia. *Major depression* is also called *clinical depression* and is associated with persistent feelings of sadness, emptiness, or hopelessness. These feelings must persist for several weeks and are usually accompanied by a lack of interest in activities that were previously thought to be enjoyable, fatigue, irritability, and insomnia or hypersomnia. Sometimes the depression manifests itself in other physical ailments for which no treatments are able to cure or reduce symptoms. *Bipolar disorder,* formerly called manic-depressive disorder, is associated with sudden swings in mood between depression and periods of mania. Mania is associated with hyperactivity, racing thoughts, insomnia, distractibility, and increased goal-directed behavior. Manic periods can last for 1 or more weeks, during which time the person may sleep little and produce a prolific amount of work. Several well-known people such as Vincent Van Gogh are believed to have had bipolar disorder. *Dysthymia* produces symptoms that are similar to major depression; however, the symptoms are less severe. People diagnosed with dysthymia have symptoms that are chronic and, while not typically debilitating, keep the person from functioning well and feeling good.

The causes of depression are not completely known, but a deficiency of certain neurotransmitters is involved. This explains why people with depression cannot "pull themselves together" to get better. Drug treatment is aimed at restoring depleted neurotransmitters to normal levels.

Neurochemistry of Depression

BIOGENIC AMINE THEORY

According to the biogenic amine theory, clinical depression results from a decrease in monoamine neurotransmitters in the brain. This hypothesis was made upon the discovery that patients treated with drugs that deplete monoamine neurotransmitters stores in the neuron develop depression. Other evidence for the monoamine theory of depression is the laboratory finding that the concentration of monoamines and their metabolites is minimal in the cerebral spinal fluid of patients diagnosed with clinical depression. Evidence exists to support the fact that adrenergic receptors and serotonergic receptors are less sensitive in depressed persons so norepinephrine (NE) and serotonin (5-hydroxytryptamine [5-HT]) binding is decreased even when levels are normal. The γ-aminobutyric acid receptor (GABA) may also be involved in depression.

If depletion of monoamine neurotransmitters causes depression, what effects are caused by excessive levels of these neurotransmitters? Bipolar affective disorder (BPAD), also known as *mania,* is believed to be associated with increased levels of monoamine neurotransmitters (Figure 6-1). The complete neurochemistry of BPAD is unclear.

The monoamine neurotransmitters that are depleted in clinical depression are NE, 5-HT, and dopamine (DA). All currently marketed antidepressants act to increase the levels of NE, 5-HT, or DA released into synapses within the brain or to increase neurotransmitter binding. Antidepressants are categorized according to the method that they use to potentiate the actions of NE, 5-HT, and DA. Some antidepressants are nonspecific, increasing the binding

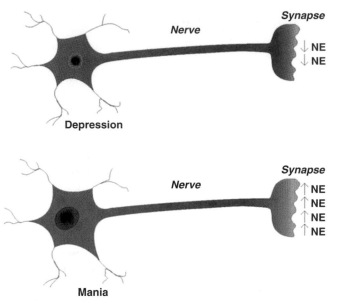

FIGURE 6-1 Biologic amine hypothesis. NE, norepinephrine. *(From Lilley LL, Harrington S, Snyder JS: Pharmacology and the nursing process, ed 5, St Louis, 2007, Mosby.)*

of more than one monoamine neurotransmitter, while other antidepressants are specific and increase the binding of only one of the neurotransmitters.

ROLE OF NOREPINEPHRINE

The neurotransmitter NE plays an important role in the treatment of depression. It is widely distributed in the brain and in the periphery. Decreased levels in the brain are responsible for depression and increased levels in the periphery can cause serious effects such as hypertension. Adrenergic neurons release NE. Most of the adrenergic neurons found in the central nervous system are found in the pons/midbrain. The antidepressant effects of NE are believed to be mediated by downregulation in postsynaptic β-receptors.

ROLE OF SEROTONIN

Antidepressants that potentiate the activity of the neurotransmitter 5-HT play an important role in the treatment of depression. Serotonin is an excitatory neurotransmitter. Serotonin receptors that have been well studied are 5-HT$_{1A}$, 5-HT$_{2A}$, 5-HT$_{2C}$, and 5-HT$_3$. More than nine 5-HT receptors have been identified. These 5-HT receptors influence G protein coupling and Na$^+$/K$^+$ channel operation. Drugs that antagonize 5-HT$_{2A}$ and 5-HT$_{2C}$ receptors are used in the treatment of depression and negative-symptom schizophrenia. Drugs that antagonize 5-HT$_3$ receptors are used to treat nausea. In addition to improved mood, 5-HT is involved in regulation of the sleep/wake cycle and pain perception.

ROLE OF DOPAMINE

There are five types of DA receptors. Binding to D$_2$, D$_3$, and D$_4$ receptors is inhibitory, while binding to D$_1$ and D$_5$ is excitatory. Dopamine binding plays a lesser role in the treatment and management of depression compared with the neurotransmitters NE and 5-HT. Drugs that are used in the treatment of Parkinson's disease and schizophrenia potentiate the activity of DA (see Chapter 8).

Drugs Used to Treat Depression

The mechanism of action for drugs used to treat depression may differ, but all antidepressants are equally effective (Figure 6-2). Inhibition of the reuptake of specific monoamine neurotransmitters is one of the ways in which antidepressants produce their effects. The other mechanism of action is to block the degradation of monoamine neurotransmitters.

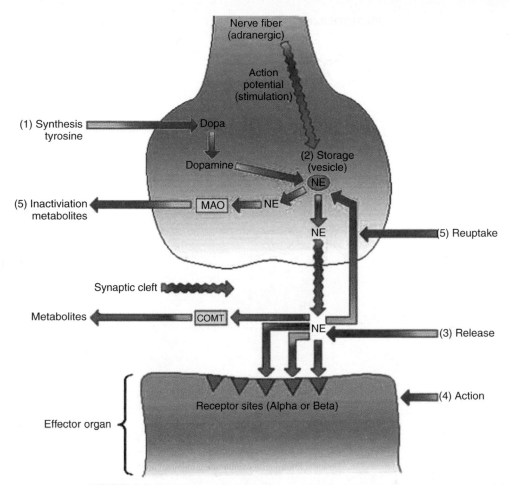

FIGURE 6-2 Site of neurotransmitter synthesis, storage, release, action and Inactivation. *(From Lilley LL, Harrington S, Snyder JS:* Pharmacology and the nursing process, *ed 5, St Louis, 2007, Mosby.)*

Selection of one antidepressant over another is based on the patient's ability to tolerate drug side effects.

TRICYCLIC ANTIDEPRESSANTS

Tricyclic antidepressants (TCAs) are the oldest class of medication used in the treatment of depression. The effectiveness of newer agents is compared with that of TCAs. As the name implies, all TCAs have a three-ring chemical structure (Figure 6-3). Because they all have a similar structure, they produce similar effects and similar side effects. The side chains attached to the rings affect the structure-activity relationship (SAR) and account for differences in duration of action and adverse reactions.

TCAs are used for the treatment and management of several medical conditions in addition to depression. They are also prescribed for *enuresis,* commonly known as bedwetting (imipramine and nortriptyline). Moreover, they are prescribed for the treatment of obsessive-compulsive disorder (clomipramine) and as an *adjunct* to other drug therapy for chronic pain (amitriptyline, nortriptyline). An adjunct is a drug that is used to complement the effects of another drug.

MECHANISM OF ACTION

In depression, sufficient neurotransmitters may be released into the synaptic cleft; however, the neurotransmitters may be returned to the neuron before binding occurs. TCAs work by producing a nonspecific blockade of the reuptake of monoamine neurotransmitters. TCAs block the reuptake of NE and 5-HT in the presynaptic neuron and in postsynaptic receptors.

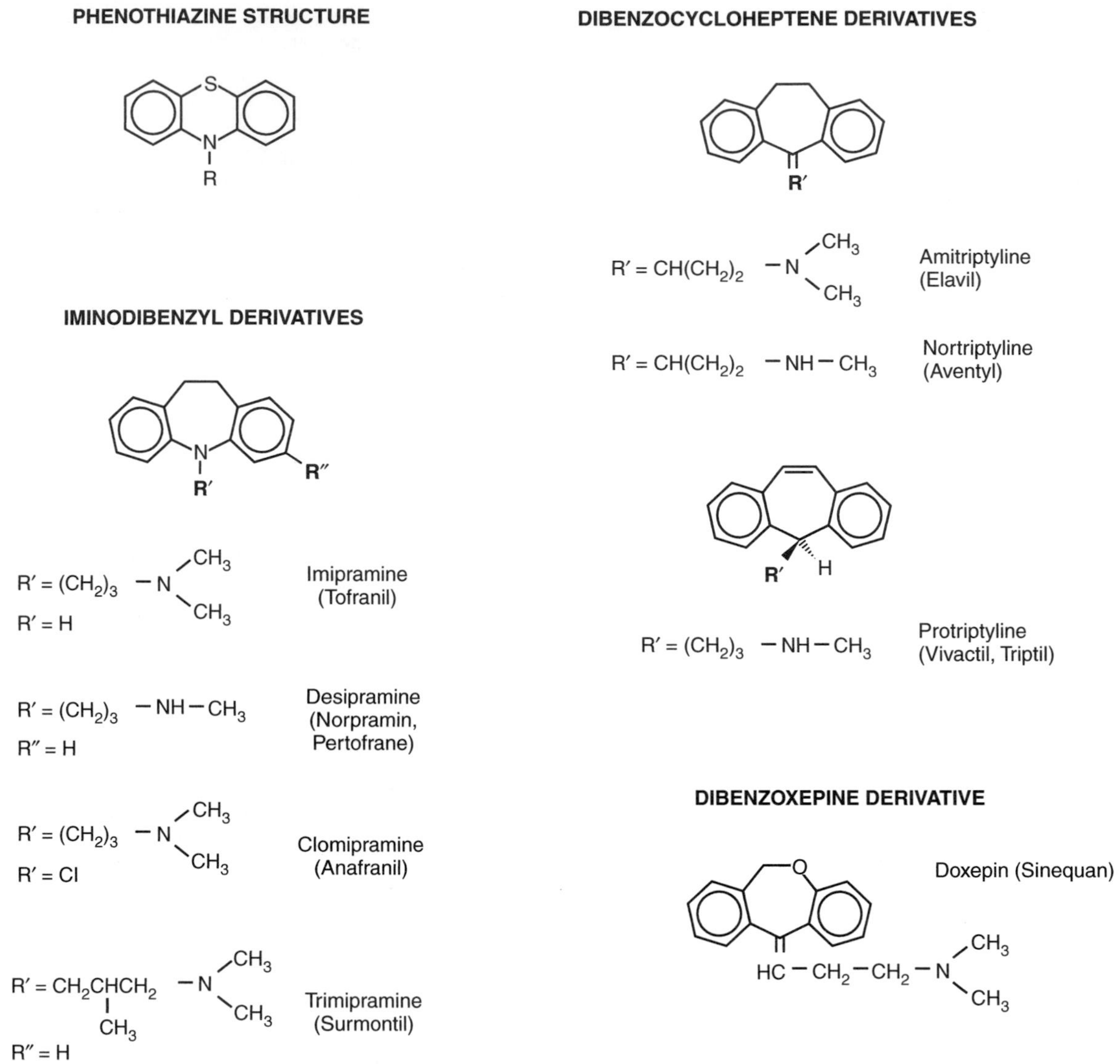

PHENOTHIAZINE STRUCTURE

DIBENZOCYCLOHEPTENE DERIVATIVES

$R' = CH(CH_2)_2$ $-N\diagup^{CH_3}_{\diagdown CH_3}$ Amitriptyline (Elavil)

$R' = CH(CH_2)_2$ $-NH-CH_3$ Nortriptyline (Aventyl)

IMINODIBENZYL DERIVATIVES

$R' = (CH_2)_3$ $-N\diagup^{CH_3}_{\diagdown CH_3}$ Imipramine (Tofranil)
$R' = H$

$R' = (CH_2)_3$ $-NH-CH_3$ Desipramine (Norpramin, Pertofrane)
$R'' = H$

$R' = (CH_2)_3$ $-N\diagup^{CH_3}_{\diagdown CH_3}$ Clomipramine (Anafranil)
$R' = Cl$

$R' = CH_2CHCH_2$ $-N\diagup^{CH_3}_{\diagdown CH_3}$ Trimipramine (Surmontil)
$\quad\quad |$
$\quad\quad CH_3$
$R'' = H$

$R' = (CH_2)_3$ $-NH-CH_3$ Protriptyline (Vivactil, Triptil)

DIBENZOXEPINE DERIVATIVE

Doxepin (Sinequan)

$HC-CH_2-CH_2-N\diagup^{CH_3}_{\diagdown CH_3}$

FIGURE 6-3 The three-ring structure of tricyclic antidepressants. *(From: Kalant H, Grant DM, Mitchell J: Principles of medical pharmacology, ed 7, Philadelphia, 2007, WB Saunders.)*

TCAs also have some affinity for adrenergic, cholinergic (muscarinic), and histaminic postsynaptic receptors.

When the reuptake of NE and 5-HT back into the neuron is blocked, the neurotransmitters remain in the synaptic cleft longer. The longer the neurotransmitter remains in the synaptic cleft, the greater is the opportunity for binding of the neurotransmitter to its receptor (Figure 6-4).

PHARMACOKINETICS

TCAs are readily absorbed by the oral route of administration. They are lipophilic so are widely distributed within the central nervous system. Their onset of action and duration of action and half-life (T½) vary. The T½ of TCAs can be as short as 4 hours (imipramine) and as long as 96 hours (nortriptyline). Their long half-life is associated with their high degree of lipid solubility. The long duration of action of these agents permits once-daily dosing.

TCAs are metabolized by microsomal enzymes in the liver. Several of the TCAs are metabolized to active metabolites. Amitriptyline is metabolized to nortripyline, and desipramine is a metabolite of imipramine. They are ultimately eliminated in the urine.

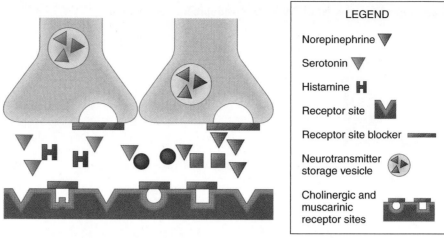

FIGURE 6-4 Mechanism of action for tricyclic antidepressants.

Although the onset of action may be relatively short with TCAs, maximum antidepression benefit from their administration may take up to 6 weeks to be achieved.

ADVERSE REACTIONS

TCAs all have a similar structure, so side effects of the drugs are similar. What varies is the degree to which a particular TCA will produce the side effect. For an example, all TCAs can produce sedation, but some TCAs, such as amitriptyline, have high sedative activity, whereas other TCAs, like desipramine, have low sedative activity.

Adverse reactions of TCAs are related to effects produced by increased binding to adrenergic, cholineric, serotonergic, and histaminic receptors. A rise in NE levels is responsible for the increased cardiovascular activity caused by TCAs. On the other hand, postsypnaptic adrenergic blockade is responsible for hypotension and reflex tachycardia caused by TCAs. Blockade of histaminic receptors can lead to sedation, weight gain, and hypotension. Blockade of cholinergic (muscarinic) receptors can lead to blurred vision, dry mouth, constipation, urinary retention, confusion, and delirium. TCAs may also produce photosensitivity.

TECH NOTE!
Dry mouth may be relieved by sucking on sugarless candy. TCAs can also increase cravings for sweets!

Comparison of Properties of Tricyclic Antidepressants

	Generic name	Sedative effects	Anticholinergic activity	Hypotensive effects	Cardiac effects	T½ (hr)	Reuptake inhibition	
							NE	5-HT
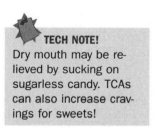	amitriptyline	High	High	Moderate-high	Moderate	8 to 24	++	++
	clomipramine	Low	High	Moderate	Moderate	17 to 28	++	++++
	desipramine	Low	Low-moderate	Moderate	Low	7 to 60	++++	+
	doxepin	High	High	High	Moderate	6 to 28	++	+
	imipramine	Moderate	Moderate	High	Moderate	4 to 18	++	+++

Continued

Comparison of Properties of Tricyclic Antidepressants—cont'd

Generic name	Sedative effects	Anticholinergic activity	Hypotensive effects	Cardiac effects	T½ (hr)	Reuptake inhibition NE	Reuptake inhibition 5-HT
nortriptyline	Low-moderate	Low-moderate	Slight	Low	18 to 96	+++	+
protriptyline	Slight	Low-moderate	Low	Moderate	55 to 125	++++	+
trimipramine	High	Moderate-high	Moderate	Moderate	20 to 26	+	+

Key: + Low
++ Low-moderate
+++ Moderate
++++ High

Adapted from Table 25-1. Relative Effects of Antidepressants, Kalant H. et al., Principles of Medical Pharmacology (p. 321), ed 7. Toronto, 2007, Fig 14-41 Pharmacokinetic considerations with antide pressants, Page C, et al. Integrated Pharmacology (p. 249) Philadelphia 2005, Table 1. Pharmacology/Pharmacokinetics http://www.drugs.com accessed Feb 15, 2008 and Clinical Pharmacology.com accessed Feb 16, 2008.

TECH NOTE!

Prescriptions for small quantities of TCAs may be written for depressed patients who are believed to be suicidal.

PRECAUTIONS

Hypotension produced by TCAs is a problem for the elderly because they are at increased risk for fainting or falling. TCAs have a narrow therapeutic index and can produce cardiotoxicity at doses that are 6 to 8 times higher than the therapeutic dose.

Tricyclic Antidepressants

Generic name	U.S. brand name(s) / Canadian brand(s)	Dosage forms and strengths
amitriptyline*	Generics / Levate	**Tablet:** 10 mg, 20 mg, 50 mg, 75 mg, 100 mg, 150 mg
desipramine*	Norpramin / Norpramin	**Tablet:** 10 mg, 25 mg, 50 mg, 75 mg, 100 mg, 150 mg
doxepin*	Prudoxin, Sinequan, Zonalon+ / Sinequan, Zonalon+	**Capsules:** 10 mg, 25 mg, 50 mg, 75 mg, 100 mg, 150 mg **Solution, oral concentrate:** 10 mg/ml **Cream:** 5% (Zonalon)
imipramine*	Tofranil, Tofranil-PM / Tofranil	**Capsule (Tofranil-PM):** 75 mg, 100 mg, 125 mg, 150 mg **Tablet (Tofranil):** 10 mg, 25 mg, 50 mg
nortriptyline*	Pamelor / Aventyl	**Capsule:** 10 mg, 25 mg, 50 mg, 75 mg **Solution:** 10 mg/5 ml
protriptyline	Vivactil / Not available	**Tablet:** 5 mg, 10 mg
trimipramine	Surmontil / Surmontil	**Capsules:** 25 mg, 50 mg, 100 mg

*Generic available
+Prudoxin and Zonalon are topical dosage forms used for the treatment of itching

SELECTIVE SEROTONIN REUPTAKE INHIBITORS

Selective serotonin reuptake inhibitors (SSRIs) are the most widely prescribed antidepressants. They are categorized by their mechanism of action rather than by their chemical structure. All are potent inhibitors of 5-HT and have little to no action on the reuptake of NE or DA.

MECHANISM OF ACTION

SSRIs work by producing selective blockade of the reuptake of 5-HT at the synaptic cleft. Serotonin reuptake requires a specific transporter to move 5-HT across cell membranes, allowing for the specificity of the SSRIs. When 5-HT reuptake is blocked, 5-HT (serotonin) remains in the synaptic cleft longer and a greater opportunity for receptor binding exists.

SSRIs are equally effective as TCAs yet they lack the cardiotoxic effects associated with TCAs. This makes them the drugs of choice when heart disease is present.

PHARMACOKINETICS

SSRIs are well absorbed from the gastrointestinal tract. They exhibit a high degree of protein binding. Fluoxetine, paroxetine, and sertraline are more than 94% protein bound. SSRIs are also extensively metabolized via the cytochrome P-450 (CYP450) isoenzyme system. Fluoxetine is metabolized to an active metabolite, which accounts for its long duration of action and relative increased length in time before reaching peak plasma levels. SSRIs interact with other drugs that are highly metabolized by CYP450 enzymes or exhibit extensive protein binding. These drug interactions may interfere with the rate of drug clearance of either the SSRI or drug that is administered with it.

ADVERSE REACTIONS

Insomnia is one of the more common side effects of SSRI administration. Fluoxetine and other SSRIs are dosed once daily in the morning to minimize nighttime sleeplessness. Other side effects include decreased appetite, nausea, agitation or anxiety, and diarrhea. Sexual dysfunction may occur as well. The most serious side effects are *serotonin syndrome* and *suicide ideation*. Both conditions are potentially fatal. Suicide ideation is persistent thoughts of suicide. Symptoms of serotonin syndrome are confusion, agitation, diarrhea, tremors, increased blood pressure, and seizures.

PRECAUTIONS

The effects of SSRIs are fairly well tolerated, but to avoid adverse reactions, increase dose gradually to desired levels and taper dose to discontinue the drug. Serotonin syndrome can result from coadministration with MAOIs. Use cautiously in patients with liver disease.

Comparison of Properties of Selective Serotonin Reuptake Inhibitors

Generic name	Sedative effects	Anti-cholinergic activity	Cardiac effects	T½ (hr)	Receptor blockade			Reuptake inhibition	
					α_1	α_2	D_2	NE	5-HT
citalopram	Low	Low	Negligible	24 to 48	+	+/−	+/−	+	++++
fluoxetine	Low	Low	Negligible	48 to 72	+	+/−	+/−	+	+++
fluvoxamine	Low	Low	None	13 to 15	+	+/−	+	+/−	+++
paroxetine	Low	Low	Negligible	21	+	+/−	+	+	++++
sertraline	Low	Low	Negligible	24	++	+	+	+/−	++++

Selective Serotonin Reuptake Inhibitors (SSRIs)

Generic name	U.S. brand name(s) / Canadian brand(s)	Dosage forms and strengths
citalopram*	Celexa	**Solution, oral:** 10 mg/5 ml (240 ml)
	Celexa	**Tablet:** 10 mg, 20 mg, 40 mg
escitalopram	Lexapro	**Solution, oral:** 1 mg/ml (240 ml)
	Not available	**Tablet:** 5 mg, 10 mg, 20 mg
fluoxetine*	Prozac, Prozac Weekly, Serafem	**Capsule (Prozac):** 10 mg, 20 mg, 40 mg; (Serafem) 10 mg, 40 mg
	Prozac	**Capsule, delayed release (Prozac Weekly):** 90 mg **Solution, oral (Prozac):** 20 mg/5 ml Tablet (Prozac): 10 mg, 20 mg
fluvoxamine*	Generic only	**Tablet:** 25 mg, 50 mg, 100 mg
	Luvox	
paroxetine*	Paxil, Paxil CR, Pexeva	**Suspension, oral:** 10 mg/5 ml (250 ml)
	Paxil, Paxil CR	**Tablet, as hydrochloride (Paxil):** 10 mg, 20 mg, 30 mg, 40 mg **Tablet, as mesylate (Pexeva):** 10 mg, 20 mg, 30 mg, 40 mg **Tablet, as controlled release (Paxil CR):** 12.5 mg, 25 mg, 37.5 mg
sertraline*	Zoloft	**Solution, oral concentrate:** 20 mg/ml
	Zoloft	**Tablet:** 25 mg, 50 mg, 100 mg

*Generic available.

TECH ALERT
The following drugs have look-alike/sound-alike issues:
Celexa and Zyprexa;
fluoxetine and fluvoxamine;
Luvox, Levoxyl, and Lovenox;
Paxil and Taxol;
Paxil and Plavix

MONOAMINE OXIDASE INHIBITORS

MECHANISM OF ACTION

MAOIs interfere with the degradation of monoamine neurotransmitters and dietary amines (e.g., tyramine). Their mechanism of action is to block the action of the enzyme MAO (Figure 6-5). This enzyme is found in the terminal neuron, liver, and intestines. When no MAO drugs are present, most of the NE, 5-HT, and DA that are released into the synaptic cleft is returned to the terminal neuron and inactivated by the enzyme MAO. When MAOIs are administered, this inactivation is blocked, which results in more NE, 5-HT, and DA being available to bind at receptor sites.

There are two forms of MAO: subtype A (MAO_A) and subtype B (MAO_B). Drugs that primarily interfere with the action of MAO_A are used in the treatment of major depression and preferentially interfere with the metabolism of NE and 5-HT. MAO_B is predominantly found in the brain. MAOIs that preferentially interfere with MAO_B are used in the treatment of Parkinson's disease because they interfere with the metabolism of DA.

PHARMACOKINETICS

MAOIs are readily absorbed when taken orally, but elimination is slow. The drugs are categorized as reversible or irreversible inhibitors of MAO according to the time it takes for enzyme levels to return to normal once the drug is discontinued. It takes approximately 3 to 5 days for MAO levels to return to normal on discontinuation of reversible MAOIs. Recovery takes up to 2 weeks when irreversible MAOIs are administered.

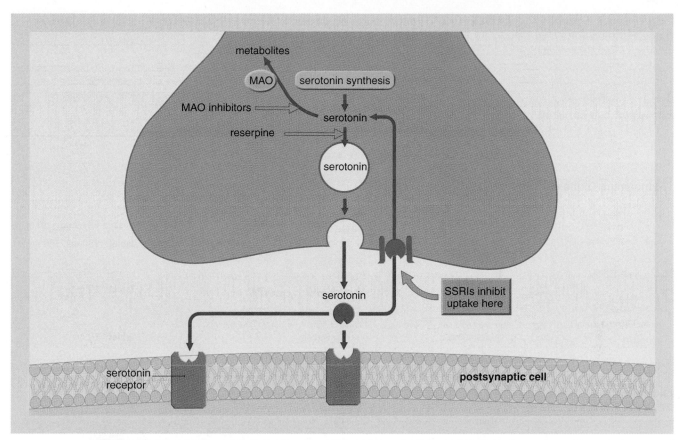

FIGURE 6-5 Mechanism of action of monoamine oxidase inhibitors (MAOIs). *(From Page C, et al.: Integrated pharmacology, ed 3, Philadelphia, 2006, Mosby.)*

TECH NOTE!
Symptoms of hypertensive crisis are throbbing headache, neck stiffness, and palpitations.

ADVERSE REACTIONS

MAOIs were first discovered in the 1950s, but the risk for serious side effects has limited their widespread use. Adverse reactions include sedation, dry mouth, urinary retention, constipation, orthostatic hypotension, impotence, and weight gain. The severity of these side effects is equal to or less than that of most TCAs. The most serious adverse reaction is hypertensive crisis.

Hypertensive crisis can be fatal and is caused by drug-drug and drug-food interactions with MAOIs. When MAOIs are not present, dietary amines (e.g., tyramine) are absorbed from the intestine and transported to the liver, where they are inactivated by the enzyme MAO in the liver. When MAOIs are administered, the effect of MAO in the liver is blocked and tyramine is able to reach the general circulation. Tyramine travels to peripheral sympathetic nerve terminals, where it promotes the release of NE stores. Excess circulating NE causes blood pressure to rise to dangerously high levels and produces excessive stimulation of the heart.

TECH NOTE!
Patients should be given a list of tyramine-containing foods to avoid and a list of drugs to avoid.

PRECAUTIONS

To avoid the risk of hypertensive crisis, patients on MAOIs are advised to avoid eating certain foods and beverages (Table 6-1).

SECOND- AND THIRD-GENERATION ANTIDEPRESSANTS

TCAs and MAOIs are effective antidepressants; however, alternatives were desired that had fewer side effects and less potentially dangerous adverse reactions. The second- and third-generation antidepressants are effective without risk for cardiotoxicity or hypertensive crisis. Serotonin-noradrenaline reuptake inhibitors (SNRIs), noradrenaline-dopamine reuptake inhibitors (NA/DRIs), and antidepressants that act on specific adrenergic or serotonergic receptors are all categorized as second- and third-generation agents.

TABLE 6-1   Foods and Beverages to Avoid While Taking Monoamine Oxidase Inhibitors (MAOIs)

Beverages	Chianti, and other red wines; alcohol-free beer, caffeine
Food	Cheeses (especially strong, aged, or processed varieties); sauerkraut; yogurt; raisins; bananas; sour cream; pickled herring; liver (especially chicken liver); dry sausage (including hard salami and pepperoni); canned figs; avocados; turkey; yeast extracts; fava beans; and broad bean pods; chocolate
Seasonings	Soy sauce; papaya products (including certain meat tenderizers)

Monoamine Oxidase Inhibitors (MAOIs)

Generic name	U.S. brand name(s) Canadian brand(s)	Dosage forms and strengths
moclobemide*†	Not available	**Tablet:** 150 mg, 300 mg
	Manerix	
phenelzine‡	Nardil	**Tablet:** 15 mg
	Nardil	
tranylcypromine*‡	Parnate	**Tablet:** 10 mg
	Parnate	

*Generic available.
†Reversible MAOI.
‡Irreversible MAOI.

TECH NOTE!
Remeron SolTab contains phenylalanine. Avoid if patient has phenylketonuria (PKU).

TECH NOTE!
Contents of Effexor-XR capsules can be sprinkled onto food.

TECH ALERT
The following drugs have look-alike/sound-alike issues: Wellbutrin, Wellbutrin SR, and Wellbutrin XL; bupropion and buspirone; Remeron, Zamuron, and Premarin; Effexor and Effexor XR

Bupropion was introduced in the 1970s as an alternative to TCAs that did not cause drowsiness. It is rapidly absorbed and has weak effects of DA and NE reuptake. Although it is well tolerated, doses of bupropion that are greater than 450 mg/day or 150 mg/dose increase the risk for seizures in people who are diagnosed with seizure disorders. Mirtazapine is a TCA that increases NE and 5-HT release. The drug exhibits a high degree of protein binding (85%) and moderate bioavailability (50%). Mirtazapine is metabolized by hepatic microsomal enzymes and is subject to drug interactions involving activation and inhibition of CYP450 isozymes. Adverse reactions of mirtazapine are sedation, dry mouth, urinary retention, blurred vision, increased appetite, weight gain, and agranulocyctosis. Trazodone is a weak inhibitor of 5-HT. When compared with TCAs, it produces moderate sedation and low anticholinergic activity. It does produce some cardiac stimulation. Side effects of trazodone are sedation, hypotension, nausea, and priapism (painful erection). Venlafaxine is an SNRI. It inhibits the reuptake of 5-HT more than NE, especially in the low therapeutic dosage range. Its side effects are similar to those of SSRIs but, unlike SSRIs, venlafaxine produces anticholinergic side effects, a modest increase in blood pressure, and hepatotoxicity. Common side effects of venlafaxine are sedation, nausea, headache, dry mouth, and dizziness.

Drugs Used to Treat Bipolar Disorder

Mood stabilizers are used in the treatment of bipolar disorder. All drugs currently indicated for the treatment of bipolar disorder have antimanic actions. Lithium is the oldest of these agents, introduced more than 50 years ago. Recently, selected medications used in the treatment of seizure, have been discovered to exhibit antimanic properties. Most of the drugs currently indicated for the treatment of bipolar disorder are listed in U.S. Food and Drug Administration pregnancy category D.

Lithium is administered to reduce current symptoms of mania and depression as well as to prevent recurrence of future episodes. Lithium is thought to produce its effects by regulating cAMP, phosphoinositide (PI), and calcium signal pathways. When signaling disturbances occur, lithium acts to restore order.

Serotonin-Noradrenaline Reuptake Inhibitors (SNRIs), and Noradrenaline-Dopamine Inhibitors (NA/DRI), and Other Antidepressants

	Generic name	U.S. brand name(s) / Canadian Brand (s)	Dosage forms and strengths
	bupropion*	Wellbutrin, Wellbutrin SR, Wellbutrin XL, Zyban† / Wellbutrin, Zyban	**Tablet, as immediate release (Wellbutrin):** 75 mg, 100 mg **Tablet, as extended release (Wellbutrin XL):** 150 mg, 300 mg **Tablet, as sustained release (Wellbutrin SR):** 100 mg, 150 mg, 200 mg
	mirtazapine*	Remeron, Remeron SolTab / Remeron	**Tablet:** 15 mg, 30 mg, 45 mg **Tablet, orally disintegrating (Remeron SolTab):** 15 mg, 30 mg, 45 mg
	trazodone*	Desyrel / Desyrel	**Tablet:** 50 mg, 100 mg, 150 mg, 300 mg
	venlafaxine*	Effexor, Effexor-XR / Effexor, Effexor-XR	**Capsule, as extended release (Effexor-XR):** 37.5 mg, 75 mg, 150 mg **Tablet (Effexor):** 25 mg, 37.5 mg, 50 mg, 75 mg, 100 mg

*Generic available.
†Zyban is indicated for smoking cessation.

Lithium is rapidly absorbed from the gastrointestinal tract, which accounts for its rapid onset of action. The drug has a long T½ (24 hours), which increases the longer the patient is on lithium therapy. The T½ can double over the course of 1 year's continuous therapy. Lithium is not metabolized and is eliminated unchanged in the urine. Lithium has a narrow therapeutic index. A competitive interaction may occur between lithium and sodium in the kidneys that may result in lithium toxicity. Increased sodium intake can decrease lithium reabsorption and dehydration and increase lithium reabsorption. Plasma lithium levels and renal function should be monitored regularly to avoid the development of lithium toxicity.

Early-onset effects associated with lithium carbonate are sedation, nausea, increased urination, dry mouth, difficulty concentrating, and tremor. Adverse reactions associated with long-term use include weight gain, acne, impotence, hypothyroidism, rash, and hair loss.

Valproic acid, carbamazepine, and lamotrigine are anticonvulsant drugs with demonstrated efficacy in the treatment of bipolar disorder. They are indicated as an adjunct to lithium therapy or when lithium administration has not produced desired results. Side effects of valproic acid and its salts, divalproex sodium and sodium valproate, include sedation, nausea, ataxia, and liver dysfunction. Side effects of carbamazepine include sedation, dizziness, ataxia, and visual disturbances. Lamotrigine is used in the treatment of bipolar disorder and seizures, and side effects include sedation, nausea, ataxia, blurred vision, double vision, and rash.

TECH ALERT
The following drugs have look-alike/sound-alike issues: Eskalith and Eskalith CR; Depakote and Depakene

Drugs Used in the Treatment of Bipolar Disorder

	Generic name	U.S. brand name(s) Canadian brand(s)	Dosage forms and strengths
	lithium*	Eskalith, Eskalith CR, Lithobid Carbolith, Duralith, Lithane	**Capsule (Eskalith):** 150 mg, 300 mg, 600 mg **Syrup:** 300 mg/5 ml **Tablet (immediate release):** 300 mg **Tablet, controlled release (Eskalith CR):** 450 mg **Tablet, slow release (Lithobid):** 300 mg
	divalproex sodium*	Depakote, Depakote ER, Depakote Sprinkle Epival ER	**Capsule, sprinkles (Depakote Sprinkle):** 125 mg **Tablet, delayed (Depakote):** 125 mg, 250 mg, 500 mg **Tablet, extended release (Depakote ER):** 250 mg, 500 mg
	carbamazepine*	Carbatrol, Equetro, Tegretol, Tergretol-XR Tegretol	**Capsule, extended release (Equetro):** 100 mg, 200 mg, 300 mg **Tablet, extended release (Tegretol-XR):** 100 mg, 200 mg, 400 mg
	lamotrigine	Lamictal Lamictal	**Tablet:** 25 mg, 100 mg, 150 mg, 200 mg **Tablet, as chewable:** 2 mg, 5 mg, 25 mg

*Generic available.

Summary of Drugs Used in the Treatment of Depression

	Generic name	U.S. brand name	Usual adult oral dose and dosing schedule	Warning labels
	Tricyclic Antidepressants (TCAs)			
	amitriptyline	Generic	50 mg to 150 mg as a single daily dose (oral); 20 mg to 30 mg four times a day (IM)	MAY CAUSE DROWSINESS; ALCOHOL MAY INTENSIFY THIS EFFECT
	desipramine	Norpramin	**Usual adult dosage:** 150 mg to 200 mg/day (Maximum dose: 300 mg/day in a single or divided doses)	MAY IMPAIR ABILITY TO DRIVE DO NOT DISCONTINUE WITHOUT MEDICAL SUPERVISION
	doxepin	Sinequan	Initiate with 25 mg to 150 mg per day and gradually increase to 300 mg/day	AVOID PROLONGED EXPOSURE TO SUNLIGHT
	imipramine	Tofranil	Start with 25 mg 3 to 4 times a day (Maximum dose: 300 mg per day)	MAY DISCOLOR URINE (BLUE-GREEN)—amitriptyline
	nortriptyline	Pamelor	25 mg 3 to 4 times per day up to 150 mg/day	
	protriptyline	Vivactil	15 mg to 60 mg daily in 3 to 4 divided doses	
	trimipramine	Surmontil	50 mg to 150 mg/day as a single bedtime dose	

Summary of Drugs Used in the Treatment of Depression—cont'd

Generic name	U.S. brand name	Usual adult oral dose and dosing schedule	Warning labels
Selective serotonin reuptake inhibitors (SSRIs)			
citalopram	Celexa	20 mg to 40 mg/day (maximum 60 mg/day)	MAY IMPAIR ABILITY TO DRIVE
escitalopram	Lexapro	20 mg/day	AVOID ALCOHOL MAY CAUSE DIZZINESS
fluoxetine	Prozac	20 mg to 40 mg/day or 90 mg/week (Prozac Weekly)	SWALLOW WHOLE; DON'T CRUSH OR CHEW (delayed release)
fluvoxamine	Generic	100 mg to 300 mg daily (divide into 2 doses with larger dose at bedtime)	DO NOT DISCONTINUE WITHOUT MEDICAL SUPERVISION
paroxetine	Paxil	20 mg/day (Paxil) Maximum dose: 50 mg/day 25 mg once daily (Paxil CR) Maximum dose: 62.5 mg/day	
sertraline	Zoloft	50 mg/day	
Monoamine oxidase inhibitors (MAOIs)			
moclobemide	Manerix (Canada)	300 mg to 600 mg/day divided into two doses per day.	TAKE WITH FOOD—moclobemide AVOID ALCOHOL
phenelzine	Nardil	15 mg to 90 mg three times a day	MAY CAUSE DIZZINESS OR DROWSINESS
tranylcypro-mine	Parnate	10 mg twice a day (maximum dose 60 mg/day)	DO NOT DISCONTINUE WITHOUT MEDICAL SUPERVISION
Serotonin-noradrenaline reuptake inhibitors (SNRIs), noradrenaline-dopamine reuptake inhibitors (NA/DRIs), and other antidepressants			
bupropion	Wellbutrin	Usual adult dosage for depression: 100 mg 2 to 3 times a day (immediate release); 150 mg twice a day (sustained release); 300 mg daily (extended release)	MAY CAUSE DIZZINESS OR DROWSINESS
mirtazapine	Remeron	15 mg to 45 mg/day (dosed at bedtime)	MAY IMPAIR ABILITY TO DRIVE AVOID ALCOHOL TAKE WITH FOOD—trazodone, venlafaxine
trazodone	Desyrel	150 mg 3 times a day (maximum dose 600 mg/day)	SWALLOW WHOLE; DON'T CRUSH OR CHEW (extended/sustained release)
venlafaxine	Effexor	75 mg to 375 mg 2 to 3 times a day (immediate-release) or 75 mg to 225 daily (extended release)	DO NOT DISCONTINUE WITHOUT MEDICAL SUPERVISION

Summary of Drugs Used in the Treatment of Bipolar Affective Disorder

	Generic name	U.S. brand name	Usual adult oral dose and dosing schedule	Warning labels
	lithium	Lithonate	900 mg to 2400 mg/day in 3 to 4 divided doses (immediate-release) or 900 mg to 1800 mg/day in 2 divided doses (sustained release)	MAY CAUSE DIZZINESS OR DROWSINESS; MAY IMPAIR ABILITY TO DRIVE AVOID ALCOHOL
	divalproex sodium	Depakote	750 mg to 1500 mg/day in divided doses	TAKE WITH FOOD DRINK LOTS OF FLUIDS-lithium SWALLOW WHOLE; DON'T CRUSH OR CHEW (controlled/slow release)
	carbamezepine	Tegretol	400 mg/day in 2 divided doses (maximum 1600 mg per day)	
	lamotrigine	Lamictal	100 mg to 200 mg/day	AVOID PREGNANCY DO NOT DISCONTINUE WITHOUT MEDICAL SUPERVISION

CHAPTER SUMMARY

- Depressive illness affects nearly 20 million American and 1.2 million Canadian men, women, and children each year.
- Depression affects self-esteem, moods, thoughts, eating, and sleeping; reduces the ability to think and concentrate; and produces feelings of worthlessness or guilt.
- Major depression is associated with persistent feelings of sadness, emptiness, or hopelessness.
- Bipolar disorder is associated with sudden swings in mood between depression and periods of mania.
- Dysthymia produces symptoms that are chronic and keep the person from functioning well.
- According to the biogenic amine theory, clinical depression results from a decrease in monoamine neurotransmitters in the brain.
- Bipolar affective disorder (mania) is believed to be associated with increased levels of monoamine neurotransmitters.
- Monoamine neurotransmitters associated with depression and bipolar disorder are norepinephrine (NE), serotonin (5-HT), and dopamine (DA).
- The mechanism of action for drugs used to treat depression may differ; however, all antidepressants are equally effective.
- Inhibition of the reuptake of specific monoamine neurotransmitters is one of the ways antidepressants produce their effects. The other mechanism of action is to block the degradation of monoamine neurotransmitters.
- Selection of one antidepressant over another is based on the patient's ability to tolerate drug side effects.
- Tricyclic antidepressants (TCAs) are the oldest class of medication used in the treatment of depression.
- TCAs are nonspecific reuptake inhibitors of monoamine neurotransmitters.
- Selective serotonin reuptake inhibitors (SSRIs) work by producing selective blockade of the reuptake of serotonin at the synaptic cleft.
- SSRIs are equally effective as TCAs yet lack the cardiotoxic effects associated with TCAs.
- Monoamine oxidase inhibitors (MAOI) interfere with the degradation of monoamine neurotransmitters and dietary amine (e.g., tyramine).
- Hypertensive crisis is a life-threatening adverse reaction caused by drug-drug and drug-food interactions with MAOIs.
- Lithium is administered to reduce current symptoms of mania and depression as well as to prevent recurrence of future episodes.
- Lithium has a narrow therapeutic index.

Anticonvulsants are used in the treatment of bipolar disorder

Multiple Choice

1. A mental health illness associated with persistent feelings of sadness, emptiness, or hopelessness that persists for several weeks is _____.
    a. bipolar disorder
    b. obsessive-compulsive disorder
    c. major depression
    d. schizophrenia

2. Antidepressants are categorized according to the method that they use to potentiate the actions of _____ neurotransmitters.
    a. norepinephrine
    b. serotonin
    c. dopamine
    d. a, b, and c

3. Tricyclics that are prescribed for enuresis, commonly known as bedwetting, are
    a. SSRIs
    b. TCAs
    c. MAOIs
    d. GABAs

4. The most widely prescribed class of antidepressants is
    a. TCAs
    b. SSRIs
    c. MAOIs
    d. PPIs

5. The brand name for citalopram is
    a. Celexa
    b. Celebrex
    c. Cerebryx
    d. none of the above

6. This SSRI is indicated for the treatment of major depression, binge-eating, obsessive-compulsive disorder, premenstrual dysphoric disorder, and panic disorder.
    a. Sertraline
    b. Lexapro
    c. Celexa
    d. Prozac

7. To avoid the risk of hypertensive crisis, patients on _____ are advised to avoid eating certain foods containing tyramine.
    a. SSRIs
    b. TCAs
    c. MAOIs
    d. A and b

8. Two examples of MAOIs are
    a. Nardil
    b. Parnate
    c. Tofranil
    d. A and b

9. Bupropion is indicated for the treatment of depression and smoking cessation.
    a. true
    b. false

10. **An example of a serotonin-noradrenaline reuptake inhibitor (SNRI) is**
   a. fluoxetine
   b. setraline
   c. venlafaxine
   d. nortriptyline

11. **Valproic acid, carbamazepine, and lamotrigine are _____ drugs with demonstrated efficacy in the treatment of bipolar disorder.**
   a. anticonvulsant
   b. antidepressant
   c. antimania
   d. antianxiety

12. **The oldest drug used to treat bipolar disorder is**
   a. Prozac
   b. Parnate
   c. lithium
   d. Lexapro

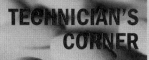

TECHNICIAN'S CORNER

1. For patients on MAOI antidepressants, what kinds of foods can they eat?
2. What is the difference between "feeling blue" and major depression?

BIBLIOGRAPHY

Kalant H, Grant D, Mitchell J: *Principles of medical pharmacology* (pp 316-333), ed 7. Toronto, 2007, Elsevier Canada, A Division of Reed Elsevier Canada.

Lance L, Lacy C, Armstrong L, Goldman M: *Drug information handbook for the allied health professional,* ed 12. Hudson, OH, 2005, APhA Lexi-Comp.

National Institute of Mental Health: *Depression.* Bethesda, MD, 2002, National Institute of Mental Health, National Institutes of Health, U.S. Department of Health and Human Services. NIH Publication No. 02-3561.

Page C, Curtis M, Sutter M, Walker M, Hoffman B: *Integrated pharmacology* (pp 239-241), Philadelphia, 2005, Elsevier Mosby.

Statistics Canada: *Mental health profiles.* Retrieved from http://www.statcan.ca/english/freepub/82-617-XIE/tables.htm. Updated 2004. Accessed November 1, 2007.

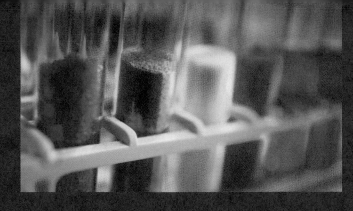

Treatment of Schizophrenia and Other Psychoses

- Describe the symptoms of schizophrenia.
- List and describe the function of neurotransmitters associated with symptoms of schizophrenia and other psychoses.
- Classify medications used to treat schizophrenia and other psychoses.
- Describe the mechanism of action for each class of drugs used to treat schizophrenia and other psychoses.
- Identify warning labels and precautionary messages associated with medications used to treat schizophrenia and other psychoses.
- Identify significant drug look-alike/sound-alike issues.

KEY TERMS

Catatonia: Symptom of schizophrenia associated with unresponsiveness and immobility.

Delusion: Irrational thoughts or false beliefs that dominate a person's behavior and viewpoint and do not change even when evidence is provided that beliefs are not valid.

Extrapyramidal symptoms: Excessive muscle movement (motor activity) associated with use of neuroleptics that includes muscular rigidity, tremor, bradykinesia (slow movement), and difficulty in walking.

Hallucination: Visions or voices that exist only in the mind and cannot be seen or heard by others.

Negative symptoms: Sign of schizophrenia that is associated with decreased ability to think, plan, or express emotion.

Neuroleptic: Drug used to treat schizophrenia or other psychosis.

Neuroleptic malignant syndrome: Potentially fatal reaction to administration of neuroleptics. Symptoms include stupor, muscle rigidity, and high temperature.

Positive symptoms: Hallucinations, delusions, or other unusual thoughts or perceptions that are symptoms of schizophrenia.

Postural hypotension: Drop in blood pressure due to a change in posture.

Pseudoparkinsonism: Adverse reaction to the administration of neuroleptics characterized by symptoms mimicking Parkinson's disease.

Psychosis: Mental state characterized by disorganized behavior and thought, delusions, hallucinations, and a loss of touch with reality.

Schizophrenia: Type of psychosis characterized by delusions of thought, visual and/or auditory hallucinations, and speech disturbances. Paranoid schizophrenia is characterized by delusions of persecution.

Tardive dyskinesia: Inappropriate postures of the neck, trunk, and limbs accompanied by involuntary thrusting of the tongue.

Overview

Schizophrenia is a chronic and major psychosis that is characterized by delusions of thought, visual and/or auditory hallucinations, and speech disturbances. Persons diagnosed with schizophrenia often see visions or hear voices that cannot be seen or heard by others. Paranoid schizophrenia is characterized by delusions of persecution. Paranoid schizophrenia is particularly challenging because the patient may believe that the health care team is prescribing medicines and therapies intended to cause him or her.

Schizophrenia affects about 1% of the population worldwide. The onset typically occurs in the late teens, after puberty begins, to the mid-20s; onset in men is slightly earlier than in women, who may not develop symptoms until the mid-20s to the early 30s. Onset of symptoms after age 45 is rare. Schizophrenia runs in families. The prevalence of schizophrenia in families where a sibling or relative has schizophrenia is about 10 times higher (10%) than in the general population. Other factors that may influence the likelihood of development of schizophrenia are environmental factors, exposure to viruses, fetal malnutrition, and substance abuse.

People diagnosed with schizophrenia often exhibit negative symptoms, positive symptoms, and cognitive symptoms. *Negative symptoms* are associated with a flat affect. This means that no visible sign of emotion is exhibited. Speech is monotonous and no facial expressions are apparent. People exhibiting negative symptoms do not interact socially with others and communicate infrequently. *Positive symptoms* may appear as bizarre behavior. People diagnosed with untreated schizophrenia have lost touch with reality. They may have delusions. *Delusions* are irrational thoughts or false beliefs that dominate the person's behavior. The person's viewpoint is unlikely to change even when evidence is provided that the beliefs are not valid. An example of a delusion is the belief that television characters are broadcasting personal messages to the person with schizophrenia. People with schizophrenia may also have visual or auditory *hallucinations*. They respond to visions and voices that only they can see. They may talk to themselves or, when speaking to others, may fail to complete sentences (their thoughts may be finished in their mind). Their thoughts are often disorganized. Cognitive symptoms associated with schizophrenia may interfere with the performance of routine activities of daily living. Memory loss may impede the person's ability to function on a job. *Cognitive symptoms* also decrease the person's capacity to interpret information and make decisions.

Schizophrenia also produces physical symptoms. The person may be clumsy and appear catatonic or make repetitive movements. People who exhibit symptoms of *catatonia* are unresponsive and immobile.

Neurochemistry of Schizophrenia and Other Psychoses

Schizophrenia is thought to be associated with excess dopamine levels. Drugs capable of blocking transmission of signals in the dopaminergic system, located in the midbrain and hypothalamus, are used in the treatment of schizophrenia. Mesocortical dopamine tracts project to various emotional areas of the brain, involved in cognition and regulation of motivation and emotion. The nigrostriatal pathway also originates in the midbrain and is involved in the control of excessive muscle movement. Treatments for schizophrenia that involve dopamine blockade can produce excessive motor movement as a side effect.

It is now known that other mechanisms of action may be involved in the treatment of schizophrenia. Other neurotransmitters that have been identified as playing a role in symptoms of schizophrenia include serotonin, cholecystokinin, neurotensin, γ-aminobutyric acid (GABA), and glutamate (Figure 7-1).

ROLE OF DOPAMINE

Of all the neurotransmitters involved in symptoms and treatment of schizophrenia, dopamine is most significant. All neuroleptic agents bind to dopamine receptors. Blockade of dopamine (D_2) receptors remains the primary mechanism of action for drugs used in the

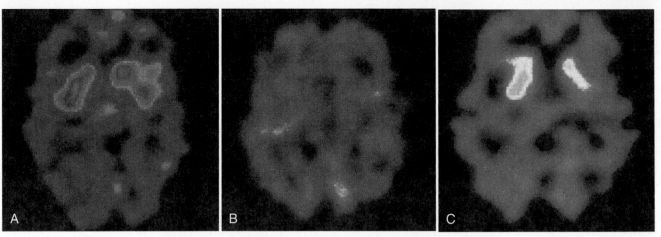

FIGURE 7-1 The cerebral distribution of dopamine receptors in treated and untreated schizophrenia. **A,** Striatal dopamine receptors in untreated schizophrenia **B,** Complete blockade of receptors with typical neuroleptic **C,** Partial blockade of receptors with equally effective dose of clozapine. *(Page C, et al.:* Integrated pharmacology, *ed 3. Philadelphia, 2006, Mosby.)*

treatment of schizophrenia. The greater the affinity the drug has for D_2 receptors, the more effective is the drug. Unfortunately, dopamine receptor blockade in the nigrostriatal tract produces Parkinson's disease-like symptoms (parkinsonism) and is associated with treatment with some classifications of neuroleptics. Some of the newer, atypical neuroleptics have a low affinity for D_2 receptors yet are clinically effective.

ROLE OF SEROTONIN

Serotonin (5-hydroxytryptamine [5-HT]) receptor blockade is a mechanism of action for some classifications of neuroleptics. Drugs that antagonize 5-HT_{2A} and 5-HT_{2C} receptors are useful in the treatment of negative symptoms of schizophrenia. Antagonism of 5-HT_{2A} receptors protects against long-term motor effects associated with some neuroleptic agents. Drugs that antagonize 5-HT_3 receptors are also used to treat schizophrenia.

ROLE OF CHOLECYSTOKININ

Cholecystokinin (CCK) is a peptide neurotransmitter. Peptide neurotransmitters are synthesized as part of larger protein molecules called preprohormones that are cleaved (cut) into smaller neuroactive peptides. Cholecytokinin coexists with the neurotransmitters dopamine and GABA and is involved in signaling mechanisms.

ROLE OF NEUROTENSIN

Neurotensin is a peptide neurotransmitter. It coexists with norepinephrine and dopamine. Neurotensin acts on the G protein receptors that are located in the area of the cortex associated with schizophrenia.

ROLE OF γ-AMINOBUTYRIC ACID

The role of GABA is not fully understood; however, abnormalities of the GABA system are believed to be associated with schizophrenia.

ROLE OF GLUTAMATE

Glutamate is an amino acid that acts as an excitatory neurotransmitter in the central nervous system. It is a principal neurotransmitter within the corticostriatal projections in the region of the brain associated with schizophrenia.

Drugs Used to Treat Schizophrenia and Psychosis

Neuroleptics are classified by structure and function. Structurally, these agents are classified as phenothiazines, thioxanthines, butyrophenones, diphenylbutylpiperidines, dibenzodiazepines, benzixasoles, benzothiazolylpiperazines, thienobenzodiazepines, dibenzothiazepines, and imidazolidinones. Functionally, all of these agents fall into two classes. The classes are based upon affinity for dopamine receptors. High-potency neuroleptics have a strong affinity for dopamine receptors. "Atypical" and low-potency neuroleptics have a weaker affinity for dopamine receptors and produce fewer side effects associated with blockade. Regardless of their potency, all of the neuroleptic agents are equally effective. Selection of agents is based on a balance between the achievement of the desired response and the patient's ability to tolerate drug side effects.

TRADITIONAL "TYPICAL" NEUROLEPTICS AND "ATYPICAL" NEUROLEPTICS

Phenothiazines, butyrophenones, and thioxanthines are categorized as "traditional" neuroleptics. They are classified as low, medium, and high potency. The prototype for low-potency neuroleptics is chlorpromazine; medium potency, fluphenazine; and high potency, haloperidol. All other neuroleptics are categorized as atypical. Clozapine and risperidone are prototypes for the atypical neuroleptics.

Phenothiazines may also be prescribed for the treatment of nausea and vomiting (chlorpromazine, perphenazine, promethazine) and of agitation, combativeness, or explosive behavior (thioridazine).

MECHANISM OF ACTION

Traditional neuroleptics block dopamine at postsynaptic receptor sites located in the basal ganglia, hypothalamus, limbic system, brainstem, and medulla. They have a strong α-adrenergic blocking action that accounts for the hypotension produced by traditional neuroleptics (Figure 7-2).

Atypical neuroleptics such as clozapine show strong affinity for serotonin receptors in addition to the dopaminergic receptor blockade.

PHARMACOKINETICS

Traditional neuroleptics are well absorbed orally, rectally, and parenterally. They readily cross the blood-brain barrier due to their lipid solubility and are up to 90% bound to plasma proteins. They are rapidly metabolized in the liver and produce active metabolites that are

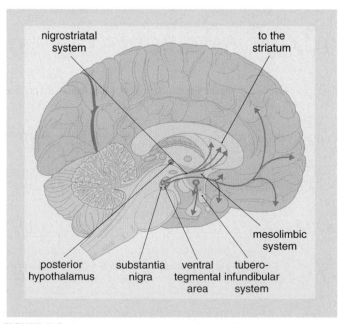

FIGURE 7-2 Dopamine pathways. *(From Page C, et al.:* Integrated pharmacology, *ed 3, Philadelphia, 2006, Mosby.)*

stored in fatty tissue (tissue binding). This reduces the bioavailability for oral routes of administration. Rectal and parenteral routes of administration have increased bioavailability. Neuroleptics are eliminated in the urine.

Several of the phenothiazines are available in slow release depot formulations for intramuscular injection. The therapeutic effects of fluphenazine deconoate and haloperiodol deconoate persist for up to 3 weeks after injection.

ADVERSE REACTIONS

Up to 80% of the people who are prescribed neuroleptics will experience adverse reactions (Table 7-1). Most adverse reactions are predictable and associated with dopaminergic, serotonergic, cholinergic, α-adrenergic, or histaminergic blockade (H$_1$). Adverse effects are classified as central effects and peripheral effects. Sedation (histamine blockade), confusion, decreased ability to regulate body temperature, weight gain, increased appetite, and increased release of some endocrine hormones are central effects. Increased release of prolactin can produce pseudopregnancy-type symptoms. Extrapyramidal effects and tardive dyskinesia are associated with dopaminergic blockade and occur more frequently in the elderly. *Extrapyramidal symptoms* are exhibited as excessive muscle movement. *Tardive dyskinesia* causes inappropriate postures of the neck, trunk, and limbs and is accompanied by involuntary thrusting of the tongue and lip smacking. There is no effective prevention or treatment for tardive dyskinesia.

Peripheral adverse effects include blurred vision, dry mouth and urinary retention (cholinergic blockade), postural hypotension (α-adrenergic blockade), hepatotoxicity and jaundice, bone marrow depression, photosensitivity, and failure to ejaculate.

PRECAUTIONS

Neuroleptic malignant syndrome (NMS) is a life-threatening side effect of neuroleptic administration. It produces symptoms of muscle rigidity, increased body temperature (hyperthermia), fluctuating consciousness, and renal failure. Clozapine use is restricted because it can produce a fatal drop in white blood cells (neutropenia). Patients on clozapine therapy are required to have white blood cell levels monitored weekly.

TECH ALERT!
The following drugs have look-alike/sound-alike issues: chlorpromazine, clomipramine, and chlorpropamide; fluphenazine, fluoxetine, and trifluoperazine; fluphenazine elixir and fluphenazine oral concentrate; Serentil, Seroquel, Serevent, and Serzone; thioridazine and thorazine

TECH ALERT!
Chlorpromazine oral concentrate and thioridiazine oral concentrate are incompatible in enteral formulas (tube feeding).

TABLE 7-1   Comparison of Side Effects of Neuropleptics

Generic name	Sedative effects	Anticholinergic activity	Hypotensive effects	Extrapyramidal effects	Neutropenia	Drug-induced jaundice
High Potency						
Fluphenazine	+	+	+	+++	–	++
Thiothixene	+	+	+	+++	–	–
Trifluoperazine	+	+	+	+++	–	++
Medium Potency						
Loxapine	+		+	++	–	
Molindone	+		+	++	–	
Perphenazine	+		+	++	–	++
Low Potency						
Chlorpromazine	+++	+++	+++	+	–	++
Mesoridazine	+++	+++	+++	+	–	++
Thioridazine	+++	+++	+++	+	–	++
"Atypical"						
Clozapine	+++	++	+++	+	+++	–
Risperidone	+	+	+	++	–	–
Olanzapine	+++	+	+++	+/–	–	–

Neuroleptic agents should be used cautiously in patients who have seizure disorders. Low-potency agents and clozapine are most likely to induce seizures. Atypical neuroleptics are associated with increased risk for diabetes and cardiovascular morbidity and mortality.

Typical Neuroleptics

Phenothiazines

Generic name	U.S. brand name(s) Canadian brand(s)	Dosage forms and strengths
chlorpromazine*	Generic only	**Injection, solution:** 25 mg/ml
	Largactil	**Tablet:** 10 mg, 25 mg, 50 mg, 100 mg, 200 mg
fluphenazine*	Prolixin Decanoate	**Elixir, as hydrochloride:** 2.5 mg/5 ml
	Modecate	**Injection, in oil as deconoate:** 25 mg/ml **Injection, hydrochloride solution:** 2.5 mg/ml **Solution, oral concentrate:** 5 mg/ml **Tablet:** 1 mg, 2.5 mg, 5 mg, 10 mg
mesoridazine*	Not available	**Tablet:** 25 mg
	Serentil	
perphenazine*	Generic only	**Tablet:** 2 mg, 4 mg, 8 mg, 16 mg
	Trilafon	
thioridazine*	Thioridazine Intensol	**Solution, oral concentrate (Thioridazine Intensol):** 30 mg/ml and 100 mg/ml
	Mellaril	**Tablet:** 10 mg, 15 mg, 25 mg, 50 mg, 100 mg, 150 mg, 200 mg
trifluoperazine*	Generic only	**Injection, solution:** 2 mg/ml
	Generic only	**Tablet:** 1 mg, 2 mg, 5 mg, 10 mg

*Generic available.

Butyrophenones

Generic name	U.S. brand name(s) Canadian brand(s)	Dosage forms and strengths
haloperidol*	Haldol, Haldol Deconoate	**Injection, oil, as deconoate:** 50 mg/ml; 100 mg/ml
	Generic only	**Injection, solution, as lactate:** 5 mg/ml **Solution, oral concentrate:** 2 mg/ml **Tablet:** 0.5 mg, 1 mg, 2 mg, 5 mg, 10 mg, 20 mg

*Generic available.

Thioxanthenes

Generic name	U.S. brand name(s) Canadian brand(s)	Dosage forms and strengths
thiothixene*	Navane	**Capsule:** 1 mg, 2 mg, 5 mg, 10 mg
	Navane	**Solution, oral concentrate:** 5 mg/ml

*Generic available.

Atypical Neuroleptics
Adverse reactions for clozapine are sedation, headache, dizziness, nausea, weight gain, hypotension, and tachycardia. Neutropenia occurs in 1% to 2% of patients.

Dibenzodiazepines

Generic name	U.S. brand name(s)	Dosage forms and strengths
	Canadian brand(s)	
clozapine*	Clozaril, Fazaclo	**Tablet (Clozaril):** 25 mg, 100 mg
	Clopsine, Leponex	**Tablet, oral disintegrating (Fazaclo):** 25 mg, 100 mg

*Generic available.

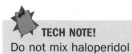

TECH NOTE!
Do not mix haloperidol oral concentrate with coffee or tea.

Thienobenzodiazepines

Thienobenzodiazepines are used in the treatment and management of schizophrenia and bipolar disorder. Adverse reactions are sedation, headache, dizziness, nausea, weight gain, hypotension, and tachycardia. Extrapyramidal symptoms occur rarely at high doses.

Thienobenzodiazepines

Generic name	U.S. brand name(s)	Dosage forms and strengths
	Canadian brand(s)	
olanzapine	Zyprexa, Zyprexa Zydis	**Injection, powder for reconstitution (Zyprexa Intramuscular):** 10 mg
	Zyprexa, Zyprexa Zydis	**Tablet:** 2.5 mg, 5 mg, 7.5 mg, 10 mg, 15 mg, 20 mg
		Tablet, oral disintegrating (Zyprexa Zydis): 5 mg

*Generic available.

TECH ALERT!
The following drugs have look-alike/sound-alike issues: Navane, Nubain, and Norvasc
These drugs may also increase vitamin B_2 requirements.

Benzixasoles

Risperidone is used in the treatment and management of schizophrenia and bipolar disorder. Side effects include sedation, dizziness, dry mouth, nausea, tremor, postural hypotension, urinary retention, sexual dysfunction, restlessness, and extrapyramidal symptoms (occurs rarely at high doses).

Benzixasoles

Generic name	U.S. brand name(s)	Dosage forms and strengths
	Canadian brand(s)	
risperidone*	Risperdal, Risperdal Consta, Risperdal M-tabs	**Injection (Risperdal Consta):** 25 mg, 37.5 mg, 50 mg (vials and prefilled syringes)
	Risperdal	**Solution, oral:** 1 mg/ml
		Tablet: 0.25 mg, 0.5 mg, 1 mg, 2 mg, 3 mg, 4 mg
		Tablet, oral disintegrating (Risperdal M-tabs): 0.5 mg, 1 mg, 2 mg

*Generic available.

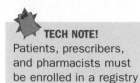

TECH NOTE!
Patients, prescribers, and pharmacists must be enrolled in a registry to dispense clozapine.

Dibenzothiazepines

Quetiapine is used in the treatment and management of schizophrenia and bipolar disorder. Side effects include sedation, headache, dizziness, hypotension, and impaired thermoregulation.

Dibenzothiazepines

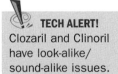

Generic name	U.S. brand name(s)	Dosage forms and strengths
	Canadian brand(s)	
quetiapine	Seroquel	**Tablet:** 25 mg, 100 mg, 200 mg, 300 mg
	Seroquel	

*Generic available.

Benzothiazolylpiperazines

Ziprasidone is used in the treatment and management of schizophrenia and bipolar disorder. Side effects include sedation, headache, weight gain, dizziness, hypotension, and impaired thermoregulation.

Benzothiazolylpiperazines

Generic name	U.S. brand name(s)	Dosage forms and strengths
	Canadian brand(s)	
ziprasidone	Geodon	**Injection, powder for reconstitution:** 20 mg
	Not available	**Tablet:** 20 mg, 40 mg, 60 mg, 80 mg

*Generic available.

TECH ALERT!
Clozaril and Clinoril have look-alike/ sound-alike issues.

Dibenzoxazepine

Loxapine is an atypical antipsychotic drug that is structurally similar to the antidepressant amoxapine. Adverse reactions include drowsiness, dizziness, photosensitivity, and hypotension.

Dibenzoxezepines

Generic name	U.S. brand name(s)	Dosage forms and strengths
	Canadian brand(s)	
loxapine*	Loxitane, Loxitane C	**Capsule:** 5 mg, 10 mg, 25 mg, 50 mg
	Generic	**Solution, oral concentrate (Loxitane C):** 25 mg/ml

*Generic available.

Summary of Drugs Used in the Treatment of Psychosis

Generic name	U.S. brand name	Usual adult oral dose and dosing schedule	Warning labels
Phenothiazines			
hlorpromazine	Generics	30 mg to 2000 mg/day in 1 to 4 divided doses (oral) or 300 mg to 800 mg/day IM or IV (maintenance dose)	MAY CAUSE DROWSINESS; MAY IMPAIR ABILITY TO DRIVE; AVOID ALCOHOL MAINTAIN ADEQUATE HYDRATION
fluphenazine	Prolixin	(Oral) 0.5 mg–10 mg/day dosed every 6 to 8 hours (maximum 10 mg/day) IM (as hydrochloride) 2.5 mg to 10 mg/day or IM (as deconoate) 12.5 mg every 3 weeks	AVOID PROLONGED EXPOSURE TO SUNLIGHT DO NOT DISCONTINUE WITHOUT MEDICAL SUPERVISION DILUTE ORAL CONCENTRATE BEFORE ADMINISTERING— chlorpromazine, fluphenazine
mesoridazine	Serentil (Canada)	25 mg to 50 mg 3 times a day (maximum 100 mg to 400 mg/day)	MAY DISCOLOR URINE (PINK-REDDISH BROWN)—thioridazine
perphenazine	Generics	4 to 16 mg 2 to 4 times a day (maximum 64 mg/day)	
thioridazine	Thioridazine Intensol	50 mg to 100 mg 3 times a day up to 800 mg/day divided in 2 to 4 doses	
trifluoperazine	generics	**Oral:** 1 to 2 mg twice daily (maximum 40 mg), **IM:** 1 to 2 mg every 4 to 6 hours (maximum 10 mg/24 hours)	
Butyrophenones			
haloperidol	Haldol	**Oral:** 0.5 mg to 5 mg 2 to 3 times/day (maximum 30 mg/day) **IM (lactate):** 2 mg to 5 mg every 4 to 8 hours **IM (deconoate):** 15 mg to 150 mg once every 4 weeks.	MAY CAUSE DROWSINESS; MAY IMPAIR ABILITY TO DRIVE; AVOID ALCOHOL DO NOT DISCONTINUE WITHOUT MEDICAL SUPERVISION DILUTE ORAL CONCENTRATE BEFORE ADMINISTRATION MAINTAIN ADEQUATE HYDRATION AVOID PROLONGED EXPOSURE TO SUNLIGHT
Thioxanthenes			
thiothixene	Navane	2 mg 3 times a day (maximum 60 mg/day)	MAY CAUSE DROWSINESS; MAY IMPAIR ABILITY TO DRIVE; AVOID ALCOHOL DO NOT DISCONTINUE WITHOUT MEDICAL SUPERVISION MAINTAIN ADEQUATE HYDRATION AVOID PROLONGED EXPOSURE TO SUNLIGHT

Continued

Summary of Drugs Used in the Treatment of Psychosis—cont'd

	Generic name	U.S. brand name	Usual adult oral dose and dosing schedule	Warning labels
Dibenzodiazepines				
	clozapine	Clozaril	Begin 12.5 mg 1 to 2 times a day; increase to 300 mg to 400 mg/day (maximum 600 mg to 900 mg/day)	MAY CAUSE DROWSINESS; MAY IMPAIR ABILITY TO DRIVE; AVOID ALCOHOL MAINTAIN ADEQUATE HYDRATION DO NOT DISCONTINUE WITHOUT MEDICAL SUPERVISION
Thienobenzodiazepines				
	olanzapine	Zyprexa	Start with 5 to 10 mg daily; increase to 10 to 30 mg daily (maximum 50 mg/day)	MAY CAUSE DROWSINESS; MAY IMPAIR ABILITY TO DRIVE; AVOID ALCOHOL MAINTAIN ADEQUATE HYDRATION DO NOT DISCONTINUE WITHOUT MEDICAL SUPERVISION
Benzixasoles				
	risperidone	Risperdal	3 mg to 6 mg/day (oral) or 25 mg every 2 weeks (IM)	MAY CAUSE DROWSINESS; MAY IMPAIR ABILITY TO DRIVE; AVOID ALCOHOL DILUTE SOLUTION BEFORE ADMINISTRATION MAINTAIN ADEQUATE HYDRATION DO NOT DISCONTINUE WITHOUT MEDICAL SUPERVISION
Dibenzothiazepines				
	quetiapine	Seroquel	Start with 25 mg twice a day; increase to 300 mg to 800 mg/day dosed 2 to 3 times a day.	MAY CAUSE DROWSINESS: MAY IMPAIR ABILITY TO DRIVE; AVOID ALCOHOL MAINTAIN ADEQUATE HYDRATION DO NOT DISCONTINUE WITHOUT MEDICAL SUPERVISION
Benzothiazolylpiperazines				
	ziprasidone	Geodon	**Oral:** 20 mg twice daily (maximum 100 mg twice daily) **IM:** 10 mg every 2 hours (maximum 40 mg/day)	MAY CAUSE DROWSINESS; MAY IMPAIR ABILITY TO DRIVE; AVOID ALCOHOL DO NOT DISCONTINUE WITHOUT MEDICAL SUPERVISION TAKE WITH FOOD AVOID GRAPEFRUIT JUICE MAINTAIN ADEQUATE HYDRATION
Dibenzoxezepines				
	loxapine	Loxitane	20 to 100 mg/day divided into 2 to 4 doses per day	MAY CAUSE DROWSINESS; MAY IMPAIR ABILITY TO DRIVE; AVOID ALCOHOL DO NOT DISCONTINUE WITHOUT MEDICAL SUPERVISION AVOID PROLONGED EXPOSURE TO SUNLIGHT MAINTAIN ADEQUATE HYDRATION

TECH ALERT!
Zyprexa, Celexa, and Zyrtec have look-alike/sound-alike issues.

TECH NOTE!
Zyprexa use in smoking cessation is unlabeled (not U.S. Food and Drug Administration approved).

TECH NOTE!
Oral solution should not be diluted with cola or tea.

TECH ALERT!
Seroquel and Serentil have look-alike/sound-alike issues.

TECH NOTE!
Dispense loxapine oral concentrate with the dropper provided with packaging.

CHAPTER SUMMARY

- Schizophrenia is a chronic and major psychosis characterized by delusions of thought, visual and/or auditory hallucinations, and speech disturbances.
- Schizophrenia affects about 1% of the population worldwide.
- The onset typically occurs in the late teens, after the puberty begins, to the mid-20s.
- Symptoms of schizophrenia in women may not develop until mid-twenties to early thirties.
- Schizophrenia is thought to be associated with excess dopamine levels.
- Drugs capable of blocking transmission of signals in the dopaminergic system, located in the midbrain and hypothalamus, are used in the treatment of schizophrenia.
- Other neurotransmitters that have been identified as playing a role in symptoms of schizophrenia include serotonin, cholecystokinin, neurotensin, GABA, and glutamate.
- The greater the affinity the drug has for D_2 receptors, the more effective is the drug.
- Dopamine receptor blockade in the nigrostriatal tract produces Parkinson's disease–like symptoms (pseudoparkinsonism) and is associated with treatment with some classifications of neuroleptics.
- Some of the newer, atypical neuroleptics have a low affinity for D_2 receptors yet are clinically effective.
- Neuroleptics are classified by structure and function.
- Structural classification includes phenothiazines, thioxanthines, butyrophenones, diphenylbutylpiperidines, dibenzodiazepines, benzixasoles, benzothiazolylpiperazines, thieno-benzodiazepines, dibenzothiazepine, and imidazolidinone.
- Functional classifications for neuroleptics are based on affinity for dopamine receptors. High-potency neuroleptics have a strong affinity for dopamine receptors. "Atypical" and low-potency neuroleptics have a weaker affinity for dopamine receptors and produce fewer side effects associated with blockade.
- The prototype for low-potency neuroleptics is chlorpromazine; medium potency, fluphenazine; and high potency, haloperidol.
- Clozapine and risperidone are prototypes for the atypical neuroleptics.
- Atypical neuroleptics such as clozapine show strong affinity for serotonin receptor in addition to dopaminergic receptor blockade.
- Traditional neuroleptics are well absorbed orally, rectally, and parenterally; readily cross the blood-brain barrier; are up to 90% bound to plasma proteins; are rapidly metabolized in the liver to active metabolites; and are stored in fatty tissue.
- Several of the phenothiazines are available in slow release depot formulations for intramuscular injection, and the therapeutic effects persist for up to 3 weeks after injection.
- Up to 80% of the people who are prescribed neuroleptics will experience adverse reactions.
- Extrapyramidal effects and tardive dyskinesia are associated with dopaminergic blockade and occur more frequently in the elderly.
- Neuroleptic malignant syndrome is a life-threatening side effect of neuroleptic administration.
- Clozapine use is restricted because it can produce a fatal drop in white blood cell levels (neutropenia).

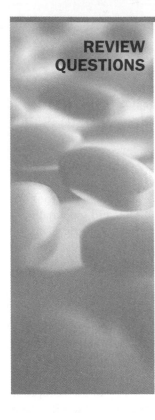

REVIEW QUESTIONS

Multiple Choice

1. A symptom of schizophrenia that is associated with unresponsiveness and immobility is termed
   a. dystonia
   b. ataxia
   c. catatonia
   d. neurolepnia

2. Schizophrenia runs in families.
   a. true
   b. false

3. Of all the neurotransmitters involved in symptoms and treatment of schizophrenia, _____ is most significant.
   a. norepinephrine
   b. dopamine
   c. serotonin
   d. epinephrine

4. Phenothiazines, butyrophenones, and thioxanthines are categorized as "_____" neuroleptics.
   a. traditional (typical)
   b. nontraditional (atypical)

5. What causes inappropriate postures of the neck, trunk, and limbs and accompanied by involuntary thrusting of the tongue and lip smacking?
   a. extrapyramidal symptoms
   b. tardive dyskinesia
   c. hyperkinesia
   d. catatonia

6. The use of _____ is restricted because it can produce a fatal drop in white blood cells (neutropenia). Patients on _____ therapy are required to have white blood cell levels monitored weekly.
   a. quetiapine
   b. clozapine
   c. olanzapine
   d. nifedipine

7. Which drug is used for the treatment of schizophrenia, tics, intractable hiccups, and Tourette's syndrome?
   a. haloperidol
   b. Mellaril
   c. Clozaril
   d. Seroquel

8. Hallucinations, delusions, or other unusual thoughts or perceptions are _____ symptoms of schizophrenia.
   a. positive
   b. negative

9. Selection of schizophrenia agents is based on a balance between achievement of desired response to the drug and the patient's ability to tolerate drug side effects.
   a. true
   b. false

10. Fluphenazine is available in which dosage forms?
    a. elixir, solution
    b. injection
    c. tablet
    d. a, b, and c

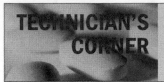

TECHNICIAN'S CORNER

1. The prevalence of schizophrenia in families where a sibling or relative has schizophrenia is about 10 times higher than in the general population. What kind of genetic implications does this statement have?
2. Can one live a "normal" life when diagnosed with schizophrenia?

BIBLIOGRAPHY

Kalant H, Grant D, Mitchell J: *Principles of medical pharmacology* (pp 303-315), ed 7. Toronto, 2007, Elsevier Canada, A Division of Reed Elsevier Canada.

Lance L, Lacy C, Armstrong L, Goldman M: *Drug information handbook for the allied health professional,* ed 12, Hudson, OH, 2005, APhA Lexi-Comp.

National Institute of Mental Health: *Schizophrenia,* Bethesda, MD, National Institute of Mental Health, National Institutes of Health, U.S. Department of Health and Human Services; Revised September 2005. Available at http://www.nimh.nih.gov/publicat/schizoph.cfm.

Page C, Curtis M, Sutter M, Walker M, Hoffman B: *Integrated pharmacology* (pp 242-247), Philadelphia, 2005, Elsevier Mosby.

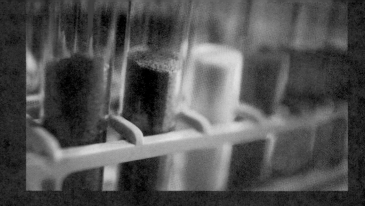

CHAPTER

8

Treatment of Parkinson's Disease and Huntington's Disease

LEARNING OBJECTIVES

- Compare and contrast the etiology of Parkinson's disease and Huntington's disease.
- Compare and contrast the function of neurotransmitters associated with symptoms of Parkinson's disease and Huntington's disease.
- Identify medications used to treat Parkinson's disease and Huntington's disease.
- Describe mechanism of action for each class of drugs used to treat Parkinson's disease and Huntington's disease.
- Identify warning labels and precautionary messages associated with medications used to treat Parkinson's disease and Huntington's disease.
- Identify significant drug look-alike/sound-alike issues.

KEY TERMS

Acetylcholinesterase: Enzyme that degrades the neurotransmitter acetylcholine.

Basal ganglia: Subcortical nuclei located in the forebrain and brainstem that initiate, control, and modulate movement and posture.

Bradykinesia: Slowness in initiating and carrying out voluntary movements.

Cognitive functions: The ability to take in information via the senses, process the details, commit the information to memory, and recall it when necessary.

Huntington's disease: Progressive and degenerative disease of neurons that affects muscle movement, cognitive functions, and emotions.

Neurodegerative disease: Disorder that results in progressive destruction of neurons.

Nigrostriatal pathways: Pathways located in the substantia nigra that stimulate and inhibit movement.

Parkinson's disease: Progressive disorder of the nervous system involving degeneration of dopaminergic neurons and causing impaired muscle movement.

Pseudoparkinsonism: Drug-induced condition that resembles Parkinson's disease.

Substantia nigra: Part of the basal ganglia containing clusters of dopamine-producing neurons.

PARKINSON'S DISEASE

Parkinson's disease is a progressive disorder of the nervous system involving degeneration of dopaminergic neurons in the basal ganglia and ***nigrostriatal pathways*** in the brain (Figure 8-1). The ***basal ganglia*** are composed of subcortical nuclei located in the forebrain (striatum and globus pallidus) and brainstem (substantia nigra and subthalamic nucleus). The basal ganglia are part of the extrapyramidal system that initiates, controls, and modulates movement and posture.

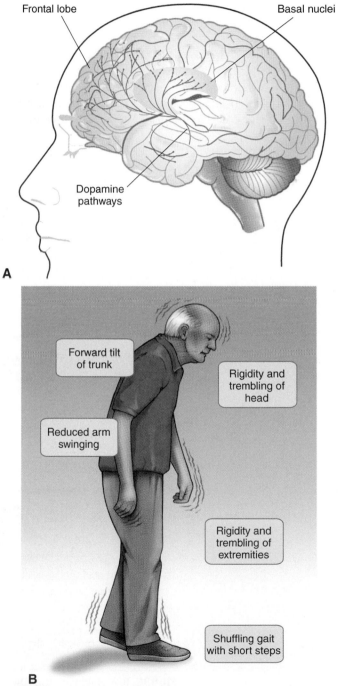

FIGURE 8-1 Dopaminergic pathways and signs of Parkinson's disease. *(From Thibodeau GA, Patton KT: Anatomy and physiology, ed 6, St Louis, 2007, Mosby.)*

Loss of dopaminergic neurons results in reduction of available dopamine. Symptoms of Parkinson's disease are a result of an imbalance between dopamine and acetylcholine (ACh) (Figure 8-2). As the loss of dopaminergic neurons progresses, voluntary muscle movement diminishes.

At least 1 to 1.2 million people in the United States have Parkinson's disease (2007). Approximately 50,000 new cases are reported annually. The disease disproportionately affects elderly men. The average age at onset of Parkinson's disease is 60 years. The prevalence and incidence (number of new cases) increase with age. Onset of Parkinson's disease in persons under 40 years old is rare and has been associated with ingestion of drugs contaminated with MPTP (1-methyl-4-phenyl-1,2,3,6-tetrahydropyridine), a byproduct of illicit synthesis of meperidine.

The etiology of Parkinson's disease is thought to be environmental; however, recent studies with twins have shown a familial inheritance of the chromosome 4 gene. Environmental causes are associated with pesticide exposure and exposure to drugs that destroy dopaminergic neurons in nigrostriatal pathways. Exposure to pesticides may increase the long-term risk for development of Parkinson's disease from 3% to 5%, according to a cohort study that reviewed surveys of 143,000 participants in the U.S. "Cancer Prevention Study II Nutrition Cohort" begun in 1982. The risks appear to be greater in men than in women. Other environmental toxins that may cause development of Parkinson's disease are carbon monoxide poisoning and heavy metal

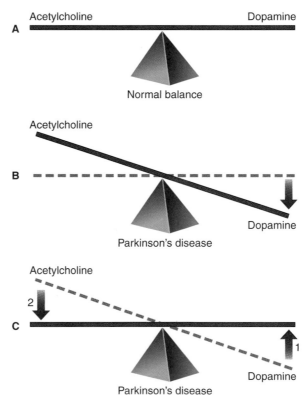

A. Normal balance of acetylcholine and dopamine in the CNS.
B. In Parkinson's disease, a decrease in dopamine results in an imbalance.
C. Drug therapy in Parkinson's disease is aimed at correcting the imbalance between acetylcholine and dopamine. This can be accomplished by either
  1. increasing the supply of dopamine or
  2. blocking or lowering acetylcholine levels.

FIGURE 8-2 Balance ACh/DA versus Parkinson's disease. *(From Lilley LL, Harrington S, Snyder JS:* Pharmacology and the nursing process, *ed 5, St Louis, 2007, Mosby.)*

poisoning (mercury). Infectious diseases such as viral encephalitis and syphilis as well as metabolic disorders such as Wilson's disease are also thought to cause Parkinson's disease.

Pseudoparkinsonism is a drug-induced condition that resembles Parkinson's disease. It is caused by administration of drugs that block dopaminergic receptors in nigrostriatal pathways located in the basal ganglia. Examples of drugs that produce pseudoparkinsonism are neuroleptics (e.g., phenothiazines), administered to treat schizophrenia, and reserpine, a drug that is used to treat hypertension.

Characteristic signs of Parkinson's disease are *bradykinesia*, slowness in initiating and carrying out voluntary movements, accompanied by muscle rigidity and tremors. When a person wishes to move forward her or his arm, the onset of movement will be delayed. Once the forward motion begins, movements will be slow, rigid, and shaking. Tremors are usually present at rest and may reduce the person's ability to perform skilled tasks. Postural and gait abnormalities are also typically present. The person walks with a characteristic shuffle. Other visible signs of Parkinson's disease are blank facial expression, drooling, and speech impairment.

Cognitive functions may be impaired as well as motor functions. Parkinson's disease can cause memory loss, and affected persons may exhibit signs of dementia. Parkinson's disease can cause depression, too.

Parkinson's disease is treated by the administration of pharmaceuticals, exercise, and nutritional support.

NEUROCHEMISTRY OF PARKINSON'S DISEASE

Symptoms of Parkinson's disease are associated with an imbalance between dopamine and ACh (Figure 8-3). The amount of dopamine available for release diminishes as the disease progresses and degeneration of dopaminergic neurons increases. This results in unopposed cholinergic excitation and produces the tremors, muscle rigidity, and immobility associated with Parkinson's disease.

ROLE OF DOPAMINE

Dopaminergic neurons in the substantia nigra are involved in motor coordination. Dopamine regulates direct and indirect extrapyramidal pathways in the substantia nigra that modulate input to the motor cortex. As Parkinson's disease progresses, degeneration of dopaminergic neurons in nigrostriatal pathways increases, thereby reducing dopamine levels and dopamine action on GABAergic neurons. Compensatory systems in the basal ganglia involving GABAergic neurons are stimulated.

ROLE OF γ-AMINOBUTYRIC ACID

Stimulation of GABAergic neurons by dopamine (D_1) sends signals that allow thalamic feedback to the motor cortex via the direct pathway that facilitate muscle movement. Stimulation of GABAergic neurons by dopamine (D_2) sends inhibitory feedback to the motor cortex via the indirect pathway. This results in impaired voluntary muscle movement.

ROLE OF GLUTAMATE

Large quantities of glutamate neurons are found in the cerebral cortex and exhibit excitatory control in the basal ganglia. Indirect and direct pathways are activated by glutamate neurons.

ROLE OF ACETYLCHOLINE

Cholinergic receptors are located at the neuromuscular junction, at parasympathetic synapses, and in the brain and spinal cord. There are two types of cholinergic receptors: nicotinic and muscarinic. Muscarinic receptors are found in the basal ganglia and substantia nigra. Nicotinic receptors are found in nigrostriatal dopaminergic pathways. Simulation of muscarinic and nicotinic receptors causes depolarization. Excessive stimulation of cholinergic neurons causes immobility and is what occurs in Parkinson's disease when the effects of ACh are unopposed. Acetylcholinesterase (AChE) is the enzyme that degrades ACh.

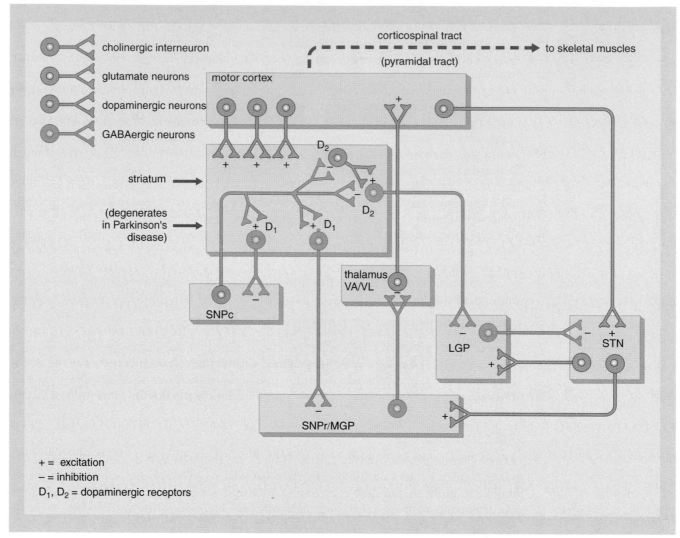

FIGURE 8-3 Summary of basal ganglia systems involved in Parkinson's disease. *(From Page C, et al.:* Integrated pharmacology, *ed 6, Philadelphia, 2006, Mosby.)*

DRUGS USED TO TREAT PARKINSON'S DISEASE

MECHANISM OF ACTION

The strategy for treatment of Parkinson's disease is to restore the balance between dopamine (inhibitory neurotransmitter) and ACh (excitatory neurotransmitter). This can be accomplished by administering drugs that are synthesized to dopamine, promote the release of existing stores of dopamine, directly stimulate dopamine receptors, or inhibit the degradation of dopamine in the terminal neuron. Anticholinergics may be administered to decrease ACh levels.

There is a decrease in the effectiveness of most anti-Parkinson drugs over time because of the disease's progressive neurodegeneration. The efficacy of levodopa and amantidine also declines with long-term therapy because of desensitization of dopamine receptors.

PHARMACOKINETICS

The absorption, distribution, metabolism, and elimination of drugs used to treat Parkinson's disease vary. Levodopa is a prodrug and is a dopamine precursor. It is administered rather than dopamine (which is available for use as a cardiac stimulant) because dopamine does

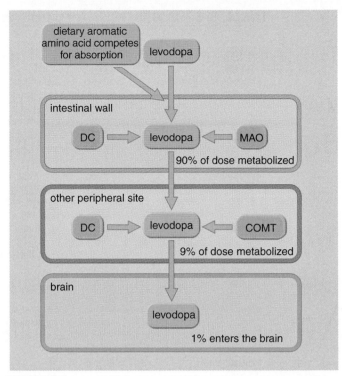

FIGURE 8-4 Disposition of orally administered levodopa. *(From Page C, et al.: Integrated pharmacology, ed 3, Philadelphia, 2006, Mosby.)*

not cross the blood-brain barrier. Although levodopa readily crosses the blood-brain barrier, much of the orally administered drug is metabolized in the gastrointestinal tract and in peripheral tissues (Figure 8-4). Only a small percentage actually reaches the neuron to be converted to dopamine. Sustained-release preparations of levodopa can further reduce the bioavailability of levodopa by as much as 30%.

Carbidopa is an adjuvant that boosts the effectiveness of levodopa. Carbidopa inhibits the metabolism of levodopa in the gastrointestinal tract and peripheral tissues. The bioavailability of levodopa is increased by 75% when combined with carbidopa. Catechol-*O*-methyltransferase (COMT) is the enzyme responsible for peripheral and central metabolism of catecholamines, and metabolizes levodopa. Tolcapone is a COMT inhibitor that boosts the bioavailability of levodopa by up to 50%.

A comparison of agents according to their mechanism of action is given in Table 8-1.

ADVERSE REACTIONS

Some side effects are common to all of the drugs used in the treatment of Parkinson's disease. Most agents produce central nervous system effects that include dizziness or lightheadedness, insomnia, and confusion. Antiparkinson drugs can produce auditory and visual hallucinations. People over the age of 65 years are most susceptible.

Gastrointestinal distress is a common side effect of most of the drugs used to treat Parkinson's disease; effects include nausea, vomiting, and decreased appetite. Hypotension and tachycardia are adverse reactions associated with most of the drugs used to treat Parkinson's disease.

Drugs that are administered to reduce ACh activity produce anticholinergic effects such as dry mouth, blurred vision, constipation, and urinary retention.

PRECAUTIONS

Selegiline and rasagiline are monoamine oxidase type B inhibitors (MAOI$_B$) and have the risk for hypertensive crisis (Figure 8-5).

TECH ALERT!
The following drugs have look-alike/sound-alike issues: amantadine, rimantidine, and ranitidine; Sinemet and Sinemet CR; Permax and Bumex; Mirapex and Miralax; pramipexole and pramoxine; selegiline and sertraline; Eldepryl, Elavil, and enalapril

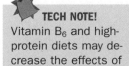

TECH NOTE!
Vitamin B$_6$ and high-protein diets may decrease the effects of Sinemet.

TABLE 8-1   Comparison of Antiparkinson Drugs

Drug	Mechanism of action	Time to peak concentration (hr)	Half-life (T½) (hr)
levodopa	Dopamine precursor	0.5 to 2	1 to 3
levodopa and carbidopa	Synthesis of dopamine inside the brain and blocking conversion outside the brain	1 to 2	
levodopa, carbidopa, and entacapone	Synthesis of dopamine inside the brain plus catechol-O-methyltransferase (COMT) inhibition	Unavailable	2.4
tolcapone	COMT inhibitor	2	2 to 3
amantadine	Stimulates release of dopamine from neuronal stores and decreases presynaptic reuptake; may have some anticholinergic activity	4 to 8	9.5 to 14.5
bromocriptine	Direct stimulation of dopamine receptors	1 to 3	48
pergolide	Direct stimulation of dopamine receptors	2	8
pramipexole	Dopamine agonist	1 to 2	8 to 12
ropinirole	Dopamine agonist	1 to 2	6
selegiline	Blocks degradation of dopamine by inhibition of monoamine oxidase type B ($MAOI_B$)	0.5 to 2	20
benztropine	Anticholinergic	Unknown	Unknown
trihexyphenidyl	Anticholinergic	1	5 to 10

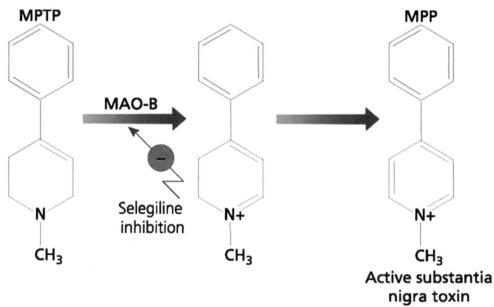

FIGURE 8-5 Selegiline inhibition. *(From Lilley LL, Harrington S, Snyder JS: Pharmacology and the nursing process, ed 4, St Louis, 2005, Mosby.)*

Drugs That Enhance Dopaminergic Activity

Generic name	U.S. brand name(s) / Canadian brand(s)	Dosage forms and strengths
amantadine*	Symmetrel	**Capsule:** 100 mg
	Symmetrel	**Syrup:** 50 mg/5 ml **Tablet:** 100 mg
bromocriptine*	Parlodel	**Capsule:** 5 mg
	Parlodel	**Tablet:** 2.5 mg
levodopa and carbidopa*	Parcopa, Sinemet, Sinemet CR	**Tablet, immediate release (Sinemet):** 10 mg/100 mg, 25 mg/100 mg, 25 mg/250 mg carbidopa/levodopa
	Sinemet, Sinemet CR	**Tablet, immediate oral disintegrating (Parcopa):** 10 mg carbidopa/100 mg levodopa
levodopa, carbidopa and entacapone	Stalevo	**Tablet:** carbidopa 12.5 mg, levodopa 50 mg, and entacapone 200 mg carbidopa 25 mg, levodopa 100 mg, and entacapone 200 mg
	Not available	carbidopa 37.5 mg, levodopa 150 mg, and entacapone 200 mg
pergolide*	Permax	**Tablet:** 0.05 mg, 0.25 mg, 1 mg
	Permax	
pramipexole	Mirapex	**Tablet:** 0.125 mg, 0.25 mg, 0.5 mg, 1 mg, 1.5 mg
	Mirapex	
ropinerole	ReQuip	**Tablet:** 0.25 mg, 0.5 mg, 1 mg, 2 mg, 3 mg, 4 mg, 5 mg
	ReQuip	
selegiline* (L-deprenyl)	Eldepryl	**Capsule (Eldepryl):** 5 mg **Tablet:** 5 mg
	Eldepryl	
tolcapone	Tasmar	**Tablet:** 100 mg, 200 mg
	Not available	

*Generic available.

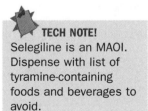

TECH NOTE!
Selegiline is an MAOI.
Dispense with list of
tyramine-containing
foods and beverages to
avoid.

Drugs That Reduce Cholinergic Activity

Anticholinergics are administered as adjunctive treatment of Parkinson's disease and to lessen drug-induced extrapyramidal symptoms. Side effects are dizziness, sedation, confusion, dry mouth, blurred vision, constipation, urinary retention, heat intolerance, hypotension, and hallucinations.

Drugs That Reduce Cholinergic Activity

Generic name	U.S. brand name(s) / Canadian brand(s)	Dosage forms and strengths
benztropine*	Cogentin	**Injection:** 1 mg/ml
	Cogentin	**Tablet:** 0.5 mg, 1 mg, 2 mg
trihexyphenidyl*	Generic only	**Elixir:** 2 mg/5 ml
	Generic only	**Tablet:** 2 mg, 5 mg

*Generic available.

Summary of Drugs Used in the Treatment of Parkinson's Disease

	Generic name	U.S. brand name	Usual adult oral dose and dosing schedule	Warning labels
Drugs that affect dopamine levels				
	amantadine	Symmetrel	100 mg twice a day up to 300 mg to 400 mg/day	MAY CAUSE DIZZINESS; MAY IMPAIR ABILITY TO DRIVE; LIMIT ALCOHOL
	bromocriptine	Parlodel	Start 1.25 mg twice/day; increase to 30 mg to 90 mg/day in 3 divided doses	
	levodopa and carbidopa	Sinemet	**Immediate release:** carbidopa 25 mg/levodopa 100 mg 3 to 4 times a day (maximum carbidopa 200 mg/levodopa 2000 mg) **Sustained release:** carbidopa 50 mg/levodopa 200 mg 2 times a day (maximum carbidopa 400 mg/ levodopa 1600 mg)	DO NOT DISCONTINUE WITHOUT MEDICAL SUPERVISION AVOID VITAMINS AND IRON SUPPLEMENTS WITHIN 2 HOURS OF DOSE— levodopa/carbidopa
	levodopa, carbidopa and entacapone	Stalevo	Individualized (maximum 1600 mg/day)	SWALLOW WHOLE; DON'T CRUSH OR CHEW (sustained release)
	pergolide	Permax	2 mg to 3 mg/day in 3 divided doses.	TAKE WITH FOOD— bromocriptine, pergolide
	pramipexole	Mirapex	Start 0.375 mg/day in 3 divided doses; increase to 1.5 mg to 4.5 mg/day	MAY DISCOLOR URINE— Stavelo, tolcapone
	ropinerole	ReQuip	Start 0.25 mg 3 times/day; increase weekly to a maximum 24 mg/day	
	selegiline	Eldepryl	5 mg twice a day or 10 mg once daily	
	tolcapone	Tasmar	100 mg to 200 mg 3 times a day	
Anticholinergics				
	benztropine	Cogentin	0.5 mg to 6 mg/day in 1 to 2 divided doses	MAY CAUSE DROWSINESS; MAY IMPAIR ABILITY TO DRIVE
	trihexyphenidyl	generic	5 mg to 15 mg/day in 3 to 4 divided doses	AVOID ALCOHOL MAINTAIN ADEQUATE HYDRATION DO NOT DISCONTINUE WITHOUT MEDICAL SUPERVISION

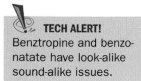

TECH ALERT!
Benztropine and benzonatate have look-alike sound-alike issues.

HUNTINGTON'S DISEASE

Huntington's disease is a progressive and degenerative disease of neurons that affects muscle movement, cognitive functions, and emotions. Huntington's disease is similar to Parkinson's disease in that it is associated with defects in the basal ganglia. Unlike Parkinson's disease, it produces excessive, abnormal muscle movement rather than immobility.

Huntington's disease is a hereditary disorder. It affects approximately 1 person in every 10,000. Children born to a parent who has Huntington's disease have a 50:50 chance of inheriting the gene for the disease. If the gene is inherited, the child will develop Huntington's disease at some point in his or her lifetime.

Characteristic symptoms of Huntington's disease are tremors, rhythmic oscillations or circular movements around the ankles or wrists, and sudden abnormal movements. Movements are typically repetitive. The person may have speech impairment and difficulty swallowing and may exhibit facial grimaces. Choreiform movements are associated with Huntington's disease. *Choreiform movements* are unpredictable, irregular, and jerking.

Huntington's disease also causes emotional and intellectual changes. The person has difficulty concentrating, which worsens as the disease progresses. Irritability, mood swings, and depression are other symptoms of the disease. Cognitive impairment may appear as fixation on an idea, slowed thinking and responses, memory problems, and difficulty sequencing activities.

NEUROCHEMISTRY OF HUNTINGTON'S DISEASE

Huntington's disease causes defects in the basal ganglia that result in increased concentrations of dopamine coupled with a decrease in the activity of the enzymes glutamic acid decarboxylase and choline acetyltransferase. *Glutamic acid decarboxylase* is the enzyme that synthesizes GABA. *Choline acetyltransferase* is involved in the production of ACh. Deficient levels of ACh and GABA lead to hyperactivity of dopaminergic neurons in nigrostriatal pathways. The balance between GABA, ACh, and dopamine is upset, and this produces the excessive muscle movement associated with Huntington's disease.

DRUGS USED TO TREAT HUNTINGTON'S DISEASE

MECHANISM OF ACTION

Huntington's disease is primarily treated with drugs that decrease excessive dopaminergic activity. This is accomplished by depleting stores of dopamine in the neuron (e.g., tetrabenazine). This means less dopamine is released when the neuron is stimulated. The other mechanism of action for drugs used to treat Huntington's disease is blockade of dopamine receptors (e.g., butyrophenones).

Drugs That Deplete Stores of Dopamine in the Neuron

Drugs that deplete stores of dopamine are used for the treatment of Huntington's disease, Gilles de la Tourette syndrome, and tardive dyskinesia. Side effects of tetrabenazine are hypotension, sedation, dizziness, and depression.

Drugs That Deplete Stores of Dopamine

Generic name	U.S. brand name(s) Canadian brand(s)	Dosage forms and strengths
tetrabenazine	Not available	**Tablet:** 25 mg
	Nitoman	

Drugs That Block Dopamine Receptors

Haloperidol is indicated for the treatment of Huntington's disease, Tourette's syndrome, and schizophrenia (see Chapter 7). Other neuroleptics have been administered to control choreiform movements but are not U.S. Food and Drug Administration approved for this purpose, including pimozide and fluphenazine. Side effects include sedation, confusion, weight gain, increased appetite, blurred vision, dry mouth, urinary retention, postural hypotension, extrapyramidal symptoms, tardive dyskinesia, photosensitivity, and sexual dysfunction.

Drugs That Block Dopamine Receptors

Generic name	U.S. brand name(s) Canadian brand(s)	Dosage forms and strengths
haloperidol*	Haldol Haldol Deconoate	**Injection, oil, as deconoate:** 50 mg/ml; 100 mg/ml **Injection, solution, as lactate:** 5 mg/ml
	generics	**Solution, oral concentrate:** 2 mg/ml **Tablet:** 0.5 mg, 1 mg, 2 mg, 5 mg, 10 mg, 20 mg

*Generic available.

Summary of Drugs Used in the Treatment of Huntington's Disease

Generic name	U.S. brand name	Usual adult oral dose and dosing schedule	Warning labels
Drugs that affect dopamine levels			
tetrabenazine*	Nitoman (Canada)	25 mg 3 times/day (maximum 200 mg/day)	MAY CAUSE DROWSINESS; MAY IMPAIR ABILITY TO DRIVE; LIMIT ALCOHOL
haloperidol	Haldol	**Oral:** 0.5 mg to 5 mg 2 to 3 times/day (maximum 30 mg/day) **IM, as lactate:** 2 mg to 5 mg every 4 to 8 hours **IM, as deconoate:** 15 mg to 150 mg once every 4 weeks	DO NOT DISCONTINUE WITH MEDICAL SUPERVISION DILUTE ORAL CONCENTRATE BEFORE ADMINISTRATION—haloperidol MAINTAIN ADEQUATE HYDRATION—haloperidol AVOID PROLONGED EXPOSURE TO SUNLIGHT—haloperidol

CHAPTER SUMMARY

- Parkinson's disease is a progressive disorder of the nervous system involving degeneration of dopaminergic neurons in the basal ganglia of the brain.
- The basal ganglia are part of the extrapyramidal system that initiates, controls, and modulates movement and posture.
- Symptoms of Parkinson's disease are a result of an imbalance between dopamine and acetylcholine.
- The average age at onset of Parkinson's disease is 60 years. Men are more often affected than women.
- Environmental exposures to pesticides, carbon monoxide poisoning, and heavy metal poisoning (mercury) can increase risk for Parkinson's disease.
- Infectious diseases, such as viral encephalitis and syphilis, and metabolic disorders, such as Wilson's disease, are also thought to cause Parkinson's disease.
- Neuroleptic drugs can cause pseudoparkinsonism, a drug-induced condition that resembles Parkinson's disease.
- Physical signs of Parkinson's disease are bradykinesia, muscle rigidity, tremors, postural and gait abnormalities, and walking with a characteristic shuffle. Other visible signs of Parkinson's disease are blank facial expression, drooling, and speech impairment.
- Parkinson's disease can cause memory loss, dementia, and depression.
- Symptoms of Parkinson's disease are associated with an imbalance between dopamine and acetylcholine.
- Levodopa is a prodrug and is a dopamine precursor.
- Carbidopa is an adjuvant that is added to levodopa to inhibit the metabolism of levodopa in the gastrointestinal tract and peripheral tissues.
- The bioavialability of levodopa is increased up to 50%, and the elimination half-life is doubled when tolcapone is added to therapy.
- Tolcapone inhibits catechol-O-methyltransferase (COMT), the enzyme responsible for metabolizing levodopa.
- Bioavailability is decreased by as much as 30% when sustained-release preparations are administered.
- People over the age of 65 years are most susceptible to dizziness, lightheadedness, insomnia, and confusion, and hallucinations are side effects of anti-Parkinson's drugs.
- Gastrointestinal distress is a common side effect of most of the drugs used to treat Parkinson's disease.

- Anticholinergic drug effects are dry mouth, blurred vision, constipation, and urinary retention.
- The efficacy of levodopa and amantidine also declines with long-term therapy because of desensitization of dopamine receptors.
- Selegiline and rasagiline are monoamine oxidase type B inhibitors ($MAOI_B$) and have the risk for hypertensive crisis.
- Huntington's disease is a progressive and degenerative disease of neurons that affects muscle movement, cognitive functions, and emotions.
- Huntington's disease is similar to Parkinson's disease in that it is associated with defects in the basal ganglia.
- Huntington's disease is a hereditary disorder.
- Characteristic symptoms of Huntington's disease are tremors, rhythmic oscillations or circular movements around ankles or wrists, and sudden abnormal movements.
- Choreiform movements are unpredictable, irregular, and jerking.
- Cognitive impairment may appear as fixation on an idea, slowed thinking and responses, memory problems, along with difficulty sequencing activities.
- The balance between GABA, acetylcholine, and dopamine is upset, which produces the excessive muscle movement associated with Huntington's disease.
- Huntington's disease is primarily treated with drugs that decrease excessive dopaminergic activity.

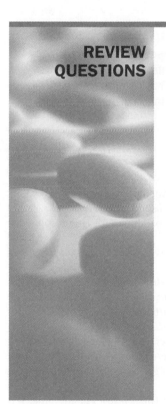

REVIEW QUESTIONS

Multiple Choice

1. **Parkinson's disease is a progressive disorder of the nervous system involving degeneration of dopaminergic neurons in the basal ganglia and nigrostriatal pathways in the brain.**
   1. true
   2. false

2. **Approximately 5000 new cases of Parkinson's disease are reported annually.**
   a. true
   b. false

3. **Characteristic signs of Parkinson's disease are _____ and slowness in initiating and carrying out voluntary movements, accompanied by muscle rigidity and tremors.**
   a. hyperkinesia
   b. tardive dyskinesia
   c. bradykinesia
   d. neurokinesia

4. **Symptoms of Parkinson's disease are associated with an imbalance between _____ and _____.**
   a. epinephrine, dopamine
   b. dopamine, serotonin
   c. acetylcholine, norepinephrine
   d. dopamine, acetylcholine

5. **_____ is a prodrug and is a dopamine precursor.**
   a. Levodopa
   b. Carbidopa
   c. Cogentin
   d. ReQuip

6. **The bioavailability of levodopa is increased by _____% when combined with carbidopa.**
   a. 25
   b. 50
   c. 75
   d. 95

7. _____ is a common side effect of most of the drugs used to treat Parkinson's disease.
   a. Headache
   b. Gastrointestinal distress
   c. Muscle spasms
   d. Flu-like symptoms

8. Huntington's disease is similar to Parkinson's disease in that it is associated with defects in the brainstem.
   a. true
   b. false

9. Huntington's disease is treated with drugs that _____ excessive dopaminergic activity.
   a. increase
   b. decrease

10. This drug is indicated in the treatment of Huntington's disease, Gilles de la Tourette syndrome, and tardive dyskinesia.
   a. tetrabenazine
   b. benztropine
   c. fexofenadine
   d. a, b, and c

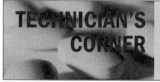

TECHNICIAN'S CORNER

1. What is the location of the basal ganglia? How can one disease be caused by excessive dopamine and another disease be caused by a deficiency of dopamine?
2. The average age at onset of Parkinson's disease is 60 years. Have there been any cases of patients younger than 60 years contracting Parkinson's disease?

BIBLIOGRAPHY

Ascherio A, et al.: Pesticide exposure and risk for Parkinson's disease, Annals of Neurology, Wiley-Liss, Inc., A Wiley Company, 2006: article online in advance of print, published 26 Jun 2006.

Bourne C, et al.: Cognitive impairment and behavioural difficulties in patients with Huntinton's disease, Nursing Standard, May 2006, vol. 20, pp 41-44.

Lance L, Lacy C, Armstrong L, Goldman M: Drug information handbook for the allied health professional, ed 12, Hudson, OH, 2005, APhA Lexi-Comp.

National Institute of Neurological Disorders and Stroke: Huntington's disease, Bethesda, MD, NINDS, National Institutes of Health, U.S. Department of Health and Human Services. Updated January 2006. Retrieved at http://www.ninds.nih.gov/disorders/huntington/huntington.htm.

National Institute of Neurological Disorders and Stroke: Parkinson's disease, Bethesda, MD, NINDS, National Institutes of Health, U.S. Department of Health and Human Services. Updated October 2004. Retrieved at http://www.ninds.nih.gov/disorders/parkinsons_disease/parkinsons_disease.htm.

Page C, Curtis M, Sutter M, Walker M, Hoffman B: Integrated pharmacology (pp 242-247), Philadelphia, 2005, Elsevier Mosby.

Raffa RB, Rawls SM, Beyzarov EP: Netter's illustrated pharmacology (pp 77-78), Philadelphia, WB Saunders, 2005.

U.S. Food and Drug Administration, U.S. Department of Health and Human Services, FDA News: FDA approves new treatment for Parkinson's disease, Press releases P06-68, May 17, 2006. Retrieved at http://www.fda.gov/bbs/topics/NEWS/2006/NEW01373.html.

USP Center for Advancement of Patient Safety: Use caution: avoid confusion. USP Quality Review No. 79, Rockville, MD, April 2004, USP Center for Advancement of Patient Safety.

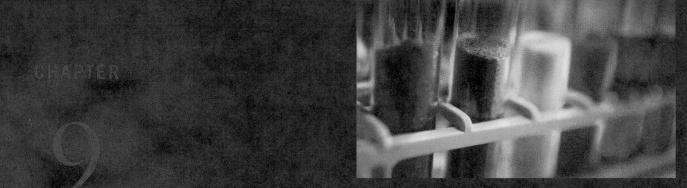

CHAPTER

9

Treatment of Seizure Disorders

LEARNING OBJECTIVES

- Describe the etiology of seizure disorders.
- Compare and contrast the function of neurotransmitters associated with symptoms of seizure disorders.
- Classify medications used in the treatment of seizure disorders.
- Describe mechanism of action for each class of drugs used to treat seizure disorders.
- Identify warning labels and precautionary messages associated with medications used to treat seizure disorders.
- Identify significant drug look-alike/sound-alike issues.
- Identify significant drug interactions.
- Learn the terminology associated with seizures.

KEY TERMS

Anoxia: Lack of oxygen to the brain.

Aura: Unusual sensation, auditory, visual, or olfactory hallucination that is experienced just before the onset of a seizure.

Complex focal seizures: Seizure disorder that produces a blank stare, disorientation, repetitive actions, and memory loss.

Convulsions: Sudden contraction of muscles that is caused by seizures.

Epilepsy: Recurrent seizure disorder characterized by a sudden, excessive, disorderly discharge of cerebral neurons.

Febrile seizure: Seizure associated with a sudden spike in body temperature.

Generalized seizures: Seizures that spread across both cerebral hemispheres and include tonic-clonic, myoclonic, and petit mal seizures.

Gingival hyperplasia: Excess growth of gum tissue that may overgrow the teeth.

Hirsutism: Excessive growth of body hair (especially in women).

Myoclonic seizure: Seizure that is characterized by jerking muscle movements and is caused by contraction of major muscle groups.

Petit mal seizure: Absence seizure in which the person experiences a brief period of unconsciousness and stares vacantly into space.

Seizure threshold: Term that refers to a person's susceptibility to seizures.

Simple focal seizures: Seizure that affects only one part of the brain and causes the person to experience unusual sensations or feelings.

Status epilepticus: Medical emergency brought on by repeated generalized seizures that can deprive the brain of oxygen.

Tonic-clonic (grand mal) seizures: Generalized seizure that causes stiffening of the limbs, difficulty breathing, and jerking movements and is followed by limbs that become limp and disorientation.

Overview

Epilepsy is one of the oldest known brain disorders and was described as early as 3000 years ago in ancient Babylon. The word epilepsy is derived from the Greek word for "attack," because ancient Greeks believed the person was being attacked by demons. Approximately 2 million people in the United States have experienced at least one seizure. ***Epilepsy*** is a type of seizure disorder. It is characterized by a sudden, excessive, disorderly discharge of cerebral neurons. The onset of a seizure may be preceded by an aura. An ***aura*** is an unusual sensation, auditory, visual, or olfactory hallucination that is experienced just before the onset of a seizure. In other words, the person may hear, see, or smell something distinctive immediately before the seizure activity begins. These signs of an upcoming seizure are important because it indicates the location of abnormal neuronal firing in the cerebrum.

About 1% of the population has epilepsy, a disorder associated with having experienced two or more seizures. Seizures are caused by a wide range of conditions that range from injury to illness; however, half of all seizures have no known cause. When the cause is known, the origin may be internal or external. Some of the more common internal or intracranial causes for seizures are birth defects, infection (meningitis, AIDS), prenatal or perinatal injury, malignant tumors, and head trauma. The incidence of seizures caused by head injury can be reduced by wearing seat belts, motorcycle helmets, or bike helmets. ***Febrile seizures*** in children are associated with an infection causing a sudden spike in temperature; aggressive treatment with fever reducers is indicated to prevent more seizures. Most children who have febrile seizures will not develop epilepsy.

External causes include metabolic disturbance, hypoglycemia, electrolyte imbalance, drug and alcohol withdrawal, and use of drugs that lower the ***seizure threshold***. Stroke and heart attack can cause seizures because the brain becomes deprived of oxygen (***anoxia***). There is a 32% incidence of seizures in the elderly caused by anoxia resulting from cerebral vascular disease.

TECH NOTE!

Flashing or strobe lights like those used in fire alarms systems can trigger a seizure in individuals with epilepsy.

Seizure Classifications

There are two major seizure classifications (Figure 9-1): generalized seizures and focal or partial seizures. ***Generalized seizures*** spread across both of the cerebral hemispheres while partial seizures are confined to a single hemisphere. Tonic-clonic (grand mal) (Figure 9-2), myoclonic, and petit mal seizures are generalized seizures. ***Tonic-clonic*** and ***myoclonic*** seizures start with a stiffening of the limbs and difficulty breathing; are followed by jerking movements, loss of bladder and bowel control; and, on conclusion (postictal phase), the limbs become limp and the person may be disoriented. The jerking muscle movement associated with grand mal seizures is sometimes referred to a ***convulsion***.

Petit mal seizures are also called absence seizures. This type of seizure is associated with a characteristic vacant or absent stare during a seizure. Absence seizures occur more commonly in children. They are barely noticeable to onlookers because no major muscle twitching is exhibited. ***Status epilepticus*** is a medical emergency and results from repeated, generalized seizures that deprive the brain of oxygen. Antiseizure medicines must be administered intravenously to persons with status epilepticus.

Approximately 60% of people with epilepsy have focal seizures. ***Focal (partial) seizures*** involve only one cerebral hemisphere. Focal seizures are classified as simple or complex. Simple focal seizures may cause the arms, face, or legs to twitch, and visual, olfactory, or auditory hallucinations may occur. ***Complex focal seizures*** often begin with a blank stare. The person becomes disoriented and engages in repetitive actions during the seizure. Once the seizure is over, the person does not have any memory of the seizure. Psychomotor and temporal lobe seizures are complex partial seizures.

Neurochemistry of Seizures

When there is an abnormality in nerve signaling by neurotransmitters, seizures result. People with epilepsy have an abnormally high level of excitatory neurotransmitters coupled with a low level of inhibitory neurotransmitters. This accounts for the excess neuronal firing that occurs with seizure disorders. γ-Aminobutyric acid (GABA) is an inhibitory

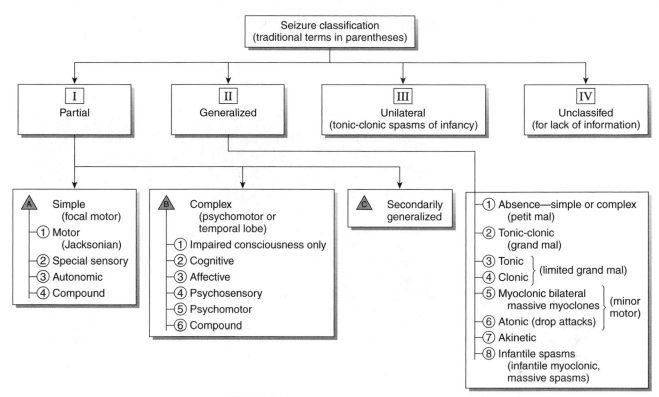

FIGURE 9-1 Classifications of seizures. *(From Clayton BD, Stock YN: Basic pharmacology for nurses, ed 12, St Louis, 1997, Mosby.)*

neurotransmitter that plays an important role in epilepsy. An excitatory neurotransmitter that plays a role in epilepsy is the amino acid glutamate. Some seizures are linked to a defect in the genes that control the ion channels that open and close to regulate the influx of chloride, sodium, and calcium into the neuron.

ION CHANNEL REGULATION

The aim of pharmaceutical treatment of seizure is to suppress seizure activity. This is accomplished by control of the voltage-dependent sodium channel. In the resting state, the neuron is more negative inside the cell and is surrounded by positive sodium, potassium, and calcium ions. Neuronal firing begins when the positive ions move from outside the neuron into the neuron. Neuronal firing is inhibited by drugs that delay the inflow of sodium ions. T-type voltage-dependent calcium channels are believed to be involved in initiation of seizure activity. Drugs that bind to T-type calcium channels inhibit absence (petit mal) seizures.

THE ROLE OF γ-AMINOBUTYRIC ACID

GABA is an inhibitory neurotransmitter. The GABA receptor regulates the movement chloride ion into the neuron. Chloride ions are negatively charged. The influx of chloride ions inhibits formation of action potentials, therefore, neuronal hyperactivity and seizures are suppressed. GABAergic receptors are stimulated by dopamine (D_2), another inhibitory neurotransmitter.

Other neurotransmitters that play a role in the initiation of seizures are acetylcholine, norepinephrine, histamine, and glutamate.

Drugs Used to Treat Seizure Disorders

The goal of treatment of epilepsy and other seizure disorders is to reduce the incidence of seizures by suppressing seizure activity. Successful achievement of this therapeutic goal is dependent on correctly classifying the seizure type and selecting an appropriate drug for seizure type, with optimal drug administration and serum monitoring. Monodrug therapy

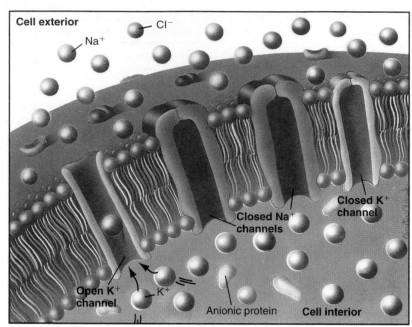

FIGURE 9-2 Role of ion channels. *(From Thibodeau GA, Patton KT: Anatomy and physiology, ed 6, St Louis, 2007, Mosby.)*

TECH NOTE!

Therapeutic blood levels for phenytoin are best maintained by dispensing the same manufacturer's formulation each time a prescription is filled. Avoid switching if possible.

TECH ALERT!

The following drugs have look-alike/sound-alike issues: Cerebyx, Celebrex, and Celexa; phenytoin and fosphenytoin; Dilantin and Diflucan

TECH NOTE!

Cerebyx, is compatible in normal saline and dextrose.

TECH NOTE!

Dilantin is compatible in normal saline. Intravenous solution is stable for 14 hours at room temperature when diluted to 2 mg/ml. Dilantin chewable tablets should be followed by a glass of water.

is preferred to lower the incidence of adverse effects, reduce the incidence of drug interactions, improve adherence to drug therapy, and lower medication costs. Medications reduce seizure activity in approximately 80% of people diagnosed with epilepsy. The remaining 20% of people will continue to experience seizures.

HYDANTOINSdes

Phenytoin (formerly diphenylhydantoin) was first introduced in 1938. It is used for the treatment of generalized (tonic-clonic) seizures, partial seizures, and status epilepticus. Fosphenytoin is used to treat status epilepticus and seizures occurring during neurosurgery.

MECHANISM OF ACTION

Phenytoin and fosphenytoin suppress seizure activity by binding to receptors on voltage dependent sodium channels. They also reduce neuronal membrane permeability to calcium.

PHARMACOKINETICS

Absorption of phenytoin is variable and is influenced by particle size as well as by inactive ingredients in manufacturers' formulations. This influences bioavailability, which may result in an increase or a decrease in blood levels when switching between different manufacturers' formulations. Ninety percent of the drug is protein bound, so drug interactions involving protein binding are common. Phenytoin is primarily metabolized in the liver by cytochrome P450 enzymes. If enough phenytoin is administered to saturate metabolic enzymes, a secondary metabolic pathway is used. When this occurs, elimination is slowed and excessive adverse reactions or toxicity can occur. Patients taking phenytoin must periodically have their blood levels monitored. Phenytoin acts as an inducer of metabolic enzymes in the liver; therefore, it can alter the rate of metabolism of other coadministered drugs that use the same metabolic system. For example, phenytoin can reduce the effectiveness of oral contraceptives as well as other antiseizure drugs. Drug interactions can also occur between phenytoin and erythromycin, isoniazid, and warfarin.

Fosphentoin is converted to phenytoin by enzymes in the blood (phosphatases). It has a short half-life of approximately 8 minutes. Unlike phenytoin, which can be administered orally or parenterally, fosphentoin is only available for parenteral use and is administered intravenously or intramuscularly. Its advantage is that it produces more predictable serum concentrations when administered intramuscularly than phenytoin and is 100% bioavailable.

ADVERSE REACTIONS

Adverse reactions are dose dependent and are similar for phenytoin and fosphenytoin. Common side effects include nausea and vomiting, *hirsutism* (excessive growth of body hair, especially in women), *gingival hyperplasia* (excessive growth of gum tissue), ataxia, and sedation. The hydantoins can also produce slowed thinking. Infants born to women who took phenytoin during pregnancy may be born with cleft palate. Hydantoins may decrease folic acid, calcium, and vitamin D absorption; it may be necessary to supplement with vitamins.

Hydantoins

	Generic name	U.S. brand name(s) Canadian brand(s)	Dosage forms and strengths
	fosphenytoin	Cerebyx	**Injection, solution:** 75 mg/ml [phentoin equivalent (PE) is 50 mg/ml]
		Cerebyx	
	phenytoin*	Dilantin	**Capsule, extended release:** 30 mg, 100 mg
		Dilantin	**Capsule, prompt release:** 100 mg
			Injection, solution: 50 mg/ml
			Suspension: 125 mg/5 ml
			Tablet, chewable: 50 mg

*Generic available.

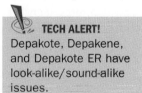

TECH ALERT!
Depakote, Depakene, and Depakote ER have look-alike/sound-alike issues.

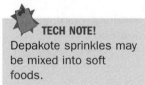

TECH NOTE!
Depakote sprinkles may be mixed into soft foods.

VALPROATES

Valproates are described as "broad-spectrum" antiseizure drugs because they are effective in treating all types of seizures. They are one of the few antiseizure drugs indicated for the treatment of absence seizures. Valproates are also effective for treating general and focal (partial) seizures.

MECHANISM OF ACTION

One of the mechanisms of action for valproates and their derivatives is to enhance the inhibitory actions of GABA. Other mechanisms of action may be involved, including actions on potassium channels that result in membrane stabilization.

PHARMACOKINETICS

The effectiveness of all valproic acid derivatives is expressed as valproic acid activity. All are rapidly absorbed when administered orally and have 100% bioavailability. Valproates are up to 95% protein bound, so drug interactions involving protein binding must be considered when dispensing other drugs with them, including other antiseizure medicines like phenobarbital and phenytoin.

ADVERSE REACTIONS

Common adverse reactions are gastrointestinal upset and sedation, although the valproates are less sedating than other drugs used to treat seizures. Other adverse effects are weight gain, hair loss, tremor, diplopia (double vision), bruising, irregular menstruation, and hepatotoxicity. Hepatotoxicity is rare, but when it occurs in children, it is potentially fatal.

PRECAUTIONS

Valproates should be used cautiously in people with a history of liver disease. Up to 10% of the drug is passed in breast milk, limiting the use of valproates during lactation.

Valproates

	Generic name	U.S. brand name(s) Canadian brand(s)	Dosage forms and strengths
	valproic acid and its derivatives*	Depacon, Depakene, Depakote Delayed Release, Depakote ER, Depakote Sprinkle	**Capsule, as valproic acid (Depakene):** 250 mg **Capsule, as sprinkles (Depakote Sprinkle):** 125 mg **Injection, solution: (Depacon):** 100 mg/ml **Syrup, as valproic acid (Depakene):** 250 mg/5 ml
		Depakene, Epival ER, Epival IV	**Tablet, as divalproex sodium delayed release (Depakote):** 125 mg, 250 mg, 500 mg **Tablet, as divalproex sodium extended release (Depakote ER):** 250 mg, 500 mg

*Generic available.

IMIONSTILBENES

There are only two antiseizure medications in this class: carbamazepine and oxcarbazepine. They are used to treat generalized and complex focal seizures. Neither drug is useful in the management of absence seizures. Carbamazepine is also used in the management of pain due to trigeminal neuralgia (see Chapter 10) and bipolar disorder (see Chapter 6).

MECHANISM OF ACTION

Carbamazepine is structurally similar to tricyclic antidepressants. The mechanism of action is not completely understood; however, it is believed to work by binding to voltage-dependent sodium channels.

PHARMACOKINETICS

Oral absorption and distribution of carbamazepine are moderately slow and are influenced by drug formulation. Differences in inactive ingredients and particle size can alter rates of absorption. Peak levels of the drug are not achieved until 6 to 8 hours after administration. Carbamazepine is metabolized in the liver. Over time, it begins to induce the same enzymes that metabolize it, causing serum levels to fluctuate. Erratic serum blood levels can result in poor seizure control. This may be minimized by administration of controlled release formulations.

ADVERSE REACTIONS

Side effects of carbamazepine and oxcarbazepine include nausea, vomiting, dizziness, sedation, unsteadiness (ataxia), bruising, jaundice, and double vision (diplopia).

PRECAUTIONS

Carbamazepine should be protected from light and moisture. Moisture can decrease the potency by as much as 30%.

Imionstilbenes

	Generic name	U.S. brand name(s) Canadian brand(s)	Dosage forms and strengths
	carbamazepine*	Carbatrol, Equetro, Tegretol, Tegretol-XR	**Capsule, extended release (Equetro):** 100 mg, 200 mg, 300 mg **Tablet, extended release (Tegretol-XR):** 100 mg, 200 mg, 400 mg
		Tegretol	
	oxcarbazepine	Trileptal	**Suspension:** 300 mg/5 ml **Tablet:** 150 mg, 300 mg, 600 mg
		Trileptal	

*Generic available.

γ-AMINOBUTYRIC ACID ANALOGS

Gabapentin, prebablin, tiagabine, and vigabatrin are administered for the treatment of general and partial (focal) seizures. All are ineffective in treating absence seizures. Gabapentin and pregablin are also used to treat herpes-related nerve pain (see Chapter 10).

MECHANISM OF ACTION

Gabapentin was structurally designed to bind to $GABA_A$ receptors and act as an agonist; however, it turns out that this is not the mechanism of action for the drug. Gabapentin binds to voltage-dependent sodium channels and increases GABA turnover without binding to the GABA receptor. Pregabalin is structurally related to gabapentin, but its mechanism of action is different. Pregabalin reduces neuronal calcium currents by binding to calcium channels rather than to sodium channels. Tiagabine blocks the reuptake of GABA in the synapse, and vigabatrin enhances GABA activity by binding to GABA transaminase (GABA-T), the enzyme that inactivates GABA.

PHARMACOKINETICS

The oral absorption of gabapentin and tiagabine is rapid. Gabapentin has lower bioavailability (60%) than tiagabine (90%) and has little protein binding, whereas tiagabine in nearly 95% protein bound (i.e., making it susceptible to drug interactions involving protein binding). Gabapentin is primarily eliminated by the kidneys. Vigabatrin has a short half-life, but the effects of GABA-T binding persist even after blood levels of the drug declines.

ADVERSE REACTIONS

Drug-related side effects for gabapentin and tiagabine are dizziness, confusion, fatigue, ataxia, and nausea. Tiagabine may cause anorexia, whereas gabapentin may increase appetite. Double vision, blurred vision, dry mouth, and constipation are also associated with gabapentin. Vigabatrin can cause irreversible tunnel vision, limiting its use.

PRECAUTIONS

Antacids decrease the absorption of gabapentin by 20%. The absorption of tiagabine is reduced by foods that have a high fat content.

GABA Analogs

Generic name	U.S. brand name(s) / Canadian brand(s)	Dosage forms and strengths
gabapentin*	Neurontin	**Capsule:** 100 mg, 300 mg, 400 mg **Solution, oral:** 250 mg/5 ml
	Neurontin	**Tablet:** 100 mg, 300 mg, 400 mg, 600 mg, 800 mg
pregabalin	Lyrica	**Capsules:** 25 mg, 50 mg, 75 mg, 100 mg, 150 mg, 200 mg, 225 mg, 300 mg
	Not available	
tiagabine	Gabatril	**Tablet:** 2 mg, 4 mg, 12 mg, 16 mg
	Gabatril	
vigabatrin	Not available	**Powder for oral suspension:** 0.5-g packets **Tablet:** 500 mg
	Sabril	

*Generic available.

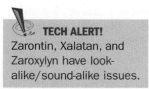

SUCCINIMIDES

Ethosuximide is the only drug in this class. It is one of the few drugs indicated for the treatment of absence seizures.

MECHANISM OF ACTION AND PHARMACOKINETICS

Ethosuximide inhibits T-type voltage-dependent calcium channels. The drug is well absorbed orally and reaches peak plasma concentrations within 3 to 7 hours after administration. Unlike many of the other antiseizure drugs, it is not protein bound and is completely metabolized by the liver. It has a long elimination half-life, approximately 40 hours. Drug interactions with phenytoin result in increased phenytoin levels, and interactions with valproic acid cause decreased ethosuximide clearance.

ADVERSE REACTIONS

Common side effects associated with ethosuximide are sedation, dizziness, unsteadiness, nausea, vomiting, and photophobia. Rarely, the drug causes liver and kidney damage.

Succinimides

Generic name	U.S. brand name(s)	Dosage forms and strengths
	Canadian brand(s)	
ethosuximide*	Zarontin	**Capsule:** 250 mg
	Zarontin	**Syrup:** 250 mg/5 ml

*Generic available.

BARBITURATES

Phenobarbital was the first drug that was used to treat seizures. It is indicated in the treatment of generalized tonic-clonic seizures and partial seizures and is administered to children to control febrile seizures. Amobarbital, mephobarbital, and primidone are also administered to treat tonic-clonic seizures. Pentobarbital is indicated for the treatment of status epilepticus and acute control of tonic-clonic seizures from meningitis, tetanus, ethanol withdrawal, eclampsia, or poisons.

MECHANISM OF ACTION

Barbiturates enhance GABA at GABA$_A$ receptors by binding to a barbiturate receptor linked to chloride ion channels. This results in an influx of chloride ions into the neuron, which inhibits neuronal excitability.

PHARMACOKINETICS

Oral absorption of phenobarbital is moderately slow; however, the drug is readily distributed throughout the central nervous system due to its high degree of lipid solubility. It has 100% bioavailability. It is metabolized in the liver, as is primidone, another barbiturate that is administered to treat seizures. Primidone is metabolized to phenobarbital. Phenobarbital is capable of self-inducing the enzymes that metabolize it and many other drugs such as phenytoin and valproic acid. It is implicated in many drug interactions involving enzyme induction.

ADVERSE REACTIONS

Sedation, unsteadiness, confusion, nausea, hypotension, tolerance, and dependence are adverse effects associated with barbiturates. Serious side effects are megaloblastic anemia and respiratory depression. Phenobarbital may produce hyperactivity, rather than sedation, in children.

BENZODIAZEPINES

Benzodiazepines are indicated for the treatment of status epilepticus (intravenous diazepam), absence seizures and myoclonic seizures (clonazepam), and partial seizures (clorazepate). Benzodiazepines bind to receptor sites on the GABA$_A$ complex. This increases the affinity of GABA to the GABA receptor. GABA receptor binding reduces neuronal excitability

Barbiturates

Generic name	U.S. brand name(s)	Dosage forms and strengths
	Canadian brand(s)	
amobarbital	Amytal	**Powder for injection:** 500 mg
mephobarbital	Mebaral	**Tablet:** 32 mg, 50 mg, 100 mg
	Not available	
pentobarbital	Nembutal	**Injection, solution:** 50 mg/ml
phenobarbital*	Luminal	**Elixir:** 20 mg/5 ml
	Generics	**Injection, solution:** 60 mg/ml, 130 mg/ml **Tablet:** 15 mg, 30 mg, 32 mg (gr ½), 60 mg, 65 mg (gr 1), 100 mg (gr 1½)
primidone*	Mysoline	**Tablet:** 50 mg, 250 mg
	Mysoline	

*Generic available.

by opening chloride (Cl⁻) ion channels and lowering the neuronal membrane resting potential. The mechanism of action and pharmacokinetics of benzodiazepines are discussed in detail in Chapter 5. Sedation, unsteadiness, confusion, impaired learning, tolerance, and dependence are adverse effects common to benzodiazepines. Intravenous diazepam can cause respiratory depression.

Benzodiazepines Used in the Treatment of Seizures

Generic name	U.S. brand name(s)	Dosage forms and strengths
	Canadian brand(s)	
clonazepam*	Klonopin	**Tablet:** 0.5 mg, 1 mg, 2 mg
	Klonopin	**Tablet, disintegrating:** 0.125 mg, 0.25 mg, 0.5 mg, 1 mg, 2 mg
clorazepate*	Tranxene, Tranxene SD, Tranxene SD Half Strength	**Tablet (Tranxene):** 3.75 mg, 7.5 mg, 15 mg **Tablet, sustained release (Tranxene SD):** 22.5 mg **Tablet, sustained release (Tranxene SD Half Strength):** 11.25 mg
	Generics	
diazepam	Diastat, Diazepam Intensol, Valium	Injection, solution 5 mg/ml **Solution, oral:** 5 mg/5 mg **Rectal gel (Diastat):** 10 mg, 20 mg
	Diastat, Diazemuls, Valium	**Tablet:** 2 mg, 5 mg, 10 mg

*Generic available.

TECH ALERT!
The following drugs have look-alike/sound-alike issues:
Keppra and Kaletra;
Lamictal, Lamisil, and Lomotil;
lamotrigine and lamivudine;
Topamax and Toprol-XL

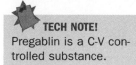

TECH NOTE!
Pregablin is a C-V controlled substance.

OTHER BROAD-SPECTRUM ANTISEIZURE DRUGS

Lamotrigine, levetiracetam, topiramate, and zonisamide are newer broad-spectrum antiseizure drugs. They are indicated for the treatment of generalized (tonic-clonic) and focal (partial) seizures.

MECHANISM OF ACTION AND PHARMACOKINETICS

Lamotrigine, zonisamide, and topiramate act by inhibiting voltage-dependent sodium channels. Additional mechanisms of action for zonisamide are inhibition of T-type calcium channels and GABA binding. Additional mechanisms of action for topiramate include antagonism of non-NMDA glutaminergic receptors and acting as a GABA agonist. The mechanism of action for levetiracetam is not fully known.

Lamotrigine, levetiracetam, and topiramate are rapidly absorbed orally. Oral absorption of zonisamide is slow to moderate. All of the drugs have greater than 95% bioavailability. Protein binding is less than 50% for all of these drugs, so there are fewer drug interactions than with some of the other antiseizure medications. Lower doses of lamotrigine are required when taken with valproic acid. Higher doses are required when taken with enzyme-inducing drugs.

Lamotrigine, leveiracetam, topiramate, and zonisamide may produce sedation and dizziness. Lamotrigine and topiramate also produce nausea and ataxia. Additional side effects of lamotrigine are blurred vision, double vision, and rash. Levetiracetam and topiramate may also produce weakness. Side effects of topiramate also include lack of concentration, headache, and heart palpitations. Zonisamide may produce nausea, rash, and kidney stones, in addition to sedation.

Broad-Spectrum Antiseizure Drugs

	Generic name	U.S. brand name(s) Canadian brand(s)	Dosage forms and strengths
	lamotrigine	Lamictal / Lamictal	**Tablet:** 25 mg, 100 mg, 150 mg, 200 mg **Tablet, as chewable:** 2 mg, 5 mg, 25 mg
	levetiracetam	Keppra / Keppra	**Solution, oral:** 100 mg/ml **Tablet:** 250 mg, 500 mg, 750 mg
	topiramate	Topamax / Topamax	**Capsule, sprinkle:** 15 mg, 25 mg **Tablet:** 25 mg, 50 mg, 100 mg, 200 mg
	zonisamide	Zonegran / Zonegran	**Capsule:** 25 mg, 50 mg, 100 mg

Summary of Drugs Used for the Treatment of Seizures

Seizure type	First choice	Second choice	Third choice	Fourth choice
Generalized (myclonic and tonic-clonic)	phenytoin	carbamazepine	valproic acid	lamotrigene topirimate tiagabine phenobarbital
Simple focal	carbamazepine	phenytoin oxcarbazepine	primidone vigabatrin	gabapentin lamotrigene levetiracetam zonisamide
Complex focal	carbamazepine	phenytoin oxcarbazepine	phenobarbital vigabatrin	valproic acid lamotrigene levetiracetam primidone tiagabine topiramate zonisamide
Psychomotor	phenytoin			
Absence seizures	clonazepam ethosuximide valproic acid			
Status epilepticus	diazepam IV fosphenytoin IV lorazepam IV*	pentobarbital IV phenobarbital IV		

*Not FDA approved.

Summary of Drugs Used in the Treatment of Seizures

	Generic name	U.S. brand name	Usual adult oral dose and dosing schedule	Warning labels
Hydantoins				
	fosphenytoin	Cerebyx	**Status epilepticus:** IV loading dose: 15 mg to 20 mg/kg (PE) administered at rate of 100 mg to 150 mg/min **Nonemergent maintenance dose:** 4 mg to 6 mg/kg (PE)/ day administered IM or IV	MAY CAUSE DROWSINESS; MAY IMPAIR ABILITY TO DRIVE AVOID ALCOHOL DO NOT DISCONTINUE WITHOUT MEDICAL SUPERVISION
	phenytoin	Dilantin	**Status epilepticus:** IV loading dose: 15 mg to 25 mg/kg; maintenance 300 mg/day in 3 divided doses **Neurosurgery:** 100 mg to 200 mg administered every 4 hours during surgery **Generalized/partial seizures (oral):** Loading dose: 10 mg to 20 mg/kg in 3 divided doses; Maintenance: 300 mg/ day in 3 divided doses (immediate release) or 1 to 2 doses (extended release)	SWALLOW WHOLE; DON'T CRUSH OR CHEW (sustained release) TAKE WITH FOOD—phenytoin AVOID PREGNANCY AVOID ANTACIDS AND CIMETIDINE— phenytoin SHAKE WELL (suspension)
Valproates				
	valproic acid and derivatives	Depakene, Depakote	**Seizures (oral):** Start 10 mg to 15 mg/kg/day in 1 to 3 divided doses, increase up to 1000 mg to 2500 mg/day. Note: regular and delayed release formulations dosed 2 to 4 times a day. Extended release formulations are dosed once daily. **Status epilepticus* (IV):** Loading dose: 15 mg to 25 mg/kg administered at 3 mg/kg/m; maintenance: infusion: 1 mg to 4 mg/kg/hr	MAY CAUSE DIZZINESS OR DROWSIINESS; MAY IMPAIR ABILITY TO DRIVE AVOID ALCOHOL TAKE WITH FOOD AVOID PREGNANCY SWALLOW WHOLE; DON'T CRUSH OR CHEW (extended release) DO NOT DISCONTINUE WITHOUT MEDICAL SUPERVISION
Imionstilbenes				
	carbamazepine	Tegretol	Start 200 mg twice a day; increase to 1200 mg to 1600 mg/day in 3 to 4 divided doses (maximum 2400 mg/day)	MAY CAUSE DIZZINESS OR DROWSINESS; MAY IMPAIR ABILITY TO DRIVE AVOID ALCOHOL TAKE WITH FOOD
	oxcarbazepine	Tripleptal	Start 600 mg twice a day; increase to 2400 mg/day	SWALLOW WHOLE; DON'T CRUSH OR CHEW (extended release) TAKE WITH A FULL GLASS OF WATER (chewable tablets) SHAKE WELL (suspension) DO NOT DISCONTINUE WITHOUT MEDICAL SUPERVISION MAY DECREASE THE EFFECTIVENESS OF ORAL CONTRACEPTIVES

Continued

Summary of Drugs Used in the Treatment of Seizures—cont'd

Generic name	U.S. brand name	Usual adult oral dose and dosing schedule	Warning labels
GABA analogs			
gabapentin	Neurontin	Start 300 mg 3 times/day; increase to 900 mg to 1800 mg/day	MAY CAUSE DIZZINESS OR DROWSINESS; MAY IMPAIR ABILITY TO DRIVE
pregabalin	Lyrica	150 to 600 mg dosed 2 to 3 times a day	AVOID ALCOHOL TAKE WITH FOOD
tiagabine	Gabatril	Start 4 mg once daily; increase up to 56 mg/day in 2 to 4 divided doses	AVOID ANTACIDS WITHIN 2 HOURS OF DOSE—gabapentin
vigabatrin	Sabril (Canada)	Start 1 g once daily; increase up to 2 to 3 g/day	DO NOT DISCONTINUE WITHOUT MEDICAL SUPERVISION SHAKE WELL; DISCARD WITHIN 30 DAYS OF RECONSTITUTION—vigabatrin suspension
Succinimides			
ethosuximide	Zarontin	Start 250 mg twice a day; increase up to 1500 mg/day	MAY CAUSE DIZZINESS OR DROWSINESS; MAY IMPAIR ABILITY TO DRIVE AVOID ALCOHOL TAKE WITH FOOD DO NOT DISCONTINUE WITHOUT MEDICAL SUPERVISION
Barbiturates			
amobarbital	Amytal	65 mg to 500 mg administered as a single IV dose	MAY CAUSE DROWSINESS
pentobarbital	Nembutal	**For mechanically ventilated patients only:** 10 mg to 15 mg/kg IV over 1 hour (maximum total loading dose 30 mg/kg) **Maintenance infusion:** 0.5 mg to 1 mg/kg/hr IV titrated by 0.5 mg/kg/hr, as needed	MAY CAUSE DROWSINESS
mephobarbital	Mebaral	32 mg to 100 mg 3 to 4 times daily	MAY CAUSE DROWSINESS; MAY IMPAIR ABILITY TO DRIVE
phenobarbital	Luminal	**Status epilepticus:** 300 mg to 800 mg IV loading dose; 120 mg to 240 mg/dose every 20 minutes until seizure is controlled (maximum dose 1000 mg to 2000 mg) **Seizure maintenance:** Oral 1 mg to 3 mg/kg/day dosed 2 to 3 times a day	AVOID ALCOHOL MAY BE HABIT FORMING DON'T DISCONTINUE WITHOUT MEDICAL SUPERVISION
primidone	Mysoline	750 mg to 1500 mg/day in 3 to 4 divided doses	

Summary of Drugs Used in the Treatment of Seizures—cont'd

	Generic name	U.S. brand name	Usual adult oral dose and dosing schedule	Warning labels
	Benzodiazepines			
	clonazepam	Klonopin	1.5 mg 3 times a day (maximum 20 mg/day)	MAY CAUSE DROWSINESS; MAY IMPAIR ABILITY TO DRIVE
	clorazepate	Tranxene	**Partial seizures:** 7.5 mg 2 to 3 times a day up to 90 mg daily	AVOID ALCOHOL MAY BE HABIT FORMING
	diazepam	Valium	**For status epilepticus and drug induced seizures:** 5 mg to 10 mg every 10 to 15 minutes IV up to 30 mg per 8-hour period	DO NOT CRUSH, BREAK OR CHEW— extended release clorazepate
	Broad-spectrum antiseizure drugs			
	lamotrigine	Lamictal	300 mg to 500 mg/day in 2 divided doses (maximum 700 mg/day)	MAY CAUSE DIZZINESS OR DROWSINESS; MAY IMPAIR ABILITY TO DRIVE
	levetiracetam	Keppra	Start 500 mg twice daily; increase to 3000 mg/day	AVOID ALCOHOL DO NOT DISCONTINUE WITHOUT MEDICAL SUPERVISION
	topiramate	Topamax	Start 25 mg to 50 mg/day in 2 divided doses; increase to 400 mg/day (maximum 1600 mg/day)	MAINTAIN ADEQUATE HYDRATION— zonisamide
	zonisamide	Zonegran	Start 100 mg/day; increase to 400 mg/day (maximum 600 mg/day)	

CHAPTER SUMMARY

- Epilepsy was described as early as 3000 years ago in ancient Babylon.
- About 1% of the population has epilepsy.
- Epilepsy is a type of seizure disorder that is characterized by a sudden, excessive, disorderly discharge of cerebral neurons.
- People with epilepsy have an abnormally high level of excitatory neurotransmitters coupled with a low level of inhibitory neurotransmitters.
- Half of all seizures have no known cause.
- Causes of seizures include birth defects, infection (meningitis, AIDS), tumors, head trauma, high fevers, hypoglycemia, drug and alcohol withdrawal, and cerebrovascular disease.
- The incidence of seizures caused by head injury can be reduced by wearing seat belts, motorcycle helmets, and bike helmets.
- Generalized seizures spread across both of the cerebral hemispheres, whereas partial seizures are confined to a single hemisphere.
- Status epilepticus is a medical emergency that results from repeated generalized seizures that deprive the brain of oxygen.
- Status epilepticus is treated with intravenous medications.
- Some seizures are linked to a defect in the genes that control the ion channels that open and close to regulate the influx of chloride, sodium, and calcium into the neuron.
- Neuronal firing is inhibited by drugs that delay the inflow of sodium ions. Drugs that bind to T-type calcium channels inhibit absence (petit mal) seizures.

- The GABA receptor regulates the movement of chloride ion into the neuron, which inhibits the formation of action potentials, neuronal hyperactivity, and seizures.
- The goal of treatment of epilepsy and other seizure disorders is to reduce the incidence of seizures by suppressing seizure activity.
- Medications reduce seizure activity in approximately 80% of people diagnosed with epilepsy.
- Therapeutic blood levels for phenytoin are best maintained by dispensing the same manufacturer's formulation each time a prescription is filled.
- Carbamazepine should be protected from light and moisture. Moisture can decrease the potency by as much as 30%.
- Antacids decrease the absorption of gabapentin by 20%. The absorption of tiagabine is reduced by foods that have a high fat content.
- Few drugs are effective for treating absence seizures; they are ethosuximide, valproic acid, and clonazepam.
- Barbiturates and benzodiazepines used in the treatment of seizures are controlled substances.
- Lamotrigine, levetiracetam, topiramate, and zonisamide are newer broad-spectrum antiseizure drugs.

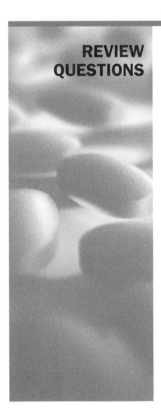

REVIEW QUESTIONS

Multiple Choice

1. One of the oldest known brain disorders described as early as 3000 years ago in ancient Babylon is
   a. schizophrenia
   b. epilepsy
   c. depression
   d. fainting

2. Febrile seizures in children are associated with an _____, causing a sudden spike in temperature.
   a. injury
   b. injection
   c. infection
   d. a, b, and c

3. The only major seizure classification is generalized seizures.
   a. true
   b. false

4. A medical emergency that results from repeated generalized seizures and deprives the brain of oxygen is called
   a. status epilepticus
   b. myoclonic epilepticus
   c. grand mal epilepticus
   d. tonic-clonic status

5. The goal of treatment of epilepsy and other seizure disorders is to reduce the incidence of seizures by _____ seizure activity.
   a. stopping
   b. sedating
   c. suppressing
   d. shocking

6. This drug is used in the management of generalized and partial seizures, status epilepticus, and seizures following head trauma or neurosurgery.
   a. phenytoin
   b. carbamazepine
   c. valproic acid
   d. fosphenytoin

7. **One of the few drugs indicated for the treatment of absence seizures is**
   a. phenytoin
   b. gabapentin
   c. carbamazepine
   d. ethosuximide

8. **What benzodiazepine is indicated for the treatment of status epilepticus, drug-induced seizures, and anxiety?**
   a. diazepam
   b. clonazepam
   c. lorazepam
   d. alprazolam

9. **Phenytoin was the first drug that was used to treat seizures.**
   a. true
   b. false

10. **An unusual sensation, auditory, visual, or olfactory hallucination that is experienced just before the onset of a seizure is called a(n)**
    a. halo
    b. aura
    c. vision
    d. hallucination

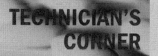

TECHNICIAN'S CORNER

1. Should you see someone experiencing a seizure, what would you do?
2. What would be the best advice you can give an epileptic patient about his or her medication?

BIBLIOGRAPHY

Kalant H, Grant D, Mitchell J: *Principles of medical pharmacology* (pp 223-235), ed 7. Toronto, 2007, Elsevier Canada, A Division of Reed Elsevier Canada.

Lance L, Lacy C, Armstrong L, Goldman M: *Drug information handbook for the allied health professional,* ed 12, Hudson, OH, 2005, APhA Lexi-Comp.

National Institute of Neurological Disorders and Stroke: *Seizures and epilepsy: Hope through research,* Bethesda, MD, National Institute of Neurological Disorders and Stroke, National Institutes of Health, U.S. Department of Health and Human Services. Updated June 2008. NIH Publication No. 04-156.

Page C, Curtis M, Sutter M, Walker M, Hoffman B: *Integrated pharmacology* (pp 257-259), Philadelphia, 2005, Elsevier Mosby.

Raffa RB, Rawls SM, Beyzarov EP: *Netter's illustrated pharmacology* (pp 67-70), Philadelphia, WB Saunders, 2005.

USP Center for Advancement of Patient Safety: *Use caution: avoid confusion.* USP Quality Review No. 79, Rockville, MD, April 2004, USP Center for Advancement of Patient Safety.

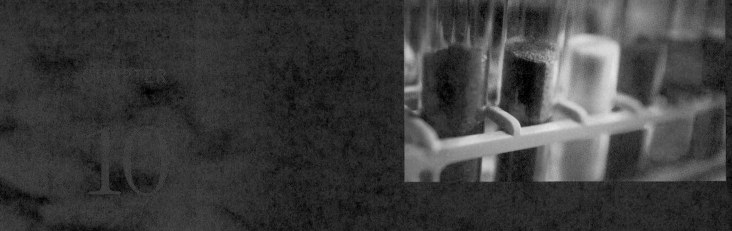

Treatment of Pain

CHAPTER 10

LEARNING OBJECTIVES

- Describe the etiology of pain.
- Compare and contrast the function of neurotransmitters associated with pain symptoms.
- Compare and contrast the treatment of nociceptive pain and neuropathic pain.
- Classify medications used in the treatment of pain.
- Describe mechanism of action for each class of drugs used to treat pain.
- Identify warning labels and precautionary messages associated with medications used to treat pain.
- Identify significant drug look-alike/sound-alike issues.
- Identify significant drug interactions.
- Learn the terminology associated with the treatment of pain.

KEY TERMS

Acute pain: Sudden pain that results from injury or inflammation and is usually self-limiting.

Acupuncture: Nonpharmacological treatment for pain that involves the application of needles to precise points on the body.

Analgesic: Drug that reduces pain.

Arthritis: Condition that is associated with joint pain.

Biofeedback: Nonpharmacological treatment for pain that involves relaxation techniques and gaining self-control over muscle tension, heart rate, and skin temperature.

Chronic pain: Pain that persists for a long period of time that is worsened by psychological factors and is resistant to many medical treatments.

COX-2 inhibitor: Analgesic, antiinflammatory drug that blocks cyclooxygenase-2, an enzyme that produces prostaglandin, which is a substance involved in mediating pain.

Diabetic neuropathy: Peripheral nerve disorder caused by diabetes and causing numbness, pain, or tingling in the feet or legs.

Dysphoria: Feeling of emotional and/or mental discomfort, restlessness, and depression; the opposite of euphoria.

Endorphins, enkephalins, and dynorphin: Substances released by the body in response to painful stimuli that act as natural painkillers.

Euphoria: State of intense happiness or well-being; the opposite of dysphoria.

Neuropathic pain: Type of pain associated with nerve injury caused by trauma, infection, or chronic diseases such as diabetes.

Nociceptors: Thin nerve fibers in skin, muscle, and other body tissues that carry pain signals.

NSAID: Nonsteroidal antiinflammatory drug.

Opiate naïve: No current exposure to opioids.

Opioid: Synthetically derived analgesic having properties similar to morphine.

PCA: Patient-controlled analgesia.

Plasticity: Ability of the brain to restructure itself and adapt to injury.

Shingles: Reoccurring and painful skin rash caused by the herpes zoster virus.

Substance P: Peptide that is involved in the production of pain sensations and controls pain perception.

Trigeminal neuralgia: Painful condition that produces intense, stabbing pain in areas of the face innervated by branches of the trigeminal nerve.

Overview

Most people will experience some type of physical pain in their lifetime. *Acute pain* is triggered by an injury, burn, infection, or some other stimuli and is self-limiting. *Chronic pain* may persist for years and is inadequately controlled by pharmaceuticals or other pain management therapies. There is a strong psychological component to pain that is often underestimated. Psychological factors can influence a person's tolerance for pain and can determine whether the outcome of treatment is successful. To reduce anxieties associated with pain that result in higher doses of pain medications, patients may be permitted to control the frequency of administration of their dose of pain medications. Patient-controlled analgesia (*PCA*) is done using a device that is connected to the patient's intravenous line. The patient pushes a button to deliver a measured dose of pain medication.

Pain is often categorized into mechanism-based categories. *Neuropathic pain* is associated with a nerve injury caused by trauma, infection, or chronic disease such as diabetes. Chronic pain is often of neuropathic origin. Pain with a nociceptive origin is caused by stimulation of nociceptors by natural substances released in response to painful stimuli. *Nociceptors* are thin nerve fibers located in the skin, muscle, and other body tissues that carry pain signals. The division of pain into distinct categories is somewhat simplistic because multiple pathophysiological mechanisms are probably involved. It is important to determine whether the pain has a neuropathic origin because the response to opioid analgesics is less with neuropathic pain than with nociceptive pain.

Pain may be *referred.* This means that the place where pain symptoms are most strongly felt may be different than the actual origin of the painful stimuli. Pain can also be triggered as part of an immune system response to fighting disease. Cytokines are a type of protein that is released as a response to nervous system injury. Cytokines produce pain-causing inflammation.

Conditions That Produce Pain

NOCICEPTIVE ORIGIN

INFLAMMATION

Inflammation is an important source of pain. *Inflammation* is a response to tissue irritation or injury that is marked by signs of redness, swelling, heat, and pain. When an injury occurs, phospholipase A_2 enzyme activity increases, stimulating the release of arachidonic acid from tissue membrane phospholipids. Arachidonic acid is activated by cyclooxygenase, an enzyme involved in the biosynthesis of prostaglandins. Prostaglandins are important mediators of pain. Arthritis, muscle or nerve damage, and even infection can produce painful inflammation.

ARTHRITIS

Arthritis is a condition that produces joint pain. Rheumatoid arthritis, osteoarthritis, and gout are all arthritic conditions. The cause and treatment of each of these arthritic conditions vary. Osteoarthritis is the most common of all arthritic conditions. It is the leading cause of musculoskeletal pain. Symptoms of osteoarthritis are joint pain, stiffness, swelling, and crepitus (creaking joints). Pain may occur after activity or at rest. Risk factors for osteoarthritis are previous joint injury or surgery, obesity, increasing age, muscle weakness, and occupations that involve excessive joint use. Inflammation of the fluid that surrounds the joint (synovial fluid) contributes to the pain associated with osteoarthritis.

LOW BACK PAIN

Nearly one third of adults will experience low back pain in any given year, making it one of the most common types of pain. Despite its high prevalence, only 20% of people experiencing low back pain will seek medical attention.

Acute low back pain produces symptoms that last less than 6 weeks. Chronic low back pain can persist indefinitely and may produce leg pain or widespread body pain or restrict spinal movement.

HEADACHE

Nonvascular

Tension headaches produce pain in both sides of the head that is mild to moderate in intensity and is described as have a pressing or tightening quality. Left untreated, tension headaches may last for 30 minutes to up to 7 days.

BURNS

Severe burns can produce excruciating pain. Third-degree burns are the most severe, because the skin has been destroyed. First-degree burns are less severe than second- or third-degree burns.

TRAUMA

Musculoskeletal pain may be caused by trauma. Sport injuries, motor vehicle accidents, and workplace or home accidents can result in painful sprains, fractures, burns, cuts, and bruises.

NEUROPATHIC ORIGIN

DIABETIC NEUROPATHY

Diabetes can cause damage to peripheral nerves. Nerve damage results in numbness, pain, or tingling of the feet or legs. Symptoms of diabetic neuropathy become more severe as the disease progresses.

PHANTOM LIMB

Patients who have had a limb amputated may describe pain in the area where the limb was removed. It is believed that although the limb is no longer present, the nerves that innervated the limb are remapped or rewired, permitting nerve messages to continue to be received. The ability of the brain to restructure itself and adapt to injury is called *plasticity*.

SHINGLES

Shingles produces a reoccurring and painful skin rash and is caused by the herpes zoster virus. The herpes zoster virus lays dormant in nerve endings until activated. Shingles cannot be cured.

TRIGEMINAL NEURALGIA

Trigeminal neuralgia produces headache and intense stabbing pain in areas of the face innervated by branches of the trigeminal nerve (lips, eyes, nose, scalp, forehead, upper jaw, and lower jaw). Approximately 1% to 2% of persons with multiple sclerosis will develop trigeminal neuralgia.

Mechanism of Pain Signal Transmission

Painful stimuli trigger the release of neurotransmitters, amino acids, and peptides that carry signals to increase sensitivity to the pain or to dull the painful sensations (Figure 10-1). The transmission of the pain message begins with activation of nociceptors in peripheral tissues.

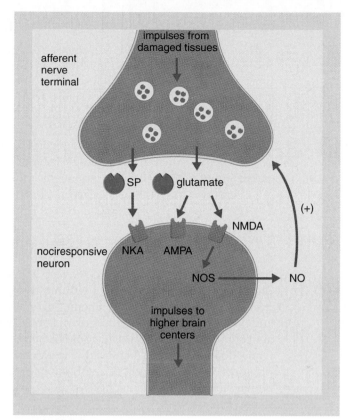

SP = substance P
NO = nitric oxide
NKA = neurokinin A

FIGURE 10-1 Mechanism of pain perception. *(From Page C, et al: Integrated Pharmacology, ed. 3, Philadelphia, Mosby, 2006.)*

The message travels rapidly to the dorsal horn of the spinal cord, where it is blocked, modified, or enhanced before carrying the pain message to the brain.

Neurochemistry of Pain

ROLES OF HISTAMINE, BRADYKININ, AND SEROTONIN

Histamine and bradykinin are released in response to tissue injury and are part of the immune system response. They produce inflammation, vasodilation, and pain. ***Bradykinin*** activates the enzyme (phospholipase A_2) that leads to the biosynthesis of prostaglandins. Prostaglandins are hormones that trigger pain response from peripheral nociceptors. Serotonin also stimulates nociceptors and causes pain when it is released by mast cells as part of the inflammatory response.

ROLE OF GLUTAMATE

Glutamate is an amino acid neurotransmitter that binds to nociceptors carrying the pain message to higher brain centers. Glutamate enhances the response to painful stimuli.

ROLE OF SUBSTANCE P

Substance P is a peptide that is involved in the production of pain sensations and controls pain perception. It acts as a neurotransmitter at the junction between nociceptors in the dorsal route of the spinal cord and afferent nerve terminals that will transmit the pain message to the brain. Neurokinin A is another neuropeptide that is involved in pain perception and the transmission pain sensations.

ROLES OF ENDORPHINS, ENKEPHALIN, AND DYNORPHIN

Endorphins, enkephalin, and *dynorphin* are opioid peptides released by the body in response to painful stimuli. They bind to opioid receptors in the brain and spinal cord and block or dull the pain sensations by inhibiting the release of substance P and glutamate. They act like natural painkillers (Figure 10-2).

ROLE OF γ-AMINOBUTYRIC ACID

GABA also plays a role in controlling pain. When GABA binds to $GABA_B$ receptors located on presynaptic afferent nerve fibers, it reduces the release of glutamate and substance P. The effect of GABA is inhibitory on nociceptors, and pain sensations are reduced.

Drugs Used to Treat Pain

OPIOIDS

Opiates are naturally occurring substances that are derived from the opium poppy and have been used for more than 2000 years to induce sleep and euphoria and to relieve diarrhea. Morphine and heroin are examples of opiates. *Opioid* is a term used to describe a drug that acts like morphine, whether naturally occurring or synthetically derived. Opiates and opioid drugs produce *analgesia*. Drugs that produce analgesia reduce pain sensations and alter pain perception. Some opioid analgesics are also used to treat opioid dependence. Once detoxification is achieved a maintenance dose is continued. Methadone and buprenorphine are examples of opioid agonists that are administered for management of drug dependence. Opioid antagonists such as naltrexone are used to treat drug and alcohol dependence, too.

MECHANISM OF ACTION

Opioids bind to opioid receptors located in the dorsal route of the spinal cord, brainstem, thalamus, hypothalamus, and limbic system. When naturally occurring peptides endorphin, enkephalin, and dynorphin or drugs bind to opioid receptors, nociceptive stimulation is reduced, decreasing pain sensation and raising the threshold for pain.

There are several types of opioid receptors: μ_1 and μ_2, κ_1, κ_2, and κ_3, and δ_1 and δ_2 receptors. The response to receptor stimulation is specific for each receptor type. Mu (μ) receptor stimulation produces analgesia, *euphoria*, respiratory depression, pupil constriction, decreased gastrointestinal motility and physical dependence. Kappa (κ) receptor binding

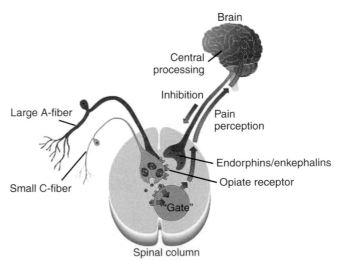

FIGURE 10-2 The role of endorphins/enkephalins in inhibiting pain perception. *(Modified from Lilley LL, Harrington S, Snyder JS:* Pharmacology and the nursing process, *ed 5, St Louis, 2007, Mosby.)*

produces analgesia, sedation, and pupil constriction, ***dysphoria,*** and hallucinations. Delta (δ) receptor stimulation produces analgesia and decreases contractions of smooth muscle.

CLASSIFICATION OF OPIOIDS

Agonists

Opioids are categorized according to their action at the opioid receptor. Opioid agonists activate μ, κ, or δ receptors. They produce analgesia and other adverse effects associated with stimulation of the specific opioid receptor. Partial agonists produce incomplete activation of the opioid receptor, producing less than maximum response.

Antagonists

Antagonists bind to the opioid receptor but do not activate it. They interfere with agonist binding. Antagonists are administered when reversal of the action of an opioid agonist is desired.

Mixed Agonist/Antagonists

The response produced by some opioids is mixed. Sometimes the opioid behaves like an agonist and sometimes it behaves like an antagonist. Agonist activity is exhibited if the patient has had no recent exposure to an opioid agonist (***opiate naïve***). If the patient is currently taking an opioid agonist, the mixed agonist/antagonist exhibits antagonist activity.

PHARMACOKINETICS

Oral absorption of opioid agonists, partial agonists, and mixed agonist/antagonist is varied and the potency of parenterally administered opioids is always superior to that of orally administered agents. Many orally administered opioids exhibit significant first-pass metabolism. Parenterally administered morphine is twice as potent as morphine that is administered orally. The average onset of action of orally administered opioids is approximately 30 minutes after administration. The onset of action of most parenterally administered opioids occurs within 10 to 15 minutes. A few opioids (meperidine, pentazocine, and butorphanol) begin working in less than 5 minutes. Peak effects are achieved between 30 minutes and 2 hours. The duration of action ranges between 2 and 6 hours for most opioid analgesics (Table 10-1).

ADVERSE REACTIONS

Adverse effects of opioid agonists, partial agonists, and mixed agonist/antagonists are determined by the extent to which they bind to specific opioid receptors. Morphine, codeine, and fentanyl act as agonists primarily at mu (μ) receptors, producing euphoria, respiratory depression, pupil constriction, constipation, and physical dependence. Pentazocine is a mixed agonist/antagonist that is a partial agonist at kappa (κ) receptors and a weak antagonist at mu (μ) receptors. It produces sedation and pinpoint pupils (Table 10-2).

PRECAUTIONS

All opioid agonists, partial agonists, and most mixed agonist/antagonists are controlled substances because they produce tolerance and dependence.

OPIOID ANTAGONISTS

Opioid antagonists are indicated for reversal of respiratory depression caused by opioid use. Respiratory depression may be produced by drugs administered during surgery for general anesthesia or may occur in infants born to opioid-dependent women. The opioid antagonist naltexone is also indicated for the treatment of opioid overdose and the management of drug and alcohol dependence. Naltrexone may produce drowsiness. The warning labels MAY CAUSE DROWSINESS; MAY IMPAIR ABILITY TO DRIVE and AVOID ALCOHOL should be applied to prescription vials. Both naltrexone and naloxone can precipitate withdrawal symptoms in patients that are opioid dependent.

TABLE 10-1   Comparison of Opioid Equivalent Doses, Onset, Peak, and Duration of Action

Drug and route	Equivalent dose*	Onset (min)	Peak (min)	Duration (hr)
Buprenorphine				
IM	0.3 mg	15	60	Up to 6
IV	0.3 mg	<15	<60	Up to 6
SL	—	—	—	—
Butorphanol				
IM	2 mg	10 to 30	30 to 60	3 to 4
IV	2 mg	2 to 3	30	2 to 4
Nasal spray	2 mg	—	—	—
Codeine				
PO	200 mg	30 to 45	60 to 120	4
IM	120 mg	10 to 30	30 to 60	4
SC	120 mg	10 to 30	30 to 60	4
Fentanyl				
IV	0.1 mg	—	—	1 to 1½
Transdermal	—	—	—	72
Hydromorphone				
PO	7.5 mg	30	90 to 120	4
IM	1.5 mg	15	30 to 60	4 to 5
IV	1.5 mg	10 to 15	15 to 30	2 to 3
SC	1.5 mg	15	30 to 90	4
Levorphanol				
PO	4 mg	10 to 60	90 to 120	4 to 5
IM	2 mg	—	60	4 to 5
IV	2 mg	—	<20	4 to 5
SC	2 mg	—	60 to 90	4 to 5
Meperidine				
PO	300 mg	15	60 to 90	2 to 4
IM	75 mg	10 to 15	30 to 50	2 to 4
IV	75 mg	1	5 to 7	2 to 4
SC	75 mg	10 to 15	30 to 50	2 to 4
Methadone				
PO	20 mg	30 to 60	90 to 120	4 to 6
IM	10 mg	10 to 20	60 to 120	4 to 5
IV	10 mg	—	15 to 30	3 to 4
Morphine				
PO	60 mg	—	10 to 120	4 to 5
IM	10 mg	10 to 30	30 to 60	4 to 5
IV	10 mg	—	20	4 to 5
SC	10 mg	10 to 30	50 to 90	4 to 5
Oxycodone				
PO	30 mg	—	60	3 to 4
Pentazocine				
PO	180 mg	15 to 30	60 to 90	3
IM	60 mg	15 to 20	30 to 60	2 to 3
IV	60 mg	2 to 3	15 to 30	2 to 3
SC	60 mg	15 to 20	30 to 60	2 to 3

*Dose in mg that produces an equivalent degree of analgesia as 10 mg of morphine.

TECH ALERT!
The following drugs have look-alike/sound-alike issues: codeine, Cardene, and Lodine; Lortab and Lorabid; Vicodin, Hycomine, and Hycodan; hydrocodone and hydromorphone Demerol and Demadex; meperidine and morphine; Roxanol and Roxicet; Avinza, Evista, and Invanz

TECH NOTE!
Duragesic patches are worn for 72 hours and should be dispensed with instructions on proper storage and disposal to prevent accidental poisoning.

TECH ALERT!
Product selection errors are common due to many strength combinations for hydrocodone and acetaminophen.

NONOPIOID ANALGESICS

NONSTEROIDAL ANTIINFLAMMATORY DRUGS AND ASPIRIN

Nonsteroidal antiinflammatory drugs (NSAIDs) and aspirin (ASA) are widely used in the treatment of pain with or without inflammation. They have analgesic, antiinflammatory, and antipyretic properties. An antipyretic is a drug that is capable of reducing fever. Their action and effectiveness are similar to those of salicylates (aspirin) but they have greater potency.

TABLE 10-2 Opioid-Induced Side Effects and Adverse Effects by Body System

Body System	Side Effect or Adverse Effect
Central nervous system	Sedation, disorientation, euphoria, ligh-headedness, dysphoria, lowered seizure threshold, and tremors
Cardiovascular system	Hypotension, palpitations, and flushing
Respiratory tract	Respiratory depression and aggravation of asthma
Gastrointestinal tract	Nausea, vomiting, constipation, and biliary tract spasm
Genitourinary tract	Urinary retention
Other	Itching, rash, and wheal information

From Lilley LL, Harrington S, Snyder JS: *Pharmacology and the Nursing Process,* 5th ed. St. Louis, Mosby, 2007.

Opioid Agonists

Generic name	U.S. brand name(s) / Canadian brand name(s)	Dosage forms and strengths	Controlled substance schedule
codeine*	Generics / Codeine Contin	**Injection:** 15 mg/ml and 30 mg/ml **Solution, oral:** 16 mg/5 ml **Tablet, controlled release (Codeine Contin):** 50 mg, 100 mg, 150 mg, 200 mg **Tablet, as phosphate:** 30 mg, 60 mg **Tablet, as sulfate:** 15 mg, 30 mg, 60 mg	C-II
codeine and acetaminophen (APAP)*	Tylenol with Codeine No. 2, Tylenol with Codeine No. 3, Tylenol with Codeine No. 4, / Tylenol with Codeine No. 1, Tylenol with Codeine No. 2, Tylenol with Codeine No. 3, Tylenol with Codeine No. 4	**Elixir:** APAP 120 mg and codeine 12 mg **Suspension:** APAP 120 mg and codeine 12 mg **Tablet, (Tylenol with Codeine No. 1):** acetaminophen 300 mg and codeine phosphate 8 mg **Tablet, (Tylenol with Codeine No. 2):** APAP 300 mg and codeine 15 mg **Tablet, (Tylenol with Codeine No. 3):** APAP 300 mg and codeine 30 mg **Tablet, (Tylenol with Codeine No. 4):** APAP 300 mg and codeine 60 mg	C-V C-III C-III C-III
fentanyl*	Actiq, Duragesic, Sublimaze / Actiq, Duragesic	**Injection, solution (Sublimaze):** 0.05 mg/ml **Lozenge (Actiq):** 200 mcg, 400 mcg, 600 mcg, 800 mcg, 1200 mcg, 1600 mcg **Transdermal (Duragesic):** 25 mcg, 50 mcg, 75 mcg, 100 mcg	C-II
hydrocodone and acetaminophen*	Anexsia, Lorcet 10/650, Lorcet-HD, Lortab, Stagesic, Vicodin, Vicodin ES, Vicodin HP, Zydone / Generics	**Capsule (Lorcet-HD, Stagesic):** 5 mg hydrocodone and 500 mg APAP **Elixir (Lortab):** 7.5 mg hydrocodone and 500 mg APAP/15 ml **Tablet (Anexsia):** 5 mg hydrocodone and 500 mg APAP; 7.5 mg/650 mg APAP **(Lorcet):** 10 mg/650 mg **(Lorcet Plus):** 7.5 mg/650 mg **(Lortab):** 2.5 mg/500 mg, 5 mg/500 mg, 7.5 mg/500 mg, 10 mg/500 mg **(Vicodin):** 5 mg/500 mg **(Vicodin ES):** 7.5 mg/750 mg **(Vicodin HP):** 10 mg/660 mg; (Zydone): 5 mg/400 mg, 7.5 mg/400 mg, 10 mg/400 mg	C-III
hydrocodone and ibuprofen*	Vicoprofen / Vicoprofen	**Tablet:** 5 mg/200 mg, 7.5 mg/200 mg hydrocodone/ibuprofen	C-III

Continued

Opioid Agonists—cont'd

Generic name	U.S. brand name(s) / Canadian brand name(s)	Dosage forms and strengths	Controlled substance schedule
hydromorphone*	Dilaudid, Dilaudid-HP, Palladone	**Capsule, controlled release (Hydromorph Contin):** 3 mg, 6 mg, 12 mg, 18 mg, 24 mg, 30 mg **Capsule, extended release (Pallidone):** 12 mg, 16 mg, 24 mg, 32 mg **Injection, powder for reconstitution (Dilaudid-HP):** 250 mg **Injection, solution:** 1 mg/ml, 2 mg/ml, 4 mg/ml, 10 mg/ml (Dilaudid-HP) **Liquid, oral (Dilaudid):** 1 mg/ml **Tablet, immediate release (Dilaudid):** 2 mg, 4 mg, 8 mg **Suppository (Dilaudid):** 3 mg	C-II
	Dilaudid, Dilaudid-HP, Dilaudid-HP Plus, Dilaudin-XP, Hydromorph Contin		
levorphanol*	Levo-Dromoran	**Injection, solution:** 2 mg/ml **Tablet:** 2 mg	C-II
	Not available		
meperidine*	Demerol, Meperitab	**Injection, solution (vials and prefilled syringe):** 25 mg/ml, 50 mg/ml, 75 mg/ml, 100 mg/ml **Injection, PCA:** 10 mg/ml (30 ml, 50 ml, 60 ml) **Syrup:** 50 mg/5 ml (500 ml) **Tablet:** 50 mg, 100 mg	C-II
	Demerol		
methadone*	Dolophine, Methadone Intensol, Methadose	**Injection, solution:** 10 mg/ml **Solution, oral:** 5 mg/5 ml, 10 mg/5 ml **Solution, oral concentrate (Methadose, Methadone Intensol):** 10 mg/ml **Tablet (Dolophine):** 5 mg, 10 mg **Tablet, dispersible (Methadose, Methadone Diskets):** 40 mg	C-II
	Dolophine, Metadol, Methadose		
morphine*	Astramorph/PF, Avinza, Duramorph, DepoDur, Kadian, MS Contin, Oramorph SR, Roxanol, Roxanol-T	**Capsule, extended release (Avinza):** 30 mg, 60 mg, 90 mg, 120 mg **Capsule, sustained release (Kadian):** 20 mg, 30 mg, 50 mg, 60 mg, 100 mg **Injection, extended release for epidural (DepoDur):** 10 mg/ml (1 ml, 1.5 ml, 2 ml) **Injection, epidural, intrathecal (Astramorph/PF, Duramorph):** 0.5 mg/ml, 1 mg/ml **Injection, solution:** 2 mg/ml, 4 mg/ml, 5 mg/ml, 8 mg/ml, 10 mg/ml, 15 mg/ml, 25 mg/ml **Solution, oral (Roxanol):** 20 mg/ml **Tablet, controlled release (MS Contin):** 15 mg, 30 mg, 60 mg, 100 mg, 200 mg **Tablet, sustained release (Oramorph SR):** 15 mg, 30 mg, 60 mg, 100 mg	C-II
	Kadian, MS Contin		
oxycodone*	OxyContin, Oxydose, OxyFast, Oxy IR Roxicodone Intensol	**Capsule, immediate release (Oxy IR):** 5 mg **Solution, oral (Roxicodone):** 5 mg/5 ml **Solution, oral concentrate (Oxydose, OxyFast, Roxicodone Intensol):** 20 mg/ml **Tablet, immediate release:** 5 mg, 15 mg, 30 mg **Tablet, controlled release:** 10 mg, 20 mg, 40 mg, 80 mg, 160 mg **Tablet, extended release:** 80 mg	C-II
	OxyContin, Oxy IR		

© 2005 GB

Opioid Agonists—cont'd

	Generic name	U.S. brand name(s) Canadian brand name(s)	Dosage forms and strengths	Controlled substance schedule
	oxycodone and acetaminophen*	Endocet, Percocet, Roxicet, Tylox Endocet, Oxycocet, Percocet, Percocet-Demi	**Capsule (Tylox):** 5 mg oxycodone/500 mg acetaminophen **Solution, oral (Roxicet):** 5 mg/325 mg/5 ml **Tablet (Endocet, Percocet):** 2.5 mg/325 mg, 5 mg/325 mg, 7.5 mg/325 mg, 7.5 mg/500 mg, 10 mg/325 mg, 10 mg/650 mg	C-II
	oxymorphone	Numorphan Numorphan	**Injection, solution:** 1 mg/ml, 1.5 mg/ml **Suppository, rectal:** 5 mg	C-II

*Generic available.

Mixed Agonist/Antagonists

	Generic name	U.S. brand name(s) Canadian brand(s)	Dosage forms and strengths	Controlled substance schedule
	buprenorphine	Buprenex, Subutex Buprenex	**Injection, solution (Buprenex):** 0.3 mg/ml **Tablet, sublingual (Subutex):** 2 mg, 8 mg	C-III
	buprenorphine and naloxone	Suboxone Not available	**Tablet, sublingual:** 2 mg buprenorphine and 0.5 mg naloxone, 8 mg buprenorphine and 2 mg naloxone	C-III
	butorphanol*	Stadol, Stadol NS Stadol NS	**Injection (Stadol):** 2 mg/ml **Intranasal solution (Stadol):** 10 mg/ml	C-IV

*Generic available.

Opioid Antagonists

	Generic name	U.S. brand name(s) Canadian brand(s)	Dosage forms and strengths	Usual adult dose
	naloxone*	Narcan Narcan	Injection, solution 0.4 mg/ml and 1 mg/ml	0.4 mg to 2 mg IV every 2 to 3 minutes. (Repeat every 20 to 60 minutes)
	naltrexone*	ReVia ReVia	50 mg tablet	Start 25 mg; 50 mg/day or 100 mg to 150 mg 3 times a week (up to 800 mg/day)

*Generic available.

Summary of Drugs Used to Manage Drug Dependence or Reverse Effects of Opioids

	Generic name	Dose	Onset (min)	Duration (min/hr)	Route
	buprenorphine buprenorphine and naloxone	Opioid dependence Opioid dependence	30 to 60 PO	12 hours (2 mg) up to 72 hours (>16 mg)	IV, PO PO
	methadone	Opioid dependence	30	24 to 36 hours	PO
	naloxone	Reverse opioid-induced respiratory depression of overdose	2	30 minutes	IV
	naltrexone	Alcohol dependence	15 to 30	50 mg (24 hours) 100 mg (48 hours) 150 mg (72 hours)	PO

*varies according to dose and route of administration

Summary of Opioid Analgesics

Generic name	U.S. brand name	Usual adult oral dose and dosing schedule	Warning labels
Opioid agonists			
codeine	Generics	**Immediate release, IM and subcutaneous injection:** 15 mg to 120 mg every 4 to 6 hours **Controlled release:** 50 mg to 300 mg every 12 hours	MAY CAUSE DROWSINESS; MAY IMPAIR ABILITY TO DRIVE
codeine and acetaminophen	Tylenol with Codeine #3	1 to 2 tablets every 4 hours (maximum 4 g daily)	AVOID ALCOHOL TAKE WITH FOOD
fentanyl	Duragesic	**For pain (opiate naïve):** 25 mcg to 100 mcg/hr system every 72 hours	MAY BE HABIT FORMING
hydrocodone and acetaminophen	Vicodin	2.5 to 10 mg every 4 to 6 hours (maximum dose: hydrocodone 60 mg and APAP 4 g/day)	TAKE EACH DOSE WITH A FULL GLASS OF WATER
hydrocodone and ibuprofen	Vicoprofen	1 to 2 tablets every 4 to 6 hours	
hydromorphone	Dilaudid	**For pain (opiate naïve):** **IV:** 0.2 mg to 0.6 mg every 2 to 3 hours; **PCA:** 0.2 mg/ml **Epidural:** 1 mg to 1.5 mg (bolus); 0.05 mg to 0.075 mg/ml (infusion) **Oral, controlled release:** 3 mg to 30 mg every 12 hours **Oral (immediate release):** 2 to 8 mg every 3 to 4 hours	SWALLOW WHOLE; DON'T CRUSH OR CHEW ROTATE SITE OF APPLICATION (Transdermal)
levorphanol	Levo-Dromoran	**For pain (opiate naïve):** **Oral:** 2 mg to 4 mg every 6 to 8 hours **IM and SC:** 1 mg to 2 mg every 6 to 8 hours	
meperidine	Demerol	**For pain (opiate naïve):** **Oral, IM, and SC:** 50 mg to 150 mg every 2 to 4 hours **IV:** 5 mg to 10 mg every 5 minutes **PCA:** 5 mg to 25 mg on demand	
methadone	Dolophine	**For pain (opiate naïve):** **Oral:** 2.5 mg to 10 mg every 3 to 4 hours **IV, IM, SC:** 2.5 mg to 10 mg every 8 to 12 hours **Detoxification (oral):** 15 mg to 40 mg daily	
morphine	MS Contin	**For pain (opiate naïve):** **Oral (prompt release):** 10 mg to 30 mg every 3 to 4 hours; Oral (extended release and sustained release capsules): dosed 1 to 2 times daily Controlled release (tablet) dosed every 8 to 12 hours **IV:** Start 2.5 mg to 5 mg every 3 to 4 hours; continuous infusion up to 80 mg/hour **PCA:** 0.5 mg to 2.5 mg, lock out interval: 5 to 10 minutes **IM, SC:** 5 to 10 mg every 3 to 4 hours **Epidural:** 10 mg as a single dose	

Summary of Opioid Analgesics—cont'd

Generic name	U.S. brand name	Usual adult oral dose and dosing schedule	Warning labels
Oxycodone	OxyContin	**For pain (opiate naïve):** Immediate release: 5 mg every 6 hours **Controlled release:** 10 mg to 40 mg every 12 hours	
oxycodone and acetaminophen	Percocet, Tylox	1 to 2 tablets every 4 to 6 hours (maximum 4 g APAP daily)	
oxymorphone	Numorphan	**IM, IV, SC:** Start 0.5 mg; 1 mg to 1.5 mg every 4 to 6 hours **Rectal:** 5 mg every 4 to 6 hours	
Mixed agonist/antagonists			
buprenorphine	Buprenex	**For pain (opiate naïve):** IM, IV: 0.3 mg every 6 to 8 hours	MAY CAUSE DROWSINESS; MAY IMPAIR ABILITY TO DRIVE
buprenorphine and naloxone	Suboxone	**Opioid dependence:** 4 mg to 24 mg/day titrated according to avoid withdrawal symptoms	
butorphanol	Stadol	**Acute pain (IM, IV):** 1 mg to 4 mg every 3 to 4 hours; labor pain 1 mg to 2 mg within 4 hours of anticipated delivery **Migraine (nasal spray):** 1 spray in 1 nostril, may repeat in 60 to 90 minutes if needed (maximum 4 doses/day)	AVOID ALCOHOL MAY BE HABIT FORMING

TECH NOTE!

Buprenorphine tablets may only be prescribed for the treatment of opioid dependency. Valid prescriptions are written by prescribers that have a DEA No. specifically for buprenorphine.

TECH NOTE!

Butorphanol is prescribed for migraine headache pain.

TECH ALERT!

Naloxone and naltrexone have look-alike/sound-alike issues.

Mechanism of Action

Like aspirin, NSAIDs decrease prostaglandin synthesis by inhibiting the action of cyclooxygenase (COX). Most NSAIDs are not selective. They inhibit COX-1 and COX-2. COX-1 is found throughout the body and is important for control of blood flowing through the vasculature and regulation of platelet aggregation. COX-2 is formed in selected cells as part of the immune response. COX-2 is involved in the biosynthesis of prostaglandins at the site of injury.

Pharmacokinetics

Aspirin and NSAIDs are well absorbed orally. Aspirin is a weak acid (acetylsalicyclic acid), and the rate of absorption varies according to the pH of stomach, small intestine, and urine. Enteric-coated aspirin is released in the pH of the intestine rather than in the stomach. Acidification of the urine with vitamin C can increase rate of reabsorption and sodium bicarbonate enhances elimination (see Chapter 2). Aspirin is eliminated in the urine.

NSAIDs are structurally dissimilar; however, they are biologically similar. Oral absorption is good and bioavailability ranges between 80% and 99%. They are all highly protein bound, more than 97%, and they all are primarily eliminated in the urine.

Adverse Reactions

All of the NSAIDs and aspirin can produce nausea, gastrointestinal bleeding, and ulceration. Some NSAIDs can produce dizziness. Serious side effects include salicylism (aspirin), hepatoxicity (ketorolac), and agranulocytosis (indomethocin, flurbiprofen). Recently, selective COX-2 inhibitors rofecoxib (Vioxx) and valdecoxib (Bextra) were withdrawn from the market because of increased risk for heart attack and stroke. Celecoxib (Celebrex) remains the only selective COX-2 inhibitor currently in use.

Commonly used nonopioid analgesics

	Generic name	Brand name	Usual adult dose	Side effects	Warning labels
	Salicylates				
	aspirin	Ecotrin, Bayer, Anacin	325 mg to 650 mg every 4 to 6 hours (maximum 4 g/day)	Gastrointestinal upset, bleeding, tinnitus, salicylism	TAKE WITH FOOD
	diflunisal	Dolobid	250 mg to 500 mg twice a day	Gastrointestinal upset, rash, drowsiness, jaundice	TAKE WITH FOOD MAY CAUSE DIZZINESS OR DROWSINESS AVOID ASPIRIN AND RELATED DRUGS
	p-Aminophenol				
	acetaminophen		325 mg to 650 mg every 4 to 6 hours (maximum 4 g/day)	Skin, liver toxicity, kidney toxicity	
	Indoles				
	indomethacin	Indocin	25 mg to 50 mg 2 to 3 times a day	Gastrointestinal upset, headache, dizziness, (drowsiness—sulindac) tinnitus, agranulocytosis (fatigue, apnea—indomethacin)	TAKE WITH FOOD MAY CAUSE DIZZINESS OR DROWSINESS AVOID ASPIRIN AND RELATED DRUGS
	sulindac	Clinoril	150 mg to 200 mg twice a day or 300 mg to 400 mg once a day		
	etodolac	Lodine Lodine XL	200 mg to 400 mg every 6 to 8 hours 400 mg to 1000 mg once a day	Gastrointestinal upset, dizziness, drowsiness, palpitations	
	phenylpropionic acid				
	flurbiprofen	Ansaid Ocufen	200 mg to 300 mg every 6 to 12 hours (maximum 300 mg/day) 1 drop every 30 minutes starting 2 hours before surgery	Gastrointestinal upset, headache, tinnitus, dizziness, kidney toxicity (ibuprofen)	TAKE WITH FOOD MAY CAUSE DIZZINESS OR DROWSINESS AVOID ASPIRIN AND RELATED DRUGS
	ibuprofen	Motrin	200 mg to 800 mg every 4 to 8 hours (maximum 3200 mg/day)		
	ketoprofen	Orudis Oruvail (extended release)	50 mg to 75 mg 3 to 4 times a day 200 mg once a day		
	oxaprozin	Daypro	600 mg to 1200 mg once a day		
	Naphthylpropionic acids				
	naproxen	Naproxen Naproxen DS	Start 500 mg to 750 mg; then 250 mg every 6 to 8 hours (naproxen base)*	Gastrointestinal upset, headache, tinnitus, rash, dizziness	TAKE WITH FOOD MAY CAUSE DIZZINESS OR DROWSINESS AVOID ASPIRIN AND RELATED DRUGS
	naproxen naand	Anaprox Anaprox DS			

Commonly used nonopioid analgesics—cont'd

	Generic name	Brand name	Usual adult dose	Side effects	Warning labels
	Naphthyalkanones				
	nabumetone	Relafen	1000 mg to 1500 mg/day dosed 1 to 2 times/day	Gastrointestinal upset, dizziness, agranulocytosis	TAKE WITH FOOD MAY CAUSE DIZZINESS OR DROWSINESS AVOID ASPIRIN AND RELATED DRUGS
	Anthranilic acids				
	meclofenamate	Meclomen (Canada)	50 mg to 100 mg every 4 to 6 hours (maximum: 400 mg/day)	Gastrointestinal upset, headache, dizziness, increased urination	TAKE WITH FOOD MAY CAUSE DIZZINESS OR DROWSINESS AVOID ASPIRIN AND RELATED DRUGS
	Pyrroleacetic acid				
	tolmetin	Tolectin	400 mg to 600 mg 3 times a day	Gastrointestinal upset, headache, dizziness, rash, liver toxicity (ketorolac), palpitations (tolmetin)	TAKE WITH FOOD MAY CAUSE DIZZINESS OR DROWSINESS AVOID ASPIRIN AND RELATED DRUGS
	ketorolac	Toradol Acular	**PO:** Start 20 mg then 10 mg every 4 to 6 hour (maximum: 40 mg/day) IM or IV 30 mg every 6 hours **Ophthalmic:** 1 drop 4 times a day		
	Phenylacetic acid				
	diclofenac	Voltaren Voltaren XR Voltaren Rapide (Canada)	100 mg to 200 mg 2 to 4 times a day (oral)	Gastrointestinal upset, pain, nausea and vomiting, ulceration	TAKE WITH FOOD MAY CAUSE DIZZINESS OR DROWSINESS AVOID ASPIRIN AND RELATED DRUGS
	Oxicams				
	meloxicam	Mobic	7.5 mg to 15 mg once daily	Gastrointestinal upset, constipation or diarrhea, gas, dizziness, edema, gastrointestinal bleeding, hypertension	TAKE WITH FOOD MAY CAUSE DIZZINESS OR DROWSINESS AVOID ASPIRIN AND RELATED DRUGS SWALLOW WHOLE; DON'T CRUSH OR CHEW TAKE WITH A FULL GLASS OF WATER SHAKE WELL— SUSPENSION
	piroxicam	Feldene	10 mg to 20 mg once a day		

Continued

Commonly used nonopioid analgesics—cont'd

	Generic name	Brand name	Usual adult dose	Side effects	Warning labels
Coxibs					
	celecoxib	Celebrex	200 mg twice a day	Gastrointestinal upset, ulceration, heart attack, stroke	TAKE WITH FOOD MAY CAUSE DIZZINESS OR DROWSINESS AVOID ASPIRIN AND RELATED DRUGS

*550 mg naproxen Na$^+$ = 500 mg naproxen base.

Drug Treatment for Neuropathic Pain

Neuropathic pain is associated with nerve injury caused by trauma, infection, or chronic diseases such as diabetes and is treated with different drugs than are used other types of pain. This pain is unique because pain sensations are felt even though the injury is healed. When nerves are damaged, the body may make adaptations to compensate for the nerve damage. These changes can lead to persistent nerve pain. Nerve injury can led to sensitization of nerve terminals. This lowers the threshold for neuron firing (action potential) and increases the response to stimuli. Nerve damage can result in a reorganization of nerves. The rewiring sometimes goes haywire, causing painful sensations even after limbs have been amputated. Another cause for neuropathic pain is changes in the sodium and calcium ion channels that result in increasing or decreasing levels of ions involved in neuronal firing. Last, nerve injuries can cause a loss of inhibitory pathways such as the GABA pathways (described in Chapter 8).

Drugs used in the treatment of neuropathic pain include antidepressants (amitriptyline), antiseizure drugs (gabapentin, lamotrigine), local anesthetics (lidocaine, mexilitine), and capsaicin. Tricyclic antidepressants are the first choice for the treatment of neuropathic pain. They inhibit the reuptake of neurotransmitters (e.g., norepinephrine and serotonin) at receptor sites in the spinal cord that are responsible for modulating pain sensation. Selective serotonin reuptake inhibitors are less effective than tricyclic antidepressants.

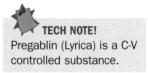

TECH NOTE!
Pregablin (Lyrica) is a C-V controlled substance.

Gabapentin, pregabalin, and carbamazepine are antiseizure drugs that are used for the treatment of diabetic neuropathy, nerve pain caused by herpes virus infection, and trigeminal neuralgia. Topiramate enhances inhibitory effects of GABA in addition to its action on voltage-dependent sodium channels. These drugs are discussed in detail in Chapter 9.

Lidocaine and mexilitine are local anesthetics used in the treatment of neuropathic pain, but the use of mexilitine is not U.S. Food and Drug Administration approved. Both drugs block sodium channels. Lidocaine may be administered intravenously or topically. Lidocaine patches are indicated for the treatment of nerve pain caused by herpes infection (shingles). Capsaicin is derived from chili peppers. It is applied topically and it depletes substance P from nerve terminals. It is indicated for the treatment of diabetic neuropathy and shingles.

Nondrug Treatment of Pain

The treatment of pain, especially chronic pain, requires a multifaceted approach that includes drug therapy and nondrug therapy. Nondrug therapies that may be supportive are education, physical therapy, occupational therapy, cognitive behavioral therapy (counseling), acupuncture, chiropractic, and transcutaneous electrical stimulation (TENS) (Figure 10-3). The transcutaneous electrical stimulation device delivers electrical impulses through the skin that cause contraction and numbness. This blocks the transmission of pain messages to the spinal cord by peripheral nerves. Cryotherapy (cold packs) and heat packs can reduce swelling, which can also decrease pain.

Commonly Used to Treat Neuropathic Pain

	Generic name	Brand name	Usual adult dose	Side effects	Warning labels
	Antidepressants				
	amitriptyline	Levate (Canada)	25 mg to 100 mg at bedtime	Sedation, dry mouth, urinary retention, nausea, blurred vision, photosensitivity	MAY CAUSE DROWSINESS
	desipramine	Norpramin	150 to 200 mg/day in 1 to 2 doses		ALCOHOL MAY INTENSIFY THIS EFFECT
	imipramine	Tofranil	1 to 3 mg/kg/dose at bedtime		MAY IMPAIR ABILITY TO DRIVE
					DO NOT DISCONTINUE WITHOUT MEDICAL SUPERVISION
					MAY DISCOLOR URINE (BLUE-GREEN)
					AVOID PROLONGED EXPOSURE TO SUNLIGHT
	Antiseizure drugs				
	gabapentin	Neurontin	300 to 1800 mg in 3 divided doses	Dizziness, confusion, fatigue, ataxia and nausea, double vision, blurred vision, dry mouth, and constipation	MAY CAUSE DROWSINESS; MAY IMPAIR ABILITY TO DRIVE
	pregabalin	Lyrica	50 to 100 mg 3 times a day		AVOID ALCOHOL
					TAKE WITH FOOD
	carbamazepine	Tegretol	400 mg to 800 mg twice a day	Nausea, vomiting, sedation, dizziness, ataxia, bruising, jaundice, and visual disturbances	DO NOT DISCONTINUE WITHOUT MEDICAL SUPERVISION
					SHAKE WELL
					SWALLOW WHOLE; DON'T CRUSH OR CHEW
					AVOID ANTACIDS WITHIN 2 HOURS OF DOSE—gabapentin, phenytoin AVOID
					PREGNANCY—phenytoin
	Local anesthetics				
	lidocaine	generic only	Nerve block and post herpetic neuralgia[+] Maximum 4.5 mg/kg/dose	Drowsiness, dizziness numbness, agitation, hypotension, heart block	MAY CAUSE DROWSINESS; MAY IMPAIR ABILITY TO DRIVE
					AVOID ALCOHOL
	Topicals				
	lidocaine	Lidoderm	1 to 3 patches up to 12 hours/day	Numbness, local irritation	ROTATE SITE OF APPLICATION
	capsaicin	Zostrix	Apply 3 to 4 times a day	Burning, stinging	WASH HANDS AFTER USE

[+]not FDA approved.

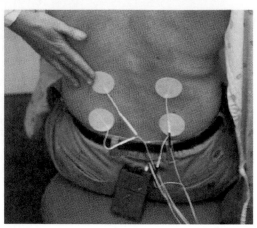

FIGURE 10-3 Transcutaneous nerve stimulation unit. *(From Ignatavicius D, workman L:* Medical-surgical nursing, *ed 5, Philadelphia, 2006, WB Saunders.)*

CHAPTER SUMMARY

- Acute pain may triggered by an injury, burn, infection, or some other stimuli and be self-limiting.
- Chronic pain may persist for years and is inadequately controlled by pharmaceuticals.
- Psychological factors can influence a person's tolerance for pain and can determine whether the outcome of treatment is successful.
- Patient-controlled analgesia permits patients to control the frequency of administration of their dose of pain medications.
- Neuropathic pain is associated with nerve injury caused by trauma, infection, or chronic diseases such as diabetes and is treated with different drugs than other types of pain.
- Osteoarthritis, gout, headache, burns, trauma, and low back pain are examples of pain with a nociceptor origin.
- Painful stimuli trigger the release of neurotransmitters, amino acids, and peptides that carry signals to increase sensitivity to the pain or to dull the painful sensations.
- Histamine, bradykinins, serotonin, prostaglandins, glutamate, and substance P are involved in the transmission of signals for pain sensation and pain perception.
- Endorphans, enkephalin, and dynorphin bind to opioid receptors and act like natural pain killers.
- Opioids are naturally occurring or synthetically derived drugs the act like morphine and are used to treat pain.
- Opioid receptors are mu (μ), kappa (κ), and delta (δ) and stimulation produces analgesia. The euphoria, dysphoria, respiratory depression, pupil constriction, decreased gastrointestinal motility, and physical dependence associated with opioid use are linked to specific receptors.
- Opioid agonists activate μ, κ, or δ receptors.
- Antagonists bind to the opioid receptor but do not activate it.
- Mixed agonist/antagonists behave like an agonist when the patient has had no recent exposure to an opioid agonist (opiate naïve).
- The potency of parenterally administered opioids is always superior to orally administered agents.
- All opioid agonists, partial agonists, and most mixed agonist/antagonists are controlled substances because they produce tolerance and dependence.
- Opioid antagonists and some mixed agonist/antagonists are used to treat drug dependence and opioid-induced respiratory depression.
- Nonsteroidal antiinflammatory drugs (NSAIDs) and aspirin are widely used in the treatment of pain with or without inflammation.
- NSAIDs have analgesic, antiinflammatory, and antipyretic properties.

- Aspirin and NSAIDs decrease prostaglandin synthesis by inhibiting the action of cyclo-oxygenase (COX), an enzyme involved in the biosynthesis of prostaglandins. Protaglandins are important mediators of pain.
- Most NSAIDs are not selective. They inhibit COX-1 and COX-2.
- COX-1 controls the flow of blood through the vasculature and regulates platelet aggregation. COX-2 is formed in selected cells as part of the immune response and is involved in the biosynthesis of prostaglandins at the site of injury.
- Recently, selective COX-2 inhibitors rofecoxib and valdecoxib were withdrawn from the market because of increased risk for heart attack and stroke.
- All of the NSAIDs and aspirin can produce nausea, gastrointestinal bleeding, and ulceration.
- Enteric-coated aspirin is released in the pH of the intestine rather than in the stomach.

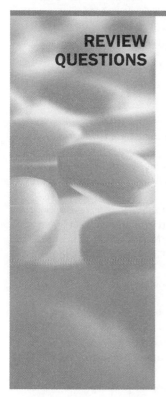

REVIEW QUESTIONS

Multiple Choice

1. _____ pain may triggered by an injury, burn, infection, or some other stimuli and be self-limiting.
   - a. chronic
   - b. dull
   - c. acute
   - d. nerve

2. The most common of all arthritic conditions is
   - a. gout
   - b. osteoarthritis
   - c. rheumatoid arthritis
   - d. ankylosis

3. _____ are hormones that trigger pain response from peripheral nociceptors.
   - a. histamines
   - b. serotonins
   - c. prostaglandins
   - d. norepinephrines

4. *Opiate* is a term used to describe _____ derived drugs that act like morphine.
   - a. naturally
   - b. synthetically
   - c. both a and b
   - d. none of the above

5. Is the following statement true or false? "Agonists activate a receptor and antagonists do not activate a receptor."
   - a. true
   - b. false

6. What controlled substance schedule does oxycodone fall into?
   - a. C-II
   - b. C-III
   - c. C-IV
   - d. C-V

7. Naloxone (Narcan), which is indicated for reversal of respiratory depression caused by opioid use and opioid overdose, is an example of an
   - a. agonist
   - b. antagonist

8. **NSAIDs have analgesic, antiinflammatory, and antipyretic properties.**
    a. true
    b. false

9. **The only COX-2 inhibitor that remains currently in use is**
    a. Vioxx
    b. Bextra
    c. acetaminophen
    d. Celebrex

10. **Acupuncture, chiropractic, and transcutaneous electrical stimulation are all drug treatments for pain.**
    a. true
    b. false

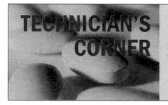
TECHNICIAN'S CORNER

1. Describe the difference between neuropathic and muscular pain. Can they be intertwined?
2. When a patient who has suffered for years with chronic pain asks, "Is there anything else I can do besides take pain medicines for my pain?" What can you tell the patient?

BIBLIOGRAPHY

Adelman J, Lewit E: Comparative aspects of triptans in treating migraine, *Clin Cornerstone,* 4:1-19, 2001.

Bennett M, Smith S, Torrance N, Lee A: Can pain be more or less neuropathic? Comparison of symptom assessment tools with ratings of certainty by clinicians, International Association for the Study of Pain, *Pain,* 122:289-294, 2006.

Freeman-Wilson K: *Methadone maintenance and other pharmacotherapeutic interventions in the treatment of opioid dependence,* National Drug Institute, Drug Court Practitioner: Fact Sheet, April 2002, vol. III No.1. Retrieved from http://www.ndci.org/publication/MethadoneFactSheet.pdf.

Kalant H, Grant D, Mitchell J: *Principles of medical pharmacology* (pp 236-251), ed 7. Toronto, 2007, Elsevier Canada, A Division of Reed Elsevier Canada.

Kidd B: Osteoarthritis and joint pain: Topical review, International Association for the Study of Pain, *Pain,* 123:6-9, 2006.

Lance L, Lacy C, Armstrong L, Goldman M: *Drug information handbook for the allied health professional,* ed 12, Hudson, OH, 2005, APhA Lexi-Comp.

Lintzeris N, et al: *National clinical guidelines and procedures for use of buprenorphine in the treatment of opioid dependency.* Retrieved from http://www.nationaldrugstrategy.gov.au/pdf/buprenorphine_guide.pdf.

Macfarlane G, Jones G, Hannaford P: Managing low back pain presenting in primary care: Where do we go from here? International Association for the Study of Pain, *Pain,* 122:219-222, 2006.

Marcus D: Treatment of nonmalignant chronic pain, *Am Fam Phys,* 61:1-8, 2000.

National Institute of Neurological Disorders and Stroke: *Pain: Hope through research,* Bethesda, MD, NINDS, National Institutes of Health, U.S. Department of Health and Human Services. Updated June 2006. NIH Publication No. 01-2406.

Page C, Curtis M, Sutter M, Walker M, Hoffman B: *Integrated pharmacology* (pp 272-247), Philadelphia, 2005, Elsevier Mosby.

Raffa RB, Rawls SM, Beyzarov EP: *Netter's Illustrated pharmacology* (p 85), Philadelphia, Saunders, 2005

Teng J, Mekhail N: Neuropathic pain: Mechanisms and treatment options, World Institute of Pain, *Pain Pract,* 3:8-21, 2003.

USP Center for Advancement of Patient Safety: *Use caution: avoid confusion.* USP Quality Review No. 79, Rockville, MD, April 2004, USP Center for Advancement of Patient Safety.

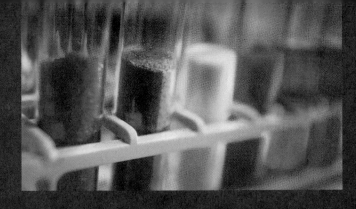

Treatment of Migraine Headache and Alzheimer's Disease

LEARNING OBJECTIVES

- Describe the cause of migraine headaches.
- Describe the function of neurotransmitters associated with symptoms of migraines.
- Describe the etiology of Alzheimer's disease.
- Describe the function of neurotransmitters associated with symptoms of Alzheimer's disease.
- Classify medications used in the treatment of migraines and Alzheimer's disease.
- Describe mechanism of action for each class of drugs used to treat migraines and Alzheimer's disease.
- Identify warning labels and precautionary messages associated with medications used to treat migraines and Alzheimer's disease.
- Identify significant drug look-alike/sound-alike issues.
- Learn the terminology associated with the treatment of migraine headaches and Alzheimer's disease.

KEY TERMS

Acetylcholinesterase: Enzyme that degrades the neurotransmitter acetylcholine.

Alzheimer's disease: Neurodegenerative disease that causes memory loss, behavioral changes, and immobility.

ApoE4 allele: Defective form of apolipoprotein E that is associated with Alzheimer's disease.

Cluster headache: Intensely painful vascular headache that occurs in groups and produces pain on one side of the head.

Dementia: Condition associated with a loss of memory and cognition.

Migraine: Vascular headache that is often accompanied by nausea and visual disturbances.

Neurodegeneration: Destruction of nerve cells.

Neuroprotective: Protects nerve cells from damage.

Plaques: Sticky, dense substances composed of a protein called beta amyloid that fill the spaces between neurons and interfere with the transmission of signals between neurons.

Tangles: Twisted fibers made up of clumps of a protein called tau that interfere with nerve signal transmission.

Migraine Headache

Approximately 10% of the population or nearly 29 million Americans and 3.4 million Canadians experience migraine headaches. Migraines and cluster headaches are vascular headaches. *Migraine* headaches are typically unilateral; affecting only one side of the head, however, the headache can spread to the opposite side. They may be preceded by an aura. An *aura* is an unusual sensation that is experienced just before the onset of the migraine headache. Severe throbbing pain is characteristic of migraines, as are nausea, photophobia (eyes are sensitive to the light), and phonophobia (sensitivity to noise). Resting in a quiet area with the lights off can sometimes improve migraine symptoms. Physical activity worsens migraine symptoms. Acute migraine attacks can last between 4 and 72 hours; the average is 29 hours. Migraine headaches occur more frequently in women than in men. A *cluster headache* is a frequently reoccurring vascular headache that produces pain on one side of the head. Cluster headaches occur more frequently in men.

PATHOPHYSIOLOGY OF MIGRAINE HEADACHES

Migraine headaches are triggered by numerous events, including stress, consumption of certain foods, red wine, caffeinated beverages, and exposure to bright or flashing lights. The trigger sets off a series of events that starts with the release of vasoactive neuropeptides that cause blood vessels in the brain to first constrict and then dilate. The trigger produces vasospasms, which reduce blood flow to the brain. Platelets in the blood clump together and cause the release of serotonin, which further constricts blood vessels. This triggers sets off afferent signals via the trigeminal nerve to release prostaglandins and other neurochemicals that dilate blood vessels, produce inflammation, and stimulate nociceptors. This causes the throbbing head pain characteristic of migraine headaches.

DRUG TREATMENT FOR MIGRAINE HEADACHE

Treatment of migraines is aimed at stopping the current migraine attack and preventing future migraines. Serotonin (5-hydroxytryptamine [5-HT]) agonists, ergot alkaloids, antidepressants (norepinephrine [NE] and serotonin reuptake inhibitors and monoamine oxidase [MAOIs]), β-blockers, and antiseizure drugs are used in the treatment and prevention of migraine headaches.

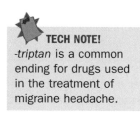

TECH NOTE!
-triptan is a common ending for drugs used in the treatment of migraine headache.

TRIPTANS

The triptans are the most widely prescribed drugs for the treatment of migraine headaches. They are administered during an acute attack to lessen symptoms and to stop the headache from progressing to more severe migraine symptoms. They are administered at the first sign of an impending migraine (aura).

Mechanism of Action

The triptans are selective serotonin (5-HT) receptor agonists. They have a high affinity for $5-HT_{1B}$ and $5-HT_{1D}$ receptors, which stimulate vasoconstriction (Figure 11-1).

Pharmacokinetics

The triptans are available for administration via mouth, subcutaneously, and intranasally. Subcutaneous injection produces the most rapid response and is the most effective route of administration; however, intranasal administration is also rapid and has fewer adverse reactions. Oral formulations have a slower onset of action. The half-life of triptans ranges between 2 hours and 25 hours. Triptans that have a long half-life, such as frovatriptan ($T\frac{1}{2} = 24$ hours) and naratriptan ($T\frac{1}{2} = 8$ hours) are more effective in preventing headache reoccurrence.

Adverse Reactions

The vasoconstriction caused by triptans is responsible for their therapeutic effects but can result in serious cardiac side effects, including arrhythmia, angina, coronary vasospasm, and myocardial infarction (heart attack). Vasoconstriction can also cause high blood pressure

Triptan Drugs: Mechanism of Action

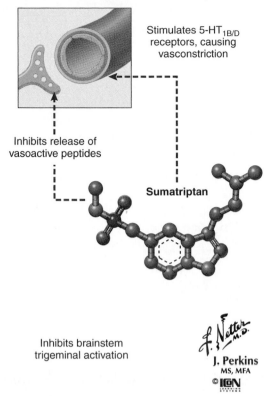

Stimulates 5-HT$_{1B/D}$ receptors, causing vasconstriction

Inhibits release of vasoactive peptides

Sumatriptan

Inhibits brainstem trigeminal activation

J. Perkins
MS, MFA

FIGURE 11-1 Mechanism of action for triptan drugs. *(From Raffa RB, Rawls SM, Beyzarov EP: Netter's illustrated pharmacology, Philadelphia, 2005, WB Saunders.)*

and stroke. Less serious and more common side effects are pain, tightness, and burning at the site of injection; dizziness; nausea; hot flashes; dry mouth; and fatigue.

Precautions

The use of triptans is limited. Nearly all triptans are restricted to a maximum of two doses per 24 hours. Frovatriptan is restricted to three doses per 24 hours. The safety of treating more than four migraines per month has not been established for most of the triptans.

OTHER PHARMACEUTICAL TREATMENTS FOR MIGRAINE HEADACHES

Ergot alkaloids, β-blockers, tricyclic antidepressants, and antiseizure drugs are also prescribed for the treatment of migraine headaches. A summary of these agents is found in the following table.

Alzheimer's Disease

Alzheimer's disease is a neurodegenerative disease that causes memory loss, behavioral changes, and immobility. According to the NIH National Insitute on Aging, 4.5 million Americans have Alzheimer's disease. Nearly 290,000 Canadians also have the disease. The risk for Alzheimer's disease increases with advancing age. In fact, nearly 5% of the adult population aged 65 years will have Alzheimer's disease. That percentage will double by age 70 years, and by age 85, nearly half of all men and women will have the disease. Although advancing age is an important risk factor for the development of Alzheimer's disease, *dementia* is not a normal part of the aging process.

Another risk factor for developing Alzheimer's disease is family history. Early-onset, familial Alzheimer's disease affects adults between 30 years and 60 years and is associated with the gene that makes the protein apolipoprotein E (*ApoE*). *Apoliprotein E* helps carry cholesterol in the blood. Approximately 40% of people with Azheimer's disease have a defective

Comparison of Triptans

Generic name (brand name)	Onset (min)	Repeat time (hr)	Route	Headache* effectiveness (%)	Dose (mg)**
almotriptan (Axert)	30	2	PO, tablet	57 to 68	25
eletriptan (Relpax)	30	2	PO, tablet	54 to 65	40
				68 to 77	80
frovatriptan (Frova)	30	2	PO, tablet	40	2.5
naratriptan (Amerge)	30	4	PO, tab	48	2.5
rizatriptan (Maxalt, Maxalt-MLT)	30	2	PO, tablet	73	10
		2	Wafer		
sumatriptan (Imitrex)	10 to 15	1	SC	80 to 85	6
	15	2	Nasal	60 to 86	20
	30	2	PO, tablet	51 to 61	50
zolmitriptan (Zomig)	30	2	PO, tablet	59 to 69	2.5
		2	Wafer		
	10 to 15		Nasal	24 to 61	5

*% patients reporting pain relief at 2 hr after dosing
**Dose associated with headache effectiveness (%)

Drugs Used in the Treatment of Migraine Headache: "Triptans" Dosage Forms and Strength

Generic name	U.S. brand name(s) / Canadian brand(s)	Dosage forms and strengths
almotriptan	Axert	**Tablet:** 6.25 mg, 12.5 mg
	Axert	
eletriptan	Relpax	**Tablet:** 20 mg, 40 mg
	Relpax	
frovatriptan	Frova	**Tablet:** 2.5 mg
	Frova	
naratriptan	Amerge	**Tablet:** 1 mg, 2.5 mg
	Amerge	
rizatriptan	Maxalt, Maxalt-MLT	**Tablet (Maxalt):** 5 mg, 10 mg **Tablet, disintegrating (Maxalt-MLT, Maxalt-RPD):** 5 mg, 10 mg
	Maxalt, Maxalt-RPD	
sumatriptan	Imitrex	**Injection, as solution:** 12 mg/ml (0.5 ml) **Intranasal solution:** 5 mg, 20 mg (100 μL unit dose spray device) **Tablet:** 25 mg, 50 mg, 100 mg
	Imitrex	
zolmitriptan	Zomig, Zomig-ZMT	**Nasal solution:** 5 mg/0.1 ml (0.1 ml) **Tablet:** 2.5 mg, 5 mg **Tablet, disintegrating (Zomig-ZMT, Zomig-Rapimelt:** 2.5 mg, 5 mg
	Zomig, Zomig-Rapimelt	

form of ApoE, although not everyone with the ***ApoE4 allele*** will develop the disease. Only 15% of people with the defective *ApoE4* allele will develop Alzheimer's disease. Other possible risk factors for the development of Alzheimer's disease are high blood pressure, high cholesterol, and low folate levels (vitamin B$_9$).

Summary of Triptans Used in the Treatment of Migraine Headaches

Generic name	U.S. brand name	Usual adult oral dose and dosing schedule	Warning labels
almotriptan	Axert	**Oral:** 6.25 mg to 12.5 mg as a single dose; repeat dose in 2 hours if needed	DO NOT TAKE MORE THAN 2 DOSES IN 24 HOURS
eletriptan	Relpax	**Oral:** 20 mg to 40 mg as a single dose; repeat dose in 2 hours if needed	DO NOT TAKE MORE THAN 2 DOSES IN 24 HOURS
frovatriptan	Frova	**Oral:** 2.5 mg as a single dose; repeat dose in 2 hours if needed	DO NOT TAKE MORE THAN 3 DOSES IN 24 HOURS
naratriptan	Amerge	**Oral:** 1 mg to 2.5 mg as a single dose; repeat dose in 4 hours if needed	DO NOT TAKE MORE THAN 5 MG IN 24 HOURS
rizatriptan	Maxalt	**Oral:** 5 mg to 10 mg as a single dose; repeat dose in 2 hours if needed	DO NOT TAKE MORE THAN 3 DOSES IN 24 HOURS
sumatriptan	Imitrex	**Oral:** 25 mg, 50 mg, or 100 mg as a single dose; repeat dose in 2 hours if needed **Nasal spray:** 5 mg, 10 mg, or 20 mg as a single dose; repeat dose in 2 hours if needed **Subcutaneous injection:** 6 mg as a single injection; repeat dose in 1 hour if needed	DO NOT TAKE MORE THAN 2 DOSES IN 24 HOURS
zolmitriptan	Zomig	**Oral:** 2.5 mg to 5 mg as a single dose; repeat dose in 2 hours if needed. **Nasal solution:** 1 spray as a single dose; repeat dose in 2 hours if needed	DO NOT TAKE MORE THAN 2 DOSES IN 24 HOURS

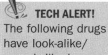

TECH ALERT!
The following drugs have look-alike/sound-alike issues: Axert and Antivert; Amerge and Amaryl; sumatriptan and zolmitriptan; Maxalt and Maxair

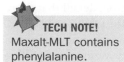

TECH NOTE!
Maxalt-MLT contains phenylalanine.

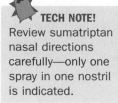

TECH NOTE!
Review sumatriptan nasal directions carefully—only one spray in one nostril is indicated.

The most commonly reported symptom of Alzheimer's disease is forgetfulness. The person may not recall recent events or names of familiar people or things. This increases as the disease progresses and may interfere with the performance of activities of daily living such as personal hygiene. In the mid- to late stages of Alzheimer's disease, the person may have difficulty reading, speaking, writing, and moving. They may become anxious, angry, and aggressive. In addition, the person may be confused and wander, unable to find his or her way back to where he or she started.

PATHOPHYSIOLOGY OF ALZHEIMER'S DISEASE

Alzheimer's disease causes damage to the hippocampus, the part of the brain that is involved in memory. The disease causes cholinergic nerve cells in the brain to die. The cerebral cortex shrinks in size and the ability to think and function diminishes. Abnormal structures, called plaques and tangles, develop in the brain (Figure 11-2). ***Plaques*** are sticky, dense substances composed of a protein called beta amyloid. The plaques fill the spaces between neurons in the brain and interfere with the transmission of signals between the neurons. ***Tangles*** look like twisted fibers and are made up of clumps of a protein called tau. Tangles also block the transmission of messages between neurons. The accumulation of plaques and tangles also produces inflammation, which further damages neurons.

Summary of Nontriptan Drugs Used to Treat Migraine Headaches

	Generic name	Brand name	Usual adult dose	Side effects	Warning labels
Ergot alkaloids					
	dihydroergotamine mesylate	D.H.E.	1 mg IM; repeat in 1 hour if needed (maximum 6 mg/week)	Numbness	DON'T EXCEED RECOMMENDED DOSAGE
		Migranal	1 spray in each nostril; repeat after 15 minutes if needed (maximum 8 sprays/week)		DON'T ASSEMBLE SPRAYER UNTIL READY TO USE
	ergotamine tartrate	Ergomar Caferegot	2 mg every 30 minutes until relief (maximum 6 mg/day or 10 mg/week)	Nausea, vomiting, numbness, chest pain, abdominal pain	DON'T EXCEED RECOMMENDED DOSAGE
β-Blockers					
	propranolol	Inderal Inderal-LA	80 mg to 240 mg daily every 6 to 8 hours or 80 mg to 240 mg daily (long acting)	Hypotension, lethergy	MAY CAUSE DIZZINESS OR DROWSINESS AND IMPAIR ABILITY TO DRIVE
Tricyclic antidepressants					
	amitriptyline	Generic only	150 mg at bedtime	Sedation, dry mouth, urinary retention, blurred vision, hypotension	MAY CAUSE DROWSINESS AND IMPAIR ABILITY TO DRIVE DO NOT DISCONTINUE ABRUPTLY MAY DISCOLOR URINE AVOID PROLONGED EXPOSURE TO SUNLIGHT
Valproates					
	divalproex Na$^+$	Depakote	250 mg twice daily up to 1000 mg/day	Sedation, nausea, ataxia, and liver dysfunction	MAY CAUSE DROWSINESS AND IMPAIR ABILITY TO DRIVE AVOID ALCOHOL TAKE WITH FOOD

ROLE OF NEUROTRANSMITTERS

Several neurotransmitters play a significant role in Alzheimer's disease. The most significant is acetylcholine (ACh). ACh levels gradually decline as the disease progresses producing the symptoms associated with Alzheimer's disease. Cholinergic pathways are involved in all aspects of *cognition,* or the ability to absorb, process, and use information. Recall that there are two types of cholinergic receptors, muscarinic and nicotinic (Figure 11-3). (See Unit 2) Stimulation of nicotinic receptors has been shown to play a role in Alzheimer's disease. Reduced nicotinic receptor function is correlated to impaired memory. Memory and attention are increased when the number of nicotinic receptors is increased.

Glutamate also plays a role in the development of Alzheimer's disease. Glutamate is an excitatory amino acid that is particularly active in the cerebral cortex and hippocampus (Figure 11-4) where binding to glutamatergic receptors is involved in memory formation and learning. There are three classes of glutamatergic receptors. The *N*-methyl-D-aspartate (NMDA) receptor is associated with memory and learning. Excess activity of this receptor is linked to Alzheimer's disease and causes ***neurodegeneration***.

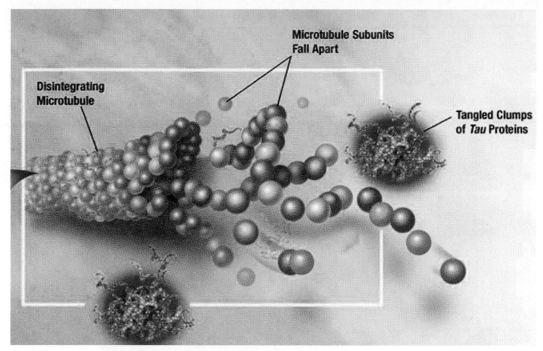

FIGURE 11-2 Disintegrating neurons and tangles. *(Courtesy The Alzheimer's Disease Education and Referral Center, National Institute on Aging, Bethesda, MD.)*

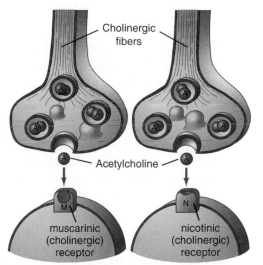

FIGURE 11-3 Muscarinic and nicotinic receptors. *(From Thibodeau GA, Patton KT: Anatomy and physiology, ed 6, St. Louis, 2007, Mosby.)*

Other neurotransmitters that are believed to play a part in Alzheimer's disease are dopamine, norepinephrine, and serotonin.

DRUG TREATMENT FOR ALZHEIMER'S DISEASE

Drugs that increase ACh levels at the synapse are used to treat Alzheimer's disease. Drugs that block glutamate activity, if administered early enough, may be able to slow the progression of Alzheimer's disease.

Acetylcholinesterase (AChE) is an enzyme that degrades ACh. There are several types of AChEs. Two forms that are important to the treatment of Alzheimer's disease are AChE-S and AChE-R. AChE-R has been shown to be neuroprotective in human and animal studies.

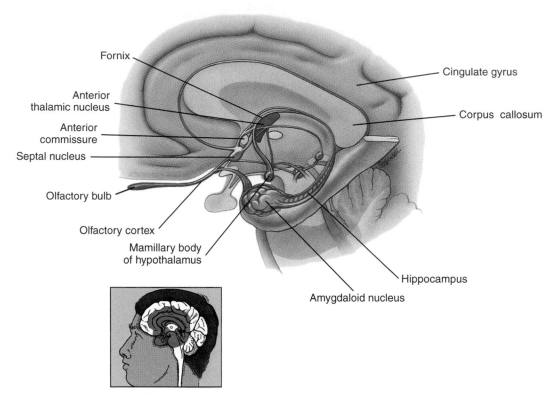

FIGURE 11-4 Parts of the brain controlling memory. *(From Thibodeau GA, Patton KT: Anatomy and physiology, ed 6, St. Louis, 2007, Mosby.)*

Neuroprotective agents protect nerve cells from damage. AChE-S appears to enhance the degeneration of cholinergic nerurons. AChE inhibitors increase levels of ACh. They also increase the number and the activity of nicotinic receptors.

There are five drugs currently approved for the treatment of Alzheimer's disease. Four of them are AChE inhibitors: tacrine (Cognex), donepezil (Aricept), rivastigmine (Exelon), and galantamine (Reminyl). Memantine (Namenda) has recently been approved; it blocks the actions of glutamate at NMDA receptor sites. Recent studies show that this mechanism of action may protect the neuron from further damage. Galantamine has a dual mechanism of action. It blocks AChE and slightly increases glutamate activity. This dual action appears to closely mimic normal body functions and enhances the drug's effectiveness.

ADVERSE REACTIONS

Donepezil, galantamine, rivastigmine, tacrine, and memantine can all produce abdominal pain and cramping, dizziness, and diarrhea. All except memantine produce nausea, and all except donepezil produce sedation and hypotension. Donepezil can additionally produce increased urination. Tacrine causes elevated liver enzymes in up to 49% of patients that may lead to hepatoxicity. Liver enzymes should be monitored every other week beginning week 4 of therapy and continuing through week 16 and every 3 months thereafter. If levels rise above acceptable levels the drug is discontinued.

Drugs Used in the Treatment of Alzheimer's Disease: Acetylcholinesterase Inhibitors

Generic name	U.S. brand name(s) Canadian brand(s)	Dosage forms and strengths
donepezil	Aricept	**Tablet:** 5 mg, 10 mg
	Aricept	
galantamine	Reminyl	**Solution, oral:** 4 mg/ml (100 ml) **Tablet:** 4 mg, 8 mg, 12 mg
	Reminyl	
rivastigmine	Exelon	**Capsule:** 1.5 mg, 3 mg, 4.5 mg, 6 mg **Solution:** 2 mg/ml (120 ml)
	Exelon ·	
tacrine	Cognex	**Transdermal patch:** 4.6 mg, 9.5 mg/24 hr
	Cognex	**Capsule:** 10 mg, 20 mg, 30 mg, 40 mg

Drugs Used in the Treatment of Alzheimer's Disease: N-Methyl-D-Aspartate Receptor Inhibitor

Generic name	U.S. brand name(s) Canadian brand(s)	Dosage forms and strengths
memantine	Namenda	**Tablet:** 5 mg, 10 mg
	Not available	

Summary of Drugs Used in the Treatment of Alzheimer's Disease

Generic name	U.S. brand name	Usual adult oral dose and dosing schedule	Warning labels
donepezil	Aricept	5 mg to 10 mg at bedtime	MAY CAUSE DIZZINESS OR DROWINESS: LIMIT ALCOHOL
galantamine	Reminyl	4 mg to 16 mg twice a day	TAKE WITH FOOD
rivastigmine	Exelon	1.5 mg to 6 mg twice a day	DON'T DISCONTINUE WITH MEDICAL SUPERVISION
tacrine	Cognex	10 mg to 40 mg 4 times a day	MAINTAIN ADEQUATE HYDRATION— galantamine SWALLOW WHOLE; DON'T CRUSH OR CHEW—rivatigmine
memantine	Namenda	5 mg to 10 mg twice a day	MAY CAUSE DIZZINESS OR DROWINESS DON'T DISCONTINUE WITHOUT MEDICAL SUPERVISION

 TECH ALERT!

The following drugs have look-alike/sound-alike issues: Donepezil and Benazepril; Reminyl and Amaryl; Tacrine and Tequin; Cognex and Corgard

CHAPTER SUMMARY

- Migraine headaches are triggered by numerous events, including stress, consumption of certain foods, red wine, caffeinated beverages, and exposure to bright or flashing lights.
- A migraine is a vascular headache.
- During a migraine, blood vessels in the brain dilate, produce inflammation, and stimulate nociceptors causing the throbbing head pain characteristic of migraine headaches.
- Treatment of migraines is aimed at stopping the current migraine attack and preventing future migraines.
- Serotonin agonists, ergot alkaloids, antidepressants (norepinephrine and serotonin reuptake inhibitors and monoamine oxidase inhibitors), β-blockers, and antiseizure drugs are used in the treatment and prevention of migraine headaches.
- Triptans are the most widely prescribed drugs for the treatment of acute migraine headaches.

- The triptans are selective serotonin receptor agonists and stimulate vasoconstriction.
- Triptans that have a long half-life, frovatriptan, and naratriptan, are more effective in preventing headache reoccurrence.
- The use of triptans is restricted to a maximum of two or three doses per 24 hours. The safety of treating more than four migraines per month has not been established for most of the triptans.
- The vasoconstriction caused by triptans is responsible for their therapeutic effects but can result in serious effects, including arrhythmia, angina, myocardial infarction, and stroke.
- Nearly 4.5 million Americans and 290,000 Canadians have Alzheimer's disease.
- Alzheimer's disease is a neurodegenerative disease that causes memory loss, behavioral changes, and immobility.
- Risk factors for Alzheimer's disease are age and heredity.
- Fifteen percent of people with the defective gene *ApoE4* allele will develop Alzheimer's disease. ApoE is involved in cholesterol transport.
- Alzheimer's disease causes damage to the part of the brain that is involved in memory.
- Abnormal structures called plaques and tangles form and interfere with the transmission of messages between neurons.
- Alzheimer's disease causes cholinergic nerve cells in the brain to die.
- The primary neurotransmitters involved in Alzheimer's disease are acetylcholine and glutamate.
- Alzheimer's disease is treated with drugs that increase acetylcholine levels that block glutamate activity.
- Acetylcholinesterase is an enzyme that degrades acetylcholine.
- Acetylcholinesterase inhibitors increase levels of acetylcholine.
- Four of the drugs approved for the treatment of Alzheimer's disease are acetylcholinesterase inhibitors. They are tacrine (Cognex), donepezil (Aricept), rivastigmine (Exelon), and galantamine (Reminyl).
- Memantine (Namenda) blocks the actions of glutamate.

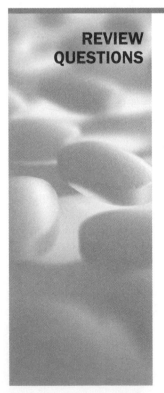

REVIEW QUESTIONS

Multiple Choice

1. The most commonly reported symptom of Alzheimer's disease is _____.
    a. pain
    b. forgetfulness
    c. heart problems
    d. incontinence

2. Several neurotransmitters play a significant role in Alzheimer's disease. The most significant is _____.
    a. epinephrine
    b. serotonin
    c. norepinephrine
    d. acetylcholine

3. Drugs that increase _____ levels at the synapse are used to treat Alzheimer's disease.
    a. dopamine
    b. acetylcholine
    c. serotonin
    d. glutamate

4. **Of the five drugs currently approved for the treatment of Alzheimer's disease, four of them are _____ inhibitors.**
   a. acetylcholinesterse
   b. acetylcholine
   c. glutamate
   d. dopamine
5. **Migraines and cluster headaches are _____ headaches.**
   a. allergy
   b. muscular
   c. vascular
   d. stress
6. **Migraine headaches are triggered by numerous events, including _____.**
   a. stress or consumption of certain foods
   b. red wine or caffeinated beverages
   c. exposure to bright or flashing lights
   d. all of the above
7. **A cluster headache is an intensely painful vascular headache that occurs in groups and produces pain on _____ of the head.**
   a. one side
   b. both sides
8. **_____ are the most widely prescribed drugs for the treatment of migraine headaches.**
   a. Ergot alkaloids
   b. Antiseizure
   c. Antidepressants
   d. Triptans
9. **Family history is not a factor for developing Alzheimer's disease.**
   a. true
   b. false
10. **Which Alzheimer drug blocks the actions of glutamate?**
    a. Aricept
    b. Namenda
    c. Imitrex
    d. Cognex

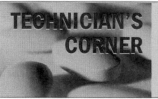

TECHNICIAN'S CORNER

1. Your friend has a throbbing migraine headache and nothing he has done has alleviated the pain. What would you recommend for relief from the pain?
2. Family history is one of the contributing factors in Alzheimer's disease. Knowing that your uncle has Alzheimer's disease, what can you do to prevent this disease from affecting you?

BIBLIOGRAPHY

Adelman, J., Lewit, El: *Comparative aspects of triptans in treating migraines,* Clinical Cornerstone, vol. 4 no. 3. January 2001, Elsevier.

Bren L: *Alzheimer's: searching for a cure,* FDA Consumer magazine, US Food and Drug Administration, US Department of Health and Human Services, March and May 2004, FDA publication No. 04-1318C rev.

Gawel, M., Aschoff, J., May, A., Charlesworth, B., Zolmitriptan 5 mg nasal spray: *Efficacy and onset of action in the acute treatment of migraine* — Results from Phase I of the REALIZE study. Headache 2005:7-16.

Geerts H: Pharmacology of acetylcholinesterase inhibitors and *N*-methyl-D-aspartate receptors for the combination therapy in the treatment of Alzheimer's disease, *J Clin Pharmacol,* 46:8S-16S, 2006.

Kelmann L: *Pain characteristics of acute migraine attack, headache,* Ames, IA, 2006, Blackwell Publishing.

Lance L, Lacy C, Armstrong L, Goldman M: *Drug information handbook for the allied health professional,* ed 12. Hudson, OH, 2005, APhA Lexi-Comp.

National Institute on Aging: *Alzheimer's disease: fact sheet.* Bethesda, MD, 2005, ADEAR, National Institutes of Health, US Department of Health and Human Services, NIH publication No. 03-3431.

Nordberg A: Mechanisms behind the neuroprotective actions of cholinesterase inhibitors in Alzheimer's disease, *Alzheimer Dis Assoc Disord,* 20(suppl 1):S12-S18, 2006.

Page C, Curtis M, Sutter M, Walker M, Hoffman B: *Integrated pharmacology* (pp 261-262), Philadelphia, 2005, Mosby.

Raffa R, Rawls S, Beyzarov E: *Netter's illustrated pharmacology* (pp 80-82), Philadelphia, 2005, WB Saunders.

USP Center for Advancement of Patient Safety: *Use caution–avoid confusion,* USP Quality Review No. 79, Rockville, MD, April 2004, USP Center for Advancement of Patient Safety.

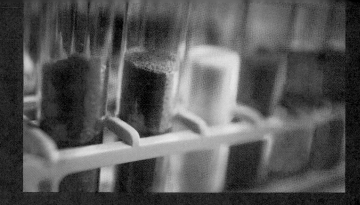

Treatment of Sleep Disorders and Attention-Deficit Hyperactivity Disorder

LEARNING OBJECTIVES

- Discuss the reasons why sleep is necessary.
- Describe the phases of a normal sleep cycle.
- Describe symptoms associated with sleep deprivation.
- Describe the types of sleep disorders.
- Describe the etiology of attention-deficit/hyperactivity disorder (ADHD).
- Describe the function of neurotransmitters associated with symptoms of sleep and ADHD.
- Classify medications used in the treatment of sleep disorders and ADHD.
- Describe mechanism of action for each class of drugs used to treat sleep disorders and ADHD.
- Identify warning labels and precautionary messages associated with medications used to treat sleep disorders and ADHD.
- Identify significant drug look-alike/sound-alike issues.
- Identify significant drug interactions.
- Learn the terminology associated with sleep disorders and ADHD.

KEY TERMS

Circadian rhythms: Biological change that occurs according to time cycles.

Depressant: Drug that decreases activity in the brain and is used as a sedative or hypnotic to promote drowsiness and relaxation.

Disinhibition: Opposite of inhibited.

Hypnotic: Drug that induces sleep.

Insomnia: Condition characterized by difficulty falling asleep and/or staying asleep.

Melatonin: Hormone that is released by the pineal gland that makes a person feel drowsy.

Non-REM sleep: Stage 1 through Stage 4 of the sleep cycle.

Rebound hypersomnia: Condition associated with excessive sleep that follows long-term insomnia or the use of drugs that depress REM and non-REM sleep.

REM sleep: Rapid eye movement sleep. The stage of sleep when dreaming occurs.

Sedative: Drug that causes relaxation and promotes drowsiness.

Stimulant: Drug that increases activity in the brain and is used to treat ADHD and narcolepsy.

Sympathomimetic: Drug whose effects mimic the effects produced by stimulation of the sympathetic nervous system.

OVERVIEW

Sleep is a necessary biological function for the growth and maintenance of a healthy body. Sleep is needed for a healthy immune system and nervous system and for emotional and social functioning, as well as for physical and mental agility. Our memory is also improved when we get sufficient sleep.

The body's sleep cycle is influenced by circadian rhythms. Circadian rhythms are biological changes that occur according to time cycles. The human body operates on a 24-hour clock; however, this clock can be manipulated by external time cues. Sunlight is the primary external time cue. Changes in sunlight and darkness are picked up by the retina in the back of the eye. The retina sends signals to the pineal gland in the brain. The pineal gland controls the release of melatonin, a hormone that makes people feel drowsy in addition to regulating body temperature and hormone secretion. The fact that our normal sleep-wake cycle is linked to sunlight explains why people who work the night shift may feel uncontrollably drowsy in the middle of the night, and it explains why workplace accidents occur more frequently in the middle of the night than during the day.

The amount of time a person needs to sleep ranges between 5 and 16 hours per day. The amount of sleep needed can vary according to age. Infants may sleep up to 16 hours per day, teenagers require as much as 9 hours, and adults need as little as 5 to 8 hours. The patterns of sleep change as people age. The elderly often sleep for shorter time spans, sleep more lightly, and dream less than they did as young adults, although their overall sleep requirement may not change.

The normal sleep pattern involves five stages of sleep (Figure 12-1). *Stage 1* occurs first; during this stage, the person sleeps lightly and can be awakened easily. Sudden muscle contractions of the limbs may occur similar to when a person is startled while awake, and the eyes move slowly back and forth. In *stage 2*, sleep eye movements stop and brain activity decreases. *Stage 3* and *stage 4* sleep are deep sleep. Brain activity slows (delta waves). It is difficult to wake someone from stage 3 or stage 4 sleep; if awakened, the person feels disoriented. The final stage of sleep is known as *rapid eye movement* (REM) sleep because of the characteristic eye movements that occur. This is the sleep cycle where dreaming occurs, and it lasts between 90 minutes and 110 minutes. REM sleep is crucial to normal emotional and physical functioning. Approximately 2 hours per night is spent in REM sleep. The thalamus and cerebral cortex actively communicate with each other during REM sleep. The cortex is the region of the brain involved in learning and interpretation of information.

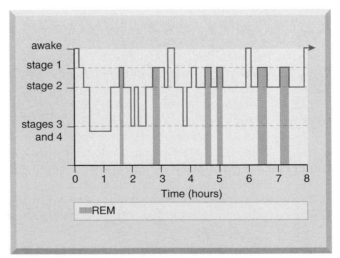

FIGURE 12-1 Normal sleep cycle. *(From Page C, et al.* Integrated pharmacology, *ed 3. Philadelphia, 2006, Mosby.)*

Too little sleep causes symptoms of sleep deprivation. A drowsy feeling during the day with or without micro-sleeps and falling asleep within 5 minutes of lying down are signs of sleep deprivation. Studies show that sleep deprivation is dangerous and can cause motor vehicle accidents at a rate similar to driving under the influence of alcohol. As many as 100,000 motor vehicle accidents in the United States each year are attributed to sleep deprivation. Sleep deprivation can also trigger seizures, paranoia, and hallucinations.

Factors that contribute to the inability to get adequate sleep are numerous and include sleep apnea, restless leg syndrome, consumption of caffeinated beverages and foods, use of prescription and nonprescription drugs and chronic illness. Chronic illnesses that can interfere with sleep are gastroesophageal reflux disorder, angina, and chronic pain.

Sleep Disorders

Millions of Americans suffer from sleep disorders. The most common sleep disorders are insomnia, restless leg syndrome, sleep apnea, and narcolepsy. *Insomnia* affects nearly 60 million Americans each year and up to one-third of the world population. It is categorized according to the length of time the symptoms persist. Transient insomnia lasts less than 7 days, short-term insomnia lasts up to 3 weeks, and long-term insomnia lasts longer than 3 weeks and is often associated with a chronic condition such as pain.

As many as 12% of the people who say they have insomnia complain about *periodic leg movements.* Restless leg syndrome is reported in up to 12 million Americans and is more common in the elderly. Diabetes, pregnancy, and anemia can also cause restless leg syndrome. *Sleep apnea* affects up to 18 million people. The condition is associated with an interruption in the supply of oxygen during sleep, which causes the person to awaken. Rarely, sleep apnea is fatal. Sudden death occurs from respiratory arrest during sleep.

Narcolepsy is the least common of the sleep disorders. It is characterized by falling asleep suddenly and without warning. Attacks may last between a few seconds and 30 minutes. The disorder is usually heredity but can be caused by brain trauma.

TREATMENT OF SLEEP DISORDERS

INSOMNIA

Pharmacological treatments for insomnia are recommended only for short-term use. Prescription drugs, nonprescription drugs, and natural remedies are commercially available, and all produce drowsiness that enables the person to drift off to sleep and stay asleep. Prescription drugs that are used to treat insomnia are barbiturates, benzodiazepines, and other sedative-hypnotics. It is important to note that drugs that promote sleep do not result in a normal pattern of sleep. They alter non-REM and REM sleep. This can result in *rebound hypersomnia* and increased dreaming once the drugs are discontinued.

Barbiturates

Barbiturates are *sedative-hypnotics* and are the oldest class of drugs prescribed to promote relaxation and sleep.

Mechanism of Action. The mechanism of action for barbiturates is to enhance binding of the γ-aminobutyric acid (GABA), a neurotransmitter, to $GABA_A$ and $GABA_B$ receptors (Figure 12-2). GABA is the major inhibitory neurotransmitter in the nervous system. $GABA_A$

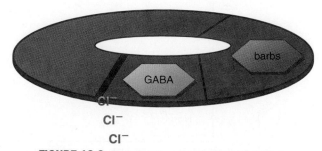

FIGURE 12-2 Barbiturate mechanism of action.

receptor binding causes chloride ion (Cl⁻) channels to open. GABA$_B$ receptor binding is coupled to G proteins. The influx of Cl⁻ results in hyperpolarization, which reduces neuronal excitability and nerve impulse transmission. Like benzodiazepines, barbiturates bind to a specific receptor, which in turn increases binding of GABA to the GABA receptors. In addition to GABA receptor binding, barbiturates are believed to have a direct action on Cl⁻ channels.

Pharmacokinetics. Barbiturates are highly lipid soluble. This accounts for the ease in which they cross the blood-brain barrier and for their rapid redistribution out of the brain to other lipid compartments in the body. Barbiturates with the highest lipid solubility have the greatest degree of redistribution and the shortest duration of effect. An example is the general anesthetic thiopental. It is categorized as an ultra-rapid-acting barbiturate and its effects last about 20 minutes.

Barbiturates are metabolized in the liver and are able to induce the hepatic enzymes of drugs that use the same metabolic enzyme pathway. They can also induce their own metabolic enzymes. Barbiturates are weak acids. They are eliminated in the urine; however, their elimination is influenced by the pH of the urine.

Adverse Reactions. The effects of barbiturates are dose dependent (Figure 12-3). Low doses produce decreased anxiety. As the dose increases, *disinhibition* occurs. This is followed by sedation. Higher doses produce somnolence or hypnosis. Increasing the dose produces general anesthesia. Toxic doses produce coma and death. Other adverse effects of barbiturates include ataxia, confusion, reduced motor performance, and hypotension.

Barbiturates can produce tolerance and dependence (see Chapter 5). When tolerance develops, the patient must take increasing doses to achieve the same effects as were achieved previously at lower doses. Barbiturates also produce drug dependence, causing the person taking the drug to continue to take the drug in order to avoid the onset of physical and/or psychological withdrawal symptoms. For this reason, barbiturates are scheduled controlled substances. The controlled substance schedule is related to their abuse potential and their potential to produce physical and/or psychological dependence (see Chapter 1, Table 1-3). Amobarbital, pentobarbital, and secobarbital are C-II controlled substances, and mephobarbital and phenobarbital are C-IV controlled substances (see Chapter 9).

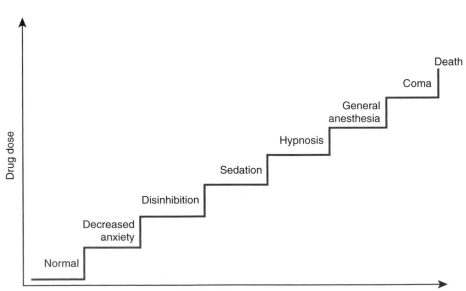

FIGURE 12-3 Dose effects of barbiturates.

Barbiturates Used in the Treatment of Insomnia

Generic name	U.S. brand name(s) Canadian brand(s)	Dosage forms and strengths
amobarbital	Amytal	**Injection, powder for reconstitution:** 500 mg
	Amytal	
pentobarbital	Nembutal	**Injection, solution:** 50 mg/ml
	Nembutal	
secobarbital	Seconal	**Capsule:** 100 mg
	Seconal	

Benzodiazepines

The use of barbiturates has been largely replaced by benzodiazepines and other miscellaneous agents, which has increased safety. Like barbiturates, benzodiazpines decrease neuronal excitability by opening Cl^- channels. The mechanism of action, pharmacokinetics, and adverse reactions of benzodiazepines are discussed in detail in Chapter 5. Drugs with a long half-life ($T\frac{1}{2}$) may cause the user to feel groggy the following morning.

Benzodiazepines Used in the Treatment of Insomnia

Generic name	U.S. brand name(s) Canadian brand(s)	Dosage forms and strengths
flurazepam*	Dalmane	**Capsule:** 15 mg, 30 mg
	Dalmane	
temazepam*	Restoril	**Capsule:** 15 mg, 30 mg
	Restoril	
triazolam*	Halcion	**Tablet:** 0.125 mg, 0.25 mg
	Halcion	

*Generic available.

Miscellaneous Drugs Used for the Treatment of Insomnia

Several newer agents are available for the treatment of insomnia that have a mechanism of action similar to that of benzodiazepines but are not benzodiazepines. Zaleplon and zolpidem are classified as imidazopyridines (also called enzodiazepines). Eszopiclone and zopiclone are classified as cyclopyrrolone derivatives. They act on benzodiazepine receptors subtype v-1. It is claimed that zaleplon and zolpidem have less disruption of the normal stages of REM and non-REM sleep than do traditional benzodiazepines and barbiturates.

Miscellaneous Drugs Used for the Treatment of Insomnia

	Generic name	U.S. brand name(s) Canadian brand(s)	Dosage forms and strengths
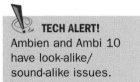	eszopiclone	Lunesta	**Tablet:** 1 mg, 2 mg, 3 mg
		Not available	
	zaleplon	Sonata	**Capsule:** 5 mg, 10 mg
		Starnoc	
	zolpidem	Ambien, Ambien CR	**Tablet:** 5 mg, 10 mg **Tablet, controlled release:** 6.25 mg, 12.5 mg
		Not available	
	zopiclone	Not available	**Tablet:** 5 mg, 7.5 mg
		Imovane	

✏ **TECH ALERT!**
Ambien and Ambi 10 have look-alike/ sound-alike issues.

Adverse Effects of Miscellaneous Agents. All of the miscellaneous agents used in the treatment of insomnia are controlled substances and can produce tolerance and dependence. Sedation and dizziness are other side effects common to all. Zaleplon may also produce photosensitivity, and eszopiclone and zopiclone can produce a bitter or metallic taste.

Half-life and Time to Peak Effect of Benzodiazepines and Miscellaneous Drugs Used in the Treatment of Insomnia

Generic name	Time to peak effect (hr)	Half-life (T½)
Benzodiazepines		
flurazepam	1 to 2	1.5
nitrazepam (Canada)	2	15 to 40
temazepam	0.8 to 1.4	10 to 20
triazolam	1 to 2	1.5 to 5
Miscellaneous		
eszopiclone	1	**6**
zaleplon	1	1
zolpidem	1.6	2.5
zopiclone	<2	3.5 to 6

Natural Remedies for Insomnia

Several natural remedies have proven effectiveness for promoting sleep; they are melatonin and valerian root. Melatonin is a hormone that is produced by the pineal gland; it is sensitive to light changes and tells the body it is time to sleep. Doses of 3 mg to 5 mg have been shown to be effective for treatment of short-term insomnia, enhancement of sleep, and prevention of jet lag. The use of valerian root dates back more than 2000 years. Galen recommended it for the treatment of insomnia. A dose of 600 mg aqueous extract, taken 1 hour before bedtime, has been shown to be effective.

Nonpharmacological Treatments

It is best to avoid the things that can cause sleeplessness, when possible. Insomnia prevention tips include the following:

- Avoid stimulants close to bedtime.

  Colas, tea, chocolate, fortified water, Mountain Dew, OTC decongestants, etc. are stimulants and can cause insomnia if consumed near bedtime.

- Adopt a regular sleeping schedule.

  A routine sleep schedule is like an external cue that sleeping time is approaching.

- Avoid daytime naps.

  Naps disrupt the normal sleep cycle.

- Create a safe comfortable sleeping environment, if possible.

  Fears about safety and extremes in temperature can prevent sleep.

- Do not go to bed hungry, if possible.

  Hunger can prevent sleep.

- Exercise 20 to 30 minutes each day (not at bedtime).

  Maximum benefits are achieved if exercise is performed 5 to 6 hours before bedtime. Exercise before bedtime can interfere with sleep.

- Do not lie in bed awake.

  If you do not fall asleep, get up and engage in a nonstimulating activity such as reading. Try to go to sleep again in about 10 minutes.

Summary of Drugs Used in the Treatment of Insomnia

Generic name	U.S. brand name	Usual adult oral dose and dosing schedule	Warning labels	Controlled substance schedule
Barbiturates				
amobarbital	Amytal	65 mg to 200 mg IM at bedtime	MAY CAUSE DROWSINESS; MAY IMPAIR ABILITY TO DRIVE	C-II
pentobarbital	Nembutal	150 mg to 200 mg (IM) or 100 mg every 1 to 3 minutes up to 200 mg to 500 mg (IV)	AVOID ALCOHOL	C-II
secobarbital	Seconal	100 mg to 200 mg at bedtime	MAY BE HABIT FORMING	C-II
Benzodiazepines				
flurazepam	Dalmane	15 mg to 30 mg at bedtime	MAY CAUSE DROWSINESS; MAY IMPAIR ABILITY TO DRIVE	C-IV
temazepam	Restoril	15 mg to 30 mg at bedtime	AVOID ALCOHOL	C-IV
triazolam	Halcion	0.125 mg to 0.25 mg at bedtime	MAY BE HABIT FORMING	C-IV
Miscellanous				
zaleplon	Sonata	5 mg to 20 mg at bedtime	MAY CAUSE DROWSINESS; MAY IMPAIR ABILITY TO DRIVE	C-IV
zolpidem	Ambiem	10 mg at bedtime	AVOID ALCOHOL	C-IV
			MAY BE HABIT FORMING	
			AVOID PROLONGED EXPOSURE TO SUNLIGHT—zaleplon only	
eszopiclone	Lunesta	1 mg to 3 mg at bedtime		C-IV
zopiclone	Imovane	5 mg to 7.5 mg at bedtime		C-IV

NARCOLEPSY

Narcolepsy is a relatively rare condition in which a person suddenly falls asleep, often in response to an emotional stimulus such as laughter or fear. The primary treatment for narcolepsy is the administration of stimulants. The loss of muscle tone that often accompanies the overwhelming feeling of sleepiness can be treated using anticholinergics and selective serotonin reuptake inhibitors (SSRIs).

Stimulants used in the treatment of narcolepsy include amphetamine, methylphenidate, and modafinil. Modafinil is a nonamphetamine stimulant; the mechanism of action is not fully known, but it is believed to stimulate α_1-adrenergic receptor sites. Modafinil is also prescribed for the treatment of sleep apnea. Amphetamine and methylphenidate are *sympathomimetics.* A sympathomimetic is a drug whose effects mimic the effects produced by stimulation of the sympathetic nervous system. A detailed discussion of amphetamine and methylphenidate is described in the section on treatment for attention-deficit/hyperactivity disorder (ADHD).

Modafinil Use for the Treatment of Narcolepsy

		U.S. brand name(s)			Controlled substance schedule
	Generic name	Canadian brand(s)	Dosage forms and strengths	Usual adult dose	
	modafinil	Provigil	**Tablet:** 100 mg, 200 mg	200 mg every morning	C-IV
		Not available			

Side Effects and Precautions

Adverse effects produced by modafinil include stimulation, insomnia, tolerance, and dependence. Modafinil may also decrease the effect of oral contraceptives. Warning labels listed below should be affixed to prescription vials for modafinil:

AVOID ALCOHOL

MAY DECREASE EFFECT OF ORAL CONTRACEPTIVES

MAY BE HABIT FORMING

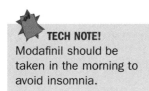

TECH NOTE!
Modafinil should be taken in the morning to avoid insomnia.

Attention-Deficit/Hyperactivity Disorder

ADHD is the most commonly diagnosed childhood behavioral disorder. The percentage of school-age children reported to have ADHD in U.S. communities varies between 3% and 8%; in Canada, the percentage ranges between 5% and 10%. Although most statistics are gathered about children, ADHD affects adolescents and adults, too.

Symptoms of ADHD are commonly observed in children without ADHD, making diagnosis challenging (Figure 12-4). These symptoms are hyperactivity, restlessness, inability to sit still when required, impulsiveness, inattention, distractibility, forgetfulness, and inability to complete tasks. All children sometimes exhibit these behaviors. A diagnosis of ADHD should only be made when these behaviors occur more frequently than would be expected for the child's age and if the behavior interferes with two or more areas of the child's life. These areas are defined as school, playground, home, community, and social relationships.

There are three subtypes of ADHD: they are predominantly hyperactive-impulsive, predominantly inattentive, and combined type. It is important to note that children who are diagnosed with predominantly inattentive type (attention deficit disorder [ADD]) rarely exhibit hyperactivity and impulsiveness. Learning disorders such as dyslexia occur in approximately 20% to 30% of children with ADHD.

There is no single cause for ADHD. Genetics is most strongly linked to ADHD. Up to 25% of children who have a parent, sibling, or other close family relative with ADHD also have ADHD. The rate is only 5% in the general population.

Look for signs of ADHD.

Put a check mark next to each one that sounds like your child. ☑

My child often…
- ☐ is moving something—fingers, hands, arms, feet, or legs.
- ☐ walks, runs, or climbs around when others are seated.
- ☐ has trouble waiting in line or taking turns.
- ☐ doesn't finish things.
- ☐ gets bored after just a short while.
- ☐ daydreams or seems to be in another world.
- ☐ talks when other people are talking.
- ☐ gets frustrated with schoolwork or homework.
- ☐ acts quickly without thinking first.
- ☐ is sidetracked by what is going on around him or her.

FIGURE 12-4 Signs of ADHD checklist. *(Courtesy National Institute of Mental Health, Bethesda, MD.)*

Exposure to environmental agents such as cigarette smoke and alcohol during pregnancy has shown to increase the risk for ADHD. Exposure to high levels of lead-based paint also increases risk. This is an important risk factor for children who live in older urban cities and attend school in old buildings that were painted with lead-based paint before it was banned. There is also an increased risk of ADHD in children who live in developing countries that still use leaded gasoline.

Some people believe that consumption of food additives and sugar can make ADHD worse. When placed on a diet that restricted these food additives, approximately 5% of children with ADHD showed improvement in symptoms.

PATHOPHYSIOLOGY OF ATTENTION-DEFICIT/HYPERACTIVITY DISORDER

The part of the brain that is affected by ADHD is the frontal lobes of the cerebrum and the basal ganglia (see Unit 2, page 72). The frontal lobe is the area of the brain involved in problem solving and planning. The basal ganglia are structures that transmit messages between the cerebrum and the cerebellum and are involved in motor movement. Brain scans of children with ADHD show that these areas of the brain are smaller than those in children without ADHD.

TREATMENTS FOR ATTENTION-DEFICIT/HYPERACTIVITY DISORDER

A variety of drug treatments are available for treating ADHD; however, medications cannot cure ADHD. They only control symptoms. Therefore, the most effective therapy for ADHD involves drug treatment in addition to behavioral therapy. The goal of behavioral therapy is to decrease anxiety and improve relationships and social skills.

Pharmaceutical treatment of ADHD is achieved with the administration of amphetamines and nonamphetamine stimulants. Amphetamines behave differently in people who have ADHD than they do in people without ADHD. They decrease hyperactivity and improve focus rather than produce hyperactivity and lack of focused behavior.

TECH ALERT!
The following drugs have look-alike/ sound-alike issues: Adderall and Inderal; Ritalin, Ritalin SR, and Ritalin LA

TECH NOTE!
Adderall should be taken in the morning to avoid insomnia.

TECH NOTE!
The following warning labels should be affixed to prescription vials for amphetamines:
TAKE WITH FOOD
MAY BE HABIT-FORMING
SWALLOW WHOLE; DO NOT CRUSH OR CHEW (sustained-release and extended-release).

MECHANISM OF ACTION AND PHARMACOKINETICS

Amphetamines are sympathomimetics. They are structurally similar to norepinephrine. They work via three primary mechanisms. They stimulate the release of norepinephrine, block monoamine oxidase (further increasing catecholamine levels), and stimulate the release of dopamine. Increased stimulation of adrenergic receptors by norepinephrine is responsible for the increased alertness, responsiveness, wakefulness, and reduced awareness of fatigue associated with amphetamines.

Amphetamines are well absorbed from the gastrointestinal tract, and their lipid solubility enables them to cross the blood-brain barrier. They are metabolized in the liver and eliminated in the urine. Amphetamines are manufactured in immediate release, sustained release, and extended release dosage forms. The duration of action varies according to the dosage form administered. Atomoxetine is a nonamphetamine stimulant. It inhibits the reuptake of norepinephrine.

ADVERSE REACTIONS

The most common side effects produced by amphetamines are decreased appetite, nausea, stomachache, anxiety, and irritability. They can also cause insomnia. Insomnia can be minimized if the last dose is taken before 6 PM. The sympathetic nervous system stimulation produced by amphetamines is responsible for the drug's cardiovascular effects. Amphetamines can cause increased heart rate, palpitations, and arrhythmia. Other side effects produced by amphetamines are dizziness and tremor. Doses greater than therapeutic doses can produce *amphetamine syndrome,* a type of drug-induced psychosis.

PRECAUTIONS

Amphetamines have a high abuse potential. They are all Schedule C-II controlled substances. Atomoxetine is not a controlled substance.

Drugs Used for the Treatment of Attention-Deficit/Hyperactivity Disorder (ADHD)

Generic name	U.S. brand name(s) / Canadian brand(s)	Dosage forms and strengths
amphetamine + dextroamphetamine*	Adderall, Adderall XR ——— Adderall XR	**Capsule, extended release (Adderall XR):** 5 mg, 10 mg, 15 mg, 20 mg, 25 mg, 30 mg **Tablet: immediate release (Adderall):** 5 mg, 7.5 mg, 10 mg, 12.5 mg, 15 mg, 20 mg, 30 mg
dextroamphetamine*	Dexedrine ——— Dexedrine, Dexedrine Spansule	**Capsule, sustained release (Dexedrine spansule):** 5 mg, 10 mg, 15 mg **Tablet: immediate release (Dexedrine):** 5 mg, 10 mg
dexmethylphenidate	Focalin, Focalin XR ——— Not available	**Tablet:** 2.5 mg, 5 mg, 10 mg
methylphenidate*	Concerta, Daytrana, Metadate CD, Metadate ER, Ritalin, Ritalin LA, Ritalin SR ——— Concerta, Ritalin, Ritalin SR	**Capsule, extended release (Metadate CD):** 10 mg, 20 mg, 30 mg; **(Ritalin LA):** 10 mg, 20 mg, 30 mg, 40 mg, 50 mg, 60 mg **Tablet, extended release (Concerta):** 18 mg, 27 mg, 36 mg, 54 mg **Tablet, extended release (Metadate ER):** 10 mg, 20 mg **Tablet, immediate release (Ritalin):** 5 mg, 10 mg, 20 mg **Tablet, sustained release (Ritalin SR):** 20 mg **Transdermal patch (Daytrana):** 1.1 mg/hr, 1.6 mg/hr, 2.2 mg/hr, 3.3 mg/hr

Drugs Used for the Treatment of Attention-Deficit/Hyperactivity Disorder (ADHD)—Cont'd

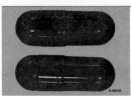

Generic name	U.S. brand name(s) Canadian brand(s)	Dosage forms and strengths
Atomoxetine	Strattera Strattera	**Capsule:** 10 mg, 18 mg, 25 mg, 40 mg, 60 mg, 80 mg, 100 mg

*Generic available.

Summary of Drugs Used in the Treatment of Attention-Deficit/Hyperactivity Disorder

Generic name	Brand name	Duration of action (hr)	Usual child dosage	Approved age
Amphetamines				
amphetamine + dextroamphetamine				3+ years
Immediate release	Adderall	6	5 to 20 mg/day (1 to 3 doses/day)	
Extended release	Adderall XR	12	5 to 10 mg every morning	
dextroamphetamine				3+ years
Immediate release	Dexedrine	4	2.5 mg to 20 mg 1 to 2 times per day	
	Dextrostat	4		
dexmethylphenidate	Focalin	6	2.5 mg to 20 mg/day given as 2 doses/day	6+ years
methylphenidate				6+ years
Immediate release	Ritalin	3 to 6	10 mg to 20 mg twice a day up to 90 mg/day	
Extended release	Concerta	12	18 mg to 54 mg/day	6 to 12 years
			18 mg to 72 mg/day	13 to 17 years
	Ritalin LA	12	20 mg once a day	
	Metadate CD	8	20 mg once a day	
	Metadate ER	8	20 mg once a day	
Sustained release	Ritalin SR	6 to 8	10 to 20 mg every 8 hours	
Nonamphetamine				
atomoxetine	Strattera	24	40 to 100 mg/day in 1 to 2 divided doses	70 kg+

CHAPTER SUMMARY

- Sleep is needed for a healthy immune system and nervous system and emotional and social functioning, as well as physical and mental agility.
- The body's sleep cycle is influenced by circadian rhythms.
- Our normal sleep-wake cycle is linked to changes in sunlight.
- The pineal gland controls the release of melatonin, a hormone that makes people feel drowsy.
- Workplace accidents occur more frequently in the middle of the night than during the day.
- Infants may sleep up to 16 hours per day, teenagers require as much as 9 hours, and adults need as little as 5 to 8 hours.
- The patterns of sleep change as people age.
- There are five stages of sleep.
- Dreaming occurs during rapid eye movement (REM) sleep and is crucial to normal emotional and physical functioning.

- As many as 100,000 motor vehicle accidents in the United States each year are attributed to sleep deprivation.
- Sleep apnea, restless leg syndrome, consumption of caffeinated beverages and foods, use of prescription and nonprescription drugs, and chronic illness can cause insomnia.
- Pharmacological treatment for insomnia is recommended for short-term use.
- Prescription drugs, nonprescription drugs, and herbal remedies are commercially available, and all produce drowsiness that enables the person to drift off to sleep and stay asleep.
- Prescription drugs used to treat insomnia are barbiturates, benzodiazepines, and other sedative hypnotics.
- Drugs that promote sleep do not result in a normal pattern of sleep. They alter non-REM and REM sleep.
- Rebound hypersomnia and increased dreaming occur once the drugs are discontinued.
- Barbiturates decrease neuronal excitability by increasing GABA binding. In addition to GABA receptor binding, barbiturates are believed to have a direct action on chloride ion channels.
- Barbiturates can produce tolerance and dependence.
- Several newer agents are available for the treatment of insomnia that have a mechanism of action similar to that of benzodiazepines e.g., zaleplon, zolpidem, eszopiclone, and zopiclone.
- Melatonin and valerian root are herbal remedies that have proven effectiveness for promoting sleep.
- Insomnia prevention tips include (1) avoid stimulants close to bedtime, (2) adopt a regular sleeping schedule, (3) avoid daytime naps, (4) create a safe comfortable sleeping environment, if possible, (5) do not go to bed hungry, if possible, (6) exercise, and (7) do not lie in bed awake.
- Stimulants are administered for the treatment of narcolepsy.
- Attention-deficit/hyperactivity disorder (ADHD) is the most commonly diagnosed childhood behavioral disorder.
- Symptoms of ADHD are hyperactivity, restlessness, inability to sit still when required, impulsiveness, inattention, distractibility, forgetfulness, and inability to complete tasks.
- Genetics and environmental factors are risk factors for ADHD.
- The most effective therapy for ADHD involves a combination of drug treatments and behavioral therapy.
- Pharmaceutical treatment of ADHD is achieved with the administration of amphetamines and nonamphetamine stimulants.
- Amphetamines behave differently in people who have ADHD than they do in people without ADHD.
- Amphetamines stimulate the release of norepinephrine, block monoamine oxidase, and stimulate the release of dopamine.
- The most common side effects produced by amphetamines are decreased appetite, nausea, stomachache, anxiety, insomnia, and irritability.
- Amphetamines have a high abuse potential and are Schedule C-II controlled substances.

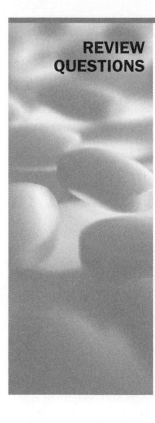

REVIEW QUESTIONS

Multiple Choice

1. Not getting enough sleep does not affect the immune system, nervous system, or emotional and social functioning of the body.
    a. true
    b. false

2. Circadian rhythms are biological changes that occur according to _____ cycles.
    a. growth
    b. age
    c. time
    d. health

3. The pineal gland controls the release of _____, a hormone that makes people feel drowsy in addition to regulating body temperature and hormone secretion.
    a. serotonin
    b. melatonin
    c. dopamine
    d. acetylcholine

4. Narcolepsy is the most common of the sleep disorders:
    a. true
    b. false

5. Pharmacological treatment for insomnia is recommended for long-term use.
    a. true
    b. false

6. What dose of barbiturates produces sedation?
    a. low
    b. medium
    c. high
    d. it does not matter

7. Zaleplon and zolpidem are classified as _____.
    a. barbiturates
    b. benzodiazepines
    c. enzodiazepines
    d. amphetamines

8. The primary treatment for narcolepsy is administration of stimulants.
    a. true
    b. false

9. Pharmaceutical treatment of ADHD is achieved with the administration of _____.
    a. amphetamines
    b. nonamphetamine stimulants
    c. antianxiety
    d. both a and b

10. Amphetamines have a high abuse potential and are classified as Schedule _____ controlled substances.
    a. C-I
    b. C-II
    c. C-IV
    d. C-III

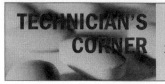

TECHNICIAN'S CORNER

1. Do diet and lack of exercise or lack of attention have anything to do with the number of children diagnosed with ADHD?
2. What would you recommend to someone with a sleep disorder who does not want to take any sleep aids?

BIBLIOGRAPHY

Kalant H, Grant D, Mitchell J: *Principles of medical pharmacology* (pp 339-342), ed 7, Toronto, 2007, Elsevier Canada, A Division of Reed Elsevier Canada.

Lance L, Lacy C, Armstrong L, Goldman M: *Drug information handbook for the allied health professional,* ed 12. Hudson, OH, 2005, APhA Lexi-Comp.

National Institute of Mental Health: *Attention deficit hyperactivity disorder,* Bethesda (MD): February 2006, National Institute of Mental Health, National Institutes of Health, US Department of Health and Human Services. NIH publication No. 03-3572.

National Institute of Neurological Disorders and Stroke, National Institute of Health, U.S. Department of Health and Humans Services: *Brain basics: understanding sleep,* Bethesda, 2007. National Institute of Neurological disorders and stroke,. NIH publication no. 06-3440-c.

Raffa R, Rawls S, Beyzarov E: *Netter's illustrated pharmacology* (pp 80-82), Philadelphia, 2005, WB Saunders.

Romano E, Baillargeon R, Tremblay R: Prevalence of hyperactivity-impulsivity and inattention among Canadian children: findings from the first data collection cycle (1994-1995) of the National Longitudinal Survey of Children and Youth–Applied Research Branch, Strategic Policy, Human Resources Development–Canada, June 2002. Retrieved from http://www.sdc.gc.ca/en/cs/sp/sdc/pkrf/publications/research/2002-000170/page02.shtml.

USP Center for Advancement of Patient Safety: *Use caution–avoid confusion,* USP Quality Review No. 79, Rockville, MD, April 2004, USP Center for Advancement of Patient Safety.

Drugs Affecting the Musculoskeletal System

- List the divisions of the human skeleton.
- Describe the basic structure of the human skeleton.
- Explain the differences in the types of joints of the skeleton.
- Demonstrate a knowledge of how muscles move the skeleton.
- Describe the different arrangements of muscles.
- Explain how the heart muscle works.
- Learn the terminology associated with the musculoskeletal system.

Anatomy and Physiology of the Skeleton

The human skeleton consists of two main divisions: the axial skeleton and the appendicular skeleton. The *axial skeleton* consists of the cranium or brain case, bones of the face and ear, the vertebral column, ribs, and sternum, and the hyoid. The *appendicular skeleton* contains the bones of the upper extremities (e.g., wrist and hand) and the lower extremities (e.g., hip, kneecap, and ankles).

SINUS CAVITY

The cranial and facial bones contain the **frontal** and **paranasal sinuses.** Another sinus cavity, the mastoid sinuses, is found in the middle and inner ear structures.

THE FETAL SKULL

The skull of the fetus and newborn infant has unique anatomical features not seen in the adult. The *fontanels,* or "soft spots," provide additional space, which allows for molding of head shape as the baby passes through the birth canal and for rapid brain growth that occurs in infancy without causing damaging increases in intracranial pressure. The fontanels close and the cranial bones fuse together as the skull reaches adult size.

VERTEBRAL COLUMN

The vertebral, or spinal, column forms the longitudinal axis of the skeleton. Joints between the vertebrae permit forward, backward, and sideways movement of the column. The vertebral column is divided into cervical vertebrae, thoracic vertebrae, lumbar vertebrae, and the sacrum.

RIBS

Twelve pairs of ribs together with the vertebral column and sternum form the thorax that protects the heart and lungs. The ribs are named according to their articulation with the sternum (i.e., true ribs, false ribs, and floating ribs). The first seven ribs attach to the sternum and are known as true ribs. The lower five ribs do not directly connect to the sternum and are known as false ribs. The last two false ribs have no ventral attachment and are called floating, fluctuating, or vertebral ribs.

APPENDICULAR SKELETON

The appendicular skeleton is divided into the upper and lower extremities. The upper extremities consist of the following bones: clavicle, scapula, humerus, radius and ulna, carpus (wrist), metacarpals (hand), and phalanges (fingers). The lower extremities consist of the following bones: hip, femur, tibia, fibula, patella (kneecap), tarsals (ankle), metatarsals, and phalanges (toes). The structure of the foot is similar to the hand. Strong ligaments and leg muscle tendons hold together the foot bones.

ARTICULATIONS

Articulations are joints or points of contact between two bones. Joints are classified on the basis of the amount of movement allowed. There are three major categories of joints: *synarthroses*—immovable (skull), *amphiarthroses*—slightly moveable (symphysis pubis in pelvic area), and *diarthroses*—freely moveable (knee, hip, elbow, shoulder). Ligaments, bands of fibrous tissue that connect bones to bones, are also present.

The Muscular System

There are more than 600 muscles in the human body, which make up 40% to 50% of the body weight. This large mass of muscles is responsible for movement of the skeleton, heat production, and posture. Contraction or shortening of individual muscle cells is ultimately responsible for purposeful movement. There are three types of muscles: **skeletal**, **smooth**, and **cardiac**. Their movements power vital homeostatic mechanisms such as breathing, blood flow, digestion, and urine flow. A number of body systems support the function of muscle tissues.

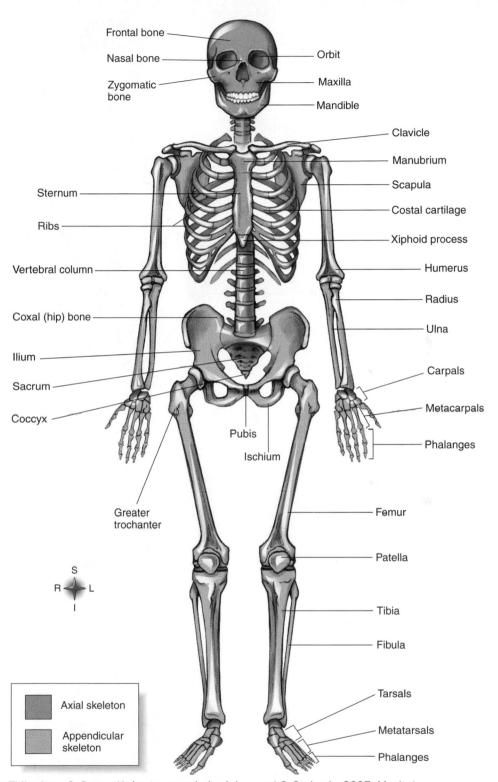

(From Thibodeau G, Patton K: Anatomy and physiology, *ed 6, St. Louis, 2007, Mosby.)*

Continued

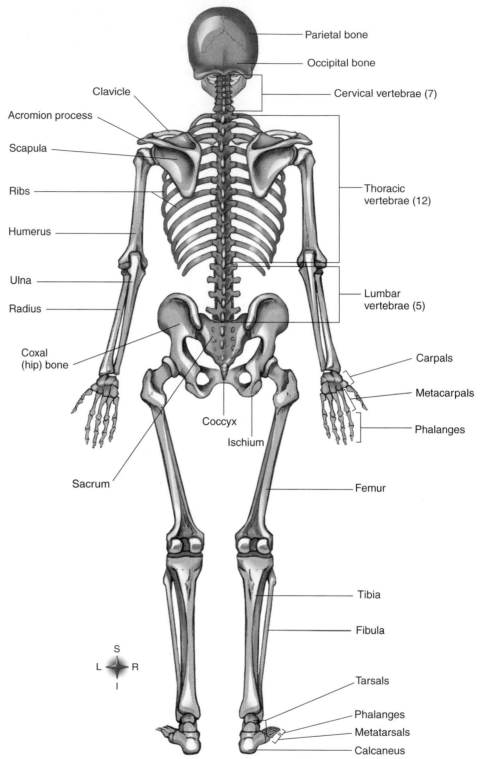

Parietal bone

Occipital bone

Cervical vertebrae (7)

Clavicle

Acromion process

Scapula

Ribs

Humerus

Ulna

Radius

Coxal
(hip) bone

Thoracic
vertebrae (12)

Lumbar
vertebrae (5)

Carpals

Metacarpals

Phalanges

Coccyx

Ischium

Sacrum

Femur

Tibia

Fibula

Tarsals

Phalanges

Metatarsals

Calcaneus

S

L   R

I

(From Thibodeau G, Patton K: Anatomy and physiology, *ed 6, St. Louis, 2007, Mosby.)*

GENERAL FUNCTIONS OF MUSCLES

Muscles are named as a result of location, points of attachment, and size. Energy for contractions comes from the nucleotide adenosine triphosphate (ATP). Glucose and oxygen are required for efficient nutrient catabolism of muscle fibers. Without the presence of glucose and oxygen in the muscle cells, lactic acid is produced, which causes pain and stiffness in the joints.

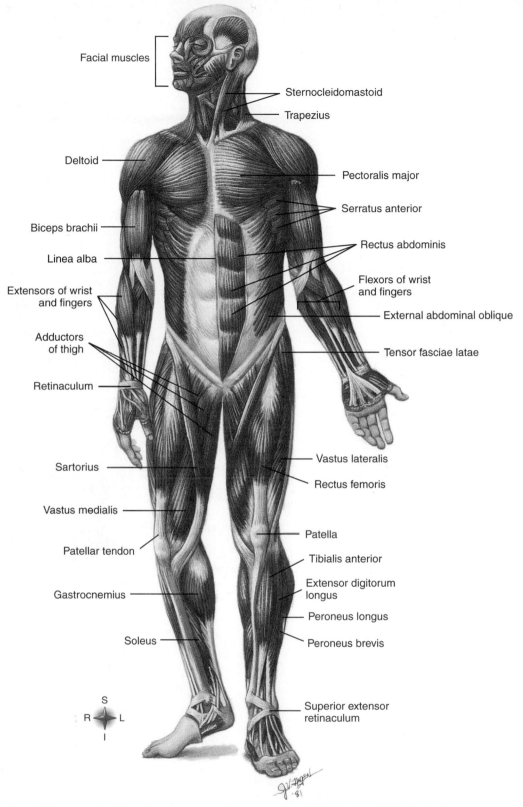

Facial muscles

Sternocleidomastoid

Trapezius

Deltoid

Pectoralis major

Serratus anterior

Biceps brachii

Rectus abdominis

Linea alba

Flexors of wrist and fingers

Extensors of wrist and fingers

External abdominal oblique

Adductors of thigh

Tensor fasciae latae

Retinaculum

Sartorius

Vastus lateralis

Rectus femoris

Vastus medialis

Patella

Patellar tendon

Tibialis anterior

Extensor digitorum longus

Gastrocnemius

Peroneus longus

Peroneus brevis

Soleus

Superior extensor retinaculum

S
R — L
I

(From Thibodeau G, Patton K: Anatomy and physiology, *ed 6, St. Louis, 2007, Mosby.)*

Continued

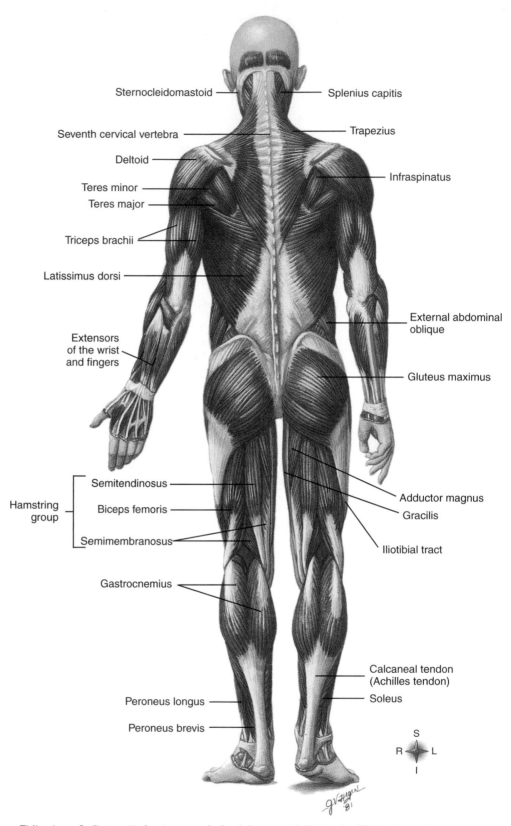

(From Thibodeau G, Patton K: Anatomy and physiology, ed 6, St. Louis, 2007, Mosby.)

FUNCTION OF SKELETAL MUSCLE TISSUE

Skeletal muscle tissue has three primary functions. They are:

Excitability: Ability of the muscle to be stimulated by a nervous impulse

Contractility: Ability to contract or shorten allows muscle tissue to pull on bones and thus produce body movement

Extensibility: Ability to extend or stretch allows muscles to return to their resting length after having contracted

CARDIAC MUSCLE

Cardiac muscle is found only in one organ of the body—the heart. Forming the bulk of the wall of each heart chamber, cardiac muscle contracts rhythmically and continuously to provide the pumping action necessary to maintain a relative constancy of blood flow through the internal environment.

SMOOTH MUSCLE

Smooth muscle cells form the muscular layer in the walls of many hollow structures like the digestive, urinary and reproductive tracts, and walls of large blood vessels. They cause *peristalsis* (waves of contraction) to move food along the digestive tract, assist the flow of urine to the bladder, and push a baby out of the womb during labor.

BIBLIOGRAPHY

Chabner E: *The language of medicine,* ed 8, St. Louis, 2007, WB Saunders.
Patton K: *Survival guide for anatomy and physiology,* St. Louis, 2006, Mosby.
Thibodeau G, Patton K: *Anatomy and physiology,* ed 6, St. Louis, 2007, Mosby.

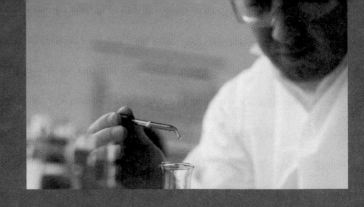

Neuromuscular Blockade

CHAPTER 13

LEARNING OBJECTIVES

- Discuss the process of neuromuscular transmission.
- List and classify drugs that cause skeletal muscle relaxation.
- Describe the mechanism of action for peripheral acting skeletal muscle relaxants.
- List uses for neuromuscular blocking drugs.
- Describe the mechanism for reversal of neuromuscular blockade.
- List strategies for safe management of neuromuscular blocking drugs in the pharmacy.
- Learn the terminology associated with the neuromuscular blockade and skeletal muscle relaxants.

KEY TERMS

Acetylcholinesterase: Enzyme that degrades acetylcholine and reverses acetylcholine-induced depolarization.

Anaphylactic shock: Acute, life-threatening allergic reaction that produces peripheral vasodilation, bronchospasm, and laryngeal edema and airway obstruction.

Blepharoptosis: Condition that causes eyelid muscles to droop.

Botulinum toxin: Poison produced by the bacterium *Clostridium botulinum* that causes muscle paralysis.

Central acting muscle relaxants: Drugs that produce relaxation of muscles through central nervous system depression blocking nerve transmission between the spinal cord and muscles.

Depolarizing neuromuscular blockers: Drugs that act as agonists at acetylcholine receptor sites and produce sustained depolarization; causing the receptors to convert to an inactive state.

Diaphoresis (hyperhydrosis): Excessive sweating.

Endotracheal intubation: Process of inserting a tube down into the trachea or windpipe to facilitate mechanical ventilation.

Endplate: Projection extending off the end of a motor neuron where the neurotransmitter acetylcholine is released.

Neuromuscular junction: Space between motor neuron endplate and the muscle soleplate that neurotransmitters must cross.

Nondepolarizing competitive blockers: Drugs that compete with acetylcholine for binding sites. When acetylcholine binding is inhibited, muscle contraction is blocked.

Peripheral acting muscle relaxants: Drugs that block nerve transmission between the motor endplate and skeletal muscle receptors.

Soleplate: Portion of the membrane of muscle cells that receives messages transmitted by motor neurons.

Tetanus: Fatal condition, characterized by continuous muscle spasm, caused by exposure to the nerve toxin produced by the bacterium *Clostridium tetani.* It is also known as "lockjaw."

Overview

Skeletal muscle contraction occurs as a response to communication between peripheral nerves and muscles. The neurotransmitter that is primarily responsible for transmitting messages between nerve cells and muscle cells is acetylcholine (ACh). The process of neuromuscular transmission begins with the release of ACh from vesicles located in the motor neuron endplate. The *endplate* is projection extending off the end of one of the branches of the motor neuron. The end of the motor neuron may be divided into as many as 200 branches. ACh that is released from the neuron endplate binds to nicotinic receptor sites located in the muscle soleplate. The *soleplate* is the portion of the membrane of muscle cells that receives messages transmitted by motor neurons. The neuronal endplate does not physically touch the soleplate so messages must travel across a 60-nm-wide space called the *neuromuscular junction* (Figure 13-1). The neuromuscular junction functions

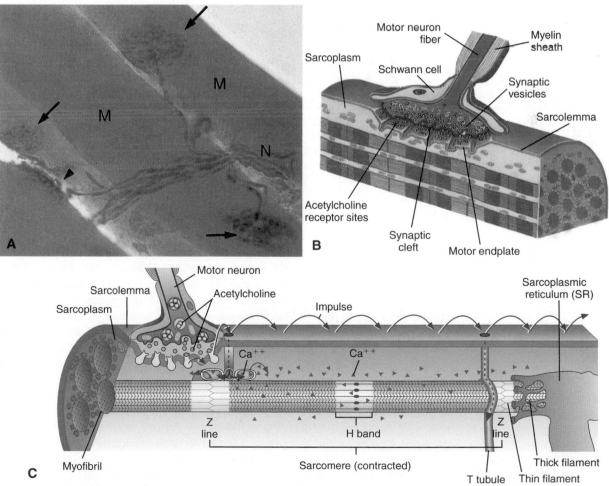

FIGURE 13-1 Excitation at the neuromuscular junction. (*A from Leeson TS:* Text/atlas of histology. *Philadelphia, 1988, Saunders. B and C from Thibodeau GA, Patton KT:* Anatomy and physiology, *ed 6, St Louis, 2007, Mosby.*)

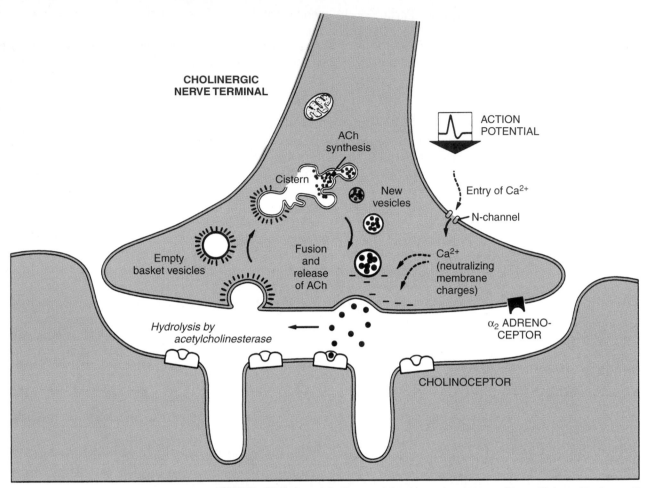

FIGURE 13-2 Acetylcholine synthesis and release. *(From Kalant H, Grant D, Mitchell J:* Principles of medical pharmacology, *ed 7, Toronto, 2007, Elsevier Canada, A Division of Reed Elsevier Canada.)*

like the synaptic cleft Central Nervous System). Approximately 90% of the soleplate is composed of nicotinic receptors that bind ACh.

ACh synthesis and release is a cyclical process (Figure 13-2). The process is stimulated by an influx of calcium into the neuronal endplate. Calcium entry occurs through voltage-regulated N channels. The influx of calcium raises the positive ions inside the cell, causing changes in the presynaptic membrane that result in the release of ACh from its storage vesicle. After ACh is released into the neuromuscular junction, a new vesicle begins to form in the presynaptic neuron. New ACh is synthesized in this vesicle. When the process is complete, the new vesicle filled with ACh buds off, awaiting a signal to release its contents.

ACh binding to nicotinic receptors opens sodium (Na^+), calcium (Ca^{2+}), and potassium (K^+) channels, increasing the endplate potential. Once endplate potential exceeds 15 mV, an action potential is produced (Figure 13-3).

Disassociation or unbinding of ACh from receptor sites inactivates and desensitizes the receptor site. The receptors are desensitized to further nerve contraction messages during the time it takes for the receptors to return to their preactivated state. Normally, between 10% and 20% of the nicotinic receptors are in an inactive state. Administration of neuromuscular blocking drugs leads to an increase in the percent of ACh receptor sites that are inactivated and results in relaxation of skeletal muscles. Drugs that decrease ACh release or deplete the neuron of ACh will also cause relaxation of muscles. Examples of drugs or substances that decrease ACh release are **botulinum toxin** and magnesium. Black widow

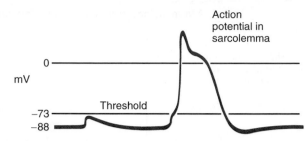

FIGURE 13-3 Diagram of an action potential. *(From Kalant H, Grant D, Mitchell J: Principles of medical pharmacology, ed 7, Toronto, 2007, Elsevier Canada, A Division of Reed Elsevier Canada.)*

spider venom depletes the neuron of ACh. High doses of ethanol will decrease ACh release, whereas low levels stimulate the release of ACh. Increased release of ACh produces skeletal muscle contraction. Calcium increases ACh release.

Skeletal Muscle Relaxants

Skeletal muscle relaxants are categorized by their site of action and mechanism of action. Drugs that produce relaxation of muscles by central nervous system depression (i.e., block nerve transmission between the spinal cord and muscles) are called ***central acting muscle relaxants***. Drugs that block nerve transmission between the motor endplate and skeletal muscle receptors are classified as ***peripheral acting muscle relaxants***. Peripheral acting drugs are further classified according to their mechanism of action. They are classified as *nondepolarizing competitive blockers* and *depolarizing blockers.* Direct-acting agents bind to and block calcium channels. Central acting muscle relaxants are discussed in Chapter 14.

INDICATION

Neuromuscular blocking agents have been used historically by indigenous peoples of South America. They were first used in surgery in 1942 and continue to be used today to induce a controlled, temporary state of paralysis. They are most commonly used in general anesthesia for ***endotracheal intubation*** to facilitate mechanical ventilation. Endotracheal intubation is the process of inserting a tube down into the trachea or windpipe. Endotracheal tubes are inserted whenever complete blockade of muscle movement is required as in ocular surgery. Other uses include to avoid intracranial pressure "spikes" in patients with increased cranial pressure, status epilepticus, status asthmaticus, strychinine poisoning, prevention of shivering in patients with severe burns, and ***tetanus***. Botulinum toxin type A, commonly known as Botox, is a neuromuscular blocking drug. Its use is becoming widespread, and it has been U.S. Food and Drug Administration (FDA) approved for a variety of conditions, including cosmetic use to temporarily remove wrinkles and treatment of excessive sweating. It has been administered for the treatment of uncontrollable blinking and spasticity associated with cerebral palsy, but this use is not FDA approved.

When neuromuscular blocking drugs are used during surgery, they should always be administered with analgesics to prevent pain. Their use should be closely monitored as these drugs can cause severe injury or death if misused. The degree of effectiveness of neuromuscular blockade should be measured using peripheral nerve stimulation using devices are made for monitoring of muscle twitching.

MECHANISM OF ACTION

The site of action of peripheral acting muscle relaxants is the neuromuscular junction (Figure 13-4). Nerve transmission between the motor endplate and skeletal muscle receptors located at the soleplate is blocked and results in the inhibition of depolarization and repolarization activity in muscles.

TECH NOTE!

The FDA has issued a warning that botulinum toxin Type A (Botox) and botulinum Type B (Myobloc) have been linked to respiratory failure and death (2008).

Pharmacology of Neuromuscular Transmission

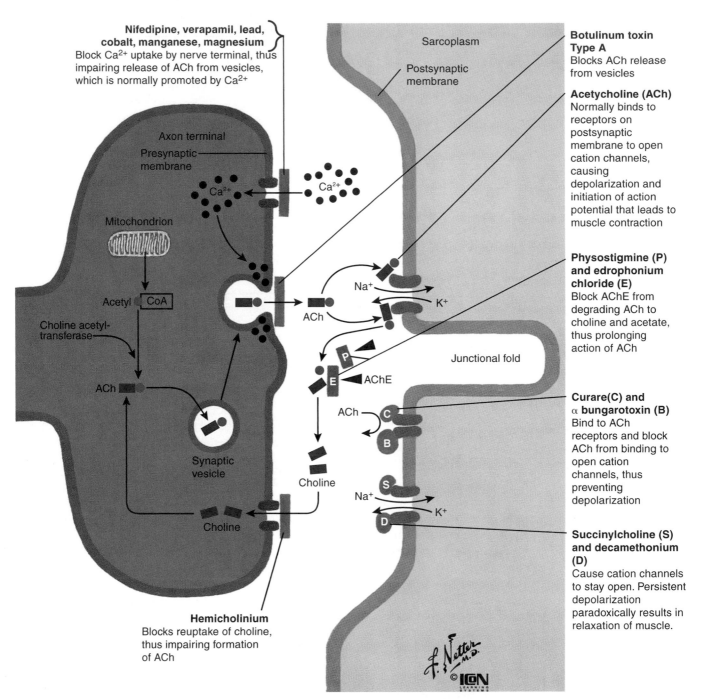

FIGURE 13-4 Mechanism of action of neuromuscular blocking drugs. *(From Raffa R, Rawls S, Beyzarov E:* Netter's illustrated pharmacology *(pp 80-82), Philadelphia, 2005, WB Saunders.)*

Depolarizing Blockers

Depolarizing neuromuscular drugs are agonists at nicotinic receptors. They bind to ACh receptors, where they produce sustained depolarization, causing receptors to convert to their inactive state. The receptors become desensitized and additional action potentials are prevented until the receptors return to their preactivated state. This prevents additional muscle contractions.

Succinylcholine is the only drug in this class. Like ACh, it is rapidly inactivated by cholinesterase enzymes. Cholinesterase enzymes are synthesized in the liver and are responsible for the breakdown of succinylcholine.

Nondepolarizing Neuromuscular Blockers

TECH NOTE!

"-curonium" and *"-curium"* are common endings for nondepolarizing neuromuscular blockers.

Most nondepolarizing neuromuscular blockers are competitive antagonists at prejunctional and postjunctional receptors. At low doses, they produce no effects of their own when they bind to receptor sites; instead, they compete with ACh for binding sites. When ACh binding is inhibited, muscle contraction is blocked. At high doses, nondepolarizing drugs interfere with Na^+, Ca^{2+}, and K^+ channels that increase endplate potential. This further weakens neuromuscular transmission and reduces the actions of acetylcholinesterase, the enzyme that reverses ACh-induced depolarization. Botulinum toxin type A, Botox, blocks the release of ACh from storage vesicles in the presynaptic neuron.

PHARMACOKINETICS

TECH NOTE!

Botox injections are made from a substance derived from botulinum toxin that works by preventing nerve impulses from reaching the muscle, causing the muscle to relax.

Most neuromuscular blocking drugs are poorly absorbed from the gastrointestinal tract, so they are administered parenterally (Table 13-1). They have low lipid solubility and they do not easily cross the blood-brain barrier. Their distribution into the central nervous system is low. They are highly water soluble and therefore are primarily eliminated in the urine. Aminosteroid-type neuromuscular blocking drugs (vecuronium) are also metabolized in the liver, and their rate of elimination may be decreased if the patient has liver disease. The onset of action is rapid (1 to 4 minutes) and duration of action is short (10 to 90 minutes). This requires a continuous infusion to be administered. An exception is botulinum toxin type A; its actions last up to 120 days. Nondepolarizing neuromuscular blocking drugs have a longer onset and longer duration of action than depolarizing neuromuscular blocking drugs. Nondepolarizing neuromuscular blocking drugs are not broken down by the enzyme acetylcholinesterase.

TABLE 13-1 Comparison of Central Acting Skeletal Muscle Relaxant Pharmacokinetics

Generic	Brand	Onset (min)	Duration of action (min)	Route of elimination (%)	
				Renal	Hepatic
Depolarizing neuromuscular blocking drugs					
succinylcholine	Quelicin	1	2 to 3	<10	–
Nondepolarizing neuromuscular blocking drugs					
atracurium	Tracrium	2 to 2.5	20 to 35	<10	0
botulinum toxin*	Botox	–	Up to 120 days	–	–
metocurine	Metubine	4	>180	43	2
Mivacurium		1 to 2	10 to 20	<10	–
pancuronium	(formerly Pavulon)	3 to 4	45 to 90 dose dependent	30 to 80	10
rocuronium	Zemuron	1 to 1.5	30 to 45	10 to 20	80 to 90
vecuronium	Norcuron	2.5 to 3	25 to 40	>25	20

*No available data.

ADVERSE REACTIONS

Allergic actions are common with the use of neuromuscular blocking drugs. These drugs have been shown to stimulate the release of histamine, a neurotransmitter involved in allergic reactions. Allergic reactions may appear as rash and redness on the face and neck or may be serious enough to produce bronchospasm, laryngospasm, and *anaphylatic shock*. Another common side effect is muscle pain. Other life-threatening adverse reactions that may be produced by neuromuscular blocking drugs are respiratory depression and cardiac arrest.

Additional adverse reactions associated with the use of neuromuscular blocking drugs are itching or burning at the injection site, hypotension, flushing (vasodilation), tachycardia or bradycardia, and pulmonary edema. Depolarizing neuromuscular blockers (succinylcholine) cause potassium channels to remain open, producing hyperkalemia and cardiac arrest. The administration of botulinum toxin type A injections may cause droopy eyelid muscles (*blepharoptosis*), headache, nausea, flu-like syndrome, redness, and muscle weakness.

Depolarizing Neuromuscular Blocking Drugs

Generic name	U.S. brand name(s) Canadian brand(s)	Dosage forms and strengths
succinylcholine*	Quelicin	**Injection, solution:** 20 mg/ml; 50 mg/ml; 100 mg/ml
	Quelicin	
Nondepolarizing neuromuscular blocking drugs		
atracurium*	Tracrium	**Injection, solution:** 10 mg/ml
	Generic	
botulinum toxin type A	Botox, Botox Cosmetic	100 units (as powder for reconstitution)
	Botox, Botox Cosmetic	
botulinum toxin type B	Myobloc	**Injection, solution:** 2500 units/0.5 ml 5000 units/1 ml 10,000 units/2 ml
	not available in Canada	
cisatracurium	Nimbex	**Injection, solution:** 2 mg/ml, 10 mg/ml
	Nimbex	
mivacurium	discontinued	**Injection, solution:** 2 mg/ml
	Mivacron	
pancuronium*	Generics	**Injection, solution:** 1 mg/ml
	Pavulon	
rocuronium	Zemuron	**Injection, solution:** 10 mg/ml
	Zemuron	
vecuronium	Norcuron	**Powder for injection:** 10 mg, 20 mg
	Norcuron	

*generic available

Reversal of Neuromuscular Blockade

Drugs that reverse the effects of neuromuscular blockade must always be readily available any time neuromuscular blocking drugs are administered. Anticholinesterase drugs inhibit the action of ACh esterase at the neuromuscular junction. This causes ACh to accumulate and compete with the administered neuromuscular blocking drug for available receptor sites. Anticholinesterase drugs are most effective once the process of spontaneous recovery from neuromuscular blocking drugs has begun.

ADVERSE REACTIONS

Edrophonium and neostigmine may produce salivation, muscle twitching, muscle weakness, abdominal cramping, nausea, increased bronchial secretions, and difficulty breathing.

Drugs That Reverse the Effects of Neuromuscular Blockade

Generic name	U.S. brand name(s) / Canadian brand(s)	Dosage forms and strengths
edrophonium	Enlon, Reversol	**Injection, solution:** 10 mg/ml
	Enlon	
neostigmine	Prostigmin	**Injection, solution:** 0.5 mg/ml
	Prostigmin	**Tablet:** 15 mg

Summary of Neuromuscular Blocking Drugs

Generic name	U.S. brand name	Usual adult oral dose and dosing schedule	Warning labels
succinylcholine	Quelicin	**Short surgeries IM: 3-4mg/kg** **rapid IV:** 0.3 mg to 1.1 mg/kg over 10-30 seconds **Continuous infusion:** 0.5 mg to 10 mg/min	KEEP REFRIGERATED After dilution to a concentration of 0.1% to 0.2%, the solution is stable for 4 weeks in the refrigerator and 1 week at room temperature.
atracurium	Tracrium	**IV:** 0.4 mg to 0.5 mg/kg; then 0.08 mg to 0.1 mg/kg 20 to 45 minutes after initial dose, and repeated every 15-25 minutes as needed **Continuous infusion:** 9 mcg to 10 mcg/kg/min **Continuous infusion:** 11 mcg to 13 mcg/kg/min	Keep refrigerated (2 °C to 8 °C); protect from freezing **After dilution:** Infusion solutions should be used within 24 hours of preparation
botulinum toxin type A	Botox	**Blepharospasm:** 1.25 units to 2.5 units IM every 1 to 3 months **Strabismus:** 1.25 units to 5 units IM **Diaphoresis:** 50 units intradermal into armpit **Wrinkles:** 0.1 ml in five designated injection sites (maximum 0.5 ml)	Keep refrigerated (2 °C to 8 °C); protect from freezing **After dilution:** refrigerated solutions should be used within 4 hours of preparation
botulinum toxin type B	Myobloc	**Usual adult dose for botulinum toxin type B for treatment of cervical dystonia is:** 2500 to 5000 unit IM divided among affected muscles	
cisatracurium	Nimbex	0.15 mg to 0.2 mg/kg IV	Refrigerate in the carton (2 °C to 8 °C); protect from freezing Protect from light **Once warmed to room temperature:** use within 21 days (even if re-refrigerated)

Continued

Summary of Neuromuscular Blocking Drugs—cont'd

Generic name	U.S. brand name	Usual adult oral dose and dosing schedule	Warning labels
mivacurium	Mivacron	**IV:** Initiate 0.15 mg to 0.25 mg/kg over 5 to 30 seconds; maintenance 0.1 mg/kg every 15 minutes **Continuous infusion:** 6 μg to 7 μg/kg/min	STORE AT ROOM TEMPERATURE
pancuronium	Pavulon (Canada)	**IV:** Initiate 0.04 mg to 0.1 mg/kg or 0.05 mg/kg after succinylcholine **Maintenance:** 0.01 mg/kg 60 to 100 minutes after initial dose, then every 25 to 60 minutes	KEEP REFRIGERATED (5°C); PROTECT FROM FREEZING DO NOT STORE IN PLASTIC SYRINGE
rocuronium	Zemuron	**Intubation:** 0.6 mg to 1.2 mg/kg IV **Continuous infusion:** Initial 0.01 mg to 0.012 mg/kg/min up to 0.04 mg to 0.016 mg/kg/min	KEEP REFRIGERATED; PROTECT FROM FREEZING AFTER RECONSTITUTION USE WITHIN 24 HOURS
vecuronium	Norcuron	**Intubation:** 0.08 mg to 0.1 mg/kg (IV); prolonged surgery 0.01 mg to 0.015 mg 25 to 40 minutes after initial dose **Continuous infusion:** 0.0008 mg to 0.0012 mg/kg/min or 1 mcg/kg/min	STORE POWDER AT ROOM TEMPERATURE PROTECT FROM LIGHT POST RECONSTITUTION (WITH BACTERIOSTATIC WATER FOR INJECT): USE WITHIN 5 DAYS REFRIGERATE AND USE WITHIN 24 HOURS AFTER RECONSTITUTION (WITH OTHER IV SOLUTIONS)

TECH NOTE!

Tubocurarine, formerly used in anesthesia, is the synthetic version of curare, a natural paralytic drug used by South American Indian hunters to immobilize prey.

Strategies for Safe Use of Neuromuscular Blocking Agents

Neuromuscular blocking drugs are classified "High Alert" by the Interdisciplinary Safe Medication Use Expert Committee of the United States Pharmacopoeia because improper use can result in permanent injury, respiratory arrest, and death. Problems associated with neuromuscular blocking drugs have been attributed to improper product selection, improper storage conditions, inappropriate dosing, improper labeling, and inadequate patient monitoring. Improper product selection is caused by similar product packaging and sound-alike

Summary of Drugs Used to Reverse the Effects of Neuromuscular Blocking Drugs

Generic name	U.S. brand name	Usual adult oral dose and dosing schedule	Warning labels
edrophonium	Enlon	10 mg over 30 to 35 seconds (IV); repeat in 5 to 10 minutes if needed up to 40 mg	STORE BELOW 25°C PROTECT FROM LIGHT
neostigmine	Prostigmin	**Reversal of neuromuscular blockade:** 0.5 mg to 2.5 mg (IV) to maximum 5 mg **Bladder atony:** 0.25 mg to 1 mg SC or IM every 3 hours for 5 doses	STABLE AT ROOM TEMPERATURE

BOX 13-1 SAFE MANAGEMENT OF NEUROMUSCULAR BLOCKING AGENTS: RECOMMENDATIONS FOR PHARMACY PRACTICE

PRODUCT SELECTION
- Procurement managers should select products that have distinctive names and packaging to avoid sound-alike/look-alike issues.

PRODUCT STORAGE
- Neuromuscular blocking drugs should be stored apart from other drugs.
- Storage of neuromuscular blocking drugs should be confined to primary care areas and pharmacy areas that care for mechanically ventilated patients.

LIMIT ACCESS
- Neuromuscular blocking drugs should be kept in sealed "intubation kits" or "anesthesia kits" until use is needed.
- Opened vials should be immediately discarded or returned to the seal kit after use.
- Neuromuscular blocking drugs should NOT be dispensed in unit dose carts or delivered to general nursing units unless in a sealed kit.
- Neuromuscular blocking drugs should be stored in a single access drawer when stored in drug storage devices like Pyxis and AccuDose-Rx.

- Neuromuscular blocking drugs requiring refrigeration should be stored in a separate area away from other refrigerated drugs.

AUXILIARY LABELS OR WARNING LABELS
- Neuromuscular blocking drugs should always be dispensed with the auxiliary label "WARNING: Paralyzing agent (Use requires mechanical ventilatory assistance)."
- Overwraps should be considered for individual vials of neuromuscular blocking drugs stored outside of pharmacy and anesthesiology areas, especially drugs stored in the refrigerator.
- Affix preprinted syringe labels to syringes filled with neuromuscular blocking drugs at the time the drug is drawn up to avoid risks associated with unlabeled syringes.

ORDERING PRACTICES AND DISPENSING
- Contact prescriber for complete directions when medication orders for neuromuscular blocking agents are written with PRN directions.
- Verify patient identity and drug identity with bar-code readers when available.

*Adapted from United States Pharmacopoeia Interdisciplinary Safe Medication Use Expert Committee recommendations.

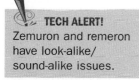

TECH ALERT!
Zemuron and remeron have look-alike/sound-alike issues.

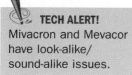

TECH ALERT!
Mivacron and Mevacor have look-alike/sound-alike issues.

drug names. Drug names that sound alike pose problems in dispensing regardless of the type of drug. Look-alike packaging is a problem that can be attributed to drug manufacturers as well as pharmacies dispensing drugs (see Chapter 4). Neuromuscular blocking drugs may be repackaged for unit of use in institutional care settings. Infusion bags and syringes that have been prepared by the pharmacy look alike. Neuromuscular blocking drugs have been administered in the place of vaccines, intravenous flush solutions, and antibiotics by mistake. A pharmacy that fails to securely affix the label onto the infusion bag or syringe of a neuromuscular blocking drug has created a potentially life-threatening situation for a patient. Inaccurate sterile compounding has resulted in the dispensing of incorrect drug concentrations and incorrect doses placed in automated dispensing machines.

To prevent possible injury or death, the United States Pharmacopoeia Interdisciplinary Safe Medication Use Expert Committee has compiled a list of recommendations for the safe use of neuromuscular blocking agents. The recommendations listed in Box 13-1 are modified for pharmacy-specific application.

CHAPTER SUMMARY

- Skeletal muscle contraction occurs as a response to communication between peripheral nerves and muscles.
- The process of neuromuscular transmission begins with the release of acetylcholine (ACh) from vesicles located in the motor neuron endplate.
- ACh that is released from the nerve endplate binds to nicotinic receptor sites located in the muscle soleplate.
- The neuromuscular junction is the space between the neuron endplate and receptor sites in the muscle cell.
- Approximately 90% of the soleplate is composed of nicotinic receptors that bind ACh.
- ACh binding to nicotinic receptors opens sodium, calcium, and potassium channels, increasing the endplate potential.
- Unbinding of ACh from receptor sites desensitizes them to further nerve conduction messages during the time it takes for the receptors to return to their preactivated state.
- Neuromuscular blocking drugs cause skeletal muscle relaxation by increasing the percent of ACh receptor sites that are inactivated.
- Drugs that decrease ACh release or deplete the neuron of ACh will also cause relaxation of muscles.
- Examples of drugs or substances that decrease ACh release are botulinum toxin, magnesium, and high doses of ethanol.
- Peripheral acting drugs are classified as nondepolarizing competitive blockers and depolarizing blockers.
- Depolarizing neuromuscular drugs are agonists at nicotinic receptors.
- Most nondepolarizing neuromuscular blockers are competitive antagonists at prejunctional and postjunctional receptors.
- Neuromuscular blocking drugs are most commonly used in general anesthesia for endotracheal intubation to facilitate mechanical ventilation.
- Botulium toxin type A has been FDA approved for cosmetic use to temporarily remove wrinkles, treat excessive sweating, and treat uncontrollable blinking.
- The onset of action of neuromuscular blocking drugs is rapid (1 to 4 minutes), and the duration of action is short (10 to 90 minutes).
- Adverse reactions associated with the use of neuromuscular blocking drugs are hypotension, tachycardia, pulmonary edema, hyperkalemia cardiac arrest, bronchospasm, and anaphylactic shock.
- Botulinum toxin type A injections can cause droopy eyelid muscles, headache, nausea, flu-like syndrome, redness, muscle weakness, and pain at the injection site.
- Drugs that reverse the effects of neuromuscular blockade must always be readily available any time neuromuscular blocking drugs are administered.
- Anticholinesterase drugs cause ACh to accumulate and compete with the administered neuromuscular blocking drug for available receptor sites.
- Neuromuscular blocking drugs are classified "High Alert" by the Interdisciplinary Safe Medication Use Expert Committee of the United States Pharmacopoeia because improper use can result in permanent injury, respiratory arrest, and death.
- To prevent possible injury or death, the United States Pharmacopoeia Interdisciplinary Safe Medication Use Expert Committee has compiled a list of recommendations for the safe use of neuromuscular blocking agents that includes suggestions for product selection, storage, limited access, auxiliary label use, ordering, and dispensing practices.

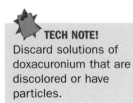

TECH NOTE!
Discard solutions of doxacuronium that are discolored or have particles.

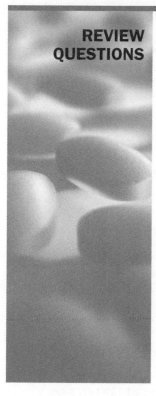

REVIEW QUESTIONS

Multiple Choice

1. The neurotransmitter that is primarily responsible for transmitting messages between nerve cells and muscle cells is _____.
   a. dopamine
   b. epinephrine
   c. acetylcholine
   d. GABA

2. Administration of neuromuscular _____ drugs leads to an increase in the percent of acetylcholine receptor sites that are inactivated and results in relaxation of skeletal muscles.
   a. blocking
   b. stimulating
   c. enhancing
   d. stabilizing

3. Botox has not been FDA approved for cosmetic use.
   a. true
   b. false

4. Most neuromuscular blocking drugs are poorly absorbed from the gastrointestinal tract so they are administered _____.
   a. topically
   b. enterally
   c. parenterally
   d. transdermally

5. Allergic actions may occur with the use of neuromuscular blocking drugs.
   a. true
   b. false

6. Neuromuscular blocking drugs are classified "_____" by the Interdisciplinary Safe Medication Use Expert Committee of the United States Pharmacopoeia.
   a. Dangerous
   b. High Alert
   c. Low Alert
   d. Use with caution

7. How should neuromuscular blocking drugs be stored?
   a. in alphabetical order on the shelf
   b. in the IV room
   c. with the fast movers
   d. apart from other drugs

8. Neuromuscular blocking drugs should always be dispensed with what auxillary label?
   a. WARNING: Paralyzing agent (Use requires mechanical ventilatory assistance)
   b. WARNING: Allergic reactions possible
   c. KEEP IN REFRIGERATOR UNTIL READY TO USE
   d. FOR ONE TIME USE ONLY

9. Which of the following is Botox *not* indicated for?
   a. blepharospasms
   b. diaphoresis
   c. cosmetic wrinkle removal
   d. cervical dystonia

10. Medication errors can easily happen with nondepolarizing neuromuscular blocking drugs because _____.
    a. All packages look the same.
    b. Some drugs have look-alike/sound-alike names.
    c. Doses are all the same.
    d. All are made by same manufacturer.

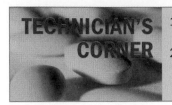

TECHNICIAN'S CORNER

1. Everyone wants to keep looking young. What solutions can you give a client other than using Botox for wrinkles?
2. You are in charge of inventory in the pharmacy and need to alert everyone about the potential of medication errors that can occur with neuromuscular blocking drugs. What would be the best way to alert everyone?

BIBLIOGRAPHY

Harboe, T., Guttormsen, A., Irgens, A., *Anaphylaxis during anesthesia in Norway*-A 6-year single center Follow-up study. Anesthesiology 2005; 102:897-903.

Kalant H, Grant D, Mitchell J: *Principles of medical pharmacology* (pp 176-180), ed 7, Toronto, 2007, Elsevier Canada, A Division of Reed Elsevier Canada.

Lance L, Lacy C, Armstrong L, Goldman M: *Drug information handbook for the allied health professional,* ed 12. Hudson, OH, 2005, APhA Lexi-Comp.

Lewis C: *Botox cosmetic: a look at looking good,* U.S. Food and Drug Administration, FDA Consumer Magazine. Retrieved from http://www.fda.gov/fdac/features/2002/402_botox.html.

Matthey, P., Wang. P., Finegan, B., Donnelly, M., Rocuronium anaphylaxis and multiple neuromuscular blocking drug sensitivities. CJA 2000; 47:9, pp. 890-893.

Mehta S, et al. Canadian survey of the use of sedatives, analgesics, and neuromuscular blocking agents in critically ill patients, *Crit Care Med,* 34:374-380, 2006.

Parenteral drug therapy manual, Pharmaceutical Sciences, Vancouver General Hospital, Vancouver, BC. Retrieved from http://www.vhpharmsci.com/PDTM/.

Phillips M, Williams R: Improving the safety of neuromuscular blocking agents: a statement from the USP Safe Medication Use Expert Committee, *Am J Health Syst Pharm,* 63:139-142, 2006.

Shapiro B, et al. Practice parameters for sustained neuromuscular blockade in the adult critically ill patient, *Crit Care Med,* 23:1601-1605, 1995.

Wood A: New neuromuscular blocking drugs, *N Engl J Med,* 332, 1995.

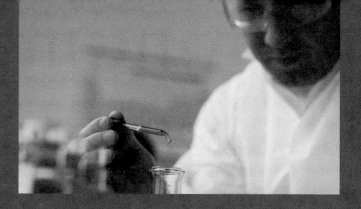

CHAPTER 14

Treatment of Muscle Spasms

LEARNING OBJECTIVES

- Describe the signs and symptoms of spasticity.
- List medical conditions that cause spasticity.
- Classify medications used in the treatment of spasticity.
- Describe the function of neurotransmitters associated with antispasticity drugs.
- Describe the mechanism of action for each class of drugs used in the treatment of spasticity.
- Identify warning labels and precautionary messages associated with medications used to treat spasticity.
- Identify significant drug look-alike/sound-alike issues.
- Learn the terminology associated with spasticity and its treatment.

KEY TERMS

Amyotrophic lateral sclerosis (ALS): Degenerative disease that causes muscle wasting and muscle weakness. ALS is also known as Lou Gehrig's disease.

Cerebral palsy: Neurological disorder that affects muscle movement and coordination.

Clonus: Involuntary rhythmic muscle contraction that causes the feet and wrists to involuntarily flex and relax.

Lower motor neurons: Neurons that branch out from the spinal cord to the muscles and tissues of the body.

Multiple sclerosis: Autoimmune disease that causes progressive damage to nerves resulting in spasticity, pain, mood changes, and other physical symptoms.

Negative symptoms: Spasticity symptoms that can produce muscle weakness, decreased endurance, and reduction in the ability to make voluntary muscle movements.

Phenylketonuria (PKU): A disease marked by failure to metabolize the amino acid phenylalanine to tyrosine. It results in severe neurological deficits in infancy if untreated.

Positive symptoms: Spasticity symptoms that cause muscle spasms and hyperexcitable reflexes.

Sarcomere: Contracting unit of muscle fibers.

Spasticity: Motor disorder that causes increased muscle tone, exaggerated tendon jerks, and hyperexcitable muscles.

Upper motor neurons: Neurons that carry messages from the brain down to the spinal cord.

Overview

Spasticity is a debilitating motor disorder that affects up to 12 million people worldwide. Symptoms of *spasticity* are an increase in muscle tone, exaggerated tendon jerks, and hyperexcitability of the stretch reflex. These symptoms are collectively known as muscle spasms and are *positive symptoms* of spasticity. *Negative symptoms* associated with spasticity include muscle weakness, decreased endurance, and reduction in the capacity to make voluntary muscle movements. Spasticity interferes with the normal performance of activities of daily living. The ability for self-care is significantly impaired, and it can inhibit effective walking, cause fatigue, cause stiffness, disturb sleep, and increase risk for pressure ulcers and infections.

Stroke, spinal cord injury, cerebral palsy, muscle trauma (e.g., whiplash), multiple sclerosis, head injury, and metabolic diseases such as amyotrophic lateral sclerosis (Lou Gehrig's disease), multiple sclerosis, and phenylketonuria can all cause spasticity. In fact, 65% to 78% of people with spinal cord injuries and 65% of people who have had a stroke will develop spasticity.

Spasticity can be aggravated by a variety of factors. Fatigue, pain, stress, fever, cold constipation, immobility, and hormonal changes can all worsen symptoms of spasticity.

Pathophysiology of Spasticity

Any condition that can damage the brain or spinal cord can cause spasticity. Regardless of the cause, the progression to spasticity follows a specific pattern and the degree of spasticity is related to the duration since the original injury. The four phases are (1) decreased muscle contractility, (2) excessive muscle tone and increased reflex activity lasting from days to years, (3) decreased reflex excitability, and, finally, (4) stiff, contracted muscles.

Conditions That Produce Spasticity

SPINAL CORD INJURY

Spinal cord injury may produce muscle paralysis and loss of tendon reflexes in the region below the level of spinal cord injury immediately following the injury. Within a few weeks, this period of spinal shock ends and is followed by a period of increased muscle tone, exaggerated tendon jerks and involuntary muscle spasms. It is believed that spasticity develops because the neurons that branch out from the spinal cord to the muscles and tissues of the body (*lower motor neurons*) grow new synapses. The increase in the number of synapses causes a stronger reflex connection and a greater response to stretching of the muscle. Moreover, normal inhibitory control of sustained neuron firing is lost during the recovery period after spinal cord injury. What follows is unopposed motor neuron excitability and changes in endplate potential (see Chapter 13). Receptors become more sensitive to neurotransmitters, but at the same time, muscle changes cause altered contractility. Muscle fibers atrophy and the number of sarcomeres decrease; however, connective tissue increases. *Sarcomeres* are units within muscle fibers responsible for muscle contraction (Figure 14-1).

Spinal cord injury also results in *clonus*, involuntary rhythmic muscle contraction that produces involuntarily flexing and relaxation of the feet and wrists.

STROKE

Stroke can cause a lesion to form in the brain or spinal cord that results in unopposed motor neuron excitability by normal inhibitory mechanisms.

CEREBRAL PALSY

Spasticity caused by cerebral palsy follows the same pathophysiological pathway as stroke and spinal cord injury. Treatment is complicated because spasticity impairs effective muscle movement in some people with cerebral palsy and helps maintain posture, making walking easier in other people.

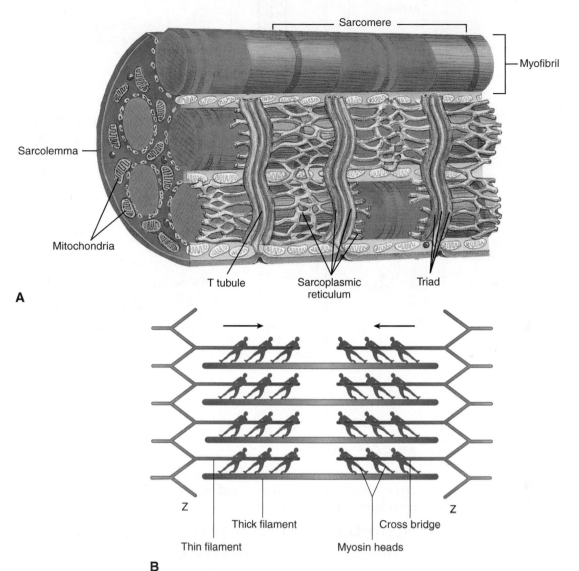

A

B

FIGURE 14-1 **A**, Sarcomere. **B**, Simplified sarcomere. *(From Thibodeau GA, Patton KT:* Anatomy and physiology, *ed 6, St Louis, 2007, Mosby.)*

AMYTROPHIC LATERAL SCLEROSIS

People who have ***amyotrophic lateral sclerosis (ALS)*** exhibit predominantly negative symptoms of spasticity. Damage to upper motor neurons is caused by decreased reuptake of the excitatory amino acid glutamate. This causes glutamate levels to accumulate and calcium to flood into motor neurons (Figure 14-2). Recall that the influx of calcium raises the positive ions inside the cell, causing changes in the presynaptic membrane that result in the release of ACh from its storage vesicle (see Chapter 13). This ultimately causes desensitization of motor nerves, muscle weakness, and cell death.

MULTIPLE SCLEROSIS

Multiple sclerosis is an autoimmune disease that causes damage to myelinated nerves (Figure 15-2). Lesions damage nerves in the central nervous system and cause spasticity, pain, fatigue, bladder dysfunction, cognitive dysfunction, sexual dysfunction, bowel dysfunction, and changes in mood or depression. Nerve damage and symptoms get progressively worse over time.

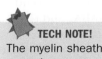

TECH NOTE!
The myelin sheath around neurons acts as an electrical insulator and increases the velocity of impulse transmission.

At Rest   **Impulse**

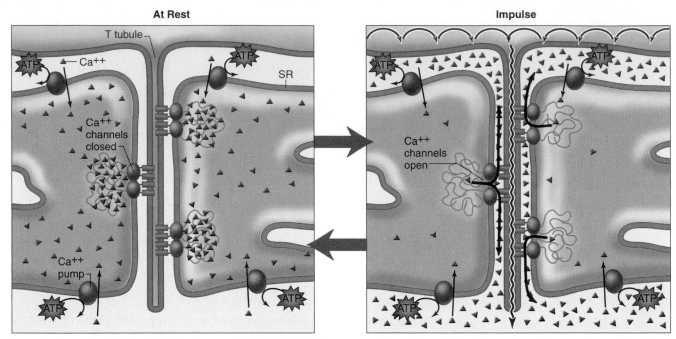

FIGURE 14-2 Storage and release of calcium ions in muscle cells. *(From Thibodeau GA, Patton KT: Anatomy and physiology, ed 6, St Louis, 2007, Mosby.)*

MUSCLE STRAIN

Muscle strain, sprains, fibromyalgia, tension headache, low back pain, and neck pain can cause muscles spasm, stiffness, and pain. When spasms are present, it is typically related to local injury or irritation of a specific muscle group.

Neurotransmitters Involved in Spasticity

Spasticity is a symptom of upper motor neuron syndrome. Upper motor neurons carry messages from the brain down to the spinal cord. Spasticity may be due to excess of neurotransmitters that carry excitatory messages, like glutamate, or decreased activity or a deficiency of inhibitory transmitters, like γ-aminobutyric acid and glycine. Spasticity also may be accompanied by pain.

ROLE OF ACETYLCHOLINE

Acetylcholine (ACh) is the neurotransmitter that is primarily responsible for transmitting messages between nerve cells and muscle cells. ACh binding to nicotinic receptors opens sodium (Na^+), calcium (Ca^{2+}), and potassium (K^+) channels, increasing the endplate potential and producing muscle contraction (see Figure 13-2).

ROLE OF γ-AMINOBUTYRIC ACID

Another mechanism of action for drugs used to treat spasticity is (1) to directly bind to GABA type B receptors ($GABA_B$) or (2) to enhance GABA binding to $GABA_A$ and $GABA_B$ receptors. GABA is the major inhibitory neurotransmitter in the nervous system. $GABA_A$ receptor binding causes chloride ion (Cl^-) channels to open. The influx of chloride ions results in hyperpolarization and inhibits formation of action potentials. $GABA_B$ receptor binding inhibits the release of excitatory neurotransmitters and substance P. Ultimately, neuronal excitability is reduced and nerve impulse transmission is decreased. GABAergic receptors are stimulated by dopamine (D_2), another inhibitory neurotransmitter.

ROLE OF GLYCINE

Glycine is an inhibitory neurotransmitter. Defects of receptors for glycine are associated with a rare disease that causes an exaggerated startle reflex called hyperekplexia. This produces intense muscle contractions known as *hypertonia*.

ROLE OF GLUTAMATE

Voltage-dependent calcium channels are believed to be involved in spasticity. Glutamate is an excitatory amino acid responsible for the flow of calcium into motor neurons. Drugs that decrease glutamate availability are used to treat amytrophic lateral sclerosis (ALS).

Drugs Used to Treat Spasticity

To manage spasticity, a variety of nonpharmaceutical treatments have been tried. Electrical stimulation, cold packs (cryotherapy), biofeedback, splinting, positioning, and physical therapy have all been proposed. These nondrug therapies may support pharmacological treatments.

Drugs used in the treatment of spasticity are grouped according to the site of action and are classified as centrally acting and peripheral acting. Peripheral acting drugs act directly on contractile mechanisms in the muscle. Central acting drugs may be further categorized according to their mechanism of action. Some drugs are GABAergic. They act on GABA receptors in the central nervous system. Another group of drugs act at α_2-adrenergic receptor sites. Regardless of their mechanism of action, the goal of most drug treatments is to reduce the positive symptoms of spasticity.

PERIPHERAL ACTING DRUGS

BOTULINUM TOXIN TYPE A

The use of botulinium toxin for the treatment of spasticity is unlabeled and investigational. It is injected locally to inhibit presynaptic release of acetylcholine at the neuromuscular junction. This causes paralysis in the muscle(s) that have received the injections. The paralysis is reversed when the motor neuron sprouts new terminals that begin to release acetylcholine. The effectiveness of botulinum toxin type A injections begin 3 to 7 days after administration and last 3 to 6 months. Resistance develops with repeated use and injections, and the frequency of injection should be limited to no sooner than every 3 months. Botulinum toxin type A was discussed in more detail in Chapter 13.

DANTROLENE

Dantrolene is indicated for the treatment of spasticity associated with spinal cord injury, stroke, cerebral palsy, multiple sclerosis, and malignant hyperthermia. It reduces spasticity by weakening hyperexcited muscles. It acts directly on contractile mechanisms in skeletal muscle. Dantrolene inhibits the release of calcium from structures found in the muscle called the sarcoplasmic reticulum (see Figure 14-1), inhibiting calcium-dependent excitation-contraction (see Figure 14-2). The use of dantrolene in the treatment of some spastic conditions is limited because the drug produces muscle weakness. Muscle weakness is undesirable when treating spasticity associated with spinal cord injury or ALS. Other adverse effects produced by dantrolene include sedation, fatigue, diarrhea, and hepatoxicity.

Peripheral Acting Drugs Used for the Treatment of Spasticity

Generic name	U.S. brand name(s) / Canadian brand(s)	Dosage forms and strengths
dantrolene*	Dantrium	**Capsule:** 25 mg, 50 mg, 100 mg
	Dantrium	**Injection, powder for reconstitution:** 20 mg

*Generic available.

CENTRAL ACTING DRUGS

Central acting skeletal muscle relaxants reduce spasticity by binding to receptors sites that control motor movement in the brain and spinal cord. The mechanism of action of these drugs is to enhance the actions of GABA, an inhibitory neurotransmitter or to stimulate α_2-adrenergic receptors.

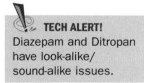

TECH ALERT!

The following drugs have look-alike/sound-alike issues: baclofen and bactroban; Lioresal, Lotensin, and Lisinopril

GABAergic DRUGS

Drugs That Bind Directly to GABA Receptors

Baclofen is structurally similar to the neurotransmitter GABA. It acts as an agonist at $GABA_B$ receptor sites and is particularly useful in treatment of spasticity associated with spinal cord injury. By mimicking a naturally occurring inhibitory neurotransmitter, baclofen screens out unnecessary sensory messages coming from the environment and effectively decreases spasticity. Baclofen is indicated for the treatment of spasticity associated with spinal cord injury and multiple sclerosis.

Mechanism of Action and Pharmacokinetics. Baclofen decreases the release of excitatory neurotransmitters that cause muscle contractions and reduces pain linked to spasticity by inhibiting the release of substance P. The site of action for baclofen is the spinal cord where it binds to presynaptic and postsynaptic receptors. GABA binding interrupts of the flow of calcium and potassium ions into the nerve terminal, causing hyperpolarization of the nerve membrane and reduction of spinal reflexes. The ability of baclofen to cross the blood-brain barrier is limited, so its effectiveness is augmented by administering the drug intrathecally. Intrathecal solutions are injected directly into the cerebrospinal fluid, so the level of the drug in the cerebral spinal fluid is increased. Surgery is required to implant the intrathecal delivery system. The pump needs to be refilled every 2 to 3 months and must be replaced every 4 to 5 years.

Adverse Reactions. Adverse reactions include dizziness, drowsiness, headache, nausea, orthostatic hypotension, confusion, and weakness. Sudden discontinuation can cause withdrawal symptoms. Rebound spasticity, hallucinations, itching, hyperthermia, and seizures are signs and symptoms of withdrawal syndrome.

Central Acting Drugs Used for the Treatment of Spasticity (Bind to GABA Receptors)

Generic name	U.S. brand name(s) Canadian brand(s)	Dosage forms and strengths
baclofen*	Lioresal	**Injection, solution:** 50 mcg/ml, 500 mcg/ml, 2000 mcg/ml
	Lioresal	**Tablet:** 10 mg, 20 mg

*Generic available.

TECH ALERT!

Diazepam and Ditropan have look-alike/sound-alike issues.

Drugs That Enhance GABA Binding

Diazepam is classified as a central acting agent because its site of action is the reticular formation of the brainstem and polysynaptic pathways in the spinal cord. Diazepam increases the binding of GABA to GABA receptors, decreasing the excitability of nerve terminals and hyperpolarizing the nerve. Diazepam is the most commonly used benzodiazepine for the treatment of spasticity, and it is effective in treating hyperactive reflexes and painful muscle spasms. At therapeutic doses, diazepam improves range of motion. Diazepam decreases anxiety and sleeplessness—both conditions that can aggravate spasticity. A detailed discussion of the pharmacokinetics and adverse reactions of benzodiazepines is found in Chapters 5 and 9.

Central Acting Drugs Used for the Treatment of Spasticity (Enhance GABA Binding)

Generic name	U.S. brand name(s) Canadian brand(s)	Dosage forms and strengths
diazepam*	Diastat, Diazepam Intensol, Valium	**Rectal gel (Diastat):** 5 mg/ml **Injection, solution:** 5 mg/ml **Oral, solution:** 5 mg/5ml
	Diastat, Diazemuls, Valium	**Oral concentrate (Diazepam Intensol), solution:** 5 mg/ml **Tablet (Valium):** 2 mg, 5 mg, 10 mg

*Generic available.

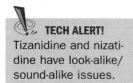

TECH ALERT!
Tizanidine and nizatidine have look-alike/sound-alike issues.

α₂-Adrenergic Drugs

α_2-Adrenergic agonists act like naturally occurring neurotransmitters. When α_2-adrenergic drugs are administered, they screen out unnecessary sensory messages that cause spasticity. They reduce muscle tone and the frequency of muscle spasms in people who have had spinal cord injuries, cerebral palsy, and stroke.

Mechanism of Action and Pharmacokinetics. Spasticity is reduced when α_2-adrenergic drugs are administered because the drugs prevent the release of excitatory neurotransmitters in the spinal cord and increase the actions of the inhibitory neurotransmitter glycine. α_2-Adrenergic agonists also cause hyperpolarization of motor neurons. Painful muscle spasms are diminished because α_2-adrenergic drugs interfere with the release of substance P, the neurotransmitter involved in the production of pain sensations and controlling pain perception (see Chapter 10).

Tizanidine is classified as an α_2-adrenergic agonist. Tizanidine is structurally similar to the antihypertensive drug clonidine, but it produces less effects on the cardiovascular system.

Adverse Reactions. Tizanidine produces sedation, hypotension, and dizziness. The incidence of sedation is less with tizanidine than with clonidine. The drug reportedly can cause hepatotoxicity but is not associated with decreased muscle strength.

Central Acting Drugs Used for the Treatment of Spasticity (α₂-Adrenergic Drugs)

Generic name	U.S. brand name(s) Canadian brand(s)	Dosage forms and strengths
tizanidine*	Zanaflex	**Tablet:** 2 mg, 4 mg
	Zanaflex	

*Generic available.

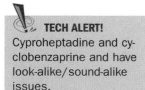

TECH ALERT!
Cyproheptadine and cyclobenzaprine and have look-alike/sound-alike issues.

Miscellaneous

Cyproheptadine is an antihistamine that is used in the treatment of spasticity associated with spinal cord injury as well as to treat baclofen withdrawal symptoms; however, this use is not approved by the FDA. Its mechanism of action appears to be linked to its effects on the neurotransmitters serotonin, histamine, and ACh.

Drugs Used to Treat Muscle Strain

Skeletal muscle relaxants are used to treat muscle stiffness, pain, and spasms associated with muscle tension, strain, sprains, or injury. Some, such as methocarbamol and orphenadrine, are additionally indicated for supportive therapy in tetanus. Drugs in this category include carisoprodol, chlorzoxazone, cyclobenzaprine, metaxalone, methocarbamol, and orphenadrine. These skeletal muscle relaxants are centrally acting; however, the mechanism of action is unknown. It is believed their actions may be related to their sedative effects on the central nervous system.

Common adverse effects associated with drugs used to treat muscle strain are dizziness, drowsiness, and blurred vision. Additional adverse effects are discoloration of urine—chlorzoxazone (orange to reddish purple) and methocarbamol (black, brown, or green).

Skeletal muscle relaxants should be used along with nonpharmaceutical therapies such as rest, exercise, cryotherapy, heat, and physical therapy.

Central Acting Drugs Used for the Treatment of Muscle Strain

	Generic name	U.S. brand name(s) / Canadian brand(s)	Dosage forms and strengths
	carisoprodol*	Soma, Soprodal-350, Vanadom, / Not available	**Tablet:** 250 mg, 350 mg
	chlorzoxazone*	Parafon Forte DSC / Parafon Forte	Caplet (Parafon Forte DSC) **Tablet:** 250 mg, 500 mg
	cyclobenzaprine*	Flexeril, Amrix / generics	**Tablet:** 5 mg, 10 mg **Capsule, extended release:** 15 mg, 30 mg
	methocarbamol*	Robaxin / Robaxin	**Injection, solution:** 100 mg/ml **Tablet:** 500 mg, 750 mg
	orphenadrine*	Norflex / Norflex, Orphenace	**Injection, solution:** 30 mg/ml (2 ml) **Tablet, extended release:** 100 mg
COMBINATION PRODUCTS			
	carisoprodol + aspirin*	Soma Compound / Not available	**Tablet:** 200 mg carisoprodol + 325 mg aspirin
	carisoprodol + aspirin + codeine*	Soma Compound with Codeine / Not available	**Tablet:** 200 mg carisoprodol + 325 mg aspirin + 16 mg codeine
	methocarbamol + aspirin	Robaxisal	**Tablet:** 400 mg methocarbamol + 325 mg aspirin
		Extra Strength Muscle and Backache Relief	**Tablet:** 400 mg methocarbamol + 500 mg aspirin
	methocarbamol + acetaminophen	Not available / Robaxacet	**Tablet:** 400 mg methocarbamol + 325 mg aspirin

Central Acting Drugs Used for the Treatment of Muscle Strain—cont'd

Generic name	U.S. brand name(s) Canadian brand(s)	Dosage forms and strengths
ophenadrine + caffeine + aspirin	Norgesic, Orphengesic; Norgesic Forte	**Tablet:** 25 mg orphenadrine + 30 mg caffeine + 385 mg aspirin;
	Not available	**Tablet:** 50 mg orphenadrine + 60 mg caffeine + 770 mg aspirin

*Generic available.

Summary of Drugs Used in the Treatment of Spasticity

Generic name	U.S. brand name	Usual adult oral dose and dosing schedule	Warning labels
Central acting skeletal muscle relaxants			
baclofen	Lioresal	**Oral:** 5 mg 3 times a day (maximum 80 mg/day) **Intrathecal:** 25 mcg to 100 mcg test dose, then 50 mcg to 200 mcg infused via intrathecal pump over 24 hours	MAY CAUSE DIZZINESS OR DROWSINESS MAY IMPAIR ABILITY TO DRIVE AVOID ALCOHOL TAKE WITH FOOD—baclofen
carisoprodol	Soma	250-350 mg 4 times a day	MAY DISCOLOR URINE—chlorzoxazone, methocarbamol
chlorzoxazone	Parafon Forte	250 mg to 500 mg 3 to 4 times a day	
cyclobenzaprine	Flexeril	5 mg to 10 mg 3 times a day	MAY BE HABIT FORMING—diazepam
diazepam	Valium	**Oral:** 2 mg to 10 mg 2 to 4 times a day **IM, IV:** 2 mg to 10 mg every 3 to 4 hours	SWALLOW WHOLE; DON'T CRUSH OR CHEW—orphenadrine extended release
methocarbamol	Robaxin	**Oral:** 1.5 g 4 times a day (up to 8 g/day) **IM, IV:** 1 g every 8 hours	
orphenadrine	Norflex	**Oral:** 100 mg twice a day **IM, IV:** 60 mg every 12 hours	
tizanidine	Zanaflex	2 mg to 4 mg 3 times a day (maximum 36 mg/day)	
Direct acting skeletal muscle relaxants			
dantrolene	Dantrium	25 mg to 100 mg 2 to 4 times a day	MAY CAUSE DIZZINESS OR DROWSINESS MAY IMPAIR ABILITY TO DRIVE AVOID ALCOHOL PROTECT FROM LIGHT AND MOISTURE

TECH NOTE!

Skeletal muscle relaxants should not be combined with alcohol. Alcohol increases the central nervous system depression produced by the skeletal muscle relaxants, which is exhibited as excessive drowsiness and decreased alertness.

TECH ALERT!

When carisoprodol is combined with codeine, it is a Schedule C-III controlled substance.

TECH ALERT!

The following drugs have look-alike/ sound-alike issues: cyclobenzaprine, cyproheptadine, and cycloserine; metaxalone and metalazone

CHAPTER SUMMARY

- Spasticity is a debilitating motor disorder that affects up to 12 million people worldwide.
- Symptoms of spasticity are an increase in muscle tone, exaggerated tendon jerks, and hyperexcitable reflexes.
- Spasticity interferes with the normal performance of activities of daily living.
- Stroke, spinal cord injury, cerebral palsy, muscle trauma, multiple sclerosis, head injury, and amyotrophic lateral sclerosis can all cause spasticity.
- Between 65% and 78% of people with spinal cord injuries and 65% of people who have had a stroke will develop spasticity.
- The progression to spasticity follows a specific pattern, and the degree of spasticity is related to the duration since the original injury.
- There are four phases to the development of spasticity: (1) decreased muscle contractility, (2) excessive muscle tone and increased reflex activity lasing from days to years, (3) decreased reflex excitability, and, finally, (4) stiff, contracted muscles.
- After a spinal cord injury, spasticity develops because the neurons that branch out from the spinal cord to the muscles and tissues of the body grow new synapses and the increase in the number of synapses causes a stronger reflex response to stretching of the muscle.
- Spasticity impairs effective muscle movement in some people and helps maintain posture making walking easier in other people.
- Spasticity may be due to excess of neurotransmitters that carry excitatory messages, like glutamate, or decreased activity or a deficiency of inhibitory transmitters, like GABA and glycine.
- Acetylcholine, GABA, glycine, and glutamate are neurotransmitters that play a role in spasticity.
- Nonpharmaceutical treatments of spasticity are electrical stimulation, cold packs (cryotherapy), biofeedback, splinting, positioning, and physical therapy.
- Drugs used in the treatment of spasticity are grouped according to the site of action and are classified as centrally acting and peripheral acting.
- Peripheral acting drugs act at the neuromuscular junction or directly on contractile mechanisms in the muscle.
- Botulinum toxin type A is injected locally to inhibit presynaptic release of acetylcholine at the neuromuscular junction. This causes paralysis in the muscle(s) that received the injections.
- The paralysis produced by botulinum toxin type A is reversed when the motor neuron sprouts new terminals that begin to release acetylcholine.
- Dantrolene is a peripheral acing drug that acts directly on contractile mechanisms in skeletal muscle.
- Central acting drugs primarily act on GABA receptors in the central nervous system or act at α_2-adrenergic receptor sites.
- Baclofen is a central acting drug that looks and acts like GABA, a naturally occurring neurotransmitter.
- The ability of baclofen to cross the blood-brain barrier is limited, so its effectiveness is augmented by administering directly into cerebral spinal fluid via a surgically implanted pump.
- Skeletal muscle relaxants are used to treat muscle stiffness, pain, and spasms associated with muscle tension, strain, sprains, or injury.

REVIEW QUESTIONS

Multiple Choice

1. Negative symptoms of spasticity are an increase in muscle tone, exaggerated tendon jerks, and hyperexcitability of the stretch reflex.
   a. true
   b. false

2. Any condition that can damage the _____ can cause spasticity.
   a. brain
   b. spinal cord
   c. motor neurons
   d. a, b, and c

3. People who have amyotrophic lateral sclerosis exhibit predominantly _____ symptoms of spasticity.
   a. positive
   b. negative
   c. no
   d. both b and c

4. The mechanism of action for drugs used to treat spasticity is to directly bind to and/or enhance the binding of _____.
   a. $GABA_A$ receptors
   b. $GABA_B$ receptors
   c. $GABA_A$ and $GABA_B$ receptors
   d. $GABA_D$ receptors

5. The use of botulinium toxin for the treatment of spasticity has been approved by the FDA.
   a. true
   b. false

6. The ability of baclofen to cross the blood-brain barrier is limited so its effectiveness is augmented by administering the drug _____.
   a. intravenously
   b. intrapleurally
   c. intrathecally
   d. intraocularly

7. _____ is the most commonly used benzodiazepine for the treatment of spasticity and it is effective in treating hyperactive reflexes and painful muscle spasms.
   a. alprazolam
   b. diazepam
   c. clonazepam
   d. lorazepam

8. Spasticity is reduced when α_2-adrenergic drugs are administered because the drugs prevent the release of inhibitory neurotransmitters in the spinal cord by increasing the actions of the excitatory neurotransmitter glycine.
   a. true
   b. false

9. Chlorzoxazone (Paraforon forte) discolors urine to what color?
   a. orange
   b. red
   c. reddish purple
   d. a and c

10. The brand name for cyclobenzaprine is
    a. Benezil
    b. Flexeril
    c. Cyclodril
    d. Skelaxin

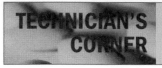

1. Why does the blood-brain barrier prevent some drugs from entering the brain?
2. When should nonpharmaceutical treatments of spasticity be discontinued in favor of pharmaceutical treatments?

BIBLIOGRAPHY

Adams MM, Hicks AL: Spasticity after spinal cord injury, *Spinal Cord,* 43:577-586, 2005.

Gallichio J: Pharmacologic management of spasticity following stroke, *Phys Ther,* 84:973-981, 2004.

Honda M, Sekiguchi Y, Sato N, Ono H: Involvement of imidazoline receptors in the centrally acting muscle-relaxant effects of tizanidine, *Eur J Pharmacol,* 445:187-193, 2002.

Lance L, Lacy C, Armstrong L, Goldman M: *Drug information handbook for the allied health professional,* ed 12. Hudson, OH, 2005, APhA Lexi-Comp.

Patel D, Soyode O: Pharmacologic interventions for reducing spasticity in cerebral palsy, *Indian J Pediatr,* 72:869-872, 2005.

USP Center for Advancement of Patient Safety: *Use caution–avoid confusion,* USP Quality Review No. 79, Rockville, MD, April 2004, USP Center for Advancement of Patient Safety.

Zafonte R, Lombard L, Elovic E: Antispasticity medications: uses and limitations of enteral therapy, *Am J Phys Med Rehabil,* 83(suppl):S50-S58, 2004.

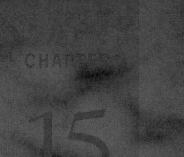
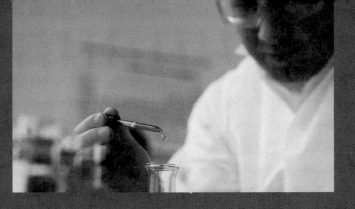

Treatment of Autoimmune Diseases That Affect the Musculoskeletal System

LEARNING OBJECTIVES

- Describe the process of autoimmunity.
- List triggers for autoimmune diseases that affect the musculoskeletal system.
- Describe characteristics of autoimmune diseases of the musculoskeletal system.
- List and categorize medications used In the treatment of myasthenia gravis, myositis, multiple sclerosis, rheumatoid arthritis, and systemic lupus erythematosus.
- Describe mechanism of action for each class of drugs used in the treatment of myasthenia gravis, myositis, multiple sclerosis, rheumatoid arthritis, and systemic lupus erythematosus.
- Identify warning labels and precautionary messages associated with medications used in the treatment of myasthenia gravis, myositis, multiple sclerosis, rheumatoid arthritis, and systemic lupus erythematosus.
- Identify significant drug look-alike/sound-alike issues.
- Learn the terminology associated with the autoimmune diseases affecting the musculoskeletal system.

KEY TERMS

Antinuclear antibody: Autoantibody or abnormal antibody that attacks the nucleus of normal cells in the body.

Autoantibody: Abnormal antibody that attacks healthy cells and tissue.

Autoimmune disease: Disease that occurs when the immune system turns against the parts of the body it is designed to protect.

Ataxia: Condition that causes the muscles to fail to function in a coordinated manner.

Demyelination: Damage caused by recurrent inflammation of myelin that results in nervous system scars that interrupt communication between the nerves and the rest of the body.

Dermatomyositis: Form of myositis that affects muscles and the skin.

Interferons: Antiviral proteins that enhance T-cell recognition of antigens (γ-interferon) and produce immune system suppression (α-interferon, β-interferon).

Multiple sclerosis: Autoimmune disease that causes progressive damage to nerves, resulting in spasticity, pain, mood changes, and other physical symptoms.

Myasthenia gravis: Autoimmune disease in which the immune system attacks the muscle cells at the neuromuscular junction and is characterized by muscle weakness.

Myelin: Fatty covering that insulates nerve cells in the brain and spinal cord.

Myelin basic protein: Major component of myelin that can be detected in the cerebrospinal fluid of people with multiple sclerosis.

Myositis: Autoimmune disease that causes chronic inflammation of the muscles.

Plaques: Patchy areas of inflammation and demyelination that disrupt nerves signals between the brain and the rest of the body.

Polymyositis: Form of myositis that affects multiple muscles, particularly the muscles closest to the trunk.

Rheumatoid arthritis: Chronic disease characterized by inflammation of the joints.

Rheumatoid factor: Immunoglobulin (antibody) that is present in many people who have rheumatoid arthritis.

Synovium: Thin layer of tissue that lines the joint space.

Systemic lupus erythematosus: Autoimmune disease that affects nearly all body systems.

Tumor necrosis factor: Inflammatory cytokine released as part of the immune response and found in synovial fluid of people with rheumatoid arthritis.

Trigger: Something that stimulates the onset of symptoms or disease in people.

Overview

Myasthenia gravis, multiple sclerosis, rheumatoid arthritis, and systemic lupus erythematosus (SLE) are examples of autoimmune diseases that affect the musculoskeletal system. An ***autoimmune disease*** occurs when the immune system turns against the parts of the body it is designed to protect. The body attacks its own cells, thinking they are germs or a harmful substance.

No one knows exactly why ***autoimmunity*** develops. It is believed that several factors may be involved. The ***triggers*** may be exposure to a virus, environmental toxins, the sun, genetics, hormonal changes, drugs, pregnancy, or some combination of any of these things. What is known is that autoimmunity can affect any organ of the body. Autoimmune diseases that involve the muscles are dermatomyositis, myasthenia gravis, and polymyositis. Multiple sclerosis is an autoimmune disease that affects the nerves and causes muscle weakness and spasticity in addition to central nervous system effects. Ankylosing spondylitis, rheumatoid arthritis, and SLE are autoimmune diseases involving the joints. SLE also commonly attacks the blood vessels, heart, lungs, nerves, brain, and skin in addition to the joints.

Description of Autoimmune Diseases Affecting the Musculoskeletal System

MYASTHENIA GRAVIS

Myasthenia gravis is an autoimmune disease that causes muscle weakness. The muscles are easily fatigued after even brief activity. Muscle weakness improves after periods of rest. Myasthenia gravis typically affects skeletal muscles of face, neck, and limbs. Sometimes the muscles involved in breathing are affected.

Approximately 20 people per 100,000 worldwide have been diagnosed with myasthenia gravis. The onset of the disease typically occurs in women under 40 years and men older than 60 years; however, the onset can be triggered at any age, including infancy.

In myasthenia gravis, the body attacks and destroys receptor sites in the neuromuscular junction (Figure 15-1) that bind acetylcholine (ACh) (see Chapter 13). Fewer nicotinic receptor sites mean that there will be fewer muscle contractions, and when contractions occur, they will not be as strong. This is because the action potentials needed to generate contractions, as well as the strength of contractions generated, are dependent on the number of interactions between ACh and nicotinic receptors (see Chapter 13).

MYOSITIS

Myositis is an autoimmune disease that causes chronic inflammation of the muscles. It often begins with pain in the shoulders and hips, interferes with walking, and can progress to involve the muscles that affect breathing, swallowing, and speech. Dermatomyositis and

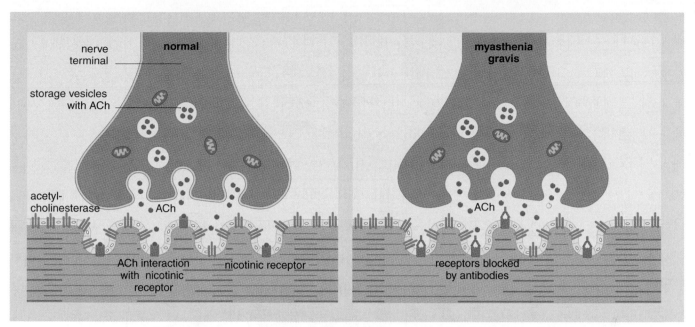

FIGURE 15-1 The effects of antibodies on the neuromuscular junction in myasthenia gravis. *(From Page C, et al.* Integrated pharmacology, *ed 3, Philadelphia, 2006, Mosby.)*

polymyositis are specific forms of myositis. ***Polymyositis***, as its name describes, affects muscles in multiple parts of the body. Inflammation of muscles closest to the trunk is most common, and the disease causes weakness, fatigue, and pain in the joints and muscles. ***Dermatomyositis*** causes inflammation and damage to muscles and skin. People with dermatomyositis develop a distinctive patchy, reddish rash on the eyelids, cheeks, bridge of the nose, back or upper chest, elbows, knees, and knuckles. It also causes fatigue and painful muscles and joints.

MULTIPLE SCLEROSIS

Nearly 350,000 people in North America have been diagnosed with multiple sclerosis. As with many autoimmune diseases, multiple sclerosis is caused by some trigger that causes the body to start attacking its own cells. Some of the risk factors and triggers that are associated with multiple sclerosis are exposure to a virus, environmental factors, genetics, and malfunction of the blood-brain barrier that permits entry of antimyelin T cells produced by the immune system.

In ***multiple sclerosis,*** the insulating coating of nerves (myelin) is attacked (Figure 15-2). Reoccurring attacks of inflammation causes ***demyelination*** of nerves and results in lesions and scarring of the white matter of the brain. The scarring, known as plaques, is responsible for the signs and symptoms of multiple sclerosis.

Initial symptoms are associated with inflammation of the optic nerves and present as visual changes (color distortions, blurred or double vision, or blindness). Muscle weakness and fatigue are also early symptoms. As the disease progresses, difficulty with coordination (ataxia), spasticity, and tremor may develop. Other symptoms of multiple sclerosis are pain, vertigo, bladder, bowel and sexual dysfunction, speech disturbances, impaired temperature and touch senses, cognitive abnormalities, and depression.

RHEUMATOID ARTHRITIS

Rheumatoid arthritis is an autoimmune disease that is characterized by inflammation of the lining of the joints. In addition to chronic inflammation, rheumatoid arthritis produces pain, joint damage, and disability. According to the Arthritis Foundation (2007), 2.1 million Americans suffer from rheumatoid arthritis. Slightly less than 300,000 Canadians are living

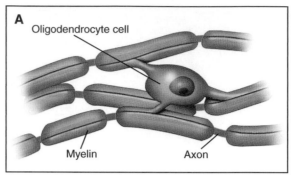

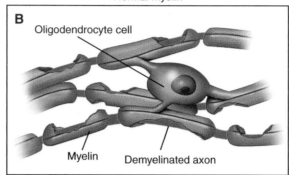

FIGURE 15-2 Effects of multiple sclerosis. *(From Thibodeau GA, Patton KT: Anatomy and physiology, ed 6, St Louis, 2007, Mosby.)*

with rheumatoid arthritis. Rheumatoid arthritis is far more common in women than in men, with women accounting for more than 70% of the people with the disease. Although children have been diagnosed with rheumatoid arthritis, the onset of the disease is usually between 30 and 50 years.

Most people who have rheumatoid arthritis have high levels of ***rheumatoid factor***, an immunoglobulin (antibody) that regulates other antibodies made by the body. Rheumatoid factor is not usually found in people who do not have rheumatoid arthritis, so its presence is part of the diagnosis for rheumatoid arthritis.

There are three distinct phases of the disease. In phase 1, the joint lining ***(synovium)*** or synovial membrane becomes inflamed, causing swelling, pain, and stiffness (Figure 15-3). In phase 2, rapid cell growth causes the synovium to thicken. In phase 3, inflamed cells in the synovium release enzymes that digest bone and cartilage. This results in more pain and disability. The damaging, chronic cycle of inflammation is stimulated by proinflammatory cytokines (interleukins) (Figure 15-4) and tumor necrosis factor (TNF-α).

Rheumatoid arthritis causes more than joint problems. Other symptoms of rheumatoid arthritis are fatigue, weakness, flu-like symptoms, lumps that form under the skin, muscle pain, decreased appetite, depression, and dry mouth.

SYSTEMIC LUPUS ERYTHEMATOSUS

SLE is an autoimmune disease that affects nearly all parts of the body. The prevalence of SLE worldwide is approximately 250 per 100,000 people. Women between the ages of 15 and 25 years are more likely to get SLE than are men, and African American women are three times more likely to get SLE than are women of European descent.

It is not known what triggers the onset of SLE. As with other autoimmune diseases, it is likely that a combination of factors is responsible. Triggers include stress, viral infection, certain drugs, and sunlight. Heredity also plays a role. Once SLE is triggered, the body produces antibodies that cause inflammation and damage healthy cells and organs. ***Antinuclear antibody (ANA)*** levels

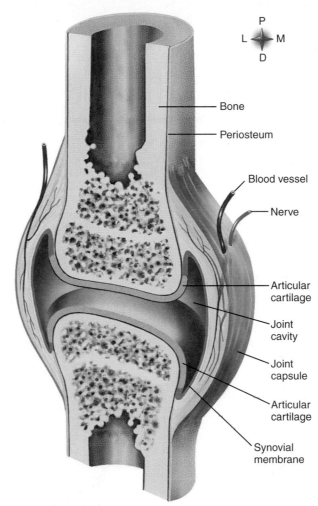

P
L ← → M
D

— Bone

— Periosteum

— Blood vessel

— Nerve

— Articular cartilage

— Joint cavity

— Joint capsule

— Articular cartilage

— Synovial membrane

FIGURE 15-3 Synovial joint. *(From Vidic B, Suarez FR: Photographic atlas of the human body, St Louis, 1984, Mosby.)*

are elevated in people who have SLE. ANA attaches to the cell nucleus, causing the body's immune system to attack it as if it were a harmful bacteria or virus (Figure 15-5).

SLE causes swollen and painful joints like rheumatoid arthritis. Unlike rheumatoid arthritis, it affects most other regions of the body, too, including the kidneys, heart, lungs, blood vessels, and skin. Inflammation of the kidney interferes with waste removal and causes swelling in legs and feet. Inflammation of the lungs causes pain when breathing. Other signs and symptoms of SLE are muscle pain, fever, red rashes, hair loss, sun sensitivity, swollen glands, extreme fatigue, seizures, mouth ulcers, and poor circulation in fingers and toes.

Treatment of Autoimmune Diseases That Affect the Musculoskeletal System

Multiple sclerosis, myasthenia gravis, SLE, myositis, rheumatoid arthritis, and other autoimmune diseases that affect the musculoskeletal system are treated using pharmacological and nonpharmacological therapies. Drug therapy is aimed at suppressing inflammation, pain, and immune system response. Treatment goals are also aimed at minimizing further nerve or joint destruction, preservation of body functions, and prevention of disability. Additional medications are administered to control disease specific symptoms such as spasticity, muscle weakness, fatigue, nerve pain, or rashes.

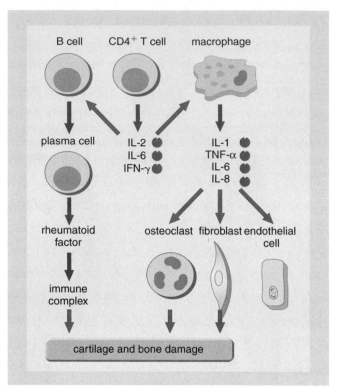

FIGURE 15-4 Cytokine network in the pathogenesis of RA. *(From Page C, et al. Integrated pharmacology, ed 6, Philadelphia, 2006, Mosby.)*

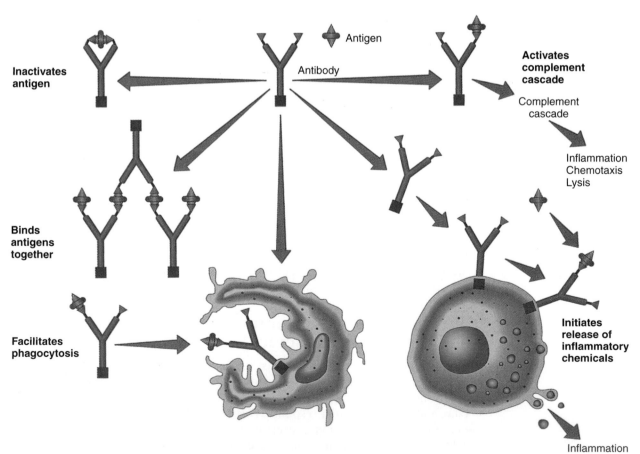

FIGURE 15-5 Actions of antibodies. *(From Thibodeau GA, Patton KT: Anatomy and physiology, ed 3, St Louis, 2007, Mosby.)*

TECH ALERT!

The following drugs have look-alike/sound-alike issues: hydrocortisone, cortisone, and hydrocodone; Medrol and Mebaral; methyprednisolone and medroxyprogesterone; prednisone, prednisolone, Pramosone, and primodone

ANTIINFLAMMATORIES AND ANALGESICS

GLUCOCORTICOSTEROIDS

Glucocorticosteroids are prescribed commonly to suppress inflammation, reduce flare-ups, and treat pain associated with multiple sclerosis, myasthenia gravis, systemic eythematosus, myositis, and rheumatoid arthritis (Figure 15-6). They may also be prescribed for the treatment of ulcerative colitis, allergic reactions, cerebral edema, or septic shock or used as a diagnostic agent for endocrine disorders (see Unit 9, Introduction to the Endocrine System). Glucocorticosteroids have immunosuppressive actions, and they inhibit the synthesis of antibodies that are responsible for attacking the body's healthy cells. They decrease the accumulation of cells that mobilize to fight when the body believes it is under attack, such as leukocytes and T cells. They interfere with the binding of antibodies to receptor sites on the cell surface. Glucocorticosteroids are also used to restore the effectiveness of the blood-brain barriers to screen out antibodies harmful to brain cells and nerves. Glucocorticosteroids are potent antiinflammatory drugs, too. They decrease the synthesis of proinflammatory substances—prostaglandins (see Chapter 10), leukotrienes, cytokines, arachidonic acid, and macrophages—that are released as part of the inflammatory response. These substances cause swelling, pain, irritation, and other effects.

Pharmacokinetics

The absorption, distribution, metabolism, and elimination of glucocorticosteroids used in the treatment of multiple sclerosis, myasthenia gravis, systemic eythematosus, myositis, and rheumatoid arthritis vary according to the dosage form administered. In general, oral dosage forms are well absorbed in the gastrointestinal tract and are readily distributed. Metabolism occurs in the liver, and they are eliminated by the kidneys in urine.

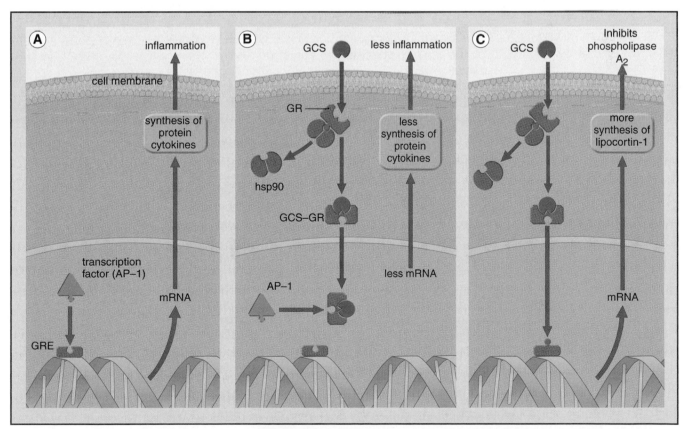

FIGURE 15-6 Suppressive effects of glucorticosteroids on immune and inflammatory response. *(From Page C, et al.* Integrated pharmacology, *ed 3, Philadelphia, 2006, Mosby.)*

Adverse Reactions

The adverse effects produced by glucocorticosteroids are numerous and affect all body systems. In the central nervous system, they cause insomnia and euphoria. In the cardiovascular system, they produce edema and hypertension. Glucocorticosteroids can cause nausea, weight gain, and ulceration in the gastrointestinal tract. Other adverse drug effects are osteoporosis, acne, cataracts, poor wound healing, and infection.

Precautions

Glucocorticosteriods may initially produce muscle weakness. This is a serious problem for people with myasthenia gravis given that muscle weakness is a symptom of the disease. Some of the adverse effects of glucocorticosteroids can be minimized by administering the drugs using alternate-day therapy. Long-term use of glucocorticosteroids may cause a need for increased potassium; vitamins A, B_6, C, and D; folate; calcium; zinc; and phosphorous.

Glucocorticoids Used in the Treatment of Myasthenia Gravis, Multiple Sclerosis, Rheumatoid Arthritis, and Systemic Lupus Erythematosus

Generic name	U.S. brand name(s) / Canadian brand(s)	Dosage forms and strengths
dexamethasone*	Decadron, Dexamethasone Intensol, DexPak, TaperPak Decadron, Dexasone	**Elixir:** 0.5 mg/5 ml **Injection, solution (Decadron):** 4 mg/ml, 10 mg/ml, 24 mg/ml **Solution, oral:** 0.5 mg/ml **Solution, oral concentrate (Dexamethasone Intensol):** 1 mg/ml **Tablet:** 0.25 mg, 0.5 mg, 0.75 mg, 1 mg, 1.5 mg, 2 mg, 4 mg, 6 mg **Tablet (DexPak, TaperPak):** 1.5 mg (51 tablets on taper dose card)
hydrocortisone*	A-Hydrocort, Cortef, Hydrocortone Phosphate, Solu-Cortef Cortef, Solu-Cortef	**Injection, powder for reconstitution (A-Hydrocort):** 100 mg, 250 mg, (Solu-Cortef): 100 mg, 250 mg, 500 mg, 1000 mg **Injection, solution:** 50 mg/ml **Tablet:** 5 mg, 10 mg, 20 mg
methylprednisolone*	A-Methapred, Depo-Medrol, Medrol, Medrol Dosepak, Solu-Medrol Depo-Medrol, Medrol, Medrol Dosepak, Solu-Medrol	**Injection, powder for reconstitution (A-Methapred, Solu-Medrol):** 40 mg, 125 mg, 500 mg, 1000 mg **Injection, suspension (Depo-Medrol):** 20 mg/ml, 40 mg/ml, 80 mg/ml **Tablet:** 2 mg, 4 mg, 8 mg, 16 mg, 32 mg **Tablet (Medrol Dosepak):** 4 mg (21 tablet taper dose)
prednisone*	Deltasone, Prednisone Intensol, Sterapred, Sterapred DS Winpred	**Solution, oral:** 1 mg/ml **Solution, oral concentrate (Prednisone Intensol):** 5 mg/ml **Tablet:** 1 mg, 2.5 mg, 5 mg, 10 mg, 20 mg, 50 mg **Tablet (Sterapred):** 5 mg (21 tablet 6-day unit dose pack or 48 tablet 12-day pack)

*Generic available.

NONSTEROIDAL ANTIINFLAMMATORY DRUGS

Nonsteroidal antiinflammatory drugs (NSAIDs) and aspirin (ASA) are widely used in the treatment of pain and inflammation associated with rheumatoid arthritis, myasthenia gravis, SLE, myositis, and multiple sclerosis. Aspirin and NSAIDs inhibit the release of prostaglandin, an important mediator of pain (see Chapter 10). Prostaglandin is a substance that stimulates a cascade of events that result in inflammation. Aspirin and NSAIDs block the activity of the enzyme cyclooxygenase (COX-1 and COX-2), interfering with the synthesis of prostaglandin.

The U.S. Food and Drug Administration (FDA) recently requested the removal of all selective COX-2 inhibitors except celecoxib (Celebrex) in the United States. Celecoxib is also the only COX-2 inhibitor available for sale in the Canada, and market authorization is conditional (i.e., its use is restricted). As per FDA requirements, manufacturers of all NSAIDs must print a "black box" warning in the package insert describing risk for cardiovascular toxicity and gastrointestinal ulceration. The pharmacokinetics, adverse reactions, and precautions for NSAIDs are discussed in detail in Chapter 10.

Selected Nonsteroidal Antiinflammatory Drugs Used in the Treatment of Myasthenia Gravis, Multiple Sclerosis, Rheumatoid Arthritis, and Systemic Lupus Erythematosus

	Generic name	U.S. brand name(s) / Canadian brand(s)	Dosage forms and strengths
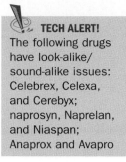	celecoxib *	Celebrex Celebrex	**Capsule:** 100 mg, 200 mg, 400 mg
	ibuprofen*	Advil [OTC], Motrin, Motrin IB [OTC] Advil, Motrin	**Caplet, Capsule, Gelcap, Tablet (Advil, Motrin IB [OTC]):** 200 mg **Suspension, oral:** 100 mg/5 ml **Suspension, oral drops:** 40 mg/ml **Tablet, chewable:** 50 mg, 100 mg **Tablet (Motrin):** 400 mg, 600 mg, 800 mg
	naproxen*	Aleve [OTC], Anaprox, Anaprox DS, EC-Naprosyn, Naprosyn SR, Naprelan Anaprox, Anaprox DS, Naprosyn	**Caplet, Gelcap, Tablet (Aleve [OTC]):** 220 mg **Tablet (Naprosyn):** 250 mg, 375 mg, 500 mg **Tablet, enteric coated (EC-Naprosyn):** 375 mg, 500 mg **Tablet (as sodium):** 275 mg (Anaprox), 550 mg (Anaprox DS), 421.5 mg (Naprelan)

*Generic available.

ANTIMALARIALS

Antimalarials have antiinflammatory and analgesic properties that are useful in the management of rheumatoid arthritis and SLE. They are used to treat joint pain, skin rashes, and inflammation of the lungs associated with SLE. Hydroxychloroquin has been shown to reduce SLE flare-ups.

Although the exact mechanism of action is unknown, antimalarials are known to accumulate inside cell structures, where they raise the pH and interfere with processes that are normally stimulated when the body thinks its own cells are harmful antigens. An antigen is a substance that stimulates an immune response (antigen) (see Figure 15-5).

The most common adverse reaction is gastrointestinal irritation; however, chloroquine and hydroxychloroquine can cause permanent damage to the retina, resulting in blindness. This adverse reaction is associated with long-term chronic use (greater than 10 years) at doses greater than 400 mg/day. Additional adverse reactions include nausea, stomach pain, visual disturbances, and tinnitus.

Antimalarials Used in the Treatment of Systemic Lupus Erythematosus

Generic name	U.S. brand name(s)	Dosage forms and strengths
	Canadian brand(s)	
chloroquine*⊥	Aralen	**Tablet:** 250 mg, 500 mg (Aralen 500 mg)
	Aralen	
hydroxychloroquine*	Plaquenil	**Tablet:** 200 mg (155 mg base)
	Plaquenil	

*Generic available.
⊥unlabeled use.

IMMUNOSUPPRESSIVES

Immunosuppressive drugs interfere with the formation of immune cells by damaging RNA and DNA needed for cell replication. They may also block immune system response to autoantibodies.

IMMUNOSUPPRESSIVES USED IN TREATMENT

Azathioprine

Azathioprine is used in the treatment of multiple sclerosis, rheumatoid arthritis, myasthenia gravis, and SLE. The mechanism of action is to block purine synthesis and cause DNA damage. Purine is an amino acid needed in the synthesis of RNA and DNA. Azathioprine also suppresses T-cell–mediated immune system response. Adverse reactions to azathioprine include nausea, vomiting, infections, hepatoxicity, cytopenias, and myelosuppression.

TECH NOTE!
Reconstituted solution of azathioprine must be mixed by gently swirling, not shaking.

Cyclophosphamide

Cyclophosphamide interferes with DNA synthesis and cell replication. It inhibits B-cell antibody production and T-cell activity, suppresses cytokine and immunoglobulin production, and suppresses the antigen-induced response to T cells. Cyclophosphamide is more toxic than most of the drugs used in the treatment of rheumatoid arthritis, SLE, myasthenia gravis, and multiple sclerosis, so its use is reserved for severe, active disease. Adverse reactions of cyclophosphamide include alopecia, nausea, infertility, infections, hemorrhagic cystitis, bladder cancer, hypoglycemia, and bone marrow depression.

Cyclophosphamide is also prescribed for the treatment of leukemia, lymphomas, and multiple cancers (breast, ovarian, endometrial, and testicular) and to prevent rejection of bone marrow transplants.

TECH NOTE!
Cyclosporine oral solution must be dispensed in a glass container. Dispense the same manufacturer's product each time (bioavailability issues).

Cyclosporine

Cyclosporine is used with azathioprine or glucocorticosteroids to treat severe rheumatoid arthritis and severe corticosteroid-resistant SLE, myasthenia gravis, and other autoimmune diseases affecting the musculoskeletal system. It is also prescribed for the prevention of organ transplant rejection, for psoriasis, and to increase tear production in patients with keratoconjunctivitis sicca. Cyclosporine selectively interferes with T-cell proliferation and interleukin production. The result is a decreased immune system response to autoantibodies. Adverse reactions include kidney toxicity, infections, nausea, abdominal pain, mouth sores, gingival hyperplasia, headache, hirsuitism, weight gain, hepatoxicity, and hypertension.

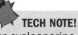

TECH NOTE!
For cyclosporine solution for injection:
Do not refrigerate.
Protect from light.
DILUTE SOLUTION AND USE IMMEDIATELY
Stable for 6 hours in plastic IV bags or 24 hours in glass.

Mitoxantrone

Mitoxantrone in used in the treatment of multiple sclerosis and interferes with DNA repair and RNA synthesis, which effectively reduces the growth and spread of immune cells and thereby decreases the progression of the disease. It is also prescribed for the treatment of leukemia, breast and prostate cancer, and pediatric sarcoma. Mitoxane is listed in FDA pregnancy category D. Adverse reactions include nausea and vomiting, hair loss, palpitations, leukopenia, blue urine and/or sclera (white part of the eye), menstrual irregularities, skin rash, mouth sores, dizziness, and drowsiness.

Immunosuppressives

Generic name	U.S. brand name(s) / Canadian brand(s)	Dosage forms and strengths
azathioprine*	Azasan, Imuran	**Injection, powder for reconstitution:** 100 mg
	Imuran	**Tablet:** 25 mg, 50 mg, 75 mg, 100 mg (Imuran only available as 50 mg)
cyclophosphamide*	Cytoxan	**Injection, powder for econstitution:** 500 mg, 1 g, 2 g
	Cytoxan, Procytox	**Tablet:** 25 mg, 50 mg
cyclosporine*	Gengraf, Neoral, Restasis, Sandimmune	**Capsule, modified (Gengraf, Neoral):** 25 mg, 100 mg **Capsule, nonmodified (Sandimmune):** 25 mg, 100 mg **Emulsion, ophthalmic (Restasis):** 0.05%
	Neoral, Sandimmune	**Injection, solution (Sandimmune):** 50 mg/ml **Solution, oral, modified (Gengraf, Neoral):** 100 mg/ml **Solution, nonmodified (Sandimmune):** 100 mg/ml
Mitoxantrone	Novantrone	**Injection, solution:** 2 mg/ml
	Novantrone	

TECH ALERT!

The following drugs have look-alike/sound-alike issues: cyclosporine, cycloserine, and cyclophosphamide; Gengraf and Prograf; Neural and Nizoral

TECH NOTE!

Drug vials and cytotoxic waste including bags, sets, tubing, gloves, etc. must be properly disposed of in the cytotoxic waste containers. e.g., cyclophosphamide, mitoxamtrone, methotrexate, and azathioprine.

BIOLOGICAL RESPONSE MODIFIERS

Autoimmune diseases are caused by a defective immune system response that causes the body to attack its own normal healthy cells. Biological response modifiers act to inhibit or modify immune system response. They inhibit the release of cells that mobilize to fight what the body believes is a harmful invasion and inhibit the release of substances that produce inflammation. Recall that chronic inflammation can result in degeneration of nerves, bones, and muscles. Biological response modifiers interfere with the activity of cytokines, leukocytes, B cells, and T cells.

INTERFERONS

There are approximately 2000 interferon receptors on each normal and malignant cell. These receptors recognize and bind interferons, proteins with antigenic properties. Interferon β1a and interferon β1b are first-line therapies for the treatment of multiple sclerosis. They alter the actions of T cells and B cells and other cytokines that produce immune response and inflammation. They reduce the development of the brain lesions that cause disability in people that have multiple sclerosis. Adverse reactions of interferon β1a and interferon β1b include flu-like symptoms, headache, fatigue, weight loss, anorexia, and neutropenia.

MYASTHENIA GRAVIS, MULTIPLE SCLEROSIS, RHEUMATOID ARTHRITIS, OR SYSTEMIC LUPUS ERYTHEMATOSUS

Interferons

Generic name	U.S. brand name(s) / Canadian brand(s)	Dosage forms and strengths
interferon β1a	Avonex, Rebif	**Injection, powder for reconstitution (Avonex):** 33 mcg
	Avonex, Rebif	**Injection, solution (Avonex):** 30 mcg/0.5 ml (0.5 ml prefilled syringe) **Injection, solution (Rebif):** 22 mcg/0.5 ml and 44 mcg/0.5 ml (0.5 ml prefilled syringe)
interferon β1b	Betaseron	**Injection, powder for reconstitution:** 0.3 mg
	Betaseron	

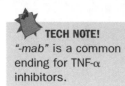

Tumor Necrosis Factor α Inhibitors

TNF is a cytokine that is released by cells that mobilize to fight what the body believes is a harmful invasion. High levels of TNF are found in the synovial fluid of people with rheumatoid arthritis and the factor is responsible for damaging inflammation.

TNF-α inhibitors are genetically engineered drugs that block the inflammatory process triggered by high concentrations of TNF. They prevent cell lysis (destruction) and release of the substances that cause inflammation. Currently, there are three TNF-α inhibitors available for use in the treatment of rheumatoid arthritis. Infliximab and adalimumab are monoclonal antibodies that bind to TNF-α and produce inhibitory effects. Infliximab is created by incorporating mouse protein into the DNA strand for IgG1 monoclonal antibody. In some cases, the body recognizes the nonhuman proteins and produces antibodies to the drug, resulting in allergic and immune system reactions to infliximab. All TNF-α inhibitors increase the risk for opportunistic infections. The most commonly reported opportunistic infection associated with TNF-α inhibitors is tuberculosis. TNF-α inhibitors are known to cause the onset of multiple sclerosis in susceptible people and should be avoided if preexisting multiple sclerosis is suspected. Adverse reactions of adalimumab and etanercept are nausea, stomach pain, headache, opportunistic infections, redness, and itching at injection site.

Tumor Necrosis Factor α Inhibitors

Generic name	U.S. brand name(s) / Canadian brand(s)	Dosage forms and strengths
adalimumab	Humira	**Injection, solution:** 40 mg/0.8 ml (1 ml prefilled syringe)
	Humira	
etanercept	Enbrel	**Injection, powder for reconstitution:** 25 mg
	Enbrel	**Injection, solution:** 50 mg/ml (0.98 ml prefilled syringe)
infliximab	Remicade	**Injection, powder for reconstitution:** 100 mg
	Remicade	

INTERLEUKIN ANTAGONISTS

Multiple sclerosis, rheumatoid arthritis, SLE, and other autoimmune diseases have been associated with increased serum levels of interleukins. Anakinra is a genetically engineered interleukin 1 (IL-1) receptor antagonist. Anakinra interferes with the binding of interleukins that promote inflammatory responses. Drug-receptor binding results in fewer lymphocytes and macrophages in synovial fluid. Adverse reactions to anakinra include redness or irritation at injection site, infections, and bone or muscle weakness.

Interleukin antagonists

Generic name	U.S. brand name(s) / Canadian brand(s)	Dosage forms and strengths
anakinra	Kineret	**Injection, solution:** 100 mg/0.67 ml (1 ml prefilled syringe)
	Kineret	

DISEASE-MODIFYING ANTIRHEUMATIC DRUGS (DMARDs)

METHOTREXATE

Methotrexate was one of the first drugs used for the treatment of rheumatoid arthritis, and it continues to be a principal treatment, used solo or along with other DMARDs. It works by inhibiting the formation of folates that are needed for purine synthesis. Recall that purine is an amino acid needed in the synthesis of RNA and DNA and lymphocyte proliferation. Methotrexate also decreases cytokine and immunoglobulin production and COX-2 activity, reducing both inflammation and immune system activity. In addition to rheumatoid arthritis, methotrexate is prescribed for the treatment of leukemias; neoplasms; psoriasis; breast, lung, and head and neck cancer; gastrointestinal tract and testes cancers; and osteosarcoma. Adverse effects include nausea, vomiting, diarrhea, gastrointestinal ulceration, rash, photosensitivity, hair loss, bone marrow depression, hepatoxicity, renal toxicity, and stomach pain.

LEFLUNOMIDE

Leflunomide selectively blocks the replication of lymphocytes by interfering with pyrimidine synthesis. Leflunomide's effectiveness is enhanced when used along with methotrexate. Additive effects are achieved because together they block both pathways in the cell division process for lymphocytes (purine and pyrimidine synthesis). Adverse reactions include nausea, diarrhea, rash, hair loss, liver dysfunction, and fetal toxicity.

SULFASALAZINE

Sulfasalazine is used in the treatment of rheumatoid arthritis. It is classified as a DMARD and was developed by combining an antiinfective agent (sulfapyridine) with an aspirin-like antiinflammatory agent (5-aminsalicylic acid). It was once believed that rheumatoid arthritis was caused by a bacterial infection. Sulfasalazine slows the progression of rheumatoid arthritis.

Sulfasalazine takes about 2 to 3 months to produce maximum effects. Common side effects are gastrointestinal upset, increased sensitivity to sunlight, allergy, crystalluria, impaired folic acid absorption, and damage to white blood cells (cytopenias).

GOLD

Gold compounds are used in the treatment of rheumatoid arthritis; however, their use is limited due to side effects, cost, and lack of sustained effectiveness. Gold compounds are believed to affect the function of B cells and macrophages, part of the immune system response. They decrease the release of antibodies and cytokines and inhibit the action of collagenase.

Gold compounds may be delivered by mouth or intramuscular injection. The onset of action is slow, and it can take 4 to 6 months before maximum effectiveness is achieved. Gold compounds can produce temporary remission in about 50% of the people who respond favorably to the drug. The drug is most effective when administered along with other DMARDs such as methotrexate. Adverse reactions to auranofin and gold sodium thiomalate include itching rash, metallic taste, sore mouth, photosensitivity, cytopenias, interstitial pneumonia, and proteinuria.

PENICILLAMINE

Penicillamine has antiinflammatory actions and alters immune system response. This makes it useful in the treatment of rheumatoid arthritis. It inhibits T-cell function and blocks collagen cross-linking. Adverse reactions include rash, gastrointestinal upset, and nephrotoxicity.

Disease-Modifying Antirheumatic drugs (DMARDs)

Generic name	U.S. brand name(s) Canadian brand(s)	Dosage forms and strengths
methotrexate*	Rheumatrex, Trexall Methotrexate	**Injection, powder for reconstitution:** 20 mg, 1000 mg **Injection, solution:** 25 mg/ml **Tablet:** 2.5 mg (Rheumatrex), 5 mg, 7.5 mg, 10 mg, 15 mg (Trexall) **Tablet (Rheumatrex Dose Pack):** 2.5 mg (4 cards with 2, 3, 4, 5, or 6 tablets each)
leflunomide	Arava Arava	**Tablet:** 10 mg, 20 mg

Continued

Summary of Neuromuscular Blocking Drugs—cont'd

Generic name	U.S. brand name(s) Canadian brand(s)	Dosage forms and strengths
sulfasalazine*	Azulfadine, Azulfadine EN-tabs	**Tablet (Azulfidine):** 500 mg Tablet, enteric coated (Azulfidine EN-tab)
	Salazopyrin, Salazopyrin EN-tabs	
auranofin	Ridura	**Capsule:** 3 mg
	Ridura	
gold sodium thiomalate	Aurolate	**Injection, solution:** 50 mg/ml
	Myochrysine	
penicillamine	Cupramine, Depen	**Capsule (Cupramine):** 125 mg, 250 mg **Tablet (Depen):** 250 mg
	Cupramine, Depen	

*Generic available.

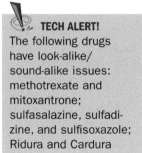

TECH ALERT!

The following drugs have look-alike/sound-alike issues: methotrexate and mitoxantrone; sulfasalazine, sulfadizine, and sulfisoxazole; Ridura and Cardura

CONTROL OF DISEASE-RELATED SYMPTOMS IN AUTOIMMUNE DISEASES AFFECTING THE MUSCULOSKELETAL SYSTEM

Multiple sclerosis, myasthenia gravis, rheumatoid arthritis, SLE, and myositis produce symptoms secondary to inflammation, brain lesions, and nerve degeneration. Multiple sclerosis can cause spasticity, fatigue, optic neuritis, trigeminal neuralgia, bladder, and sexual dysfunction. Drug therapy for spasticity is covered in detail in Chapter 14, fatigue in Chapter 12, and trigeminal neuralgia in Chapter 10. A summary of the drugs used to treat secondary symptoms of autoimmune diseases affecting the musculoskeletal system is given in Table 15-1.

TABLE 15-1   Drugs Used to Treat Specific Symptoms of Myasthenia Gravis, Multiple Sclerosis, Rheumatoid Arthritis, and Systemic Lupus Erythematosus

Acute symptom	Drug	Disease
Inflammation	**Glucocorticosteroids** dexamethasone hydrocortisone methylprednisolone prednisone	Myasthenia gravis (MG), multiple sclerosis (MS), rheumatoid arthritis (RA), systemic lupus erythematosus (SLE), myositis - all glucocorticosteroids listed
	NSAIDs celecoxib ibuprofen naproxen	MG, MS, RA, SLE - all NSAIDS listed
	Antimalarials hydroxychloroquine chloroquine	RA, MS RA, MS
Pain	aspirin acetaminophen opioids antidepressants	MS, RA, SLE, myositis, MG - all agents listed
Immune response	**Immunosuppressives** azathioprine cyclophosphamide cyclosporine mitoxantrone	RA (SLE, MG)* (RA, SLE, myositis)* RA MS
	Interferons interferon β1a interferon β1b	MS MS

TABLE 15-1 **Drugs Used to Treat Specific Symptoms of Myasthenia Gravis, Multiple Sclerosis, Rheumatoid Arthritis, and Systemic Lupus Erythematosus—cont'd**

Acute symptom	Drug	Disease
Spasticity	**Peripheral acting skeletal muscle relaxants**	
	dantrolene	MS
	Central acting skeletal muscle relaxants	
	baclofen	MS
	diazepam	MS
	tizanidine	MS
Fatigue	amantadine*	MS
	pemoline*	MS
	antidepressants*	MS
Trigeminal neuralgia	carbamazepine	MS
Muscle weakness	neostigmine	MG
	pyridostigmine	MG
Slow Progression of Disease		
Disease modifying antirheumatic drugs (DMARDs)	methotrexate	MS, SLE, RA, myositis
	gold salts	RA
	lefluonomide	RA
	penicillamine	RA
	sulfasalazine	RA
Biologic response modifiers	**Tumor necrosis factor inhibitors**	RA
	etanercept	RA
	infliximab	RA
	adaliumumab	RA
	Interleukin atagonists	RA
	anakinra	

*Unlabeled use.

Usual Dosage and Warnings for Drugs Used in the Treatment of Myasthenia Gravis, Multiple Sclerosis, Rheumatoid Arthritis, and Systemic Lupus Erythematosus

Generic name	U.S. brand name	Usual adult oral dose and dosing schedule	Warning labels
dexamethasone	Decadron	**Multiple sclerosis:** **Oral:** 16 mg daily, given in 4 divided doses for 5 days **Myasthenia gravis, RA, SLE:** **Oral:** 0.75 mg to 9 mg/day, given in 2-4 divided doses	TAKE WITH FOOD DON'T DISCONTINUE ABRUPTLY TAKE AT THE SAME TIME EACH DAY TAKE WITH A FULL GLASS OF WATER
hydrocortisone	Cortef	**Myasthenia gravis, MS, SLE:** **Oral:** 25 mg to 300 mg once daily or on alternate days. **IM:** 20 mg to 300 mg once daily or on alternate days	

Continued

Usual Dosage and Warnings for Drugs Used in the Treatment of Myasthenia Gravis, Multiple Sclerosis, Rheumatoid Arthritis, and Systemic Lupus Erythematosus—cont'd

Generic name	U.S. brand name	Usual adult oral dose and dosing schedule	Warning labels
methylprednisolone	Medrol	**Multiple sclerosis:** **Oral:** 200 mg once daily for 7 days, followed by 80 mg every other day for 1 month IV or IM: 160 mg daily for 1 week followed by 64 mg PO, IV, or **IM:** every other day for 1 month **Myasthenia gravis:** **Oral:** 12 mg to 20 mg/day **Rheumatoid arthritis, SLE:** **Oral:** 4 mg to 48 mg/day **IM:** 10 mg to 120 mg **Intraarticular:** 10 mg to 80 mg **IV:** 10 mg to 40 mg IV infused over several minutes	
prednisone	Deltasone	**Myasthenia gravis:** **Oral:** Initially, 15 mg to 20 mg/day Increase by 5 mg every 2 to 3 days as needed (maximum 60 mg/day) **Immunosuppression:** 5 mg to 60 mg/day in 1 to 4 divided doses **Rheumatoid arthritis:** **Oral:** 5 mg to 30 mg once daily **Systemic lupus erythematosus:** **Oral:** 20 mg to 300 mg/day in 2 to 3 divided doses (acute); **maintenance:** 10 mg to 20 mg once daily or 20 mg to 40 mg every other day	
NSAIDs			
celecoxib	Celebrex	**Osteoarthritis:** 200 mg/day in 1 to 2 divided doses **Rheumatoid arthritis:** 100 mg to 200 mg twice a day	TAKE WITH FOOD AVOID ASPIRIN AND RELATED PRODUCTS
ibuprofen	Motrin	**Inflammatory disease/rheumatoid arthritis:** 400 mg to 800 mg 3 to 4 times a day (maximum 3200 mg/day)	MAY CAUSE DIZZINESS OR DROWSINESS SWALLOW WHOLE; DON'T CRUSH OR CHEW (EC-Naprosyn)
naproxen	Anaprox, Naprosyn	**Rheumatoid arthritis, osteoarthritis, ankylosing spondylitis:** 500 mg to 1000 mg/day in 2 divided doses up to 1500 mg	
Antimalarials			
chloroquine	Aralen	**Rheumatoid arthritis:** 250 mg (150 mg base) daily until maximal response, then taper to discontinue (usually 3 to 6 weeks)	AVOID ANTACIDS TAKE WITH FOOD AVOID PROLONGED EXPOSURE TO SUNLIGHT

Usual Dosage and Warnings for Drugs Used in the Treatment of Myasthenia Gravis, Multiple Sclerosis, Rheumatoid Arthritis, and Systemic Lupus Erythematosus—cont'd

Generic name	U.S. brand name	Usual adult oral dose and dosing schedule	Warning labels
hydroxychloroquine	Plaquenil	**Rheumatoid arthritis:** 400 mg to 600 mg/day. Once optimal response is reached (4 to 12 weeks); reduce dose to 200 mg to 400 mg/day **Systemic lupus erythematosus:** Begin 400 mg (310 mg base) 1 to 2 times daily; maintenance 200 mg to 400 mg/day	
Immunosuppressives			
azathioprine	Imuran	**Rheumatoid arthritis:** 1 mg/kg/day for 6 to 8 weeks; increase every 4 weeks up to 2.5 mg/kg/day	TAKE WITH FOOD AVOID PREGNANCY
cyclophosphamide	Cytoxan	**Oral:** 50 mg to 100 mg/m^2/day or 400 mg to 1000 mg/m^2 dosed over 4 to 5 days **I.V.:** 400 mg to 1800 mg/m^2 as a single dose repeated at 2- to 4-week intervals	TAKE WITH A FULL GLASS OF WATER TAKE AT THE SAME TIME EACH DAY SWALLOW WHOLE; DON'T CRUSH OR CHEW—cyclosporine, cyclophosphamide
cyclosporine	Neoral, Sandimmune	**Rheumatoid arthritis:** Begin 2.5 mg/kg/day in 2 divided doses; increase 0.5 mg to 0.75 mg/kg/day after 8 weeks if inadequate response. Maximum dose 4 mg/kg/day	AVOID ASPIRIN and NSAIDs—cyclophosphamide AVOID ALCOHOL—cyclosporine AVOID GRAPEFRUIT JUICE-cyclosporine
mitoxantrone	Novantrone	12 mg/m^2 IV infused once every 3 months	AVOID ASPIRIN and NSAIDs MAY DISCOLOR URINE, NAILS, OR THE WHITES OF THE EYES—blue-green AVOID PREGNANCY
Biologic response modifiers			
interferon β1a	Avonex, Rebif	**IM (Avonex):** 30 mcg once weekly **SC (Rebif):** 44 mcg 3 times a week	REFRIGERATE; DON'T FREEZE WARM PREFILLED SYRINGES TO ROOM TEMP BEFORE USING
interferon β1b	Betaseron	**SC:** 0.25 mg every other day	AVOID PREGNANCY
adalimumab	Humira	**SC:** 40 mg every other week (if not taking methotrexate 40 mg/week)	PROTECT FROM LIGHT
anakinra	Kineret	**SC:** 100 mg once daily	REFRIGERATE; DON'T FREEZE
etanercept	Enbrel	25 mg twice weekly or 50 mg once weekly	
infliximab	Remicade	**Rheumatoid arthritis:** 3 mg/kg at 2 and 6 weeks after first dose. Repeat in 8 weeks. If IV infusion: 3 mg to 10 mg/kg. Repeat at 4-week or 8-week intervals	REFRIGERATE; DON'T FREEZE GENTLY SWIRL RECONSTITUTED PRODUCT; DO NOT SHAKE AFTER RECONSTITUTION, DISCARD ANY UNUSED PORTION

Continued

Usual Dosage and Warnings for Drugs Used in the Treatment of Myasthenia Gravis, Multiple Sclerosis, Rheumatoid Arthritis, and Systemic Lupus Erythematosus—cont'd

Generic name	U.S. brand name	Usual adult oral dose and dosing schedule	Warning labels
DMARDs			
methotrexate	Rheumatrex	**Rheumatoid arthritis:** SC/ **IM:** 7.5 mg to 40 mg once weekly **Oral:** 7.5 mg once a week or 2.5 mg every 12 hours for 3 doses/week	TAKE WITH FOOD AVOID ALCOHOL
leflunomide	Arava	Start 100 mg/day for 3 days; decrease to 20 mg/day	AVOID ASPIRIN and NSAIDs— methotrexate AVOID PROLONGED EXPOSURE TO SUNLIGHT— methotrexate AVOID PREGNANCY
sulfasalazine	Azulfadine	**Rheumatoid arthritis:** Start 500 mg to 1000 mg/day; increase to 2000 mg to 3000 mg/day in 2 divided doses (enteric coated tablets)	TAKE WITH FOOD AVOID PROLONGED EXPOSURE TO SUNLIGHT MAINTAIN ADEQUATE HYDRATION MAY DISCOLOR URINE (or skin)— orange-yellow
auranofin	Ridura	**Rheumatoid arthritis:** 6 mg/day in 1 to 2 divided doses (maximum 9 mg/day)	TAKE WITH FOOD AVOID PROLONGED EXPOSURE TO SUNLIGHT
gold sodium thiomalate	Aurolate	**Rheumatoid arthritis:** Start 10 mg/ week (IM); increase to 25 mg to 50 mg/week until 1000 mg cumulative dose has been reached. If effective, continue 25 mg to 50 mg every 2 to 3 weeks for 2 to 20 weeks, then once every 3 to 4 weeks indefinitely	
penicillamine	Cupramine	**Rheumatoid arthritis:** 125 mg to 250 mg/day (maximum 1500 mg/day)	TAKE ON AN EMPTY STOMACH

CHAPTER SUMMARY

- An autoimmune disease occurs when the immune system attacks its own cells, thinking they are germs or a harmful substance.
- Triggers for autoimmunity may be exposure to a virus, environmental toxins, the sun, genetics, hormonal changes, drugs, pregnancy, or some combination of any of these things.
- Myasthenia gravis, multiple sclerosis, rheumatoid arthritis, and systemic lupus erythematosus are examples of autoimmune diseases that affect the musculoskeletal system.
- Myasthenia gravis is an autoimmune disease that causes muscle weakness.
- In myasthenia gravis, the body attacks and destroys receptor sites in the neuromuscular junction that bind acetylcholine.
- Myositis is an autoimmune disease that causes chronic inflammation of the muscles.
- In multiple sclerosis, myelin, the insulating coating of nerves, is attacked.
- Multiple sclerosis causes muscle weakness, fatigue, spasticity, pain, bladder, bowel and sexual dysfunction, speech disturbances, and depression.

- Rheumatoid arthritis is an autoimmune disease that is characterized by inflammation of the lining of the joints.
- Rheumatoid arthritis is far more common in women than in men.
- Systemic lupus erythematosus (SLE) is an autoimmune disease that affects nearly all parts of the body.
- SLE causes swollen and painful joints like rheumatoid arthritis.
- Other signs and symptoms of SLE are muscle pain, fever, red rashes, hair loss, sun sensitivity, swollen glands, extreme fatigue, seizures, mouth ulcers, and poor circulation in fingers and toes.
- Drug therapy for autoimmune diseases affecting the musculoskeletal system is aimed at suppressing inflammation, pain, and immune system response. Treatment goals are also aimed at minimizing further nerve or joint destruction, preservation of body functions, and prevention of disability.
- Glucocorticosteroids are prescribed commonly to suppress inflammation, reduce flare-ups, and treat pain.
- Glucocorticosteroids have immunosuppressive actions and they inhibit the synthesis of antibodies that are responsible for attacking the body's healthy cells.
- Nonsteroidal antiinflammatory drugs (NSAIDs) and aspirin (ASA) are widely used in the treatment of pain and inflammation.
- Celecoxib is the only selective COX-2 inhibitors still available for use in the United States and Canada. Its use is restricted in Canada.
- Selective COX-2 inhibitors increase the risk for cardiovascular toxicity and gastrointestinal ulceration.
- Antimalarials have antiinflammatory and analgesic properties that are useful in the management of rheumatoid arthritis and SLE.
- Biological response modifiers act to inhibit the release of cells that mobilize to fight what the body believes is a harmful invasion and inhibit the release of substances that produce inflammation.
- Biological response modifiers interfere with the activity of cytokines, leukocytes, B cells, and T cells.
- Immunosuppressive drugs interfere with the formation of immune cells by damaging RNA and DNA needed for cell replication.
- Interferon β1a and interferon β1b are first-line therapies for the treatment of multiple sclerosis, and they alter the actions of T cells and B cells and other cytokines that produce immune response and inflammation.
- Tumor necrosis factor α inhibitors are genetically engineered drugs that block the inflammatory process triggered by high concentrations of TNF.
- Multiple sclerosis, rheumatoid arthritis, systemic lupus erythematosus, and other autoimmune diseases have been associated with increased serum levels of interleukins.
- Interleukin 1 receptor antagonists interfere with the binding of interleukins that promote inflammatory responses.
- Methotrexate blocks purine synthesis needed for lymphocyte cell proliferation, reducing inflammation and immune system activity.
- Leflunomide interferes with pyrimidine synthesis, and when used along with methotrexate, both pathways in the cell division process for lymphocytes are blocked.
- Sulfasalazine is a combination of an antiinfective agent and an aspirin-like antiinflammatory agent, and it is used to treat rheumatoid arthritis.
- Gold compounds are used in the treatment of rheumatoid arthritis and work by decreasing the release of antibodies and cytokines and inhibiting the action of collagenase, actions that are part of the immune response.
- Penicillamine is used in the treatment of rheumatoid arthritis because it has antiinflammatory actions and alters immune system response.

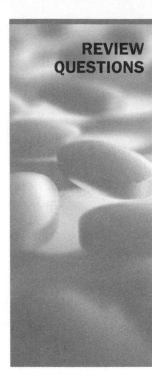

REVIEW QUESTIONS

Multiple Choice

1. A disease that occurs when the immune system turns against the parts of the body it is designed to protect is called a(an) _____.
   a. autoimmune disease
   b. viral disease
   c. immune disease
   d. bacterial disease

2. Which of the following is *not* an example of an autoimmune disease
   a. myasthenia gravis
   b. rheumatoid arthritis
   c. osteoarthritis
   d. systemic lupus erythematosus

3. In myasthenia gravis, the body attacks and destroys receptor sites in the neuromuscular junction that bind _____.
   a. dopamine
   b. epinephrine
   c. GABA
   d. acetylcholine

4. Systemic lupus erythematosus is an autoimmune disease that affects nearly _____ parts of the body.
   a. one-fourth of the
   b. all
   c. the trunk
   d. one-half of the

5. _____ are prescribed commonly to suppress inflammation, reduce flare-ups and treat pain associated with multiple sclerosis, myasthenia gravis, systemic erythematosus, myositis, and rheumatoid arthritis.
   a. mineralocoricoids
   b. glucocorticosteroids
   c. anabolic steroids
   d. all of the above

6. Aspirin and NSAIDs inhibit the release and block the activity of _____.
   a. prostaglandins
   b. COX-1
   c. COX-2
   d. all of the above

7. _____ response modifiers interfere with the activity of cytokines, leukocytes, B cells, and T cells.
   a. Biological
   b. Microbiological
   c. Neurological
   d. Protein

8. Tumor necrosis factor α inhibitors are _____ engineered drugs that block the inflammatory process triggered by high concentrations of tumor necrosis factor.
   a. chemically
   b. biologically
   c. genetically
   d. neurologically

9. **Which of the following drugs is indicated for the treatment of active rheumatoid arthritis, ankylosing spondylitis, and chronic plaque psoriasis?**
   a. Enbrel
   b. Remicade
   c. Humira
   d. Kineret

10. **Gold compounds can produce permanent remission in about 50% of the people who respond favorably to the drug.**
    a. true
    b. false

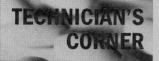
TECHNICIAN'S CORNER

1. Celebrex is the only prescriptive COX-2 inhibitor left on the market. How can we ensure it is not taken off the market?
2. What are some nonpharmacological therapies for autoimmune diseases?

BIBLIOGRAPHY

Arthritis Foundation Disease Center: *Rheumatoid arthritis: overview.* Retrieved from http://www.arthritis.org/conditions/DiseaseCenter/RA/ra_overview.asp.

Crayton H, Rossman H: Managing the symptoms of multiple sclerosis: a multimodal approach, *Clin Therap,* 28, 2006.

Doan T, Massarotti E: Rheumatoid arthritis: an overview of new emerging therapies, *J Clin Pharmacol,* 45:751-762, 2005.

Fox R, Bethoux F, Goldman M, Cohen J: Multiple sclerosis: Advances in understanding, diagnosing, and treating the underlying disease, *Cleve Clin J Med,* 73:91-102, 2006.

Kalant H, Grant D, Mitchell J: *Principles of medical pharmacology* (pp 548-549, 553-554, 595-596), ed 7, Toronto, 2007, Elsevier Canada, A Division of Reed Elsevier Canada.

Lance L, Lacy C, Armstrong L, Goldman M: *Drug information handbook for the allied health professional,* ed 12. Hudson, OH, 2005, APhA Lexi-Comp.

National Institute of Arthritis and Musculoskeletal and Skin Diseases: *Autoimmunity,* Bethesda, MD, 2002, NIAMS, National Institutes of Health, U.S. Department of Health and Human Services. NIH Publication No. 02-4858. Retrieved from http://www.niams.nih.gov/hi/topics/autoimmune/autoimmunity.htm.

National Institute of Arthritis and Musculoskeletal and Skin Diseases: *Systemic lupus erythematosus,* Bethesda, MD, 2003, NIAMS, National Institutes of Health, U.S. Department of Health and Human Services. NIH publication No. 03-4178. Retrieved from http://www.niams.nih.gov/hi/topics/lupus/slehand-out/index.htm.

National Institute of Neurological Disorders and Stroke: *Multiple sclerosis: hope through research,* Bethesda, MD, 2006, NINDS, National Institutes of Health, U.S. Department of Health and Human Services. NIH publication No. 96-75. Retrieved from http://www.ninds.nih.gov/disorders/multiple_sclerosis/multiple_sclerosis_pr.htm.

National Institute of Neurological Disorders and Stroke: *Myasthenia gravis fact sheet,* Bethesda, MD, 2006, NINDS, National Institutes of Health, U.S. Department of Health and Human Services. Retrieved from http://www.ninds.nih.gov/disorders/myasthenia_gravis/myasthenia_gravis.htm.

Page C, Curtis M, Sutter M, Walker M, Hoffman B: *Integrated pharmacology* (pp 228-233, 336-341, 445-452), Philadelphia, 2005, Mosby.

Pharmaceutical Sciences, Vancouver General Hospital, Vancouver, British Columbia, Canada: *Parenteral drug therapy manual,* Retrieved from http://www.vhpharmsci.com/PDTM/.

Raffa R, Rawls S, Beyzarov E: *Netter's illustrated pharmacology* (pp 79), Philadelphia, 2005, WB Saunders.

Torpy J: Myasthenia gravis, *JAMA,* 293:1940, 2005.

USP Center for Advancement of Patient Safety: *Use caution–avoid confusion,* USP Quality Review No. 79, Rockville, MD, April 2004, USP Center for Advancement of Patient Safety.

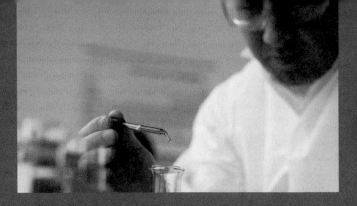

CHAPTER 16

Treatment of Osteoporosis and Paget's Disease of the Bone

LEARNING OBJECTIVES

- Describe the signs and symptoms of osteoporosis.
- List causes of osteoporosis.
- List and classify medications used in the treatment of osteoporosis.
- Describe the mechanism of action for each class of drug used in the treatment of osteoporosis.
- Describe the signs and symptoms of Paget's disease of the bone.
- List and classify medications used in the treatment of Paget's disease of the bone.
- Describe mechanism of action for each class of drugs used to treat Paget's disease of the bone.
- Identify warning labels and precautionary messages associated with medications used to treat osteoporosis and Paget's disease of the bone.
- Identify significant drug look-alike/sound-alike issues.
- Learn the terminology associated with osteoporosis and Paget's disease of the bone.

KEY TERMS

Bone mineral density (BMD): Test measurement that is taken to determine the degree of bone loss.

Osteoblasts: Cells responsible for bone formation, deposition, and mineralization of the collagen matrix of bone.

Osteoclasts: Cells responsible for bone resorption.

Osteolysis: Dissolution or degradation of bone.

Osteopenia: Decrease in bone mineral density that is the precursor of osteoporosis.

Osteoporosis: Chronic, progressive disease of bone characterized by loss of bone density and bone strength and resulting in increased risk for fractures.

Remodeling: Process of continual turnover of bone.

Resorption: Process where bone is broken down into mineral ions (calcium).

Osteoporosis

Osteoporosis is a chronic, progressive disease of bone characterized by loss of bone density and bone strength and resulting in increased fracture risk. Osteoporosis affects between 13% and 18% of women older than 50 years and 3% and 6% of men older than 50 years, making it the most common disease of bone in the United States. *Osteopenia* is a condition whereby **bone mineral density (BMD)** is decreased, and it is the precursor of osteoporosis. Osteopenia affects an additional 37% to 59% of women and 28% to 47% of men.

Osteoporosis is responsible for more than 1.5 million fractures annually in the United States. The most common are fractures of the vertebrae of the spine (700,000) and hips (300,000 in hips), although fractures of the wrists, feet, toes, and forearm are also common. The lifetime risk for fractures in people over 50 years is 1:2 women and 1:4 men, regardless of ethnic background. Fractures caused by osteoporosis are classified according to health outcomes—as low impact or fragility fractures. Low-impact osteoporosis fractures are due to falls or trauma. Fragility fractures may occur in the absence of trauma and can occur from coughing or sneezing.

PATHOPHYSIOLOGY OF OSTEOPOROSIS

Primary osteoporosis is associated with the aging process. Up until the age of 30 or 40 years, the percentage of bone formed is greater than the percentage of bone lost. After menopause, women have a dramatic shift in the ratio between bone formation and bone loss, with bone loss exceeding bone formed. In men, this process is more gradual until the age 65 or 70; then, the rates of bone loss for men and women are about equal.

Bone formation and loss is a carefully controlled process and is regulated from birth to death. The process is called *remodeling* (Figure 16-1). Osteoclasts and osteoblasts are cells that are involved in the bone turnover process. *Osteoblasts* are responsible for bone formation, deposition, and mineralization of the collagen matrix of bone. *Osteoclasts* are responsible for bone resorption. Resorption is the process whereby bone is broken down **(osteolysis)** into mineral ions (calcium).

Bone turnover is linked to levels of calcium in the blood (Figure 16-2). Ninety-nine percent of total body calcium in located in the skeleton; therefore, bones are a reservoir for calcium when serum levels are too low.

If serum calcium levels are too low, hormones are released to transfer calcium stored in bones back into serum. When blood levels are too high, hormones are released to reduce

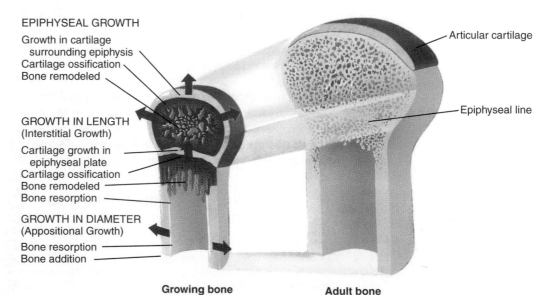

EPIPHYSEAL GROWTH

Growth in cartilage
  surrounding epiphysis
Cartilage ossification
Bone remodeled

GROWTH IN LENGTH
(Interstitial Growth)

Cartilage growth in
  epiphyseal plate
Cartilage ossification
Bone remodeled
Bone resorption

GROWTH IN DIAMETER
(Appositional Growth)

Bone resorption
Bone addition

Articular cartilage

Epiphyseal line

Growing bone   **Adult bone**

FIGURE 16-1 Bone remodeling. *(From Thibodeau GA, Patton KT:* Anatomy and physiology, *ed 6, St Louis, 2007, Mosby.)*

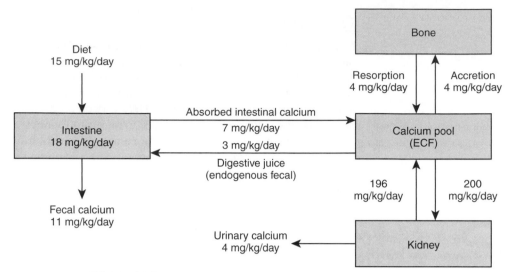

FIGURE 16-2 Calcium level fluctuations between bone, kidneys, intestines, and calcium reservoirs. *(From Kalant H, Grant D, Mitchell J:* Principles of medical pharmacology, *ed 7, Toronto, 2007, Elsevier Canada, A Division of Reed Elsevier Canada.)*

serum calcium and deposit excess in bones. The hormones principally responsible for regulation of serum calcium levels are parathyroid hormone, calcitonin, and vitamin D. Parathyroid hormone is secreted by the parathyroid gland when intestinal absorption of calcium and renal reabsorption of calcium are insufficient to maintain the required calcium balance. Parathyroid hormone mobilizes calcium from bone, increasing serum calcium levels by transferring calcium from bone to blood. Calcitonin reduces serum calcium levels by storing excess in the bone. Vitamin D enhances calcium absorption and is one of the hormones involved in the formation of osteoclasts. Parathyroid hormone and sex hormones are also associated with osteoclast formation. Other hormones linked to the regulation of bone formation and bone loss are estrogen, progesterone, luteinizing hormone, and androgens. Estrogen and progesterone levels are lowered in postmenopausal women and testosterone levels are reduced in men as part of the normal aging process, which in part explains why calcium absorption decreases as men and women age.

CONDITIONS THAT PRODUCE OSTEOPOROSIS

Osteoporosis can be classified as primary or secondary. Secondary osteoporosis may be related to another disease process or is drug induced. Some of the diseases that can produce secondary osteoporosis include hyperthyroidism, hyperparathyroidism, rheumatoid arthritis, systemic lupus erythematosus, multiple myeloma, inflammatory bowel disease, renal insufficiency, Parkinson's disease, multiple sclerosis, and AIDS.

Drugs that can induce osteoporosis are administered for a wide variety of diseases. They are used in the treatment of autoimmune diseases of the musculoskeletal system, seizures, prostate cancer, bipolar disorder, hypothyroidism, kidney disease, and other conditions. Alcohol abuse can also produce osteoporosis. Examples of some of the drugs that can produce bone loss leading to osteoporosis are shown in Box 16-1.

BOX 16-1 DRUGS THAT CAN PRODUCE BONE LOSS

- Antiandrogens (flutamide and nilutamide)
- Cyclosporine
- Depo-medroxyprogesterone acetate
- Gonadotropin-releasing hormone agonists (leuprolide)
- Glucocorticosteroids
- Lithium
- Methotrexate
- Phenytoin

TECH NOTE!
Physical activity can improve bone health, but most people are not active enough.

PREVENTION TIPS

It is best to lay the foundation for healthy dense bones early in life, although bone health can be improved at any age. Mild weight-bearing exercise along with a diet rich in vitamin D and calcium is key to strong bones that resist fractures. Lifestyle changes that reduce alcohol consumption and smoking are also important.

Recommended daily allowances (RDAs) for calcium are listed in Table 16-1. The Osteoporosis Society of Canada and the National Osteoporosis Foundation (U.S.) recommend that postmenopausal women and men at risk for fractures ingest 1500 mg of calcium and 800 IU of vitamin D each day.

Milk, leafy green vegetables, and soybeans contain calcium, and vitamin D is produced by the skin upon exposure to sunlight. Foods rich in calcium and vitamin D are given in Table 16-2.

Calcium can be obtained from calcium supplements in addition to food. Calcium supplements are available as calcium chloride, calcium citrate, calcium carbonate, calcium lactate, and calcium gluconate. The amount of elemental calcium contained in these calcium salts varies (Table 16-3). Calcium citrate is most absorbable and easiest to tolerate; however, calcium carbonate provides the greatest amount of elemental calcium per tablet. Calcium should be taken on a full stomach. Food increases absorption and decreases upset stomach.

Paget's Disease of Bone

Paget's disease is most common in men older than 55 years. The disease is most common in the United Kingdom, Australia, New Zealand, and North America and is uncommon in Africa, Asia, and Scandinavia. Approximately 2% of American men over the age of 60 years have Paget's disease. The cause is unknown, yet it is believed that genetics, viral infection (paramyxoviruses), and environmental factors are involved.

PATHOPHYSIOLOGY OF PAGET'S DISEASE OF THE BONE

Paget's disease is a progressive disease of bone. The disease produces irregular activity of osteoclasts and osteoblasts. Excessive bone resorption in focal areas is followed by increased bone formation, resulting in enlarged bones that are structurally weak. Effects of the disease tend to be localized and most commonly affect the pelvis, lumbar sacral spine, skull, femur, or tibia; however, Paget's disease may be widespread throughout the body, and the entire skeleton may be affected.

Paget's disease causes deformities such as bowed legs, pain, arthritis, deafness, and, rarely, cranial nerve palsies. Pain may be constant or intermittent. Intermittent pain is typically associated with weight bearing or localized microfractures. When pain is constant, it may even occur at rest.

TABLE 16-1   Your Body Needs Calcium

If This Is Your Age,	Then You Need This Much Calcium Each Day (mg)
0 to 6 months	210
6 to 12 months	270
1 to 3 years	500
4 to 8 years	800
9 to 18 years	1300
18 to 50 years	1000
Over 50 years	1200

(A cup of milk or fortified orange juice has about 300 mg of calcium.)
Courtesy of NIH, *The 2004 Surgeon General's Report on Bone Health and Osteoporosis.*

TABLE 16-2   Calcium Calculator

Help your bones. Choose foods that are high in calcium. Here are some examples.

Food	Calcium (mg)	Points
Fortified oatmeal, 1 packet	350	3
Sardines, canned in oil, with edible bones, 3 oz.	324	3
Cheddar cheese, 1½ oz. shredded	306	3
Milk, nonfat, 1 cup	302	3
Milkshake, 1 cup	300	3
Yogurt, plain, low-fat, 1 cup	300	3
Soybeans, cooked, 1 cup	261	3
Tofu, firm, with calcium, 6 oz.	204	2
Orange juice, fortified with calcium, 6 oz.	200-260 (varies)	2-3
Salmon, canned, with edible bones, 3 oz.	181	2
Pudding, instant, (chocolate, banana, etc.) made with 2% milk, ½ cup	153	2
Baked beans, 1 cup	142	1
Cottage cheese, 1% milk fat, 1 cup	138	1
Spaghetti, lasagna, 1 cup	125	1
Frozen yogurt, vanilla, soft-serve, ½ cup	103	1
Ready-to-eat cereal, fortified with calcium, 1 cup	100-1000 (varies)	1-10
Cheese pizza, 1 slice	100	1
Fortified waffles, 2	100	1
Turnip greens, boiled, ½ cup	99	1
Broccoli, raw, 1 cup	90	1
Ice cream, vanilla, ½ cup	85	1
Soy or rice milk, fortified with calcium, 1 cup	80-500 (varies)	1-5

Points Needed   Your Total Today

Babies/toddlers (ages 0 to 3) need .... 2 to 5
Children (ages 4 to 8) need 8
Teens need 13
Adults under 50 need 10
Adults over 50 need 12

Courtesy of NIH, *The 2004 Surgeon General's Report on Bone Health and Osteoporosis.*

TABLE 16-3   Percent Elemental Calcium per Calcium Salt

Calcium salt	Percent elemental calcium per tablet	Strength commercially available (mg)	No. of tablets needed to obtain recommended dose of 1200 to 1500 mg/day
Calcium carbonate	40%	500 to 600	2-3
Calcium chloride	27%	—	—
Calcium citrate	21%	—	8
Calcium lactate	13%	42.25 to 84.5	16
Calcium gluconate	9%	45 to 90	16
Calcium phosphate	—	600	2 to 3
Oyster shell (calcium carbonate)	—	250 to 1250	1 to 6

Drugs Used for the Treatment of Osteoporosis and Paget's Disease of Bone

The goals of pharmacological treatment for osteoporosis are to increase bone density and to reduce risks for future fractures. Pharmacological agents are categorized as *antiresorptive* (inhibit bone resorption) or *anabolic* (promote bone formation).

Paget's disease is also treatable; however, treatment is recommended for patients who have symptoms of bone pain and localized neurological involvement. Treatment is also recommended when the vertebrae, femur, and base of the skull are involved because of risks for fractures and deafness.

ANTIRESORPTIVE AGENTS

The majority of the drugs used to treat osteoporosis and Paget's disease are antiresorptive agents. They suppress bone turnover and loss. Antiresorptive agents are further classified by their structure and mechanism of action. Classifications of antiresorptive agents are biphosphonates, calcitonin, and estrogens.

BIPHOSPHONATES

Mechanism of Action and Pharmacokinetics

All of the biphosphonates are used for the treatment of Paget's disease and osteoporosis. However, ibandronate is not FDA approved for Paget's disease and etidronate, pamidronate, and zoledronic acid are not FDA approved for treatment of osteoporosis. Biphosphonates inhibit osteoclast activity. Recall that osteoclasts are cells responsible for bone resorption. Biphosphonates interfere with recruitment, differentiation, and action of osteoclasts. There are two groups of biphosphonates. The nitrogen-containing biphosphonates (alendronate, pamidronate, risedronate) are more potent than the non–nitrogen-containing agents (etidronate, tiludronate). Pamidronate, and zoledronic acid are biphosphonates used for the treatment of Paget's disease that are administered via intravenous infusion.

The biphosphonates are poorly absorbed in the gastrointestinal tract, and food further reduces absorption. They must be taken on an empty stomach, at least 30 minutes before the first meal or beverage of the day. Between 50% and 80% of the drug is eliminated unchanged in the urine within 24 hours of dosing. The remainder permanently binds to bone. Alendronate and risedronate are available in dosage forms for daily and weekly dosing. Patient adherence is improved when the medication is dosed once weekly. Zolendronic acid is administered as a single dose and in one study was shown to be effective as a daily risedronate therapy at 6 months after the drug was infused.

Adverse Reactions

Common adverse effects associated with biphosphonates are painful swallowing, heartburn, diarrhea, nausea, and vomiting. Less common adverse reactions are musculoskeletal pain, necrosis or erosion of the jaw bone (rare), and eye inflammation.

Precautions

To prevent injury to the esophagus by biphosphonates, the patient should sit or stand upright for 30 to 60 minutes after taking their medicine. Each tablet should be taken with 6 to 8 ounces of water. Calcium and vitamin D supplementation is recommended when biphosphonates are administered; however, supplements should be avoided within 2 hours of administration of the prescribed biphosphonate dose.

> **✎ TECH ALERT!**
> The following drugs have look-alike/ sound-alike issues: Fosamax and Flomax; Aredia and Adriamycin; Actonel and Actos

---

Biphosphonates

	Generic name	U.S. brand name(s) / Canadian brand(s)	Dosage forms and strengths
	alendronate	Fosamax ——————— Fosamax	**Solution, oral:** 70 mg/75 ml **Tablet:** 5 mg, 10 mg, 35 mg, 40 mg, 70 mg
	etidronate	Didronel ——————— Didronel	**Injection:** 50 mg/ml (6 ml) **Tablet:** 200 mg, 400 mg
	ibandronate	Boniva ——————— Not available	**solution for injection:** 1 mg/ml **Tablet:** 2.5 mg, 150 mg

Continued

Biphosphonates—cont'd

	Generic name	U.S. brand name(s) / Canadian brand(s)	Dosage forms and strengths
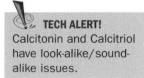	pamidronate	Aredia / Aredia	**Injection, powder for reconstitution:** 30 mg, 90 mg / **Injection, solution:** 3 mg/ml, 6 mg/ml, 9 mg/ml
	risedronate	Actonel / Actonel	**Tablet:** 5 mg, 30 mg, 35 mg, 75 mg
	tiludronate	Skelid / Not available	**Tablet:** 200 mg
	zoledronic acid	Reclast, Zometa / Zometa	**Injection, powder for reconstitution:** 4 mg / **Injection, solution:** 4 mg/5 ml (Zometa), 5 mg/100 mg (Reclast)
Combinations			
	alendronate + cholecalciferol	Fosamax Plus D	70 mg alendronate + 2800 international units vitamin D
	risedronate + calcium carbonate	Actonel with Calcium	35 mg risedronate + 1250 mg calcium carbonate

SELECTIVE ESTROGEN RECEPTOR MODULATORS

Mechanism of Action and Pharmacokinetics

Raloxifene is indicated for the treatment and prevention of osteoporosis in postmenopausal women. It is a selective estrogen receptor modulator, and it binds to estrogen receptors to produce an agonist effect in bone and lipid metabolism and an antagonist effect in the breast and uterus. It has been shown to reduce new fractures of the vertebrae by up to 68%.

Only 2% of the amount of raloxifene administered is bioavailable. First-pass metabolism and protein binding limit the amount of drug that can produce effect.

Adverse Reactions

Side effects common to raloxifene are hot flashes, leg cramps, and venous thromboembolism.

Selective Estrogen Receptor Modulators (SERMs)

	Generic name	U.S. brand name(s) / Canadian brand(s)	Dosage forms and strengths
	raloxifene	Evista / Evista	**Tablet:** 60 mg

TECH ALERT!
Calcitonin and Calcitriol have look-alike/sound-alike issues.

CALCITONIN

Calcitonin is a hormone that is secreted by the thyroid gland and inhibits the rate of bone turnover stimulated by release of parathyroid hormone. It lowers serum calcium levels by decreasing intestinal absorption of calcium and increasing renal elimination of calcium. These actions make calcitonin useful for the treatment of Paget's disease. The effectiveness of calcitonin in the treatment of osteoporosis is related to its ability to increase BMD. Postmenopausal women tend to have reduced calcitonin levels.

Absorption of calcitonin from intramuscular and subcutaneous injection sites is rapid, and the half-life of calcitonin is short (20 minutes). The availability of calcitonin when administered intranasally is 3% to 50%. Local adverse reactions are mainly irritation of the nose or injection site.

Miscellaneous

Generic name	U.S. brand name(s) Canadian brand(s)	Dosage forms and strengths
calcitonin	Fortical, Miacalcin	**Injection, solution:** 200 units/ml
	Calcimar, Miacalcin NS	**Nasal solution:** 200 units per actuation (spray)

HORMONE REPLACEMENT THERAPY

Estrogen and progesterone decrease bone turnover, bone loss, and fractures; however, hormone replacement therapy (HRT) is not a first-line therapy for the prevention of osteoporosis because of the increased risk for coronary heart disease, stroke, thromboembolism, and breast and uterine cancer.

Estrogen deficiency occurs postmenopause and increases osteoclast activity. Osteoclasts are responsible for bone resorption. Hormone replacement restores estrogen levels and inhibits the effects of estrogen deficiency on cytokines that regulate the formation of osteoclasts. Cytokines involved in osteoclast regulation are interleukins (IL-1, IL-6) and tumor necrosis factor. HRT also has beneficial effects on BMD. Increases in BMD are dose dependent; higher doses produce increased BMD. Increases in BMD occur with oral and transdermal dosage forms.

Hormone Replacement Therapy (HRT)

Generic name	U.S. brand name(s) Canadian brand(s)	Dosage forms and strengths
estradiol*	Alora, Climara, Esclim, Estrace, Estraderm, Gynodiol, Menostar, Vivelle-Dot	**Tablet, oral (Estrace, Gynodiol):** 0.5 mg, 1 mg, 2 mg (1.5 mg Gynodiol only)
		Transdermal patch: Alora (once weekly patch): 0.05 mg/24 hr and 0.1 mg/24 hr (box of 4)
	Climara, Estrace, Estraderm, Estradot, Oesclim, Vivelle	**(twice weekly patch):** 0.025 mg/24 hr (9 cm^2), 0.05 mg/24 hr (18 cm^2), 0.075 mg/24 hr (27 cm^2), 0.1 mg/24 hr (36 cm^2) box of 8
		Climara (once weekly patch): 0.025 mg/24 hr (6.5 cm^2), 0.0375 mg/24 hr (9.375 cm^2), 0.05 mg/24 hr (12.5 cm^2), 0.06 mg/24 hr (15 cm^2), 0.075 mg/24 hr (18.75 cm^2), 0.1 mg/24 hr (25 cm^2) box of 4
		Esclim (twice weekly patch): 0.025 mg/24 hr (11 cm^2), 0.0375 mg/24 hr (16.5 cm^2), 0.05 mg/24 hr (22 cm^2), 0.075 mg/24 hr (33 cm^2), 0.1 mg/24 hr (44 cm^2) box of 8
		Estraderm (twice weekly patch): 0.05 mg/24 hr (10 cm^2), 0.1 mg/24 hr (20 cm^2) box of 8
		Menostar (once weekly patch): 0.014 mg/24 hr (3.25 cm^2) box of 4
		Vivelle (twice weekly patch): 0.025 mg/24 hr (7.25 cm^2), 0.0375 mg/24 hr (11 cm^2), 0.05 mg/24 hr (14.5 cm^2), 0.075 mg/24 hr (22 cm^2), 0.1 mg/24 hr (29 cm^2) box of 8
		Vivelle-Dot (twice weekly patch): 0.0375 mg/24 hr (3.75 cm^2), 0.05 mg/24 hr (5 cm^2), 0.075 mg/24 hr (7.5 cm^2), 0.1 mg/24 hr (10 cm^2) box of 8
		See Chapter 34 for other dosage form strengths

Continued

Hormone Replacement Therapy (HRT)—cont'd

	Generic name	U.S. brand name(s) Canadian brand(s)	Dosage forms and strengths
	estradiol + levonorgestrol	Climara Pro	**Transdermal patch:** estradiol, 0.045 mg + levonorgestrel, 0.015 mg per 24 hr
	estradiol + norethindrone	Activella, CombiPatch Estalis,	**Combination pack (Estalis Sequi) 140/50:** estradiol 50 mcg/day (as Vivelle patch) plus norethindrone acetate 140 mcg and estraciol 50 mcg/day (as Estalis patch) box of 4
		Estalis-Sequi	**Estalis Sequi 250/50:** estradiol 50 mcg/day (as Vivelle patch) plus norethindrone acetate 250 mcg and estradiol 50 mcg/day (as Estalis patch) box of 4 **Tablet: (Activella):** Estradiol 1 mg and norethindrone 0.5 mg (28s) **Transdermal patch (CombiPatch, Estalis):** estradiol 50 mcg + norethindrone 140 mcg/day (9 cm^2), estradiol 50 mcg + norethindrone 250 mcg/day (16 cm^2)
	estradiol + norgestimate	Prefest Not available	**Tablet:** Estradiol 1 mg (15 pink tablets) and estradiol 1 mg plus norgestimate 0.09 mg (15 white tablets)
	conjugated estrogens	Premphase, Prempro Premphase, Premplus Prempro	**Tablet (Premphase):** conjugated estrogens 0.625 mg (14 maroon tablets) and 0.625 mg conjugated estrogen plus 5 mg medroxyprogesterone (14 blue tablets) **Tablet (Prempro):** 0.3 mg conjugated estrogen plus 1.5 mg medroxyprogesterone (28s) 0.45 mg conjugated estrogen plus 1.5 mg medroxyprogesterone (28s) 0.625 mg conjugated estrogen plus 2.5 mg medroxyprogesterone (28s) 0.625 mg conjugated estrogen plus 5 mg medroxyprogesterone (28s)
	estrogens + medroxyprogesterone	Premarin Premarin	**Tablet:** 0.3 mg. 0.45 mg, 0.625 mg, 0.9 mg, 1.25 mg, 2.5 mg See Chapter 34 for other dosage form strengths
	estrogens esterified	Menest Estratab, Menest	**Tablet:** 0.3 mg, 0.625 mg, 1.25 mg, 2.5 mg
	estropipate	Ogen, Ortho-Est Ogen	**Tablet:** 0.625 mg (0.75 mg estropipate), 1.25 mg (1.5 mg estropipate), 2.5 mg (3 mg estropipate)

> **TECH ALERT!**
> The following drugs have look-alike/sound-alike issues: Alora and Aldara; Estraderm and Testoderm; Estratab and Estratest

Pharmaceuticals that are prescribed for HRT in the treatment of osteoporosis are estradiol, estradiol and norethindrone, estradiol and norgestimate, estrogens and medroxyprogesterone, conjugated estrogens, esterified estrogens, and estropipate. HRT is also indicated for the treatment of treatment of menopausal symptoms (hot flashes, vaginal dryness and atrophy), postmenopausal urogenital symptoms (urgency, dysuria), abnormal uterine bleeding, hypoestrogenism, and breast and prostate cancer (palliation). These drugs are discussed in detail in Unit 9. Adverse reactions include headache, nausea, rash at site of patch application, coronary heart disease, depression, stroke, thromboembolism, and breast and uterine cancer.

ANABOLIC AGENTS

Parathyroid hormone analogues increase the rate of bone remodeling, thicken structural units of bone (ostens), and produce bone architecture that closely resembles normal bone. They decrease osteoblast cell death, allowing the balance between bone formation and bone resorption to shift toward bone formation. This is an improvement over biphosphonates because alendronate, risedronate, and etidronate only prevent further destruction of bone architecture. They do not restore normal structure. Despite the benefits of teriparatide, a genetically engineered form of human parathyroid hormone and the only drug currently available in this category, its use is limited because of risks for osteosarcoma. Other adverse reactions associated with teriparatide use are orthostatic hypotension, dizziness, headache, hypercalcemia, leg cramps, nausea, arthralgias, hyperuricemia, and gout.

Anabolic Agents

Generic Name	U.S. brand name(s) / Canadian brand(s)	Dosage forms and strengths
teriparatide	Forteo Not available	**Injection, solution:** 20 mg/dose (prefilled syringe)

Usual Dosage and Warnings for Drugs Used in the Treatment of Osteoporosis and Paget's Disease

Generic name	U.S. brand name	Usual adult oral dose and dosing schedule	Warning Labels
Biphosphonates			
alendronate	Fosamax	**Osteoporosis, prevention:** 5 mg once a day or 35 mg once weekly **Osteoporosis, treatment:** 10 mg once a day or 70 mg once weekly **Paget's disease:** 40 mg once daily for 6 months	TAKE 30 MINUTES BEFORE THE FIRST MEAL OF THE DAY WITH 6 TO 8 OUNCES OF WATER AVOID DAIRY PRODUCTS AND SUPPLEMENTS CONTAINING CALCIUM, MAGNESIUM, VITAMIN D, OR IRON WITHIN 2 HOURS OF DOSE
ibandronate	Boniva	**Osteoporosis:** 2.5 mg once a day or 150 mg once monthly, or administer 3 mg IV bolus every 3 months	
etidronate	Didronel	**Paget's disease:** 5 mg to 10 mg/kg/day for up to 6 months or 11 mg to 20 mg/kg/day up to 3 months. Retreat if needed after a drug-free period of 90 days	REDUCE SMOKING AND ALCOHOL CONSUMPTION SIT OR STAND UPRIGHT FOR AT LEAST 30 MINUTES AFTER DOSE
pamidronate	Aredia	**Paget's disease:** 30 mg infused in 500 ml ½ NS or NS over 4 hours for 3 days in a row	TAKE ON AN EMPTY STOMACH—etidronate, tiludronate
risedronate	Actonel	**Osteoporosis:** 5 mg once a day, 35 mg once weekly, 75 mg once daily for 2 days a month or 150 mg once a month **Paget's disease:** 30 mg once a day for 2 months. Retreat if needed after a 2-month drug-free period	
tiludronate	Skelid	**Paget's disease:** 400 mg daily for 3 months	
zoledronic acid	Zometa	**Paget's disease:** 5 mg as a single dose infused over at least 15 minutes **Osteoporosis*:** 5 mg IV once yearly	
Biphosphonate combinations			
alendronate + cholecalciferol	Fosamax Plus D	1 tablet once weekly	
risedronate + calcium carbonate	Actonel with Calcium	1 tablet risedronate once weekly + daily calcium	

Continued

Usual Dosage and Warnings for Drugs Used in the Treatment of Osteoporosis and Paget's Disease—cont'd

	Generic name	U.S. brand name	Usual adult oral dose and dosing schedule	Warning Labels
	Selective estrogen receptor modulators			
	raloxifene	Evista	60 mg/day	TAKE WITH OR WITHOUT FOOD
	Hormone replacement therapy (HRT)			
	estradiol	Estrace	**Prevention of osteoporosis:** **Oral:** 0.5 mg/day (3 weeks on and 1 week off) **Transdermal patch, as Climara, Menostar:** 1 patch once weekly **Transdermal patch, as Alora, Estraderm, Vivelle-Dot or Vivelle:** 1 patch twice weekly	TAKE WITH FOOD ROTATE SITE OF APPLICATION (patch) STORE IN SEALED FOIL POUCH AT ROOM TEMPERATURE— CombiPatch
	estradiol + levonorgestrol	Climara Pro	**Prevention of osteoporosis:** One patch weekly	
	estradiol + norethindrone	Activella, CombiPatch	**Prevention of osteoporosis:** **Tablet (Activella):** 1 tablet daily Transdermal patch **(CombiPatch, Estalis):** 1 patch twice a week **Sequential regimen (Estalis Sequi):** 1 estradiol only patch for first 14 days of cycle followed by 1 Combipatch (or Estalis) twice weekly for remainder of cycle	
	conjugated estrogens	Premarin	**Prevention of osteoporosis:** 0.3 mg cyclically or daily	
	estrogens esterified	Menest	**Prevention of osteoporosis:** 0.3 mg cyclically or daily (maximum 1.25 mg/day)	
	estropipate	Ogen	**Prevention of osteoporosis:** 0.75 mg daily for 25 days of a 31-day cycle	
	estradiol + norgestimate	Prefest	**Prevention of osteoporosis:** 1 mg estradiol daily for 3 days (pink tablet), followed by 1 mg estradiol + norgestimate 0.09 mg once daily for 3 days (white tablet). Repeat continuously	
	estrogens + medroxyprogesterone	Premphase Prempro	**Prevention of osteoporosis:** Premphase: 0.625 mg conjugated estrogen days 1 through 14 (maroon tablet), 0.625 mg conjugated estrogen + 5 mg medroxyprogesterone days 15 through 28 (blue tablet) **Prempro:** 0.3 mg conjugated estrogen + 1.5 mg medroxyprogesterone daily up to 0.625 mg conjugated estrogen + 5 mg medroxyprogesterone daily	
	Calcitonin hormone			
	calcitonin	Miacalcin	**Osteoporosis:** 100 units/day (IM, SC) or 1 spray in 1 nostril (200 units/day) (intranasal) **Paget's disease:** Start 100 units/day (IM, SC); maintenance 50 to 100 units every 1 to 3 days	ALTERNATE SPRAY IN NOSTRILS (1 SPRAY EVERY OTHER DAY)

Usual Dosage and Warnings for Drugs Used in the Treatment of Osteoporosis and Paget's Disease—cont'd

Generic name	U.S. brand name	Usual adult oral dose and dosing schedule	Warning Labels
Parathyroid hormone analogue			
teriparatide	Forteo	**SC:** 20 mcg once a day	store in the refrigerator; do not freeze DISCARD AFTER 28 DAYS OF OPENING

*Not FDA approved

CHAPTER SUMMARY

- Osteoporosis is a chronic, progressive disease of bone characterized by loss of bone density and bone strength and resulting in increased fracture risk.
- The lifetime risk for fractures in people over 50 years is 1:2 women and 1:4 men.
- Low impact osteoporosis fractures can occur from falls or trauma; fragility fractures may occur from coughing or sneezing.
- Primary osteoporosis is associated with the aging process.
- Secondary osteoporosis may be caused by diseases or drugs.
- Glucocorticoids use can cause osteoporosis.
- After menopause, women's rate of bone loss exceeds the rate of bone formed. The rate of bone loss for men and women is equal after age 65 to 70 years.
- Bone formation and loss is a carefully controlled process and is regulated from birth to death.
- Osteoblasts are responsible for bone formation, and osteoclasts are responsible for bone resorption.
- 99% of total body calcium in located in the skeleton; therefore, bones are a reservoir for calcium when serum levels are too low.
- The hormones principally responsible for regulation of serum calcium levels are parathyroid hormone, calcitonin, and vitamin D.
- Other hormones linked to the regulation of bone formation and bone loss are estrogen, progesterone, luteinizing hormone, and androgens.
- Paget's disease is a progressive disease of bone.
- Paget's disease is characterized by excessive bone resorption in focal areas followed by increased bone formation that results in enlarged bones that are structurally weak.
- Paget's disease causes bone deformities, pain, fractures, and deafness.
- The disease is most common in men older than 55 years.
- A three-point program is recommended to prevent and treat osteoporosis: lifelong nutritional calcium and vitamin D intake, exercise (weight bearing and strength training), and pharmacotherapy.
- Pharmacologic agents used in the treatment of osteoporosis or Paget's disease are categorized as antiresorptive (inhibit bone resorption) or anabolic (promote bone formation).
- Biphosphonates, calcitonin, selective estrogen receptor modulators, and estrogen are antiresorptive agents.
- Parathyroid hormone is an anabolic agent.
- Biphosphonates must be taken on an empty stomach, at least 30 minutes before the first meal or beverage of the day, or 2 hours before or after meals.
- Patients taking alendronate and risedronate must sit upright or stand for at least 30 minutes after dosing to avoid possible esophageal ulceration.
- Calcium and vitamin D supplementation is recommended when biphosphonates are administered.
- Mild weight-bearing exercise along with a diet rich in vitamin D and calcium is key to strong bones that resist fractures.
- Lifestyle changes that reduce alcohol consumption and smoking are also important.

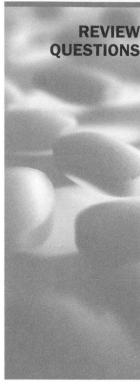

REVIEW QUESTIONS

1. A chronic, progressive disease of bone characterized by loss of bone density and bone strength and resulting in increased fracture risk is called _____.
   a. rheumatoid arthritis
   b. osteoporosis
   c. brittle bone disease
   d. osteosarcoma

2. Alcohol abuse can also produce osteoporosis.
   a. true
   b. false

3. Paget's disease is most common in women older than 55 years.
   a. true
   b. false

4. The goals of treatment are to _____ bone density and to _____ risks for future fractures.
   a. decrease, reduce
   b. increase, reduce
   c. reduce, remove
   d. decrease, reduce

5. The majority of the drugs used to treat osteoporosis and Paget's disease are _____ agents.
   a. absorption
   b. antifracture
   c. antiresorptive
   d. anticalcium

6. Only some of the biphosphonates are indicated for the treatment of Paget's disease.
   a. true
   b. false

7. _____ is a selective estrogen receptor modulator indicated for the treatment and prevention of osteoporosis in postmenopausal women and prevents further destruction of bone architecture.
   a. Fosamax
   b. Evista
   c. Boniva
   d. Osteo-cal

8. Hormone replacement therapy (HRT) is the first-line therapy for the prevention of osteoporosis because of the increased risk for coronary heart disease, stroke, thromboembolism, and breast and uterine cancer.
   a. true
   b. false

9. A diet rich in vitamin _____ and _____ is key to strong bones that resist fractures.
   a. C, calcium
   b. D, sodium
   c. D, calcium
   d. B, iron

10. The use of teriparatide, a genetically engineered form of human parathyroid hormone and the only drug currently available in this category, is limited because of risks for _____.
    a. fractures
    b. osteosarcoma
    c. pituitary tumors
    d. all of the above

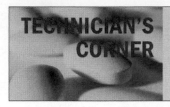

TECHNICIAN'S CORNER

1. Mild weight-bearing exercise along with a diet rich in vitamin D and calcium is key to strong bones that resist fractures. Come up with a 10-day plan of meals and exercises for a client who is menopausal and overweight.
2. Why are lifestyle changes that reduce alcohol consumption and smoking so important to prevent osteoporosis or Paget's disease?

BIBLIOGRAPHY

Alibhai S, Rahman S, Warde P, Jewett M, Jaffer T, Cheung A: Prevention and management of osteoporosis in men receiving androgen deprivation therapy: a survey of urologists and radiation oncologists, *Urology,* 68:126-131, 2006.

Cranney A, Papaioannou A, Zytaruk N, Hanley D, Adachi J, Goltzman D, Murray T, Hodsman A, for the Clinical Guidelines Committee of Osteoporosis Canada: Parathyroid hormone for the treatment of osteoporosis: a systematic review, *CMAJ,* 175:52-59, 2006.

Gold D, Alexander I, Ettinger M: How can osteoporosis patients benefit more from their therapy? Adherence issues with bisphosphonate therapy, *Ann Pharmacother,* 40:1143-1150, 2006.

Kalant H, Grant D, Mitchell J: *Principles of medical pharmacology* (pp 860-861, 878-889), ed 7, Toronto, 2007, Elsevier Canada, A Division of Reed Elsevier Canada.

Lance L, Lacy C, Armstrong L, Goldman M: *Drug information handbook for the allied health professional,* ed 12. Hudson, OH, 2005, APhA Lexi-Comp.

Langston A, Ralston S: Management of Paget's disease of bone, *Rheumatology,* 43:955-959, 2004.

Mauck K, Clarke B: Diagnosis, screening, prevention, and treatment of osteoporosis, *Mayo Clin Proc,* 81:662-672, 2006.

Newman E, Matzko C, Olenginski T, Perruquet J, Harrington T, Maloney-Saxon G, Culp T, Wood G: Glucocorticoid-Induced Osteoporosis Program (GIOP): a novel, comprehensive, and highly successful care program with improved outcomes at 1 year, *Osteoporos Int,* 17:1428–1434, 2006.

Reid I, Miller P, Lyles K, et al. Comparison of a single infusion of zoledronic acid with risedronate for Paget's disease, *N Engl J Med,* 353;898-908, 2005.

U.S. Department of Health and Human Services: *The 2004 Surgeon General's Report on bone health and osteoporosis: what it means to you.* Washington, DC, 2004, U.S. Department of Health and Human Services, Office of the Surgeon General.

Walsh J: Paget's disease of bone: clinical update, *MJA,* 181:262-265, 2004.

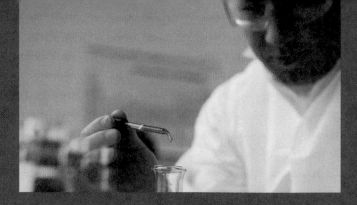

Treatment of Hyperuricemia and Gout

LEARNING OBJECTIVES

- List medical conditions that are associated with hyperuricemia.
- Describe the signs and symptoms of gout.
- List and classify medications used in the treatment of hyperuricemia and gout.
- Describe the mechanism of action for each class of drugs used in the treatment of hyperuricemia and gout.
- Identify warning labels and precautionary messages associated with medications used in the treatment of hyperuricemia and gout.
- Identify significant drug look-alike/sound-alike issues.
- Learn the terminology associated with drugs used in the treatment of hyperuricemia and gout.

KEY TERMS

Gout: Disease associated with deposits of urate crystals in the joints that produces inflammation and is caused by hyperuricemia.

Hyperuricemia: Condition in which urate levels build up in the blood serum.

Urates: Product of purine metabolism that produces inflammation when crystals accumulate in joints.

Uricosuric: Drug that increases the renal clearance of urates.

Overview

Hyperuricemia is a condition in which urate levels build up in the blood serum. *Urates* are the product of the metabolism of the amino acid purine. Between 5% and 8% of men in the United States have asymptomatic hyperuricemia (serum urate in excess of 6.8 mg/dl). Population studies show that the rate of hyperuricemia in men is greater than in women until menopause, when the rates equalize. Before puberty, boys and girls both have low serum urate levels.

Medical Conditions Associated with Hyperuricemia

Hyperuricemia is associated with several medical conditions. *Gout* is the primary disease associated with hyperuricemia, but it is not the only medical condition associated with increased serum urates. Hyperuricemia is associated with cardiovascular disease, chronic kidney disease, hyperlipidemia, insulin resistance, and obesity. Pain is the most common symptom associated with increased serum urate levels.

Up to 12% of persons with hypertension have gout, and between 20% to 40% of people with untreated hypertension have hyperuricemia. It is likely that relationship between hypertension and hyperuricemia is due to decreased renal clearance associated with hypertension. Decreased clearance causes urate to accumulate. Resistance to the flow of blood through vessels, peripheral resistance, and renal vascular resistance is increased in hypertension and gout. Hyperuricemia can cause kidney disease and make preexisting kidney disease worse.

Hyperuricemia has been shown to increase the risk of coronary heart disease and stroke, partly because of its role in producing hyperlipidemia. Hyperlipidemia causes atherosclerosis, a buildup of lipids in arteries that results in arterial occlusion. Patients with congestive heart failure do worse if they have hyperuricemia.

The relationship between hyperuricemia, obesity, and insulin resistance is interesting. Serum urate levels tend to be elevated in obesity due to increased production of urates accompanied by decreased renal clearance. Hyperuricemia is a risk factor for diabetes, and obesity is associated with increased insulin resistance. Weight loss reduces hyperuricemia and insulin resistance.

PATHOPHYSIOLOGY OF GOUT

Gout affects about 1% of the population and is more common in men than in women. In fact, gout is rare in premenopausal women. Gout or gouty arthritis accounts for 5% of all arthritis and is the disease most commonly associated with hyperuricemia. The disease is caused when urate crystals are deposited in joints where they produce inflammation. Deposits of uric acid are called tophi (singular: tophus) and look like lumps under the skin around the joints and at the rim of the ear (Figure 17-1).

The joints most commonly affected are the big toe, foot, ankle, knee, wrist, finger, and elbow. Obesity increases risk for the disease. Beer consumption also increases risks of an

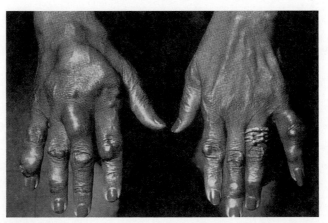

FIGURE 17-1 Gouty arthritis. *(Courtesy Lanny L. Johnson, MD, East Lansing, MI. From Thibodeau GA, Patton KT: Anatomy and physiology, ed 6, St Louis, 2007, Mosby.)*

acute attack, perhaps because beer contains high levels of purine. Exposure to lead in the environment can also increase the risk for development of gout.

Some people with gout will experience sharp needle-like painful symptoms, while some people will have no symptoms at all. Acute gout attacks will resolve spontaneously in 7 to 10 days without treatment; however, people with symptoms may benefit from treatment. Chronic gout develops over a period of years and may cause permanent joint or kidney damage. Treatment is recommended when patients have symptoms, are being treated for malignancy, or are at risk for development of kidney stones.

DRUGS USED TO TREAT GOUT

Drugs prescribed for the treatment of gout include analgesics, antiinflammatories, uricosurics, and inhibitors of uric acid synthesis. A *uricosuric* is a drug the increases the renal clearance of urates.

ANALGESICS AND ANTIINFLAMMATORY DRUGS

The principal antiinflammatories and analgesics used for the treatment of acute gout are NSAIDs, corticosteroids and colchicine. Colchicine is one of the oldest agents use to treat gout but it is most commonly used today when NSAIDs and corticosteroids do not control symptoms. Colchicine may be used in chronic gout to prevent symptoms. Colchicine penetrates inflammatory cells and inhibits their ability to respond normally to the site of irritation. It inhibits histamine release and blocks cell division. Common adverse reactions associated with the use of colchicine include nausea, vomiting, and diarrhea. Other adverse reactions are alopecia, bone marrow suppression, renal failure, intravascular coagulation, and death.

Antiinflammatories Used in the Treatment of Gout

Generic name	U.S. brand name(s) / Canadian brand(s)	Dosage forms and strengths
colchicine*	Generics	Injection, solution: 0.5 mg/ml
	Generics	Tablet: 0.6 mg
NSAIDs, COX-2 inhibitors (see Chapters 10 and 15)		
indomethacin	Indocin	
sulindac	Clinoril	
etodolac	Lodine, Lodine XL	
flurbiprofen	Ansaid	
ibuprofen	Motrin	
ketoprofen	Orudis, Oruvail (extended release)	
oxaprozin	Daypro	
naproxen	Naproxen, Naproxen DS	
naproxen Na$^+$	Anaprox, Anaprox DS	
nabumetone	Relafen	
meclofenamate	Meclomen (Canada)	
tolmetin	Tolectin	
ketorolac	Toradol	
diclofenac	Voltaren, Voltaren XR	
	Voltaren Rapide (Canada)	

Antiinflammatories Used in the Treatment of Gout—cont'd

Generic name	U.S. brand name(s) Canadian brand(s)	Dosage forms and strengths
meloxicam	Mobic	
piroxicam	Feldene	
celecoxib	Celebrex	
Glucocorticosteroids (see Chapter 15)		
dexamethasone*	Decadron, Dexamethasone Intensol, DexPak, TaperPak, Dexasone (Canada)	
hydrocortisone*	A-Hydrocort (US), Hydrocortone Phosphate (US), Cortef, Solu-Cortef	
methylprednisolone*	A-Methapred, Depo-Medrol, Medrol, Medrol Dosepak, Solu-Medrol	
prednisone*	Deltasone, Prednisone Intensol, Sterapred, Sterapred DS, Winpred (Canada)	

*Generic available.

Nonsteroidal anti-inflammatory drugs (NSAID) and glucocorticosteroids are used in the treatment of gout. The most commonly prescribed NSAID is indomethacin; however, diclofenac, ketoprofen, tolmetin, and naproxen are also administered. The COX-2 inhibitor celecoxib may be prescribed for the treatment of acute gout. Oral prednisone and intraarticular injections of corticosteroids may sometimes be given when only one or two joints are involved. NSAIDs and glucocorticosteroids are discussed in depth in Chapters 10 and 15.

URICOSURICS

Uricosurics are drugs that increase the clearance of uric acid. Probenicid is a uricosuric used in the treatment of gout. It inhibits the reabsorption of uric acid in the renal tubules and thereby promotes the elimination of urates. Nausea, vomiting, and worsening of preexisting kidney stones are adverse reactions to probenicid.

Uricosurics Used in the Treatment of Gout

Generic name	U.S. brand name(s) Canadian brand(s)	Dosage forms and strengths
probenecid*	Generics	**Tablet:** 500 mg
	Benuryl	
Combination		
probenecid + colchine*	Generics	**Tablet:** 500 mg probenecid + 0.5 mg colchine
	Not available	

*Generic available.

INHIBITORS OF URIC ACID SYNTHESIS

Xanthine oxidase inhibitors block the final enzymatic step in the synthesis of uric acid. Urate lowering drugs are indicated for patients that experience frequent attacks of gout. Allopurinol is a xanthine oxidase inhibitor and is effective in reducing hyperuricemia produced by gout, secondary to malignancy or drug induced. Thiazide diuretics (such as hydrochlorothiazide) and aspirin are known to increase urate levels. Allopurinol is readily absorbed when administered orally and is easily eliminated in the urine. Nausea, drowsiness, headache, diarrhea, and itchy skin rash are adverse reactions linked to allopurinol use.

Inhibitors of Uric Acid Synthesis

	Generic name	U.S. brand name(s)	Dosage forms and strengths
		Canadian brand(s)	
	allopurinol*	Aloprim, Zyloprim	**Injection, powder for reconstitution (Aloprim):** 500 mg
		Zyloprim	**Tablet (Zyloprim):** 100 mg, 300 mg

*Generic available.

Usual Dosage and Warnings for Drugs Used in the Treatment of Gout

	Generic name	U.S. brand name	Usual adult oral dose and dosing schedule	Warning labels
	Antiinflammatories			
	colchine	Generics	**Oral, prevention:** Begin 0.6 mg twice a day; decrease to 0.6 mg every other day or 3 times a week. **Oral, acute attack:** 0.6 mg to 1.2 mg every 1 to 2 hours until relief or 3 doses. Wait 3 days before retreatment. **IV, acute attack:** Begin 1 mg to 2 mg, decrease to 0.5 mg every 6 hours until relief (maximum 4 mg). Wait 7 days before another treatment with any dosage form of colchicine	AVOID ALCOHOL TAKE WITH LOTS OF WATER
	Uricosurics			
	probenecid	Generics	250 mg twice a day for 1 week; increase as frequently as 250 mg to 500 mg/day up to maximum 2 to 3 g/day if needed	TAKE WITH FOOD TAKE WITH LOTS OF WATER AVOID ASPIRIN
	Inhibitors of uric acid synthesis			
	allopurinol	Zyloprim	**Gout:** 200 mg to 600 mg/day orally. Start with 100 mg/day and increase weekly **Hyperuricemia:** 600 mg to 800 mg/day orally in 2 to 3 divided doses for 2 to 3 days before starting chemotherapy. **IV:** 200 mg to 400 mg/m^2/day as single IV infusion or divided at 6-, 8-, or 12-hour intervals	TAKE WITH FOOD AVOID ALCOHOL MAY CAUSE DIZZINESS OR DROWSINESS TAKE WITH LOTS OF WATER (10-12 GLASSES/DAY)

NONPHARMACOLOGICAL THERAPY

A diet low in purine has been recommended to prevent gout attacks (Box 17-1). Foods high in the amino acid purine are meat (especially liver), fish (anchovies), dried beans and peas, and gravies. Beer and spirits are also known to increase purine levels. Low-fat dairy products have low purine levels. Prevention tips include weight loss, decrease meat consumption, drink skim milk daily, and reduce alcohol consumption (especially beer).

BOX 17-1 PURINE CONTENT OF FOODS

Foods considered high in purine content include
- Alcoholic beverages
- Fish, seafood, and shellfish, including anchovies, sardines, herring, mussels, codfish, scallops, trout, and haddock
- Meats, such as bacon, turkey, veal, and venison, and organ meats like liver and sweetbreads

Foods considered moderate in purine content include
- Meats such as beef, chicken, duck, pork, and ham
- Crab, lobster, oysters, and shrimp

- Vegetables and beans such as asparagus, cauliflower, kidney beans, lentils, lima beans, peas, mushrooms, and spinach
- Grains: oatmeal, whole wheat bread, and cereal

Foods considered low in purine content include:
- Dairy products: Skim milk and cheese
- Eggs
- Fruit and most vegetables (except those listed above)
- Grains: enriched bread and cereal
- Butter or margarine

CHAPTER SUMMARY

- Hyperuricemia is a condition in which urate levels build up in the blood serum.
- Hyperuricemia is more common in men than in women. It is rare in children before puberty or in women before menopause.
- Gout is the primary disease associated with hyperuricemia.
- Gout affects about 1% of the population and is more common in men than in women.
- Hyperuricemia is also associated with cardiovascular disease, chronic kidney disease, hyperlipidemia, insulin resistance, and obesity.
- Acute gout attacks will resolve spontaneously in 7 to 10 days without treatment.
- In gout, urate crystals are deposited in joints, where they produce inflammation.
- The joints most commonly affected by gout are the big toe, foot, ankle, knee, wrist, finger, and elbow.
- Drugs prescribed for the treatment of gout include analgesics, antiinflammatories, uricosurics, and inhibitors of uric acid synthesis.
- A uricosuric is a drug the increases the renal clearance of urate.
- NSAIDS and glucocorticosteroids are used to reduce pain and inflammation in gout.
- Colchicine is the oldest drug used for the treatment of acute gouty arthritis pain.
- Probenicid is a uricosuric used in the treatment of gout.
- Allopurinol, a xanthine oxidase inhibitor, blocks the final enzymatic step in the synthesis of uric acid.
- Diets low in purine have been recommended to prevent gout attacks. Meat, fish, beer, and spirits are known to increase purine levels.
- Beer consumption also increases risks of an acute attack, perhaps because beer contains high levels of purine.

REVIEW QUESTIONS

Multiple Choice

1. _____ is the most common symptom associated with increased serum urate levels.
   a. Pain
   b. Bladder infection
   c. Nausea
   d. Vomiting

2. _____ is the primary disease associated with hyperuricemia.
   a. Arthritis
   b. Gout
   c. Osteoporosis
   d. Kidney stones

3. There is a relationship between hypertension and hyperuricemia.
   a. true
   b. false

4. Weight loss has no effect on hyperuricemia and insulin resistance.
   a. true
   b. false

5. Drugs prescribed for the treatment of gout include _____.
   a. analgesics
   b. antiinflammatories
   c. uricosurics and inhibitors of uric acid synthesis
   d. all of the above

6. The most commonly prescribed NSAID for gout is _____.
   a. indomethacin
   b. diclofenac
   c. ketoprofen
   d. tolmetin

7. The oldest drug used in the treatment of gout is _____.
   a. naproxen
   b. allupurinol
   c. colchicine
   d. ketoprofen

8. Diets _____ in purine have been recommended to prevent gout attacks.
   a. high
   b. low

9. The brand name for allopurinol is _____.
   a. Zyban
   b. Zomig
   c. Zyloprim
   d. Zyrtec

10. A uricosuric is a drug the decreases the renal clearance of urates.
    a. true
    b. false

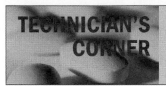

TECHNICIAN'S CORNER	1. Beer consumption increases risks of an acute gout attack, perhaps because beer contains high levels of purine. Will nonalcoholic beer have the same effect? 2. Diets that are low in purine have been recommended to prevent gout attacks. What would you recommend patients with gout eat as part of their diet?

BIBLIOGRAPHY

Becker M, Jolly M: Hyperuricemia and associated diseases, *Rheum Dis Clin North Am,* 32:275-293, 2006.

Kalant H, Grant D, Mitchell J: *Principles of medical pharmacology* (p 381), ed 7, Toronto, 2007, Elsevier Canada, A Division of Reed Elsevier Canada.

Lance L, Lacy C, Armstrong L, Goldman M: *Drug information handbook for the allied health professional,* ed 12. Hudson, OH, 2005, APhA Lexi-Comp.

National Institute of Arthritis and Musculoskeletal and Skin Diseases: *Questions and answers about gout,* Bethesda, MD, 2002, NIAMS, National Institutes of Health, US Department of Health and Human Services. NIH publication No. 02-5027. Retrieved at www.niams.nih.gov/hi/topics/gout/gout.htm.

Page C, Curtis M, Sutter M, Walker M, Hoffman B: *Integrated pharmacology* (pp 450-451), Philadelphia, 2005, Mosby.

Underwood M: Diagnosis and management of gout, *BMJ,* 332:1315-1319, 2006.

USP Center for Advancement of Patient Safety: *Use caution–avoid confusion,* USP Quality Review No. 79, Rockville, MD, April 2004, USP Center for Advancement of Patient Safety.

Treatment of Diseases of the Ophthalmic and Otic Systems

- Learn the basic anatomy and physiology of the eye and ear.
- Differentiate between the different parts of the eye and the ear.
- Understand the function of the accessory structures of the eye.
- Describe the process of seeing and the process of hearing.
- Differentiate between the process of hearing and the sense of balance.

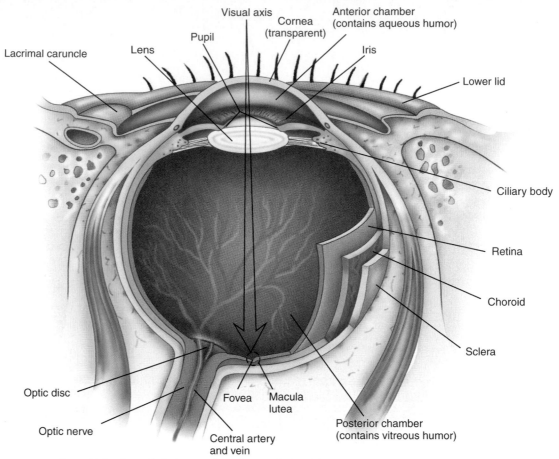

(From Thibodeau G, Patton K: Anatomy and physiology, *ed 6, St. Louis, 2007, Mosby.)*

Overview of Anatomy and Physiology of the Eye

One of the most important sensations involved in maintaining homeostasis is vision. Vision allows us to activate and respond to a multitude of warning systems and provides us with almost constant feedback in an ever-changing environment.

STRUCTURE OF THE EYE

The eye is divided into different parts and layers. Three layers of tissue compose the eyeball: the ***fibrous layer***—sclera and cornea; the ***vascular layer***—the choroids, ciliary body, and iris; and the ***inner layer***—retina, optic nerve, and retinal blood vessels.

The fibrous layer or the anterior portion of the sclera is called the ***cornea*** and lies over the colored portion of the eye, the **iris**. The cornea is transparent, but the rest of the ***sclera*** is white and opaque and is known as the "white" of the eye. No blood vessels are found in the cornea or in the lens.

The vascular layer of the eye is characterized by many blood vessels and a large amount of pigment and contains the ciliary body, pupil, and retina. The ***ciliary body*** is composed of ciliary muscles and ciliary processes and functions to hold and suspend the lens in place; the iris, or colored portion of the eye, has an opening in the middle called the ***pupil*** that controls the amount of light entering the eye by adjusting its size. The inner layer contains the ***retina***, the innermost coat of the eyeball, which is made up of three layers of neurons that constitute our visual receptors. One type of receptor contains rods and cones. ***Rods*** function best for night vision and ***cones*** help to see color. The ***optic disc,*** or blind spot, contains no rods or cones and is located at the posterior end of the eyeball.

CAVITIES AND HUMORS

The eyeball is also divided into two cavities: the anterior and posterior cavities. The anterior cavity lies at the front of the lens and is filled with a clear watery liquid called *aqueous humor*. The posterior cavity lies at the back of the lens and contains a soft gelatin-like material called the *vitreous humor*. Both the aqueous and vitreous humors help to maintain the intraocular pressure of the eye to keep it from collapsing.

MUSCLES

There are two types of eye muscles: extrinsic and intrinsic. The *extrinsic eye muscles* are skeletal and voluntary muscles that move the eyeball in any desired direction. Four of them are straight (superior, inferior, medial, and lateral rectus) and two of them are oblique (superior and inferior). *Intrinsic eye muscles* are smooth muscles located within the eye that control involuntary movement. The iris and ciliary muscles are intrinsic eye muscles. The iris regulates the size of the pupil and the ciliary controls the shape of the lens.

ACCESSORY STRUCTURES

Accessory structures of the eye include the eyebrows, eyelashes, eyelids, and lacrimal apparatus. The eyebrows and eyelashes give some protection against the entrance of foreign objects into the eye and help to shade the eye and provide at least minimal protection from direct light. The eyelids consist mainly of voluntary muscles and skin, with a border of thick connective tissue. A mucous membrane called the *conjunctiva* lines each lid and continues over the surface of the eyeball where it is transparent. The *lacrimal apparatus* secretes tears and drains them from the surface of the eyeball and consists of the lacrimal glands, lacrimal ducts, lacrimal sacs, and nasolacrimal ducts. *Tear deficiency*, also known as dry eyes, is a common disorder and is associated with aging, environmental conditions, and disease (e.g., rheumatoid arthritis). It causes eye irritation, blurred vision, redness, excessive tearing, and a "gritty" feeling in the eye. Dry eyes can be treated with nonprescription drugs.

TECH NOTE!
Pharmacy technicians are susceptible to "dry eyes" while performing sterile preparation of IV products in the Laminar Flow Hood. Application of eye products such as Fresh Tears, Lacrilube, or other istonic solutions can help to prevent discomfort caused by the constant flow of air from the hood.

THE PROCESS OF SEEING

For vision to occur, an image must be formed on the retina and nerve impulses must be conducted to the visual areas of the cerebral cortex for interpretation. Formation of retinal image involves four processes that focus light rays so that they form a clear image on the retina:

- **Refraction:** (deflection) or bending of light rays through the cornea, aqueous humor, lens, and vitreous humor. Nearsightedness (*myopia*), farsightedness (*hyperopia*), and *astigmatism* are errors of refraction.
- **Accommodation of the lens:** The ability of the lens to contract and relax to adjust for vision to see things from a distance of close up. For near vision, the ciliary muscle is contracted and the lens is bulging; for far vision, the ciliary muscle is relaxed and the lens is comparatively flat. As people grow older, they tend to become farsighted (*presbyopia*) because lenses lose their elasticity and therefore their ability to bulge and accommodate for near vision.
- **Constriction of the pupil:** Muscles of the iris play an important part in the formation of clear retinal images. Constriction of the pupil occurs simultaneously with accommodation of the lens for near vision. The pupil also constricts in bright light to protect the retina from stimulation that is too intense or too sudden, and convergence of the eye, single binocular vision, occurs when light rays from an object fall on the corresponding points of the two retinas.
- **Convergence:** The movement of the two eyeballs inward so that the visual axes come together at the object viewed.

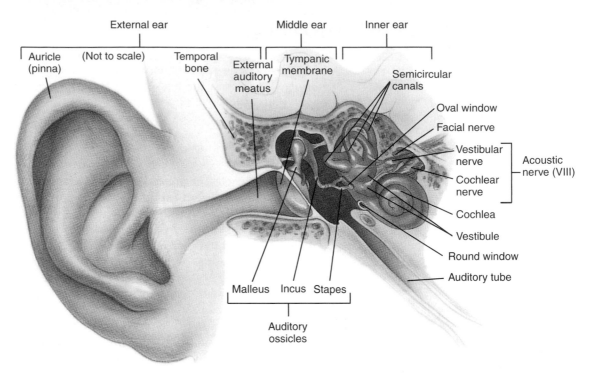

(From Thibodeau G, Patton K: Anatomy and physiology, *ed 6, St. Louis, 2007, Mosby.)*

Overview of the Anatomy and Physiology of the Ear

The ear is divided into three anatomical parts: external ear, middle ear, and inner ear.

The ear has dual sensory functions: **hearing** and balance or **equilibrium**. The stimulation or "trigger" for hearing and balance is the activation of hair cells, receptors that transmit nerve impulses and are perceived in the brain as sound or balance.

EXTERNAL EAR

The external ear or outer ear has two divisions: the auricle or pinna and the **external auditory *meatus*** (ear canal). The auricle is the visible appendage on the side of the head and surrounding the opening of the external auditory meatus. The external auditory meatus travels into the temporal bone ending at the ***tympanic membrane*** or eardrum that stretches across the inner end of the canal, separating it from the middle ear. ***Cerumen***, a wax-like substance is secreted by modified sweat glands in the auditory canal.

MIDDLE EAR

The middle ear (tympanic cavity), a tiny epithelia-lined cavity hollowed out of the temporal bone, contains the three auditory ossicles: the ***malleus*** (hammer), ***incus*** (anvil), and ***stapes*** (stirrup). The "handle" of the malleus is attached to the surface of the tympanic membrane, and the "head" is attached to the incus, which in turn attaches to the stapes. There are two openings into the inner ear: the oval window into which the stapes fit and the round window, which is covered by a membrane, and one into the auditory (eustachian) tube. The ***eustachian tube*** is composed partly of bone, cartilage, and fibrous tissue and lined with mucus. It extends from the middle ear into the ***nasopharynx*** and functions to equalize pressure between the inner and outer surfaces of the tympanic membrane.

INNER EAR

The inner ear, or ***labyrinth,*** consists of two main parts: the bony labyrinth and a membranous labyrinth. The bony labyrinth consists of the **vestibule, cochlea**, and the **semicircular canals**. The membranous labyrinth consists of the **utricle** and **saccule** inside the vestibule, the cochlear duct inside the cochlea, and the membranous semicircular canals inside the bony ones. The vestibule and the semicircular canals are involved in balance; the cochlea is involved in hearing. The membranous labyrinth is filled with a clear fluid called **endolymph** and is surrounded by another fluid called the **perilymph.**

COCHLEA AND COCHLEAR DUCT

The word *cochlea* means "snail," and inside the cochlea is the membranous cochlear duct—the only part of the inner ear concerned with hearing. The hearing sense organ named the ***organ of Corti*** contains sensory neurons that extend to form the cochlear nerve that conduct impulses to the brain and produce the sensation of hearing. Hearing results from the stimulation of the auditory area of the cerebral cortex.

HEARING IMPAIRMENT

Hearing problems can be divided into two basic categories: conduction impairment and nerve impairment. ***Conduction impairment*** refers to the blocking of airwaves as they are conducted through the external and middle ear to the sensory receptors of the inner ear. Causes of conduction impairment are waxy buildup of cerumen, foreign objects in external auditory meatus, tumors, and other matter. ***Nerve impairment*** may be inherited or acquired and results in insensitivity to sound. ***Presbycusis***, common in the elderly, causes degeneration of nerve tissue in the ear and vestibular nerve. Chronic exposure to loud noise damages receptors in the organ of Corti.

BIBLIOGRAPHY

Chabner E: *The language of medicine,* ed 8, St. Louis, 2007, Saunders.
Patton K: *Survival guide for anatomy and physiology,* St. Louis, 2006, Mosby.
Thibodeau G, Patton K: *Anatomy and physiology,* ed 6, St. Louis, 2007, Mosby.

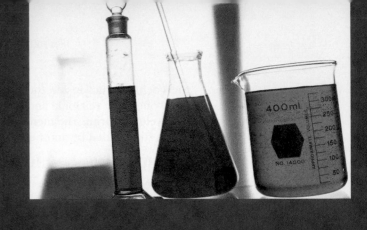

Treatment of Glaucoma

LEARNING OBJECTIVES

- Learn the terminology associated with the eye.
- List and categorize medications used in the treatment of glaucoma.
- Describe mechanism of action for each class of drugs used in the treatment of glaucoma.
- Identify warning labels and precautionary messages associated with medications used in the treatment of glaucoma.
- Identify significant drug look-alike/sound-alike issues.
- Learn the terminology associated with the treatment of glaucoma.

KEY TERMS

Aqueous humor: Fluid made in the front part of the eye.

Central vision: What is seen when you look straight ahead or when you read.

Conjunctiva: Transparent mucous membrane that lines each lid and continues over the surface of the eyeball.

Cornea: Clear part of the eye located in front of the iris.

Glaucoma, angle closure: Sudden increase in intraocular pressure caused by obstruction of the drainage portal between the cornea and iris (angle) that can rapidly progress to blindness.

Glaucoma, open angle: Disorder characterized by elevated pressure in the eye that can lead to permanent blindness.

Intraocular pressure (IOP): Inner pressure of the eye. Normal intraocular pressure usually ranges from 12 to 22 mm Hg.

Iris: Colored part of the eye that can expand or contract to allow the right amount of light to enter the eye.

Keratotomy: Incision of the cornea to correct myopia.

Lacrimal apparatus: Structures that keep the surface of the eye moistened with lacrimal fluid (tears).

Optic disk: Ocular end of the optic nerve where the retinal nerve fibers from the eye exit and the blood vessels enter the eye.

Optic nerve: Bundle of nerve fibers located in the back of the eye that connects the retina to the brain.

Peripheral vision: Sometimes called "side vision," this is usually the first area of vision to be lost with glaucoma.

Tonometry: Use of a device to measure the pressure in the eye.

Trabecular meshwork: Small openings around the outer edge of the iris that form meshlike drainage canals surrounding the iris and sometimes referred to as Schlemm's canal.

Glaucoma

Approximately 2.2 million Americans were diagnosed with glaucoma in 2004. According to the 2002-2003 National Population Health and Community Health Survey in Canada, approximately 409,000 Canadians over the age of 20 years had glaucoma. The global prevalence of glaucoma is predicted to be greater than 60.5 million people by the year 2010, according to World Health Organization estimates, United Nations world population data, and reviews of published data. This number is expected to increase to 79.6 million by 2020. Advancing age and diabetes increase the risk for glaucoma. The prevalence of glaucoma in the United States in 2002 rose from 1.9% for persons between the age of 50 to 64 years and without diabetes to 7% by the age of 65 years. This trend was true for Canada, where the prevalence of glaucoma among persons over 40 years increased from 2.7% to 3.9% by the age of 50 years.

Nearly one-sixth of the population with glaucoma will develop bilateral blindness (4.5 million persons with open angle glaucoma and 3.9 million persons with angle closure glaucoma). This makes glaucoma the second leading cause of blindness worldwide.

PATHOPHYSIOLOGY

There are actually several types of glaucoma; and all are associated with progressive damage to the structures in the eye responsible for vision. *Peripheral vision* is first to be lost. The person gradually loses the ability to see images from the sides, top, or bottom of the eye(s). Eventually, only central vision remains (Figure 18-1).

Open angle glaucoma is the most common and results from abnormal accumulation of *aqueous humor* (Figure 18-2). This in turn causes excessive *intraocular pressure (IOP)* and causes degeneration of the optic nerve. Sometimes, damage to the optic nerve can occur in the absence of increased IOP. When this happens, low tension or normal tension glaucoma is said to be the cause. The unit of measure for intraocular pressure is mm Hg, or millimeters of mercury.

IOP rises rapidly to dangerously high levels when a person has narrow angle or *angle closure glaucoma*. Normally, aqueous fluids drain from the eye through an opening in the eye where the cornea and iris meet. This region is called the *angle* (see Figure 18-2). When the angle becomes obstructed as occurs with inflammation or partial blockage of *trabecular meshwork*, aqueous humor drainage is impaired and there is a sudden increase in eye pressure. Pain and nausea may occur. If untreated, blindness can result in a little as a few days. Children born with defects in the structure of the angle of the eye may develop congenital glaucoma. Children with congenital glaucoma often have cloudy eyes, light sensitivity, and excessive tearing. If treated promptly, impaired vision may be avoided. Neovascular glaucoma is associated with diabetes, which is discussed in Chapter 33.

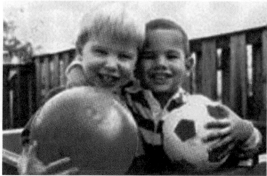
Normal vision

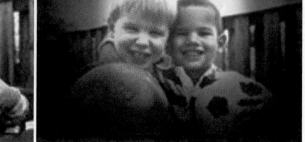
Glaucoma

FIGURE 18-1 Glaucoma. *(Courtesy of U.S. National Institutes of Health National Eye Institute.)*

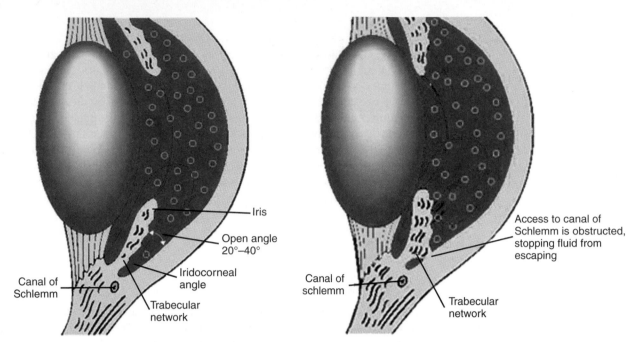

FIGURE 18-2 A, Aqueous humor: flow. **B,** Aqueous humor: obstruction. *(From Clayton BD, Stock YN, Harroun RD:* Basic pharmacology for nurses, *ed 14, St Louis, 2007, Mosby.)*

DIAGNOSIS

Tonometry is a diagnostic test that is performed to measure IOP. There are two types of devices used to perform tonometry. A tonometer may be placed on the cornea, and gentle pressure is applied, after numbing drops and a stain have been applied to the eye. Another type of tonometry device releases a puff of air into the eye.

TREATMENT

Drugs used in the treatment of glaucoma can be divided into two main classifications according to their method of action. They may lower IOP by decreasing the formation of fluids that build up in the eye, or they may promote drainage of fluids that accumulate. This is accomplished by actions on parasympathetic or sympathetic nerves that control secretion of fluids and contraction of muscles the block fluid drainage.

DRUGS THAT DECREASE AQUEOUS HUMOR FORMATION

β-Adrenergic Antagonists

TECH NOTE!
"-olol" is a common ending for β-adrenergic antagonists (also known as β-blockers).

β-Adrenergic antagonists are the classification of most drugs commonly used for the treatment of open angle glaucoma. They are also administered for the treatment on intraocular hypertension. Stimulation of β-adrenergic receptors on ciliary cells increases secretion of aqueous humor. β-Adrenergic antagonists decrease aqueous humor formation by inhibiting the action of epinephrine and norepinephrine on β-adrenergic receptors located on the muscle and on blood vessels within the ciliary body. β-Adrenergic antagonists vary in potency, with betaxolol being the least potent and levobunolol being the most potent. Betaxolol, however, is the only β-adrenergic antagonist that is selective for β_1-receptor sites. This means that betaxolol may be safer for use in patients who have asthma, congestive heart failure, or other conditions where blockade of β_2-receptor sites is undesirable. Adverse reactions produced by betaxolol are blurred vision, light sensitivity (photophobia), dizziness, and nausea. Local adverse reactions of carteolol, levobunolol, and timolol include burning, pain, and itching in addition to blurred vision. Systemic effects are less common and include dizziness, weakness, depression, hypotension, decreased heart rate, and difficulty breathing.

β-Adrenergic Antagonists

Generic name	U.S. brand name(s) Canadian brand (s)	Dosage forms and strengths
betaxolol*	Betoptic S	**Suspension, ophthalmic:** 0.25%
	Betoptic S	**Tablet:** 10 mg, 20 mg
carteolol*	Generics	**Solution, ophthalmic:** 1%
	Not available	
levobunolol*	Betagan	**Solution, ophthalmic:** 0.25%, 0.5%
	Betagan	
timolol hemihydrate*	Betimol	**Solution, ophthalmic:** 0.25%, 0.5%
	Not available	
timolol maleate*	Isatol, Timoptic, Timoptic OcuDose, Timoptic Ocumeter, Timoptic XE	**Solution, gel forming (Timoptic XE):** 0.25%, 0.5%
	Timoptic, Timoptic XE	**Solution, ophthalmic (Timoptic, Istalol):** 0.25%, 0.5% **Solution, preservative free (Timoptic OcuDose):** 0.25%, 0.5%
Combinations		
timolol + lantanoprost	Xalcom	**Solution, ophthalmic:** 0.5% timolol + 0.005% latanoprost
	Xalcom	

*Generic available.

α-Adrenergic Agonists

α-Adrenergic receptor agonists are used for the prevention and treatment of IOP. There are two α-adrenergic receptors in the eye (α_1 and α_2). Administration of α_1-adrenergic receptor agonists reduces blood flow in the ciliary body, and administration of α_2-adrenergic receptor agonists reduces the formation of aqueous humor. Administration of α_2-adrenergic agonists produces effects similar to administration of β-adrenergic antagonists. Adverse reactions produced by apraclonidine and brimonidine may be systemic as well as local. Local reactions include blurred vision, decreased night and distance vision, dry eyes, and irritated eyelids. Systemic effects are drowsiness and headache.

α-Adrenergic Agonists

Generic name	U.S. brand name(s) Canadian brand(s)	Dosage forms and strength
apraclonidine	Iopidine	**Solution, ophthalmic:** 0.5%, 1%
	Iopidine	
brimonidine*	Alphagan P	**Solution, ophthalmic:** 0.15%, 0.1%, 0.2%
	Alphagan	

*Generic available.

TECH NOTE!
Generic brimonidine 0.2% is *NOT* substitutable for Alphagan P which is currently only available in 0.1% and 0.15% strengths.

TECH NOTE!
"-zolamide" is a common ending for carbonic anhydrase inhibitors.

Carbonic Anhydrase Inhibitors

Carbonic anhydrase inhibitors are indicated for the treatment of open angle glaucoma. Acetazolamide and methazolamide are also indicated for prevention of secondary acute angle closure glaucoma and short-term treatment of angle closure glaucoma when surgery must be delayed. Oral and parenteral dosage forms are used for the treatment of edema and centrencephalic epilepsy and prevention of altitude sickness. Their use in the treatment of glaucoma is based on the fact that they inhibit carbonic anhydrase, an enzyme responsible for speeding up the first step in the process of the conversion of carbon dioxide and water to bicarbonate. It is found in many parts of the body, including the ciliary structures of the eye. The production of aqueous humors depends on the transport of bicarbonate and sodium ions. Administration of carbonic anhydrase inhibitors decreases the rate of production of aqueous humors, thereby decreasing intraocular pressure. Adverse effects of acetazolamide and methazolamide include dizziness, drowsiness, potassium loss, frequent urination, kidney stones, tingling sensation in fingers and toes, bitter or metallic taste, nausea, impotence, and depression. Brimzolamide and dorzolamide produce primarily local adverse effects that include blurred vision, bitter taste in the mouth, and burning or stinging, dry eyes. Less common reactions are irritation, discharge from eyes, soreness, headache, and dizziness.

Carbonic Anhydrase Inhibitors

Generic name	U.S. brand name(s) Canadian brand(s)	Dosage forms and strength
acetazolamide*	Diamox Sequels	**Capsule, sustained release (Diamox Sequels):** 500 mg **Injection, powder for reconstitution:** 500 mg **Tablet:** 125 mg, 250 mg
	Diamox	
brinzolamide	Azopt	**Suspension, ophthalmic:** 1%
	Azopt	
dorzolamide	Trusopt	**Solution, ophthalmic:** 2%
	Trusopt	
methazolamide*	Neptazane	**Tablet:** 25 mg, 50 mg
	Not available	
Carbonic anhydrase inhibitor combination		
dorzolamide and timolol	Cosopt	**Solution, ophthalmic:** 2% dorzolamine and 0.5% timolol
	Cosopt	

*Generic available.

TECH NOTE!
Carbonic anhydrase inhibitors may cause allergic reactions in people who have allergies to sulfonamide antiinfective agents.

DRUGS THAT INCREASE AQUEOUS HUMOR DRAINAGE

Miotics are drugs that are used to increase the drainage of the aqueous humor. They produce this effect via a variety of mechanisms of action. They are categorized as adrenergic agonists, cholinergic agonists, and acetylcholinesterase inhibitors. The prostaglandin analog latanoprost is also used for its ability to promote drainage of accumulated levels of aqueous humor and reduce IOP.

Adrenergic Agonists

Sympathetic nervous system and parasympathetic nervous system stimulation of the of ciliary muscles control the expansion and contraction of the iris and the size of the pupil's opening. Sympathetic nervous system stimulation dilates the pupil, and parasympathetic nervous

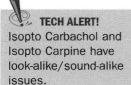

TECH ALERT!
Acetazolamide and acetohexamide have look-alike/sound-alike issues.

system stimulation makes the pupil smaller. This is important because blockage of the angle formed by the iris and the cornea impedes drainage of ocular fluids (see Figure 18-2, *B*).

Dipivefrin is an adrenergic agonist and a prodrug; this means that it is inactive until it is metabolized in the body to an active substance (see Chapter 2). Dipivefrin is metabolized to epinephrine. It has a greater bioavailabilty and a longer duration of action than epinephrine, which is rapidly metabolized by the enzyme monoamine oxidase. The mechanism of action for adrenergic agonists is to constrict blood vessels in the ciliary body and thereby decrease the rate of aqueous humor formation. Adrenergic agonists may also desensitize β-adrenergic receptors after prolonged use, explaining why their use lowers IOP rather than raises IOP. Adverse reactions are primarily local. Local effects are stinging or burning, red eye, blurred vision, twitching eyelids, watering eyes, and decreased night vision. Less common systemic effects are headache, increased blood pressure, palpitations, tremor, and anxiety.

Adrenergic Agonists

Generic name	U.S. brand name(s)	Dosage forms and strength
	Canadian brand(s)	
dipivefrin*	Propine	Solution, ophthalmic: 0.1%
	Propine	

*Generic available.

TECH ALERT!
Isopto Carbachol and Isopto Carpine have look-alike/sound-alike issues.

Cholinergic Agonists and Cholinesterase Inhibitors

Cholinergic agonists are indicated for the treatment of glaucoma, intraocular hypertension, and production of miosis during surgery. Pilocarpine can be used in the treatment of open and closed angle glaucoma. Cholinergic agonists bind to receptors sites and produce effects that mimic the neurotransmitter acetylcholine. Binding produces parasympathetic nervous system effects in the eye such as contraction of ciliary muscles resulting in contraction of the pupil (miosis). Cholinergic agonists also produce dilation of the trabecular meshwork and decreased IOP (see Figure 18-2, *B*).

Echothiophate iodide is a cholinesterase inhibitor. Cholinesterase inhibitors block the enzyme that deactivates acetylcholine (see Chapter 13). This prolongs the effects of acetylcholine and administered cholinergic agonists. Adverse reactions include blurred vision, change in near or distance vision, difficulty in seeing at night or in dim light, headache, twitching of eyelids, and watering of eyes. For preparation instructions, see Box 18-1.

Cholinergic Agonists

Generic name	U.S. brand name(s)	Dosage forms and strength
	Canadian brand(s)	
carbachol	Isopto Carbachol, Carboptic	Solution, ophthalmic (Isopto Carbachol): 1.5%, 3%
	Isopto Carbachol, Miostat	
pilocarpine*	Isopto Carpine, Pilopine HS, Piloptic, Salagen	Gel, ophthalmic (Pilopine HS): 4% Solution, ophthalmic (Isopto Carpine): 1%, 2%, 4% Solution, ophthalmic (Piloptic): 0.5%, 1%, 2%, 3%, 4%, 6% Tablet (Salagen): 5 mg, 7.5 mg
	Akarpine, Diocarpine, Isopto Carpine, Pilopine HS, Salagen	
Cholinesterase inhibitor		
echothiophate iodide	Phospholine Iodide	Powder for reconstitution: 0.125% (6.25 mg)
	Not available	

*Generic available.

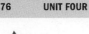

TECH NOTE!

"-*prost*" is a common ending for drugs that are prostaglandin analogs.

Prostaglandin Analogs

Latanoprost is a prostaglandin analog. It mimics the action of prostaglandin $F_{2\alpha}$ and therefore relaxes the ciliary muscle to permit drainage of aqueous humors. Lantanoprost and other prostaglandin analogs directly dilate the trabecular meshwork to promote drainage. The use of latanoprost can cause changes in the color or pigmentation of the eyes. Lantanoprost and other prostaglandin analogs may produce decreased vision, eye irritation, eye pain, itching eye, redness of eye, dry eyes, sun sensitivity, watery eyes, and permanent changes in eye pigmentation.

Proastaglandin Analogs

Generic name	U.S. brand name(s)	Dosage forms and strength
	Canadian brand(s)	
bimatoprost	Lumigan	**Solution, ophthalmic:** 0.03%
	Lumigan	
latanoprost	Xalatan	**Solution, ophthalmic:** 0.005%
	Xalatan	
travoprost	Travatan	**Solution, ophthalmic:** 0.004%
	Travatan	

*Generic available.

BOX 18-1 DIRECTIONS FOR PREPARING ECHOTHIOPATE IODIDE EYE DROPS

- Use aseptic technique.
- Tear off aluminum seals, and remove and discard rubber plugs from both drug and diluent containers.
- Pour diluent into drug container.
- Remove dropper assembly from its sterile wrapping. Holding dropper assembly by the screw cap and, WITHOUT COMPRESSING RUBBER BULB, insert into drug container and screw down tightly.
- Shake for several seconds to ensure mixing.
- Do not cover nor obliterate instructions to patient regarding storage of eye drops.

MISCELLANEOUS

The use of marijuana is controversial. Some studies have shown it can reduce intraocular pressure. Marijuana is a Schedule I (C-I) controlled substance and possession is a federal crime, despite passage of regulation authorizing medical use in some states.

Summary of Drugs Used to Treat Glaucoma

	Generic	Brand name	Usual dose	Warning labels
Decrease aqueous humor formation				
β-Adrenergic antagonists				
	betaxolol	Betoptic	**Open angle glaucoma:** Instill one drop twice a day in affected eye(s)	WASH HANDS BEFORE USE; AVOID CONTAMINATION OF TIP
	carteolol	Ocupress	**Open angle glaucoma:** Instill one drop twice a day in affected eye(s)	REMOVE CONTACT LENSES BEFORE USE; RE-INSERT AFTER 15 MINUTES
	levobunolol	Betagan	**Open angle glaucoma:** Instill one drop in affected eye(s) 1 to 2 times a day	
	timolol maleate	Timoptic, Timoptic XE	**Open angle glaucoma:** (Timoptic): Instill one drop twice daily in affected eye(s) **(Timoptic XE, Istalol):** Instill one drop daily in the morning	DON'T DISCONTINUE WITHOUT MEDICAL SUPERVISION
	timolol hemihyrate	Betimol	**Open angle glaucoma:** Instill one drop twice daily in affected eye(s)	
α-Adrenergic agonists				
	apraclonidine	Iopidine	Instill 1 to 2 drops 3 times a day	WASH HANDS BEFORE USE; AVOID CONTAMINATION OF TIP
	brimonidine	Alphagan	Instill 1 drop 3 times a day	REMOVE CONTACT LENSES BEFORE USE; RE-INSERT AFTER 15 MINUTES
				DON'T DISCONTINUE WITHOUT MEDICAL SUPERVISION
Carbonic anhydrase inhibitors				
	acetozolamide	Diamox Sequels	**Oral (sustained release):** 500 mg twice daily	TAKE WITH FOOD
		Diamox	**Oral:** 250 mg 1 to 4 times a day	SWALLOW WHOLE; DON'T CRUSH OR CHEW (sustained release capsule)
			IV: 250 mg to 500 mg may repeat in 2 to 4 hours up to a maximum of 1 g/day (acute angle closure)	MAY CAUSE DIZZINESS OR DROWSINESS
	brinzolamide	Azopt	Instill 1 drop 3 times a day	WASH HANDS BEFORE USE; AVOID CONTAMINATION OF TIP
	dorzolamide	Trusopt	Instill 1 drop 3 times a day	REMOVE CONTACT LENSES BEFORE USE; RE-INSERT AFTER 15 MINUTES
	dorzolamide and timolol	Cosopt	Instill 1 drop twice a day	DON'T DISCONTINUE WITHOUT MEDICAL SUPERVISION
	methazolamide	Formerly Neptazane	50 mg to 10 mg 2 to 3 times a day	TAKE WITH FOOD MAY CAUSE DIZZINESS OR DROWSINESS

Continued

Summary of Drugs Used to Treat Glaucoma—cont'd

	Generic	Brand name	Usual dose	Warning labels
	Increase drainage of aqueous humor			
	Adrenergic agonists			
	dipivefrin	Propine	**Open angle glaucoma:** Instill 1 drop every 12 hours	DON'T DISCONTINUE WITHOUT MEDICAL SUPERVISION
				WASH HANDS BEFORE USE; AVOID CONTAMINATION OF TIP
				DISCARD DISCOLORED SOLUTION
				REMOVE CONTACT LENSES BEFORE USE; RE-INSERT AFTER 15 MINUTES
	Cholinergic agonists			
	carbachol	Isopto Carbachol	**Glaucoma:** Instill 1 to 2 drops up to 3 times a day	WASH HANDS BEFORE USE; AVOID CONTAMINATION OF TIP
	pilocarpine	Pilocar Pilopine HS	Instill 1 to 2 drops up to 6 times a day	REFRIGERATE; DO NOT FREEZE—pilocarpine gel
			Apply 0.5 inch in lower conjunctival sac at bedtime	
	Cholinesterase inhibitor			
	echothiophate	Phospholine Iodide	Open angle glaucoma: Instill 1 drop twice a day	REFRIGERATE OR STORE RECONSTITUTED SOLUTION FOR UP TO 4 WEEKS AT ROOM TEMPERATURE
	Prostaglandin analogs			
	bimatoprost	Lumigan	Instill 1 drop once daily in the evening	WASH HANDS BEFORE USE
	latanoprost	Xalatan	Instill 1 drop once daily in the evening	REMOVE CONTACT LENSES BEFORE USE; RE-INSERT AFTER 15 MINUTES
	travoprost	Travatan	Instill 1 drop once daily in the evening	DON'T DISCONTINUE WITHOUT MEDICAL SUPERVISION
				REFRIGERATE; DO NOT FREEZE-latanoprost STORE UNOPENED BOTTLES UNDER REFRIGERATOR ONCE OPENED MAY STORE AT ROOM TEMP FOR 6 WKS
				PROTECT FROM HEAT AND LIGHT

NONDRUG TREATMENT

Laser Surgery

Laser surgery may be performed to reduce IOP. There are three forms of laser surgery for glaucoma. Laser peripheral iridotomy creates a new drainage hole in the iris, permitting fluids to drain out of the eye. Laser trabeculoplasty unblocks existing channels, and laser cyclophotocoagulation is indicated for people who have severe glaucoma and have not responded to standard glaucoma surgery. Laser cyclophotocoagulation partially destroys the tissues that make the fluid in the eye.

TECH NOTE!

To minimize systemic side effects, patients are advised to apply gentle pressure to lacrimal sac for 1 to 2 minutes following the administration of eye drops.

CHAPTER SUMMARY

- Glaucoma is the second leading cause of blindness worldwide.
- The percentage of the population who will develop glaucoma increases with advancing age.
- The prevalence of glaucoma in persons with diabetes is greater than that in persons without diabetes, yet for both groups, the prevalence increases with advancing age.
- There are actually several types of glaucoma: open angle, angle closure, and secondary glaucoma.
- The most common form is open angle glaucoma.
- Glaucoma may result in degeneration of the optic nerve.
- Increased intraocular pressure is caused by a buildup of aqueous humor and is a symptom of glauoma.
- The aqueous humor accumulates when the angle formed by the iris and the cornea is reduced and drainage of fluid is blocked.
- Drugs used in the treatment of glaucoma can be divided into two main classifications according to their method of action: drugs that decrease formation of aqueous humor and drugs that promote drainage of aqueous humor.
- Drug classifications that decrease formation of the aqueous humor are β-blockers, α-adrenergic agonists, and carbonic anhydrase inhibitors.
- Drug classifications that promote drainage of the aqueous humor are adrenergic agonists, cholinergics, cholinesterase inhibitors, and prostaglandin analogs.
- Miotics are drugs that cause contraction of the pupil. Drugs that promote drainage of the aqueous humor produce miosis.

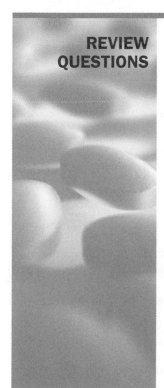

REVIEW QUESTIONS

Multiple Choice

1. Glaucoma is the leading cause of blindness worldwide.
   a. true
   b. false
2. The most common form of glaucoma is _____.
   a. open angle
   b. closed angle
   c. narrow angle
   d. wide angle
3. Drugs used in the treatment of glaucoma can be divided into two main classifications.
   a. lower intraocular pressure by decreasing the formation of fluids
   b. they may promote drainage of fluids that accumulate
   c. lower intraocular pressure by increasing the formation of fluids
   d. a and b
4. The classification of the drug(s) most commonly used for the treatment of glaucoma is _____.
   a. α-adrenergic antagonists
   b. β-adrenergic antagonists
   c. carbonic anhydrase inhibitors
   d. prostaglandins
5. "-zolamide" is a common ending for which class of drugs?
   a. α-adrenergic antagonists
   b. β-adrenergic antagonists
   c. carbonic anhydrase inhibitors
   d. prostaglandins

6. **Miotics are drugs that are used to decrease the drainage of the aqueous humor.**
   a. true
   b. false

7. **This drug is β-adrenergic antagonist indicated for the treatment of open angle glaucoma.**
   a. betalol
   b. acetazolamide
   c. epinephrine
   d. timolol

8. **Cholinergic agonists produce constriction of the trabecular meshwork and decrease intraocular pressure.**
   a. true
   b. false

9. **Tear deficiency, also known as dry eyes, is a common disorder and is associated with _____.**
   a. aging
   b. environmental conditions
   c. disease
   d. all of the above

10. **Laser surgery is not recommended to reduce intraocular pressure.**
    a. true
    b. false

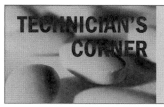

TECHNICIAN'S CORNER

1. The medical use of marijuana is controversial. What are your views on this subject? Give three pros and three cons for the medical use of marijuana.
2. The prevalence of glaucoma in person with diabetes is greater than in persons without diabetes. What can be done to help diabetic patients to decrease the chance of developing glaucoma?

BIBLIOGRAPHY

Bourne R: Worldwide glaucoma through the looking glass, *Br J Ophthalmol,* 90:253-254, 2006.

Centers for Disease Control and Prevention: Prevalence of visual impairment and selected eye diseases among persons aged ≥50 years with and without diabetes–United States 2002, *MMWR Morb Mortal Wkly Rep,* 53:1069-1071, 2004.

Chabner D: *The language of medicine,* ed 8, Philadelphia, 2007, WB Saunders.

Lance L, Lacy C, Armstrong L, Goldman M: *Drug information handbook for the allied health professional,* ed 12. Hudson, OH, 2005, APhA Lexi-Comp.

National Eye Institute: *Glaucoma: what you should know,* Bethesda, MD, 2006, NEI, National Institutes of Health, U.S. Department of Health and Human Services. NIH publication No. 03-651. Retrieved from http://www.nei.nih.gov/health/glaucoma/glaucoma_facts.asp.

Page C, Curtis M, Sutter M, Walker M, Hoffman B: *Integrated pharmacology* (pp 523-534), Philadelphia, 2005, Mosby.

Patton K: *Survival guide for anatomy and physiology,* St Louis, 2006, Mosby.

Quigley H, Broman A: The number of people with glaucoma worldwide in 2010 and 2010, *Br J Ophthalmol,* 90:262-267, 2006.

Raffa R, Rawls S, Beyzarov E: *Netter's illustrated pharmacology* (p 48), Philadelphia, 2005, WB Saunders.

The Glaucoma Foundation: *About glaucoma, 2006.* Retrieved from http://www.glaucomafoundation.org/education_content.php?i=7.

Thibodeau GA, Patton KT: *Anatomy and physiology,* ed 6, St Louis, 2007, Mosby.

USP Center for Advancement of Patient Safety: *Use caution–avoid confusion,* USP Quality Review No. 79, Rockville, MD, April 2004, USP Center for Advancement of Patient Safety.

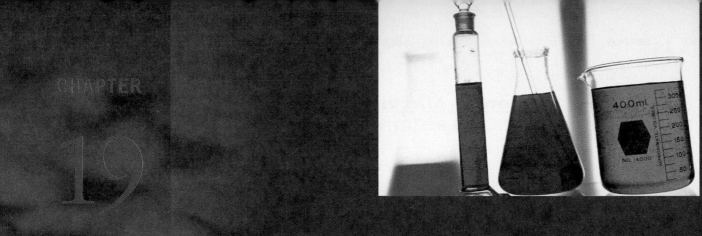

Treatment of Vertigo and Other Disorders of the Ear

LEARNING OBJECTIVES

- Learn the terminology associated with the ear.
- Become familiar with the disorders of the ear.
- Describe factors that influence the sense of balance.
- List and categorize medications used in the treatment of disorders of the ear.
- Identify warning labels and precautionary messages associated with medications used in the treatment of disorders of the ear.
- Identify significant drug look-alike/sound-alike issues.

KEY TERMS

Cerumen: Waxlike substance secreted by modified sweat glands in the ear.

Cochlea: Portion of the inner ear involved in hearing.

Conductive hearing loss: Hearing loss caused by abnormalities of the outer ear or middle ear that interfere with transmission of sound between inner and outer ear.

Equilibrium: Steadiness or balance accompanied by a sense of knowing where the body is in relationship to surroundings.

Labyrinth: Bony structure in the inner ear consisting of three parts (vestibule, cochlea, and the semicircular canals) and involved in balance.

Ménière's disease: Chronic inner ear disease associated with intermittent build up of fluid in the inner ear that causes hearing loss and vertigo.

Otitis: Inflammation of the ear.

Otitis media: Infection of the middle ear.

Otoliths: Calcium carbonate crystals found in the utrical and saccule of the inner ear.

Otosclerosis: Hardening of the bones of the middle ear.

Ototoxicity: Damage or toxicity to the ear or eighth cranial nerve (associated with hearing).

Presbycusis: Bilateral hearing loss linked to aging and often accompanied by tinnitus.

Saccule: Saclike inner ear structure that senses vertical motion of the head.

Tinnitus: Intermittent or continuous whistling, crackling, squeaking, or ringing noise in the ears.

Tympanic membrane: Eardrum.

Utricle: Saclike inner ear structure that senses forward and backward motion and side-to-side motion of the head.

Vertigo: Feeling of spinning in space (dizziness and loss of balance).

Disorders Affecting Hearing

DISORDERS RESULTING IN HEARING LOSS

OTOSCLEROSIS

Otosclerosis is a disorder that causes destruction of bones in the ear (see Figure 19-1 for the anatomy of the ear). Bones that are typically affected are the stapes. Fixation of the stapes footplate causes conduction-hearing loss. Otosclerosis appears as tinnitus in childhood or early adulthood. The incidence of otosclerosis is lower in areas that have fluoridated drinking water, according to some epidemiological studies. Fluoride increases bone density by increasing bone mineralization.

SUDDEN SENSORINEURAL HEARING LOSS

Sudden sensorineural hearing loss (SSHL) progresses rapidly (hours to days) and typically causes hearing loss in only one ear. Other symptoms of SSHL may be vertigo and tinnitus. The exact cause of SSHL is unknown; however, it is believed it may be caused by a viral infection, vascular disorder, tumor, or rupture of the inner ear membrane or be drug induced. Drugs that can cause SSHL are loop diuretics, aminoglycoside antiinfectives, and antineoplastic agents.

Treatment of SSHL involves the use of glucocorticosteroids (see Chapters 15). The best response occurs when hearing loss is moderate. Mild hearing loss resolves spontaneously without treatment and no benefit is observed when hearing loss is severe. Vasodilating drugs and plasma expanders (e.g., normal saline, 5% glucose) may also be prescribed.

AUTOIMMUNE HEARING LOSS

Autoimmune diseases like multiple sclerosis can cause SSHL, but sometimes autoimmune hearing loss occurs in the absence of any other disease. Progression occurs over several months and hearing loss may occur in both ears. Glucocorticosteroids such as prednisone are used in treatment (see Chapter 15).

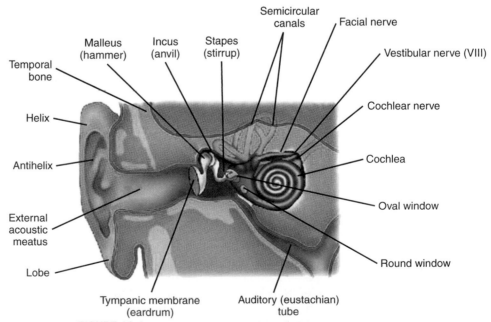

FIGURE 19-1 Anatomy of the ear. *(From Lilley LL, Harrington S, Snyder JS: Pharmacology and the nursing process, 5th ed. St. Louis, 2007, Mosby.)*

DISORDERS RESULTING IN IMPAIRED PERCEPTION OF SOUND

TINNITUS

Tinnitus is a condition that can cause intermittent or continuous whistling, crackling, squeaking, or ringing noise in the ears. Sometimes it is described as ringing in the ear. It may be caused by disease, ***presbycusis*** (bilateral hearing loss due to aging), or it may be induced by drugs or noise. Tinnitus may be the first sign of ototoxicity. Alcohol and salicylates (aspirin) are the most common cause for drug-induced tinnitus.

Tinnitus is treated by masking the noise using a noise generator or by administering drugs. Drugs used to treat tinnitus are local anesthetics, benzodiazepines (see Chapter 5), baclofen (see Chapter 15), and tricyclic antidepressants (see Chapter 6).

Sense of Balance

The sense organs involved in the sense of balance or equilibrium are found in the vestibule and the three semicircular canals of the labyrinth (see Figure 19-1). The sense organs located in the utricle and saccule function in static equilibrium. They sense the position of the head relative to gravity, acceleration, or deceleration of the body. The sense organs associated with the semicircular canals function in dynamic equilibrium to maintain balance when the head or body itself is rotated or suddenly moved. Fluids in the semicircular canals shift when the body is in motion to inform the direction and speed of rotation. The superior, posterior, and horizontal semicircular canals inform whether movement is up or down and side to side.

Disorders of Sense of Balance and Motion

DISORDERS RESULTING IN IMPAIRED PERCEPTION OF MOTION

VERTIGO

Our perception of balance and movement is a function of input from our eye, inner ear, and sense receptors on the skin and skeleton. The body integrates the input it gets from these three sources and compares it to previous experience. ***Vertigo*** is a balance disorder that is caused by a neural mismatch or sensory conflict. When our eyes tell us our body should be moving, yet our body remains still, such as when we watch a movie of a roller coaster, a sensory conflict occurs. Similarly, when we read a book in a car that is moving, our inner ear and skin receptors tell us we are in motion, yet our eyes are fixed on the book that is not moving. Once again, a sensory conflict occurs. Sensory conflicts may also occur from inner ear infection, especially if only one ear is involved. If one ear receives motion signals and the other ear receives none or a different signal, a sensory conflict occurs. Head trauma, degeneration of otolith organs (benign positional vertigo), inflammation of the vestibular nerve, bacterial infection of the labyrinths, brainstem or cerebral pathology, Ménèire's disease, or motion sickness may also produce vertigo.

Vertigo and other balance disorders produce symptoms of dizziness or spinning, nausea and vomiting, blurred vision, disorientation, and a feeling of falling.

BENIGN PAROXYSMAL POSITIONAL VERTIGO

Benign paroxysmal positional vertigo (BPPV) is the number 1 cause of vertigo, accounting for approximately 20% of all cases. It follows trauma to the inner ear, infection, or degeneration of otolith organs. Otoliths are calcium carbonate crystals found in the utricle and saccule of the inner ear. When otoliths dislodge, the debris moves to the lowest part of the posterior semicircular canal each time the head shifts position. The shifting of the otoliths produces vertigo, nausea, and nystagmus.

MÉNÈIRE'S DISEASE

Ménèire's disease is the second most common cause of vertigo. It is a chronic inner ear disease associated with intermittent buildup of fluid in the inner ear. It is characterized by tinnitus, progressive nerve deafness, and vertigo. The cause is unknown.

Ménèire's disease is treated by administering medicines and with diet and lifestyle changes. Reducing sodium, caffeine, nicotine. and alcohol consumption may be helpful. Aminoglycoside antiinfectives such as gentamicin and streptomycin are sometimes used, but their use is controversial because they can cause ototoxicity.

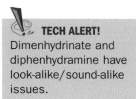

TECH ALERT!
Dimenhydrinate and diphenhydramine have look-alike/sound-alike issues.

TREATMENT OF VERTIGO AND OTHER DISORDERS OF THE EAR

Many of the treatments for vertigo, Ménèire's disease, and other balance disorders do not involve drug therapy. Physical therapy is the treatment of choice for benign paroxysmal positional vertigo (BPPV). Physical therapy is used to manipulate the head and shift otoliths that have dislodged. A low-sodium diet and lifestyle changes that restrict alcohol consumption are useful for the treatment of Ménèire's disease.

When drug therapy is indicated, antihistamines are most widely prescribed. This is most likely because centrally acting antihistamines have anticholinergic actions that can moderate symptoms of motion sickness. Acetylcholine and histamine are excitatory neurotransmitters involved in the control of vomiting (emesis). Nausea and vomiting are common symptoms of vertigo. Moreover, antihistamines and anticholinergics are vestibular suppressants. Vestibular suppression is useful because it reduces the eye activity responsible for symptoms of vertigo. Administration of vestibular suppressants is not recommended when treatment for vertigo involves physical manipulation of the head and "retraining" of vestibular pathways.

Agents used to manage vertigo and Ménèire's disease are betahistine, dimenhydrinate, diphenhydramine, and meclizine. Side effects common to all of these drugs are sedation, dry mouth, urinary retention, and blurred vision. Transdermal scopolamine patches may produce local irritation, burning, or pain at the site where the patch is applied. Dry mouth, thickened bronchial secretions, and urinary retention may be produced and limits their use in patients with prostate disease, asthma, and other conditions. Use should be limited in lactating women as the drugs may reduce the supply of breast milk.

Agents Used to Manage Vertigo and Ménèire's Disease

Generic name	U.S. brand name(s) / Canadian brand(s)	Dosage forms and strengths
betahistine*	Not available	**Tablet:** 16 mg, 24 mg
	Serc	
dimenhydrinate*	Dramamine [OTC], Trip Tone [OTC]	**Caplet (Trip Tone):** 50 mg **Capsule (Gravol):** 50 mg, 100 mg **Tablet (Dramamine):** 50 mg
	Gravol	**Tablet, chewable:** 50 mg
meclizine*	Antivert, Bonine [OTC], Dramamine Less Drowsy Formula [OTC]	**Tablet:** 12.5 mg, 25 mg, 50 mg (Antivert only) **Tablet, chewable:** 25 mg
	Antivert, Bonamine, Bonine	
scopolamine hydrobromine*	Scopace, Transderm Scop	**Tablet:** 0.4 mg (Scopace) **Transdermal (Transderm Scop):** ≈1 mg/72 hr (4s)
	Transderm V	

*Generic available.

Usual Dosage and Warning Labels for Agents Used to Treat Vertigo and Ménèire's Disease

	Generic	Brand	Usual dose	Warning labels
	betahistine	Serc (Canada only)	8 mg to 16 mg 3 times a day	MAY CAUSE DROWSINESS; MAY IMPAIR ABILITY TO DRIVE AVOID ALCOHOL MAINTAIN ADEQUATE FLUID INTAKE
	dimenhydrinate	Dramamine	**Vertigo, motion sickness, nausea, and vomiting:** 50 mg to 100 mg every 4 to 6 hours (maximum 400 mg/day)	OBSERVE GOOD ORAL HYGEINE ROTATE SITE OF PATCH APPLICATION —scopolamine
	meclizine	Antivert	**Motion sickness:** 12.5 mg to 25 mg 1 hour before travel; repeat in 12 to 24 hours as needed **Vertigo:** 25 mg to 100 mg daily in divided doses	TAKE WITH FOOD—betahistine
	scopolamine hydrobromlne	Transderm Scop	**Motion sickness:** Place one patch behind ear every 72 hours as needed	

Other Disorders of the Ear

AURALGIA

Ear pain, also called auralgia or otalgia, is a symptom of otitis externa, otitis media, swimmer's ear, and many other disorders, including viral myringitis, temporomandibular joint (TMJ) disorders, referred pain from abscessed teeth, and others. It is treated by administration of topical analgesics, local anesthetics, and/or oral analgesics. Corticosteroids such as hydrocortisone are combined with otic agents to reduce inflammation and pain. Local anesthetics numb or anesthetize the ear canal and tympanic membrane, further reducing pain and irritation.

When the ear is inflamed, otic drops can produce stinging. This can be minimized by administering suspensions rather than solutions containing alcohol, if this option is available. Otic drops should also be warmed to room temperature before administering into the ear. Sweet olive oil is a home remedy for ear pain. The oil has no analgesic properties, but the warmed oil may be soothing and dislodge cerumen, which may be the cause of the pain.

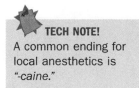

TECH NOTE!
A common ending for local anesthetics is *"-caine."*

Pharmacological Treatments for Miscellaneous Ear Conditions

	Generic name	U.S. brand name(s) Canadian brand(s)	Dosage forms and strengths
Analgesics			
	antipyrine and benzocaine *	Aurodex, Oto Care Otic Liquid, Otalgan Auralgan	**Solution, otic:** antipyrine 5.4% and benzocaine 1.4%

*Generic available.

WATER-CLOGGED EARS AND SWIMMER'S EAR

Water-clogged ears and swimmer's ear are different conditions that are sometimes confused. Water-clogged ears are caused by fluids that accumulate in the ear after swimming or showering. Swimmer's ear produces inflammation and infection of the external ear following prolonged exposure to water, along with damage to the lining of the ear canal. Damage to the lining typically occurs when the person uses a rigid object to remove water from the ears. Swimmer's ear produces acute pain, itching, and a foul-smelling discharge from the ear.

Both conditions cause earache. Nonprescription drying agents are safe and effective for treatment of water-clogged ears. Alcohol (Auro Dri) and mild acidic solutions of vinegar or boric acid dry excess water and soothe the eardrum. Ear drops that contain alcohol such as boric acid solution and alcohol may produce stinging if the ears are inflamed.

Treatments for Water-Clogged Ears and Swimmer's Ear

Generic name	U.S. brand name(s)	Dosage forms and strength
	Canadian brand name(s)	
acetic acid solution*	Generics only	Solution, otic: 2%
	Not available	
boric acid solution*	Dri Ear Otic [OTC], Ear Dry [OTC]	Solution, otic: 2.75%
	Not available	
Combination otic drops		
acetic acid + hydrocortisone solution*	Acetasol	Solution, otic: 2% acedtic acid + 1% hydrocortisone
	Not available	
isopropyl alcohol + glycerin*	Auro-Dri Ear-Water Drying Aid [OTC], Swim-Ear Ear-Water Drying Aid [OTC]	Solution, otic: 95% isopropyl alcohol and glycerin 5%
	Auro-Dri Ear-Water Drying Aid [OTC]	

*Generic available.

TECH NOTE!

The *pH* is a measure of how acidic or alkaline (or basic) a solution is. A pH of 1 indicates the solution is very acidic (e.g., stomach acids [HCl]). A pH of 7 is neutral. Plasma has a pH between the range of 7.35 to 7.45. A pH of greater than 7 is alkaline.

CERUMEN IMPACTION

Cerumen (earwax) is a normal and necessary substance produced by the ear. It functions to reduce the risk for bacterial infections in the ear because earwax has a pH of 6.5 and is bactericidal. Cerumen repels water and helps to keep the ear dry during swimming and bathing. It provides a barrier to entry of airborne substances (dust, insects) into the ear canal. Last, it lubricates the skin of the external ear canal.

The healthy ear continuously replaces old cerumen. If cerumen becomes impacted, it can produce hearing loss, pressure, and ear pain. This condition is more common in people who wear hearing aids or regularly place earplugs and earphones in the ear. A cotton-tipped applicator or other small sharp object should never be used to remove earwax. These objects can cause accidental perforation of the eardrum (tympanic membrane).

Agents used to remove excess cerumen are called cerumenolytics. Emollients and carbamide peroxide are the principal ingredients found in cerumenolytics. Emollients are used to soften the wax, enabling it to slide out of the ear. Olive oil, mineral oil, and glycerin are emollients found in otics for earwax removal.

Peroxide-based products are used to break up the earwax and bubble away the debris. Carbamide peroxide 6.5% is the only approved agent for earwax removal.

After administration of emollients or peroxide-based agents, the affected ear is gently cleansed (irrigated) with warm water to remove cerumen that has become dislodged. Ear irrigation is performed using a bulb syringe.

Cerumenolytics Used to Aid in Earwax Removal

Generic name	U.S. brand name(s) / Canadian brand name(s)	Dosage forms and strength
carbamide peroxide (also known as urea hydrogen peroxide)*	Auro-Dri, Debrox [OTC], Earwax Removal System [OTC] / Murine Earwax Removal System	**Solution, otic:** 6.5%
triethanolamine polypeptide oleate-condensate	Generics only / Cerumenex	**Solution, otic:** 10%

*Generic available.

Summary of Drugs Used to Treat Miscellaneous Conditions of the Ear

Generic	Brand	Usual dose	Warning labels
Analgesics			
antipyrine and benzocaine	Aurodex	Fill ear canal and place a cotton pledgette in external ear every 1 to 2 hours until pain relieved.	FOR THE EAR
Drying agents			
acetic acid solution	Generics	Insert a saturated wick into affected ear. Keep moist for 24 hours; then instill 5 drops 3 to 4 times a day	FOR THE EAR
boric acid solution	Drl Ear Otic	**Prevention of swimmer's ear:** Instill 2 to 4 drops in affected ear(s) as needed	
Isopropyl alcohol and glycerin	Auro-Dri Ear-Water Drying Aid	**Water-clogged ears:** Instill 4 to 5 drops in affected ear(s)	
Cerumenolytics			
carbamide peroxide	Debrox [OTC]	**Earwax removal:** Instill 5 to 10 drops twice daily for up to 4 days.	FOR THE EAR
triethylanolamine polypeptide oleate-condensate	generics	**Earwax removal:** Fill ear canal. Insert cotton pledgette. Leave in for 15 to 30 minutes; then flush with warm water	FOR THE EAR

CHAPTER SUMMARY

- The ear provides a sense of hearing and equilibrium or balance.
- The semicircular canals are located in the inner ear. Their positioning provides a sense of balance.
- Otosclerosis, autoimmune diseases like multiple sclerosis, and sudden sensorineural hearing loss are conditions that can cause hearing loss.
- Otosclerosis is a disorder that causes destruction of bone in the ear, hearing loss, and ringing in the ears (tinnitis).
- Sudden sensorineural hearing loss is treated with glucocorticosteroids.
- Tinnitus is a condition that produces ringing in the ear.
- Tinnitus may be drug induced. Aspirin and alcohol are common drugs that can cause tinnitus.

- Aminoglycoside antiinfectives (gentamicin) and loop diuretics can cause ototoxicity.
- Benign paroxysmal positional vertigo (BPPV) is the number 1 cause of vertigo.
- Ménèire's disease is the second most common cause of vertigo.
- Our perception of balance and movement is a function of input from our eye, inner ear, and sense receptor on the skin and skeleton.
- Vertigo is a balance disorder that is caused by a neural mismatch or sensory conflict.
- Vertigo can occur from head trauma or degeneration of otolith organs (benign positional vertigo), inflammation of the vestibular nerve, bacterial infection of the labyrinths, brainstem or cerebral pathology, or Ménèire's disease.
- Vertigo and other balance disorders produce symptoms of dizziness or spinning, nausea and vomiting, blurred vision, disorientation, and a feeling of falling.
- Treatment of balance disorders may involve physical therapy diet and lifestyle changes.
- When drug therapy is indicated, antihistamines are most widely used.
- Antihistamines have anticholinergic actions that can moderate symptoms of motion sickness but produce urinary retention and other side effects that limit their use in patients with prostate disease or asthma or in women who are lactating.
- Other side effects that are common to all antihistamine drugs are sedation, dry mouth, and blurred vision.
- One scopolamine transdermal patch placed behind the ear prevents motion sickness for up to 3 days.
- Ear pain, also called auralgia or otalgia, is a symptom of otitis externa, otitis media, and many disorders of the ear such as viral myringitis, temporomandibular joint disorders, referred pain from abscessed teeth, and others.
- Ear pain is treated by administration of topical analgesics, local anesthetics, and/or oral analgesics.
- When the ear is inflamed, otic suspensions are more soothing than are solutions that contain alcohol.
- Water-clogged ears and swimmer's ear are different conditions that are sometimes confused.
- Swimmer's ear produces inflammation and infection of the external ear.
- Nonprescription drying agents are safe and effective for treatment of water-clogged ears.
- Cerumen (earwax) is a normal and necessary substance produced by the ear.
- Cerumen is bactericidal and water repellant, and it provides a barrier to entry of airborne substances and lubricates the skin of the external ear canal.
- A cotton-tipped applicator or other small sharp object should never be used to remove earwax.
- Emollients and carbamide peroxide are the principal ingredients found in cerumenolytics.
- After administration of emollients or peroxide-based agents, the affected ear is gently cleansed (irrigated) with warm water to remove cerumen that has become dislodged.

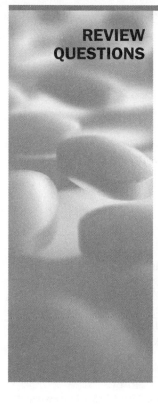

REVIEW QUESTIONS

Multiple Choice

1. **The number 1 cause of vertigo accounting for approximately 20% of all cases is _____.**
   a. overdose of aspirin and alcohol
   b. water in the ear
   c. benign paroxysmal positional vertigo
   d. constant diving

2. **Presbycusis, common in (the) _____, causes degeneration of nerve tissue in the ear and vestibular nerve.**
   a. diabetic patient
   b. elderly
   c. middle aged
   d. children with birth defects

3. **Treatment of sudden sensorineural hearing loss involves the use of what type of medications?**
   a. antiinflammatories
   b. mineralocorticoids
   c. glucocorticosteroids
   d. stimulants

4. **The most common cause for drug-induced tinnitus is _____.**
   a. noise
   b. aspirin
   c. alcohol
   d. b and c

5. **Which drug treatment for vertigo is available in a "patch"?**
   a. diphenhydramine
   b. scopolamine hydrobromine
   c. dimenhydrinate
   d. betahistine

6. **Corticosteroids such as hydrocortisone are combined with _____ agents to reduce inflammation and pain in the ear.**
   a. optic
   b. otic
   c. glaucoma
   d. ocular

7. **Swimmer's ear produces inflammation and infection of the _____ ear following prolonged exposure to water, along with damage to the lining of the ear canal.**
   a. internal
   b. inner
   c. external
   d. semicircular canals

8. **A cotton-tipped applicator or other small sharp object should always be used to remove earwax.**
   a. true
   b. false

9. **Olive oil, mineral oil, and glycerin are emollients found in otics for removal of _____.**
   a. ear wax
   b. fluid
   c. bacteria
   d. foreign material

10. **Carbamide peroxide 6.5% is the only approved agent for _____ removal.**
    a. earwax
    b. fluid
    c. bacteria
    d. foreign material

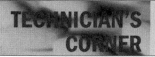

TECHNICIAN'S CORNER

1. How does ear candling work to remove unwanted cerumen or debris from the ear?
2. What other home remedies have you heard of for helping with ear pain?

BIBLIOGRAPHY

Chabner D: *The language of medicine,* ed 8, Philadelphia, 2007, WB Saunders.

Hain T, Uddin M: Pharmacological treatment of vertigo, *CNS Drugs,* 17:85-100, 2003.

National Institute on Deafness and Other Communication Disorders: *Balance disorders,* Bethesda, MD, 2006, NIDCD, National Institutes of Health, US Department of Health and Human Services. Retrieved from http://www.nidcd.nih.gov/health/balance/balance_disorders.asp.

Page C, Curtis M, Sutter M, Walker M, Hoffman B: *Integrated pharmacology* (pp 539-544), Philadelphia, 2005, Mosby.

Patton K: *Survival guide for anatomy and physiology,* St Louis, 2006, Mosby.

Thibodeau GA, Patton KT: *Anatomy and physiology,* ed 6, St Louis, 2007, Mosby.

USP Center for Advancement of Patient Safety: *Use caution–avoid confusion,* USP Quality Review No. 79, Rockville, MD, April 2004, USP Center for Advancement of Patient Safety.

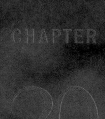

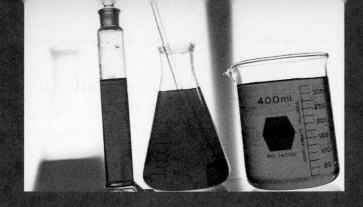

CHAPTER

20

Treatment of Ophthalmic and Otic Infections

LEARNING OBJECTIVES

- Learn the terminology associated with the eye and ear infections.
- List and describe infections of the eye.
- List and describe infections of the ear.
- List and categorize medications used in the treatment of eye and ear infections.
- Identify significant drug look-alike/sound-alike issues.

KEY TERMS

Blepharitis: Chronic disease of the eye that produces distinctive flaky scales that form on the eyelids and eyelashes.

Conjunctivitis (pink eye): Common, self-limiting ailment that causes itching, burning, and teary outflow.

Cytomegalovirus retinitis: Viral opportunistic infection of the eye that can cause pain and blindness.

Floaters: Particles that float in the vitreous and cast shadows on the retina and appear as spots, cobwebs, or spiders.

Fusarium keratitis: Rare fungal infection that occurs in soft contact lens wearers and can result in blindness.

Helminthes: Parasitic worms that can cause eye infection and blindness.

Herpes simplex keratitis: Painful eye infection caused by herpes virus that can lead to blindness.

Herpes zoster ophthalmicus: Painful eye infection caused by herpes virus that can lead to blindness.

Iritis: Condition associated with inflammation of the iris.

Keratitis: Severe infection of the cornea that may be caused by bacteria or fungi.

Otitis externa: Inflammation of the ear canal or external ear.

Otitis media: Inflammation of the middle ear typically caused by viral or bacterial infection.

Otorrhea: Discharge coming from the external auditory canal or inside of the canal.

Photopsia: Condition similar to floaters and associated with flashes of light.

Stye: Painful lump located on the eyelid margin caused by an acute self-limiting infection of the oil glands of the eyelid.

Uveitis: Serious eye condition that produces inflammation of the uvea and can cause scarring of the eye and blindness if untreated.

Bacterial Infections of the Eye

BLEPHARITIS

Blepharitis is a chronic disease of the eye. It is also known as *granulated eyelids,* because of the distinctive flaky scales on the eyelids and eyelashes produced by the condition. There are two forms of blepharitis: anterior blepharitis and posterior blepharitis. Anterior blepharitis affects the outside of the lid where the eyelashes are attached and is caused by bacteria (*Staphyloccocus*) and scalp dandruff. Posterior blepharitis affects the inside of the eyelid and is caused by dysfunction of the oil glands in the eyelid, seborrhea, psoriasis (Figure 20-1), and acne rosacea.

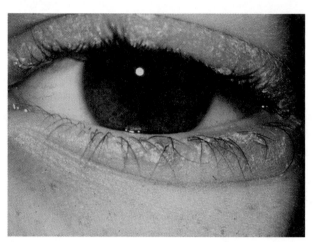

FIGURE 20-1 Psoriatic blepharitis. *(Courtesy of the Cogan Collection, National Eye Institute/National Institutes of Health.)*

Symptoms of blepharitis are eye pain or burning, excessive tearing, feeling of "something in the eye," light sensitivity, blurred vision, dry eye, and flaky scales on the eyelids and lashes. Complications of blepharitis are stye and tear film abnormalities.

Blepharitis is self-treated by applying clean warm compresses to the eyelids to loosen the scales followed by cleansing the lids with a mild lid scrub. Antiinfective ointments, corticosteroid eye drops, and artificial tears may also be used to manage the symptoms of blepharitis. Aminoglycoside antiinfectives are used in the treatment of blepharitis and include gentamicin, neomycin, and tobramycin.

CONJUNCTIVITIS

Conjunctivitis (pink eye) is a common ailment that causes itching, burning, and teary outflow. It may be caused by allergies, a virus, or bacteria. Conjunctivitis in adults is often caused by a virus and is self-limiting without treatment with antiinfective agents. Conjunctivitis of bacterial origin is contagious and must be treated with antibiotic eye drops or orally administered antiinfectives. Various pathogens such as the bacterium *Chlamydia trachomatis, Staphylococcus aureus, Streptococcus pneumoniae* and *Haemophilus influenzae* may be the causative agent for bacterial infections. Antibacterial agents are used to treat conjunctivitis of bacterial origin and include aminoglycosides, sulfonamides, quinolones, and macrolides. The antiviral trifluridine is used to treat keratoconjunctivitis due to herpes simplex type 1 virus (Figure 20-2).

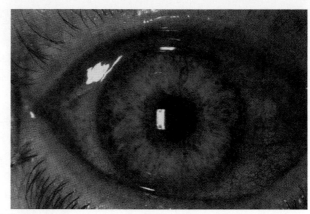

FIGURE 20-2 Viral conjunctivitis. *(Courtesy of the Cogan Collection, National Eye Institute/National Institutes of Health.)*

IRITIS

Iritis is a condition associated with inflammation of the iris (Figure 20-3). Most causes of iritis are unknown; however, known causes have been a herpes virus, autoimmune disease, eye trauma, and gout.

Symptoms of iritis include redness, blurred vision, inflammation, pain, and light sensitivity. Iritis is treated with the administration of corticosteroids (to reduce inflammation), mydriatics (to reduce painful swelling), and antivirals as appropriate.

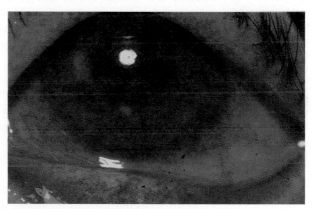

FIGURE 20-3 Iritis with Rosacea Keratitis. *(Courtesy of the Cogan Collection, National Eye Institute/National Institutes of Health.)*

KERATITIS

Keratitis is a severe infection of the cornea and may be caused by bacteria or fungi. If untreated, the infection can cause permanent loss of vision. Microbial keratitis and fungal keratitis are most commonly caused by trauma, immunodeficiency, and chronic eye surface diseases. Contact lens use can also cause microbial and fungal keratitis. Soft contact lens wearers, especially those who wear their contact lenses overnight, are at greater risk for eye infection. Of the approximately 30 million soft contact lens wearers in the United States, up to 21 persons of 10,000 will develop microbial keratitis. The incidence of fungal keratitis varies according to geographic region. The incidence is higher in the southern United States (up to 35% of microbial keratitis cases) and lowest in the northeastern United States (up to 1% of microbial keratitis cases).

STYE

A *stye* (hordeolem) is a small, painful lump located on the eyelid margin (Figure 20-4). It is caused by an acute self-limiting infection of the oil glands of the eyelid and will typically resolve on its own in a few days. When more than one stye is present at the same time, the

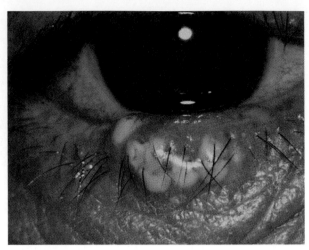

FIGURE 20-4 Stye. *(Courtesy of the Cogan Collection, National Eye Institute/National Institutes of Health.)*

condition is called blepharitis. Styes are can be self-managed and are treated by applying warm compresses to the area.

UVEITIS

Uveitis is a serious eye condition that results in inflammation of the uvea and can cause scarring of the eye and blindness if untreated. There are three kinds of uveitis, each associated with a different part of the eye. Inflammation of the uvea in the area of the iris is called *iritis.* Inflammation in the middle of the eye is called *cyclitis,* and inflammation in the back of the eye is called *choroiditis.*

Most causes of uveitis are unknown; however, known causes have been herpes virus, histoplasmosis (fungus), toxoplasmosis (parasite), autoimmune disease, eye trauma, or other eye disease. Other eye conditions that may cause uveitis are glaucoma, cataracts, and abnormal growth of new blood vessels in the eye.

Symptoms of uveitis include redness, blurred vision, pain, inflammation, and light sensitivity. These symptoms may develop suddenly or over a prolonged time period, as occurs with choroiditis.

Uveitis is treated with the administration of corticosteroids (to reduce inflammation), mydriatics (to reduce painful swelling), and antiinfective, antivirals, or antifungals as appropriate. Drugs used in the treatment of uveitis are listed in the drug tables in this chapter.

TECH ALERT!

The following drugs have look-alike/sound-alike issues: Bleph-10 and Blephamide; gentamicin and tobramycin; Tobrex and Tobradex

Topical Ophthalmics Used to Treat Bacterial Infections

Generic name	U.S. brand name(s)	Dosage forms and strengths
	Canadian brand(s)	
Aminoglycosides		
gentamicin*	Genoptic SOP, Gentak, Gentasol	**Ointment, ophthalmic:** 0.3% **Solution, ophthalmic:** 0.3%
	Alcomicin, Garamycin	
tobramycin*	Tobrasol, Tobrex	**Ointment, ophthalmic:** 0.3% **Solution, ophthalmic:** 0.3%
	Tobrex	
neomycin sulfate + bacitracin zinc + polymyxin B sulfate*	Generics only	**Ointment, ophthalmic:** 400 units/g bacitracin zinc + 0.5% neomycin + 10,000 units/ml polymyxin B
	Not available	

Topical Ophthalmics Used to Treat Bacterial Infections—cont'd

Generic name	U.S. brand name(s) Canadian brand(s)	Dosage forms and strengths
neomycin sulfate + polymyxin B sulfate + gramicidin*	Neocidin, Neosporin Ophthalmic solution	**Solution, ophthalmic:** 1.75 mg/ml neomycin + 10,000 units/ml polymyxin B + 0.025 mg/ml gramicidin
	Optimyxin Plus Oto-Opth Gtte	
Sulfonamides		
sulfacetamide Na⁺*	Bleph-10	**Ointment, ophthalmic:** 10% (generic) **Solution, ophthalmic:** 10%
	Bleph-10, Cetamide oint.	
trimethoprim + polymyxin B sulfate*	Polytrim	**Solution, ophthalmic:** 1 mg/ml trimethoprim + 10,000 units/ml polymyxin B
	Polytrim	
Quinolones		
ciprofloxacin*	Ciloxan	**Ointment, ophthalmic:** 0.3% **Solution, ophthalmic:** 0.3%
	Ciloxan	
levofloxacin	Iquix, Quixin	**Solution, ophthalmic:** 1.5% (Iquixin), 0.5% (Quixin)
	Not available	
ofloxacin*	Ocuflox	**Solution, ophthalmic:** 0.3%
	Ocuflox	
Macrolides		
erythromycin	Romycin	**Ointment, ophthalmic:** 0.5%
	Generics	
Antiinfective + corticosteroid		
neomycin + bacitracin + polymyxin B + hydrocortisone	Generics	**Ointment, ophthalmic:** 0.35% neomycin + 400 units/g bacitracin + 10,000 units/g polymyxin B + 1% hydrocortisone
	Not available	
neomycin + polymyxin B + dexamethasone*	Dexasporin, Maxitrol, Poly-Dex	**Ointment, ophthalmic:** 0.35% neomycin + 10,000 units/g polymyxin B + 0.1% dexamethasone **Suspension, ophthalmic:** 0.35% neomycin + 10,000 units/ml polymyxin B + 0.1% dexamethasone
	AK Trol, Maxitrol†	
neomycin + polymyxin B + prednisolone	Poly-Pred	**Suspension, ophthalmic:** 0.35% neomycin + 10,000 units/ml polymyxin B + 0.5% prednisolone
	Not available	
gentamicin + prednisolone*	Pred-G	**Suspension, ophthalmic:** 0.3% gentamicin + 1% prednisolone **Ointment, ophthalmic:** 0.3% gentamicin + 0.6% prednisolone
	Not available	
sulfacetamide + prednisolone acetate*	Blephamide	**Ointment, ophthalmic:** 10% sulfacetamine + 0.2% prednisolone **Solution, ophthalmic:** 10% sulfacetamine + 0.2% prednisolone
	Blephamide	
sulfacetamide + fluorometholone*	generics	**Solution, ophthalmic:** 10% sulfacetamide + 0.1% fluorometholone
	Not available	

Continued

Topical Ophthalmics Used to Treat Bacterial Infections—cont'd

Generic name	U.S. brand name(s)	Dosage forms and strengths
	Canadian brand(s)	
tobramycin + dexamethasone	Tobradex	**Ointment, ophthalmic:** 0.3% tobramycin + 0.1% dexamethasone
	Tobradex	**Suspension, ophthalmic:** 0.3% tobramcyin + 0.1% dexamethasone

*Generic available.
†The product formulations for Maxitrol (U.S.) and Maxitrol (Canada) are different. The formulation in Canada contains only 6000 units of polymyxin B sulfate.

Viral Infections of the Eye

CYTOMEGALOVIRUS RETINITIS

Most adults throughout the world have been exposed to cytomegalovirus (CMV). It is estimated that 50% to 85% of adults in the United States harbor anti-CMV antibodies. In healthy individuals, exposure to CMV does not cause active disease. The virus remains dormant unless the immune system becomes depressed, and then infections of the eyes, gastrointestinal tract, lungs, and central nervous system may develop.

Cytomegalovirus retinitis is an opportunistic infection in the eye that occurs in patients who have HIV infection/AIDS or take immunosuppressive drugs. The infection can lead to hemorrhage, cell death, and blindness. The most common symptoms of CMV retinitis are decreased vision, eye pain, floaters, and photopsia. *Floaters* are particles that cast shadows on the retina and appear as spots, cobwebs, or spiders. *Photopsia* is a condition similar to floaters and is associated with flashes of light.

Cytomegalovirus retinitis is treated by administration of antivirals such as ganciclovir, valganciclovir, foscarnet, and cidofovir. Valganciclovir is the only drug that can be taken orally for the induction phase of therapy (initial therapy). Oral ganciclovir is only approved for maintenance therapy. Drugs used in the treatment of cytomegalovirus retinitis are cidofovir, ganciclovir, foscarnet, and valganciclovir.

HERPETIC EYE DISEASE

The herpes virus is the cause of many infections throughout the body. Herpetic corneal disease is the cause of more than 500,000 cases of blindness annually. Two strains of the virus are responsible for infections of the eye. *Herpes zoster ophthalmicus* is caused by the virus that is responsible for chickenpox and shingles (varicella-zoster). *Herpes simplex keratitis* is caused by the same virus that produces cold sores on the lips and mouth (herpes simplex 1).

Herpes simplex virus (HSV) can cause blepharitis, conjunctivitis, dendritic epithelial keratitis, corneal ulceration, stromal keratitis, endothelilitis, trabeculitis, scleritis, iridocyclitis, acute retinal necrosis syndrome, and other conditions (Figure 20-5).

Both herpes zoster ophthalmicus and herpes simplex keratitis produce eye pain, redness, and cloudiness of the cornea. The virus lives around nerve fibers and, when activated, produces painful symptoms. Symptoms only associated with herpes zoster ophthalmicus are swelling and rash or sores around the eye, lids, or forehead. Symptoms of herpes simplex keratitis are excessive tearing, decreased vision, gritty feeling in the eye, and pain when looking at bright light.

Herpes zoster ophthalmicus and herpes simplex keratitis are treated by administering antiviral eye drops and/or pills. Acyclovir is used to prevent and suppress recurrent herpetic eye disease, but its use for herpes simplex ocular infection prophylaxis is not U.S. Food and Drug Administration approved. Corticosteroids are used to reduce inflammatory cells that can block the trabecular meshwork, impede the outflow of eye fluids, and may lead to increased intraocular pressure and pain. Use of corticosteroids must be carefully monitored because the drugs can also increase intraocular pressure. Mydriatics may be administered to maintain the normal flow of eye fluids and prevent buildup of intraocular pressure. Drugs used in the treatment of herpetic eye disease are listed the following table. A detailed discussion of antivirals is found in Chapter 36.

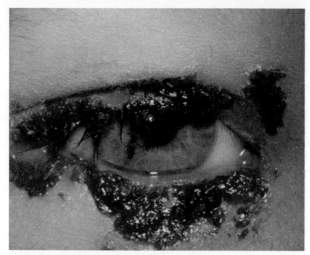

FIGURE 20-5 Herpetic blepharitis. *(Courtesy of David G. Cogan Ophthalmic pathology collection http://cogancollection.nei.nih.gov/.)*

Drugs Used to Treat Viral Infections in the Eye

Generic name	U.S. brand name(s) Canadian brand (s)	Dosage forms and strengths
cidofovir	Vistide	**Solution, for injection:** 75 mg/ml
	Not available	
ganciclovir	Cytovene	**Capsule:** 250 mg, 500 mg
	Cytovene, Vitrasert	**Powder, for injection:** 500 mg **Intravitreal Implant (Vitrasert):** 4.5 mg
foscarnet	Foscavir	**Solution, for injection:** 24 mg/ml
	Not available	
trifluridine	Viroptic	**Solution, ophthalmic:** 1%
	Viroptic	
valganciclovir	Valcyte	**Tablet:** 450 mg
	Valcyte	

*Generic available.

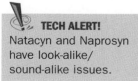

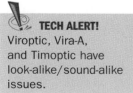

TECH ALERT!
Viroptic, Vira-A, and Timoptic have look-alike/sound-alike issues.

TECH ALERT!
Natacyn and Naprosyn have look-alike/sound-alike issues.

Fungal and Protozoal Infections of the Eye

FUSARIUM KERATITIS

Fusarium keratitis is a rare fungal infection of the eye that occasionally occurs in people who wear soft contact lenses. If untreated, it can lead to blindness. See the discussion of keratitis for more information. Fusarium keratitis and other fungal infections of the eye are treated with antifungals such as natamycin.

TOXOPLASMOSIS

Ocular toxoplasmosis is caused by protozoa and is transmitted by handling or eating raw and undercooked meat or by handling cat feces. According to the Centers for Disease Control and Prevention (CDC), there may be as many as 1.26 million people in the United States with ocular toxoplasmosis. Exposure to the protozoa causes the development of antigens that can cause ocular inflammation, vasculitis, uveitis, and retinal edema.

Drugs used in the treatment and management of toxoplasmosis are pyramethamine and sulfonamides (sulfadiazine and trimethoprim + sulthamethoxazole).

Ophthalmic Antifungals

Generic name	U.S. brand name(s)	Dosage forms and strengths
	Canadian brand(s)	
natamycin	Natacyn	Suspension, ophthalmic: 5%
	Not available	

Helminthic Infections

Helminthes are parasitic worms that can cause eye infections and blindness. Three species can cause infection in the human eye.

ONCHONOCERIASIS

Onchonoceriasis is caused by the nematode (roundworm) *O. volvulus*. The disease is also known as river blindness. Onchonoceriasis is the second leading cause of infectious blindness in the world, according the World Health Organization (WHO). Most cases of onchonoceriasis occur in Africa, Yemen, and Central and South America, where the fly that carries the disease lives.

Onchonoceriasis is treated by administering a single dose of ivermectin yearly. This antihelminthe kills living worms and prevents the inflammatory reaction and scarring in the eye that is triggered by the worms.

CYSTICERCOSIS

Cysticercosis is caused by the cestode (flat worm) *T. solium*. It is transmitted to humans who eat poorly cooked pork. Cysticercosis is most common in Andean South America, Brazil, Central America, Mexico, China, India, southeast Asia, and sub-Saharan Africa. It is treated with praziquantel (not FDA approved), corticosteroids, and surgical removal of the living worms.

TOXOCARIASIS

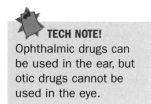

TECH NOTE!
Ophthalmic drugs can be used in the ear, but otic drugs cannot be used in the eye.

Toxocariasis is caused by a worm that is carried by dogs, cats, wolves, and foxes. The infection is most common in children because it is contracted by eating soil that is infested with feces containing the worm eggs. Toxocariasis is the fifth cause of uveitis worldwide. Infections can cause loss of vision in the affected eye and strabismus. It is treated by the administration of topical corticosteroids and systemic antihelminthics such as albendazole and thiabendazole.

The dog is also the carrier of another roundworm (*A. caninum*) that can cause diffuse unilateral subacute neuroretinitis (DUSN). The worms produce inflammation in the retina progresses to atrophy of the optic nerve and blindness. The infection is treated by administering topical corticosteroids and systemic antihelminthics such as thiabendazole.

Drugs Used to Treat Parasitic Infections of the Eye

Generic name	U.S. brand name(s)	Dosage forms and strengths
	Canadian brand(s)	
albendazole	Albenza	Tablet: 200 mg
	Not available for human use	
ivermectin	Stromectol	Tablet: 3 mg
	Not available for human use	
praziquantel*	Biltricide	Tablet: 600 mg
	Biltricide	
thiabendazole	Mintezol	Tablet, chewable: 500 mg
	Not available	

*Not FDA approved.

Summary of Treatments of Bacterial, Fungal, and Viral Infections of the Eye

Usual Dosage for Drugs Used to Treat Infections of the Eye

Generic name	Brand name	Usual dosage
Aminoglycosides		
gentamicin 0.3%	Garamycin, Genoptic	Instill 1 to 2 drops every 4 hours while awake until resolved (solution) *or* Apply ½-inch ribbon of ointment applied 2 to 3 times a day to lid margin
tobramycin 0.3%	Tobrex	Instill 1 to 2 drops in eye(s) every 4 hours *or* Apply ointment 2 to 3 times a day (every 3 to 4 hours for severe infection)
neomycin + bacitracin + polymyxin B	**Neosporin Ophthalmic:** ointment	Apply small amount to conjunctival sac every 3 to 4 hours
neomycin + polymyxin B + gramicidin	**Neosporin Ophthalmic:** solution	Instill 1 to 2 drops in eye(s) every 4 to 6 hours (or more for severe infection)
Sulfonamides		
sulfacetamide Na⁺ 10%	Sulamyd, Bleph-10	Instill 1 to 2 drops every 2 to 3 hours while awake until resolved (solution) *or* Apply a thin ribbon of ointment 1 to 4 times a day and at bedtime to lid margin
trimethoprim 1 mg + polymyxin B 10,000 units	Polytrim	Instill 1 to 2 drops into eye(s) every 4 to 6 hours
Quinolones		
ciprofloxacin 0.3%	Ciloxan	Instill 1 to 2 drops in eye(s) every 2 hours while awake for 2 days then 1 to 2 drops every 4 hours for 5 days *or* Apply ½-inch ribbon to conjunctival sac 3 times a day for 2 days, then twice daily for 5 days
levofloxacin 0.5%	Iquixin, Quixin	Instill 1 to 2 drops in eye(s) every 2 hours while awake days 1 to 2; then instill every 4 hours days 3 to 7 (up to 4 times a day)
ofloxacin 0.3%	Ocuflox	Instill 1 to 2 drops in affected eye every 2 to 4 hours for 2 days; then use 4 times a day for 5 days more
Macrolides		
erythromycin 0.5%	generics	Apply ½ inch (1.25 cm) 2 to 6 times a day until resolved
Miscellaneous		
oxytetracycline 5 mg + polymyxin B 10,000 units	Terramycin w/Polymyxin B	Apply ½ inch (1.25 cm) to the lower eyelid 2 to 4 times a day until resolved
Antiinfective + corticosteroid		
neomycin + bacitracin + polymyxin B + hydrocortisone	Cortisporin Ointment	Apply a ½-inch ribbon of ointment every 3 to 4 hours to lower lid margin until improvement

Continued

Usual Dosage and Warning Labels for Drugs Used to Treat Infections of the Eye—cont'd

Generic name	Brand name	Usual dosage
neomycin + dexamethasone	NeoDecadron	Instill 1 to 2 drops into eye(s) every 3 to 4 hours
neomycin + polymyxin B + dexamethasone	Dexasporin, Maxitrol	Apply a ½-inch ribbon of ointment 3 to 4 times a day or at bedtime **or** Instill 1 to 2 drops into eye(s) every 3 to 4 hours
neomycin + polymyxin B + prednisolone	Poly-Pred	Instill 1 to 2 drops into eye(s) every 3 to 4 hours
gentamicin 0.3% + prednisolone (0.6% ointment and 1% suspension)	Pred-G	Instill 1 drops into eye(s) every 2 to 4 hours **or** Apply a ½-inch ribbon of ointment 1 to 3 times a day
sulfacetamide 10% + prednisolone acetate 0.2%	Blephamide	Apply to lower conjunctival sac 1 to 4 times a day **or** Instill 1 to 3 drops into eye(s) every 2 to 3 hours while awake
sulfacetamide 10% + prednisolone phosphate 0.25%	generics	
sulfacetamide 10% + fluorometholone 0.1%	FML-S	Instill 1 to 3 drops into eye(s) every 2 to 3 hours while awake
tobramycin 0.3% + dexamethasone 0.1%	Tobradex	Instill 1 to 2 drops in eye(s) every 4 hours **or** Apply ointment 2 to 3 times a day (every 3 to 4 hours for severe infection)
Antivirals		
cidofovir	Vistide	Infuse 5 mg/kg IV over 1 hour once weekly for 2 weeks, then once every other week
ganciclovir	Cytovene, Vitrasert	Infuse 5 mg/kg IV every 12 hours for 14 to 21 days, then once daily 7 days/week (or 6 mg/kg/day for 5 days/week) **or** 1000 mg orally 3 times a day (or 500 mg 6 times/day) **or** One implant every 5 to 8 months (Vitrasert)
foscarnet 24 mg/ml	Foscavir	Infuse 60 mg/kg/dose every 8 hours or 100 mg every 12 hours for 14 to 21 days, then 90 to 120 mg/kg/day as a single dose
trifluridine	Viroptic	Instill 1 drop in eye(s) every 2 hours while awake up to 9 drops/day until corneal ulcer heals, then 1 drop every 4 hours for 7 days
valganciclovir 450 mg	Valcyte	900 mg twice a day for 21 days, then take once daily thereafter
Antifungals		
natamycin	Natacyn	Instill 1 drop into conjunctival sac every 1 to 2 hours for 3 to 4 days; then 1 drop every 6 to 8 hours for 2 to 3 weeks

Bacterial Infections of the Ear

OTITIS EXTERNA

Otitis externa is inflammation of the external auditory canal. It may be caused by bacterial infection, fungal infection, seborrheic dermatitis, psoriasis, and lupus erythematosus. The most common cause is bacterial infection. Fungi (candida) account for only 10% of the cases of otitis externa. Risk factors for development of otitis externa are (1) exposure to excessive moisture (swimming, humidity, sweating); (2) high environmental temperature; (3) irritation caused by earwax removal; (4) insertion of objects into the ear; and (5) chronic dermatological disease.

The most common symptoms of otitis externa are ear discomfort or pain, itchiness, and discharge (otorrhea). Topical and systemic drugs are used to treat otitis externa and control symptoms. Antiinfectives used in treatment are listed in the following drug monograph.

TREATMENT OF OTITIS EXTERNA

Topical Antiinfectives Used to Treat Otitis Externa

Generic name	U.S. brand name(s)	Usual dosage
	Canadian brand name(s)	
Aminoglycosides		
gentamicin sulfate 0.3%*⊥	generic opthalmics	Apply 3 to 4 drops in ear(s) 3 times a day
	Garamycin Otic	
Quinolones		
ofloxacin 0.3%*⊥	Floxln Otic	Instill 10 drops in affected ear(s) daily for 7 days
	Not available	
Antiinfective + corticosteroid		
ciprofloxacin 0.3%+ dexamethasone 1%	Ciprodex	Instill 4 drops in ear(s) 4 times a day
	Ciprodex	
ciprofloxacin 0.2% + hydrocortisone 1%	Cipro HC otic suspension	Instill 3 drops in affected ear(s) 2 times a day for 7 days
	Cipro HC otic suspension	
neomycin 0.35% + polymyxin B 10,000 u+ hydrocortisone 1%*	Cortisporin Otic, Pediotic	Instill 4 drops into ear(s) 3 to 4 times a day
	Cortisporin Otic	
acetic acid 2% + hydrocortisone 1%*	Aceta sol HC	Instill 4 drops in ear(s) 3 to 4 times a day
	Not available	

*generic available
⊥Tobramycin and ciprofloxacin ophthalmic solution are used off label.

OTITIS MEDIA

Otitis media is an inflammation in the middle ear. It may accompany an upper respiratory infection. Children are more susceptible to otitis media than adults because their eustachian tube is shorter and straighter than that of an adult. When the eustachian tube is blocked by swelling or mucus from a cold, fluids accumulate and collect in the normally air-filled middle ear. Bacteria may collect in the fluid along with white blood cells released by the body to fight the infection. Hearing becomes impaired because the eardrum and

TECH ALERT!
The following drugs have look-alike/sound-alike issues:
Lorabid, Levbid, and Lopid;
Pediazole and Pediapred;
cefixime, cefuroxime, cefpodoxime, and cephalexin;
amoxicillin, ampicillin, and Augmentin

middle ear bones are unable to move as freely. Pain and pressure builds, and finally the eardrum may tear to release the pressure.

Historically, otitis media has been treated aggressively with orally administered antiinfective drugs; however, new evidence shows that the infection is self-limiting in many cases and will resolve on its own without treatment. Excessive use of antiinfective agents may increase the risk of the development of bacterial resistance. Furthermore, evidence shows that prophylactic use of antihistamines and decongestants is ineffective in preventing otitis media. Antiinfective agents used in the treatment of otitis media are listed in the following drug monograph along with usual dosages for children. These agents are described fully in Unit 10.

TREATMENT

Selected Antiinfectives Used to Treat Otitis Media

Generic name	US Brand name(s) Canadian Brand name(s)	Usual child dosage
Penicillins		
amoxicillin*	Amoxil	25 to 90 mg/kg/day every 8 to 12 hours for 10 days (depending on severity)
	Generics	
amoxicillin + clavulanate*	Augmentin	90 mg/kg/day every 12 hours for 10 days (<40 kg); 250 mg to 500 mg every 8 hours or 875 mg every 12 hours (>40 kg)
	Clavulin	
pivampicillin (Canada only)	Pondocillin	40 to 60 mg/kg/day divided in 2 doses (<1 year) 35 mg/kg/day divided in 2 doses up to 500 mg 2 times a day (≤10 years)
Cephalosporins		
cefaclor*	generics	40 mg/kg/day
	Ceclor	
cefdinir	Omnicef	7 mg/kg/dose for 5 to 10 days or 14 mg daily for 10 days
	Not available	
cefixime	Suprax	8 mg/kg/day in 1 to 2 doses
	Suprax	
cefpodoxime*	Vantin	10 mg/kg/day every 12 hours for 5 day (max. 400 mg/day) [2 months to 12 yr]
	Not available	
cefprozi*	Cefzil	15 mg/kg every 12 hours for 10 days [6 months to 12 years]
	Cefzil	
ceftibuten	Cedax	9 mg/kg/day for 10 days (<12 years)
	Not available	
cefuroxime*	Ceftin	30 mg/kg/day divided in 2 doses for 10 days up to 250 mg 2 times a day
	Ceftin	
cephalexin*	Keflex	75 mg to 100 mg/kg/day in 4 divided doses
	Keflex	

Selected Antiinfectives Used to Treat Otitis Media—cont'd

Generic name	US Brand name(s) Canadian Brand name(s)	Usual child dosage
Sulfonamides		
sulfisoxizole + erythromycin ethylsuccinate*	Pediazole ———————————— Pediazole	150 mg/kg/day sulfisoxazole + 50 mg/kg/day erythromycin divided in 4 doses for 10 days
sulfamethoxazole (SMX) + trimethoprim (TMP)*	Septra, Septra DS Bactrim, Bactrim DS Sulfatrim, Sulfatrim DS ———————————— generics	40 mg SMX + 8 mg TMP/kg/day in 2 divided doses

*Generic available.

CHAPTER SUMMARY

- Blepharitis is a chronic eye disease that produces distinctive flaky scales on the eyelids and eyelashes.
- Blepharitis is self-treated by applying clean warm compresses, but in some cases antiinfective ointments, corticosteroid eye drops, and artificial tears may be administered to manage the symptoms.
- Conjunctivitis (pink eye) may be caused by a virus or bacteria.
- Uveitis is treated with the administration of corticosteroids (to reduce inflammation), mydriatics (to reduce painful swelling), and antiinfectives or antivirals as appropriate.
- Microbial keratitis and fungal keratitis are most commonly caused by trauma, immunodeficiency, and chronic eye surface diseases.
- Soft contact lens wearers, especially those who wear their contact lenses overnight, are at risk for fungal keratitis.
- A stye is a small, painful lump on the lid that is caused by an acute self-limiting infection of the oil glands of the eyelid.
- Cytomegalovirus (CMV) retinitis is an opportunistic infection in the eye that occurs in patients who have HIV infection/AIDS or who take immunosuppressive drugs.
- CMV retinitis can lead to blindness.
- Cytomegalovirus retinitis is treated by administration of antivirals such as ganciclovir, valganciclovir, foscarnet, and cidofovir.
- Herpetic corneal disease is the cause of more than 500,000 cases of blindness annually.
- Herpes virus lives around nerve fibers and, when activated, produces painful symptoms.
- Symptoms of herpes zoster ophthalmicus are swelling and rash or sores around the eye, lids, or forehead.
- Symptoms of herpes simplex keratitis are excessive tearing, decreased vision, gritty feeling in the eye, and pain when looking at bright light.
- Herpes zoster ophthalmicus and herpes simplex keratitis are treated by administering antiviral eye drops and/or orally administered drugs.
- Ocular toxoplasmosis is caused by protozoa and is transmitted by handling or eating raw and undercooked meat or by handling cat feces.
- Toxoplasmosis can cause ocular inflammation, vasculitis, uveitis, and retinal edema and is treated by administering pyramethamine and sulfonamides (sulfadiazine and trimethoprim + sulthamethoxazole).
- Helminthes are parasitic worms that can cause eye infections and blindness.
- Onchonoceriasis (river blindness) is caused by a roundworm and is the second leading cause of infectious blindness in the world.
- Onchonoceriasis is treated by administering a single dose of ivermectin yearly.
- Cysticercosis is transmitted to humans who eat poorly cooked pork.
- Cysticercosis is treated with praziquantal, corticosteroids, and surgical removal of the living worms.

- Toxocariasis is the fifth cause of uveitis worldwide.
- Toxocariasis is treated by administering topical corticosteroids and systemic antihelminthics such as thiobendazole.
- Otitis externa is inflammation of the external auditory canal and is most commonly caused by a bacterial infection.
- Risk factors for development of otitis externa are (1) exposure to excessive moisture (swimming, humidity, sweating); (2) high environmental temperature; (3) irritation caused by earwax removal; (4) insertion of objects into the ear; and (5) chronic dermatological disease.
- Otitis media is an inflammation in the middle ear.
- Excessive use of antiinfective agents to treat otitis media may increase the risk of development of bacterial resistance.

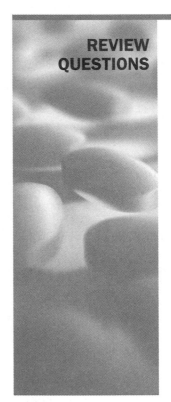

REVIEW QUESTIONS

Multiple Choice

1. A common, self-limiting ailment that causes itching, burning, and teary outflow is _____.
   a. blepharitis
   b. conjunctivitis
   c. iriditis
   d. keratitis

2. Otitis media is an inflammation in the _____ ear.
   a. inner
   b. outer
   c. middle
   d. cochlea

3. Keratitis is a severe infection of the iris and may be caused by bacteria or fungi.
   a. true
   b. false

4. The medical term for "granulated eyelids" is _____.
   a. uveitis
   b. keratitis
   c. blepharitis
   d. iriditis

5. Aminoglycoside antiinfectives are used in the treatment of blepharitis and include _____.
   a. gentamicin
   b. neomycin
   c. tobramycin
   d. all of the above

6. A stye (hordeolem) is a small, painful lump located on the _____.
   a. eyelid
   b. iris
   c. conjunctiva
   d. pupil

7. Prophylactic use of _____ is ineffective in preventing otitis media.
   a. antihistamines
   b. decongestants
   c. both a and b
   d. none of the above

8. Cytomegalovirus retinitis is treated by administration of antifungals.
   a. true
   b. false

9. **The most common cause of otitis externa is _____.**
    a. viral infection
    b. bacterial infection
    c. psoriasis
    d. lupus

10. **Children are more susceptible to otitis media than adults because their eustachian tube is longer and straighter than that of an adult.**
    a. true
    b. false

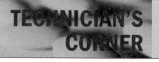
TECHNICIAN'S CORNER

1. Can putting a baby to bed with a bottle of milk contribute to otitis media?
2. Can nonsterile colored contact lenses cause eye infections?

BIBLIOGRAPHY

Ament C, Young L: Ocular manifestations of helminthic infections: onchocersiasis, cysticercosis, toxocariasis, and diffuse unilateral subacute neuroretinitis, *Int Ophthalmol Clin,* 46:1-10, 2006.

Centers for Disease Control and Prevention: Fusarium keratitis—multiple states, *MMWR Morb Mortal Wkly Rep,* 55:1-2, 2006. Retrieved from http://www.cdc.gov/mmwr/preview/mmwrhtml/mm55d410a1.htm.

Green L, Pavan-Langston D: Herpes simplex ocular inflammatory disease, *Int Ophthalmol Clin,* 46:27-37, 2006.

Health Information Center at the Cleveland Clinic: Herpetic eye disease. Retrieved from http://www.clevelandclinic.org/health/health-info/docs/3400/3433.asp?index=8861.

Koo L, Young L: Management of ocular toxoplasmosis, *Int Ophthalmol Clin,* 46:183-193, 2006.

MayoClinic.com: Iritis. Retrieved from http://www.mayoclinic.com/health/iritis/HQ00940.

MayoClinic.com: Stey. Retrieved from http://www.mayoclinic.com/health/sty/DS00257.

MEDEM Medical Library: Uveitis: a closer look, *Am Acad Ophthalmol.* Retrieved from http://www.medem.com/medlb/article_detaillb.cfm?article_ID=ZZZ622FTYIEandsub_cat=0.

National Eye Institute: *Blepharitis resource guide,* Bethesda, MD, 2006, National Institutes of Health, US Department of Health and Human Services. Retrieved from http://www.nei.nih.gov/health/blepharitis.

National Institute on Deafness and Other Communication Disorders: *Otitis media,* Bethesda, MD, 2002, NIDCD, National Institutes of Health, US Department of Health and Human Services. Retrieved from http://www.nidcd.nih.gov/health/hearing/otitism.asp.

Sander R: Otitis externa: a practical guide to treatment and prevention, *Am Fam Phys,* 63:927-936, 941-942, 2001.

US Food and Drug Administration, US Department of Health and Human Services: *Contact lenses and eye infections.* Retrieved from http://www.fda.gov/oc/opacom/hottopics/contacts.html.

Weigland T, Young L: Cytomegalovirus retinitis, *Int Ophthalmol Clin,* 46:91-110, 2006.

UNIT V

Drugs Affecting the Cardiovascular System

LEARNING OBJECTIVES

- List and describe the composition of blood.
- Describe the properties of blood cells.
- Identify the different types of white blood cells and their functions.
- Classify the different blood groups.
- Explain the Rh factor and its properties.
- Learn the terminology associated with the hematologic system.
- Demonstrate a basic knowledge of the physical structure of the heart.
- Learn and describe circulation of blood through the heart.
- Describe the conduction system of the heart.
- Describe the different types of blood vessels.

Overview of the Anatomy and Physiology of the Hematologic System

Homeostasis of the internal environment depends on continual transport of oxygen, nutrients, and biochemical messengers between the body's cells. Blood is a complex transport medium that performs vital pickup and delivery services for the body. It picks up food and oxygen from the digestive and respiratory systems and delivers them to the cells while picking up waste from the cells for delivery to the excretory organs. Blood also transports hormones, enzymes, buffers, and various other biochemical substances that serve important functions. Blood is the keystone of the body's heat-regulating mechanism and is able to absorb large quantities of heat without an appreciable increase in its own temperature, transferring it from the body's core to the surface to be dissipated.

COMPOSITION OF BLOOD

The components of blood are ***plasma*** (fluid), ***erythrocytes*** (red blood cells), ***leukocytes*** (white blood cells), and ***thrombocytes*** (platelets).

Plasma, when separated from "whole blood," is a clear straw-colored liquid that consists of about 90% water and 10% solutes. It contains many proteins such as factor VIII, which regulates blood clotting; γ-globulin, which helps a weakened immune system; and albumin, a blood volume expander. Other solutes present in smaller amounts are food substances (glucose, amino acids, and lipids), compounds formed by metabolism (urea, uric acid, creatinine, and lactic acid), respiratory gases (oxygen and carbon dioxide), and regulatory substances (hormones and enzymes).

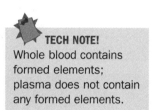

TECH NOTE!
Whole blood contains formed elements; plasma does not contain any formed elements.

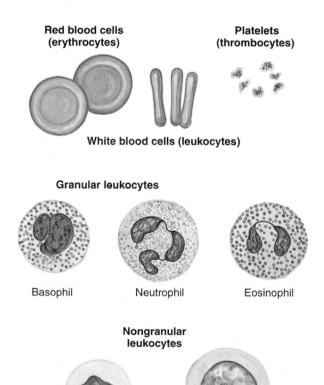

Red blood cells (erythrocytes)

Platelets (thrombocytes)

White blood cells (leukocytes)

Granular leukocytes

Basophil   Neutrophil   Eosinophil

Nongranular leukocytes

Lymphocyte   Monocyte

(From Thibodeau G, Patton K: Anatomy and physiology, *ed 6, St. Louis, 2007, Mosby.)*

RED BLOOD CELLS

Red blood cells (RBCs) are formed from stem cells in the red bone marrow in a process called *erythropoiesis*. Normal, mature RBCs have no nucleus and are shaped like biconcave discs. The primary component of each RBC is the red pigment, hemoglobin. *Hemoglobin* is made up of iron atoms. RBCs are the most numerous of the formed elements and play a critical role in the transportation of oxygen and carbon dioxide in the body. The life span of the RBC averages 105 to 120 days.

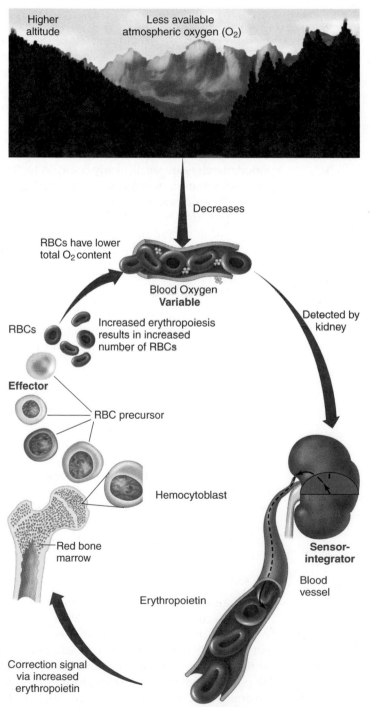

(From Thibodeau G, Patton K: Anatomy and physiology, *ed 6, St. Louis, 2007, Mosby.)*

WHITE BLOOD CELLS

White blood cells (WBCs), or *leukocytes,* are differentiated into five different types. They all have nuclei and are generally larger than RBCs. They originate in red bone marrow like erythrocytes. WBCs containing *granulocytes* are called neutrophils, eosinophils, and basophils. *Neutrophils* are highly mobile, very active phagocytic cells that can migrate out of blood vessels and enter tissue spaces. They help to fight off bacterial infections. *Eosinophils* are numerous in body areas such as the lining of the respiratory and digestive tracts and help to protect against infections caused by parasitic worms and allergic reactions. *Basophils* are the least numerous of the WBCs and are capable of migrating out of blood vessels into tissue spaces. They contain histamine (an inflammatory biochemical) and heparin (an anticoagulant).

Lymphocytes and *monocytes* are categorized as *agranulocytes* and do not contain granules. Lymphocytes are the smallest of the leukocytes and most numerous. The two types of lymphocytes, T-lymphocytes and B-lymphocytes, have an important role in immunity. T-lymphocytes function by directly attacking an infected or cancerous cell, whereas B-lymphocytes produce antibodies against specific antigens. Monocytes are the largest leukocytes. They are motile and highly phagocytic cells capable of engulfing large bacterial organisms and virus-infected cells.

PLATELETS (THROMBOCYTES)

Blood platelets are small, nearly colorless bodies that have three important physical properties: agglutination, adhesiveness, and aggregation. Platelets play an important role in *hemostasis* (the stoppage of blood flow) and coagulation (blood clotting). Within 1 to 5 seconds after injury to a blood capillary, platelets will adhere to the damaged lining of the blood vessel and to each other to form a hemostatic platelet plug that helps to stop the flow of blood into the tissues. Formation of platelets is referred to as *thrombopoeisis.* Platelets live an average of 7 days.

BLOOD VOLUME

Whole blood is about 8% of total body weight. Total blood volume is made up of 55% plasma and 45% formed elements. In females, that amounts to 4 to 5 liters, and in a male, about 5 to 6 liters. Blood volume also varies with age, body composition, and method of measurement.

BLOOD TYPES OR BLOOD GROUPS

The term *blood type* refers to the type of antigens (markers) present on RBC membranes. Antigens A, B, and Rh are the most important blood antigens as far as transfusions and newborn survival is concerned. A transfusion reaction can occur when of antigens and antibodies mix. The result is *agglutination* (clumping) of the donor and recipient blood, a potentially fatal event. Clinical laboratory tests such as blood typing and cross matching ensure proper identification of blood group antigens and antibodies in both donor and recipient blood. Every person's blood belongs to one of the four following ABO blood groups: type A—antigen A on RBCs; type B—antigen B on RBCs; type AB—both antigen A and antigen B on RBCs (universal recipients); and type O—neither antigen A nor antigen B on RBCs (universal donors).

Rh FACTOR

Blood does not normally contain anti-Rh antibodies. It can appear if an Rh-negative person has received a blood transfusion from an Rh-positive donor. The body then makes anti-Rh antibodies that stay in the blood. The other way in which Rh-positive red blood cells can enter the bloodstream of an Rh-negative person is through pregnancy. This presents danger to the baby born to an Rh-negative mother and Rh-positive father. If the baby inherits the Rh-positive trait from the father, the Rh factor may stimulate the mother's body to make anti-Rh antibodies. During a second pregnancy, if the fetus is Rh-positive, the fetus may develop a disease called *erythroblastosis fetalis.* All Rh-negative mothers who carry an Rh-positive fetus should be treated with a protein marketed as RhoGAM, which stops the mother's body from forming anti-Rh antibodies and prevents possible harm to the fetus.

BLOOD DISORDERS

Red Blood Cell Disorders

Polycythemia occurs when the bone marrow produces too many RBCs and blood becomes too thick to flow properly. Many types of anemias also affect RBCs. *Anemia* describes different disease conditions caused by the inability of the blood to carry sufficient oxygen to the body cells. *Aplastic anemia* causes an abnormally low number of RBCs; most cases result from destruction of bone marrow by drugs, toxic chemicals, or radiation and maybe even cancer. *Pernicious anemia* is characterized by a low number of RBCs and sometimes results from a dietary deficiency of vitamin B_{12}. *Folate deficiency anemia* results from a folic acid vitamin deficiency.

Blood loss anemia often occurs after a hemorrhage associated with trauma, extensive surgery, or other situation involving sudden loss of blood. ***Iron deficiency anemia*** results from an inadequate amount of iron in the diet that causes the body not to manufacture enough hemoglobin. **Hemolytic anemia** applies to a variety of inherited blood disorders characterized by an abnormal amount of hemoglobin (e.g., sickle cell anemia and thalassemia).

WHITE BLOOD CELL DISORDERS

Leukopenia is an abnormally low WBC count. The opposite of leukopenia is **leukocytosis,** an abnormally high WBC count. It is seen in most types of leukemias and nearly always accompanies bacterial infections. Blood-related cancers or malignant neoplasms constitute a majority of WBC disorders. Some examples are multiple myeloma and **leukemia**. Infectious **mononucleosis** is a common noncancerous WBC disorder that appears most often in adolescents and young adults between 15 to 25 years of age and is caused by a virus found in the saliva of infected individuals.

BONE MARROW DISORDERS

Most blood disorders are disorders of the formed elements. If the bone marrow is severely damaged, a bone marrow transplant may be offered to the patient.

CLOTTING DISORDERS

Hemophilia is an X-linked inherited disorder that affects 1 in every 10,000 males worldwide. It results from a failure to produce one or more plasma proteins responsible for blood clotting and is characterized by the inability to form blood clots. The most common form is hemophilia A (caused by an absence of factor VIII protein). Hemophiliacs can receive monthly transfusions of factor VIII to aid in blood clotting. **Thrombocytopenia** results from a deficiency in the platelet count and is characterized by bleeding from many small blood vessels throughout the body, most visibly in the skin and mucous membranes. The usual cause is bone marrow destruction by drugs, an immune system disease, or cancer. Drugs may also cause thrombocytopenia as a side effect.

Overview of the Cardiovascular System

The cardiovascular system consists of the heart and a closed system of blood vessels called **arteries, veins**, and **capillaries**. Blood contained in the circulatory system is continuously pumped by the heart around a closed circuit of vessels.

HEART

The human heart is a four-chambered muscular organ that lies in the mediastinum just behind the sternum. The heart has its own special covering. The loose-fitting sac called the ***pericardium*** is made up of two layers: the fibrous pericardium and the serous pericardium. The serous pericardium consists of two sublayers: the parietal layer and the visceral layer (***epicardium***). Between the parietal and visceral layer is a space that contains serous or pericardial fluid that helps to prevent friction as the heart beats.

> ★ **TECH NOTE!**
> Folate deficiency is linked to neural tube disorders in the fetus (e.g., spina bifida), so folic acid supplements are added to prenatal vitamins.

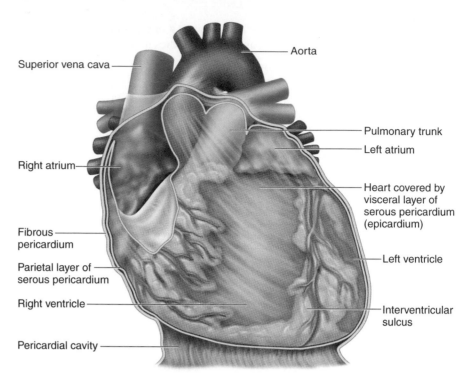

(From Thibodeau G, Patton K: Anatomy and physiology, *ed 6, St. Louis, 2007, Mosby.)*

STRUCTURE OF THE HEART

The heart wall has three distinct layers. They are the ***epicardium,*** or outer layer; the ***myocardium,*** or the middle layer and bulk of the heart wall; and the ***endocardium***. The myocardium is a muscular layer. All cardiac muscle cells can contract and produce their own slow, steady rhythm. The endocardium or the lining of the interior of the myocardial wall is made up of a delicate layer of endothelial tissue.

The interior of the heart is divided into four chambers. The two upper chambers are called ***atria.*** They receive blood from the veins. The two lower chambers are called ***ventricles*** and receive blood from the atria. Their walls are thicker than the walls of the atria because they pump blood out of the heart to the rest of the body. The heart wall is separated by a wall of muscles known as the ***interatrial septum*** and the ***interventricular septum***. Before birth, an opening is present in this wall but it closes immediately after birth when the infant takes his or her first breath. If this opening does not close, the infant will experience a mixing of deoxygenated and oxygenated blood. This condition is commonly called the "blue-baby syndrome" because the infant has too little oxygen in the blood. Infants with this condition will need surgery to correct the problem.

HEART VALVES

The heart valves are mechanical devices that permit the flow of blood in one direction only. The heart contains two sets of valves: the **atrioventricular valves** and **semilunar valves**. The bicuspid and tricuspid valves are atrioventricular valves. They guard the opening between the atria and the ventricles. They prevent the backflow of blood from the ventricle into the atria.

The pulmonary semilunar valve and the aortic semilunar valve and are located where the pulmonary artery and the aorta arise from the right and left ventricle, respectively. Their function is to prevent the flow of blood from the aorta back into the left ventricle or from the pulmonary artery back into the right ventricle.

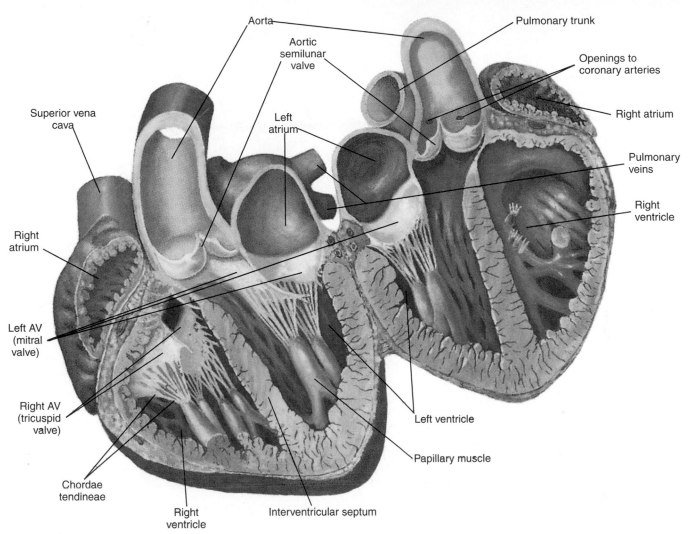

(From Thibodeau G, Patton K: Anatomy and physiology, *ed 6, St. Louis, 2007, Mosby.)*

BLOOD VESSELS

There are three major types of blood vessels in the cardiovascular system: *arteries, capillaries,* and *veins.* Arteries are larger blood vessels and carry blood away from the heart. Nearly all arteries carry oxygenated blood. The pulmonary artery is the one exception. Arterioles are smaller arteries that are important to regulate blood flow throughout the body. Capillaries are microscopic vessels that carry blood from arterioles to venules (small veins) and transfer nutrients and other vital substances between blood and tissue cells. This is the site of gas exchange in the body. Veins are blood vessels that carry blood toward the heart and contain one-way valves that prevent its potential backflow. Blood flows through smaller veins and enters progressively larger veins. All of the veins except the pulmonary vein contain deoxygenated blood.

BLOOD SUPPLY TO HEART AND THE BODY SYSTEMS

PATHWAY OF BLOOD FLOW

The flow of blood through the right and left side of the heart occurs simultaneously by the two-sided pumping action of the heart muscle, thereby providing a constant supply of blood to the heart and its accessory structures. One can trace the flow of blood on the right side (deoxygenated; indicated by the blue arrows in figure) and the left side (oxygenated; indicated by the red arrows in figure).

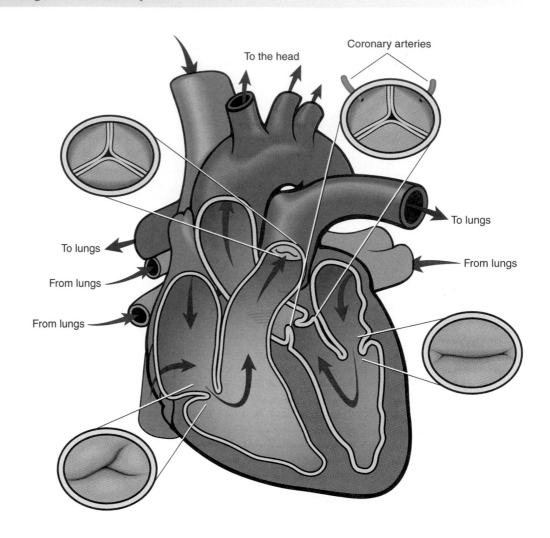

RIGHT SIDE OF THE HEART   LEFT SIDE OF THE HEART

(Modified from Damjanov I: Pathology for the health professions, *ed 3, St. Louis, 2006, WB Saunders.)*

MAJOR CIRCULATORY ROUTES IN THE BODY

Blood follows a specific pathway as it travels throughout the body. In systemic circulation, blood flows from the heart (left ventricle) through blood vessels to all parts of the body (except the lungs) and back to the heart. There are two subdivisions of systemic circulation. They are the hepatic portal and fetal circulation. In hepatic portal circulation, blood flows through systemic circulation in the abdominal cavity and then passes through the hepatic portal vein to the liver before returning to the heart. The liver detoxifies and metabolizes impurities, harmful substances, and drugs before returning the blood to systemic circulation. In the fetal circulation, fetal blood secures oxygen and food from maternal blood instead of from fetal lungs and digestive organs.

THE HEART'S BLOOD SUPPLY

The heart itself needs a constant supply of oxygen to do its work of supplying blood to the rest of the body. This is done by the ***coronary arteries***, small blood vessels that encircle the heart.

Both ventricles receive their blood supply from branches of the right and left coronary arteries. Each atrium receives blood from a small branch of the coronary artery. The most abundant blood supply goes to the myocardium of the left ventricle because the left ventricle does the most work and so needs the most oxygen and the nutrients.

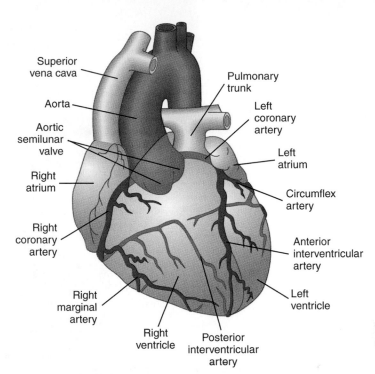

(From Thibodeau G, Patton K: Anatomy and physiology, *ed 6, St. Louis, 2007, Mosby.)*

CONDUCTION SYSTEM OF THE HEART

The conduction system of the heart is responsible to ensuring that blood is ejected out of the heart chambers in a coordinated manner that permits an effective volume of distribution of blood to be pumped from the heart to the rest of the body. Four structures make up this conduction system: the ***sinoatrial node*** or pacemaker, the ***atrioventricular node***, ***atrioventricular bundle***, and ***right and left bundle branches***.

CONDUCTION PATHWAY

The main specialty of cardiac muscle is contraction, which occurs as a result of conduction of nerve impulses. The impulse starts at the sinoatrial node (SA node) or pacemaker, which sets the rhythm of the heart. Next, it passes to the atrioventricular node (AV node), which lies in the right atrium along the lower part of the interatrial septum. Impulses travel down the middle of the heart through the atrioventricular bundle (bundle of His), which branches into right and left bundle branches. The bundle of His extends out to the lateral walls of the ventricles and papillary muscles, and innervates the whole heart.

DISORDERS OF THE HEART LINING, MUSCLE, AND VALVES

Rheumatic heart disease results from a delayed inflammatory response to streptococcal infection and occurs most often in children. ***Endocarditis*** is inflammation of the inner lining of the heart caused by a bacterial infection, and ***pericarditis*** is inflammation of the pericardium surrounding the heart. ***Mitral valve prolapse*** is a condition affecting the bicuspid or mitral valve that causes the valves to not close properly. Backflow of blood occurs from the left ventricle into the left atrium and results in turbulence, causing an "extra" heartbeat termed a *heart murmur.* ***Cardiomyopathy*** involves a number of different types of heart diseases that cause abnormal enlargement of the heart.

DISORDERS OF BLOOD VESSELS

Arteriosclerosis results from a loss of elasticity of blood vessels. ***Peripheral vascular disease*** decreases circulation to peripheral tissues such as the hands, lower legs, or feet and results in ischemia. Damage to the arterial wall can lead to the formation of an aneurysm. An ***aneurysm*** is a section of an artery that has become abnormally widened because

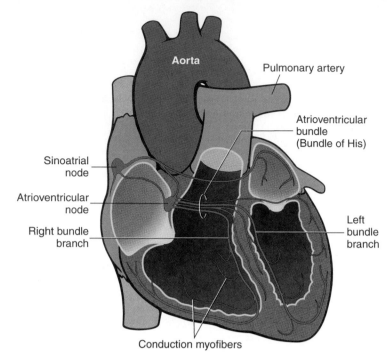

Aorta

Pulmonary artery

Atrioventricular
bundle
(Bundle of His)

Sinoatrial
node

Atrioventricular
node

Left
bundle
branch

Right bundle
branch

Conduction myofibers

(From Chabner E: The language of medicine, *ed 8, St. Louis, 2007, Saunders.)*

of the weakening in the wall. Aneurysms can be dangerous because they can rupture and cause hemorrhaging that may result in death. ***Varicose veins*** are a disorder in which the veins become enlarged and cause the blood to pool in them rather than continue toward the heart. Varicose veins of the anal canal are called ***hemorrhoids*** and may be caused by excessive straining during defecation. Several factors can cause ***phlebitis***, or vein inflammation. An example is irritation caused by an intravenous catheter. ***Thrombophlebitis*** is caused by blood clots in the veins. A clot that is formed in a deep vein is known as ***deep vein thrombosis (DVT),*** and it usually occurs in the lower legs. ***Raynaud disease*** is marked by intense constriction and vasospasm of arterioles and may be secondary to some other, more serious disorder.

BIBLIOGRAPHY

Chabner E: *The language of medicine,* ed 8, St. Louis, 2007, Saunders.
Patton K: *Survival guide for anatomy and physiology,* St. Louis, 2006, Mosby.
Thibodeau G, Patton K: *Anatomy and physiology,* ed 6, St. Louis, 2007, Mosby.

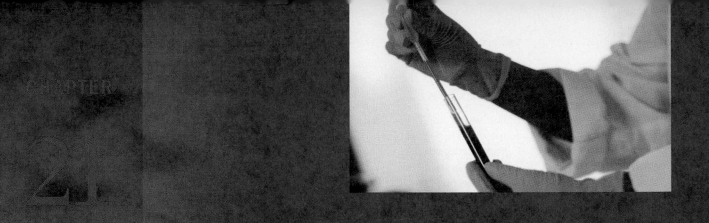

Treatment of Angina

LEARNING OBJECTIVES

- Learn the terminology associated with the treatment of angina.
- Explain the role of coronary artery disease in the development of angina.
- List the symptoms of angina.
- List risk factors for angina.
- Identify lifestyle changes that reduce the risk for angina.
- List and categorize medications used to treat angina.
- Describe mechanism of action for each classification of drugs used to treat angina.
- Identify warning labels and precautionary messages associated with medications used to treat angina.
- Identify significant drug look-alike/sound-alike issues.
- List common endings for drug classes used in the treatment of angina.

KEY TERMS

Angina pectoris: Symptomatic manifestation of ischemic heart disease characterized by a severe squeezing or pressure-like chest pain and brought on by exertion or stress.

Arteriosclerosis: Thickening and loss of elasticity of arterial walls; sometimes called "hardening of the arteries."

Atheromas: Hard plaque formed within an artery.

Atherosclerosis: Process in which plaques (atheromas) containing cholesterol, lipid material, and lipophages are formed within arteries.

Coronary artery disease: Condition that occurs when the arteries that supply blood to the heart muscle become hardened and narrowed.

Hyperlipidemia: Increased concentration of cholesterol and triglycerides in the blood that is associated with the development of atherosclerosis.

Ischemia: Deficient blood supply to an area of the body. Myocardial ischemia results in angina and myocardial infarction.

Ischemic heart disease: Any condition in which heart muscle is damaged or works inefficiently because of an absence or relative deficiency of its blood supply.

Necrosis: Cell death that may be caused by lack of blood and oxygen to the affected areas.

Plaque: Hardened lipid streak within an artery formed by deposits of cholesterol, lipid material, and lipophages.

Thrombus: Stationary blood clot.

Vasospasm: Spasms that constrict blood vessels and reduce the flow of blood and oxygen.

Overview

The word "angina" is derived form the Latin word *ango,* which means "to choke." This is an apt description of the symptoms of angina, which are described as severe squeezing or pressure-like chest pain, sometimes radiating to the arms, shoulders, neck, or jaw. The pain is sometimes described as severe heartburn or indigestion. *Angina* is a symptom of *ischemic heart disease*. Ischemia is caused by loss of blood supply to a region of the body.

Based on the 2000/2001 Canadian Community Health Survey (CCHS) data, it was estimated that among the 5% of Canadians 12 years of age and older who have heart disease, 1.9% have angina. In the United States, more than 6 million people have angina according to the National Institutes of Health (2006). Although people with a history of heart disease, hypertension, and diabetes are at risk for angina, lifestyle is also a significant risk for the condition. In fact, angina is often classified as a chronic disease of lifestyle because many of the risks for developing the condition are related to lifestyle. Risk factors associated with lifestyle include smoking, overeating, diet high in cholesterol and salt, excessive alcohol consumption, obesity, and lack of exercise. Stress is also a risk factor for angina.

High dietary cholesterol is a contributing factor for the development of coronary artery disease and causes myocardial ischemia. Cholesterol, lipid material, and lipophages are deposited within arteries. The lipid streaks harden into plaques (*atheromas*); this process is called *atherosclerosis*. An atheroma can increase in size and reduce blood flow and has the potential to result in a thrombosis formation (Figure 21-1). Thrombi can further occlude the artery in which it was formed. A thrombus that breaks off is called an emboli; it can travel to a smaller artery, where it completely occludes the blood vessel, causing ischemia. Prolonged ischemia can result in a tissue *necrosis* (death), leading to myocardial infarction (heart attack) or stroke.

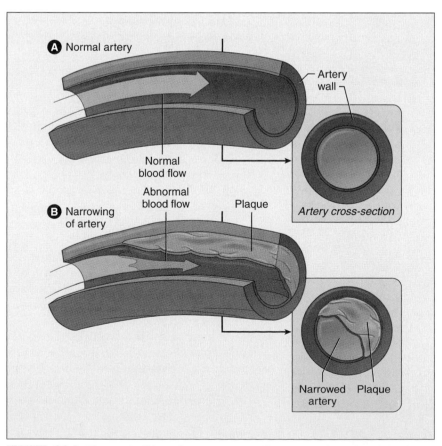

FIGURE 21-1 Plaque build-up in an artery. *(Courtesy of National Institutes of Health Bethesda, MD.)*

TYPES OF ANGINA

There are three types of angina, which vary according to their pattern and ability to be relieved by medication. They are called stable angina, unstable angina, and variant or vasospastic angina. In all types of angina, there is an imbalance between blood supplied to the heart muscle and the need for blood and oxygen. The symptoms of angina occur when the blood supplied to the heart is insufficient to meet the heart's need for oxygen (Figure 21-2).

STABLE (EXERTIONAL) ANGINA

Symptoms of stable angina are typically brought on by physical exertion, smoking, eating heavy meals, exposure to extreme changes in temperature (hot or cold), and emotional stress. Physical exertion is the most common reason for the onset of angina. Whereas the amount of blood and oxygen that is supplied to the heart meets its needs under typical conditions, it is insufficient during periods of exercise. Rest and antianginal medications adequately treat the acute symptoms of stable angina. Symptoms often subside within 5 minutes.

UNSTABLE ANGINA

Unstable angina may occur at rest, without physical exertion, and may result when an embolus partially or completely occludes an artery. Myocardial ischemia causes the symptoms of pain and chest pressure. Unstable angina is a serious condition requiring medical evaluation because it may precede a myocardial infarction. Symptoms are not relieved by rest or antianginal medicine and may last for up to 30 minutes.

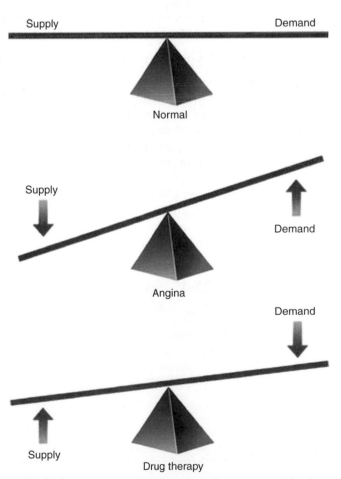

FIGURE 21-2 Imbalance between oxygen (O_2) need and blood supply. *(From Lilley LL, Harrington S, Snyder JS: Pharmacology and the nursing process, ed 5, St Louis, 2007, Mosby.)*

VARIANT ANGINA

Variant angina is also known as vasospastic angina because it is caused by vasospasm of the coronary arteries. Spasms reduce the opening of the artery, thereby decreasing the blood supply and oxygen to the heart. Like unstable angina, it occurs at rest and during the night or early morning. Unlike unstable angina, it is relieved by antianginal medicines. Symptoms often persist longer than stable angina and may exceed 5 minutes.

Nonpharmacological Treatment of Angina

LIFESTYLE CHANGE

Change in modifiable lifestyle practices is an important part of the treatment and prevention of angina and other cardiovascular diseases. Lifestyle changes can reduce the risk for angina as well as decrease the frequency and severity of symptoms and prevent or slow the progression of angina to myocardial infarction or death.

We may not be able to limit our exposure to stressful situations, but we can control the volume of food we consume, and lose weight if necessary. Increasing our level of daily activity, while avoiding overexertion, is another modifiable lifestyle change that we can make. If you smoke, you should quit.

Other lifestyle changes that should be implemented if possible include
- Taking frequent rest breaks if necessary, to avoid angina that is caused by exertion
- Avoiding foods high in salt and cholesterol
- Eating small portions rather than a heavy meal
- Learning techniques to manage stress
- Being an advocate for workplace and community-wide changes that facilitate lifestyle change (such as nutritious food choices in school and workplace cafeterias)

Drugs Used in the Treatment of Angina

Drugs used in the treatment of angina are administered to increase the blood and oxygen supply to the heart and to decrease the workload of the heart. The mechanisms of action of the drugs are varied. Increased blood supply can be accomplished by dilating blood vessels or by reducing vasospasms. When the workload of the heart is reduced, the demand for oxygen decreases. Reduction in cardiac workload is achieved by reducing heart rate.

The current focus of drug therapy for angina has shifted to emphasize reduction in cardiovascular events by treatment and prevention of cardiovascular diseases that often accompany angina. Previously, treatment was focused primarily on treatment and prevention of acute symptoms. Drugs may be administered to persons who have angina to treat comorbid conditions such as hypertension (see Chapter 22), hyperlipidemia, atherosclerosis, atherothrombosis, and myocardial infarction (see Chapter 24) (Table 21-1).

TABLE 21-1   Summary of Drug Categories Used in the Treatment of Angina and Comorbid Conditions

Drug classification	Acute use	Prevent angina	Comorbid conditions (hypertension, hyperlipidemia, myocardial infarction, etc.)
Nitrates	√	√	Hypertension, myocardial infarction
β-Adrenergic blockers		√	Hypertension
Calcium channel blockers		√	Hypertension
ACE Inhibitors		√	Hypertension, myocardial infarction
Anticoagulants, antiplatelet, glycoprotein IIb-IIIa		√	Myocardial infarction
Antihyperlipidemics		√	Myocardial infarction

NITRATES

The organic nitrates are the oldest class of drugs used to treat acute symptoms of angina. They dilate blood vessels (arteries and veins) and increase supply of oxygen to the heart. Nitrates that are commonly used in the treatment and prevention of angina are nitroglycerin, isosorbide dinitrate, and isosorbide mononitrate. Nitrates are also indicated for the treatment of congestive heart failure (intravenous), pulmonary hypertension, and hypertensive emergencies.

MECHANISM OF ACTION

Nitrates act to dilate veins, reduce heart muscle tension, and decrease oxygen demand (Figure 21-3). Most nitrates are prodrugs. They are converted in the body to nitrous oxide. Nitrous oxide acts at the cellular level to activate the enzyme guanylyl cyclase and inhibit protein kinases (cGMP PK). Inhibition of cGMP PK blocks the opening of voltage-gated calcium channels. Reduced intracellular calcium causes decreased actin/myosin combining and results in blockade of muscle contraction, relaxing blood vessels.

Nitrates relax and dilate medium- to large-size coronary arteries and veins. This increases oxygen to the heart. Nitrates produce venodilation, which decreases cardiac preload (reduces fluid back up in the ventricles) and the work needed to pump blood out of the ventricles. In the case of obstruction of a coronary artery, nitrates may cause the dilation of adjacent arteries, shifting blood supply away for the blocked region.

PHARMACOKINETICS

Nitrates are formulated for a variety of dosage delivery systems. Nitroglycerin dosage forms (Figure 21-4) include parenteral, sublingual tablets, buccal tablets, lingual spray, oral tablets and capsules, ointments, and transdermal patches. Some dosage delivery systems are designed to deliver nitroglycerin quickly and are used to treat acute symptoms. These include parenteral solution, sublingual tablets, and lingual spray. The other dosage forms of nitroglycerin deliver medication over an extended period (up to 24 hours) and are intended to prevent symptoms of angina.

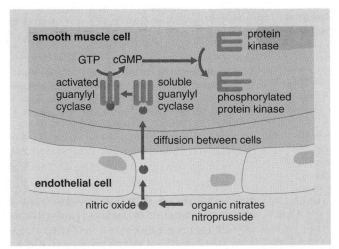

FIGURE 21-3 Mechanism of action of nitrates. *(From Page C, et al. Integrated pharmacology, ed 3, Philadelphia, 2006, Mosby.)*

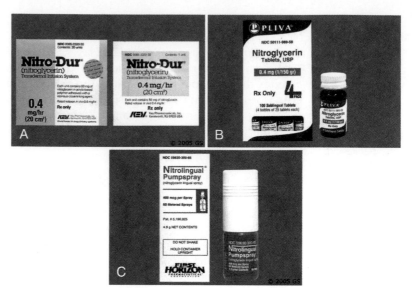

FIGURE 21-4 Nitroglycerin dosage forms. *(Drug photos provided by Gold Standard.)*

Nitroglycerin is lipid soluble and readily crosses cell membranes. It is subject to extensive first-pass metabolism, and only 10% of an oral dose is available to produce effect. This explains why parenteral and sublingual dosage forms produce actions more quickly and are more potent than enteral dosage forms (capsules, tablets).

Nitroglycerin is volatile and loses its potency on exposure to air, light, and moisture. Potency can also be lost if it is repackaged in plastic prescription vials. Nitroglycerin is packaged by manufacturers in amber glass bottles and should be dispensed in the manufacturer's original container.

Isosorbide dinitrate is formulated for acute use (sublingual and chewable tablets) and prevention (extended action tablets). Isosorbide mononitrate is not used to treat acute symptoms. It is the long-acting metabolite of isosorbide dinitrate. Isosorbide dinitrate and isosorbide mononitrate are more stable than nitroglycerin and do not need to be dispensed in the manufacturer's original container.

ADVERSE REACTIONS

Some of the adverse reactions to nitrates are dosage form dependent and other effects are common regardless the dosage delivery system. Adverse reactions associated with vasodilation are the most common and include hypotension, facial flushing, dizziness, and headache. Nausea and vomiting, weakness, and fatigue are additional side effects produced by nitroglycerin, isosorbide dinitrate, and isosorbide mononitrate. Sublingual dosage forms can cause stinging or burning under the tongue, and adhesives used in patches can produce allergic reactions.

PRECAUTIONS

Patients who use nitrates can develop tolerance to their effects. This means the drug actions are less effective over time. Tolerance is most common with long-acting nitrates. To minimize the risk for development of tolerance, it is important to avoid continuous exposure to the drug. Transdermal patches are designed to deliver their effects for 24 hours; however, the patch should never be worn for the entire 24-hour period. Patient should be instructed to remove the patch after 10 to 12 hours. The patient must be nitrate free for at least 10 to 12 hours per day (Table 21-2).

TABLE 21-2 Comparative Pharmacokinetics of Nitrates

Drug name	Dosage form	Acute use	Prevent angina	Additional use	Onset (min)	Duration (hr)
Isosorbide Dinitrate						
Dilatrate SR	Capsule, extended release		√		60	12
Isordil	Chewable		√	CHF, MI (adjunct)	2 to 5	1 to 2
Isordil	Sublingual	√		CHF, MI (adjunct)	2 to 5	1 to 2
Isordil	Tablet, immediate acting		√	CHF, MI (adjunct)	15 to 40	4 to 6
Isochron	Tablet, long acting		√		60	12
Isosorbide Mononitrate						
Imdur, Ismo, Monoket	Tablet, long acting		√		30 to 60	6 to 12
Nitroglycerin						
nitroglycerin	Injection	√		High Blood Pressure	Instant	Minutes (dose dependent)
NitroQuick, Nitrostat, Nitro-Tab	Sublingual	√		CHF, MI (adjunct)	1 to 3	½ to 1
Nitrolingual	Translingual spray	√		CHF, MI (adjunct)	2 to 4	3 to 5
Nitro-Time	Capsule, extended release		√		60	8 to 12
Nitrogard	Tablet, buccal long acting		√		2 to 3	3 to 5
Nitro-Bid	Ointment		√	CHF, MI (adjunct)	30 to 60	7 to 12
Minitran, Nitrek, Nitro-Dur	Patch		√	MI (adjunct)	30 to 60	24

Dosage Forms and Strengths of Nitrates Used in the Treatment of Angina

	Generic name	U.S. brand name(s) / Canadian brand(s)	Dosage forms and strengths
	isosorbide dinitrate*	Dilatrate-SR, Isochron, Isordil ——— Cedogard-SR	**Capsule, sustained release (Dilatrate-SR):** 40 mg **Tablet, immediate release:** 5 mg (Isordil), 10 mg, 20 mg, 30 mg, 40 mg (Isordil) **Tablet, extended release (Isochron):** 40 mg **Tablet, sublingual (Isordil):** 2.5 mg, 5 mg
	isosorbide mononitrate*	Imdur, Ismo, Monoket ——— Imdur	**Tablet (Ismo, Monoket):** 10 mg, 20 mg **Tablet, extended release (Imdur):** 30 mg, 60 mg, 120 mg

Continued

Dosage Forms and Strengths of Nitrates Used in the Treatment of Angina—cont'd

	Generic name	U.S. brand name(s) / Canadian brand(s)	Dosage forms and strengths
	nitroglycerin*	Minitran, Nitro-Bid, Nitro-Dur, Nitrol-lingual, NitroQuick, Nitrostat, NitroTime Minitran, Nitro-Dur, Nitrolingual, Nitrostat, Transderm-Nitro	**Capsule, extended release (Nitro-Time):** 2.5 mg, 6 mg, 9 mg **Infusion (premixed in D_5W):** 0.1 mg/ml, 0.2 mg/ml, and 0.4 mg/ml **Injection, solution:** 5 mg/ml **Ointment (Nitro-Bid):** 2% **Tablet, buccal, extended release (Nitrogard):** 2 mg, 3 mg **Tablet, sublingual (NitroQuick, Nitrostat, Nitro-Tab):** 0.3 mg (gr1/200), 0.4 mg (gr1/150), 0.6 mg (gr1/100) **Transdermal patch (Minitran, Nitrek, Nitro-Dur, Transderm Nitro):** 0.1 mg/hr (5 cm²), 0.2 mg/hr (10 cm²), 0.3 mg/hr (15 cm²), 0.4 mg/hr (20 cm²), 0.6 mg/hr, 0.8 mg (40 cm²) **Translingual spray (Nitrolingual):** 0.4 mg/spray (200 sprays/canister)

*Generic available.

TECH ALERT!
The following drugs have look-alike/sound-alike issues: atenolol, albuterol, and timolol; Tenormin, Norpramin, and thiamine; metoprolol, metolazone, metaproterenol, and misoprostal; Toprol-XL and Topamax; Corgard, Coreg, and Cognex; Inderal, Isordil, Toradol, Imdur, Adderall, Enduron, Enduronyl, Inderal LA, and Inderide

TECH NOTE!
β-Adrenergic blockers are easily identified because their generic name ends in "-olol."

TECH NOTE!
Calcium channel blockers (CCBs) are easily identified because their generic name ends in "-dipine."

β-ADRENERGIC BLOCKERS

Angina pectoris occurs when there is an imbalance between the heart's demand for oxygen and the oxygen supply (see Figure 21-2). β-Adrenergic blockers are administered to reduce the heart's demand for oxygen. This is achieved by decreasing the heart rate and thereby reducing the workload of the heart. β-Adrenergic blockers are also indicated for the management of hypertension and post myocardial infarction (see Chapters 22 and 24) and for the prevention of migraine headache (see Chapter 11).

MECHANISM OF ACTION

β-Adrenergic blockers decrease the frequency and severity of stable (exertional) angina. They bind to β-receptor sites and block activity of the sympathetic nervous system on cardiac smooth muscle. Heart contractility is reduced and heart rate is slowed, thereby reducing the workload of the heart. When the heart works less, its need for oxygen and blood supply is reduced.

β-Adrenergic blocking drugs, used to treat stable angina, include cardioselective β₁-adrenergic blockers and nonselective mixed β₁/β₂ blockers. (More discussion is found in Chapter 22.)

PHARMACOKINETICS

β-Adrenergic blockers are formulated in immediate- and long-acting dosage forms. The elimination half-life varies for specific agents and ranges from as short as 3 to 4 hours (propranolol) to as long as 24 hours (nadolol). Most agents are dosed once to twice a day except short-acting propranolol, which is dosed 2 to 4 times a day.

ADVERSE REACTIONS

β-Adrenergic blockers can produce dizziness, fatigue, bradycardia, hypotension, impotence, heart block, and occasionally insomnia. β-Adrenergic blockers can produce bronchospasm, so their use is contraindicated in persons with asthma. The use of β-adrenergic blockers is also contraindicated in persons with diabetes because their action to decrease heart rate masks one of the principal signs of hypoglycemia. Abrupt discontinuation of β-adrenergic blockers should be avoided as this can produce tachycardia and a sudden increase in the workload of the heart.

β-ADRENERGIC BLOCKERS USED IN THE TREATMENT OF ANGINA

β-Adrenergic Blockers

Generic name	U.S. brand name(s) Canadian brand(s)	Dosage forms and strengths
atenolol*	Tenormin	**Injection, solution:** 0.5 mg/ml mg (10 ml) **Tablet:** 25 mg, 50 mg, 100 mg
	Tenormin	
metoprolol*	Lopressor, Toprol-XL	**Injection, solution:** 1 mg/ml (5 ml) **Tablet (Lopressor):** 25 mg, 50 mg, 100 mg **Tablet, extended release (Toprol-XL):** 25 mg, 50 mg, 100 mg, 200 mg
	Betaloc, Lopressor,	
nadolol*	Corgard	**Tablet:** 20 mg, 40 mg, 80 mg, 120 mg, 160 mg
	generics	
propranolol*	Inderal, Inderal-LA, InnoPran XL	**Capsule, extended release (InnoPran XL):** 80 mg, 120 mg **Capsule, sustained release (Inderal LA):** 60 mg, 80 mg, 120 mg, 160 mg **Injection, solution (Inderal):** 1 mg/ml **Solution, oral:** 4 mg/ml **Tablet, extended release (Inderal):** 10 mg, 20 mg, 40 mg, 60 mg, 80 mg
	Inderal-LA	

*Generic available.

CALCIUM CHANNEL BLOCKERS

Calcium channel blockers are used in the treatment of variant and stable angina. They are effective in the treatment of variant angina because of their ability to reduce vasospasms that restrict the flow of blood and oxygen. In stable angina, they improve exercise tolerance by decreasing heart rate and the force of contraction of heart muscle. This decreases the workload of the heart. Calcium channel blockers are also effective in the treatment of stable angina alone and in combination with nitrates or β-blockers.

MECHANISM OF ACTION

Calcium channel blockers block L-type voltage-dependent calcium channels, suppress depolarization, and reduce contraction of the heart muscle. There are three classes of Ca^{2+} channel blockers: dihydropyridines (nifedipine, nicardipine, nimodipine), phenylalkylamines (verapamil), and benzothiazepines (diltiazem).

Phenylalkylamines and benzothiazepines reduce heart oxygen consumption during exercise by decreasing heart rate and heart contractions. Dihydropyridines are selective for blood vessels, so they are able to increase blood and oxygen supply without slowing heart rate or contractions or increasing the risk of heart block.

ADVERSE REACTIONS

Some adverse drug reactions are common to all calcium channel blockers, while other side effects are specific to drug classification. All calcium channel blockers produce hypotension, skin rash, and effects on heart rate. Dihydropyridines (e.g., nifedipine) cause adverse effects associated with vasodilation: dizziness, flushing, and tachycardia. Peripheral edema is caused by venodilation. Phenylalkylamines and benzothiazepines (e.g., diltiazem) can produce congestive heart failure (CHF), bradycardia, and constipation. Diltiazem slows conduction through the atrioventricular node and can cause heart block.

TECH ALERT!
Norvasc, Norvir, and Vasocor;
amlodipine and amiloride;
Cardizem, Cardura, Cardene, Cardizem SR, Cardene SR, and Cardizem CD;
Tiazac, Tigan, and Ziac
nicardipine, nifedipine, and nimodipine;
Procardia, Procardia XL, and Cartia XT;
Covera HS and Provera; Veralan, verapamil, and Volteran

CALCIUM CHANNEL BLOCKERS USED IN THE TREATMENT OF ANGINA

Calcium Channel Blockers (CCBs)

	Generic name	U.S. brand name(s) / Canadian brand(s)	Dosage forms and strengths
	amlodipine*	Norvasc	**Tablet:** 2.5 mg, 5 mg, 10 mg
		Norvasc	
	diltiazem*	Cardizem, Cardizem CD, Cardizem LA, Cartia XT, Dilacor XR, Diltia XT, Taztia XT, Tiazac	**Capsule, extended release (Cardizem CD, Cartia XT, Dilacor XR, Diltia XT, Taztia XT, Tiazac):** 180 mg, 240 mg, 300 mg, 360 mg
		Cardizem, Cardizem CD, Tiazac Tiazac XC	**Capsule, sustained release (Cardizem SR):** 60 mg, 90 mg, 120 mg
			Injection, solution: 5 mg/ml (5 ml, 10 ml)
			Injection, powder for reconstitution (Cardizem): 25 mg
			Tablet, immediate release (Cardizem): 30 mg, 60 mg, 90 mg, 120 mg
			Tablet, extended release (Cardizem LA): 120 mg, 180 mg, 240 mg, 300 mg, 360 mg, 420 mg
	nicardipine*	Cardene, Cardene SR	**Capsule (Cardene):** 20 mg, 30 mg
		Not available	**Capsule, sustained release (Cardene SR):** 30 mg, 45 mg, 60 mg
			Injection, solution: 2.5 mg/ml
	nifedipine*	Adalat CC, Afeditab CR, Nifediac CC , Nifedical XL , Procardia, Procardia XL	**Capsule, liquid filled (Procardia):** 10 mg
			Tablet, extended release (Adalat CC, Nifediac CC , Procardia XL): 30 mg, 60 mg, 90 mg
		Adalat XL	**(Afeditab CR, Nifedical XL):** 30 mg, 60 mg
	verapamil*	Calan, Calan SR, Covera HS, Isoptin SR, Verelan, Verelan PM	**Caplet, sustained release (Calan SR):** 120 mg, 180 mg, 240 mg
		Covera HS, Isoptin, Isoptin Inj, Isoptin SR, Verelan	**Capsule, extended release (Verelan PM):** 100 mg, 200 mg, 300 mg
			Capsule, sustained release (Verelan): 120 mg, 180 mg, 240 mg, 360 mg
			Injection, solution: 2.5 mg/ml (2 ml, 4 ml)
			Tablet, immediate release (Calan): 40 mg, 80 mg, 120 mg
			Tablet, extended release (Covera HS): 180 mg, 240 mg
			Tablet, sustained release (Isoptin SR): 120 mg, 180 mg, 240 mg

*Generic available.

Summary of Drugs Used in the Treatment of Angina

	Generic	Brand	Usual dose	Warning labels
Nitrates				
	isosorbide dinitrate	Isordil	**Angina:** 5 mg to 40 mg 4 times a day or 40 mg SR every 8 to 12 hours	TAKE ON AN EMPTY STOMACH— isosorbide dinitrate SWALLOW WHOLE; DON'T CRUSH OR CHEW (sustained and extended release)
	isosorbide mononitrate	Imdur	**Angina:** 5 mg to 10 mg twice a day (7 hours apart), 30 mg to 60 mg daily (extended release) up to maximum 240 mg/day	AVOID ALCOHOL
	nitroglycerin	Nitrostat	**Buccal:** 1 mg to 3 mg every 3 to 5 hours while awake **IV:** Infuse 5 mcg to 10 mcg/min every 3 to 5 minutes **Oral:** 2.5 mg to 9 mg 2 to 4 times a day (maximum 26 mg 4 times a day) **Ointment:** ½ inch (1.25 cm) twice a day (6 hours apart) **Transdermal patch:** Wear 1 patch (0.2 mg to 0.8 mg/hr) for 12 to 14 hr/day; patch off for 10 to 12 hr/day **Sublingual:** Dissolve 1 tablet sublingually as needed for chest pain. May repeat 1 tablet every 5 minutes if no relief up to 3 tablets (15 minutes) or dissolve 1 tablet sublingually 5 minutes prior to strenuous activity. **Translingual spray:** Place 1 to 2 sprays in mouth as needed for chest pain. May repeat every 5 minutes if no relief up to 3 doses (15 minutes) or use 5 to 10 minutes prior to strenuous activity.	STORE IN MANUFACTURER'S ORIGINAL CONTAINER (sublingual, capsules) REPLACE VIALS 3 to 6 MONTHS AFTER OPENING (sublingual) ROTATE SITE OF APPLICATION (transdermal patch) HOLD SPRAY IN MOUTH FOR UP TO 10 SECONDS BEFORE SWALLOWING. IF NO RELIEF OF SYMPTOMS AFTER 3 DOSES OF SUBLINGUAL TABS OR LINGUAL SPRAY (OR 15 MINUTES), CALL 911. SWALLOW WHOLE; DON'T CRUSH OR CHEW (sustained and extended release) AVOID ALCOHOL
β-Adrenergic Blockers				
	atenolol	Tenormin	**Angina:** 50 mg daily (may increase to 100 mg to 200 mg once daily)	MAY CAUSE DIZZINESS USE CAUTION WHEN DRIVING OR PERFORMING TASKS REQUIRING ALERTNESS
	metoprolol	Toprol XL	**Angina:** Start with 50 mg twice daily increasing to 100 mg to 450 mg/day in 2 to 3 divided doses OR 100 mg to 450 mg daily as a single dose (extended release)	AVOID ABRUPT DISCONTINUATION
	nadolol	Corgard	**Angina:** Begin at 40 mg/day increase to 160 mg to 240 mg once daily	TAKE WITH FOOD—metoprolol (immediate release)
	propranolol	Inderal, Inderal LA	**Angina:** 80 mg to 320 mg/day in 2 to 4 divided doses or 80 mg to 320 mg once daily (extended release)	SWALLOW WHOLE; DON'T CRUSH OR CHEW (sustained release)

Continued

Summary of Drugs Used in the Treatment of Angina—cont'd

	Generic	Brand	Usual dose	Warning labels
Calcium Channel Blockers				
	amlodipine	Norvasc	**Angina:** 5 mg to 10 mg daily	MAY CAUSE DIZZINESS
	diltiazem	Cardizem, Cardizem CD, Cardizem LA	**Extended release, caps:** 120 mg to 180 mg once daily (maximum 480 mg/day) **Extended release, tablet:** 180 mg once daily (maximum 360 mg/day) **Immediate release, tablet:** 30 mg 4 times a day (maximum 180 mg to 360 mg/day) **Sustained release, caps:** 60 mg to 120 mg twice a day	USE CAUTION WHEN DRIVING OR PERFORMING TASKS REQUIRING ALERTNESS AVOID ABRUPT DISCONTINUATION LIMIT CAFFEINE AND ALCOHOL
	nicardipine	Cardene, Cardene SR	**Immediate release:** 20 mg to 40 mg 3 times a day **Sustained release:** 30 mg to 60 mg twice daily	SWALLOW WHOLE; DON'T CRUSH OR CHEW (extended and sustained release)
	nifedipine	Procardia, Procardia XL	**Immediate release:** 10 mg to 30 mg 3 times a day **Sustained release:** 30 mg to 60 mg once daily (maximum 120 mg to 180 mg per day)	TAKE WITH FOOD—nicardipine (sustained release)
	verapamil	Calan	**Angina: (immediate release):** Begin 80 mg to 120 mg 3 times a day; may increase to 240 mg to 480 mg/day	

TECH NOTE!
Be careful when retrieving Cardizem from the shelf because of the many types of dosage forms available (XR, CD, SR).

OTHER DRUG CLASSIFICATIONS

Angiotensin-converting enzyme inhibitors (ACEIs), anticoagulants, antiplatelet drugs, glycoprotein IIb/IIIa drugs, and antihyperlipidemics may be administered to patients who have angina, especially when comorbid conditions (hypertension or myocardial infarction) are present. These drug classifications are discussed in Chapters 22 and 24.

CHAPTER SUMMARY

- Angina is a symptom of ischemic heart disease.
- The symptoms of angina are described as severe squeezing or pressure-like chest pain; sometimes radiating to the arms, shoulders, neck, or jaw.
- Angina pain is sometimes described as severe heartburn or indigestion.
- People with a history of heart disease, hypertension, and diabetes are at risk for angina; however, lifestyle is a significant risk for the condition.
- Risk factors associated with lifestyle include smoking, overeating, diet high in cholesterol and salt, excessive alcohol consumption, obesity, lack of exercise, and stress.
- Coronary artery disease causes myocardial ischemia.
- Atherosclerosis is a disease of the coronary arteries that results in the buildup of lipid streaks in arteries.
- Atherosclerosis can block the flow of blood through the artery, producing ischemia and cell death (necrosis).
- There are three types of angina (stable, unstable, and variant).
- In all types of angina, there is an imbalance between blood supplied to the heart muscle and the need for blood and oxygen.

- Symptoms of stable angina are typically brought on by physical exertion, smoking, eating heavy meals, exposure to extreme changes in temperature (hot or cold), and emotional stress.
- Unstable angina may occur at rest, without physical exertion, and results when an embolus partially or completely occludes an artery.
- Variant angina is also known as vasospastic angina because it is caused by vasospasm of the coronary arteries.
- Variant angina may occur at rest like unstable angina.
- Lifestyle changes can reduce risk, the frequency and severity of symptoms and prevent or slow the progression of angina to myocardial infarction or death.
- Recommended lifestyle changes are to (1) take frequent rest breaks, (2) avoid eating foods high in salt and cholesterol, (3) eat smaller portions, (4) learn techniques to manage stress, and (5) become an advocate for workplace and community-wide changes that facilitate lifestyle change.
- Drugs used in the treatment of angina are administered to increase the blood and oxygen supply to the heart and to decrease the workload of the heart.
- Drug therapy for angina is focused on treatment and prevention of symptoms and treatment and prevention of cardiovascular diseases that often accompany angina.
- The organic nitrates are the oldest class of drugs used to treat acute symptoms of angina. They dilate blood vessels (arteries and veins) and increase supply of oxygen to the heart.
- Nitrates that are commonly used in the treatment and prevention of angina are nitroglycerin, isosorbide dinitrate, and isosorbide mononitrate.
- Nitroglycerin is formulated for parenteral, oral, sublingual, and topical use.
- Dosage delivery systems that are designed to deliver nitroglycerin quickly are used to treat acute symptoms; they include parenteral solution, sublingual tablets, and lingual spray.
- Nitroglycerin in the form of buccal tablets, capsules, extended release tablets, patches, and ointments delivers medication over an extended period (up to 24 hours) and is intended to prevent symptoms of angina.
- Nitroglycerin is volatile and loses its potency when exposed to air, light, and moisture. It must be dispensed in the manufacturer's original container.
- Isosorbide dinitrate is formulated for acute use (sublingual and chewable tablets) and prevention (extended action tablets).
- Isorsorbide mononitrate is not used to treat acute symptoms.
- Adverse reactions of nitrates include hypotension, facial flushing, dizziness, headache, nausea and vomiting, weakness, and fatigue.
- Sublingual dosage forms can cause stinging or burning under the tongue, and adhesives used in patches can produce allergic reactions.
- To minimize the risk for development of tolerance to nitrates, it is important to have a 10- to 12-hour drug-free period each day.
- A fatal drop in blood pressure can occur when drugs used to treat erectile dysfunction (sildenafil [Viagra], vardenafil [Cialis], and tadalafil [Levitra]) are administered to patients who are taking nitroglycerin.
- β-Adrenergic blockers are easily identified because their generic name ends in *"-olol."*
- β-Adrenergic blockers decrease the heart rate and workload of the heart, thereby reducing the heart's demand for oxygen.
- β-Adrenergic blockers decrease the frequency and severity of stable (exertional) angina.
- Adverse reactions of β-adrenergic blockers are dizziness, fatigue, bradycardia, hypotension, impotence, heart block, and occasionally insomnia.
- β-Adrenergic blockers are contraindicated in patients with asthma and diabetes because they can produce bronchospasm and mask the signs of hypoglycemia.
- Abrupt discontinuation of β-adrenergic blockers should be avoided as this could produce tachycardia and a sudden increase in the workload of the heart.
- Calcium channel blockers are easily identified because their generic name ends in *"-dipine."*
- Calcium channel blockers are used in treatment of variant and stable angina.

- Calcium channel blockers reduce vasospasms and improve exercise tolerance by decreasing heart rate and the force of contraction of heart muscle.
- There are three classes of Ca^{2+} channel blockers: dihydropyridines (nifedipine, nicardipine), phenylalkylamines (verapamil), and benzotiazepines (diltiazem).
- Dihydropyridines are selective for blood vessels, so they are able to increase blood and oxygen supply without slowing heart rate or contractions or increasing the risk of heart block.

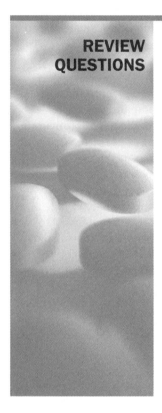

REVIEW QUESTIONS

<u>Multiple Choice</u>

1. Thickening and loss of elasticity of arterial walls that is sometimes called "hardening of the arteries" characterizes _____.
   a. atherosclerosis
   b. arteriosclerosis
   c. angiosclerosis
   d. vasosclerosis
2. People with what kind of health history are at risk for angina?
   a. heart disease
   b. hypertension
   c. diabetes
   d. all of the above
3. There are two types of angina: stable and unstable.
   a. true
   b. false
4. Which of the following is *not* true of drugs used in the treatment of angina?
   a. They are administered to increase the blood supply to the heart.
   b. They are administered to increase oxygen supply to the heart.
   c. They are administered to increase the workload of the heart.
   d. They are administered to decrease the workload of the heart.
5. The organic nitrates are the oldest class of drugs used to treat acute symptoms of angina.
   a. true
   b. false
6. Nitrates act to _____ the vein.
   a. constrict
   b. occlude
   c. dilate
   d. none of the above
7. Calcium channel blockers are used in treatment of what types of angina?
   a. variant
   b. stable
   c. unstable
   d. a and b
8. Stable angina may occur at rest, without physical exertion, and results when an embolus partially or completely occludes an artery.
   a. true
   b. false
9. The generic name for Tenormin is _____.
   a. atenolol
   b. nifedipine
   c. nadolol
   d. amlodipine

10. **Which drug must be dispensed in the manufacturer's original container?**
   a. isosorbide dinitrate
   b. isosorbide mononitrate
   c. nitroglycerin
   d. diltiazem

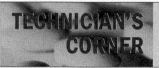

TECHNICIAN'S CORNER

1. What is the major difference between arteriosclerosis and atherosclerosis?
2. Both nitroglycerin and sildenafil have vasodilating effects on blood vessels. Why is it so important not to use these drugs at the same time?

BIBLIOGRAPHY

Chow CM, Donovan L, Manuel D, Johansen H, Tu JV: Canadian Cardiovascular Outcomes Research Team, regional variation in self-reported heart disease prevalence in Canada, *Can J Cardiol* 21:1265-1271, 2005.

Drug information online: *Nitroglycerin drug information, professional.* Retrieved from http://www.drugs.com/MMX/Nitroglycerin.html.

Fougera: *Nitro-Bid package insert.* Retrieved from http://www.fougera.com/products/documents/1114.PI.pdf#search=%22Nitro-Bid%20ointment%20duration%20of%20action%22.

Fulcher E, Soto C, Fulcher R: *Pharmacology: principles and applications: a worktext for allied health professionals* (pp 586-590). Philadelphia, 2003, Elsevier Saunders, 2003.

Kalant H, Grant D, Mitchell J: *Principles of medical pharmacology* (pp 451-453, 458-460), ed 7, Toronto, Ontario, Canada, 2007, Elsevier Canada, A Division of Reed Elsevier Canada.

Lance L, Lacy C, Armstrong L, Goldman M: *Drug information handbook for the allied health professional,* ed 12. Hudson, OH, 2005, APhA Lexi-Comp.

National Heart Lung and Blood Institute: *Angina,* Bethesda, MD, 2006, National Heart and Blood Institute, National Institutes of Health, US Department of Health and Human Services. Retrieved from http://www.nhlbi.nih.gov/health/dci/Diseases/Angina/Angina_All.html.

Page C, Curtis M, Sutter M, Walker M, Hoffman B: *Integrated pharmacology* (pp 377-383), Philadelphia, 2005, Mosby.

USP Center for Advancement of Patient Safety: *Use caution–avoid confusion,* USP Quality Review No. 79, Rockville, MD, April 2004, USP Center for Advancement of Patient Safety.

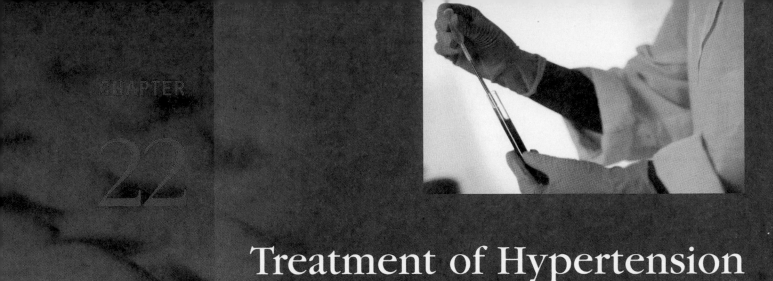

Treatment of Hypertension

**LEARNING
OBJECTIVES**

- Learn the terminology associated with the treatment of hypertension.
- Explain the role of coronary artery disease in the development of hypertension.
- List risk factors for development of hypertension.
- List complications associated with untreated or poorly controlled hypertension.
- Identify lifestyle changes that reduce the risk for hypertension.
- List and categorize medications used to treat hypertension.
- Describe mechanism of action for each class of drugs used to treat hypertension.
- Identify warning labels and precautionary messages associated with medications used to treat hypertension.
- Identify significant drug look-alike/sound-alike issues.
- List common endings for drug classes used in the treatment of hypertension.

KEY TERMS

Aldosterone: Hormone that promotes sodium and fluid reabsorption.

Angiotension II: Potent vasocontrictor that is produced when the renin-aldosterone-angiotensin system (RAAS) is activated.

Angiotensin-converting enzyme (ACE): Enzyme that catalyzes the conversion of angiotensin I to angiotensin II.

Body mass index: Measure of human body size and proportion. It is defined as the weight in kilograms divided by the square of the height in meters.

Cardiac output: Volume of blood ejected from the left ventricle in 1 minute.

Diastolic blood pressure (DBP): Measure of blood pressure when the heart is at rest (diastole).

Diuretic: Drug that produces diuresis (urination).

Gynecomastia: Painful breast enlargement in men.

Hirsutism: Excessive hair growth in women.

Hyperkalemia: Excessive serum potassium levels.

Hypokalemia: Deficient serum potassium levels.

Hypernatremia: Excessive serum sodium levels.

Hyponatremia: Deficient serum sodium levels.

Hypertension (high blood pressure): Elevated diastolic or systolic blood pressure.

Hyperuricemia: Increased uric acid levels in the blood that is produced by some diuretics and can aggravate gout.

Metabolic syndrome: Important risk factor of hypertension that promotes the development of atherosclerosis and cardiovascular disease.

Nocturia: Nighttime urination.

Orthostatic hypotension: Sudden drop in blood pressure that occurs when arising from lying down or sitting to standing.

Photosensitivity: Increased sensitivity to sun exposure that can result in sunburn.

Preeclampsia: Sudden rise in blood pressure, excessive weight gain, generalized edema, proteinuria, severe headache, and visual disturbances occurring in late pregnancy.

Prehypertension: Systolic blood pressure ranging between 120 and 139 mm Hg and diastolic blood pressure ranging between 80 and 89 mm Hg.

Peripheral vascular resistance: Resistance to the flow of blood in peripheral arterial vessels that is associated with blood vessel diameter, vessel length, and blood viscosity.

Renin-aldosterone-angiotensin system (RAAS): System that is activated when there is a drop in renal blood flow that increases blood volume, blood flow to the kidney, vasoconstriction, and blood pressure.

Systolic blood pressure (SBP): Measure of the pressure when the heart's ventricles are contracting (systole).

Blood Pressure

Blood pressure is necessary to circulate blood, oxygen (O_2), and nutrients to body organs and to remove carbon dioxide (CO_2) and waste products. Without blood pressure shock, circulatory collapse and death would result.

Blood pressure is measured using a sphygmomanometer (aneroid or mercury), or an electronic blood pressure measuring device. Two pressures are measured. They are the systolic pressure and the diastolic pressure.

$$BP = \frac{Systole}{Diastole}$$

The *systolic blood pressure (SBP)* is a measure of the pressure when the heart's ventricles are contracting (systole). The *diastolic blood pressure (DBP)* is a measure of the heart at rest (diastole).

$$Average\ normal\ blood\ pressure\ is\ \frac{120\ (systole)}{80\ (diastole)}$$

The formula for determining blood pressure is:

$$BP = CO \times PR$$

where CO is the cardiac output and PR is the peripheral resistance. Cardiac output is determined by measuring the heart rate (HR) and multiplying it by the stroke volume (volume of blood ejected by the ventricles).

Blood Pressure Control

The body sensors monitor blood flow, and when decreases are detected, regulatory mechanisms are "switched on." Sites for blood pressure control are the kidneys, heart, blood vessels, central nervous system (CNS), and sympathetic nerves.

When the kidney detects a drop in renal blood supply, the *renin-aldosterone-angiotensin-system (RAAS)* is activated (Figure 22-1). This causes levels of aldosterone (endocrine hormone) and angiotensin to rise. Aldosterone and angiotensin act to increase blood volume, blood flow to the kidney, vasoconstriction, and blood pressure.

The heart controls the *cardiac output* (the amount of blood ejected from the ventricles) by increasing or decreasing the rate of contractions. When the CNS senses a drop in blood pressure, it signals sympathetic nerves to release neurotransmitters that control

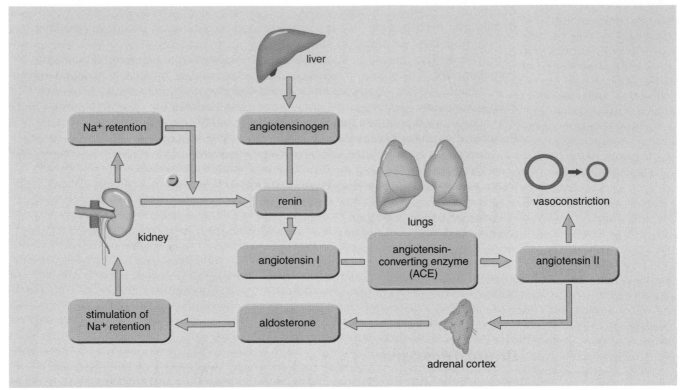

FIGURE 22-1 Renin-aldosterone-angiotensin system. *(From Page C, et al:* Integrated pharmacology, 3rd ed *Philadelphia, 2006, Mosby.)*

heart rate and blood flow through the arteries. Sympathetic nerves release norepinephrine, which causes vasoconstriction and increased peripheral vascular resistance. When ***peripheral vascular resistance*** increases, blood pressure increases. If the blood vessels lose their elasticity or if the vessel opening is narrowed, like in atherosclerosis, pressure can build, too. It is similar to a garden hose when the opening is partially closed. The water shoots out of the hose at high pressure. If blood viscosity (thickness) increases, blood pressure will also rise.

Hypertension

Hypertension is the most diagnosed medical condition in the United States, affecting more than 65 million Americans (nearly 25% of the adult population). According to Statistics Canada, more than 3 million Canadians (10% of the population) have high blood pressure. By the age of 60, 30% to 40% of people have hypertension. Diastolic hypertension is the predominant form of hypertension before age 50. Thereafter, increased DBP begins to level off. SBP increases throughout life, and after the age of 50 years, systolic hypertension is the predominant form of hypertension. It was once believed that increased SBP was benign. It is now known that SBP poses an important cardiovascular risk.

WHAT CAUSES HYPERTENSION?

In more than 90% of cases, the actual cause for hypertension is unknown, yet some risk factors for chronic elevated high blood pressure are known. ***Metabolic syndrome*** is an important risk factor of hypertension. Metabolic syndrome promotes the development of atherosclerosis and cardiovascular disease. Box 22-1 lists additional risk factors for high blood pressure.

BOX 22-1 HYPERTENSION RISK FACTORS

- Age (years) >55 in men and >65 in women
- Diabetes mellitus
- Family history of heart disease
- Metabolic syndrome
- Obesity
- Tobacco usage
- Decreased physical activity
- Increased total LDL or low HDL
- Diet high in salt and saturated fats
- Excessive alcohol consumption

BOX 22-2 DRUGS THAT CAN INCREASE BLOOD PRESSURE

- Nonsteroidal antiinflammatory drugs (COX-2 inhibitors)
- Cocaine, amphetamines
- Decongestants
- Diet pills
- Oral contraceptives
- Glucocorticosteroids (e.g., prednisone, hydrocortisone, methylprednisolone)
- Mineralocorticoids (aldosterone)
- Cyclosporine and tacrolimus
- Erythropoietin
- Licorice
- Herbals (*ma huang*, ephedra, bitter orange)

Medical conditions known to produce high blood pressure are chronic kidney disease, thyroid disease, Cushing's syndrome, and sleep apnea. Drugs may also induce high blood pressure (Box 22-2).

Blood Pressure Classifications

PREHYPERTENSION

The 7th Joint National Committee on the Prevention, Detection, Evaluation, and Treatment of High Blood Pressure defines *prehypertension* as SBP ranging between 120 and 139 mm Hg and DBP ranging between 80 and 89 mm Hg. Reduction of blood pressure to normal levels is beneficial for persons with prehypertension with and without preexisting disease. Adoption of a healthy lifestyle is often sufficient to reduce blood pressure in this population. Drug therapy should be added to the treatment program in people who have diabetes or kidney disease if lifestyle modifications do not bring blood pressure down to the normal range.

STAGE 1 HYPERTENSION

Stage 1 hypertension is classified as SBP ranging between 140 and 159 mm Hg and DBP ranging between 90 and 99 mm Hg. It should be managed with lifestyle modification and drug therapy.

STAGE 2 HYPERTENSION

Stage 2 hypertension is classified as SBP ≥160 mm Hg and DBP ≥100 mm Hg. It is the most severe stage of hypertension and should be managed with lifestyle modification and drug therapy. Two-drug combination therapy is necessary for most patients. Blood pressure greater than 180/110 mm Hg is a medical emergency and should be treated immediately.

PREECLAMPSIA AND GESTATIONAL HYPERTENSION

Hypertension during pregnancy is dangerous to the pregnant woman and the fetus. Gestational hypertension typically occurs after 20 weeks of pregnancy in susceptible women. It can progress to *preeclampsia* and cause premature delivery and fetal growth retardation. Approximately 25% of pregnant women who have chronic hypertension for more than 4 years will develop preeclampsia during pregnancy. Women with a history of gestational

TABLE 22-1   Summary of Blood Pressure Classifications

Normal	<120/80 mm Hg
Prehypertension	120 to 139/80 to 89 mm Hg
Hypertension	≥140/90 mm Hg
Stage 1	140 to 159/90 to 99 mm Hg
Stage 2	160 to 179/100 to 109 mm Hg
Stage 3	≥180/110 mm Hg

hypertension in a previous pregnancy are at risk. Preeclampsia can progress to eclampsia and cause seizures.

WHITE COAT HYPERTENSION

Some people have a condition that is known as "white coat hypertension." They have abnormally high blood pressure when the measurement is taken by a health care professional but blood pressure measurements taken in a nonclinic setting are within normal range (Table 22-1).

Complications Associated with Untreated or Poorly Controlled Hypertension

Hypertension is sometimes called the "silent killer" because it can cause damage to the body without any obvious symptoms. High blood pressure can cause damage to the kidney, heart, brain, arteries, and eyes. Hypertension can weaken arteries and cause aneurysms that can bleed and cause death if they occur in the brain, aorta, or abdomen. Hypertension can cause blindness when blood vessels to the retina are damaged and scarred. For each 20-mm Hg increase in SBP and 10-mm Hg increase in DBP, there is a 2-fold increase in risk of death due to ischemic heart disease (IHD) and stroke. This is because hypertension can damage arteries and make them stiff and thick. It can cause atherosclerosis and thrombi formation that can block the blood supply to areas of the heart and brain (see Chapter 21).

Nonpharmacological Management of Hypertension

Hypertension poses a serious public health challenge because of the risks for death and long-term disability. Hypertension is categorized as a chronic disease of lifestyle because it is associated with obesity, excess dietary sodium intake, reduced physical activity, excessive alcohol consumption, and inadequate consumption of fruits and vegetables. More than 122 million Americans are overweight and fewer than 20% engage in regular physical activity or consume adequate fruits and vegetables (5 servings per day).

Lifestyle modification is an important strategy for prevention and management of hypertension. Lifestyle changes can reduce SBP between 4 and 20 mm Hg. A reduction of as little as 5 mm Hg can lower the risk of death due to stroke by 14% and death due to coronary heart disease (CHD) by 9%. The U.S. Joint National Committee on the Prevention, Detection, Evaluation, and Treatment of High Blood Pressure recommendations for lifestyle changes are listed in Table 22-2.

Drugs Used in the Treatment of Hypertension

Lifestyle modification is the first step in prevention and management of hypertension in people with normal blood pressure or who have prehypertension; however, most people with hypertension will require a combination of drug therapy and lifestyle modification. Pharmaceutical management of hypertension can be challenging because medications prescribed to reduce blood pressure can sometimes produce more symptoms than the disease, resulting in poor adherence to drug therapy.

TECH NOTE!
Natural licorice may aggravate hypertension and interfere with the effects of antihypertensive drugs. It increases sodium and water retention and potassium depletion.

TABLE 22-2* **Lifestyle Modifications for Management and Prevention of Hypertension***

Modification	Recommendation
Weight loss	Maintain normal body weight
	Body mass index (18.5 to 24.9 kg/m^2)
Diet	Reduce salt (sodium) intake (≤2.4 g sodium)
	Reduce saturated and total fats
	Eat 5 or more servings of fruits and vegetables/day
Physical activity	Engage in 30 minutes of aerobic physical activity daily
Alcohol consumption	Drink no more than 2 alcoholic beverages† per day—men (women and light-weight persons 1 drink/day)
Tobacco usage	Stop smoking cigarettes and cigars

*Adapted from 7th Report of the Joint National Committee on Prevention, Detection, Evaluation, and Treatment of High Blood Pressure.
†Alcoholic beverage = 24 oz. beer or 10 oz. wine or 3 oz. whiskey (80 proof).

Drugs used in the treatment of hypertension work at the sites for blood pressure regulation: the kidney, heart, blood vessels, brain, and sympathetic nerves.

DIURETICS

The kidney plays a major role in regulating blood pressure and diuretics exert their effects on the kidney. They increase the elimination of water, sodium, and selected electrolytes (K^+, Cl^-, HCO_3^-), depending on their location of action in the kidney (Figure 22-2).

Diuretics lower blood pressure by decreasing peripheral resistance and cardiac output. They lower peripheral resistance by decreasing the blood volume. It is similar to a balloon filled with water. When the balloon is filled to maximum capacity, the pressure of water pushing on the walls of the balloon is high. If some of the water is let out, the pressure is lowered. The effect of diuretics on lowering the blood volume also reduces cardiac output. When cardiac output is reduced, blood pressure decreases. Recall the formula: $BP = CO \times PR$.

There are several classifications of diuretics. They are thiazide, loop, and potassium sparing. Aldosterone antagonists are sometimes classified as diuretics because their location of action is the kidney.

THIAZIDE DIURETICS

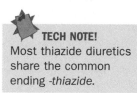

TECH NOTE!
Most thiazide diuretics share the common ending -thiazide.

Thiazide diuretics promote the elimination of water, sodium, potassium, magnesium, and chloride ions. Fluid loss decreases blood volume, yet this is not the primary mechanism of action for their effectiveness in decreasing blood pressure. Thiazides act at the distal convoluted tubule where they block the sodium-chloride cotransporter (Figure 22-2). This interferes with calcium transport into arterioles, decreasing vasoconstriction. Peripheral resistance is lowered along with blood pressure. Thiazides indirectly stimulate aldosterone secretion, causing potassium excretion. They stimulate calcium reabsorption, which makes them useful for the treatment of kidney stones that are caused by increased calcium in the urine (hypercalciuria) but at the expense of increasing blood calcium levels (hypercalcemia).

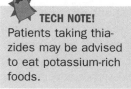

TECH NOTE!
Patients taking thiazides may be advised to eat potassium-rich foods.

Pharmacokinetics

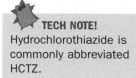

TECH NOTE!
Hydrochlorothiazide is commonly abbreviated HCTZ.

Thiazide diuretics are readily absorbed by oral administration. They are weak acids and highly protein bound. Once transported into the proximal tubule of the nephron, tubular secretion is decreased. Their lipid solubility permits reabsorption along the distal nephron. Their duration of effect varies from as little as 6 hours to as long as 48 hours depending upon the drug. Most thiazide diuretics are dosed once a day.

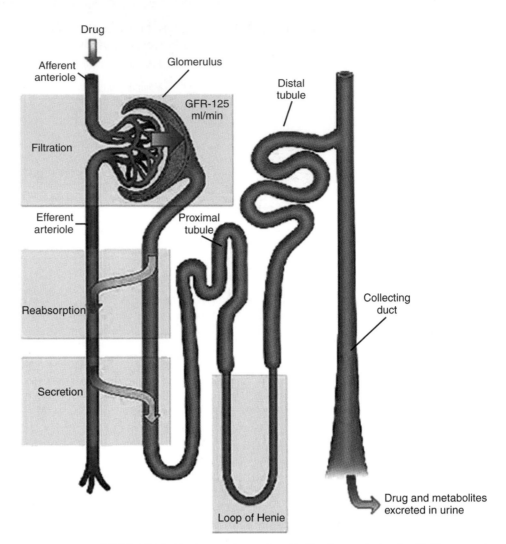

FIGURE 22-2 Nephron. *(From Lilley LL, Harrington S, Snyder JS:* Pharmacology and the nursing process, *ed 5, St Louis, 2007, Mosby.)*

Adverse Reactions

Thiazide diuretics can cause dehydration, *hyponatremia* (sodium loss), and electrolyte deficiency including *hypokalemia* (potassium loss), *hypomagnesia* (magnesium loss), and *hypochloremia* (choride loss). They can cause *hyperuricemia* (excess uric acid), precipitating a flare-up of gout. Hyperglycemia and glucose intolerance are additional adverse of thiazides. Thiazides have direct and indirect effects on insulin release. Other adverse drug reactions are gastrointestinal upset, impotence, and *photosensitivity*.

Precautions

Thiazide diuretics should be used cautiously in patients with gout and diabetes. The effect of thiazide diuretics is reduced if they are taken concurrently with NSAIDs. Diuretics should be taken in the morning to avoid the need to urinate in the middle of the night (*nocturia*).

Thiazide Diuretics

Generic name	U.S. brand name / Canadian brand(s)	Dosage forms and strengths
chlorthiazide*	Diuril	**Injection, powder for reconstitution:** 500 mg
	Diuril	**Suspension, oral:** 250 mg/5 ml (237 ml) **Tablet:** 250 mg, 500 mg (generic only)
chlorthalidone*	Thalitone	**Tablet:** 15 mg (Thalitone), 25 mg, 50 mg, 100 mg
	(various)	
hydrochlorothiazide*	Microzide	**Capsule (Microzide):** 12.5 mg **Tablet:** 25 mg, 50 mg
	(various)	
indapamide*	Lozol	**Tablet:** 1.25 mg, 2.5 mg
	Lozide	
metolazone*	Zaroxolyn	**Tablet, slow acting (Zaroxolyn):** 2.5 mg, 5 mg, 10 mg
	Zaroxolyn	
polythiazide	Generics	**Tablet:** 2 mg
	Not available	

*Generic available.

TECH ALERT!
The following drugs have look-alike/sound-alike issues: Bumex, Buprenex, Nimbex, and Permax; Lasix, Luvox, and Lanoxin; Furosemide, torsemide, fluoxetine, famotidine, and fosinopril; Demadex and Demerol; Torsemide, furosemide, and topiramate

LOOP DIURETICS

Loop diuretics also block the sodium-potassium cotransporter in the ascending loop of Henle. They are the most potent diuretics because they inhibit the reabsorption of 20% to 30% of sodium load, whereas thiazides inhibit only 5% to 10% and potassium-sparing diuretics inhibit only 1% to 3% of the sodium load. Loop diuretics increase potassium excretion and stimulate aldosterone secretion, similar to the thiazides. They also increase calcium excretion.

Pharmacokinetics

Loop diuretics are readily absorbed from the gastrointestinal tract. They are up to 98% protein bound. Differences between the loop diuretics are associated with their degree of metabolism in the liver and the extent to which they are eliminated unchanged in the urine. Bumetanide is partially metabolized in the liver and 50% is excreted unchanged in the urine, whereas torsemide's metabolism in the liver is greater and 20% is excreted unchanged. Torsemide's long half-life permits once-daily dosing.

Adverse Reactions

Loop diuretics can cause dehydration, severe hypotension, hypokalemia, hyperuricemia, and photosensitivity. Deafness has occurred when large doses are infused rapidly.

Precautions

The effect of loop diuretics is reduced if they are taken concurrently with NSAIDs. Patients taking loop diuretics should take the last dose of the day in early evening to avoid the need to urinate in the middle of the night.

POTASSIUM-SPARING DIURETICS

Potassium-sparing diuretics inhibit sodium reabsorption while avoiding potassium loss. They are less effective than loop and thiazide diuretics. Their effectiveness can be increased by combining them with a thiazide diuretic. Fixed dose potassium-sparing diuretic

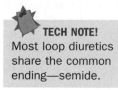

TECH NOTE!
Most loop diuretics share the common ending—semide.

combinations currently available are amiloride + hydrochlorothiazide and triamterene + hydrochlorothiazide. The usual dose prescribed to adults for the management of hypertension is listed in the mini drug monograph at the end of this chapter.

Loop Diuretics

	Generic name	U.S. brand name	Dosage forms and strengths
		Canadian brand(s)	
	bumetanide*	Bumex	**Injection, solution:** 0.25 mg/ml **Tablet:** 0.5 mg, 1 mg, 2 mg (1 mg, 5 mg Canada)
		Burinex	
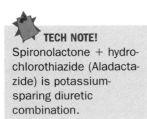	furosemide*	Lasix	**Injection, solution:** 10 mg/ml **Solution, oral:** 10 mg/ml; 40 mg/5ml **Tablet:** 20 mg, 40 mg, 80 mg
		Lasix, Lasix Special	
	torsemide*	Demadex	**Injection, solution:** 10 mg/ml **Tablet:** 5 mg, 10 mg, 20 mg, 100 mg
		Not available	

*Generic available.

Triamterene is readily absorbed in the gastrointestinal tract, and amiloride is 50% absorbed. Duration of effect ranges from 7 to 9 hours (triamterene) and 24 hours (amiloride).

Adverse Reactions
Hyperkalemia is the most serious adverse reaction of potassium-sparing diuretics, and the risk is increased if they are prescribed along with ACE inhibitors. They may also cause nausea or vomiting.

Precautions
Potassium-sparing diuretics should be used cautiously in patients with congestive heart failure who are taking digoxin. Patients should be advised to avoid salt substitutes because they contain potassium chloride (KCl).

ALDOSTERONE RECEPTOR BLOCKERS
Aldosterone is a hormone that is released when the kidney perceives a drop in blood flow and blood pressure. Aldosterone causes sodium and water reabsorption. Spironolactone is a competitive antagonist of aldosterone. It blocks the effect of aldosterone on sodium channels, decreases sodium reabsorption, and inhibits potassium elimination. Spironolactone is sometimes classified as a potassium-sparing diuretic.

Spironolactone is about as effective as triamterene and amiloride (sodium reabsorption is approximately 1% to 3%). It is readily absorbed orally and is eliminated in urine. It has a long half-life and is dosed once daily.

ADVERSE REACTIONS AND PRECAUTIONS
Hyperkalemia is a serious adverse drug reaction caused by spironolactone. Other adverse reactions are nausea, unpleasant aftertaste, gynecomastia (breast enlargement in males), hirsutism (excessive hair growth in women), impotence, and menstrual irregularities. Salt substitutes should be avoided when spironolactone is administered.

TECH NOTE!
Spironolactone + hydrochlorothiazide (Aladactazide) is potassium-sparing diuretic combination.

Aldosterone Receptor Blockers

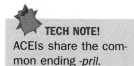

Generic name	U.S. brand name / Canadian brand(s)	Dosage forms and strengths	Other use(s)
spironolactone*	Aldactone Aldactone	**Tablet:** 25 mg, 50 mg, 100 mg	Primary aldosteronism, hypokalemia, and liver disease

© 2005 GS

*Generic available.

TECH NOTE!
ACEIs share the common ending -pril.

TECH ALERT!
The following drugs have look-alike/sound-alike issues: Benazepril and Benadryl; Lotensin, Loniten, Lioresal, and lovastatin; Capoten and Catapres; captopril and carvedilol; Vasotec and Norvasc; enalapril and Eldepryl; Univasc, Uniretic, and Urispas; Accupril, Accolate, Aciphex, Accutane, Altace, and Aricept; Altace, Accupril, Amerge, and Artane; ramipril and rifampin; Trandolapril and tramadol

ANGIOTENSION-CONVERTING ENZYME INHIBITORS

ACE inhibitors (ACEIs) lower SBP and DBP by their blocking action on angiotensin converting enzyme (ACE). ACE converts angiotensin I to angiotensin II. When angiotensin II levels rise, blood pressure increases because *angiotensin II* is a potent vasoconstrictor, stimulates the release of aldosterone, and promotes the release of norepinephrine from sympathetic neurons.

MECHANISM OF ACTION

ACEIs inhibit the activity of angiotensin converting enzyme, reducing angiotensin II and aldosterone levels. They decrease reabsorption of sodium in the renal tubules. In addition, they cause the accumulation of bradykinins (peptides that produce dilation of arteries). This reduces peripheral resistance, further lowering blood pressure.

PHARMACOKINETICS

ACEIs differ in activity, metabolism, and elimination, which may influence which ACE is prescribed. For example, enalapril, perindopril, quinapril, ramipril, and trandolapril are prodrugs. They would not be drugs of first choice for patients with decreased liver function because prodrugs have limited activity until they undergo metabolism. Enalaprilat, perindoprilat, quinaprilat, ramiprilat, and trandolaprilat are their active metabolites. Captopril and lisinopril are already active compounds. Fosinopril is a good choice for patients with decreased kidney function because it is eliminated by the liver (50%) and the kidney (50%). All other ACEIs are 90% eliminated by the kidney and can accumulate if kidney disease is present.

ADVERSE REACTIONS

Accumulation of bradykinins by ACEIs is responsible for the dry cough that is a characteristic side effect. Other adverse drug reactions are hyperkalemia, lightheadedness, hypotension, diarrhea, skin rashes, and airway obstruction (angioedema).

PRECAUTIONS

ACEIs are contraindicated in pregnancy because they can interfere with fetal development of the kidneys and fetal death has been reported. Salt substitutes should be avoided to reduce risks for hyperkalemia.

Angiotension-Converting Enzyme Inhibitors (ACEIs)

	Generic name	U.S. brand name Canadian brand(s)	Dosage forms and strengths
	benazepril*	Lotensin Lotensin	**Tablet:** 5 mg, 10 mg, 20 mg, 40 mg
	captopril*	Capoten Capoten	**Tablet:** 12.5 mg, 25 mg, 50 mg, 100 mg
	enalapril*	Vasotec Vasotec	**Injection, solution (as enalaprilat):** 1.25 mg/ml **Tablet:** 2.5 mg, 5 mg, 10 mg, 20 mg
	fosinopril*	Monopril Monopril	**Tablet:** 10 mg, 20 mg, 40 mg
	lisinopril*	Prinivil, Zestril Prinivil, Zestril	**Tablet:** 2.5 mg, 5 mg, 10 mg, 20 mg, 30 mg, 40 mg
	moexipril*	Univasc Not available	**Tablet, film-coated:** 7.5 mg, 15 mg
	perindopril	Aceon Coversyl, Coversyl Plus	**Tablet:** 2 mg, 4 mg, 8 mg
	quinapril	Accupril Accupril	**Tablet:** 5 mg, 10 mg, 20 mg, 40 mg
	ramipril	Altace Altace	**Capsule:** 1.25 mg, 2.5 mg, 5 mg, 10 mg
	trandolapril	Mavik Mavik	**Tablet:** 1 mg, 2 mg, 4 mg

Angiotension-Converting Enzyme Inhibitors (ACEIs)—cont'd

Generic name	U.S. brand name Canadian brand(s)	Dosage forms and strengths
Combination ACEIs and diuretics		
benazepril + hydrochlorothiazide*	Lotensin HCT	**Tablet:** benazepril 5 mg + hydrochlorothiazide 6.25 mg
	Not available	benazepril 10 mg + hydrochlorothiazide 12.5 mg benazepril 20 mg + hydrochlorothiazide 12.5 mg benazepril 20 mg + hydrochlorothiazide 20 mg
captopril + hydrochlorothiazide*	Capozide	**Tablet:** captopril 25 mg + hydrochlorothiazide 15 mg
	Not available	captopril 25 mg + hydrochlorothiazide 25 mg captopril 50 mg + hydrochlorothiazide 15 mg captopril 50 mg + hydrochlorothiazide 25 mg
enalapril + hydrochlorothiazide*	Vaseretic	**Tablet:** enalapril 5 mg + hydrochlorothiazide 12.5 mg
	Vaseretic	enalapril 10 mg + hydrochlorothiazide 25 mg
fosinopril + hydrochlorothiazide	Monopril HCT	**Tablet:** fosinopril 10 mg + hydrochlorothiazide 12.5 mg
	Not available	fosinopril 20 mg + hydrochlorothiazide 12.5 mg
lisinopril + hydrochlorothiazide*	Prinizide, Zestoretic	**Tablet:** lisinopril 10 mg + hydrochlorothiazide 12.5 mg
	Prinizide, Zestoretic	lisinopril 20 mg + hydrochlorothiazide 12.5 mg lisinopril 20 mg + hydrochlorothiazide 25 mg
moexipril + hydrochlorothiazide	Uniretic	**Tablet:** moexipril 7.5 mg + hydrochlorothiazide 12.5 mg
	Not available	moexipril 15 mg + hydrochlorothiazide 12.5 mg moexipril 15 mg + hydrochlorothiazide 25 mg
quinaprll + hydrochlorothiazide*	Accuretic, Quinarectic	**Tablet:** quinapril 10 mg + hydrochlorothiazide 12.5 mg
	Accuretic	quinapril 20 mg + hydrochlorothiazide 12.5 mg quinapril 20 mg + hydrochlorothlazide 25 mg
ramipril + hydrochlorothiazide	Not available	**Tablet:** ramipril 2.5 mg + hydrochlorothiazide 12.5 mg
	Altace HCT	ramipril 5 mg + hydrochlorothiazide 12.5 mg ramipril 10 mg + hydrochlorothiazide 12.5 mg ramipril 5 mg + hydrochlorothiazide 25 mg ramipril 10 mg + hydrochlorothlazide 25 mg

*Generic available.

ANGIOTENSIN II RECEPTOR ANTAGONISTS

Angiotensin II receptor blockers (ARBs) are competitive antagonists at the angiotensin II receptor site. They lower blood pressure by blocking the binding of angiotensin II. ARBs also inhibit angiotensin II–stimulated growth of smooth muscle, reducing ventricular and arterial hypertrophy that is associated with chronic hypertension. They do not inhibit angiotensin II–stimulated tissue growth and repair.

Angiotensin II receptor blockers are similar to ACE inhibitors in effectiveness but do not produce dry cough, perhaps because they do not increase bradykinin levels like ACEIs.

PHARMACOKINETICS

The plasma half-life of ARBs varies. Losartan, one of the first ARBs to be marketed, has a relatively short $T\frac{1}{2}$ (only 2 hours) but it has an active metabolite with a plasma half-life of up to 6 to 9 hours. Losartan has an active metabolite that is 10 to 40 times more potent than the parent compound. The duration of action for irbesartan, candesartan, and telmisartan is longer (12 to 18 hours) and they are administered as a single daily dose.

ADVERSE REACTIONS

Adverse drug reactions associated with ARBs are fatigue, abdominal pain, dizziness, dry mouth, constipation, impotence, and muscle cramps.

PRECAUTIONS

ARBs are contraindicated in the second and third trimester of pregnancy because they can interfere with fetal development of the kidneys and fetal death has been reported.

β-BLOCKERS

There are three specific β-receptors. β_1-Receptor binding produces cardiac stimulation, β_2-receptor binding causes bronchial relaxation, and β_3-receptor binding causes the breakdown of fat tissue. β-Blockers lower blood pressure by decreasing heart rate and peripheral resistance.

MECHANISM OF ACTION

β-Adrenergic blockers used in the treatment of hypertension may be selective (β_1) or nonselective (β_1, β_2). All β-blockers decrease blood pressure but selective β_1-adrenergic blockers are less likely to produce bronchospasm. This selectivity is lost when higher doses are prescribed.

Angiotension II Receptor Antagonists (ARBs)

	Generic name	U.S. brand name / Canadian brand(s)	Dosage forms and strengths
	candesartan	Atacand	**Tablet:** 4 mg, 8 mg, 16 mg, 32 mg
		Atacand	
	eprosartan	Teveten	**Tablet:** 400 mg, 600 mg
		Teveten	
	irbesartan	Avapro	**Tablet:** 75 mg, 150 mg, 300 mg
		Avapro	
	losartan	Cozaar	**Tablet:** 25 mg, 50 mg, 100 mg
		Cozaar	

Angiotension II Receptor Antagonists (ARBs)—cont'd

	Generic name	U.S. brand name / Canadian brand(s)	Dosage forms and strengths
	olmesartan	Benicar	**Tablet:** 5 mg, 20 mg, 40 mg
		Not available	
	telmisartan	Micardis	**Tablet:** 20 mg, 40 mg, 80 mg
		Micardis	
	valsartan	Diovan	**Tablet:** 40 mg, 80 mg, 160 mg, 320 mg
		Diovan	

Combination ARBs and diuretics

	Generic name	U.S. brand name / Canadian brand(s)	Dosage forms and strengths
	candesartan + HCTZ	Atacand HCT	**Tablet:**
		Atacand Plus	candesartan 16 mg + hydrochlorothiazide 12.5 mg candesartan 32 mg + hydrochlorothiazide 12.5 mg
	eprosartan + HCTZ	Teveten HCT	**Tablet:**
		Teveten Plus	eprosartan 600 mg + hydrochlorothiazide 12.5 mg eprosartan 600 mg + hydrochlorothiazide 12.5 mg
	irbesartan + HCTZ	Avalide	**Tablet:**
		Avalide	irbesartan 150 mg + hydrochlorothiazide 12.5 mg irbesartan 300 mg + hydrochlorothiazide 12.5 mg
	losartan + HCTZ	Hyzaar	**Tablet:**
		Hyzaar, Hyzaar DS	losartan 50 mg + hydrochlorothiazide 12.5 mg losartan 100 mg + hydrochlorothiazide 25 mg
	olmesartan + HCTZ	Benicar HCT	**Tablet:**
		Not available	olmesartan 20 mg + hydrochlorothiazide 12.5 mg olmesartan 40 mg + hydrochlorothiazide 12.5 mg olmesartan 40 mg + hydrochlorothiazide 25 mg
	telmisartan + HCTZ	Micardis HCT	**Tablet:**
		Micardis Plus	telmisartan 40 mg + hydrochlorothiazide 12.5 mg telmisartan 80 mg + hydrochlorothiazide 12.5 mg telmisartan 80 mg + hydrochlorothiazide 25 mg
	valsartan + HCTZ	Diovan HCT	**Tablet:**
		Diovan HCT	valsartan 80 mg + hydrochlorothiazide 12.5 mg valsartan 160 mg + hydrochlorothiazide 12.5 mg valsartan 160 mg + hydrochlorothiazide 25 mg

*Generic available.

All β-blockers decrease heart rate, especially during exercise, and decrease the force of contractions in the heart. This lowers the cardiac output. Chronic use produces vasodilation. This may be due to decreased renin release. Renin acts to convert the hormone angiotensinogen to angiotensin I, a precursor to angiotensin II.

ADVERSE REACTIONS

Adverse drug reactions associated with β-adrenergic blockers are dizziness, lethargy, nausea, palpitations, impotence, bradycardia, bronchoconstriction, hypoglycemia, cardiac rhythm disturbance, congestive heart failure, and depression. Their adverse effects make them contraindicated in patients who have diabetes and asthma.

PRECAUTIONS

β-Adrenergic blockers should not be discontinued abruptly because this may cause the onset of arrhythmias or angina. Important drug interactions exist between β-adrenergic blockers and cimetidine (inhibits metabolic enzymes in the liver, which increases the antihypertensive effects of drugs like propranolol and metoprolol) and salicylates (decrease the effectiveness of β_1-blockers like atenolol and metoprolol).

> **TECH ALERT!**
> The following drugs have look-alike/ sound-alike issues:
> Corgard and Cognex; nadolol and Mandol Inderal, Inderide, Enduronyl, Adderall, Isordil, Toradol, and Imdur;
> Inderal 40 and Enduronyl Forte;
> Propranol and Pravachol

β-Adrenergic Blockers: Nonselective

	Generic name	U.S. brand name / Canadian brand(s)	Dosage forms and strengths
	nadolol*	Corgard	**Tablet:** 20 mg, 40 mg, 80 mg, 120 mg, 160 mg (20 mg, 120 mg not available in Canada)
		Generics	
	penbutolol	Levatol	**Tablet:** 20 mg
		Not available	
	pindolol*	Generics	**Tablet:** 5 mg, 10 mg
		Visken	
	propranolol*	Inderal, Inderal LA, InnoPran XL,	**Capsule, extended release (InnoPran XL):** 80 mg, 120 mg **Capsule, sustained release (Inderal LA):** 60 mg, 80 mg, 120 mg, 160 mg **Injection, solution:** 1 mg/ml **Solution, oral:** 4 mg/ml and 8 mg/ml **Tablet:** 10 mg, 20 mg, 40 mg, 60 mg, 80 mg, 120 mg
		Inderal LA	
	timolol*	Generics	**Tablet:** 5 mg, 10 mg, 20 mg
		Generics	
β-Adrenergic blockers: nonselective			
	acebutolol*	Sectrol	**Capsule:** 100 mg, 200 mg, 400 mg (100 mg available in Canada only)
		Rhotral, Sectral	
	atenolol*	Tenormin	**Tablet:** 25 mg, 50 mg, 100 mg
		Tenormin	

β-Adrenergic Blockers: Nonselective—cont'd

Generic name	U.S. brand name / Canadian brand(s)	Dosage forms and strengths
betaxolol*	Kerlone	**Tablet:** 10 mg, 20 mg
	Not available	
bisoprolol*	Zebeta	**Tablet:** 5 mg, 10 mg
	Monocor	
metoprolol*	Lopressor, Toprol XL	**Injection, solution (Lopressor):** 1 mg/ml (5ml)
	Betaloc, Lopressor, Lopressor SR	**Tablet, immediate release (Betaloc, Lopressor) :** 25 mg, 50 mg, 100 mg **Tablet, extended release (Toprol XL):** 25 mg, 50 mg, 100 mg, 200 mg **Tablet, extended release (Lopressor SR):** 100 mg, 200 mg

Combination β-adrenergic blockers and diuretics

Generic name	U.S. brand name / Canadian brand(s)	Dosage forms and strengths
nadolol + bendroflumethiazide	Corzide	**Tablet:** nadolol 40 mg + bendroflumethiazide 5 mg nadolol 80 mg + bendroflumethiazide 5 mg
	Not available	
pindolol + hydrochlorothiazide	Not available	**Tablet:** pindolol 10 mg + hydrochlorothiazide 25 mg pindolol 10 mg + hydrochlorothiazide 50 mg
	Viskazide	
propranolol + hydrochlorothiazide	Inderide	**Tablet:** propranolol 40 mg + hydrochlorothiazide 25 mg propranolol 80 mg + hydrochlorothiazide 25 mg
	Not available	
timolol + hydrochlorothiazide	Timolide	**Tablet:** timolol 10 mg +hydrochlorothiazide 25 mg
	Not available	
atenolol + chlorthalidone	Tenoretic	atenolol 50 mg + chlorthalidone 25 mg atenolol 100 mg + chlorthalidone 25 mg
	Tenoretic	
bisoprolol + hydrochlorothiazide	Ziac	**Tablet:** bisoprolol 2.5 mg + hydrochlorothiazide 6.25 mg bisoprolol 5 mg + hydrochlorothiazide 6.25 mg bisoprolol 10 mg + hydrochlorothiazide 6.25 mg
	Not available	
metoprolol + hydrochlorothiazide	Lopressor HCT	**Tablet:** Metoprolol 50 mg + hydrochlorothiazide 25 mg metoprolol 100 mg + hydrochlorothiazide 25 mg
	Not available	

*Generic available.

Combination β₁- and α₁-Blockers

	Generic name	U.S. brand name / Canadian brand(s)	Dosage forms and strengths
	carvedilol	Coreg, Coreg CR / Generics	**Tablet:** 3.125 mg, 6.25 mg, 12.5 mg, 25 mg
	labetalol	Trandate / Trandate	**Injection, solution, and prefilled syringe:** 5 mg/ml (4 ml, 20 ml, 40 ml) **Tablet:** 100 mg, 200 mg, 300 mg

TECH ALERT!

The following drugs have look-alike/ sound-alike issues: Sectral, Seconal, and Septra; Tenormin, Imuran, thiamine, and Trovan; Zebeta and Diabeta; metoprolol, metoclopramide, metolazone, metronidazole, and misoprostol; Toprol XL, Topimax, and Tegretol XR

α₁-BLOCKERS

The arteries have an abundance of $\alpha\alpha_1$ receptors that mediate vasoconstriction. Administration of α_1-blockers produces vascular relaxation, which reduces peripheral resistance and lowers blood pressure. α_1-Adrenergic antagonists also reduce LDL cholesterol levels, making them useful in the treatment of ischemic heart disease. Finally, doxazosin and terazosin have the ability to reduce urethral resistance and increase urine flow, making them effective in the treatment of benign prostatic hyperplasia (BPH).

ADVERSE REACTIONS

Adverse drug effects are postural hypotension, dizziness, reflex tachycardia, headache, weakness, and fatigue.

α₁-Blockers

	Generic name	U.S. brand name / Canadian brand(s)	Dosage forms and strengths
	doxazosin*	Cardura Cardura XL / Cardura-1, Cardura-2, Cardura-4	**Tablet:** 1 mg, 2 mg, 4 mg, 8 mg (8 mg not available in Canada) **Tablet, extended release (Cardura XL):** 4 mg, 8 mg
	prazosin*	Minipress / Minipress	**Capsule:** 1 mg, 2 mg, 5 mg
	terazosin*	Hytrin / Hytrin	**Capsule (Hytrin) and Tablet:** 1 mg, 2 mg, 5 mg, 10 mg

α₁-Blockers—cont'd

Generic name	U.S. brand name Canadian brand(s)	Dosage forms and strengths
Combination α₁-blockers and diuretics		
prazosin + polythiazide	Minizide	**Capsule:** prazosin 1 mg + polythiazide 0.5 mg
	Not available	prazosin 2 mg + polythiazide 0.5 mg prazosin 5 mg + polythiazide 0.5 mg

*Generic available.

TECH ALERT!
Carvedilol, carteolol, and captopril have look-alike/sound-alike issues.

TECH NOTE!
α₁-Blockers share the common ending -zosin.

TECH ALERT!
The following drugs have look-alike/sound-alike issues: clonidine, quinidine, colchicine, clomiphene, and Klonopin; Catapres and Cataflam guanfacine and guaifenesin; methyldopa and levodopa; reserpine, resperidone, and Risperdal

CALCIUM CHANNEL BLOCKERS

Calcium channel blockers (CCBs) are effective at lowering blood pressure because of their ability to relax blood vessels. This decreases peripheral resistance. They also decrease heart rate and force of contractions, lowering the cardiac output. The exact mechanism of action, pharmacokinetics, and adverse reactions are discussed in Chapter 21. CCBs that are used in the treatment of hypertension are: amlodipine, felodipine, isradipine, nicardipine, nifedipine, and nisoldipine. The Joint National Committee on Prevention, Detection, Evaluation, and Treatment of High Blood Pressure recommended usual dose ranges for these CCBs are listed in mini drug monographs listing drugs used in the treatment and management of hypertension.

CENTRAL ACTING α₂-AGONISTS

Blood pressure is controlled by a complex feedback mechanism. Increased adrenergic stimulation in the brain results in decreased sympathetic nervous system messages flowing from the CNS. Methyldopa is a prodrug that acts like a false neurotransmitter. It is metabolized to α-methylnorepinephrine, which the body thinks is norepinephrine; however, it is selective in mimicking the autoinhibitory effects of norepinephrine. When methyldopa binds to receptors, efferent sympathetic activity is reduced, blood vessels dilate, and peripheral resistance is decreased. Clonidine inhibits norepinephrine release from the CNS and peripheral sites and reserpine depletes neuronal stores of norepinephrine at CNS and peripheral sites. Prolonged use results in decreases in heart rate and cardiac output further reducing blood pressure.

ADVERSE REACTIONS

Adverse drug effects of centrally acting α₂-agonists include sedation, dry mouth, orthostatic hypotension, impotence, and constipation. Methyldopa can also cause depression, nasal stuffiness, gastrointestinal upset. Methyldopa may produce galactorrhea, hemolytic anemia, and liver dysfunction.

α₂-Agonists

Generic name	U.S. brand name Canadian brand(s)	Dosage forms and strengths
clonidine*	Catapres, Catapres-TTS, Duraclon	**Injection, epidural solution (Duraclon):** 100 mcg/ml **Patch, transdermal:** 0.1 mg/24 hr (Catapres TTS-1),
	Catapres, Dixarit	0.2 mg/24 hr (Catapres TTS-2), 0.3 mg/24 hr (Catapres TTS-3) **Tablet:** 0.1 mg, 0.2 mg, 0.3 mg **Tablet (Dixarit):** 0.025 mg

Continued

α₂-Agonists—cont'd

Generic name	U.S. brand name	Dosage forms and strengths
	Canadian brand(s)	
guanfacine*	Tenex	**Tablet:** 1 mg, 2 mg
	Not available	
methyldopa*	Generics	**Injection, solution:** 50 mg/ml
	Generics	**Tablet:** 125 mg, 250 mg, 500 mg
reserpine*	Generics	**Tablet:** 0.1 mg, 0.25 mg
	Not available	
Combination α₂-agonist and diuretic		
clonidine + chlorthalidone	Clorpres	**Tablet:**
	Not available	clonidine 0.1 mg + chlorthalidone 15 mg
		clonidine 0.2 mg + chlorthalidone 15 mg
		clonidine 0.3 mg + chlorthalidone 15 mg
methyldopa + hydrochlorothiazide	Aldoril, Aldoril D30 Aldoril D50	**Tablet:**
		methyldopa 250 mg + hydrochlorothiazide 15 mg
	Generics	methyldopa 250 mg + hydrochlorothiazide 25 mg
		methyldopa 500 mg + hydrochlorothiazide 30 mg
		methyldopa 500 mg + hydrochlorothiazide 50 mg

*Generic available.

TECH ALERT!
The following drugs have look-alike/sound-alike issues: Cardura, Ridura, Cardene, Cordarone, Coumadin, and K-Dur; prazosin, doxazosin, and terazosin

TECH ALERT!
The following drugs have look-alike/sound-alike issues: hydralazine, hydroxyzine, and hydrochlorothiazide; minoxidil and Monopril; Loniten and Lotensin

DIRECT VASODILATORS

Hydralzine and minoxidil decrease peripheral resistance and reduce blood pressure by relaxing vascular smooth muscle. Minoxidil works by activating ATP-sensitive K^+ channels setting in motion a chain of events that decrease calcium influx through L-type calcium channels in vascular smooth muscle. This decreases arterial blood vessel contractions.

Neither hydralazine nor minoxidil is a first-line drug for the treatment of hypertension. Hydralazine is recommended for hypertensive emergencies (parenteral use) and is safe for the treatment of preeclampsia in pregnant women.

ADVERSE REACTIONS

Adverse drug reactions for hydralazine and minoxidil are orthostatic hypotension, headache, gastrointestinal upset, sodium and fluid retention, palpitations, and arrhythmia. Hydralzine can cause a lupus-like syndrome, and minoxidil causes facial hair growth. The discovery that minoxidil increases hair growth resulted in the drug being formulated for topical use for the treatment of baldness.

Vasodilators

	Generic name	U.S. brand name Canadian brand(s)	Dosage forms and strengths
	hydralazine*	Generics	**Injection, solution:** 20 mg/ml (1ml)
		Apresoline	**Tablet:** 10 mg, 25 mg, 50 mg, 100 mg
	minoxidil*	Generics	**Tablet:** 2.5 mg, 10 mg
		Loniten	
Combination vasodilator and diuretic			
	hydralazine + hydrochlorothiazide*	Hydrazide	**Capsule** hydralazine 25 mg + hydrochlorothiazide 25 mg
		Not available	hydralazine 50 mg + hydrochlorothiazide 50 mg hydralazine 100 mg + hydrochlorothiazide 50 mg

*Generic available.

Summary of Drugs Used in the Treatment and Management of Hypertension*

	Drug name	Usual Dose and Dosing Schedule	Warning label(s)
Diuretics			
	Thiazides		
	chlorothiazide	125 mg to 500 mg 1 to 2 times a day	TAKE WITH FOOD
	chlorthalidone	12.5 mg to 25 mg once daily	MAY BE ADVISABLE TO EAT BANANAS OR DRINK ORANGE JUICE
	hydrochlorothiazide (HCTZ)	12.5 mg to 50 mg once daily	AVOID PROLONGED EXPOSURE TO SUNLIGHT
	polythiazide	2 mg to 4 mg once daily	SOME OTC DRUGS CAN AGGRAVATE YOUR CONDITION
	indapamide	1.25 mg to 2.5 mg once daily	
	metolazone	0.5 mg to 5 mg once daily	
	Loop		
	bumetanide	0.5 mg to 2 mg twice daily	MAY BE ADVISABLE TO EAT BANANAS OR DRINK ORANGE JUICE
	furosemide	20 mg to 80 mg twice a day	MAY CAUSE DIZZINESS OR LIGHTHEADNESS
	torsemide	2.5 mg to 10 mg daily	AVOID PROLONGED EXPOSURE TO SUNLIGHT
			SOME OTC DRUGS CAN AGGRAVATE YOUR CONDITION
	Aldosterone receptor antagonist		
	spironolactone	25 mg to 50 mg once daily	TAKE WITH FOOD
			MAY CAUSE DIZZINESS OR LIGHTHEADNESS
			SOME OTC DRUGS CAN AGGRAVATE YOUR CONDITION

Continued

Summary of Drugs Used in the Treatment and Management of Hypertension*—cont'd

	Drug name	Usual Dose and Dosing Schedule	Warning label(s)
	Potassium-sparing combination		
	spironolactone + HCTZ	1 to 4 tablets daily in 1 to 2 divided doses 25 mg to 100 mg spironolactone + 25 mg to 100 mg HCTZ once daily	AVOID SALT SUBSTITUTES AND POTASSIUM RICH DIETS
	amiloride + HCTZ	10 mg amiloride + 100 mg HCTZ once daily	MAY CAUSE DIZZINESS OR LIGHTHEADNESS AVOID PROLONGED EXPOSURE TO SUNLIGHT
	triamterene + HCTZ	37.5 mg to 75 mg triamterene/ 25 mg to 50 mg HCTZ once daily	
β-Blockers			
	atenolol	25 mg to 100 mg once daily	DO NOT DISCONTINUE WITHOUT MEDICAL SUPERVISION
	acebutolol	200 mg to 800 mg twice daily	
	betaxolol	5 to 20 mg once daily	MAY CAUSE DIZZINESS OR LIGHTHEADNESS
	bisoprolol	2.5 mg to 10 mg once daily	TAKE WITH FOOD (immediate release metoprolol)
	metoprolol metoprolol extended release	50 mg to 100 mg 1 to 2 times a day 50 mg to 100 mg once daily	SWALLOW WHOLE; DON'T CRUSH OR CHEW (sustained release)
	nadolol	40 mg to 120 mg once daily	
	propranolol propranolol long acting	40 mg to 160 mg twice daily 60 to 180 mg once daily	
	timolol	20 to 40 mg twice daily	
	esmolol	250 mcg to 500 mcg/kg/min IV bolus; then 50 mcg to 100 mcg/kg/min IV infusion	FOR HYPERTENSIVE EMERGENCY
Combined α- and β-blockers			
	carvedilol	12.5 mg to 50 mg twice daily	TAKE WITH FOOD DO NOT DISCONTINUE WITHOUT MEDICAL SUPERVISION
	labetalol	200 mg to 800 mg twice daily	MAY CAUSE DIZZINESS OR LIGHTHEADNESS
	β-Blockers + diuretic combination		
	atenolol + chlorthalidone	50 mg to 100 mg atenolol + 25 mg chlorthalidone once daily	Same warnings for thiazides plus β-blockers
	bisoprolol + HCTZ	2.5 mg to 20 mg bisoprolol + 6.25 mg to 12.5 mg once daily	
	metoprolol + HCTZ	100 mg to 200 mg metaprolol + 25 mg to 50 mg HCTZ once daily	
	nadolol + bendroflumethiazide	40 mg to 80 mg nadolol + 5 mg bendroflumethrazide once daily	
	pindolol + HCTZ	1 to 2 tablets once daily	
	propranolol-LA + HCTZ	80 mg to 160 mg propranolol + HCTZ 50 mg once daily	
	timolol + HCTZ	1 tablet twice daily or 2 tablets once daily 10 mg timolol + 25 mg HCTZ twice daily or 20 mg timolol + 50 mg HCTZ once daily	

Summary of Drugs Used in the Treatment and Management of Hypertension*—cont'd

	Drug name	Usual Dose and Dosing Schedule	Warning label(s)
ACEIs			
	benazepril	10 mg to 40 mg once a day	DO NOT DISCONTINUE WITHOUT MEDICAL SUPERVISION
	captopril	25 mg to 100 mg twice a day	
	enalapril	5 mg to 40 mg 1 to 2 times a day	MAY CAUSE DIZZINESS OR LIGHTHEADNESS
	fosinopril	10 mg to 40 mg once a day	AVOID SALT SUBSTITUTES AND POTASSIUM-RICH DIETS
	lisinopril	10 mg to 40 mg once a day	
	moexipril	7.5 mg to 30 mg once a day	DON'T TAKE THIS DRUG IF YOU BECOME PREGNANT
			MAY CAUSE A DRY COUGH; IF IT PERSISTS REPORT IT TO YOUR DOCTOR
			TAKE ON AN EMPTY STOMACH—moexipril
			TAKE WITH FOOD—perindopril
	perindopril	4 mg to 8 mg once a day	
	quinapril	10 mg to 80 mg once a day	
	ramipril	2.5 mg to 20 mg once a day	
	trandolapril	1 mg to 4 mg once a day	
	ACEI + diuretic combination		
	benazepril + HCTZ	10 mg to 40 mg benazepril + 12.5 mg to 50 mg HCTZ once daily	Same warnings for thiazides plus ACEIs
	captopril + HCTZ	25 mg to 50 mg captopril + 15 mg to 50 mg HCTZ 2 to 3 time a day	
	enalapril + HCTZ	5 mg to 20 mg enalapril + 12.5 mg to 50 mg HCTZ once daily	
	fosinopril + HCTZ	10 mg to 80 mg/12.5 to 50 mg daily	
	lisinopril + HCTZ	10 mg to 80 mg lisinopril + 12.5 to 50 mg HCTZ once daily	
	moexipril + HCTZ	7.5 to 30 mg/12.5 to 50 mg daily	
	quinapril + HCTZ	10 mg to 40 mg quinapril + 12.5 mg to 25 mg HCTZ once daily	
Angiotensin II antagonists			
	candesartan	8 mg to 32 mg once daily	DO NOT DISCONTINUE WITHOUT MEDICAL SUPERVISION
	eprosartan	400 mg to 800 mg 1 to 2 times a day	
	irbesartan	150 mg to 300 mg once daily	MAY CAUSE DIZZINESS OR LIGHTHEADNESS
	losartan	25 to 100 mg 1 to 2 times a day	DON'T TAKE THIS DRUG IF YOU BECOME PREGNANT
	olmesartan	20 mg to 40 mg once daily	
	telmisartan	20 mg to 80 mg once daily	
	valsartan	80 mg to 320 mg 1 to 2 times a day	

Continued

Summary of Drugs Used in the Treatment and Management of Hypertension*—cont'd

	Drug name	Usual Dose and Dosing Schedule	Warning label(s)
Angiotensin II antagonist + diuretic combination			
	candesartan + HCTZ	16 mg to 32 mg/12.5–25 mg once daily	Same warnings as for ARBs and thiazide diuretics
	eprosartan + HCTZ	600 mg/12.5 mg once daily	
	irbesartan + HCTZ	150 to 300 mg/12.5 mg once daily	
	losartan + HCTZ	50 to 100 mg/12.5 to 25 mg daily	
	olmesartan + HCTZ	20 to 40 mg/12.5 to 25 mg once daily	
	telmisartan + HCTZ	80 mg/12.5 to 25 mg once daily	
	valsartan + HCTZ	80 mg to 160 mg/12.5 to 25 mg daily	
Calcium channel blockers			
	diltiazem extended release	180 mg to 420 mg once daily	MAY CAUSE DIZZINESS USE CAUTION WHEN DRIVING OR PERFORMING TASKS REQUIRING ALERTNESS
	diltiazem long acting	120 mg to 540 mg once a day	
	verapamil immediate release	80 mg to 320 mg twice daily	AVOID ABRUPT DISCONTINUATION
	verapamil long acting	120 mg to 480 mg 1 to 2 times a day	LIMIT CAFFEINE AND ALCOHOL
	verapamil extended release	120 mg to 360 mg once daily	SWALLOW WHOLE; DON'T CRUSH OR CHEW (sustained release)
	amlodipine	2.5 mg to 10 mg once a day	
	felodipine	2.5 mg to 20 mg once a day	
	isradipine	2.5 mg to 10 mg twice a day	
	nicardipine sustained release	60 mg to 120 mg twice a day	
	nicardipine IV	5 to 15 mg/hr IV	
	nifedipine long acting	30 mg to 60 mg once daily	
	Nisoldipine	10 mg to 40 mg once daily	
Calcium channel blockers + ACEI combination			
	amlodipine + benazepril	2.5 mg to 10 mg amlodipine + 10 mg to 40 mg benazepril once daily	Same warnings as CCBs plus ACEIs
	felodipine + enalapril	5 mg to 20 mg enalapril + 2.5 mg to 10 mg felodipine once daily	
	verapamil + trandolapril	2 mg to 8 mg trandolapril + 180 mg to 240 mg verapamil daily in 1 or 2 divided doses	
Centrally acting α_2-agonist and other centrally acting drugs			
	clonidine	0.1 mg to 0.8 mg twice a day	ROTATE SITE OF APPLICATION—patch
	clonidine patch	0.1 mg to 0.3 mg once a week	DO NOT DISCONTINUE WITHOUT MEDICAL SUPERVISION
	methyldopa	250 mg to 1000 mg twice daily	
	reserpine	0.1 mg to 0.25 mg once a day	MAY CAUSE DIZZINESS OR LIGHTHEADNESS
	guanfacine	0.5 mg to 2 mg once daily	

Summary of Drugs Used in the Treatment and Management of Hypertension*—cont'd

	Drug name	Usual Dose and Dosing Schedule	Warning label(s)
	Centrally acting drug + diuretic combination		
	250 mg methyldopa + 15 mg HCTZ 2 to 3 times daily	1 tablet 2 to 3 times daily	Same warnings as α_2–agonist and thiazide diuretics
	250 mg methyldopa + 25 mg HCTZ twice daily	1 tablet twice daily	
	500 mg methyldopa + 50 mg HCTZ once daily	1 tablet daily	
α_1-Antagonists			
	doxazosin	1 mg to 16 mg once a day	DO NOT DISCONTINUE WITHOUT MEDICAL SUPERVISION
	prazosin	2 mg to 20 mg 2 to 3 times a day	
	terazosin	1 mg to 20 mg 1 to 2 times a day	MAY CAUSE DIZZINESS OR LIGHTHEADNESS
Direct vasodilators			
	hydralazine	25 mg to 100 mg twice daily 10 mg to 20 mg IV or 10 mg to 40 mg IM	DO NOT DISCONTINUE WITHOUT MEDICAL SUPERVISION TAKE WITH FOOD MAY CAUSE DIZZINESS OR LIGHTHEADNESS
	minoxidil	2.5 mg to 80 mg 1 to 2 times a day	
	enalaprilat	1.25 mg to 5 mg every 6 hours IV	For hypertensive emergencies
	fenoldopam mesylate	0.1 mcg to 0.3 mcg/kg/min IV infusion	
	nitroglycerin	5 mcg to 100 mcg/min IV infusion	
	sodium nitroprusside	0.25 mcg to 10 mcg/kg/min IV infusion	
Adrenergic inhibitor			
	phentolamine	5 mg to 15 mg IV bolus	For hypertensive emergencies

*JNC 7 recommendations.

TECH NOTE!

Clonidine is also prescribed to manage heroin, nicotine, and ethanol withdrawal; glaucoma; and ADHD; and to prevent migraine headaches.

CHAPTER SUMMARY

- Systolic blood pressure (SBP) is a measure of the pressure when the heart's ventricles are contracting (systole). The diastolic blood pressure is a measure of the heart at rest (diastole).

$$BP = \frac{\text{Systolic pressure}}{\text{Diastolic pressure}}$$

- The average normal blood pressure $= \dfrac{<120 \text{ mm Hg}}{<80 \text{ mm Hg}}$

- The formula for determining blood pressure is: BP = CO × PR.
- Sites for blood pressure control are the kidneys, heart, blood vessels, CNS, and sympathetic nerves.
- The renin-aldosterone-angiotensin system (RAAS) responds to a drop in renal blood flow by increasing blood volume, blood flow to the kidney, vasoconstriction, and blood pressure.
- The CNS senses changes in blood pressure and signals sympathetic nerves to release neurotransmitters that control heart rate and blood flow through the arteries.
- When peripheral vascular resistance increases, blood pressure increases.
- Hypertension is the most diagnosed medical condition in the United States, affecting more than 65 million Americans (nearly 25% of the adult population).
- Diastolic hypertension is the predominant form of hypertension before age 50.
- Risk factors for high blood pressure are age (years) older than 55 in men and 65 in women, diabetes mellitus, family history of heart disease, metabolic syndrome, obesity, tobacco usage, decreased physical activity, increased total LDL or low HDL, diet high in salt and saturated fats, and excessive alcohol consumption.
- Metabolic syndrome promotes the development of atherosclerosis and cardiovascular disease.
- Reduction of blood pressure to normal levels is beneficial for persons with prehypertension with and without preexisting disease.
- Stage 1 hypertension is classified as systolic blood pressure ranges between 140 and 159 mm Hg and diastolic blood pressure ranging between 90 and 99 mm Hg.
- Stage 2 hypertension is classified as systolic blood pressure ≥160 mm Hg and diastolic blood pressure ≥100 mm Hg.
- Hypertension during pregnancy is dangerous to the pregnant woman and the fetus.
- White coat hypertension is an abnormally high blood pressure when the measurement is taken by a health care professional.
- Hypertension is sometimes called the "silent killer" because it can cause damage to the body without any obvious symptoms. Hypertension can weaken arteries and cause aneurysms in the brain, aorta, or abdomen; blindness; kidney disease; and ischemic heart disease.
- Adoption of a healthy lifestyle is often sufficient to reduce blood pressure in patients with prehypertension. Drug therapy should be added to the treatment program in people who have diabetes, kidney disease, or other disease.
- Lifestyle modifications include weight loss, a diet low in salt and cholesterol, increased physical activity, and decreased alcohol and tobacco consumption.
- Diuretics lower blood pressure by decreasing peripheral resistance and cardiac output.
- Diuretics are classified as thiazides, loop, and potassium sparing. Aldosterone antagonists may also be classified as diuretics.
- Thiazide diuretics promote water and sodium, potassium, and chloride ion elimination; decrease blood volume; and lower peripheral resistance.
- Thiazide diuretics should be used cautiously in patients with gout and diabetes.
- Diuretics should be taken in the morning to avoid the need to urinate in the middle of the night (nocturia).
- Loop diuretics block the sodium-potassium cotransporter in the ascending loop of Henle and are the most potent diuretics.

- Loop diuretics can cause dehydration, severe hypotension, hypokalemia, hyperuricemia, photosensitivity, and deafness.
- The effect of loop diuretics and thiazides is reduced if they are taken concurrently with NSAIDs.
- Potassium-sparing diuretics inhibit sodium reabsorption while avoiding potassium loss. They are less effective than loop and thiazide diuretics.
- Patients taking potassium-sparing diuretics should be advised to avoid salt substitutes because they contain potassium chloride (KCl).
- Spironolactone is a competitive antagonist of aldosterone. It is sometimes classified as a potassium-sparing diuretic.
- ACEIs block the conversion of angiotensin I to angiotensin II by inhibiting the activity of angiotensin converting enzyme. Angiotensin II is a potent vasoconstrictor and stimulates the release of aldosterone.
- Dry cough is a common side effect of ACEIs.
- ACEIs are contraindicated in pregnancy because they can interfere with fetal development of the kidneys.
- Angiotensin II receptor blockers are competitive antagonists at the angiotensin II receptor site.
- Angiotensin II receptor blockers are similar to ACE inhibitors in effectiveness but have fewer side effects. They do not produce dry cough.
- β-Adrenergic blockers (β-blockers) lower blood pressure by decreasing heart rate and peripheral resistance.
- β-Blockers used in the treatment of hypertension may be selective (β_1) or nonselective (β_1, β_2).
- β-Blockers are contraindicated in asthma and diabetes.
- α_1-Blockers lower blood pressure by producing vascular relaxation, which reduces peripheral resistance.
- Calcium channel blockers are effective at lowering blood pressure because of their ability to relax blood vessels. They also decrease heart rate and force of contractions, lowering the cardiac output.
- Methyldopa is a prodrug that mimics the autoinhibitory effects of norepinephrine.
- When methyldopa binds to receptors, efferent sympathetic activity is reduced, blood vessels dilate, and peripheral resistance is decreased.
- Clonidine inhibits norepinephrine release from the CNS and peripheral sites, and reserpine depletes neuronal stores of norepinephrine at CNS and peripheral sites.
- Hydralzine and minoxidil decrease peripheral resistance and reduce blood pressure by relaxing vascular smooth muscle.
- Hydralazine is recommended for hypertensive emergencies (parenteral use) and is safe for use in pregnant women.

Multiple Choice

1. _____ is the most often diagnosed medical condition in the United States.
   a. myocardial infarction
   b. hypertension
   c. diabetes
   d. cancer

2. Lifestyle modification is not an important strategy for the prevention and management of hypertension.
   a. true
   b. false

3. The _____ play a major role in regulating blood pressure, and are the site of action for diuretics.
   a. liver
   b. brain
   c. heart
   d. kidneys

4. There are several classifications of diuretics. Which of the following is *not* a class of diuretics?
   a. thiazide
   b. loop
   c. sodium sparing
   d. potassium sparing

5. Diuretics should be taken in the _____ to avoid the need to urinate in the middle of the night (nocturia).
   a. evening
   b. morning
   c. afternoon
   d. night

6. Spironolactone blocks the effect of _____.
   a. aldosterone
   b. antidiuretic hormone
   c. epinephrine
   d. norepinephrine

7. A common ending for ACEIs is
   a. *-pine*
   b. *-statin*
   c. *-pril*
   d. *-olol*

8. Doxazosin and terazosin are examples of what class of drugs?
   a. ACE inhibitors
   b. β-blocker
   c. α_1-blocker
   d. calcium channel blocker

9. Calcium channel blockers are effective at lowering blood pressure because of their ability to constrict blood vessels.
   a. true
   b. false

10. _____ is recommended for hypertensive emergencies (parenteral use) and is safe for use in pregnant women.
    a. hydralazine
    b. hydroxyzine
    c. hydrodiuril
    d. hydrocodone

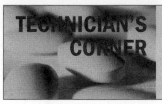

1. Patients with hypertension are often advised to "cut your salt intake in half" as part of their treatment. How much salt is too much, and what is the daily healthy limit?
2. Once a patient has been prescribed antihypertensive medications, can he or she ever be released from taking them?

BIBLIOGRAPHY

Grundy S, et al. Diagnosis and management of the metabolic syndrome: an American Heart Association/National Heart, Lung, and Blood Institute scientific statement, 2005, American Heart Association. Available at: http://www.circulationaha.org DOI: 10.1161/CIRCULATIONAHA.105.169404.

Kalant H, Grant D, Mitchell J: *Principles of medical pharmacology* (pp 157-169, 449-464), ed 7. Toronto, 2007, Elsevier Canada, A Division of Reed Elsevier Canada.

Khan N, et al. The 2006 Canadian Hypertension Education Program recommendations for the management of hypertension: Part II—Therapy. *Can J Cardiol,* 15:583-593, 2006.

Lance L, Lacy C, Armstrong L, Goldman M: *Drug information handbook for the allied health professional,* ed 12. Hudson, OH, 2005, APhA Lexi-Comp.

National Heart, Lung, and Blood Institute: The Seventh Report of the Joint National Committee on Prevention, Detection, Evaluation and Treatment of High Blood Pressure. US Department of Health and Human Services, Bethesda, MD, National Heart, Lung, and Blood Institute, National Institutes of Health, National Blood Pressure Education Program, August 2004. NIH publication No. 04-5290. Available at: http://www.nhlbi.nih.gov/guidelines/hypertension/index.htm.

Page C, Curtis M, Sutter M, Walker M, Hoffman B: *Integrated pharmacology* (pp 395-408), Philadelphia, 2005, Mosby.

USP Center for Advancement of Patient Safety: *Use caution–avoid confusion,* USP Quality Review No. 79, Rockville, MD, April 2004, USP Center for Advancement of Patient Safety.

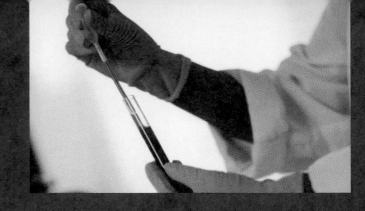

CHAPTER 23

Treatment of Heart Failure

LEARNING OBJECTIVES

- Learn the terminology associated with congestive heart failure (CHF).
- List the symptoms of CHF.
- List risk factors for CHF.
- List and categorize medications used to treat CHF.
- Describe mechanism of action for each class of drugs used to treat CHF.
- Identify warning labels and precautionary messages associated with medications used to treat CHF.
- Identify significant drug look-alike/sound-alike issues.
- List common endings for drug classes used in the treatment of CHF.

KEY TERMS

Automaticity: Spontaneous depolarization (contraction) of heart cells.

Cardioglycosides: Class of drugs, most commonly derived from the foxglove plant, that have the ability to alter cardiovascular function. Digitalis is representative of this class of drugs.

Digitalization: Process of rapidly increasing the initial dose of digoxin until the therapeutic dose is achieved.

Ejection fraction: Percentage of blood ejected from the left ventricle with each heartbeat.

Heart failure: Clinical syndrome in which the heart is unable to pump blood at a rate to meet the body's metabolic needs.

Natriuretic peptides: Hormones that play a role in cardiac homeostasis.

Positive inotropic effect: Increase in the force of myocardial contractions.

Stroke volume: Equal to the volume of blood ejected by the left ventricle during each cardiac contraction minus the volume of blood in the ventricle at the end of systole.

Overview

Heart failure is a clinical syndrome in which the heart is unable to pump blood at a rate necessary to meet the body's metabolic needs. Heart failure affects more than 5 million people in the United States and is responsible for nearly 300,000 deaths each year. More than 500,000 new cases are diagnosed annually. The syndrome primarily affects the elderly affecting more than 10% of the population over 50 years as compared to 1% of persons under the age of 50. Up to age 75, the prevalence of heart failure is higher in men, but after age 75, the prevalence is higher in women.

Disease, lifestyle, and drugs can contribute to the onset or aggravation of heart failure. Kidney dysfunction, diabetes, ischemic heart disease, hypertension, hypothyroidism, hyperthyroidism, bradyarrhythmia, tachyarrhythmia, pulmonary embolism, HIV/AIDS, and myocardial infarction contribute to heart failure. Excessive salt and alcohol consumption as well of lack of physical activity can worsen heart failure. Nonsteroidal antiinflammatory drugs worsen edema and interfere with the effect of drugs used to treat heart failure (e.g., ACE inhibitors).

Pathophysiology of Heart Failure

Heart failure may affect the left side of the heart, the right side of the heart, or both sides. Left-sided heart failure reduces the volume of oxygen and nutrient-rich blood pumped from the left ventricle to the rest of the body. Persons with left-sided heart failure may have swelling in the legs and ankles and feel fatigued. Fluid accumulation can result in weight gain and increased urination. Right sided-heart failure reduces the capacity of the heart to pump blood to the lungs. Fluids back up (venous congestion) and cause pulmonary edema and shortness of breath. Blood pressure increases.

Heart failure may be classified as systolic heart failure (SHF) or diastolic heart failure (DHF). In SHF, left ventricular contractions are reduced causing a decrease in the volume of blood ejected from the ventricles (stroke volume). The result is reduced cardiac output. In DHF, stroke volume is reduced because the left ventricle is unable to accept a sufficient volume of blood during diastole. Cardiac output is reduced, causing fatigue, dyspnea, and pulmonary hypertension.

Compensatory mechanisms are "switched on" when the heart function fails (Figure 23-1). In an attempt to satisfy the metabolic needs of the body, and to reduce elevated blood pressure, the renin-aldosterone-angiotensin system (RAAS) is activated. RAAS activation results in increases in blood volume and cardiac output because RAAS activation produces sodium and fluid retention. The RAAS is also activated by chronic sympathetic nervous system (SNS) stimulation, which is also linked to heart failure.

Natriuretic peptides are hormones that also play a role in cardiac physiology. Their release is another compensatory mechanism in heart failure. Atrial natriuretic peptide (ANP) and brain natriuretic peptide (BNP) promote sodium and water elimination by the kidneys, vasodilation, and diastolic relaxation. ANP and BNP increase with aging and heart wall stress. Levels decrease in obesity and may contribute to hypertension.

Stages of Heart Failure

There are four stages of heart failure. Heart failure may also be described by functional class. American College of Cardiology/American Heart Association (ACC/AHA) descriptions and New York Heart Association (NYHA) functional classifications are compared in Table 23-1.

Drugs Used to Treat Heart Failure

Most of the treatments used in heart failure focus on treating symptoms, underlying causes, and factors that worsen heart failure. Many of the same drugs administered in the treatment of hypertension are also used in the treatment of heart failure. They include diuretics, aldosterone antagonists, β-blockers, ACE inhibitors, and angiotensin II receptor blockers. These drugs are covered in detail in Chapter 22. Cardioglycosides are the oldest class of drugs used in the treatment of heart failure and are described following. Statins (see Chapter 24) are also administered for the treatment of heart failure.

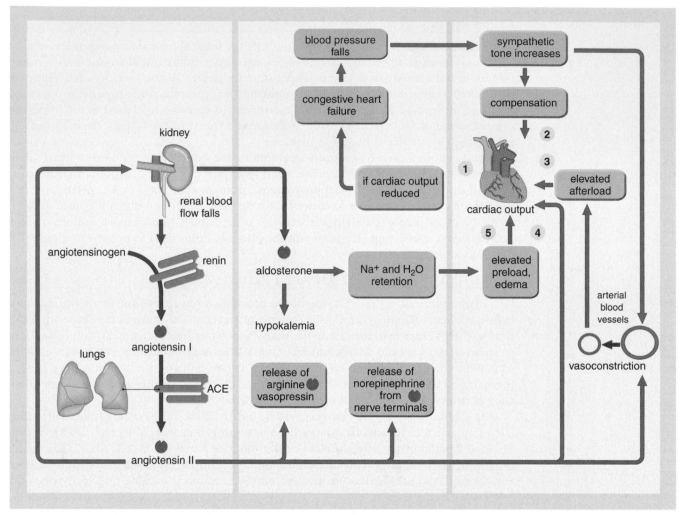

FIGURE 23-1 Compensatory mechanisms in congestive heart failure. *(From Page C, et al.* Integrated pharmacology, *ed 3 Philadelphia, 2005, Mosby.)*

TABLE 23-1 Classification* and Management of Heart Failure

ACC/AHA Stage A	No NYHA classification	High risk for developing heart failure because of: • Hypertension • Coronary artery disease • Diabetes mellitus • History of cardiotoxic drug therapy • Alcohol abuse • History of rheumatic fever • Family history of cardiomyopathy	Lifestyle modification Diuretics if patient has fluid retention ACE inhibitors β-Blockers Treatment of underlying disease (diabetes, hypertension, etc.) Antihyperlipidemics Antiarrhythmics

ACC/AHA Stage B	NYHA Class II	Structural heart disease but no prior symptoms
		  of heart failure
		Prior myocardial infarction
		Left ventricular hypertrophy
		Asymptomatic valvular disease
		Left ventricular dilation or hypocontractility
			All of Stage A treatment options plus
			Structural repairs, e.g., heart valve
			  replacement if needed

ACC/AHA Stage C	NYHA Class II and III	Current or prior symptoms of HF associated
		  with structural heart disease
			Treatment of symptoms as per Stage A
			  and B recommendations plus digoxin

ACC/AHA Stage D	NYHA Class IV	Advanced structural heart disease plus heart failure
		  symptoms at rest despite medical therapy
			Treatment of symptoms as per Stage A
			  and B recommendations plus digoxin

*American College of Cardiology/American Heart Association guidelines for evaluation and management and NHYA functional classes.

CARDIOGLYCOSIDES

Digitalis is a cardioglycoside derived from the foxglove plant. Despite its historical use, studies by the Digitalis Investigation Group (DIG) trial show that although digoxin reduces hospitalization and improves exercise tolerance in symptomatic patients, it fails to increase survival in patients with heart failure. In fact, digoxin may actually increase mortality in women. Digoxin should be administered along with ACE inhibitors, diuretics, and or β-blockers (Figure 23-2).

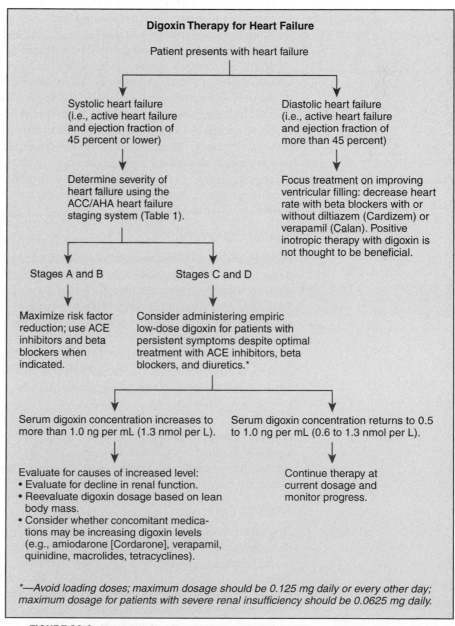

Digoxin Therapy for Heart Failure

Patient presents with heart failure

Systolic heart failure (i.e., active heart failure and ejection fraction of 45 percent or lower)

Diastolic heart failure (i.e., active heart failure and ejection fraction of more than 45 percent)

Determine severity of heart failure using the ACC/AHA heart failure staging system (Table 1).

Focus treatment on improving ventricular filling: decrease heart rate with beta blockers with or without diltiazem (Cardizem) or verapamil (Calan). Positive inotropic therapy with digoxin is not thought to be beneficial.

Stages A and B

Stages C and D

Maximize risk factor reduction; use ACE inhibitors and beta blockers when indicated.

Consider administering empiric low-dose digoxin for patients with persistent symptoms despite optimal treatment with ACE inhibitors, beta blockers, and diuretics.*

Serum digoxin concentration increases to more than 1.0 ng per mL (1.3 nmol per L).

Serum digoxin concentration returns to 0.5 to 1.0 ng per mL (0.6 to 1.3 nmol per L).

Evaluate for causes of increased level:
• Evaluate for decline in renal function.
• Reevaluate digoxin dosage based on lean body mass.
• Consider whether concomitant medications may be increasing digoxin levels (e.g., amiodarone [Cordarone], verapamil, quinidine, macrolides, tetracyclines).

Continue therapy at current dosage and monitor progress.

*—Avoid loading doses; maximum dosage should be 0.125 mg daily or every other day; maximum dosage for patients with severe renal insufficiency should be 0.0625 mg daily.

FIGURE 23-2 Algorithm for digoxin therapy for heart failure. *(Modified from Morris S, Hatcher HF: Digoxin therapy for heart failure: An update,* Am Family Phys, *August 15, 2006. Available at: http://www.aafp.org/afp/20060815/613.html.)*

BOX 23-1 LIFESTYLE MODIFICATIONS RECOMMENDED FOR PEOPLE WITH HEART FAILURE

- Follow a diet low in salt.
- Limit the amount of fluids that you drink.
- Increase physical activity.

- Lose weight if you are overweight.
- Quit smoking if you smoke.
- Limit alcohol consumption.

TECH NOTE!

Lifestyle modification is recommended for people with heart failure in order to reduce symptoms and complications.

MECHANISM OF ACTION

Cardioglycosides such as digoxin have a ***positive inotropic effect*** on the heart; they increase the force of myocardial contractions. The greater force of contractions increases the cardiac output and reduces diastolic heart size. As end-diastolic pressures decrease, pulmonary and systemic venous pressures are reduced.

The positive inotropic effect is produced by the inhibition of the Na^+/K^+ ATPase pump, leading to increased intracellular sodium, and inhibition of the Na^+/Ca^{2+} exchanger. Digoxin-induced inhibition of the Na^+/Ca^{2+} exchanger leads to increased calcium, an electrolyte involved in the contraction of cardiac smooth muscle.

Digoxin increases cardiac output and decreases compensatory sympathetic activity, which results in a slowed heart rate. Heart rate is also slowed by stimulation of parasympathetic nervous system activity (increased vagal tone). Digoxin also decreases intracellular potassium. Excessively low potassium depletion can increase ***automaticity.*** Automaticity is the spontaneous depolarization (contraction) of heart cells (see Chapter 25) and can cause arrhythmias. Moreover, digoxin produces significant effects on the heart's conduction system. It decreases conduction velocity through the atrioventricular (AV) node, prolonging the refractory period (time between contractions). The number of depolarizations is reduced, too. A further description of digoxin's effect on the conduction system is described in Chapter 25.

PHARMACOKINETICS

Digoxin is the only commercially available cardioglycoside in the United States. Available dosage forms are capsules, tablets, elixir, and parenteral solution. Oral absorption is good (60% to 85%), and bioavailability of orally administered digoxin is between 70% and 85%. The bioavailability of digoxin differs between commercial manufacturers, so attempts should be made to consistently dispense the same manufacturer's product each time. Food can decrease absorption.

The peak effect of digoxin occurs 1.5 to 5 hours after administration and the half-life of digoxin is approximately 36 hours. Between 30% and 50% is eliminated unchanged by the kidneys and clearance is reduced in heart failure.

ADVERSE REACTIONS

Adverse drug reactions produced by digoxin include diarrhea, constipation, nausea, vomiting, fatigue, weakness, visual disturbances (altered color perception, hazy vision), photophobia, impotence, and gynecomastia. Signs of digitalis toxicity are arrhythmia, dizziness, headache, convulsions, delusions, and coma.

PRECAUTIONS

Digitalization is the process of rapidly increasing the initial dose of digoxin until the therapeutic dose is achieved. The patient must be monitored carefully for signs of digitalis toxicity because digoxin has a narrow therapeutic index. Half of the total digitalizing dose should be administered as the initial dose, followed by one-fourth of the digitalizing dose in 8 to 12 hours. The final one-fourth dose is administered 8 to 12 hours later.

Switching between manufacturer's products is not recommended because of bioavailability differences. According to current AHA/ACC recommendations, digoxin is not recommended for the treatment of DHF in men or women, especially if sinoatrial or AV block is present (see Chapter 25).

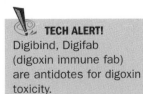

TECH ALERT!

Digibind, Digifab (digoxin immune fab) are antidotes for digoxin toxicity.

Usual Dose, Dosing Schedule, and Warnings for Digoxin

Drug name	Usual dose and dosing schedule	
Cardioglycosides		
digoxin	0.125 mg to 0.5 mg once daily	TAKE AS DIRECTED; DON'T SKIP OR EXCEED DOSAGE
		IF YOU MISS A DOSE, TAKE IT AS SOON AS YOU REMEMBER UNLESS THE NEXT DOSE IS SCHEDULED TO BE TAKEN IN FEWER THAN 12 HOURS

Cardioglycosides Used in the Treatment of Heart Failure

The only cardioglycoside currently marketed in the United States and Canada is digoxin.

Cardioglycosides

	U.S. brand name(s)	
Generic name	**Canadian brand(s)**	**Dosage forms and strengths**
digoxin*	Digitek, Lanoxin, Lanoxicaps	Capsule (Lanoxicaps): 0.1 mg, 0.2 mg
		Elixir (Lanoxin): 0.05 mg/ml
	Digibind, Lanoxin CSD	Injection, solution: 0.25 mg/ml
		Tablet (Digitek, Lanoxin): 0.125 mg, 0.25 mg, 0.5 mg

*Generic available.

DIURETICS

Diuretics are administered to treat volume overload. They also lower blood pressure. Elevated blood pressure can aggravate existing DHF or precipitate its onset. Diuretics also reduce pulmonary edema and swelling in the ankles, legs, and feet (peripheral edema). When diuretics are administered, potassium levels should be monitored, as loop and thiazide diuretics can cause hypokalemia (see Chapter 22). Hypokalemia can cause ventricular arrhythmias and increase the effects of digoxin leading to toxicity. See the following drug table for usual doses of diuretics used in the treatment of heart failure.

β-BLOCKERS

β-Blockers reduce heart rate, lower peripheral arterial resistance, and decrease the workload of your heart. They also reduce left ventricular hypertrophy, and studies show β-blockers can lower the risk of mortality associated with congestive heart failure. The mechanism of action for β-blockers use in the treatment of heart failure is to block excess sympathetic stimulation induced by heart failure. Recall that increased sympathetic tone is a compensatory mechanism commonly seen with heart failure. See the following drug table for doses used in the treatment of heart failure.

CALCIUM CHANNEL BLOCKERS

Calcium channel blockers may be used in the treatment of diastolic heart failure because they control heart rate, lower blood pressure, and treat ischemia—risk factors for congestive heart failure. Like β-blockers, calcium channel blockers reduce left ventricular hypertrophy. Exercise tolerance and diastolic filling are improved by verapamil. Calcium channel blockers should not be administered for the treatment of SHF because they can make ventricular contractions worse, further reducing cardiac output. Congestive heart failure may be induced when ventricular function is impaired. See the following drug table for doses used in the treatment of heart failure.

ACE INHIBITORS AND ANGIOTENSIN II RECEPTOR BLOCKERS

ACE inhibitors are one of the few classes of drugs used in the treatment of heart failure that have been shown to reduce mortality (prolong life). They reduce left ventricular hypertrophy, improve diastolic filling, increase cardiac output, and reduce peripheral vascular resistance. When angiotensin II levels are decreased, sympathetic tone and aldosterone-mediated sodium increase and blood volume expansion are also reduced. Angiotensin II receptor blockers (ARBs) are also administered for the treatment of heart failure. ARBs improve exercise tolerance and diastolic filling in patients with diastolic heart failure. See the following drug table for doses used in the treatment of heart failure.

STATINS

Administration of a statin (e.g., atrovastatin) is associated with increased survival in patients with heart failure with ischemic disease but increased mortality when total cholesterol levels are low and ischemic disease is absent. Heart failure is linked to inflammation and statins have been shown to reduce inflammation. Statins are discussed in depth in Chapter 24.

VASODILATORS

Isosorbide dinitrate and hydralazine are used in combination for the treatment of heart failure for their vasodilating effects. This reduces peripheral resistance along with cardiac preload and afterload. Moreover, hydralazine has been shown to indirectly increase the force of myocardial contractions (positive inotropic effect). When combined with nitrates such as isosorbide dinitrate, hydralazine can decrease mortality and effectively reduce cardiac congestion. See the following drug table for doses used in the treatment of heart failure.

Usual Dose and Dosing Schedule for Other Drugs Used in the Treatment of Heart Failure

Drug name	Usual dose and dosing schedule
Diuretics	
Thiazides	
chlorothiazide	500 mg to 1 g 1 to 2 times a day
chlorthalidone	25 mg to 100 mg/day or 100 mg 3 times/week
hydrochlorothiazide (HCTZ)	25 mg to 100 mg daily
indapamide	2.5 mg to 5 mg daily
Loop	
bumetanide	0.5 mg to 2 mg daily
furosemide	40 mg to 120 mg PO or IV per day (maximum 600 mg orally/day)
torsemide	10 mg to 20 mg PO or IV daily (maximum 200 mg/day)
Aldosterone receptor antagonist	
spironolactone	25 mg to 50 mg daily
Cardioglycosides	
digoxin	0.125 mg to 0.5 mg once daily
β-blockers	
bisoprolol	1.25 mg to 10 mg daily
metoprolol extended release	Begin 25 mg/day; increase up to 200 mg daily

Usual Dose and Dosing Schedule for Other Drugs Used in the Treatment of Heart Failure—cont'd

Drug name	Usual dose and dosing schedule	
Combined α- and β-blockers		
carvedilol	Begin 3.125 mg twice daily; increase to 25 mg to 50 mg twice daily	
ACE inhibitors		
benazepril	2 mg to 20 mg/day	
captopril	25 mg to 50 mg 2 to 3 times a day	
enalapril	2.5 mg to 20 mg PO twice daily	
lisinopril	5 mg to 40 mg daily	
quinapril	10 mg to 20 mg twice daily	
ramipril	2.5 mg to 5 mg daily	
trandolapril	1 mg to 4 mg daily	
Angiotensin II antagonists		
candesartan	Begin 4 mg daily; increase to 32 mg daily	
losartan	50 mg daily	
valsartan	40 mg to 160 mg twice daily	
Vasodilators (hydralazine + isosorbide in combination)		
hydralazine	10 mg to 25 mg 3 times a day (maximum 300 mg daily)	Systolic heart failure
isosorbide dinitrate	10 mg to 40 mg 3 times a day	

CHAPTER SUMMARY

- Heart failure is a clinical syndrome in which the heart is unable to pump blood at a rate to meet the body's metabolic needs.
- Kidney dysfunction, diabetes, ischemic heart disease, hypertension, hypothyroidism, hyperthyroidism, bradyarrhythmia, tachyarrythmia, pulmonary embolism, HIV/AIDS, and myocardial infarction contribute to heart failure.
- Lifestyle factors such as excessive salt and alcohol consumption and lack of physical activity can worsen heart failure.
- Nonsteroidal antiinflammatory drugs worsen edema and interfere with the effect of drugs used to treat heart failure such as ACE inhibitors.
- Heart failure may affect the left side of the heart, the right side of the heart, or both sides. Left-sided heart failure reduces the volume of oxygen and nutrient blood pumped from the left ventricle to the rest of the body. Right-sided heart failure reduces the capacity of the heart to pump blood to the lungs.
- Heart failure may be classified as systolic heart failure (SHF) or diastolic heart failure (DHF). The choice of drug therapy is influenced by whether the patient has SHF or DHF.
- Compensatory mechanisms are "switched on" when the heart function fails. Compensatory mechanisms attempt to satisfy the metabolic needs of the body and to reduce elevated blood pressure.
- There are four stages of heart failure: stage A, high risk for developing heart failure; stage B, structural changes without symptoms; stage C, symptomatic; and stage D, advanced structural heart disease plus heart failure symptoms.

- Lifestyle modification is recommended for all stages of heart failure.
- Drugs used in the treatment of heart failure include cardioglycosides, diuretics, aldosterone antagonists, β-blockers, ACE inhibitors, and angiotensin II receptor blockers.
- Digoxin is the only cardioglycoside currently marketed in the United States and Canada.
- Digoxin reduces hospitalization and improves exercise tolerance in symptomatic patients but fails to increase survival in patients with heart failure.
- Digoxin has a positive inotropic effect on the heart; the result is an increase in the force of myocardial contractions.
- Digoxin increases cardiac output and decreases compensatory sympathetic activity.
- Available dosage forms are capsules, tablets, elixir, and parenteral solution.
- The bioavailability of digoxin differs between commercial manufacturers and food can decrease absorption.
- Digitalization is the process of rapidly increasing the initial dose of digoxin until the therapeutic dose is achieved. The patient must be monitored carefully for signs of digitalis toxicity because digoxin has a narrow therapeutic index.
- Diuretics are administered in heart failure to reduce edema. Diuretics that produce hypokalemia can increase the effects of digoxin leading to toxicity.
- Studies show β-blockers can lower the risk of mortality associated with congestive heart failure. β-Blockers reduce excess sympathetic stimulation induced by heart failure.
- Calcium channel blockers may be used in the treatment of diastolic heart failure but should be avoided in systolic heart failure.
- ACE inhibitors reduce mortality. They reduce left ventricular hypertrophy, improve diastolic filling, increase cardiac output, and reduce peripheral vascular resistance.
- Administration of statins is associated with increased survival in patients with heart failure with ischemic disease but increased mortality when total cholesterol levels are low and ischemic disease is absent.
- Isosorbide dinitrate and hydralazine are used in combination for the treatment of heart failure to decrease mortality and effectively reduce cardiac congestion.

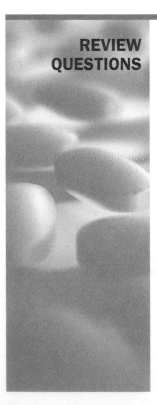

REVIEW QUESTIONS

Multiple Choice

1. **Heart failure affects only the left side of the heart.**
   a. true
   b. false
2. **Heart failure may be classified as**
   a. systolic heart failure
   b. diastolic heart failure.
   c. ventricular heart failure
   d. a and b
3. _____ **are the oldest class of drugs used in the treatment of heart failure.**
   a. aminoglycosides
   b. cardioglycosides
   c. diuretics
   d. antiobiotics
4. **Digitalis is a cardioglycoside derived from the foxglove plant.**
   a. true
   b. false

5. Digitalization is the process of rapidly _____ the initial dose of digoxin until the therapeutic dose is achieved.
    a. increasing
    b. decreasing
    c. stabilizing
    d. titrating

6. Thiazide diuretics can cause
    a. hyperkalemia
    b. hypernatremia
    c. hypokalemia
    d. hypocalcemia

7. The mechanism of action for β-blockers used in the treatment of heart failure is to block excess _____ stimulation induced by heart failure.
    a. sympathetic
    b. parasympathetic

8. Calcium channel blockers may be used in the treatment of diastolic heart failure because they _____.
    a. control heart rate
    b. lower blood pressure
    c. treat ischemia
    d. all of the above

9. ACE inhibitors are one of the few classes of drugs used in the treatment of heart failure that have been shown to _____.
    a. increase mortality
    b. reduce mortality
    c. have no effect on mortality
    d. all of the above

10. Isosorbide dinitrate and hydralazine are used in combination for the treatment of heart failure for their _____ effects.
    a. vasodilating
    b. vasoconstricting
    c. sympathetic
    d. parasympathetic

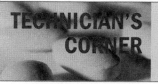

TECHNICIAN'S CORNER

1. From the time the drug digoxin was discovered, it has always been extracted from the foxglove plant. Why can't it be produced synthetically in the lab?
2. Patients with heart failure are always advised to make lifestyle modifications as part of their treatment. Why is that process so important and so difficult to do?

BIBLIOGRAPHY

Aronow W: Epidemiology, pathophysiology, prognosis, and treatment of systolic and diastolic heart failure, *Cardiol Rev,* 14:108-124, 2006.

Davies M, Gibbs C, et al. ABC of heart failure management: diuretics, ACE inhibitors, and nitrates, *BMJ.*320:428-431, 2000.

Felker M, Petersen J, Mark D: Natriuretic peptides in the diagnosis and management of heart failure, *CMAJ* 175:611-617, 2006.

Kalant H, Grant D, Mitchell J: *Principles of medical pharmacology* (pp 22-27, 451, 453-454, 503-504), ed 7. Toronto, 2007, Elsevier Canada, A Division of Reed Elsevier Canada.

Lance L, Lacy C, Armstrong L, Goldman M: *Drug information handbook for the allied health professional,* ed 12. Hudson, OH, 2005, APhA Lexi-Comp.

May H, et al. Relation of serum total cholesterol, C-reactive protein levels, and statin therapy to survival in heart failure, *Am J Cardiol*, 98:653-658, 2006.

National Heart, Lung, and Blood Institute: What is heart failure? Diseases and conditions index. Bethesda, MD, National Heart, Lung, and Blood Institute, National Institutes of Health, US Department of Health and Human Services, July 2006 Available at: http://www.nhlbi.nih.gov/health/dci/Diseases/Hf/HF_WhatIs.html.

Page C, Curtis M, Sutter M, Walker M, Hoffman B: *Integrated pharmacology* (pp 386-391, 393-395), Philadelphia, 2005, Mosby.

Shammas R, Khan N, Nekkanti R, Movahed A: Diastolic heart failure and left ventricular diastolic dysfunction: What we know, and what we don't know! *Int J Cardiol*, 2006.

USP Center for Advancement of Patient Safety: *Use caution–avoid confusion*, USP Quality Review No. 79, Rockville, MD, April 2004, USP Center for Advancement of Patient Safety.

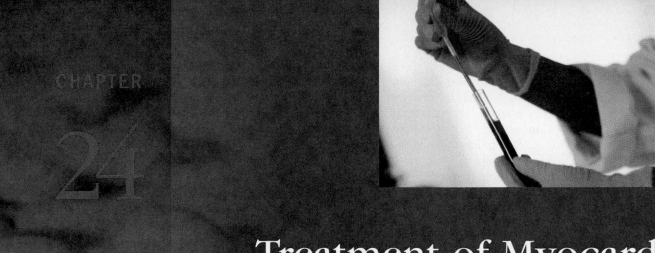

Treatment of Myocardial Infarction and Stroke

- Learn the terminology associated with myocardial infarction and stroke.
- List the symptoms of myocardial infarction and stroke.
- List risk factors for myocardial infarction and stroke.
- List and categorize medications used to treat myocardial infarction, stroke, and hyperlipidemia.
- Describe the mechanism of action for each class of drugs used to treat myocardial infarction and stroke.
- Identify warning labels and precautionary messages associated with medications used to treat myocardial infarction, stroke, and hyperlipidemia.
- Identify significant drug look-alike/sound-alike issues.
- List common endings for drug classes used in the treatment of myocardial infarction, stroke, and hyperlipidemia.

KEY TERMS

Aneurysm: Weakened spot of the artery wall that has stretched or burst filling the area with blood and causing damage. If in the brain, damage to nerves results.

Anoxia: Absence of oxygen supply to cells that results in cell damage or death.

Anticoagulant: Drug that prolongs coagulation time and is used to prevent clot formation.

Antiplatelet agent: Drug that prevents accumulation of platelets, thereby blocking an important step in the clot formation process.

Antithrombotic: Drug that inhibits clot formation by reducing the coagulation action of the blood protein thrombin.

Atherosclerosis: Buildup of lipids and plaque inside artery walls; impeding the flow of blood and oxygen.

Atherothrombosis: Formation of a blood clot in an artery.

Cholesterol: Naturally occurring, waxy substance produced by the liver and found in foods that maintains cell membranes and is needed for vitamin D production. Excess cholesterol can cause atherosclerosis.

Embolic stroke: Stroke caused by an emboli obstructing the flow of blood through an artery.

Hemorrhagic stroke: Sudden bleeding into or around the brain.

Hemostasis: Process of stopping the flow of blood.

High-density lipoprotein (HDL): "Good cholesterol"; lipoproteins that transport cholesterol, triglycerides, and other lipids from blood to body tissues.

Hyperlipidemia: Excess lipids or fatty substances in the blood.

Hypoxia: Reduced oxygen delivery to cells. Total reduction of oxygen supplied is called anoxia.

Infarction: Sudden loss of blood supply to an area that results in cell death. A myocardial infarction is known as a heart attack. A cerebral infarction is also known as a stroke.

Ischemia: Reduction of blood supplied to tissues that is typically caused by blood vessel obstruction due to atherosclerosis, stenosis, or plaque.

Ischemic stroke: Ischemia in the brain.

Lipoprotein: Small globules of cholesterol covered by a layer of protein.

Low-density lipoprotein (LDL): Compound consisting of a lipid and a protein that carries the majority of the total cholesterol in the blood and deposits the excess along the inside of arterial walls; also known as "bad cholesterol."

Mitral valve stenosis: Disease of the mitral valve involving build-up of plaque-like material around the valve.

Necrosis: Cell death.

Plaque: Fatty cholesterol deposits.

Platelets: Structures found in the blood that are involved in the coagulation process.

Partial thromboplastin time (PTT): Test given to determine effectiveness of heparin in reducing antithrombotic activity.

Prothrombin time (PT), Pro-Time, INR: Test given to determine the effectiveness of warfarin in reducing clotting time.

Rhabdomyolysis: Breakdown of muscle fibers and release of muscle fiber contents into the circulation. These muscle fibers are toxic to the kidneys.

Stenosis: Stiffening and narrowing of artery walls.

Thrombolytic: Drug used to dissolve blood clots.

Thrombosis: Formation of a blood clot.

Thrombotic stroke: Stroke caused by thrombosis.

Tissue plasminogen activator (t-PA): Naturally occurring thrombolytic substance.

Transient ischemic attack (TIA): Stroke that typically lasts for a few minutes; also known as a mini-stroke.

Triglycerides: Storage form of energy found in fat tissue muscle; metabolize to very low-density lipoproteins (VLDLs).

Overview

Americans have more than 1.2 million heart attacks annually and up to 40% of patients die from it. That makes myocardial infarction the leading cause of death in the United States, accounting for nearly 500,000 deaths. More than 600,000 Americans each year will have a stroke. Stroke is the third leading cause of death in the United States. Approximately 50,000 will have a mini-stroke (*transient ischemic attack*). Persons that have had one stroke, and recover, are more likely to have another. Nearly 25% of patients will have a second stroke within 5 years of the first stroke. Cardiovascular disease is the number one cause of death in Canada, accounting for 36% of deaths due to all causes. Acute myocardial infarction (27%), cerebral vascular disease (20%), and ischemic heart disease (27%) are the primary causes of death due to all cardiovascular disease in Canada.

Types of Stroke

Strokes occur when brain cells are deprived of oxygen or are damaged by sudden bleeding into the brain. *Ischemic strokes* account for 80% of all strokes and are caused by oxygen deprivation. *Anoxia* (absence of oxygen) occurs when arteries are obstructed and is the cause of brain infarcts. *Thrombotic stroke* is caused by an enlarged *thrombus* or blood clot. *Embolic stroke* is caused by an embolus (traveling clot) or *plaque* that has been dislodged. Blood clots (thrombi, emboli) are the most common cause of strokes.

Hemorrhagic strokes account for the remaining 20% of all strokes and are caused by bleeding in the brain. It may be the result of an *aneurysm,* a weakened spot of the artery wall that has stretched or burst filling the area with blood and causing damage.

Transient ischemic attacks (TIAs) are also known as mini-strokes. They typically last only a few minutes and symptoms usually resolve within an hour.

Symptoms of Stroke

Regardless of the cause, strokes produce similar symptoms. Symptoms appear suddenly and are listed in Table 24-1.

Symptoms of Myocardial Infarction

Myocardial infarction produces symptoms that are similar to angina. Prompt treatment of myocardial infarction is essential to persons experiencing the symptoms listed in Table 24-2. If symptoms persist beyond 15 minutes, emergency assistance (dialing 911) should be sought.

Pathophysiology of Stroke and Myocardial Infarction

Stroke and myocardial infarction occur when the blood supply to the brain (stroke) or heart (myocardial infarction) is interrupted. Cells become damaged or die when they are deprived of oxygen and nutrients. Chronic inflammation of arteries that supply the heart and brain can also lead to stroke and myocardial infarction because vascular inflammation is a cause of atherosclerosis. *Atherosclerosis* (a buildup of lipids and plaque inside of artery walls) can block bloodflow through arteries. *Atherothrombosis* (the formation of a blood clot in the artery) is triggered by atherosclerosis and can also cause clogged arteries. The risk for chronic vascular inflammation increases with age.

Risk Factors for Stroke and Myocardial Infarction

Risk factors for stroke and myocardial infarction are categorized as modifiable and non-modifiable. Nonmodifiable risk factors are age, gender, and family history. In addition, chronic diseases such as hypertension, ischemic heart disease, and diabetes place patients at increased risk for stroke.

TABLE 24-1   Symptoms of Stroke

Limbs	Numbness or weakness of arms, legs
	Difficulty walking
	Loss of balance or coordination
EENT	Facial numbness or weakness
	Impaired speech
	Impaired vision
Cognitive	Confusion
	Difficulty understanding speech
Other	Dizziness
	Severe headache

TABLE 24-2   Characteristics of Myocardial Infarction Versus Stroke

Characteristics	Myocardial infarction	Angina
Timing	Sudden onset	Often occur after exercise
	Last longer than 30 minutes	Last 1 to 5 minutes
	May occur at rest	Rest may relieve symptoms
Location	Mid-chest radiating to jaw, neck, arms, and epigastric area	Mid-chest radiating to jaw, neck, arms, and epigastric area
Quality	Severe, squeezing or heaviness in chest area	Heaviness, chest tightness, indigestion

NONMODIFIABLE RISK FACTORS

AGE

Age is a significant risk factor for stroke and myocardial infarction. Although stroke can occur at any age, the risk increases exponentially with each increasing decade. Approximately 66% of strokes occur in persons older than 65 years. Strokes that occur in persons more than 65 years old are more likely to be fatal.

GENDER

Gender is also an important risk factor for stroke. Men are 1.25 times more likely to have a stroke than are women, yet strokes in men are less likely to be fatal. This is probably because men are often younger than women when they have a stroke. As with stroke, men have a greater risk for heart attack than do women; however, the older women are more likely to die within 3 weeks of a heart attack than are men.

MODIFIABLE RISK FACTORS

Modifiable risk factors for stroke and myocardial infarction are smoking, alcohol consumption, and diet. Smoking promotes atherosclerosis, increases clotting factors in the blood (fibrinogen), stimulates vasoconstriction, and weakens the endothelial wall. These factors contribute to the risk for ischemic stroke and hemorrhagic stroke. Excessive alcohol consumption and binge drinking lead to an increase in blood pressure and can reduce platelets, which increase the risk for hemorrhagic stroke. After heavy drinking, a rebound effect occurs that increases platelets and thickens the blood significantly, increasing the risk of ischemic stroke. A diet high in cholesterol may increase the risk for atherosclerosis, and a diet high in salt can aggravate hypertension.

HYPERTENSION

Hypertension increases the risk for stroke 4 to 6 times above that of persons without hypertension, and 90% of persons who have had a stroke have hypertension.

ATRIAL FIBRILLATION

Atrial fibrillation (see Chapter 25), rapid and irregular beating of the atrium chamber of the heart, can increase the risk for clots. If the clots are dislodged, they can occlude an artery, leading to stroke or myocardial infarction. Malformations of the heart valves (mitral valve stenosis) can also lead to clot formation, increasing the risk of stroke or myocardial infarction.

HIGH CHOLESTEROL

High cholesterol levels are a risk factor for stroke and myocardial infarction. Cholesterol may be in the form of high-density lipoproteins (HDL) and low-density lipoproteins (LDL). LDL can build up within artery walls and harden. This hardened material is called ***plaque,*** and it can impede blood supply to the heart and brain. During surgery, plaque can become dislodged, interrupting blood supply and causing stroke or myocardial infarction. Diabetes also increases the development of atherosclerosis and therefore is a risk factor for stroke and myocardial infarction.

INFECTION

Infection is a risk factor for stroke and myocardial infarction. The immune system response to bacterial and viral infections is to release cytokines, leukotrienes, macrophages, and other infection-fighting substances that also increase inflammation. These substances can increase the risk for ischemic and embolic stroke.

Lifestyle Modification

Lifestyle modifications are recommended to reduce risk for stroke and myocardial infarction and are listed in Box 24-1.

BOX 24-1 LIFESTYLE MODIFICATIONS RECOMMENDED FOR PEOPLE WITH HEART FAILURE

- Follow a diet low in salt.
- Limit the amount of fluids that you drink.
- Increase physical activity.
- Lose weight if you are overweight.
- Quit smoking if you smoke.
- Limit alcohol consumption.

Drugs Used in the Treatment of Stroke and Myocardial Infarction

Given the fact that atherosclerosis and atherothrombosis are important risk factors for stroke and myocardial infarction, drugs that control the buildup of lipids and plaque and drugs that reduce the formation of blood clots are administered to prevent stroke and myocardial infarction.

DRUGS THAT CONTROL HEMOSTASIS

Drugs that control *hemostasis* (the process of stopping the flow of blood) can prevent atherothrombosis and complications associated with the formation of blood clots in arteries. Clotting is a normal process without which one would bleed to death should an injury occur (Figure 24-1). If clots form in an artery and obstruct the supply of blood and oxygen to the brain and heart, a stroke and myocardial infarction may occur. Drugs that control the rate of clot formation and clot dissolution are classified as antithrombotics and can prevent stroke and myocardial infarction. Antithrombotic drugs include (1) agents that inhibit platelets; (2) anticoagulants, which lessen coagulation; and (3) fibrinolytic agents. Fibrinolytics dissolve existing clots.

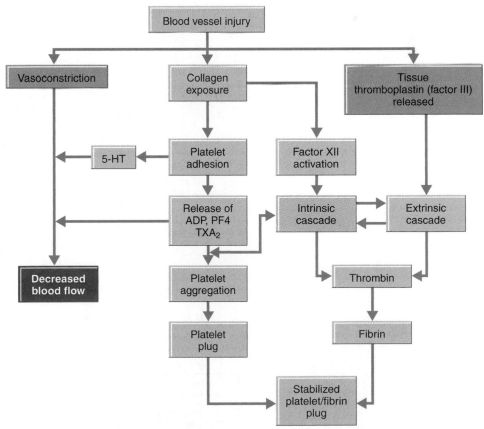

FIGURE 24-1 Clot formation. *(From Lilley LL, Harrington S, Snyder JS: Pharmacology and the nursing process, ed 5. St. Louis, 2007, Mosby.)*

ANTIPLATELET DRUGS

MECHANISM OF ACTION

Antiplatelet drugs produce their effect by interfering with steps in the clot formation process (Figure 24-2). When an injury occurs, platelets cluster at the site and start to stick to the damaged cell wall (adhesion). The platelets are activated by natural substances in the blood such as thromboxane A_2 (TXA_2), thrombin, and collagen. Once platelets are activated, a cascade of events occurs that attracts more platelets to the region (aggregation) and causes fibrin to combine with the platelets. This strengthens the clot.

Although aspirin is a nonprescription drug, it is effective for the management of post–myocardial infarction and stroke. In addition to its antiplatelet activity, aspirin blocks the enzyme cyclooxygenase (see Chapter 10), reducing plaque formation. Aspirin inhibits prostaglandin synthesis, which decreases TXA_2.

Abciximab is a glycoprotein IIb/IIIa inhibitor. It blocks the final pathway of platelet aggregation. Abciximab is the only parenteral antiplatelet drug. Ticlopidine interferes with platelet adhesion and aggregation. Ticlopidine also decreases the thickness or viscosity of blood by reducing the concentration of fibrinogen. Clopidogrel's mechanism of action is similar to ticlopidine. Dipyridamole inhibits platelet aggregation and is a coronary vasodilator.

PHARMACOKINETICS

Oral absorption of aspirin, clopidogrel, and ticlopidine is good. Bioavailability of ticlopidine is enhanced by administering the drug with food. Bioavailability of clopidogrel and aspirin is unaffected by food; however, food may decrease the bioavailabilty of dipyridamole. Abciximab must be administered parenterally.

The maximum effects on platelets occur within 30 minutes of administration of aspirin and abciximab. A continuous infusion of abciximab must be given to maintain therapeutic blood levels. The peak effect of clopidogrel and ticlopidine is delayed and may take up to 4 days to be reached.

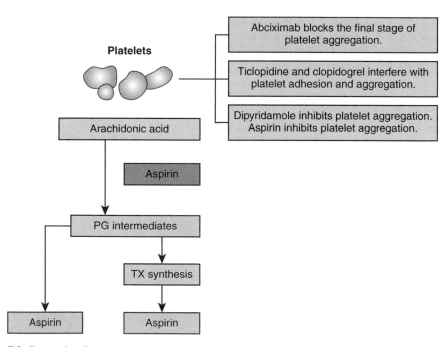

PG: Prostaglandins
TX: Thromboxane

FIGURE 24-2 Action for antiplatelet drugs. *(Modified from Lilley LL, Harrington S, Snyder JS:* Pharmacology and the nursing process, *ed 5. St. Louis, 2007, Mosby.)*

ADVERSE REACTIONS

Bleeding is a common side effect of antiplatelet drugs. Black, tarry stools; blood in vomit, urine, or stools; nosebleeds; and red or purple spots on the skin may indicate bleeding. Other side effects associated with antiplatelet drugs are skin rash or itching, stomach pain, and pain at the injection site (abciximab). Less commonly, patients may experience difficulty breathing, dizziness, weakness, joint pain, and bone marrow toxicity.

PRECAUTIONS

Many drugs can enhance the effects of antiplatelet drugs and increase the potential for bleeding or hemorrhage. Antiplatelet drugs should not be combined with anticoagulants without medical supervision. Nonprescription drugs such as NSAIDS (e.g., ibuprofen), vitamin supplements (fish oil), and herbs (feverfew, garlic, ginger) can also cause interactions.

Antiplatelet Drugs

Generic name	U.S. brand name(s) Canadian brand(s)	Dosage forms and strengths
aspirin*	Aspirin, Bayer Low Strength, Norwich Aspirin, St. Joseph Aspirin Adult Chewable Ascriptin Enteric, Bayer Adult Low Strength EC Aspirin, Bayer Ecotrin, Ecotrin Maximum-Strength, Halfprin, St. Joseph Aspirin Adult EC Asaphen, Entrophen, Novasen	**Tablet:** 81 mg, 325 mg, 500 mg **Tablet, Delayed release:** 81 mg, 325 mg
clopidogrel*	Plavix Plavix	**Tablet:** 75 mg
dipyridamole*	Permole-25, Permole-50, Permole-75, Persantine Persantine	**Injection:** 5 mg/ml **Tablet:** 25 mg, 50 mg, 75 mg
ticlopidine*	Ticlid Ticlid	**Tablet:** 250 mg
dipyridamole + aspirin	Aggrenox Not available	**Tablet:** 200 mg (dipyridamole)/ 25 mg (aspirin) 200 mg dipyridamole + 25 mg aspirin

*Generic available.

TECH ALERT!
The following drugs have look-alike/sound-alike issues: Plavix and Paxil; Ticlid and Tequin

TECH NOTE!
200 mg dipyridamole + 25 mg aspirin (Aggrenox) is a combination antiplatelet agent.

ANTICOAGULANTS

HEPARIN AND LOW-MOLECULAR-WEIGHT HEPARIN

Heparin is an anticoagulant that is derived from pig intestines or cow lungs. The extraction process results in a mixture of fragments of varied molecular weights. Low-molecular-weight heparins (LMWH) are produced by separating the heparin fragments.

Heparin and LMWH are administered to prevent the formation blood clots. Their uses include:

- Treatment of deep vein thrombosis (DVT)
- Early treatment of acute myocardial infarction and unstable angina
- Prevention of pulmonary embolism
- Prevention of secondary myocardial infarction
- Prevent clotting in indwelling catheters
- Prevent clotting in devices used in cardiac surgery (e.g., stents or prosthetic valves)

Warfarin

Warfarin is an orally administered anticoagulant that is used to prevent pulmonary embolism, thrombotic and embolic stroke, acute myocardial infarction (AMI), and atrial fibrillation.

TECH NOTE!

Warfarin is the active ingredient in rodent poisons.

MECHANISM OF ACTION OF ANTICOAGULANTS

Heparin and LMWH increase the activity of antithrombin III (ATIII). This causes the inhibition of clotting factors of the common pathway, Xa and IIa (thrombin), and prevents clot formation (Figure 24-3). To test the effectiveness of heparin and to determine whether dosage adjustments are necessary, an activated partial thromboplastin time (aPTT) test is

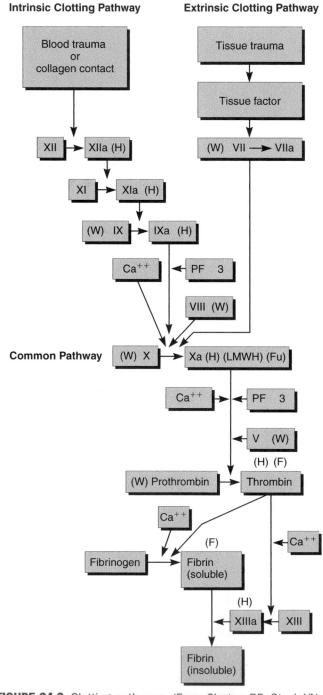

FIGURE 24-3 Clotting pathways. *(From Clayton BD, Stock YN, Harroun RD:* Basic pharmacology for nurses, *ed 14. St. Louis, 2007, Mosby.)*

performed. This test measures antithrombic activity. The test is not performed when LMWH is administered because increases in the aPPT may occur even when antithrombotic activity has not increased.

Warfarin interferes with the formation of vitamin K–dependent clotting factors. Prothrombin time (PT) or Pro-Time is a test to determine how well warfarin is working to prevent clotting and to determine whether dosage adjustments are necessary. This test may also be called an INR test. The effectiveness of warfarin may be decreased by consumption of foods rich in vitamin K and nutritional supplements with vitamin K. Foods and beverages rich in vitamin K are chickpeas, kale, turnip greens, broccoli, beef and pork liver, parsley, spinach, and green tea.

PHARMACOKINETICS

Heparin and LMWH are administered by intravenous or subcutaneous injection. Oral absorption is poor. LMWH differs from heparin in a variety of ways. LMWH can be dosed less frequently than heparin, yet they are equally effective. Heparin is dosed 2 or 3 times a day and LMWH is dosed once daily. LMWH has higher bioavailability, increased half-life (T½), fewer side effects (lower risk of thrombocytopenia and osteoporosis), and less protein binding. Higher doses of heparin must be administered because of protein binding.

Warfarin has good oral absorption and bioavailability. The maximum effects of warfarin are not achieved until 4 to 5 days after initiating therapy because warfarin does not block the activity of existing coagulation factors. Stores of existing clotting factors must be depleted before the maximum effect of warfarin on clotting is achieved. Warfarin is highly protein bound so it interacts with many other drugs. Pharmacy technicians should alert the pharmacist whenever a drug interaction is reported.

ADVERSE REACTIONS

Adverse drug reactions to administered anticoagulants include skin rash; itching; fever; pain; irritation or bleeding at the injection site; bruising; bleeding gums; bleeding in the eye; red spots on the skin; nosebleeds; back or stomach pain; cold, blue, or painful hands and feet; coughing up blood; difficulty breathing; heavy menstrual bleeding; and dizziness or fainting spells. In addition, heparin and LMWH can cause osteoporosis.

PRECAUTIONS

Pharmacy technicians should remind patients taking anticoagulants to seek the advice of the pharmacist before taking prescription and nonprescription drugs. Many drugs interact with anticoagulants causing serious bleeding or hemorrhage. Anticoagulants should not be combined with antiplatelet drugs, aspirin, NSAIDs, vitamin supplements, and herbs (e.g., feverfew, fish oil supplements, garlic, ginger, ginkgo biloba).

Warfarin can cause fetal abnormalities, so pharmacy technicians should apply the warning label **AVOID PREGNANCY** to prescription vials.

TREATING OVERDOSE

Overdose of warfarin or heparin can result in hemorrhage and death. Overdose may be treated by giving a blood transfusion. In some cases, warfarin overdose can be reversed by the administration of vitamin K. Heparin overdose may be treated by the administration of protamine sulfate.

THROMBOLYTICS

Thrombolytics, also called fibrinolytics, are drugs that can dissolve blood clots. The drugs are administered in the early stage of stroke to open blood vessels in the brain. They are also used in the treatment of acute myocardial infarction. They are derived from a variety of sources (Table 24-3).

MECHANISM OF ACTION

Only two thrombolytic agents are currently in use in the US (alteplase and tenecteplase). Streptokinase and urokinase are still available in Canada. All activate the fibrinolytic system, the body's normal system for preventing excess clotting. Just as the body has a mechanism

TECH NOTE!
Pharmacy technicians should be aware that low-molecular-weight heparins are not substitutable in accordance with product substitution laws. They must be dispensed as written. They differ in manufacturing process, molecular weight, dosage, units, and antithrombotic activity.

TECH ALERT!
Warfarin can cause fetal abnormalities so pharmacy technicians should apply the warning label **AVOID PREGNANCY** to prescription vials.

TECH NOTE!
Warfarin tablets are color coded to reduce medication errors.

Anticoagulant Drugs

	Generic name	U.S. brand name(s) / Canadian brand(s)	Dosage forms and strengths
	warfarin*	Coumadin, Jantoven — Coumadin	**Tablet:** 1 mg, 2 mg, 2½ mg, 3 mg, 4 mg, 5 mg, 6 mg, 7½ mg, 10 mg
	dalteparin	Fragmin — Fragmin	**Injection, soln:** 10,000 international units/ml **Injection, prefilled syringe:** 2500 international units/0.2 ml, 5000 international units/0.2 ml 7500 international units/0.3 ml, and 10,000 international units/ml
	enoxapari*	Lovenox — Lovenox, Lovenox HP	**Injection, solution:** 100 mg/ml **Injection, prefilled syringe:** 30 mg/0.3 ml, 40 mg/0.4 ml, 60 mg/0.6 ml, 80 mg/0.8 ml, 100 mg/1 ml, 120 mg/0.8 ml, 150 mg/ml
	heparin sodium*	Hemochron, Hep-Lock flush, HepFlush-10 — Hepalean, Heparin Leo, Heparin Lock Flush	**Injection, solution (HepFlush, Hep-Lock Flush):** 10 units/ml, 100 units/ml **Injection, solution:** 1000 units/ml, 5000 units/ml, 10,000 units/ml, 20,000 units/ml
	tinzaparin	Innohep — Innohep	**Injection, solution:** 20,000 units/ml

*Generic available.

 TECH ALERT!
The following drugs have look-alike/sound-alike issues: Lovenox, Lanoxin, Avonex, Luvox, Levaquin, and Lotronex; Coumadin, Cardura, Cordarone, Kemadrin, and Ambien

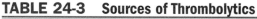

TABLE 24-3   Sources of Thrombolytics

Thrombolytic	Source
Alteplase (t-PA)	Recombinant DNA
Streptokinase	Beta-hemolytic streptococci
Anistreplase (APSAC) (not marketed)	Synthetic streptococcal culture
Tenectaplase	Human tissue plasminogen activator
Urokinase (discontinued)	Human kidney cell extracts

to form clots at the site of injury to prevent hemorrhage, the body has a system to stop excessive clot formation thereby avoiding obstructions to blood flow in blood vessels. Thrombolytics dissolve blood clots that have formed in blood vessels. They increase the activity of plasmin, an enzyme that digests fibrin and other clotting factors. Without fibrin, the structure of the thrombin clot is weakened and the clot dissolves.

PHARMACOKINETICS

Thrombolytics work rapidly. They can reopen an obstructed blood vessel within 90 minutes of administration. Alteplase, streptokinase, and tenecteplase differ in specificity and half-life (T½). The T½ for alteplase is 30 to 45 minutes, whereas the T½ of tenecteplase is 20 to 24 minutes. All thrombolytics lose shelf-life rapidly after reconstitution. They must be stored in the refrigerator and used within 24 hours.

ADVERSE REACTIONS

Thrombolytics must be administered within the first 1 to 3 hours after a stroke occurs. Thereafter, the risk of hemorrhage exceeds the benefit of administering clot-dissolving drugs. The risk of intracranial hemorrhage, leading to irreversible damage or death, increases

 TECH NOTE!
"-plase" and *"-kinase"* are common endings for thrombolytic drugs.

TECH NOTE!
Thrombolytic agents are very expensive. A single dose can cost more than $1000.

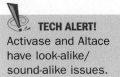

TECH ALERT!
Activase and Altace have look-alike/ sound-alike issues.

exponentially over time. Thrombolytics can cause bruising and bleeding in the gastrointestinal tract, genitourinary tract, and mouth (gums), in addition to bleeding in the brain. Other adverse reactions are nausea, vomiting, hypotension, transient arrhythmia, allergic reaction, and fever.

Thrombolytic Agents

Generic name	U.S. brand name(s) Canadian brand(s)	Dosage forms and strengths
alteplase (t-PA)	Activase, Cathflo Activase powder	**Injection, powder for reconstitution (Activase):** 50 mg (29 million international units) 100 mg (58 million international units); 2 mg (Cathflo Activase)
	Activase, Cathflo Activase	
streptokinase	Not Available	**Injection, powder for reconstitution:** 250,000 units, 750,000 units, 1,500,000 units in all strengths
	Streptase	
tenecteplase	TNKase	**Injection, powder for reconstitution:** 50 mg
	TNKase	
urokinase	Not available	**Injection, powder for reconsitution:** 250,000 units/vial (Abbokinase); 5,000 units/vial (Abbokinase Open-Catch) in for both strengths
	Abbokinase, Abbokinase Open-Catch	

Drugs That Treat Hyperlipidemia

Hyperlipidemia is a disorder associated with dysfunctional fat metabolism. While fats are necessary to form steroid hormones, bile, prostaglandins, and cell membranes, excessive buildup in the blood (hyperlipidemia) is a significant risk factor for stroke and myocardial infarction. A principle focus for prevention of cardiovascular disease and stroke is treatment of hyperlipidemia. The emphasis is on reducing LDLs and raising HDL levels.

LDLs are known as "bad cholesterol" because elevated LDL cholesterol (-C) levels promote plaque buildup in arteries, atherothrombosis, and vasoconstriction. All increase the risk of cardiovascular disease and stroke. Recent evidence has shown that increasing HDL ("good cholesterol") in addition to reducing LDL-C can further lower the risk for cardiovascular disease, even in persons who have normal HDL levels before starting HDL drug therapy. HDL controls excessive levels of LDL by transporting cholesterol from cells in the artery wall back to the liver for removal. Atherosclerosis is a chronic inflammatory disorder, and HDL has protective antiinflammatory properties. HDL acts as an antioxidant, diminishing LDL oxidation and reducing inflammation and oxidative stress. HDL also has antithrombotic, vasodilatory, and antiinfectious properties, all of which protect against cardiovascular disease.

MECHANISM OF ACTION

Lipid-lowering drugs interfere with steps in the lipid metabolism pathway (Figure 24-4). They may affect cholesterol synthesis or elimination in bile or act on LDL metabolism. Although the mechanisms of action may vary, all lipid-lowering drugs reduce LDL and triglyceride levels.

STATINS

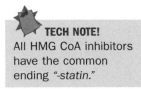

TECH NOTE!
All HMG CoA inhibitors have the common ending "-statin."

Statins are hydroxymethylglutaryl (HMG) CoA reductase inhibitors. HMG CoA reductase is an enzyme that is involved in the final step of cholesterol synthesis. Statins also increase LDL clearance. Statins are more effective than other classes of lipid-lowering drugs at lowering LDL (up to 60%). They have been shown to only minimally elevate HDL (up to 16%) above predrug levels. Simvastatin and lovastatin are prodrugs and must undergo metabolic changes before they are pharmacologically active.

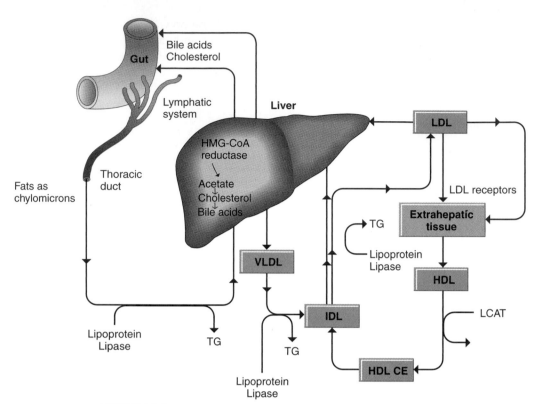

FIGURE 24-4 Lipid metabolism pathways. *(From Lilley LL, Harrington S, Snyder JS: Pharmacology and the nursing process, ed 5. St. Louis, 2007, Mosby.)*

ADVERSE REACTIONS

Myosititis (inflammation of muscle) and ***rhabdomyolysis*** (breakdown of muscle fibers and release of contents into the circulation) are serious, life-threatening muscle disorders that may be caused by statins. Statins can also elevate liver enzymes, resulting in liver dysfunction. More common and less serious side effects include diarrhea, gas, headache, joint pain, nausea, vomiting, stomach upset or pain, and tiredness.

Statins (HMG CoA Inhibitors)

	Generic name	U.S. brand name(s)	Dosage forms and strengths
		Canadian brand(s)	
	atorvastatin	Lipitor	**Tablet:** 10 mg, 20 mg, 40 mg, 80 mg
		Lipitor	
	fluvastatin*	Lescol, Lescol XL	**Capsule (Lescol):** 20 mg, 40 mg
		Lescol	**Tablet (Lescol XL):** 80 mg

Statins (HMG CoA Inhibitors)—cont'd

	Generic name	U.S. brand name(s) / Canadian brand(s)	Dosage forms and strengths
	lovastatin*	Altocor, Altoprev, Mevacor / Mevacor	**Tablet (Mevacor):** 10 mg, 20 mg, 40 mg **Tablet, extended release (Altocor, Altoprev):** 20 mg, 40 mg, 60 mg
	pravastatin*	Pravachol / Pravachol	**Tablet:** 10 mg, 20 mg, 40 mg, 80 mg
	rosuvastatin	Crestor / Crestor	**Tablet:** 5 mg, 10 mg, 20 mg, 40 mg
	simvastatin*	Zocor / Zocor	**Tablet:** 5 mg, 10 mg, 20 mg, 40 mg, 80 mg
	ezetimibe + simvastatin	Vytorin / Not available	**Tablet:** 10 mg ezetimibe + 10 mg simvastatin 10 mg ezetimibe + 20 mg simvastatin 10 mg ezetimibe + 40 mg simvastatin 10 mg ezetimibe + 80 mg simvastatin
	aspirin + pravastatin	Pravigard PAC / Not available	**Tablet:** 81 mg aspirin + 20 mg pravastatin 81 mg aspirin + 40 mg pravastatin 81 mg aspirin + 80 mg pravastatin 325 mg aspirin + 20 mg pravastatin 325 mg aspirin + 40 mg pravastatin 325 mg aspirin + 80 mg pravastatin
	niacin (extended release) + lovastatin	Advicor / Not available	**Tablet:** 500 mg niacin + 20 mg lovastatin 1000 mg niacin + 20 mg lovastatin
	atorvastatin + amlodipine	Caduet / Caduet	**Tablet:** atrovastatin 10 mg + amlodipine 2.5 mg atrovastatin 10 mg + amlodipine 5 mg atrovastatin 10 mg + amlodipine 10 mg atrovastatin 20 mg + amlodipine 2.5 mg atrovastatin 20 mg + amlodipine 5 mg atrovastatin 20 mg + amlodipine 10 mg atrovastatin 40 mg + amlodipine 2.5 mg atrovastatin 40 mg + amlodipine 5 mg atrovastatin 40 mg + amlodipine 10 mg atrovastatin 80 mg + amlodipine 5 mg atrovastatin 80 mg + amlodipine 10 mg

*Generic available.

FIBRIC ACID DERIVATIVES

Fibrates increase the clearance of very low-density lipoprotein (VLDL). Fibrates are less effective than statins at reducing LDL (approximately 10%) and in elevating HDL (up to 10% above pretherapy levels). If administered together, statins and fibrates produce a drug interaction that may increase the likelihood of development of myopathies.

Fibric Acid Derivatives

	Generic name	U.S. brand name(s)	Dosage forms and strengths
		Canadian brand(s)	
	gemfibrozil*	Lopid	**Tablet:** 600 mg
		Lopid	
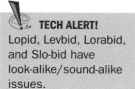	fenofibrate*	Antara, Lofibra, Tricor, Triglide	**Capsule:** 43 mg, 130 mg (Antara); 67 mg, 134 mg, 200 mg (Lofibra, Tricor) **Tablet:** 50 mg, 160 mg (Triglide); 54 mg, 67 mg, 160 mg (Lofibra); 48 mg, 54 mg, 145 mg, 160 mg (Tricor)
		Lipidil	

*Generic available.

BILE ACID SEQUESTRANTS

Bile acid sequestrants promote intestinal clearance of cholesterol. They are not absorbed and therefore are the drugs of choice for use in pregnancy. They produce bloating and gas and must be administered at least 1 hour before or 4 hours after other medications to avoid decreasing the absorption of other drugs. Bile acid sequestrants can lower body levels of fat-soluble vitamins such as vitamins A, D, E, and K.

Bile Acid Sequestrants

	Generic name	U.S. brand name(s)	Dosage forms and strengths
		Canadian brand(s)	
	cholestyramine*	LoCHOLEST, LoCHOLEST Lite, Prevalite, Questran, Questran Lite	**Powder, for reconstitution (regular and sugar-free):** 4 g/packet or scoop
		Generics	
	colesevelam	Welchol	**Tablet:** 625 mg
		Not available	
	colestipol*	Colestid	**Granules, for reconstitution:** 5 g/packet or scoop **Tablet:** 1 g
		Colestid	
	ezetimibe	Zetia	**Tablet:** 10 mg
		Ezetrol	

*Generic available.

NICOTINIC ACID DERIVATIVES

Niacin is vitamin B_3. It is less effective at decreasing LDL than statins, but it is the most effective lipid-lowering agent for increasing HDL (up to 35%). Niacin produces vasodilation, causing flushing, pruritus, headaches, or pain, which some find intolerable. Niacinamide does not produce vasodilation, but it is not effective in lowering lipid levels. Sustained release preparations may minimize vasodilation and gastrointestinal upset. Glucose intolerance and abnormal liver function may limit the use of niacin.

Nicotinic Acid

Generic name	U.S. brand name(s) / Canadian brand(s)	Dosage forms and strengths
niacin*	Niaspan, Niacor, Nico-400, Nicobid Tempules, Nicolar, Nicotinex, Slo-Niacin Generic only	**Capsule, time-released:** 125 mg, 250 mg, 500 mg (various generic) **Tablet:** 50 mg, 250 mg, 500 mg (Niacor, various) **Tablet, time-released:** 500 mg, 750 mg, 1000 mg Niaspan); 250 mg, 500 mg (Slo-Niacin)

*Generic available.

Nonprescription Drugs Used for Myocardial Infarction and Stroke

Antioxidants and other vitamins are sometimes prescribed to reduce risk of myocardial infarction and stroke. They are prescribed to protect cells and reduce inflammation and oxygen free radicals that increase plaque formation. Recommended vitamins include vitamin C (ascorbic acid), vitamin B_{12} (cyanocobalamin), vitamin B_9 (folate), vitamin B_6 (pyridoxine), vitamin E (tocopherols), vitamin A (retinoic acid), and magnesium oxide.

Summary of drugs used in the treatment and prevention of myocardial infarction and stroke

Generic name	U.S. brand name	Dosage form(s)	Usual dose and dosing schedule	Warning Labels
Drugs to control hemostasis				
Antiplatelet drugs				
abciximab	ReoPro	Injection, IV infusion	0.25 mg/kg bolus followed by 0.125 mcg/kg/min infusion for up to 12 hours	DO NOT SHAKE AVOID ASPIRIN, NSAIDs, AND OTHER OTC WITHOUT SUPERVISION REFRIGERATE AT 2°C TO 8°C DO NOT FREEZE
aspirin	Various	Tablet, enteric coated tablet	81 mg to 325 mg once daily	TAKE WITH FOOD AVOID PREGNANCY (3rd TRIMESTER)
clopidogrel	Plavix	Tablet	75 mg once daily	AVOID ASPIRIN, NSAIDs, AND OTHER OTC

Continued

Summary of drugs used in the treatment and prevention of myocardial infarction and stroke—cont'd

Generic name	U.S. brand name	Dosage form(s)	Usual dose and dosing schedule	Warning Labels
dipyridamole	Persantine	Tablet	75 mg 3 times/day up to 400 mg/day	TAKE ON AN EMPTY STOMACH TAKE WITH A FULL GLASS OF WATER AVOID ASPIRIN, NSAIDs, AND OTHER OTC
ticlopidine	Ticlid	Tablet	250 mg twice daily	AVOID ASPIRIN, NSAIDs, AND OTHER OTC TAKE WITH FOOD
Anticoagulants				
dalteparin	Fragmin	Injection SC	150 international units/ kg/day	AVOID OTC WITHOUT MEDICAL SUPERVISION (vitamins, herbals, analgesics)
enoxaparin	Lovenox	Injection IV and SC	30 mg IV bolus followed by 1 mg/kg SC every 12 hours for up to 7 days	AVOID ASA AND NSAIDS REPORT SIGNS OF BLEEDING
heparin Na$^+$	Hep-Lock Flush	Injection IV	60 international units/kg IV bolus with initial dose of thrombolytic therapy; then 12 international units/kg per hour IV	AVOID PREGNANCY (warfarin)
tinzaparin	Innohep	SC injection	175 units/kg (or 0.00875 ml/kg) SC once daily	
warfarin	Coumadin	Injection Tablet	2 mg to 5 mg daily for 2 to 4 days then adjust as required	
Thrombolytics				
alteplase (t-PA)	Activase	IV	15 mg IV bolus followed by 50 mg infused over 30 minutes, then 35 mg infused over 60 minutes	REFRIGERATE RECONSTITUTED SOLUTION (2°C TO 8°C) STABLE FOR 24 HOURS AFTER RECONSTITUTION (under refrigeration)
streptokinase	Streptase	IV	1,500,000 units by IV infusion over 60 minutes or 20,000 units intracoronary followed by 2,000 units administered over 1 hour	DO NOT SHAKE—AGITATE GENTLY STORE POWDER AT ROOM TEMPERATURE
tenectaplase	TNKase	IV	30 mg to 50 mg bolus over 5 seconds	
Combination Drugs				
aspirin + dipyridamole	Aggrenox	Capsule	Take 1 capsule twice daily	SWALLOW WHOLE; DO NOT CRUSH OR CHEW

Summary of drugs used in the treatment and prevention of myocardial infarction and stroke—cont'd

Generic name	U.S. brand name	Dosage form(s)	Usual dose and dosing schedule	Warning Labels
Drugs to Control Hyperlipidemia				
HMG CoA reductase inhibitors (statins)				
atorvastatin	Lipitor	Tablet	10 mg to 80 mg once daily	AVOID GRAPEFRUIT JUICE—atorvastatin, lovastatin, simvastatin
lovastatin	Mevacor	Tablet	10 mg to 80 mg once daily	AVOID ALCOHOL
fluvastatin	Lescol	Capsule	20 mg to 80 mg once daily	AVOID PREGNANCY
pravastatin	Pravachol	Tablet	10 mg to 40 mg once daily	SWALLOW WHOLE; DON'T CHEW (extended release)
rosuvastatin	Crestor	Tablet	10 mg to 40 mg once daily	
simvastatin	Zocor	Tablet	10 mg to 80 mg once daily	
Fibric acid derivatives				
fenofibrate	Tricor	Capsule	200 mg once daily	MAY CAUSE DROWSINESS AVOID PROLONGED EXPOSURE TO SUNLIGHT
gemfibrozil	Lopid	Capsule	600 mg twice daily	TAKE ON AN EMPTY STOMACH
Bile acid sequestrants				
cholestyramine	Questran	Powder	4 g to 8 g 2 to 3 times/day	TAKE 1 HOUR BEFORE OR 4 HOURS AFTER OTHER DRUGS
colestipol	Colestid	Granule Tablet	5 g to 15 g twice/day	RECONSTITUTE WITH 2 to 6 OUNCES LIQUID—SHAKE WELL
colesevelam	Welchol	Tablet	1.9 g to 4.4 g daily in 1 to 2 doses	SWALLOW WHOLE TAKE WITH ½ GLASS WATER AND FOOD
Miscellaneous				
ezetimibe	Zetia	Tablet	10 mg once daily	AVOID ALCOHOL
niacin (Vit. B₃)	Various Niaspan	Tablet Capsule	0.5 g to 2 g 3 times/day 1 g to 2 g once daily	AVOID ALCOHOL TAKE WITH FOOD
Combination				
ezetimibe + simvastatin	Vytorin	Tablet	1 tablet once daily in the evening	AVOID GRAPEFRUIT JUICE
niacin + lovastatin	Advicor	Tablet	1 to 2 tablets at bedtime (maximum 40 mg lovastatin + 2000 mg niacin/day)	TAKE WITH FOOD AVOID ALCOHOL
pravastatin + aspirin	Pravigard PAC	Tablets	Take 1 tablet daily	AVOID ALCOHOL

CHAPTER SUMMARY

- Myocardial infarction is the leading cause of death in the United States.
- Stroke is the third leading cause of death in the United States.
- Strokes occur when brain cells are deprived of oxygen or are damaged by sudden bleeding into the brain.
- There are four major types of stroke: ischemic stroke, thrombotic stroke, embolic stroke, and hemorrhagic stroke.
- Transient ischemic attacks are also known as mini-strokes and last only a few minutes.
- Myocardial infarction produces symptoms that are similar to angina.
- Chronic inflammation of arteries that supply the heart and brain can also lead to stroke and myocardial infarction because vascular inflammation is a cause of atherosclerosis.
- Atherosclerosis (a buildup of lipids and plaque inside of artery walls) can block blood-flow through arteries.
- Atherothrombosis (the formation of a blood clot in the artery) is triggered by atherosclerosis and can also cause clogged arteries.
- The risk for stroke and myocardial infarction is increased by nonmodifiable risk factors, modifiable risk factors, and chronic disease.
- Nonmodifiable risk factors are age, gender, and family history of stroke and myocardial infarction.
- Modifiable risk factors are smoking, heavy alcohol consumption, and diet high in cholesterol.
- Diseases that can increase risk for stroke and myocardial infarction are diabetes, hypertension, hyperlipidemia, atrial fibrillation, and infection.
- Drugs administered to prevent stroke and myocardial infarction control the buildup of lipids and plaque reduce the formation of blood clots.
- Drugs that control hemostasis (the process of stopping the flow of blood) prevent the formation of clots that can obstruct the supply of blood to the brain and heart.
- Antithrombotic drugs include (1) agents that inhibit platelets; (2) anticoagulants, which attenuate coagulation; and (3) fibrinolytic agents. Fibrinolytics dissolve existing clots.
- Antiplatelet drugs interfere with early steps in the clot formation process.
- Aspirin is a nonprescription drug that has antiplatelet activity.
- Abciximab is the only parenteral antiplatelet drug. It blocks the final pathway for platelet aggregation
- Ticlopidine, clopidogrel, and dipyridamole are orally administered antiplatelet drugs.
- Bleeding is a common side effect of all antiplatelet drugs. Other side effects associated with antiplatelet drugs are skin rash or itching, stomach pain, and pain at the injection site (abciximab).
- Nonprescription drugs, vitamin supplements, and herbs can enhance the effects of antiplatelet drugs. These drugs include NSAIDs (e.g., ibuprofen), feverfew, fish oil supplements, garlic, and ginger.
- Heparin and low-molecular-weight heparin are anticoagulants that are administered to prevent the formation of blood clots.
- Low-molecular-weight heparins are not substitutable.
- To test the effectiveness of heparin and to determine whether dosage adjustments are necessary, an activated partial thromboplastin time test is performed.
- Warfarin interferes with the formation of vitamin K–dependent clotting factors. Prothrombin time or Pro-Time is a test to determine how well warfarin is working to reduce clotting.
- Maximum effects of warfarin are not achieved until 4 to 5 days after initiating therapy.
- Warfarin can cause fetal abnormalities, so pharmacy technicians should apply the warning label AVOID PREGNANCY to prescription vials.
- Warfarin overdose is reversed by the administration of vitamin K. Heparin overdose is treated with protamine sulfate.
- Thrombolytics, also called fibrinolytics, are drugs that can dissolve blood clots and must be administered within the first few hours of a stroke.

- A principle focus for prevention of cardiovascular disease and stroke is treatment of hyperlipidemia.
- Low-density lipoproteins (LDLs) are known as "bad cholesterol" because elevated LDL-C levels promote plaque buildup in arteries, atherothrombosis, and vasoconstriction.
- Increasing HDL ("good cholesterol"), in addition to reducing LDL-C, can further lower the risk for cardiovascular disease.
- Statins are HMG CoA reductase inhibitors and block the final step of cholesterol synthesis and promote LDL elimination.
- Fibrates increase clearance of very low-density lipoproteins (VLDL). Fibrates are less effective than statins.
- Bile acid sequestrants promote intestinal clearance of cholesterol.
- Niacin is vitamin B_3. It is less effective at decreasing LDL than statins, but it is the most effective lipid-lowering agent for increasing HDL.

REVIEW QUESTIONS

Multiple Choice

1. Strokes occur when brain cells are deprived of _____ or are damaged by sudden bleeding into the brain.
   - a. carbon dioxide
   - b. oxygen
   - c. both a and b
   - d. none of the above

2. _____ last only a few minutes and symptoms usually resolve within an hour.
   - a. Embolic strokes
   - b. Hemorrhagic strokes
   - c. Transient ischemic attacks
   - d. Aneurysms

3. Age does not pose a significant risk factor for stroke or myocardial infarction.
   - a. true
   - b. false

4. Drugs that control the rate of clot formation and clot dissolution are classified as _____ and can prevent stroke and myocardial infarction.
   - a. antihyperlipidemics
   - b. antifibrinolytics
   - c. antithrombotics
   - d. antihemorrhagics

5. Aspirin is not effective for the management of post myocardial infarction and stroke.
   - a. true
   - b. false

6. _____ is the only parenteral antiplatelet drug.
   - a. Ticlopidine
   - b. Dipyridamole
   - c. Abciximab
   - d. Simvastatin

7. Warfarin interferes with the formation of vitamin _____–dependent clotting factors.
   - a. A
   - b. D
   - c. E
   - d. K

8. **Heparin and LMWH are administered to prevent the formation blood clots.**
   a. true
   b. false

9. **Thrombolytics must be administered within the first _____ hours after a stroke has occur.**
   a. 1 to 3
   b. 2 to 4
   c. 3 to 5
   d. 4 to 6

10. **Statin drugs lower what kind of cholesterol?**
    a. LDL
    b. bile
    c. HDL
    d. all of the above

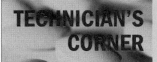

TECHNICIAN'S CORNER

1. What kind of reaction happens if aspirin and warfarin are used at the same time?
2. What kind of diet helps to lower cholesterol levels?

BIBLIOGRAPHY

Chapman J: Therapeutic elevation of HDL-cholesterol to prevent atherosclerosis and coronary heart disease, *Pharmacol Therap* 111:893-908, 2006.

Hoffman: *Hematology: Basic principles and practice,* ed 4, 2005, Figure 130-1, Chapter 130.

Kalant H, Grant D, Mitchell J: *Principles of medical pharmacology* (pp 472-482), ed 7. Toronto, 2007, Elsevier Canada, A Division of Reed Elsevier Canada.

Lance L, Lacy C, Armstrong L, Goldman M: *Drug information handbook for the allied health professional,* ed 12. Hudson, OH, 2005, APhA Lexi-Comp.

National Heart, Lung, and Blood Institute: Heart attack. Bethesda, MD, National Institutes of Health, US Department of Health and Human Services. Available at: http://www.nhlbi.nih.gov/health/dci/Diseases/HeartAttack/HeartAttack_All.html.

National Heart, Lung, and Blood Institute: High blood cholesterol. Bethesda, MD, National Institutes of Health, US Department of Health and Human Services. Available at: http://www.nhlbi.nih.gov/health/dci/Diseases/Hbc/HBC_all.html.

National Institute of Neurological Disorders and Stroke: Stroke: Hope through research. Bethesda, MD, National Institute of Mental Health, National Institutes of Health, US Department of Health and Human Services, July 2004. Last updated December 20, 2006; NIH publication No. 99-2222. Available at: http://www.ninds.nih.gov/disorders/stroke/detail_stroke.htm.

Otto M, Hochadel M: Thrombolytic agents–Overview, *Clin Pharmacol,* 2000. Available at: http://www.clinicalpharmacology.com/apps/default.asp?entry=11andrNum=791.

Ringleb, P: Thromolytics, anticoagulants, and antiplatelet agents, *Stroke,* 37:312-313, 2006. Available at: http://stroke.ahajournals.org/cgi/content/full/37/2/312.

USP Center for Advancement of Patient Safety: *Use caution–avoid confusion,* USP Quality Review No. 79, Rockville, MD, April 2004, USP Center for Advancement of Patient Safety.

Vieson, K: Low-molecular weight heparins (LMWHs), *Clin Pharmacol,* 2001. Available at: http://www.clinicalpharmacology.com/apps/default.asp?entry=11andrNum=206.

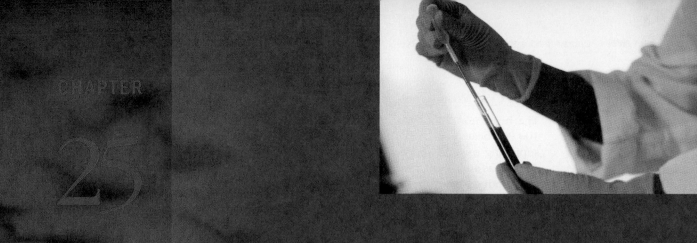

Treatment of Arrhythmia

- Learn the terminology associated with arrhythmias.
- Describe types of arrhythmias.
- List risk factors for arrhythmias.
- List and categorize medications used to treat arrhythmias.
- Describe mechanism of action for each class of drugs used to treat arrhythmias.
- Identify warning labels and precautionary messages associated with medications used to treat arrhythmias.
- Identify significant drug look-alike/sound-alike issues.
- List common endings for drug classes used in the treatment of arrhythmias.

KEY TERMS

Atrial fibrillation: Rapid and uncoordinated contractions. Heart may beat between 300 to 400 beats per minute.

Atrial flutter: Irregular heart beat in which contractions in atrium exceed the number of contractions in the ventricle (Heart rate between 160 to 350 beats per minute.) (Heart rate of 160 to 350 minutes per minute.)

Automaticity: Spontaneous contraction of heart muscle cells.

Depolarization: Process where the heart muscle conducts an electrical impulse causing a contraction.

Ectopic: Occurring in an abnormal location.

Electrical cardioversion: Process of applying an electrical shock to the heart with a defibrillator.

Refractory period: Time between contractions that it takes for repolarization to occur.

Repolarization: Period of time when the heart is recharging and preparing for another contraction.

Supraventricular tachycardia: Heart rate up to 200 beats per minute that originates in an area above the ventricles.

Ventricular tachycardia: Ventricles beat faster than 200 beats per minute.

Ventricular fibrillation: Life-threatening arrhythmia where the heart beats up to 600 beats per minute.

Overview

The heart normally beats at a rate between 60 and 100 beats per minute; approximately 100,000 beats per day. With each beat or contraction, blood is pumped throughout the body, supplying oxygen and nutrients to cells and organs, including the heart. An arrhythmia is defined as an irregular heart rhythm or a heart rate that is too rapid or too slow. Arrhythmias can produce heart rates that exceed 600 beats per minute. An arrhythmia can impair the heart's ability to distribute blood. Symptoms of arrhythmia are listed in Box 25-1.

Atrial fibrillation is the most common arrhythmia, and while not usually life threatening, it is a risk factor for stroke. It affects approximately 1% of the population and it is estimated that it will affect nearly 15 million Americans by 2050. Risk factors for atrial fibrillation are similar to risk factors for coronary heart disease (CHD) and are similarly categorized as nonmodifiable risk factors, modifiable risk factors, and disease risk factors (Table 25-1). A description of these risk factors is found in chapters on hypertension, heart failure, myocardial infarction, and stroke (see Chapters 22 through 24).

Ventricular fibrillation is the leading cause of sudden cardiac death, killing nearly 600,000 people in the United States and Europe each year.

How Arrhythmias are Formed

Heart contractions occur when cardiac cells "fire." This is known as *depolarization*. During depolarization, positively-charged ions enter the cells through specialized exchange channels and an action potential is formed (Figure 25-1). Sodium entry initiates depolarization of the atria and ventricles, and calcium entry results in depolarization of the sinoatrial and atrial ventricular nodes. Once the heart cells have fired, another contraction cannot occur until repolarization occurs. *Repolarization* is the process of returning the cells to their resting state. The time it takes for repolarization to occur is called the *refractory period*.

Arrhythmias occur when the cardiac ion exchange channels function improperly. This can result in excessive firing, extra currents during the refractory period, and establishment of sinus rhythm by nonpacemaker cells. These conditions may occur following a heart attack because fibrous scar tissue may develop in the healing process. Conduction is poor across fibrous tissue. Inflammation and oxidative stress (see Chapter 24) can cause arrhythmias, too. In addition, once arrhythmias have occurred, they may stimulate the formation of other arrhythmias. Moreover, treatment of arrhythmia can result in secondary arrhythmias.

Types of Arrhythmias

ATRIAL FLUTTER

Atrial flutter refers to an irregular heart beat in which contractions in the atrium exceed the number of contractions in the ventricle. The heart rate may be between 160 and 350 beats per minute. It usually occurs in the right atrium and is treated by inserting a catheter into the atrium (catheter ablation) rather than drug therapy.

BOX 25-1 SYMPTOMS OF ARRHYTHMIA

- Palpitations or fluttering in the chest
- Rapid heart rate
- Slow heart rate
- Chest pain
- Shortness of breath
- Lightheadedness or dizziness
- Fainting

TABLE 25-1   Risk Factors for Atrial Fibrillation

Nonmodifiable	Age, gender, low heart rate, emotional stress
Modifiable	Obesity, smoking, excessive alcohol consumption, stimulant use
Disease	Hypertension, heart failure, CHD, stroke, infection, diabetes, thyroid disease, obstructive sleep apnea

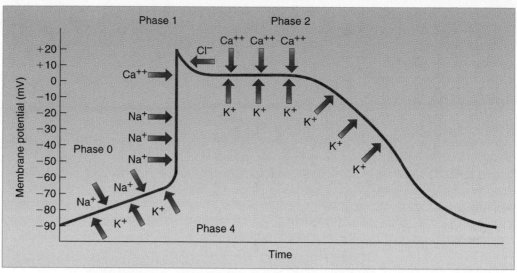

FIGURE 25-1 Action potential. *(From Lilley LL, Harrington S, Snyder JS: Pharmacology and the nursing process, ed 5. St. Louis, 2007, Mosby.)*

ATRIAL FIBRILLATION

Atrial fibrillation is defined as a rapid and uncoordinated contractions. The heart may beat between 300 to 400 beats per minute. Atrial fibrillation is the most common arrhythmia and occurs with increasing frequency as people age, affecting approximately 10% of the population over 80 years. Atrial fibrillation often accompanies other cardiac diseases such as coronary artery disease, heart failure, and hypertension.

SUPRAVENTICULAR TACHYCARDIA

Supraventricular tachycardia (SVT) occurs in areas of the heart that lay above the ventricles. SVT may occur intermittently (paroxysmal) or frequently. The heartbeat may increase up to 200 beats per minute and last several seconds to a few hours.

VENTRICULAR TACHYCARDIA

Ventricular tachycardia causes the ventricles to beat faster than 200 beats per minute. It may occur when the spread of electrical impulses between heart chambers is "short circuited" across scar tissue caused by a heart attack.

VENTRICULAR FIBRILLATION

Ventricular fibrillation may cause the ventricles to beat faster than 600 beats per minute. Ventricular fibrillation is life threatening because the ventricles are unable to fill with blood and blood is not effectively pumped throughout the body. Ventricular fibrillation is typically reversed only after electrical cardioversion. *Electrical cardioversion* is the process of applying an electrical shock to the heart with a defibrillator.

The mechanism for ventricular fibrillation is thought to be complex, and multiple mechanisms are involved, including self-generated reentry of unstable wavelets and rapid, intermittent excitation alternating with conduction block.

Treatment of Arrhythmia

Antiarrhythmic drugs are used to treat irregular heart rhythms and rate. Their use has been declining except in the treatment of supraventricular arrhythmias, such as atrial fibrillation, because studies have shown that they may cause other cardiac arrhythmias. Antiarrhythmic drugs are categorized into four classes (Class I, II, III, and IV) according to their mechanism of action and structural similarities. Class I antiarrhythmics are further subdivided into Class Ia, Ib, and Ic. Antiarrhythmic drugs are listed in Table 25-2.

TABLE 25-2   Antiarrhymic Drugs

Class	Category	Generic name	Site of action
Class IA	Na⁺ channel blocker	quinidine sulfate, quinidine gluconate, procainamide, disopyramide	Na⁺ channels
Class IB	Na⁺ channel blocker	lidocaine, mexiletine, tocainide	Na⁺ channels
Class IC	Na⁺ channel blocker	encainide, flecainide, moricizine, propafenone	Na⁺ channels
Class II	β-Blockers	propranolol, esmolol, acebutolol	β-Adrenergic receptors
Class III	K⁺ channel blocker	amiodarone, bretylium, sotalol	K⁺ channels
Class IV	Ca²⁺ channel blockers	Verapamil	Ca²⁺ channels

β-Blockers are the only class of drugs indicated for primary management of ventricular arrhythmias. They are effective in suppressing *ectopic* (occurring in an abnormal location) beats and arrhythmias.

MECHANISM OF ACTION Musculoskeletal System

Quinidine is the prototype Class IA antiarrhythmic and has been widely used since the 1920s. It is the active ingredient in cinchona bark. Class I agents act on sodium channels and slow the rate of depolarization. Recall that contractions occur as a result of depolarization. They also reduce *automaticity* (spontaneous contraction of heart muscle cells), delay conduction, and prolong the time between contractions (refractory period). Class IA agents have a moderate effect on depolarization and intermediate effects on the sodium channel. Class IB agents have a minimal effect on depolarization, and their effect on the sodium channel is rapid. The effect of Class IC antiarrhythmic drugs on sodium channels is very slow, and they produce marked effects on depolarization. They are 80% to 90% effective at suppressing arrhythmias. All Class I antiarrhythmic agents may be administered orally except lidocaine.

Class II antiarrhythmic agents are β-adrenergic antagonists. β-Blockers antagonize stimulation of the atrial ventricular (AV) and sinoatrial (SA) nodes. They increase the refractory period, decrease automaticity, and slow conduction velocity.

Amiodarone, bretylium, and sotalol are Class III antiarrhythmic agents. Class III antiarrhythmic agents block potassium channels. They prolong depolarization and prolong the refractory period. Bretylium initially causes the release of norepinephrine, which can stimulate cardiac activity, but once nerve terminals are depleted, it prevents further release. It is the most effective antifibrillatory agent. Amiodarone's effectiveness is achieved through multiple mechanisms of action, and it can suppress both supraventricular and ventricular arrhythmias, notably by increasing reentry time. Class IV antiarrhythmic agents are calcium channel blockers, although only verapamil and diltiazem are effective in treating supraventricular arrhythmias, atrial fibrillation, and atrial flutter.

ADVERSE REACTIONS

All antiarrhythmic agents are proarrhythmic (can cause other arrhythmias). They all can cause bradycardia, hypotension, and dizziness. Most antiarrhythmic agents cause nausea and vomiting, diarrhea, or constipation. Class I antiarrhymic agents can produce local anesthesia and itchy, flaky rashes. Class II antiarrhythmics can cause depression in addition to the general side effects listed. Amiodarone has many adverse effects, and up to 20% of patients will discontinue the drug because of side effects. Common side effects are photosensitivity, skin discoloration, stomach upset, visual disturbances (sun sensitivity, blurred vision, dry eyes), and corneal deposits. Calcium channel blockers (Class IV) produce headache, flushing, and peripheral edema, in addition to the adverse reactions listed earlier.

PRECAUTIONS

Tinnitus is a sign of quinidine toxicity. Quinidine and procainamide can also produce a lupus-like syndrome causing arthritis and chest pain. Class II antiarrhythmics (β-blockers) are contraindicated in patients with asthma, diabetes, and heart failure. They can cause bronchospasm and mask the signs of hypoglycemia and may increase or decrease blood sugar levels. Amiodarone may induce thyroid disease and fatal hepatotoxicity.

Class IA

	Generic name	U.S. brand name(s) / Canadian brand(s)	Dosage forms and strengths
	disopyramide*	Norpace, Norpace CR	**Capsule:** 100 mg, 150 mg
		Rythmodan, Rythmodan-LA	**Capsule, extended release:** 100 mg, 150 mg
	procainamide*	Procanbid, Pronestyl, Pronestyl SR	**Capsule:** 250 mg, 375 mg, 500 mg
			Tablet: 250 mg, 500 mg
		Procan SR	**Tablet, extended release (Procanbid):** 500 mg, 750 mg, 1000 mg
	quinidine gluconate*	Quinadure	**Solution, injection:** 80 mg/ml
		Generics	**Tablet, extended release:** 324 mg
	quinidine sulfate*	Generics	**Solution, injection (Canada only):** 190 mg/ml
			Tablet: 200 mg, 300 mg
		Generics	**Tablet, extended release:** 300 mg
	quinidine arabo-galactane sulfate	Not available	**Tablet, extended release:** 250 mg
		Biquin Durales	

*Generic available.

Class IB

	Generic name	U.S. brand name(s) / Canadian brand(s)	Dosage forms and strengths
	lidocaine*	Xylocaine	**Solution, injection:** 0.5%, 1%, 2%, 4%, 20% (Xylocard)
		Xylocard	
	mexiletine*	Mexitil	**Capsule:** 150 mg, 200 mg, 250 mg
		Generic	

*Generic available.

Class IC

	Generic name	U.S. brand name(s) / Canadian brand(s)	Dosage forms and strengths
	flecainide*	Tambocor	**Tablet:** 50 mg, 100 mg, 150 mg (150 mg not available in Canada)
		Tambocor	
	moricizine	Ethmozine	**Tablet:** 200 mg, 250 mg, 300 mg
		Not available	
	propafenone*	Rhythmol, Rhythmol SR	**Capsule, extended release:** 225 mg, 325 mg, 425 mg
		Rhythmol	**Tablet:** 150 mg, 225 mg, 300 mg

*Generic available.

Class II

| Generic name | U.S. brand name(s) | Dosage forms and strengths |
	Canadian brand(s)	
acebutolol*	Sectral	**Capsule:** 200 mg, 400 mg
	Rhotral, Sectral	
esmolol*	Brevibloc, Brevibloc Double Strength	**Solution, injection:** 250 mg/ml, 10 mg/ml, 20 mg/ml premixed solution, double strength
	Brevibloc	
propranolol*	Inderal, Inderal LA, InnoPran XL	**Capsule, extended release:** 60 mg, 80 mg, 120 mg, 160 mg **Solution, injection:** 1 mg/ml **Solution, oral:** 20 mg/5 ml
	Inderal	**Tablet:** 10 mg, 20 mg, 40 mg, 60 mg, 80 mg

*Generic available.

Class III

| Generic name | U.S. brand name(s) | Dosage forms and strengths |
	Canadian brand(s)	
amiodarone*	Cordarone, Pacerone	**Solution, injection:** 50 mg/ml **Tablet:** 100 mg, 200 mg, 400 mg
	Cordarone	
bretylium tosylate*	Not available	**Solution, injection:** 50 mg/ml **Prefilled syringe, injection:** 50 mg/ml
	Generic	
sotalol*	Betapace, Betapace AF	**Tablet:** 80 mg, 120 mg, 160 mg, 240 mg **Tablet (Betapace AF):** 80 mg, 120 mg, 160 mg
	Rylosol	

*Generic available.

Class IV

| Generic name | U.S. brand name(s) | Dosage forms and strengths |
	Canadian brand(s)	
verapamil	Calan, Calan SR, Isoptin SR, Verelan, Verelan PM Covera HS	**Capsule, extended release:** 180 mg, 240 mg, 360 mg **Solution, injection:** 2.5 mg/ml **Tablet:** 40 mg, 80 mg, 120 mg, **Tablet, extended release (Calan SR, Isoptin SR, Covera HS, Verelan, Verelan PM):** 100 mg, 120 mg, 180 mg, 200 mg, 240 mg, 300 mg
	Covera, Isoptin, Isoptin SR, Tarka	

TECH ALERT!
The following drugs have look-alike/ sound-alike issues: Procan SR and Proscar; Procanbid and probenecid; Procardia and Provera; quinidine and quinine

MISCELLANEOUS

Digoxin and phenytoin are miscellaneous drugs used in the treatment of arrhythmias. The use of phenytoin is uncommon as its use is not approved by the Food and Drug Administration. The dose for management of atrial and ventricular arrhythmias is located in the next drug table. Digoxin, on the other hand, is approved for the treatment of atrial fibrillation. It reduces arrhythmias by slowing the conduction velocity and prolonging the refractory period in the Purkinje fibers and AV node. In the atria and ventricles, digoxin shortens the refractory period. Digoxin also reduces electrical discharges from the SA node. It may be administered intravenously or orally. Digoxin has a narrow therapeutic index, so it is important to avoid excessive doses. It is administered so the first dose equals approximately one-half the total daily dose. The remainder is divided in half and given every 6 hours for two doses. Adverse effects of digoxin are described in Chapter 24.

Drug Used to Prevent Arrhythmias

Arrhythmia management is currently focused on prevention. Prevention is important because atrial fibrillation is a risk factor for stroke (see Chapter 24). Hypertension doubles the risk for atrial fibrillation therefore hypertension should be treated to reduce the risk. Angiotensin-converting enzyme inhibitors (ACEIs) and angiotensin II type 1 receptor blockers (ARBs) can significantly reduce the risk for first-time atrial fibrillation in patients with hypertension, heart failure, and post–myocardial infarction. The use of these drugs to treat hypertension is discussed in Chapter 22.

MECHANISM OF ACTION

ACEIs lengthen the refractory period and shorten conduction time. ACEIs also decrease dilatation of coronary arteries, reducing blood pressure. Angiotensin receptor blockers have a similar mechanism but also reduce inflammation and structural changes in the atria that can activate atrial fibrillation.

Summary of Drugs Used in the Treatment of Arrhythmia

	Generic name	Usual dose and dosing schedule	Warning labels
	Antiarrhythmic drugs		
	Class IA		
	disopyramide	150 mg to 200 mg every 6 hours (immediate release)	MAY CAUSE DIZZINESS OR DROWSINESS
		300 mg every 12 hours (extended release)	SWALLOW WHOLE; DON'T CRUSH OR CHEW—extended release
	procainamide	**Atrial arrhythmias:** 500 mg to 1000 mg every 4 to 6 hours *or* 750 to 1500 mg every 6 hours (extended release); for Procanbid, take every 12 hours **Ventricular arrhythmias:** 50 mg/kg every 3 to 4 hours *or* 20 mg/min IV until tachycardia resolves; then 1 to 4 mg/min as a continuous IV infusion	TAKE ON AN EMPTY STOMACH— procainamide AVOID GRAPEFRUIT JUICE—quinidine sulfate
	quinidine gluconate	324 mg to 648 mg orally every 8 to 12 hours 600 mg IM every 2 hours; 800 mg IV in 50 ml of $D_5W\%$ infused 1 ml/min	REFRIGERATE; DO NOT FREEZE— Diluted quinidine gluconate solution may be stored for up to 48 hours at 4 °C (39 °F) or 24 hours at room temperature
	quinidine sulfate	200 mg to 300 mg every 6 to 8 hours (immediate release); 300 mg to 600 mg every 8 to 12 hours (extended release)	
	Class IB		
	lidocaine	50 mg to 100 mg IV infused 25 to 50 mg/min. Repeat in 5 minutes. **Continuous infusion:** 1 mg/min to 4 mg/min **IM:** 300 mg	MAY CAUSE DIZZINESS OR DROWSINESS TAKE WITH FOOD—mexiletine
	mexiletine	200 mg to 300 mg every 8 hours	

Continued

Summary of Drugs Used in the Treatment of Arrhythmia—cont'd

	Generic name	Usual dose and dosing schedule	Warning labels
	Class IC		
	flecainide	50 mg to 150 mg every 12 hours	DON'T SKIP OR EXCEED DOSE
	moricizine	900 mg/day in 2 to 3 doses	TAKE ON AN EMPTY STOMACH
	propafenone	150 mg to 300 mg every 8 hours 225 mg to 425 mg every 12 hours (extended release)	WEAR SUNGLASSES—propafenone AVOID GRAPEFRUIT JUICE SWALLOW WHOLE; DON'T CRUSH OR CHEW
	Class II		
	acebutolol	400 mg to 1200 mg daily in 2 divided doses	MAY CAUSE DIZZINESS OR DROWSINESS
	esmolol	500 mcg/kg IV loading dose over 1 minute. Maintenance infusion rate: 50 mcg/kg/min IV for 4 minutes.	CONCENTRATE; MUST BE DILUTED— esmolol
	propranolol	30 mg to 160 mg daily	ORAL CONCENTRATE; MUST BE DILUTED—propranolol SWALLOW WHOLE; DON'T CRUSH OR CHEW DON'T SKIP DOSES
	Class III		
	amiodarone	800 mg to 1600 mg daily orally in single or divided doses; maintenance dose 400 mg/day **IV:** rapid infusion of 150 mg over first 10 minutes; then slow IV infusion of 1 mg/min for next 6 hours (total = 360 mg); then 0.5 mg/min for the next 18 hours (total dose infused = 540 mg). After 24 hours, a maintenance IV infusion of 0.5 mg/min (720 mg/day)	AVOID PROLONGED EXPOSURE TO SUNLIGHT—amiodarone MAY CAUSE DIZZINESS OR DROWSINESS AVOID GRAPEFRUIT JUICE
	bretylium	5 mg/kg to 10 mg/kg IV over 8 to 15 minutes. Repeat in 1 to 2 hours. Maintenance dose is 1 mg/min to 2 mg/min by continuous IV infusion	FOR IV USE
	sotalol	80 mg to 160 mg two times a day. Betapace is usually taken twice a day, and Betapace AF is taken once or twice a day	TAKE ON AN EMPTY STOMACH AVOID SALT SUBSTITUTES
	Class IV		
	verapamil	240 mg/day to 360 mg/day orally in 3 to 4 divided doses (immediate release) 2.5 mg to 5 mg IV over 2 to 4 minutes; may repeat 5 mg to 10 mg every 15 to 30 minutes up to 20 mg IV	TAKE WITH FOOD SWALLOW WHOLE; DON'T CRUSH OR CHEW—extended release

Summary of Drugs Used in the Treatment of Arrhythmia—cont'd

	Generic name	Usual dose and dosing schedule	Warning labels
	ACE inhibitors (ACEIs)—see Chapter 22 Angiotensin II type 1 receptor antagonists (ARBs)—see Chapter 22		
	Miscellaneous		
	digoxin	**Loading dose:** 10 mcg/kg to 15 mcg/kg orally or IV given in 3 divided doses every 6 to 8 hours **Maintenance:** 125 mcg to 500 mcg orally or IV once a day	TAKE ON AN EMPTY STOMACH AVOID HIGH-FIBER DIET ASK PHARMACIST BEFORE TAKING OTC MEDICINES

TECH ALERT!
The following drugs have look-alike/sound-alike issues: acebutolol and albuterol; esmolol and Osmitrol; Brevibloc and Brevital; propranolol and Pravachol; Inderal, Adderall, Isordil, and Toradol

TECH ALERT!
The following drugs have look-alike/sound-alike issues: amiodarone, amantadine, and trazodone; Cordarone, Cardura, and Coumadin; Betapace AF and Betapace

TECH ALERT!
The following drugs have look-alike/sound-alike issues: verapamil and Verelan; Calan SR and Calan

CHAPTER SUMMARY

- An arrhythmia is defined as an irregular heart rhythm or a heart rate that is too rapid or too slow.
- An arrhythmia can impair the heart's ability to distribute blood.
- Atrial fibrillation is the most common arrhythmia; it affects approximately 1% of the population and can increase the risk for stroke.
- Nonmodifiable risk factors for arrhythmia are age, gender, low heart rate, and emotional stress.
- Modifiable risk factors for arrhythmia are obesity, smoking, excessive alcohol consumption, and stimulant use.
- Disease risk factors for arrhythmia are hypertension, heart failure, CHD, stroke, infection, diabetes, thyroid disease, and obstructive sleep apnea.
- Ventricular fibrillation is the leading cause of sudden cardiac death.
- Arrhythmias occur when the cardiac ion exchange channels function improperly. This can result in excessive firing, extra currents during the refractory period, and establishment of sinus rhythm by nonpacemaker cells.
- Once arrhythmias form they may stimulate the formation of other arrhythmias.
- Atrial flutter refers to a heart rate of 160 to 350 beats per minute.
- Atrial fibrillation is defined as a rapid heart rate between 300 and 400 beats per minute.
- Ventricular tachycardia causes the ventricles to beat faster than 200 beats per minute.
- Ventricular fibrillation may cause the ventricles to beat faster than 600 beats per minute.
- Antiarrhythmic drugs are categorized into four classes (Class I, II, III, IV) according to their mechanism of action and structural similarities.
- Class I antiarrhythmic drugs produce a sodium channel blockade.
- Class I antiarrhythmic drugs reduce automaticity (spontaneous contraction of heart muscle cells), delay conduction, and prolong the time between contractions (refractory period).
- Class II antiarrhythmic drugs are β-adrenergic blockers.
- β-Blockers antagonize stimulation at the atrial ventricular and sinoatrial nodes. They increase the refractory period, decrease automaticity, and slow conduction velocity.
- Class III antiarrhythmic drugs produce potassium channel blockade.
- Class III antiarrhythmic drugs prolong depolarization and prolong the refractory period.
- Class IV antiarrhythmic drugs produce calcium channel blockade.
- β-Blockers are the only class of drugs indicated for primary management of ventricular arrhythmias.
- All antiarrhythmic agents are proarrhythmic (can cause other arrhythmias).
- Digoxin is approved for the treatment of atrial fibrillation. It reduces arrhythmias by slowing the conduction velocity and prolonging the refractory period in the Purkinje fibers and atrioventricular node.
- In the atria and ventricles, digoxin shortens the refractory period. Digoxin also reduces electrical discharges from the sinoatrial node.

- Angiotensin-converting enzyme inhibitors and angiotensin II type 1 receptor blockers can significantly reduce the risk for first-time atrial fibrillation in patients with hypertension, heart failure, and post–myocardial infarction.
- Angiotensin-converting enzyme inhibitors lengthen the refractory period and shorten conduction time.
- Angiotensin II type 1 receptor blockers also reduce inflammation and structural changes in the atria that can activate atrial fibrillation.

REVIEW QUESTIONS

Multiple Choice

1. Arrhythmias can produce heart rates that exceed _____ beats per minute.
   a. 200
   b. 400
   c. 600
   d. 800

2. _____ fibrillation is the most common arrhythmia.
   a. Atrial
   b. Ventricular
   c. Aortic
   d. Pulmonary

3. What kind of fibrillation is life threatening?
   a. atrial
   b. venticular
   c. aortic
   d. a and b

4. β-Blockers are the only class of drugs indicated for primary management of atrial arrhythmias.
   a. true
   b. false

5. All antiarrhythmic agents are proarrhythmic (can cause other arrhythmias). They also can cause all of the following symptoms except _____.
   a. bradycardia
   b. hypotension
   c. hypertension
   d. dizziness

6. Digoxin has a narrow therapeutic index so it is important to avoid excessive doses.
   a. true
   b. false

7. Arrhythmia management is currently focused on _____.
   a. cure
   b. prevention
   c. medication
   d. all of the above

8. A sign of quinidine toxicity is _____.
   a. fibrillation
   b. tinnitus
   c. clot formation
   d. numbness

9. Bretylium is placed in which class of drugs for arrhythmias?
   a. Class I
   b. Class II
   c. Class III
   d. Class IV

10.   **The brand name for verapamil is** _____.
   a. Covera HS
   b. Calan
   c. Isoptin
   d. all of the above

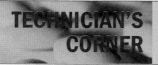

1. What is the difference between a palpitation and an arrhythmia?
2. Can an arrhythmia be controlled with medication?

BIBLIOGRAPHY

Aksnes T, Flaa A, Strand A, Kjeldsen S: Prevention of new-onset atrial fibrillation and its predictors with angiotensin II-receptor blockers in the treatment of hypertension and heart failure, *J Hypertens*, 25:15-23, 2007.

Kalant H, Grant D, Mitchell J: *Principles of medical pharmacology* (pp 366-376), ed 7. Toronto, 2007, Elsevier Canada, A Division of Reed Elsevier Canada.

Lance L, Lacy C, Armstrong L, Goldman M: *Drug information handbook for the allied health professional*, ed 12. Hudson, OH, 2005, APhA Lexi-Comp.

Nash M, et al. Evidence for multiple mechanism in human ventricular fibrillation, *Circulation*, 114:536-542, 2006. Available at: http://circ.ahajournals.org/cgi/content/full/114/6/536.

Otto M: Class 1B antiarrhythmics, *Clin Pharmacol*, 1994; revised 2003. Available at: http://www.clinicalpharmacology.com/apps/default.asp?entry=11andrNum=96.

Otto M: Class 1C antiarrhythmics, *Clin Pharmacol*, 2003. Available at: http://www.clinicalpharmacology.com/apps/default.asp?entry=11andrNum=96.

Otto M, Markowsky S: Class 1A antiarrhythmics, *Clin Pharmacol*, 2003. Available at http://www.clinicalpharmacology.com/apps/default.asp?entry=11andrNum=96.

Page C, Curtis M, Sutter M, Walker M, Hoffman B: *Integrated pharmacology* (pp 432-446), Philadelphia, 2005, Mosby.

Tveit A, et al. Candesartan in the prevention of relapsing atrial fibrillation, *Int J Cardiol*, 1-7, 2006.

Zipes, D.P, et al. ACC/AHA/ESC practice guidelines, *J Am Coll Cardiol*, 48:e268-e270, 2006.

Drugs Affecting the Gastrointestinal System

Identify the organs of the digestive system and their functions.
Explain the process of digestion: both mechanical and chemical.
Understand the support role of accessory organs in digestion.

Role of the Digestive System

The organs of the digestive system work together to perform a vital function—that of preparing food for absorption and for use by the millions of body cells. Food that is eaten must be modified in both chemical composition and physical state so that nutrients can be absorbed and used by the body cells. The complete process of altering the physical and chemical composition of ingested food materials so that it can be absorbed and used by the body cells is called *digestion*. The first step in the digestive process is called *mechanical digestion* and involves the physical breaking down of ingested food material into smaller pieces. It begins in the mouth and continues with the churning and mixing of food as it passes through the digestive system. The second phase of digestion, called *chemical digestion*, completes the breakdown process. It results in the release of nutrient "end products" such as glucose and amino acids, which can be absorbed and enter cells for use as an energy source or for other metabolic functions.

Organization of the Digestive System

ORGANS OF DIGESTION

The main organs of digestive system form a tube all the way through the ventral cavities of the body. It is open at both ends. The tube is commonly called the *alimentary canal* or *gastrointestinal (GI) tract,* and from beginning to end, it follows a specific path: oral

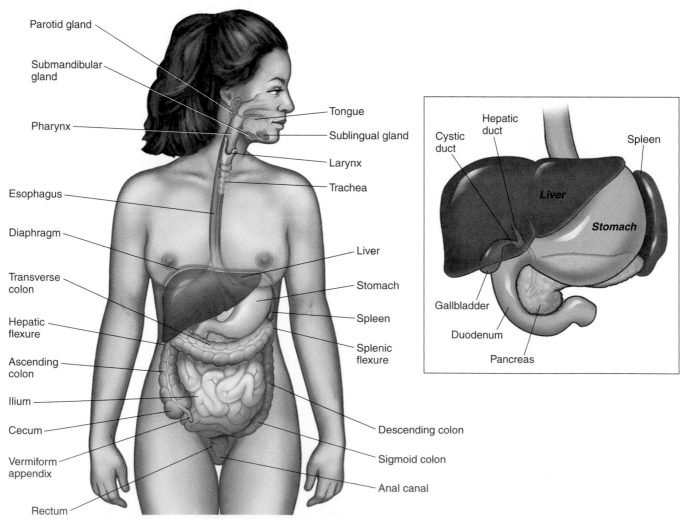

(From Thibodeau GA, Patton KT: Anatomy & physiology, ed 6. St. Louis, Mosby, 2007.)

cavity, oropharynx, esophagus, stomach, small intestine, large intestine, rectum, and anal canal. Organs not part of the alimentary tube are called *accessory organs* and play a support role in digestion. The accessory organs are the salivary glands, tongue, and teeth; liver; gallbladder; pancreas; and appendix.

STRUCTURES OF THE ORAL CAVITY

The *oral cavity* is made up of the following parts: the mouth, lips, cheeks, tongue, and the hard and soft palate. The *hard palate* and *soft palate* form a partition between the mouth and the *nasopharynx*. Suspended from the middle of the soft palate is the *uvula*. The tongue is a solid mass of skeletal muscle that assists during *mastication* (chewing), *deglutition* (swallowing), and speech. The surface of the tongue contains *papillae* and imbedded in these papillae are the *taste buds*. Three pairs of salivary glands—the *parotid, submandibular,* and *sublingual glands*—secrete the majority of saliva that is produced each day. The saliva contains enzymes and mucus, which facilitate the breakdown of food.

The *pharynx* serves as a passageway for air and food. It passes from the mouth to the pharynx and then to the esophagus.

The *esophagus* is a collapsible, muscular, mucus-lined tube that extends from the pharynx to the stomach and pierces the diaphragm. It serves as a dynamic passageway for food, pushing the food toward the stomach. Each end of the esophagus is guarded by a muscular sphincter. The *upper esophageal sphincter* helps prevent air from entering during respiration. The *lower esophageal sphincter* opens into the diaphragm.

STOMACH

Just below the diaphragm is an elongated pouch-like structure, the stomach. The stomach is divided into the *fundus, body*, and *pylorus*. Sphincter muscles guard the openings between the upper and lower ends of the stomach. The lower esophageal sphincter controls entry of contents between the esophagus and the stomach. The *pyloric sphincter* controls the opening from the pyloric portion of the stomach into the *duodenum*, the first part of the small intestine.

The epithelial lining of the stomach is composed of folds, called *rugae,* and is marked by depressions called gastric pits. *Gastric glands* are found below the *gastric pits* and secrete most of the gastric juice, a mucous fluid containing digestive enzymes and hydrochloric acid. The gastric glands also contain three major secretory cells: *chief cells, parietal cells,* and *endocrine cells.*

The stomach performs the following functions:
- Serves as a reservoir for food
- Secretes gastric juice (chief cells) and hydrochloric acid (parietal cells) to chemically break down food
- Secretes the intrinsic factor (binds to vitamin B_{12})
- Produces hormone gastrin to regulate digestion and ghrelin (endocrine cells) to increase appetite
- Helps protect the body by destroying pathogenic bacteria swallowed with food or with mucus

SMALL AND LARGE INTESTINES

The small intestine consists of three divisions: the *duodenum* (uppermost), *jejunum* (middle), and *ileum* (lowest). The lining of the intestines contain *circular plicae* (folds) that have many tiny projections called *villi.* The presence of villi and microvilli increases the surface area of the small intestine and makes this organ the main site of digestion and absorption. The large intestine is divided into the *cecum, colon,* and *rectum and anal canal.*

APPENDIX

The *appendix* is found just behind the cecum or over the pelvic rim. Its functions are not certain, and it is thought to serve as a "breeding ground" for some of the nonpathogenic intestinal bacteria thought to aid in the digestion or absorption of nutrients.

LIVER

The *liver* is the largest gland in the body and lies immediately under the diaphragm. It consists of two lobes. The functions of the liver are as follows:

- Detoxification
- Secretion of bile
- Metabolism of foods: proteins, fats, and carbohydrates
- Kupffer cells (phagocytic cells) that remove bacteria, worn red blood cells, and other particles from the bloodstream
- Storage: iron, vitamins A, B_{12}, and D
- Production of plasma proteins
- Serve as a site of hematopoiesis during fetal development

GALLBLADDER

The gallbladder lies on the undersurface of the liver. Functions of the gallbladder are to store and concentrate bile and to contract and eject concentrated bile into the duodenum.

PANCREAS

The pancreas is composed of two different types of glandular tissue: one endocrine (alpha and beta cells) and one exocrine (acinar cells). The *beta cells* secrete **insulin,** and *alpha cells* secrete **glucagon**. These hormones control carbohydrate metabolism. **Acinar** cells secrete digestive enzymes found in pancreatic juice.

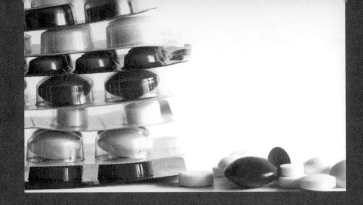

Treatment of Gastroesophageal Reflux Disease, Laryngopharyngeal Reflux, and Peptic Ulcer Disease

LEARNING OBJECTIVES

- Learn the terminology associated with gastroesophageal reflux disease (GERD), laryngopharyngeal reflux (LPR), and peptic ulcer disease (PUD).
- List the symptoms of GERD, LPR, and PUD.
- List risk factors for GERD and PUD.
- List and categorize medications used to treat GERD, LPR, and PUD.
- Describe mechanism of action for drugs used to treat GERD, LPR, and PUD.
- Identify warning labels and precautionary messages associated with medications used to treat GERD and PUD.
- Identify significant drug look-alike/sound-alike issues.
- List common endings for drug classes used in the treatment of GERD, LPR, and PUD.

KEY TERMS

Duodenal ulcer: Ulcer that is located in the upper portion of the small intestine or duodenum.

Endoscopy: Test used to look for ulcers inside of the stomach and small intestine using an endoscope. An endoscope is a thin flexible tube with a small video camera and light attached to one end.

Gastric ulcer: Ulcer that is located in the stomach.

Gastroesophageal reflux disease (GERD): Motility disorder associated with impaired peristalsis that results in the backflow of gastric contents into the esophagus.

Hiatal hernia: Condition in which the lower esophageal sphincter shifts above the diaphragm.

Laryngopharyngeal reflux (LPR): Reflux of gastric contents into the larynx and pharynx.

Lower esophageal sphincter (LES): Sphincter separating the esophagus and the stomach.

Peptic ulcer disease (PUD): Term used to describe ulcers that are located in either the duodenum or stomach.

Peristalsis: Forceful wave of contractions in the esophagus that moves food and liquids from the mouth to the stomach.

Reflux: Backflow of gastric contents into esophagus or laryngopharyngeal region.

Ulcer: Open wound or sore.

Upper esophageal sphincter (UES): Sphincter separating the pharynx and esophagus. It relaxes to permit passage of food and liquids during swallowing; prevent air from entering the esophagus during breathing; and prevent gastric secretions from entering the pharynx.

Overview

Gastroesophageal reflux disease (GERD), peptic ulcer disease (PUD), and laryngopharyngeal reflux (LPR) are diseases that affect millions of Americans and Canadians. It is estimated that 18.6 million Americans have GERD and 1 of 10 Americans has been diagnosed with PUD. The prevalence seems to be growing, and the diagnosis of GERD has tripled between 1990 and 2001. Annual health care costs attributed to PUD are estimated to be greater than $6 billion.

Although these diseases initially produce minor discomfort, they may progress to life-threatening hemorrhage or stomach cancer. GERD may increase the risk for development of chronic disease such as asthma.

Gastroesophageal Reflux Disease

GERD is a motility disorder associated with impaired peristalsis. *Peristalsis* is a forceful wave of contractions in the esophagus that moves food and other orally ingested contents from the mouth to the stomach. The *lower esophageal sphincter* (LES) is a muscle located at the junction between the esophagus and the upper stomach that relaxes to permit food and liquids to pass from the esophagus into the stomach and then contracts to prevent stomach contents from returning to the esophagus. When natural body processes fail to prevent backflow (reflux) of acidic stomach contents and digestive enzymes up into the esophagus, heartburn results. Excessive or chronic exposure to gastric acid and pepsin can lead to inflammation, ulceration, and changes to the epithelial cells that can lead to stomach cancer.

WHAT CAUSES REFLUX?

Stomach contents back up into the esophagus when there is a build-up of pressure in the stomach that causes the LES to open and leak stomach contents back up into the esophagus. Delayed gastric emptying or transient relaxation of the LES (especially after eating) may also cause gastroesophageal reflux.

Persons of any age can develop GERD. Infants may have GERD because their digestive system is immature. Many children will outgrow GERD by their first birthday. Hiatal hernia is a significant risk factor for GERD in persons over 50 years old. Normally, the LES lies below the diaphragm, which helps keep the stomach contents from flowing back into the esophagus. When a *hiatal hernia* occurs, the diaphragm muscle is unable to hold the LES in normal position and the sphincter shifts above the diaphragm. Larger hiatal hernias are linked to more severe esophagitis (Figure 26-1).

FACTORS CONTRIBUTING TO GASTROESOPHAGEAL REFLUX DISEASE

Many factors can aggravate GERD and include foods, lifestyle, prescription and OTC medicines, and even body position. Foods that can aggravate GERD are citrus fruits, chocolate, caffeinated beverages, fried and fatty food, mint flavoring, spicy food, tomato-based foods and sauces, garlic, and onions. Lifestyle factors that aggravate GERD include alcohol consumption and cigarette smoking. GERD symptoms are made worse when the body is in a prone position (lying down). Raising the head of the bed 6 to 8 inches can reduce symptoms. Pregnancy and obesity can also aggravate GERD. Many prescription and OTC medicines can worsen GERD. Some categories of drugs that worsen gastroesophageal reflux are anticholinergics (hyoscyamine), opioids (codeine), calcium channel blockers (verapamil), nonsteroidal antiinflammatory drugs (NSAIDs) (naproxen), and xanthines (theophylline). These drugs impair peristalsis, delay gastric emptying, decrease esophageal sphincter tone, decrease protective mucosal lining, and/or increase gastric acids.

Laryngopharyngeal Reflux

LPR is closely related to GERD and can occur simultaneously. When gastric contents reflux into the larynx and pharynx (located in the head and neck region), inflammation occurs that may cause hoarseness, voice fatigue, laryngitis, sore throat, chronic cough, bad breath, sinusitis, wheezing, aggravation of asthma, and even middle ear infections.

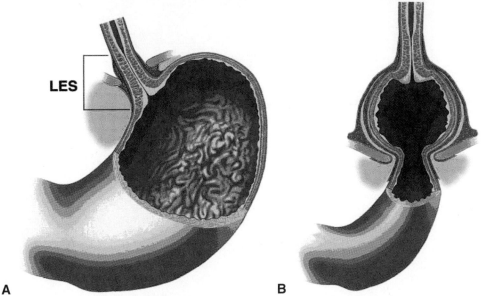

FIGURE 26-1 Gastroesophageal junction. **A,** Location of the lower esophageal sphincter (LES). **B,** Hiatal hernia. *(Courtesy of Jeffrey T. Laitman, Mount Sinai School of Medicine, Center for Anatomy and Functional Morphology, New York, NY.)*

As in GERD, LPR occurs when the normal reflux barriers fail. Anatomical barriers that protect against LPR are the gastroesophageal junction (includes the LES), esophageal motor function and acid clearance, and the upper esophageal sphincter (UES). Laryngeal mucosal resistance also protects the larynx from damage due to reflux.

The UES separates the pharynx and esophagus and relaxes to permit passage of food and liquids during swallowing, prevent air from entering the esophagus during breathing, and prevent gastric secretions entering the pharynx via the esophagus. If the UES is damaged by exposure to stomach contents, it can become less sensitive and lose its ability to function properly. This increases the likelihood of reflux and more damage (Figure 26-2).

Peptic Ulcer Disease

An *ulcer* is an open wound or sore. Ulcers can occur anywhere on the body. An ulcer that is located in the stomach is called a *gastric ulcer* (Figure 26-3). An ulcer that is located in the upper region of the small intestine is called a *duodenal ulcer*. A *peptic ulcer* is an ulcer that is located in either the stomach or the duodenum.

RISK FACTORS FOR PEPTIC ULCER DISEASE (PUD)

Nearly two-thirds of the global population is infected with *Helicobacter pylori (H. pylori)*, the number one cause of PUD. More than 90% of people who have duodenal ulcers and 80% of people who have gastric ulcers are infected with *H. pylori*. Worldwide, most of the people infected with *H. pylori* develop the infection in childhood. Infections are transmitted person-to-person by a gastro-oral route. Once the bacteria are ingested, they release buffers that enable the bacteria to survive in the acidic contents of the stomach. The bacteria also release virulence factors that are responsible for inflammation and tissue damage. Fortunately, most people who are infected with *H. pylori* will not develop chronic gastritis or PUD. Researchers are working to develop a vaccine to prevent *H. pylori* infection that can be administered in childhood.

When a person exhibits symptoms of an ulcer, several simple tests can be performed to see if the person has an *H. pylori* infection. A sample of blood may be drawn to look for antibodies and other evidence of past or current infection or a breath test may be done to check for evidence of urease, an enzyme released by *H. pylori*. An endoscopy may be performed to look for ulcers inside of the stomach and small intestine using an endoscope,

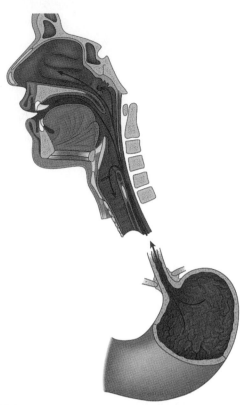

FIGURE 26-2 Laryngopharyngeal reflux. Direction of back flow into head and neck region. *(Courtesy of Jeffrey T. Laitman, Mount Sinai School of Medicine, Center for Anatomy and Functional Morphology, New York, NY.)*

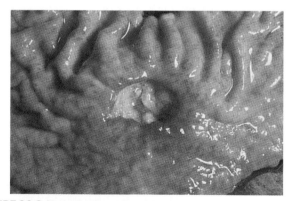

FIGURE 26-3 Gastric ulcer. *(From Rosai J: Rosai and Ackerman's surgical pathology, ed 9. Philadelphia, 2004, Mosby.)*

a thin flexible tube with a small video camera and light attached to one end that is passed down the esophagus into the stomach.

Family history of ulcers or living with close relatives who have PUD increases the risk for developing an ulcer. Age is another risk factor; and persons over the age of 50 years are at increased risk. Medicines that can cause ulcers to develop include salicylates (i.e., aspirin), NSAIDs (i.e., naproxen), and corticosteroids (i.e., prednisone). NSAIDs and salicylates reduce the protective mucus lining of the stomach or duodenum.

Symptoms of Gastroesophageal Reflux Disease, Laryngopharyngeal Reflux, and Peptic Ulcer Disease

Some of the symptoms of GERD, LPR, and PUD are common to all three conditions, while others are disease specific. Symptoms that are associated with GERD, LPR, and PUD are categorized in Table 26-1.

Lifestyle Modification

Cigarette smoking and alcohol consumption can increase the risk for PUD and can aggravate existing disease. Cigarette smoking interferes with the healing of an ulcer by constricting blood vessels to the ulcerated area. Alcohol is a gastric irritant. See Box 26-1 for lifestyle modifications recommended for people with GERD and PUD.

Drugs Used in the Treatment of Gastroesophageal Reflux Disease, Laryngopharyngeal Reflux, and Peptic Ulcer Disease

The treatment of GERD, LPR, and PUD is aimed at reducing gastrointestinal (GI) irritants (i.e., the volume of gastric acid, digestive enzymes such as pepsin) and increasing protective factors (i.e., mucus secretion by epithelial cells). There are some major differences in treatment strategies for GERD, LPR, and PUD. Treatment of PUD also involves eliminating

TECH NOTE!
It is a myth that stress and spicy foods can cause ulcers; however, some foods can aggravate existing GERD.

TABLE 26-1 **Symptoms of Gastroesophageal Reflux Disease, Laryngopharyngeal Reflux, and Peptic Ulcer Disease**

Disease	Unique symptoms	Common symptoms
Gastroesophageal reflux disease (GERD)	Difficulty swallowing Dry cough Bad breath Bloated stomach Rumbling noise in stomach Belching or burping Respiratory problems Hoarseness	Heartburn Stomachache Hunger pains Nausea or vomiting Chest pain
Laryngopharyngeal reflux (LPR)	Hoarseness Voice fatigue or breaks Sore throat Excessive phlegm or saliva Chronic cough Bad breath Middle ear infection Wheezing Chronic sinusitis	
Peptic ulcer disease (PUD)	Burning pain in the gut beginning 2 to 3 hours after a meal Weight loss Loss of appetite	

BOX 26-1 LIFESTYLE MODIFICATIONS RECOMMENDED FOR PEOPLE WITH GASTROESOPHAGEAL REFLUX DISEASE OR PEPTIC ULCER DISEASE

- Avoid lying down after eating (wait at least 3 hours).
- Elevate the head of the bed 6 to 8 inches.
- Eat small meals.
- Lose weight if you are overweight.
- Quit smoking if you smoke.
- Do not drink alcohol.
- Limit use of aspirin and NSAIDs.

H.pylori infection. Patients that have GERD and LPR may be prescribed drugs that increase GI motility. These drugs are known as prokinetic drugs.

Drugs used in the treatment of PUD, GERD, and LPR are classified according to their pharmacological effect: (1) acid-neutralizing drugs (e.g., antacids), (2) acid-suppressing drugs (e.g., histamine$_2$ receptor antagonists, proton pump inhibitors), (3) mucosal protectants (e.g., prostaglandins, sucralfate), (4) drugs that eliminate *H.pylori* (e.g., antiinfectives), and (5) prokinetic drugs (e.g., metoclopramide).

HISTAMINE$_2$ (H$_2$)-RECEPTOR ANTAGONIST DRUGS

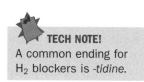

There are four H$_2$-receptor antagonists marketed in the United States and Canada. They are cimetidine, famotidine, nizatidine, and ranitidine. H$_2$-receptor antagonists are used for the treatment of GERD, LPR, and PUD. All H$_2$-receptor antagonists are available in prescription and nonprescription strengths.

MECHANISM OF ACTION

Histamine stimulates acid secretion by gastric parietal cells. Histamine$_2$-receptor antagonists competitively and reversibly bind to H$_2$-receptors, blocking histamine-mediated acid secretion. The secretion of pepsin, a digestive enzyme that is released when the volume of acid in the stomach is high, occurs when food is present in the stomach and decreases as gastric acid levels decrease. Chronic exposure to pepsin can cause inflammation and peptic ulcers.

PHARMACOKINETICS

The H$_2$-receptor antagonists have a similar time to peak plasma levels, half-life (T½), and duration of action. The time required to reach maximum effect ranges from ½ hour (nizatidine) to 2 to 3 hours (ranitidine). The elimination T½ is approximately 2 hours for all H$_2$-receptor antagonists. The effect of H$_2$-receptor antagonists on nocturnal acid secretion is significantly greater than on acid secretion after meals. The duration of effect on nocturnal secretion ranges between 8 hours (cimetidine) to 13 hours (ranitidine). The duration of effect on secretion after meals is reduced to 3 to 5 hours. There are differences in potency between the H$_2$-receptor antagonists. Ranitidine is the most potent and is up to 10 times more effective than cimetidine.

ADVERSE REACTIONS

H$_2$-receptor antagonists can produce dizziness or drowsiness, constipation or diarrhea, bloating, headache, and confusion when taken at therapeutic doses. The elderly are more susceptible to these adverse effects than are other patient populations. Other less common adverse effects include skin rash, agitation, depression, hepatitis, decreased libido, and gynecomastia (high-dose cimetidine). Males who develop ***gynecomastia*** have symptoms of breast swelling and tenderness.

PRECAUTIONS

Cimetidine inhibits several cytochrome P450 metabolic enzymes and is responsible for increasing the elimination of more than 25 different drugs. The pharmacist should be alerted to all drug interactions.

PROTON PUMP INHIBITOR DRUGS

There are five proton pump inhibitors (PPIs) currently marketed in the United States and Canada. They are esomeprazole, lansoprazole, omeprazole, pantoprazole, and rabeprazole. PPIs are effective in treating GERD, LPR, and PUD because they decrease gastric acids. They are more potent that H$_2$-receptor antagonists. Omeprazole is the only PPI that is available for OTC use. All other PPIs are only commercially available in prescription strengths.

MECHANISM OF ACTION

PPIs decrease gastric acids by interfering with the final step in gastric acid production. PPIs interfere with hydrogen and potassium ion exchange by the H$^+$/K$^+$-ATPase proton pump located on parietal cells in the stomach (Figure 26-4).

Histamine$_2$ Receptor Antagonists (H$_2$-Blockers)

Generic name	U.S. brand name(s) / Canadian brand(s)	Dosage forms and strengths
cimetidine*	Tagamet, Tagamet HB	**Tablet:** 200 mg, 300 mg, 400 mg, 600 mg, (Canada only), 800 mg
	Generics	**oral liquid:** 300 mg/5 ml **Injection, solution:** 150 mg/ml
famotidine*	Pepcid, Pepcid AC	**Tablet:** 10 mg, 20 mg, 40 mg **Injection, solution:** 20 mg/2 ml
	Pepcid	**Powder for oral suspension:** 40 mg/5 ml
nizatidine*	Axid, Axid XR	**Capsule:** 150 mg, 300 mg **Oral solution:** 15 mg/ml
	Axid	
ranitidine*	Zantac	**Capsule:** 75 mg, 150 mg, 300 mg **Tablet:** 75 mg, 150 mg, 300 mg
	Zantac	**Injection, solution:** 25 mg/ml **Oral solution:** 15 mg/ml **Effervescent tablet:** 25 mg, 150 mg

H$_2$-receptor antagonists combinations

famotidine + calcium carbonate + magnesium hydroxide	Pepcid Complete	famotidine 10 mg + 800 mg calcium carbonate + 165 mg magnesium hydroxide

*Generic available.

PHARMACOKINETICS

PPIs are acid labile, therefore, they can be destroyed in gastric acids. It is recommended they be taken on an empty stomach when gastric acid volume is lowest. Zegerid is a formulation combining an antacid with omeprazole to reduce omeprazole degradation by gastric acids. PPIs are delayed release formulations. They must not be crushed or chewed. Esomeprazole is an *S*-isomer (mirror image) of omeprazole which the manufacturer claims has greater bioavailability and is more potent. Delayed release tablets (lansoprazole) disintegrate in less than one minute.

ADVERSE REACTIONS

All of the PPIs have a similar side effect profile. More common side effects are abdominal pain, headache, diarrhea or constipation, flatulence (gas), and nausea. Less common side effects are: jaundice, skin rash, unusual tiredness or fatigue, agitation, vitamin B$_{12}$ deficiency, dark yellow or brown urine, and vomiting.

MUCOSAL PROTECTANTS

Mucosal protectants decrease the susceptibility of epithelial cells that line the stomach and small intestine to damage by gastric acids, pepsin, and *H. pylori.* Misoprostol is approved for prevention of NSAID-induced peptic ulcers. Sucralfate is approved for treatment and maintenance of duodenal ulcers.

MECHANISM OF ACTION

Misoprostol is a synthetic prostaglandin E (PGE). It stimulates the production of protective mucus and bicarbonate in the stomach. Misoprostol also increases regeneration of gastric epithelial cells and enhances blood flow to the stomach.

TECH NOTE!
Misoprostol MUST be dispensed in the manufacturer's original container.

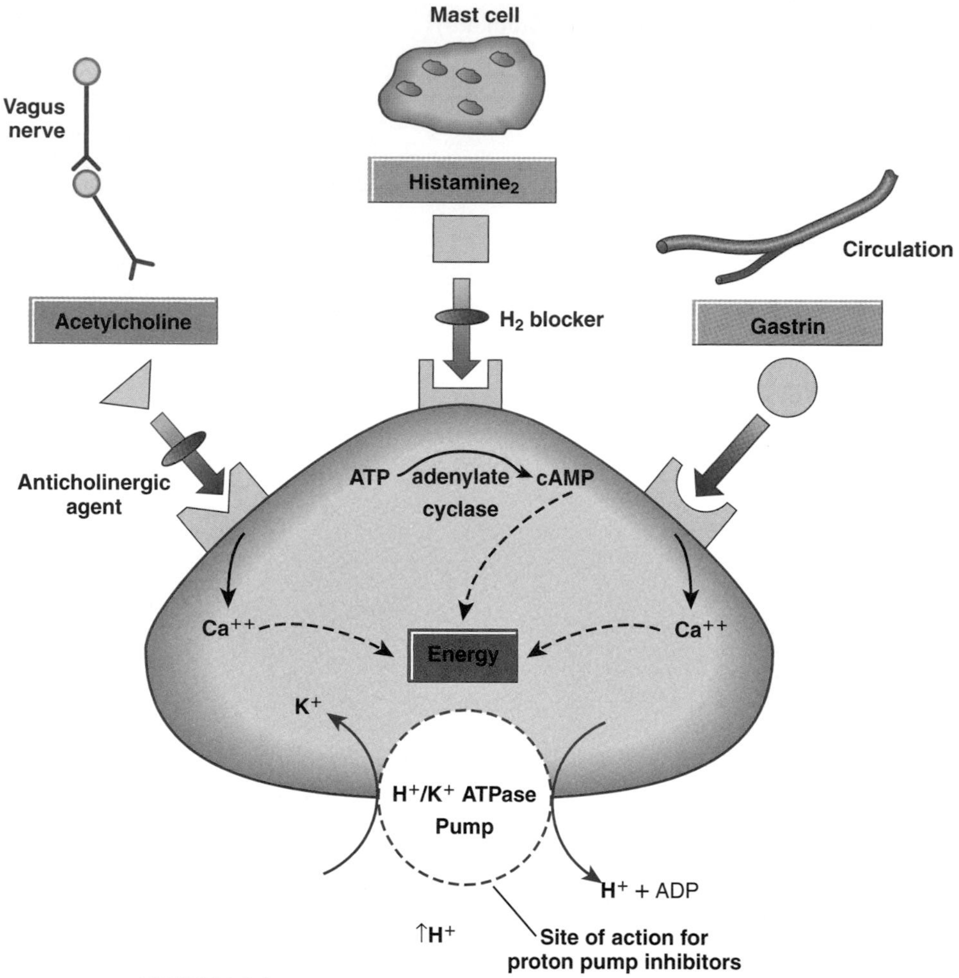

FIGURE 26-4 Mediators of gastric acid production. *(From Lilley LL, Harrington S, Snyder JS: Pharmacology and the nursing process, ed 5. St. Louis, 2007, Mosby.)*

Proton Pump Inhibitors (PPIs)

	Generic name	U.S. brand name(s) / Canadian brand(s)	Dosage forms and strengths
	esomeprazole	Nexium	**Capsules, delayed release:** 20 mg, 40 mg
			Granules for suspension: 20 mg, 40 mg per packet
		Nexium	**Powder for injection:** 20 mg
	lansoprazole	Prevacid, Prevacid SoluTab	15 mg, 30 mg DR capsules, 15 mg, 30 mg granules for suspension, 15 mg, 30 mg disintegrating tablets
		Prevacid	**Capsules, delayed release:** 15 mg, 30 mg
			Granules for suspension: 15 mg, 30 mg per packet
			Disintegrating tablets: 15 mg, 30 mg
	omeprazole*	Prilosec	**Capsules, delayed release:** 10 mg, 20 mg, 40 mg
			Tablets, delayed release: 10 mg, 20 mg, 40 mg
		Losec	

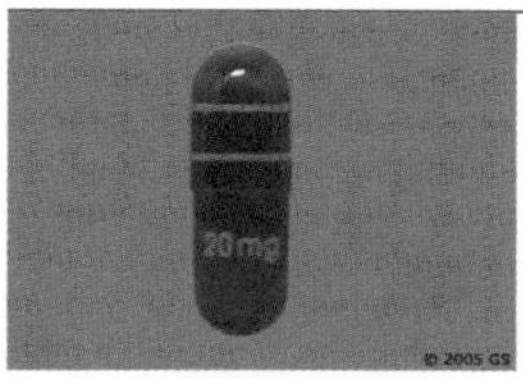

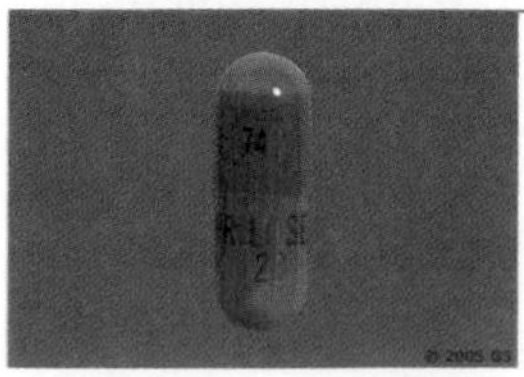

Proton Pump Inhibitors (PPIs)—cont'd

	Generic name	U.S. brand name(s Canadian brand(s)	Dosage forms and strengths
	pantoprazole	Protonix	**Tablet, delayed release:** 20 mg, 40 mg **Powder for injection:** 40 mg
		Pantoloc	
	rabeprazole	Aciphex	20 mg DR tablet **Tablet, delayed release:** 20 mg
		Pariet	
PPI combination products			
	lansoprazole + naproxen	Prevacid NapraPAC	15 mg lansoprazole capsule + 500 mg naproxen tablet
	lansoprazole + amoxicillin + clarithromycin	Prevpac	30 mg lansoprazole capsule + 500 mg amoxicillin capsule + 500 mg clarithromycin tablet
		HP-PAC	
	omeprazole + sodium bicarbonate	Zegerid	20 mg omeprazole + 1100 mg sodium bicarbonate capsule; 40 mg omeprazole + 1100 mg sodium bicarbonate capsule; 20 mg omeprazole + 1680 mg sodium bicarbonate powder for suspension; 40 mg omeprazole + 1680 mg sodium bicarbonate powder for suspension

*Generic available.

Sucralfate binds to the ulcerated area and forms a protective barrier much like a bandage protects a sore. It also promotes regeneration of stomach epithelial cells. It is a weak inhibitor of *H. pylori*.

ADVERSE REACTIONS

Misoprostol may produce abdominal cramps, diarrhea, menstrual irregularities, headache, and dizziness. Sucralfate may produce constipation, gas, dry mouth, and headache.

PRECAUTIONS

Misoprotol is contraindicated in pregnancy because it stimulates uterine contractions. Sucralfate blocks the absorption of several drugs including H_2-receptor antagonists, PPIs, and several antibiotics. To avoid drug interactions, the drugs should not be taken at the same time as sucralfate.

PROKINETIC DRUGS

Prokinetic drugs are used for the treatment of GERD and LPR. They increase peristalsis, the wave-like movement throughout the GI tract; speed gastric emptying; and improve LES tone. Metoclopramide is currently the only prokinetic drug approved by the Food and Drug Administration. Domperidone has been approved for the treatment of heartburn in Canada; however, it is primarily used in the treatment of nausea in the United States and in Canada.

ADVERSE REACTIONS

More common adverse effects associated with metoclopramide include drowsiness, dizziness, diarrhea, abdominal pain, constipation, restlessness, and headache. Less common effects are muscle twitching, skin rash, irregular heartbeat, and breast enlargement in men and women.

✎ TECH ALERT!
The following drugs have look-alike/sound-alike issues:
Prevacid, Prevpac, Prilosec, Pravachol, and Prinivil;
Prilosec, Plendil, Prozac, and prilocaine;
Protonix, Lotronex, Lovenox, and protamine
rabeprazole and aripiprazole;
Aciphex, Aricept, and Accupril

Mucosal Protectant Drugs

	Generic name	U.S. brand name(s) / Canadian brand(s)	Dosage forms and strengths
	misoprostol*	Cytotec	100 mcg, 200 mcg
		Generic	
	sucralfate*	Carafate	1 g tablet, 1 g/5 ml suspension
		Sulcrate	
	Combination products		
	misoprostol + diclofenac	Arthrotec-50; Arthrotec-75	200 mcg misoprostol + 50 mg diclofenac delayed release (DR) tablet;
		Arthrotec-50; Arthrotec-75	200 mcg misoprostol + 75 mg diclofenac DR tablet

*Generic available.

Prokinetic Drugs

	Generic name	U.S. brand name(s) / Canadian brand(s)	Dosage forms and strengths
	metoclopramide*	Reglan	**Tablet:** 5 mg, 10 mg **Oral solution:** 5 mg/5 ml **Injection/solution:** 5 mg/ml
		Generics	
	domperidone*	Motilium†	**Tablet:** 10 mg
		Generics	

*Generic available.
†Investigational use.

ANTACIDS

Antacids are the oldest drugs used in the treatment of GERD and PUD. Antacid use has declined since more potent drugs, requiring fewer daily doses, have been developed. Antacids can be obtained without prescription.

MECHANISM OF ACTION

Antacids neutralize gastric acids and decrease pepsin secretion. The acid-neutralizing capacity (ANC) is a standard used to evaluate the potency of antacids. The ANC is a measure of the ability of an antacid to (1) neutralize approximately 1 to 2 ounces hydrochloric acid (i.e., the volume of acid normally present between meals) and (2) raise the pH of the stomach to 3.5 within 10 minutes.

ADVERSE REACTIONS

The side effects of antacids are related to their active ingredient and are dose related. Magnesium-containing antacids cause diarrhea; aluminum-containing antacids cause constipation and in high doses deplete phosphates levels in blood (hypophosphatemia). Calcium-containing antacids cause constipation and in high doses produce hypercalcemia and kidney stones. Sodium bicarbonate (baking soda) has been associated with rebound hyperacidity, metabolic alkalosis, edema, and hypertension.

TECH ALERT!
The following drugs have look-alike/sound-alike issues: misoprostol and metoprolol; Cytotec, Cytoxan, and Sytobex; sucralfate and salsalate; Carafate and Cafergot

ANTIMICROBIALS

Antimicrobials are prescribed in the treatment of PUD to eradicate *H. pylori* infection. Clarithromycin, metronidazole, amoxicillin, and tetracycline are effective for eradicating *H. pylori*. They are prescribed in combination with drugs that decrease gastric acids and protect the gastric mucosa. Antimicrobials will be described in detail in Chapter 35.

Examples of Selected Antacids

Generic name	U.S. brand name(s) / Canadian brand(s)
aluminum hydroxide*	Amphojel, Alu-Tab Amphojel, Alu-Tab
aluminum hydroxide + magnesium hydroxide*	Gelusil, Maalox, Maalox Plus, Mylanta, Mylanta II Diovol EX, Gelusil, Maalox, Maalox TC
calcium carbonate*	Titralac, TUMS, Caltrate
calcium carbonate + magnesium hydroxide*	Rolaids CALMAG + D

*Generic available.

Summary of Drugs Used in the Treatment of Gastroesophageal Reflux Disease (GERD), Laryngopharyngeal Reflux (LPR), and Peptic Ulcer Disease (PUD)

Generic name	U.S. brand name	Usual adult oral dose and dosing schedule	Warning labels
H₂-receptor antagonists			
cimetidine	Tagamet	PUD 800 mg daily at bedtime, or 400 mg twice daily or 300 mg four times per day for 8 to 12 weeks GERD 800 mg twice daily or 400 mg four times per day for 12 weeks	AVOID ANTACIDS WITHIN 2 HOURS OF DOSE (cimetidine, nizatidine) AVOID ALCOHOL—All SHAKE SUSPENSION WELL
famotidine	Pepcid	PUD 40 mg once daily at bedtime. for 4 to 8 weeks GERD 20 mg to 40 mg twice daily for 6 to 12 weeks	DISCARD FAMOTIDINE ORAL SUSPENSION 30 DAYS AFTER MIXING STORE INJECTION IN THE REFRIGERATOR (famotidine, ranitidine)
nizatidine	Axid	PUD 150 mg every 12 hours or 300 mg at bedtime for up to 8 weeks GERD 150 mg every 12 hours for up to 12 weeks	STORE CIMETIDINE INJECTION AT ROOM TEMPERATURE
ranitidine	Zantac	PUD 150 mg twice daily or 300 mg once daily at bedtime for 4 to 6 weeks GERD 150 mg to 300 mg twice daily for 4 to 8 weeks	

Continued

Summary of Drugs Used in the Treatment of Gastroesophageal Reflux Disease (GERD), Laryngopharyngeal Reflux (LPR), and Peptic Ulcer Disease (PUD)—cont'd

Generic name	U.S. brand name	Usual adult oral dose and dosing schedule	Warning labels
Proton pump inhibitors			
esomeprazole	Nexium	*PUD* 40 mg once daily *GERD* 20 mg to 40 mg once daily for up to 4 to 8 weeks	SWALLOW WHOLE; DO NOT CRUSH OR CHEW (CAPSULES CAN BE SPRINKLED ONTO FOOD BUT DO NOT CRUSH THE CONTENTS INTO THE FOOD)
lansoprazole	Prevacid	*PUD* 15 mg once daily in the morning for up to 4 weeks. *GERD* 15 mg to 30 mg once daily in the morning for up to 8 weeks	TAKE ½ TO 1 HOUR BEFORE A MEAL GRANULES FOR ORAL SUSPENSION MUST BE MIXED WITH 1 TO
omeprazole	Prilosec	*PUD* 40 mg once daily for 4 to 8 weeks *GERD* 20 mg once daily for 4 to 8 weeks	2 TABLESPOONFULS OF LIQUID. ALLOW MIXTURE TO STAND FOR 2 TO 3 MINUTES, THEN IMMEDIATELY DRINK ENTIRE MIX
pantoprazole	Protonix	*PUD* 40 mg once daily after the morning meal for 2 to 4 weeks *GERD* 40 mg once daily for up to 8 weeks	DISSOLVE DISINTEGRATING TABLETS ON TONGUE; DON'T CHEW OR SWALLOW WHOLE
rabeprazole	Aciphex	*PUD* 20 mg once daily after the morning meal for 3 to 6 weeks *GERD* 20 mg once daily for 4 weeks; repeat course of treatment if necessary	
Prokinetic drugs			
metoclopramide	Reglan	*GERD* 10 mg to 15 mg up to 4 times per day	MAY CAUSE DROWSINESS AVOID ALCOHOL TAKE 15 TO 30 MIN BEFORE MEALS
Mucosal protectants			
misoprostal	Cytotec	*NSAID-induced PUD prevention* 100 mcg to 200 mcg 4 times a day	AVOID PREGNANCY
sucralfate	Carafate	Duodenal ulcer 1 g 4 times per day for 4 to 8 weeks	TAKE ON AN EMPTY STOMACH SHAKE SUSPENSION WELL

Summary of Drugs Used in the Treatment of Gastroesophageal Reflux Disease (GERD), Laryngopharyngeal Reflux (LPR), and Peptic Ulcer Disease (PUD)—cont'd

Generic name	U.S. brand name	Usual adult oral dose and dosing schedule	Warning labels
Antimicrobial combinations for *H. pylori* eradication			
metronidazole + tetracycline + bismuth	Helidac: 14-day kit	*H. pylori–associated ulcer* 1 metronidazole tablet + 1 tetracycline cap + 2 bismuth tablets four times a day for 14 days, with a H_2 receptor antagonist or proton pump inhibitor	AVOID ALCOHOL MAY CAUSE DICOLORATION OF URINE OR FECES AVOID PROLONGED EXPOSURE TO SUNLIGHT AVOID DAIRY, ANTACIDS, AND IRON PRODUCTS
lansoprazole + amoxicillin + clarithromycin	PrevPAC	*H. pylori–associated ulcer* 2 amoxicillin caps + 1 lansoprazole cap + 1 clarithromycln tablet twice daily for 14 days	SWALLOW WHOLE; DON'T CRUSH OR CHEW MAY DECREASE THE EFFECTIVENESS OF ORAL CONTRACEPTIVES

TECH ALERT!
The following drugs have look-alike/sound-alike issues: metoclopramide and metolazone; Reglan, Regonol, and Renagel

CHAPTER SUMMARY

- Gastroesophageal reflux disease (GERD), peptic ulcer disease (PUD), and laryngopharyngeal reflux (LPR) are diseases that affect millions of Americans and Canadians.
- Persons of any age can develop GERD.
- Although these diseases initially produce minor discomfort, they may progress to life-threatening hemorrhage or stomach cancer.
- GERD causes a chronic backflow (reflux) of acidic stomach contents and digestive enzymes up into the esophagus.
- Stomach contents back up into the esophagus when there is a build-up of pressure in the stomach. Pressure buildup causes the lower esophageal sphincter (LES), a muscle located at the junction between the esophagus and the upper stomach, to open and leak.
- Excessive or chronic exposure to gastric acids can lead to inflammation, ulceration, and changes to the epithelial cells that can lead to stomach cancers.
- GERD may also increase the risk for development of chronic disease such as asthma.
- Hiatal hernia is a significant risk factor for GERD in persons over 50 years old.
- Fried food, mint flavoring, spicy food, tomato-based foods, and citrus fruits are some of the foods that can aggravate GERD.
- Consumption of caffeinated beverages and alcohol and cigarette smoking are lifestyle factors that make GERD symptoms worse.
- Prescription and OTC medicines can aggravate GERD.
- Laryngopharyngeal reflux (LPR) is closely related to GERD and occurs when gastric contents reflux into the larynx and pharynx.
- LPR causes hoarseness, voice fatigue, laryngitis, sore throat, chronic cough, bad breath, sinusitis, wheezing, aggravation of asthma, and even middle ear infections.
- An ulcer is an open wound or sore. A peptic ulcer may be located in either the stomach or the duodenum.
- Nearly two-thirds of the global population is infected with *Helicobacter pylori (H. pylori)*, the number one cause of peptic ulcer disease (PUD).

- *H. pylori* releases buffers that enable the bacteria to survive in the acidic contents of the stomach. The bacteria also release virulence factors that are responsible for inflammation and tissue damage.
- Age, medicines, and family history or living with close relatives who have PUD are risk factors for developing an ulcer.
- Medicines that can cause ulcers to develop are salicylates (e.g., aspirin), nonsteroidal antiinflammatory drugs (e.g., naproxen), and corticosteroids (e.g., prednisone).
- The treatment of GERD, LPR, and PUD is aimed at reducing gastrointestinal irritants (gastric acid and digestive enzymes such as pepsin) and increasing protective factors (i.e., mucus secretion by epithelial cells).
- Acid-neutralizing drugs (antacids), acid-suppressing drugs (proton pump inhibitors and H_2-receptor antagonists), and mucosal protectants (misoprostol and sucralfate) are used to treat GERD, LPR, and PUD.
- Treatment of PUD also involves eliminating *H. pylori* infection with antimicrobials.
- Patients who have GERD and LPR may be prescribed prokinetic drugs (metoclopramide) to increase gastrointestinal motility.
- The four H_2-receptor antagonists marketed in the United States and Canada are cimetidine, famotidine, nizatidine, and ranitidine.
- Histamine$_2$-receptor antagonists competitively and reversibly bind to H_2-receptors, blocking histamine-mediated acid secretion.
- H_2-receptor antagonists can produce dizziness or drowsiness, constipation or diarrhea, bloating, headache, and confusion when taken at therapeutic doses.
- The five proton pump inhibitors (PPIs) currently marketed in the United States and Canada are esomeprazole, lansoprazole, omeprazole, pantoprazole, and rabeprazole.
- PPIs decrease gastric acids by interfering with the final step in gastric acid production.
- PPIs are delayed-release formulations and must not be crushed or chewed.
- The most common side effects linked to PPIs are abdominal pain, headache, diarrhea or constipation, flatulence (gas), and nausea.
- Misoprostol is synthetic prostaglandin E. It stimulates the production of protective mucus and bicarbonate in the stomach.
- Misoprostol may produce abdominal cramps, diarrhea, menstrual irregularities, headache, and dizziness. It is contraindicated in pregnancy.
- Sucralfate binds to the ulcerated area and forms a protective barrier much like a bandage protects a sore.
- Sucralfate may produce constipation, gas, dry mouth, and headache.
- Prokinetic drugs (metoclopramide) increase peristalsis, speed gastric emptying, and improve lower esophageal sphincter tone.
- Common adverse effects associated with metoclopramide include drowsiness, dizziness, diarrhea, abdominal pain, constipation, restlessness, and headache.
- Antacids neutralize gastric acids and decrease pepsin secretion.
- Antimicrobials are prescribed in the treatment of PUD to eradicate *H. pylori* infection. Clarithromycin, metronidazole, amoxicillin, and tetracycline are effective for eradicating *H. pylori*.

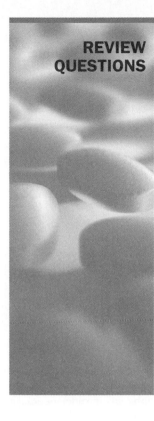

REVIEW QUESTIONS

Multiple Choice

1. **Which sphincter in the digestive system is affected by GERD?**
   a. cardiac sphincter
   b. pyloric sphincter
   c. lower esophageal sphincter
   d. laryngeal sphincter

2. **What bacteria contribute to peptic ulcer disease?**
   a. *Streptococcus*
   b. *Helicobacter pylori*
   c. *Staphylococcus*
   d. *Helicobacter spirella*

3. **Name two H$_2$-receptor antagonist drugs:**
   a. Prilosec and cimetidine
   b. Prevacid and ranitidine
   c. famotidine and diphenhyramine
   d. ranitidine and famotidine

4. **Proton pump inhibitors are effective in treating GERD, LPR, and PUD because they _____.**
   a. decrease gastric acid
   b. block histamine
   c. decrease respiratory mucus
   d. do none of the above

5. **Name two proton pump inhibitor drugs.**
   a. omeprazole and ketaconazole
   b. esomeprazole and lansoprazole
   c. pantoprazole and miconazole
   d. omeprazole and nizatadine

6. **_____ is currently the only prokinetic drug approved by the FDA.**
   a. Pantoprazole
   b. Misprostol
   c. Metoclopramide
   d. Sucralfate

7. **_____-containing antacids cause diarrhea; _____-containing antacids cause constipation.**
   a. Calcium; aluminum
   b. Magnesium; sodium
   c. Calcium; magnesium
   d. Magnesium; calcium

8. **Antacids are the oldest drugs used in the treatment of GERD and PUD. Is this statement true or false?**
   a. true
   b. false

9. **What is the brand name for pantoprazole?**
   a. Aciphex
   b. Nexium
   c. Pepcid
   d. Protonix

10. **Which drug binds to the ulcerated area and forms a protective barrier much like a bandage protects a sore?**
    a. sucralfate
    b. misoprostol
    c. Axid
    d. Nexium

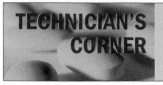

TECHNICIAN'S CORNER

1. Describe the function of the lower esophageal sphincter and how it is affected by GERD.
2. Consumption of what two products increases the risk for peptic ulcer disease and can aggravate existing disease? How does it interfere with the healing of an ulcer?

BIBLIOGRAPHY

Guimarães E, Marguet C, Moreira Camargos P: Treatment of gastroesophageal reflux disease, *J Pediatr,* 82:(Suppl), 2006.

Howden C, Blume S, de Lissovoy G: Practice patterns for managing *Helicobacter pylori* infection and upper gastrointestinal symptoms, *Am J Manag Care,* 13:37-44, 2007.

Lance L, Lacy C, Armstrong L, Goldman M: *Drug information handbook for the allied health professional,* ed 12. Hudson, OH, 2005, APhA Lexi-Comp.

Kabir S: The current status of *Helicobacter pylori* vaccines: a review, *Helicobacter,* 12:89-102,

Kalant H, Grant D, Mitchell J: *Principles of medical pharmacology* (pp 557-571), ed 7. Toronto, 2007, Elsevier Canada, A Division of Reed Elsevier Canada.

Lipan M, Reidenberg J, Laitman J: *Anatomy of reflux: a growing health problem affecting structures of the head and neck, the anatomical record (Part B: new anatomy)* (pp 261-270). New York, 2006, Wiley-Liss.

National Digestive Diseases Information Clearinghouse: Heartburn, hiatal hernia, and gastroesophageal reflux disease (GERD). Bethesda, MD, National Institute of Diabetes and Digestive and Kidney Diseases, National Institutes of Health, US Department of Health and Human Services, June 2003. NIH publication No. 03-0882. Available at: http://www.digestive.niddk.nih.gov.

Pilotto A, Francheschi M, Leandro G, et al. Clinical features of reflux esophagitis in older people: a study of 840 consecutive patients, *J Am Geriatr Soc,* 54:1537-1542, 2006.

Reents S, Prosser T: Overview: H_2 blockers, gold standard clinical pharmacology. Available at: http://www.clinicalpharmacology.com.

USP Center for Advancement of Patient Safety: *Use caution–avoid confusion,* USP Quality Review No. 79, Rockville, MD, April 2004, USP Center for Advancement of Patient Safety.

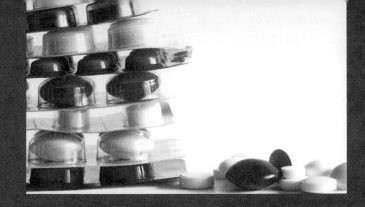

Treatment of Inflammatory Bowel Syndrome, Ulcerative Colitis, and Crohn's Disease

LEARNING OBJECTIVES

- Learn the terminology associated with inflammatory bowel syndrome (IBS), ulcerative colitis, and Crohn's disease.
- List the symptoms of IBS, ulcerative colitis, and Crohn's disease.
- List risk factors for IBS, ulcerative colitis, and Crohn's disease.
- List and categorize medications used to treat IBS, ulcerative colitis, and Crohn's disease.
- Describe mechanism of action for drugs used to treat IBS, ulcerative colitis, and Crohn's disease.
- Identify warning labels and precautionary messages associated with medications used to treat IBS, ulcerative colitis, and Crohn's disease.
- Identify significant drug look-alike/sound-alike issues.
- List common endings for drug classes used in the treatment of IBS, ulcerative colitis, and Crohn's disease.

KEY TERMS

Antidiarrheals: Drugs that prevent or relieve diarrhea.

Colonoscopy: Examination of the colon for signs of inflammation and damage that is performed by inserting a thin tube with a small light and camera at the end (i.e., an endoscope) into the anus.

Constipation: Abnormally delayed or infrequent passage of dry hardened feces.

Crohn's disease: Irritable bowel disease that produces inflammation and damage anywhere along the GI tract.

Diarrhea: Abnormally frequent passage of loose and watery stools.

Fistula: Ulcer that tunnels from the site of origin to surrounding tissues.

Gastroenteritis: Infection in the gastrointestinal tract that can cause post-infection inflammatory bowel syndrome.

Irritable bowel disease (IBD): Chronic disorder of the gastrointestinal tract, characterized by inflammation of the intestine and resulting in abdominal cramping and persistent diarrhea.

Inflammatory bowel syndrome (IBS): Condition that causes abdominal distress and erratic movement of the contents of the large bowel; resulting in diarrhea and/or constipation.

Laxative: Medicine that induces evacuation of the bowel.

Toxic megacolon: Life-threatening condition characterized by a very inflated colon, abdominal distention, and sometimes fever, abdominal pain, or shock.

Ulcer: Craterlike wound or sore.

Ulcerative colitis: Irritable bowel disease that produces inflammation, ulcers, and damage to the colon.

Overview

Inflammatory bowel syndrome (IBS), ulcerative colitis, and Crohn's disease are conditions that are linked to inflammation of the gastrointestinal (GI) tract. Many of the symptoms are similar (e.g., abdominal pain and diarrhea) and are listed in Table 27-1. A diagnosis of IBS may be made, based on symptoms, after diagnostic tests have been performed to rule out other diseases e.g., ulcerative colitis and Crohn's disease. Diagnostic tests that may be performed to diagnose ulcerative colitis and Crohn's disease include testing stool samples, taking X-rays, and performing a ***colonoscopy***. A colonoscopy is performed by inserting a thin tube with a small light and camera at the end (i.e., an endoscope) into the anus. This enables the physician to exam the colon for inflammation and damage (Figure 27-1).

Inflammatory Bowel Syndrome

Inflammatory bowel syndrome (IBS) is a condition that causes abdominal distress and erratic movement of the large bowel. As many as one in five American and Canadian adults have IBS. Symptoms commonly occur before the age of 35 years. When an individual has IBS, movement of waste through the colon (large bowel) may occur too slowly and constipation results ***or*** it occurs too rapidly, causing diarrhea. IBS is sometimes called colitis, but it is not the same condition as ulcerative colitis.

TABLE 27-1   Symptoms of Inflammatory Bowel Syndrome, Ulcerative Colitis, and Crohn's Disease

	Inflammatory bowel syndrome	Ulcerative colitis	Crohn's disease
Similar symptoms	Abdominal pain Diarrhea (mucus/pus) Cramping	Abdominal pain Diarrhea (bloody) Cramping	Abdominal pain Diarrhea Cramping
Disease-specific symptoms	Erratic bowel movements (diarrhea alternating with constipation) Abdominal pain is relieved by having a bowel movement Bloating Constipation	Rectal bleeding Anemia Weight loss and loss of appetite Fatigue Loss of vitamins and mineral Skin lesions Joint pain (arthritis) Decreased growth in children Fever	Rectal bleeding Anemia Weight loss and loss of appetite Loss of vitamins and mineral Skin lesions Joint pain (arthritis) Decreased growth in children Fever

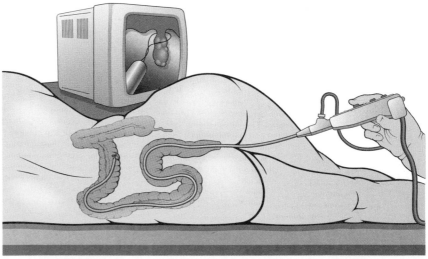

FIGURE 27-1 Colonoscopy and sigmoidoscopy. *(From Chabner DE: The language of medicine, ed 8, St. Louis, 2008, Saunders.)*

WHAT CAUSES INFLAMMATORY BOWEL SYNDROME?

There is no one specific cause for IBS. Persons with IBS have an overly sensitive colon. Food allergies, stress, antibiotic use, chronic alcohol use, and bile acid malabsorption are possible causes of IBS. *Gastroenteritis,* a stomach and intestines infection, may trigger postinfectious IBS. IBS may also be associated with abnormally low levels of the neurotransmitter serotonin. Up to 95% of the body's serotonin (5-HT) is found in the stomach epithelium. The remaining 5% is found in neurons in the brain (see Chapter 6). Low levels of serotonin can cause GI motility problems and increase the sensitivity of pain receptors in the GI tract.

Ulcerative Colitis

Ulcerative colitis is one of several irritable bowel diseases that produce inflammation and damage to the colon. Ultimately, ulcers (or sores) form in the lining of the colon and rectum. Ulcerative colitis can occur at any age, but it most commonly occurs between the ages of 15 and 30 years. The disease tends to run in families, but, unlike irritable bowel disease, it affects men and women equally.

Ulcerative colitis differs from Crohn's disease, another disease causing irritation of the bowel, in two important ways. Ulcerative colitis produces inflammation in the upper layers of the lining of the small intestine and colon, whereas Crohn's disease produces inflammation deep in the intestinal wall. Moreover, the inflammation is limited to the small intestine and colon rather than other areas of the GI tract.

WHAT CAUSES ULCERATIVE COLITIS?

The exact cause of ulcerative colitis is unknown, but it is believed to be linked to abnormal functioning of the immune system. When a person has ulcerative colitis, the body's immune system recognizes the bacteria that normally inhabit the GI tract as harmful invaders. Antitumor necrosis factor (TNF) and other substances that are released to fight the *"infection"* cause pain and inflammation.

Crohn's Disease

Crohn's disease is one of several irritable bowel diseases. Like ulcerative colitis, it causes chronic inflammation of the entire GI tract. Inflammation can occur anywhere along the entire length of the GI tube, from the mouth to the anus, although typically it affects the ileum (the lower part of the small intestine). The inflammation is formed deep within the intestinal wall causing abdominal pain.

WHAT CAUSES CROHN'S DISEASE?

The immune system in people who have Crohn's disease works abnormally. As with ulcerative colitis, the immune system attacks the bacteria normally present in the body, as well as food, thinking them to be harmful invaders. Anti-TNF and other substances released by the immune system produce the inflammation characteristic of Crohn's disease.

SYMPTOMS OF INFLAMMATORY BOWEL SYNDROME, ULCERATIVE COLITIS, AND CROHN'S DISEASE

Many of the symptoms of IBS, ulcerative colitis, and Crohn's disease are similar; however, there are some symptoms that are disease specific. Table 27-1 compares symptoms common to IBS, ulcerative colitis, and Crohn's disease.

Lifestyle Modification

People who have IBS, ulcerative colitis, or Crohn's disease can reduce their symptoms by making changes in their lifestyle. Food and beverages that aggravate diarrhea, bloating, and gas should be avoided. Stress management may reduce the frequency of symptoms even where it is not the direct cause of the disease, as with ulcerative colitis. A complete list of lifestyle modifications is given in Box 27-1.

TECH NOTE!
Drinking carbonated beverages and chewing gum can cause gas and bloating.

BOX 27-1 LIFESTYLE MODIFICATION TO REDUCE THE SYMPTOMS OF INFLAMMATORY BOWEL SYNDROME, ULCERATIVE COLITIS, AND CROHN'S DISEASE

- Eat small meals.
- Drink at least 6 to 8 glasses of water daily.
- Avoid alcohol.
- Avoid caffeinated beverages (coffee, tea, cola drinks).

- Limit carbonated beverages.
- Avoid foods that worsen symptoms.*
- Engage in stress reduction activities.

*Following a diet for celiac disease may reduce symptoms of inflammatory bowel syndrome. Avoid wheat, rye, barley, dairy, and chocolate.

Drugs Used in the Treatment of Inflammatory Bowel Syndrome

IBS is treated by administering serotonin receptor antagonists (5-HT$_3$ and 5-HT$_4$), antidiarrheals, laxatives, fiber supplements, and anticholinergics.

SEROTONIN RECEPTOR ANTAGONISTS

New medications have been developed that selectively target the serotonin receptors. The neurotransmitter serotonin (5-HT) controls GI motility. There are multiple types of serotonin receptors. Stimulation of 5-HT$_3$ receptors can cause diarrhea. Stimulation of 5-HT$_4$ receptors produces constipation.

MECHANISM OF ACTION

Alosetron is a 5-HT$_3$ receptor antagonist, and is used to control diarrhea caused by severe IBS. Tegaserod is a partial agonist at the 5-HT$_4$ receptor. It is approved for short-term use to control constipation caused by IBS. Tegaserod is sometimes classified as a prokinetic drug because it accelerates gastric emptying and speeds transit through the colon.

PHARMACOKINETICS

Tesagerod is rapidly absorbed when taken on an empty stomach. There are few drug interactions despite the fact that tesagerod is 98% protein bound.

ADVERSE REACTIONS

The most common side effects of alosetron are constipation, anxiety, difficulty sleeping or drowsiness, dry mouth, frequent urination, gas, headache, nausea, and restlessness. Alosetron side effects limit its use. Alosetron may cause severe GI obstruction or impaction leading to toxic megacolon. Tegaserod side effects are dizziness, gas, headache, heartburn, nausea or vomiting, and diarrhea.

PRECAUTIONS

TECH NOTE!
Alosetron is available only from health care providers who participate in a special Prescribing Program.

Alosetron is approved for women with severe IBS, when other therapies have failed. The drug was withdrawn from the market shortly after its introduction. The Food and Drug Administration (FDA) permitted alosetron to be reintroduced with restricted access. Refills are not permitted until the patient has a follow-up examination by their prescribing physician. Patients and physicians must agree to adhere to therapy plans. The drug must be used cautiously because it can significantly decrease blood flow to the colon causing ischemic colitis, toxic megacolon, and death.

Serotonin Receptor Antagonist

Generic name	U.S. brand name(s)	Dosage forms and strengths
	Canadian brand(s)	
alosetron	Lotronex	0.5 mg, 1 mg tablet
	Not available	

Serotonin Receptor Partial Agonist

Generic name	U.S. brand name(s)	Dosage forms and strengths
	Canadian brand(s)	
tegaserod	Zelnorm	2 mg, 6 mg tablet
	Zelnorm	

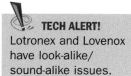

BULK-FORMING LAXATIVES AND FIBER SUPPLEMENTS

Bulk-forming laxative and fiber supplements are administered to relieve constipation and diarrhea. They are the laxative of choice for treating the symptoms of IBS. Bulk-forming laxatives swell in the presence of liquid. Bacteria normally live in the colon and digest cellulose and polysaccharide fibers. As the bacteria colony grows, colonic bulk increases. This causes the bowel to feel full and stimulates evacuation. The bulk-forming laxatives also promote fluid accumulation in the colon. Polycarbophil is the only bulk-forming laxative that is FDA approved for the treatment of IBS. It can be obtained without prescription. It is listed in the next table.

ADVERSE REACTIONS

Bulk-forming laxatives can cause bloating, gas, abdominal cramps, nausea, diarrhea, or constipation.

Bulk-Forming Laxatives

Generic name	U.S. brand name(s)	Dosage forms and strengths	OTC/prescription
	Canadian brand(s)		
polycarbophil*	Equalactin, Fiberall, Fibercon, Fibertab, Konsyl Fiber Tablet	500 mg, 1250 mg chew tablet, 625 mg tablet	OTC
	Equalactin, Prodiem Bulk Fiber Therapy		

*Generic available.

OPIOID ANTIDIARRHEALS

Opioid antidiarrheals are administered to control watery and frequent stools. They bind to opioid receptors and induce spasms that interfere with effective peristalsis. They decrease propulsive contractions by inhibiting the release of acetylcholine. Opioid antidiarrheals prescribed for the treatment of diarrhea are difenoxin, diphenoxylate, and loperamide. Difenoxin and loperamide are more potent than diphenoxylate.

ADVERSE REACTIONS

Sedation and dizziness are the most common side effects of opioid antidiarrheals. They may also produce constipation. Diphenoxylate and its metabolite diphenoxin are controlled substances and may cause tolerance and dependence. Loperamide is not habit forming and is not a controlled substance. Loperamide is available without a prescription. Antidiarrheals should be used cautiously in patients with ulcerative colitis as they can cause toxic megacolon.

Antidiarrheals

	Generic name	U.S. brand name(s) Canadian brand(s)	Dosage forms and strengths	U.S. Controlled substance schedule
	difenoxin + atropine	Motofen	**Tablet:** 1 mg difenoxin + 0.025 mg atropine	C-IV
		Not available		
	diphenoxylate + atropine*	Lomotil, Lonox	**Tablet:** 2.5 mg diphenoxylate + 0.025 mg atropine	C-V
		Lomotil		
	loperamide*	Imodium-AD	**Tablet:** 2 mg **Liquid:** 1 mg/5 ml	Not scheduled
		Imodium, Diarr-eze		

*Generic available.

ANTICHOLINERGICS

Anticholinergic drugs are used in the treatment of IBS when diarrhea is the primary symptom. Atropine and dicylomine are the only FDA-approved agents for the treatment of IBS. Other anticholinergic agents have been used despite the lack of FDA approval. Atropine and dicyclomine decrease GI muscular tone and motility by producing a nonspecific, direct spasmolytic action on GI smooth muscle.

ADVERSE REACTIONS

Anticholinergic agents may produce constipation, difficulty sleeping, dry mouth, change in taste, headache, photophobia (increased sensitivity of the eyes to light), nausea, sexual difficulty (impotence), fast or slow heartbeat, urinary retention, dizziness, or drowsiness. At higher doses, hallucinations may occur.

Antidiarrheals

	Generic name	U.S. brand name(s) Canadian brand(s)	Dosage forms and strengths
	atropine	Atreza	**Tablet:** 0.4 mg
		Not available	
	dicyclomine*	Bentyl	**Capsule:** 10 mg **Tablet:** 20 mg
		Bentylol, Formulex	**Syrup:** 10 mg/5 ml

*Generic available.

Drugs Used in the Treatment of Ulcerative Colitis

Medicines administered in the management of ulcerative colitis are used to reduce symptoms and induce remission.

AMINOSALICYLATES

Aminosalicylates are administered to patients with ulcerative colitis and Crohn's disease in order to reduce inflammation. The four aminosalicylate antiinflammatory agents available in the United States and Canada are sulfasalazine, olsalazine, mesalamine (mesalazine), and balsalazide.

MECHANISM OF ACTION

The mechanism of antiinflammatory action produced by aminosalicylates is not completely known. Sulfasalazine inhibits substances that are released by the body that produce the symptoms of inflammation (e.g., leukotrienes, prostaglandins, and cytokines). It also decreases cytokine production.

TECH ALERT!
The following drugs have look-alike/ sound-alike issues: sulfasalazine, sulfadiazine, and sulfisoxazole; Colazal and Clozaril; mesalamine and mecamylamine; Asacol and Os-Cal; olsalazine and olanzapine; Dipentum and Dilantin

PHARMACOKINETICS

Sulfasalazine, olsalazine, mesalamine, and mesalazine are all formulations that contain 5-aminosalicylic acid (5-ASA). Sulfasalazine (sulfapyridine+5-ASA) and olsalazine (two 5-ASA molecules) are prodrugs. Bacteria in the colon metabolize the drugs and release the active metabolite (5-ASA). The effectiveness of sulfasalazine and olsalazine is reduced by factors that decrease the bacteria in the colon (e.g., antibiotics). Mesalamine and mesalazine are coated with a pH-dependent resin. The 5-ASA is released in the pH of the distal ileum (mesalamine) and proximal ileum (mesalazine) rather than the colon. Pentasa is a time-release formulation.

ADVERSE REACTIONS

The most common adverse effects of sulfasalazine, olsalazine, mesalamine, and mesalazine are nausea, vomiting, heartburn, headache, and watery diarrhea. Side effects that occur less frequently are inflammation of the heart muscle and pericardium, pancreatitis, and pneumonitis. Sulfasalazine may additionally cause sunburn, impaired folic acid absorption, crystalluria, and damage to white blood cells (cytopenias).

Aminosalicylates

Generic name	U.S. brand name(s) Canadian brand(s)	Dosage forms and strengths
balsalazide	Colazal	750 mg capsules
	Not available	
mesalamine* (known as mesalazine in Canada)	Asacol, Lialda, Canasa supp. Rowasa enema	400 mg tablet, 1.2 g DR tablet, 1 g supp., 4 g/60 ml enema
	Asacol	
olsalazine	Dipentum	250 mg capsules
	Dipentum	
sulfasalazine*	Azulfadine, Azulfadine EN-tablets	500 mg tablets, 500 mg EC tablets
	Salazopyrin, Salazopyrin EN-tablets	
5-aminosalicylic acid (5-ASA)	Pentasa	250 mg, 500 mg delayed release tablet, 1 g and 4 g/100 ml enema, 500 mg, 1 g suppository
	Pentasa, Mesasal, Salofalk	

*Generic available.

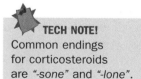

TECH NOTE!
Common endings for corticosteroids are "-sone" and "-lone".

CORTICOSTEROIDS

Glucocorticosteroids are commonly prescribed to suppress inflammation, reduce flare-ups, and treat pain associated with ulcerative colitis and Crohn's disease. Glucocorticosteroids are potent antiinflammatory drugs. They decrease the synthesis of proinflammatory substances: prostaglandins (see Chapter 10), leukotrienes, cytokines, arachidonic acid, and macrophages that are released as part of the inflammatory response. Glucocorticosteroids have immunosuppressive actions that may inhibit the abnormal immune system activity that is associated with Crohn's disease and ulcerative colitis.

ADVERSE REACTIONS

Corticosteroids prescribed to treat ulcerative colitis and Crohn's may be administered by mouth or rectally in the form of an enema or suppository. Oral administration produces systemic effects, which are described in Chapter 15. Adverse effects due to rectal administration may be local (burning and itching) or systemic (nausea, constipation or diarrhea, appetite changes, headache).

Corticosteroids

	Generic name	U.S. brand name(s) / Canadian brand(s)	Dosage forms and strengths
	hydrocortisone*	Colocort enema, Anucort-HC supp, Cortifoam, Cortef, Hydrocortone	**Tablet:** 100 mg/60 ml rectal enema; 10% rectal foam; 25 mg suppository; 5 mg, 10 mg, 20 mg
		Cortef, Cortenema susp, Cortifoam	
	prednisone*	generics	**Tablet:** 1 mg, 2.5 mg, 5 mg, 10 mg, 20 mg, 50 mg **Oral concentrate:** 5 mg/ml
		Winpred	
	dexamethasone*	Decadron	**Tablet:** 0.25 mg, 0.5 mg, 0.75 mg, 1 mg, 1.5 mg, 2 mg, 4 mg, 6 mg **Oral concentrate:** 0.5 mg/5 ml solution; 1 mg/ml
		Dexasone	
	methylprednisolone*	Medrol	**Tablet:** 2 mg, 4 mg, 8 mg, 16 mg, 32 mg
		Medrol	

*Generic available.

TECH ALERT!
Prednisone and prednisolone have look-alike/sound-alike issues.

TECH ALERT!
The following drugs have look-alike/sound-alike issues: azathioprine and Azulfidine; Imuran and Imdur

Drugs Used in the Treatment of Crohn's Disease

Given the similarity of symptoms and the similar mechanism of disease progression of Crohn's disease and ulcerative colitis, many of the medicines used in the treatment of the two diseases are the same. Aminosalicylates, corticosteroids, immunosuppressants, antidiarrheals, and nutritional supplements are used in the treatment of Crohn's disease and ulcerative colitis. Additional medications used in the treatment of Crohn's disease are immunomodulators and antibiotics.

IMMUNOSUPPRESSANTS

Azathioprine, 6-mercaptopurine, and methotrexate are classified as antimetabolites. They are used in the treatment of Crohn's disease to induce remission. Azathioprine suppresses T-cell–mediated immune system response. Methotrexate decreases cytokine and immunoglobulin production and COX-2 activity, reducing inflammation and immune system activity (see Chapter 15).

Immunosuppressants

	Generic name	U.S. brand name(s) / Canadian brand(s)	Dosage forms and strengths
	azathioprine*†	Azasan, Imuran	**Tablet:** 50 mg, 75 mg, 100 mg
		Imuran	
	6-mercaptopurine*†	Purinethol	**Tablet:** 50 mg
		Purinethol	
	methotrexate*†	Rheumatrex, Trexall	**Tablet:** 2.5 mg, 5 mg, 7.5 mg, 10 mg **Solution, injection:** 25 mg/ml **Powder, injection:** 1 g
		generics	

*Generic available.
†Not FDA approved for Crohn's disease or ulcerative colitis.

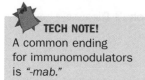

IMMUNOMODULATORS

Infliximab is an immunomodulator that has been approved for the treatment of Crohn's disease. It is administered to induce remission of active disease and then continued as maintenance therapy in patients who have had unsuccessful results with other therapies.

MECHANISM OF ACTION

Infliximab is a tumor necrosis factor-α inhibitor that is genetically engineered. Infliximab blocks the inflammatory process triggered by high concentrations of TNF. TNF levels are increased in Crohn's disease. Infliximab prevents cell lysis (destruction) and release of substances that cause inflammation. A detailed description of infliximab's mechanism of action is described in Chapter 15.

ADVERSE REACTIONS

Nausea, stomach pain, headache, redness, itching at the site of infusion, chest pain, hypertension, dyspnea, increased susceptibility to opportunistic infections, reactivation of dormant infections (e.g., tuberculosis), and worsening of existing infection are adverse reactions produced by infliximab.

Immunomodulators

Generic name	U.S. brand name(s) Canadian brand(s)	Dosage forms and strengths
infliximab	Remicade	Powder for injection: 100 mg
	Remicade	

ANTIINFECTIVES

Patients who have Crohn's disease may develop fistulas. A *fistula* forms when an ulcer tunnels from the site of origin to surrounding tissues. Fistulas may be located in the bladder, vagina, and skin surrounding the anus and rectum. Antiinfective agents may be prescribed to treat infections that develop in the fistulas. Antiinfectives that are prescribed to treat fistulas include ampicillin, sulfonamides, cephalosporins, tetracycline, or metronidazole and are described in Chapter 35.

Summary of Drugs Used in the Treatment of Irritable Bowel Disease, Ulcerative Colitis, and Crohn's Disease

Generic name	U.S. brand name	Usual adult oral dose and dosing schedule	Warning Labels
Serotonin receptor antagonist			
alosetron	Lotronex	1 mg daily for 4 weeks*	MAY CAUSE DIZZINESS OR DROWSINESS; AVOID DRIVING AVOID ALCOHOL TAKE WITH A FULL GLASS OF WATER
Serotonin receptor partial agonist			
tesagerod	Zelnorm	6 mg twice a day	TAKE ON AN EMPTY STOMACH

*alosetron is only approved for 4 weeks courses of therapy and should be discontinued if symptoms are not controlled after 4 weeks of therapy.

Continued

Summary of Drugs Used in the Treatment of Irritable Bowel Disease, Ulcerative Colitis, and Crohn's Disease—cont'd

	Generic name	U.S. brand name	Usual adult oral dose and dosing schedule	Warning Labels
Bulk-forming laxatives				
	polycarbophil	Equalactin, Fiberall, Fibercon, Fibertab	1 g 1 to 4 times per day	TAKE WITH A FULL GLASS OF WATER
Antidiarrheals				
	difenoxin + atropine	Motofen	2 tablets immediately; then 1 tablet after each loose stool	MAY CAUSE DIZZINESS OR DROWSINESS; AVOID DRIVING
	diphenoxylate + atropine	Lomotil	2 tablets 3 to 4 times a day	AVOID ALCOHOL
	loperamide	Imodium	2 tablets immediately; then 1 tablet after each loose stool	DRINK LOTS OF FLUIDS
Anticholinergics				
	atropine	Atreza	0.3 mg to 1.2 mg every 4 to 6 hours	MAY CAUSE DIZZINESS OR DROWSINESS; AVOID DRIVING
	dicyclomine	Bentyl		AVOID ALCOHOL
				DRINK LOTS OF FLUIDS
				TAKE ON AN EMPTY STOMACH
Aminosalicylates				
	balsalazide	Colazal	3 caps (2250 mg) 3 times a day	SWALLOW WHOLE; DON'T CRUSH OR CHEW
	mesalamine	Canasa	1 suppository rectally twice a day	REMOVE FOIL AND INSERT MAY DISCOLOR CLOTHING OR SKIN—orange-yellow
		Rowasa	4 g enema nightly	SHAKE WELL
		Asacol	1 tablet 3 times a day	SWALLOW WHOLE; DON'T CRUSH OR CHEW
		Lialda	1 tablet daily	
	olsalazine	Dipentum	1 g daily in 2 divided doses	SWALLOW WHOLE; DON'T CRUSH OR CHEW
				TAKE WITH FOOD
	sulfasalazine	Azulfidine	1 g 3 to 4 times a day	SWALLOW WHOLE; DON'T CRUSH OR CHEW—enteric-coated tablets
				AVOID PROLONGED EXPOSURE TO SUNLIGHT
				DRINK LOTS OF FLUIDS

Summary of Drugs Used in the Treatment of Irritable Bowel Disease, Ulcerative Colitis, and Crohn's Disease—cont'd

Generic name	U.S. brand name	Usual adult oral dose and dosing schedule	Warning Labels
5-ASA	Pentasa, Mesasal, Salofalk	1 g 4 times a day	SWALLOW WHOLE; DON'T CRUSH OR CHEW
Corticosteroids			
hydrocortisone	Cortema	100 mg rectal enema nightly for 21 days	SHAKE WELL
	Anucort	1 supp rectally 2 to 3 times a day for 2 weeks	REMOVE FOIL AND INSERT
	Cortifoam	1 applicatorful 1 to 2 times a day for 2 to 3 weeks; then every other day	SHAKE WELL
	Hydrocortone, Cortef	20 mg to 240 mg daily in 2 to 4 divided doses	TAKE WITH FOOD DON'T DISCONTINUE ABRUPTLY
dexamethasone	Decadron	0.75 mg/day to 9 mg/day in 2 to 4 divided doses	TAKE WITH FOOD DON'T DISCONTINUE ABRUPTLY
prednisone	generic	40 mg to 60 mg daily; taper over 2 to 3 months	
methylprednisolone	Medrol	4 mg to 48 mg daily in 4 divided doses	
Immunosuppressants			
azathloprine*	Azasan, Imuran	1.5 mg to 2 mg/kg/day	TAKE WITH FOOD
6-mecaptopurine*	Purinethol	1.5 mg to 2 mg/kg/day	AVOID ALCOHOL AVOID PREGNANCY
methotrexate*	Trexall	25 mg IM weekly	AVOID ALCOHOL AVOID PREGNANCY
Immunomodulators			
infliximab	Remicade	5 mg/kg IV at week 0, 2, and 6; then every 8 weeks	

*Not FDA approved.

CHAPTER SUMMARY

- Inflammatory bowel syndrome (IBS), ulcerative colitis, and Crohn's disease are conditions that are linked to inflammation of gastrointestinal (GI) tract.
- IBS is a condition that causes abdominal distress and erratic movement of the large bowel.
- Persons with IBS may have diarrhea or constipation.
- IBS may also be associated with abnormally low levels of the neurotransmitter serotonin.
- Low levels of serotonin can cause GI motility problems and increase the sensitivity of pain receptors in the GI tract.
- Ulcerative colitis and Crohn's disease are irritable bowel diseases.
- In ulcerative colitis and Crohn's disease, the body's immune system recognizes the bacteria that normally inhabit the GI tract as harmful invaders and releases tumor necrosis factor (TNF).
- Ulcerative colitis produces inflammation in the upper layers of the lining of the small intestine and colon.
- Crohn's disease may produce inflammation and can occur anywhere along the entire length of the GI tube, from the mouth to the anus, although typically it affects the ileum (the lower part of the small intestine). Inflammation occurs deep in the intestinal wall.
- Abdominal pain, diarrhea, and cramping are common symptoms of IBS, ulcerative colitis, and Crohn's disease.
- Lifestyle modification can reduce symptoms of IBS, ulcerative colitis, and Crohn's disease.
- Stress management, eating small meals, and avoiding alcohol and caffeinated and carbonated beverages are recommended lifestyle changes.
- IBS is treated by administering serotonin receptor ($5\text{-}HT_3$ and $5\text{-}HT_4$) antagonists, antidiarrheals, laxatives, fiber supplements, and anticholinergics.
- Alosetron is a $5\text{-}HT_3$ receptor antagonist that is used to control diarrhea in women caused by severe IBS when other therapies have failed.
- Tegaserod is a partial agonist at the $5\text{-}HT_4$ receptor approved for short term use to control constipation caused by IBS.
- Alosetron must be used cautiously because it can significantly decrease blood flow to the colon causing ischemic colitis, toxic megacolon, and death.
- Alosetron prescriptions may not be refilled without a follow-up examination by the physician.
- Bulk-forming laxative and fiber supplements are administered to relieve constipation and diarrhea.
- Antidiarrheals are administered to control watery and frequent stools.
- Diphenoxylate and difenoxin are controlled substances and may cause tolerance and dependence. Loperamide is not habit forming and is not a controlled substance.
- Antidiarrheals should be used cautiously in patients with ulcerative colitis as they can cause toxic megacolon.
- Atropine and dicyclomine decrease diarrhea by reducing GI muscular tone and motility.
- The aminosalicylates mesalazine, olsalazine, balsalazide, and mesalamine are administered to patients with ulcerative colitis and Crohn's disease in order to reduce inflammation.
- All commercially available aminosalicylates (5-ASA) are formulated as delayed release products.
- Glucocorticosteroids are prescribed commonly to suppress inflammation, reduce flare-ups, and treat pain associated with ulcerative colitis and Crohn's disease.
- Glucocorticosteroids also have immunosuppressive actions that may inhibit the abnormal immune system activity that is associated with Crohn's disease and ulcerative colitis.
- Azathioprine, 6-mercaptopurine, and methotrexate are prescribed for the treatment of Crohn's disease to induce remission.
- Infliximab is an immunomodulator that has been approved for the treatment of Crohn's disease and is administered to induce remission.

- Infliximab is a tissue necrosis factor-α inhibitor that is genetically engineered to block the inflammatory process.
- Patients who have Crohn's disease may develop fistulas. Antiinfective agents may be prescribed to treat fistula infections.

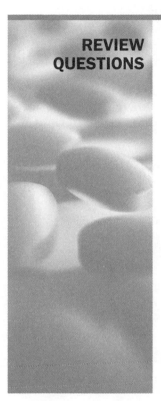

REVIEW QUESTIONS

Multiple Choice

1. **Which diseases are conditions that are linked to inflammation of gastrointestinal tract?**
   a. inflammatory bowel syndrome
   b. ulcerative colitis
   c. Crohn's disease
   d. all of the above

2. **Which tests may be performed to diagnose ulcerative colitis and Crohn's disease?**
   a. sigmoidoscopy and proctoscopy
   b. proctoscopy and colonoscopy
   c. colonscopy and sigmoidoscopy
   d. jejunoscopy and stool sample

3. **Which disease affects men and women equally?**
   a. ulcerative colitis
   b. diverticulitis
   c. Crohn's disease
   d. proctitis

4. **Name three common symptoms of inflammatory bowel syndrome, ulcerative colitis, and Crohn's disease:**
   a. bloating, constipation, cramping
   b. abdominal pain, diarrhea, cramping
   c. rectal bleeding, bloating, diarrhea
   d. cramping, abdominal pain, bloating

5. **Which of the following drugs does *not* act at the serotonin receptor?**
   a. Zelnorm
   b. Lotronex
   c. Lovenox
   d. Alosetron

6. **The laxatives of choice for treating the symptoms of inflammatory bowel syndrome are _____.**
   a. Bulk-forming laxatives
   b. fiber supplements
   c. bile acid sequestrants
   d. a and b

7. **An immunomodulator that has been approved for the treatment of Crohn's disease is _____.**
   a. infliximab
   b. methotrexate
   c. Lomotil
   d. dexamethasone

8. Patients who have Crohn's disease may develop _____, which form when an ulcer tunnels from the site of origin to surrounding tissues.
   a. ulcers
   b. fistulas
   c. diverticuli
   d. none of the above

9. Give the trade name for the corticoid dexamethasone.
   a. Dexacortef
   b. Medrol
   c. Imuran
   d. Decadron

10. These warning labels should be applied to prescription vials for which class of drugs used for IBS? MAY CAUSE DIZZINESS OR DROWSINESS; AVOID DRIVING, AVOID ALCOHOL, DRINK LOTS OF FLUIDS, TAKE ON AN EMPTY STOMACH
    a. anticholinergics
    b. bulk forming laxatives
    c. serotonin antagonists
    d. corticosteroids

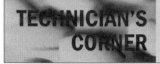

TECHNICIAN'S CORNER

1. How do opioids work as antidiarrheals?
2. What lifestyle modifications can be made to lessen the symptoms of inflammatory bowel syndrome?

BIBLIOGRAPHY

Kalant H, Grant D, Mitchell J: *Principles of medical pharmacology* (pp 572-583), ed 7. Toronto, 2007, Elsevier Canada, A Division of Reed Elsevier Canada.

Lance L, Lacy C, Armstrong L, Goldman M: *Drug information handbook for the allied health professional,* ed 12. Hudson, OH, 2005, APhA Lexi-Comp.

National Digestive Diseases Information Clearinghouse: *Crohn's disease.* Bethesda, MD, National Institute of Diabetes and Digestive and Kidney Diseases, National Institutes of Health, US Department of Health and Human Services; Publication Date February 2006; NIH publication No. 06-3410. Available at: http://www.digestive.niddk.nih.gov.

National Digestive Diseases Information Clearinghouse: *Inflammatory bowel syndrome.* Bethesda, MD, National Institute of Diabetes and Digestive and Kidney Diseases, National Institutes of Health, US Department of Health and Human Services; Publication Date February 2006; NIH publication No. 06-693. Available at: http://www.digestive.niddk.nih.gov.

National Digestive Diseases Information Clearinghouse: *Ulcerative colitis.* Bethesda, MD, National Institute of Diabetes and Digestive and Kidney Diseases, National Institutes of Health, US Department of Health and Human Services; Publication Date February 2006; NIH publication No. 06-1597. Available at: http://www.digestive.niddk.nih.gov.

USP Center for Advancement of Patient Safety: *Use caution–avoid confusion,* USP Quality Review No. 79, Rockville, MD, April 2004, USP Center for Advancement of Patient Safety.

UNIT VII

Drugs Affecting the Respiratory System

Function of the Respiratory System

The respiratory system functions as an air distributor and a gas exchanger so that oxygen may be supplied to and carbon dioxide removed from the body's cells. In addition, the respiratory system effectively filters, warms, and humidifies the air we breathe. Respiratory organs also influence sound reproduction, including speech used in communicating oral language. Specialized epithelium in the respiratory tract makes the sense of smell (*olfaction*) possible. The respiratory system also plays an important role in the regulation, or homeostasis, of pH in the body.

Structural Plan of the Respiratory System

The respiratory system is divided into upper and lower tracts, or divisions. The ***upper respiratory tract*** is composed of the nose, nasopharynx, oropharynx, laryngopharynx, and pharynx. The ***lower respiratory tract*** consists of the ***trachea,*** all segments of the ***bronchial tree,*** and the lungs. Functionally, the respiratory system also includes accessory structures, such as the oral cavity, rib cage, and respiratory muscles including the diaphragm.

UPPER RESPIRATORY TRACT

NOSE STRUCTURE

The nose consists of an internal and external portion. The internal portion, or ***nasal cavity,*** lies over the roof of the mouth where the palatine bones separate the nasal cavities from the mouth cavity. The hollow nasal cavity is separated into a right and left cavity by a midline partition called the ***septum***. The external openings into the nasal cavities (nostrils) are named the anterior ***nares*** and open into an area called the ***vestibule***. Once air passes over the vestibule, it enters the respiratory portion of each nasal passage then air passes into the ***pharynx***.

RESPIRATORY MUCOSA (NOSE)

Once air has passed over the skin of the vestibule and enters the respiratory portion of the nasal passage, it passes over the ***respiratory mucosa***. The respiratory mucosa of the nose possesses a rich blood supply and contains many olfactory nerve cells and a rich lymphatic plexus. A ciliated mucous membrane lines the rest of the respiratory tract down as far as the smaller bronchioles.

PARANASAL SINUSES

The four pairs of ***paranasal sinuses*** are air-containing spaces that open, or drain, into the nasal cavity. These paranasal sinuses are the frontal, maxillary, ethmoid, and sphenoid sinuses. Like the nasal cavity, each paranasal cavity is lined by respiratory mucosa.

Function of the Nose

The nose serves as a passageway for air going to and from the lungs. Air is filtered of impurities and chemically examined for substances that might prove irritating to the lining of the respiratory tract. The ***respiratory membrane*** produces mucus and possesses a rich blood supply, which permits rapid warming and moistening of the dry inspired air. Mucous secretions provide for removal of any particulate matter from air as it moves through the nasal passages. Fluid from the lacrimal glands (tear ducts) and mucus produced in the paranasal sinuses also help to trap particulate matter and moisten air passing through the nose. In addition, the hollow sinuses act to lighten the bones of the skull and serve as resonating chambers for speech.

PHARYNX STRUCTURE AND FUNCTION

Another name for the ***pharynx*** is the throat. The ***nasopharynx*** lies behind the nose; the ***oropharynx*** lies behind the mouth; and the ***laryngopharynx*** extends from the hyoid bone to its termination in the esophagus. The ***pharyngeal tonsils*** are located in the nasopharynx on its posterior wall. Two pairs of organs are found in the oropharynx: the

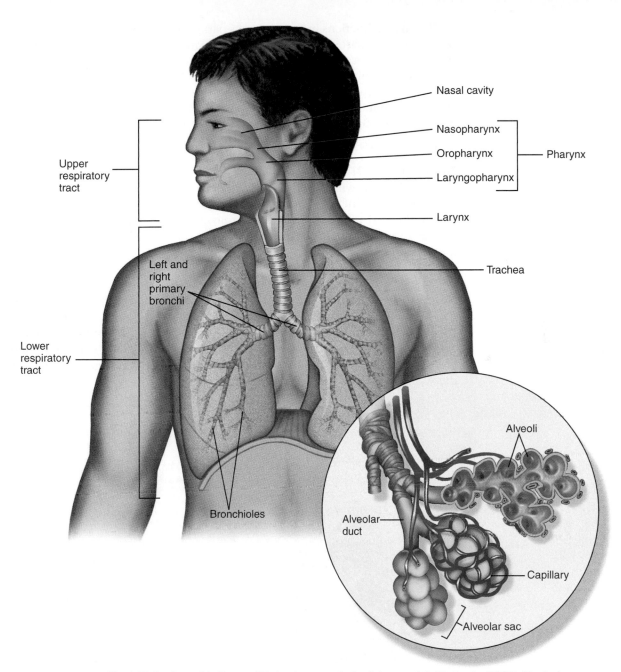

(From Thibodeau GA, Patton KT: Anatomy and physiology, *ed 6. St. Louis, 2007, Mosby.)*

palatine tonsils and the ***linguine tonsils.*** The pharynx serves as a common pathway for the respiratory and digestive tracts. It also affects ***phonation*** (speech production).

LARYNX STRUCTURE AND FUNCTION

The ***larynx,*** or voice box, consists largely of cartilages that are attached to one another and to surrounding structures by muscles and is lined by a ciliated mucous membrane. The mucous membrane of the larynx forms two pairs of folds: the upper pair or the vestibular, and the lower pair, which serve as the true vocal cords. The true vocal cords and the space between them are together designated as the glottis. Nine cartilages form the framework of the larynx. The ***thyroid cartilage*** is the largest of cartilage of the larynx. The ***epiglottis*** is attached below the thyroid and moves up and down during swallowing to prevent food or liquids from entering the trachea.

The larynx functions in respiration as part of the vital airway of the lungs. It helps in the removal of dust particles and in warming and humidification of inspired air. It also protects the airway against the entrance of solids and liquids during swallowing and serves as the instrument of voice production—hence, the name *voice box*. Air expired through the glottis and narrowed by partial adduction of the true vocal cords causes them to vibrate. Their vibration produces sound, and the size and shape of the nose, mouth, pharynx, and the bony sinuses help determine the quality of the sound or voice.

LOWER RESPIRATORY TRACT

TRACHEA STRUCTURE AND FUNCTION

The ***trachea,*** or windpipe, is a tube that extends from the larynx in the neck to the primary bronchi in the thoracic cavity. Its walls consist of C-shaped cartilages that give firmness to the wall and tend to prevent it from collapsing and shutting off the vital airway. The trachea furnishes part of the open passageway through which air can reach the lungs from the outside.

BRONCHI STRUCTURE

The trachea divides at its lower end into two ***primary bronchi***. The bronchi and trachea are lined by ciliated mucosa. The primary bronchus divides into smaller branches called ***secondary bronchi,*** which continue to branch to form ***tertiary bronchi*** and small ***bronchioles***. The bronchioles subdivide into smaller tubes, eventually terminating in microscopic branches that divide into alveolar ducts, which terminate in several alveolar sacs, the walls of which consist of numerous alveoli.

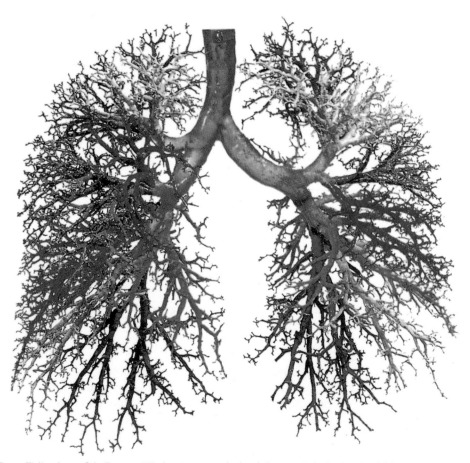

(From Thibodeau GA, Patton KT: Anatomy and physiology, *ed 6. St. Louis, 2007, Mosby.)*

ALVEOLI STRUCTURE

The alveoli are the primary gas exchange structures of the respiratory tract. Alveoli are very effective in the exchange of carbon dioxide (CO_2) and oxygen (O_2) because each alveolus is extremely thin walled and lies in contact with blood capillaries. The barrier at which gases are exchanged between alveolar air and blood is called the ***respiratory membrane***. The surface of the respiratory membrane inside each alveolus is coated with a fluid containing ***surfactant***. Surfactant helps reduce surface tension—the force of attraction between water molecules—of the fluid. This helps prevent each alveolus from collapsing and "sticking shut" as air moves in and out during respiration.

FUNCTION OF THE BRONCHI AND ALVEOLI

The tubes composing the bronchial tree distribute air to the lungs' interior. The alveoli accomplish the lungs' main and vital function, that of gas exchange between air and blood. The layer of protective mucus that covers a large portion of the membrane that lines the respiratory tree serves as the most important air purification mechanism.

LUNGS' STRUCTURE AND FUNCTION

The lungs extend from the diaphragm to slightly above the clavicles and lie against the ribs both anteriorly and posteriorly. The primary bronchi and pulmonary blood vessels enter each lung through a slit on its medial surface called the ***hilum***. Each lung is divided into lobes by fissures. The left lobe is divided into two lobes (superior and inferior) and the right lung into three lobes (superior, middle, and inferior). ***Visceral pleura*** cover the outer surfaces of the lungs and adhere to them. The lungs perform two functions—air distribution and gas exchange. Gas exchange between the air and blood is the joint function of the alveoli and the networks of blood capillaries that envelop them.

STRUCTURE AND FUNCTION OF THE THORACIC CAVITY

The thoracic cavity has three divisions, separated from each other by partition of ***pleura***. The ***parietal pleura*** line the entire thoracic cavity. A separate pleural sac encases each lung. The outer surface of each lung is covered by the ***visceral pleura***, which lies against the parietal pleura and is separated by a "potential space" (***pleural space***) that contains just enough pleural fluid for lubrication. Thus, when the lungs inflate with air the smooth, moist visceral pleura coheres (sticks together) to the smooth, moist parietal pleural. The **thorax** plays a major role in respiration. The thorax becomes larger when the chest is raised and smaller when it is lowered. An even greater change in the thorax occurs when the diaphragm contracts and relaxes. When the diaphragm contracts, it flattens out and thus pulls the floor of the thoracic cavity downward, thereby enlarging the volume of the thorax. When the diaphragm relaxes, it returns to its resting, dome-like shape, reducing the volume of the thoracic cavity.

Respiratory Physiology

The proper functioning of the respiratory system ensures the tissues of the body receive an adequate oxygen supply and prompt removal of carbon dioxide. This complex function would not be possible without integration between numerous physiological control systems, including acid-base, water, electrolyte balance, circulation, and metabolism. Functionally, the respiratory system is composed of an integrated set of regulated processes that include the following: *external respiration:* pulmonary respiration (breathing) and gas exchange in the pulmonary capillaries of the lungs; *transport of gases by blood;* and *internal respiration:* gas exchange in the systemic blood capillaries and cellular respiration; and overall regulation of respiration.

PULMONARY VENTILATION

Pulmonary ventilation is the technical term for breathing. One phase of it, ***inspiration,*** moves air into the lungs, and the other phase, ***expiration,*** moves air out of the lungs.

PULMONARY VOLUME AND CAPACITY

PULMONARY VOLUMES

An apparatus called a *spirometer* is used to measure the volume of air exchanged in breathing. A graphic recording of the changing pulmonary volumes observed during breathing is called a *spirogram.* The volume of air moved in and out of the lungs and remaining in them is of great importance. The volume must be normal so that exchanges of oxygen and carbon dioxide can occur between alveolar air and pulmonary capillary blood.

REGULATION OF PULMONARY FUNCTION

RESPIRATORY CONTROL CENTERS

Various mechanisms operate to maintain relative constancy of the blood percentage of oxygen (Po_2) and percentage of carbon dioxide (Pco_2). The main integrators that control the nerves that affect inspiratory and expiratory muscles are located in the brainstem (medulla, pons) and are simply called the respiratory centers. The apneustic and pneumotaxic centers located in the pons prevent overinflation of the lungs and permits a normal rhythm of breathing.

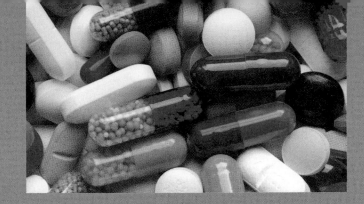

Treatment of Asthma and Chronic Obstructive Pulmonary Disease

---

LEARNING OBJECTIVES

- Learn the terminology associated with asthma and chronic obstructive pulmonary disease (COPD).
- List the symptoms of asthma.
- List symptoms of COPD.
- List risk factors for asthma and COPD.
- List and categorize medications used in the treatment of asthma and COPD.
- Describe mechanism of action for drugs used to treat asthma and COPD.
- Identify warning labels and precautionary messages associated with medications used to treat asthma and COPD.
- Identify significant drug look-alike/sound-alike issues.
- List common endings for drug classes used in the treatment of asthma and COPD.

KEY TERMS

Allergic asthma: Asthma symptoms are a hypersensitivity reaction due to overexpression of immunoglobulin E (IgE) antibodies upon exposure to environmental allergens.

Asthma: Chronic disease that affects the airways producing irritation, inflammation, and difficulty breathing.

Bronchodilator: Drug that relaxes tightened airway muscles and improves airflow through the airways.

Chronic obstructive pulmonary disease (COPD): Progressive disease of the airways that produces gradual loss of pulmonary function.

Forced expiratory volume (FEV$_1$): Maximum volume of air that can be breathed out in one second; also called forced vital capacity (FVC).

Nebulizer: Device that makes a mist out of liquid inhalant solution, making drug delivery easier.

Peak flowmeter: Hand-held device that is used to measure the volume of air exhaled and how fast the air is moved out.

Spacer: Device that is attached to the end of a metered-dose inhaler that facilitates drug delivery into the lungs (rather than to the back of the throat).

Spirometry: Test that measures the volume of air that is expired (blown out of the lungs) after taking a deep breath and how rapidly the volume of air is expired.

Overview

Asthma is a chronic disease that affects the airways producing irritation, inflammation, and difficulty breathing. According to 2005 Centers for Disease Control and Prevention statistics, approximately 11.2% of U.S. adults (32.6 million) have ever been diagnosed with asthma by a health professional; more than 7.7% (22 million) still have it. As many as 6.5 million U.S. children (8.9%) have been diagnosed with asthma, making it the number one chronic disease of childhood. In Canada in 2005, 2.2 million persons were diagnosed with asthma. The prevalence of asthma in boys is 30% greater than in girls. Gender differences are reversed in adulthood, where the prevalence in women is 31% to 40% greater than in men.

The burden of disease attributed to asthma is great, and the disease is responsible for missed days at school and work and increased health care system utilization (outpatient office visits, emergency department visits, and hospitalization) above those without asthma. Approximately 1.9 million emergency department visits were attributed to asthma in 2002. Greater than 450,000 people die each year from asthma, too.

Asthma is classified according to frequency and severity of symptoms. The four classifications for asthma are mild intermittent, mild persistent, moderate persistent, and severe persistent asthma (Box 28-1).

It is not known exactly why some people develop asthma whereas others do not; however, there are factors that can increase risk for asthma. A positive family history of asthma and exposure to tobacco smoke can increase the likelihood of developing asthma. Second-hand smoke is an important risk factor and can even affect the fetus in the uterus of a pregnant woman. Chronic exposure to other air pollution may also increase risk for developing asthma. Exposure to some allergens and infections, early in life, may also be risk factors.

Pathophysiology of Asthma

Symptoms of asthma are linked to a progression of physiological changes in airways. Initially airways (bronchial tube and bronchioles) become irritated. This causes airway constriction, which impedes the passage of air. Airways also become inflamed, which produces swelling and further restricts the flow of air through bronchial passages. Mucus production is increased, above normal levels, which can further obstruct breathing passages (Figure 28-1).

Symptoms of Asthma

Airway constriction, inflammation, and mucus produce characteristic asthma symptoms (Box 28-2) and include coughing, wheezing, shortness of breath, and chest tightness. Symptoms may be mild or severe (i.e., life-threatening) and vary for each individual. During an asthma episode, breathing may be noisy and labored. A whistling or creaking sound

BOX 28-1 CLASSIFICATIONS FOR ASTHMA*

Mild intermittent: Symptoms occur twice a week or less, nighttime symptoms are bothersome twice a month or less; and between episodes there are no symptoms and lung function is normal.

Mild persistent asthma: Symptoms occur more than twice a week, but not more than once in a single day. Nighttime symptoms are bothersome more than twice a month and symptoms affect normal activity levels.

Moderate persistent asthma: Symptoms occur daily and nighttime symptoms are bothersome more than once a week. Asthma attacks may affect normal activity levels.

Severe persistent asthma: Symptoms occur throughout the day on most days and nighttime symptoms occur frequently. Physical activity is typically limited.

*A severe asthma attack may occur with all classifications of asthma.

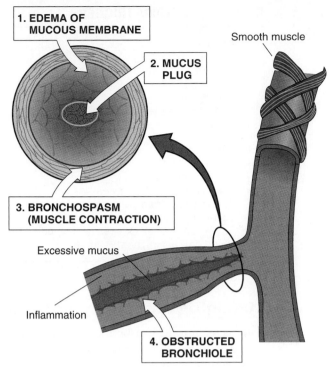

FIGURE 28-1 Airway changes during an asthma episode. *(From Gould BE: Pathio-physiology for the heart professions, ed 3, St. Louls, Saunders, 2007.)*

BOX 28-2 COMMON SYMPTOMS OF ASTHMA

Cough	Chest tightness
Wheezing	Nocturnal awakening
Shortness of Breath	Sleep deprivation

may be heard with inspiration and expiration. Patients describe chest tightness that feels as if something or someone is "squeezing or sitting on your chest." They may also describe a feeling that they cannot get enough air in the lungs. Actually, shortness of breath (SOB) is associated with reduced expiration rather than decreased inspiration. Breathing may become faster and shallow. Nocturnal asthma is a condition that is characterized by decreased FEV_1 and increased airway inflammation and hyperresponsiveness occurring in the middle of the night. Cough at night may disrupt sleep. In one study of patients with asthma, as many as 74% reported nocturnal asthma symptoms at least once per week. In nocturnal asthma, lung function and antiinflammatory hormones (cortisol) decrease and release of proinflammatory mediators (leukotrienes, cytokines) increase in the middle of the night according to circadian rhythm (biological clock).

Asthma "Triggers"

Asthma "triggers" are things that can precipitate an asthma episode in those with asthma (Box 28-3). An asthma episode is also called an asthma "attack." Exposure to allergens (especially animal dander), environmental pollutants, cleaning fluids, mold, tobacco smoke, and even cold air may trigger an asthma episode. Exposure to cockroach droppings and air pollution are believed to be important triggers for asthma that are linked to the rise of asthma in inner-city youth. An upper respiratory infection and strenuous exercise may also trigger an asthma episode. The risks for exercise-induced asthma can be minimized by taking prescribed medicines prior to exercise.

BOX 28-3 ASTHMA TRIGGERS

ALLERGENS
- Animal dander (from the skin, hair, or feathers of animals)
- Dust mites (contained in house dust)
- Cockroaches
- Pollen from trees and grass
- Mold (indoor and outdoor)

IRRITANTS
- Cigarette smoke
- Air pollution
- Cold air or changes in weather
- Strong odors from painting or cooking
- Scented products
- Strong emotional expression (including crying or laughing hard) and stress

OTHERS
- Medicines such as aspirin and β-blockers
- Sulfites in food (dried fruit) or beverages (wine)
- Gastroesophageal reflux disease and laryngopharyngeal reflux can worsen asthma symptoms.
- Irritants or allergens that you may be exposed to at your work, such as special chemicals or dusts
- Infections

Managing Asthma Symptoms

Asthma symptoms can be managed with a combination of medication, lifestyle modification, and home monitoring of breathing using a peak flow meter and medication. A peak flow meter is a hand-held device that is used to measure the volume of air exhaled and how fast the air is moved out. Regular measurements can enable a person with asthma to spot trends that signal an impending asthma attack. A peak flow meter permits self-management of asthma similar to monitoring blood glucose levels enables self-management of diabetes. Low peak flow numbers signal that asthma is not controlled.

Overview of Chronic Obstructive Pulmonary Disease

Chronic obstructive pulmonary disease (COPD) is a progressive disease of the airways that produces gradual loss of pulmonary function. Emphysema, chronic bronchitis, and chronic obstructive bronchitis are all classified under the heading of COPD. COPD is the fourth leading cause of death in the United States and is projected to become the third leading cause of death by 2010. In COPD, the lungs are chronically inflamed. Inflammatory cells such as $CD8^+$ T lymphocytes are recruited to the lung where they infiltrate airways. Interleukin (IL)-6 is also present (see Chapter 15).

RISK FACTORS FOR CHRONIC OBSTRUCTIVE PULMONARY DISEASE

Various lifestyle and environmental factors contribute to the risk for developing COPD. Cigarette smoking or exposure to second-hand smoke places one at risk. Similarly, exposure to occupational irritants to the lungs such as asbestos, industrial chemicals, and dust can increase the risk of developing COPD. Air pollution may contribute and worsen existing COPD. Viral infections also aggravate COPD, in particular, respiratory syncytial virus and adenovirus.

SYMPTOMS OF CHRONIC OBSTRUCTIVE PULMONARY DISEASE

Airflow obstruction produces shortness of breath. Persons with COPD may also exhibit a chronic persistent cough, wheezing, and increased sputum production.

TREATMENT OF CHRONIC OBSTRUCTIVE PULMONARY DISEASE

The aim for COPD management is to (1) relieve symptoms and airway obstruction, (2) correct hypoxia, and (3) treat any precipitating factors and/or comorbidities. Pharmacological treatment of COPD involves the administration of bronchodilators, glucocorticosteroids, and antibiotics, when infections are present. The use of bronchodilators and glucocorticosteroids in reducing inflammation and opening airways is described under the topic headings for asthma. Usual doses administered for the treatment of COPD are listed in the drug table at the end of this chapter. Nonpharmacological treatments include oxygen therapy and mechanical ventilation.

Drugs Used in the Treatment of Asthma

Drugs used for the treatment and management of asthma are divided into two classes. Drugs for treatment of acute symptoms are classified as "rescue" medicines. Drugs administered to prevent asthma episodes are classified as "controllers."

DRUGS USED FOR THE TREATMENT OF ACUTE SYMPTOMS

Rescue medicines, also known as "relievers," provide rapid and short-term relief of asthma symptoms. They reverse bronchospasm and open airways. Albuterol (also known as salbutamol), a short-acting β_2-adrenergic agonist, is the most frequently prescribed bronchodilator. Other β_2-adrenergic agonists currently prescribed for the treatment of asthma include levalbuterol, metaproterenol, and terbutaline. Inhaled anticholinergics such as ipratropium bromide may also be administered for relief of acute symptoms.

MECHANISM OF ACTION

Bronchial airways are composed of smooth muscle that is innervated by β_2, α_1, α_2, and muscarinic (M1 and M3) receptors. When short-acting β_2-adrenergic agonists bind to β_2-receptors, bronchial smooth muscle relaxes and bronchospasm is reversed. Stimulation of β_2-receptor activates adenylcyclase on bronchial smooth muscle, increasing intracellular cyclic AMP (cAMP), which, in turn, produces bronchodilation. Levalbuterol is an isomer of albuterol and is a moderately selective β_2-receptor agonist.

Ipratropium bromide is an example of an antimuscarinic, anticholinergic bronchodilator that is prescribed for short-term relief of asthma symptoms. Anticholinergics bind to muscarinic receptors and block the effects of acetylcholine (released by the vagus nerve) resulting in relaxation of bronchial smooth muscle. Recall that parasympathetic nervous system stimulation produces increased mucus and bronchoconstriction. Antagonism of cholinergic receptors relaxes of bronchial smooth muscle.

PHARMACOKINETICS

Short-acting β_2-adrenergic agonists have a rapid onset of action and short duration of action. The onset of action for albuterol is within 15 minutes, and the peak effect occurs within ½ to 2 hours. The duration of action of albuterol is 2 to 6 hours compared to its isomer, levalbuterol, which has a duration of action of approximately 3 to 6 hours. β_2-Adrenergic agonists are commonly administered by oral inhalation using a ***metered-dose inhaler*** or ***nebulizer***.

Ipratropium bromide is also administered by the inhalation route. Bioavailability is low, which accounts for the low incidence of adverse reactions.

ADVERSE REACTIONS

Drugs like albuterol can produce nervousness, difficulty sleeping, dry mouth, mild headache, and throat irritation (inhalants). β-Receptors are also located on the heart and skeletal muscle, so the use of β_2-agonists can increase heart rate and can lead to arrhythmias, hypertension, palpitations, tachycardia, and tremors. β_2 stimulation may also produce hyperglycemia, hypokalemia, and increased insulin secretion. Ipratropium bromide can additionally cause difficulty urinating and blurred vision.

PRECAUTIONS

Store the canister at room temperature. Exposure to excessive heat can cause the canister to explode. Excessive cold can reduce the effectiveness of albuterol. Keep DuoNeb nebulizer solution in the foil package until time of use; protect from light.

TECH NOTE!
To comply with FDA ruling that by December 31, 2008, the propellant used in metered-dose inhalers must no longer contain chlorofluorocarbons (CFCs), a compound known to deplete the ozone layer, manufacturers have begun to replace CFCs with hydrofluoroalkanes (HFAs).

TECH NOTE!
To determine whether the contents of the metered-dose inhaler canister are low, patients may suspend the canister in a glass of water. A canister that floats to the top is empty and a canister that sinks to the bottom is full.

TECH NOTE!
Excessive use of reliever medication is a sign that asthma is not well controlled.

Short-Acting β₂-Adrenergic Agonists

Generic name	U.S. brand name(s)	Dosage forms and strengths
	Canadian brand(s)	
albuterol* (salbutamol)	AccuNeb, Proair HFA, Proventil, Proventil HFA, Ventolin HFA	**Inhaler (MDI):** 90 mcg/actuation **inhalant solution (AccuNeb):** 0.63 mg/3 ml **inhalant solution (Proventil):** 2.5 mg/3 ml (0.083%), (Sandoz Salbutamol) 5 mg/ml **MDI inhaler (Airomir):** 100 mcg/actuation **inhalant powder (Ventolin Diskus):** 200 mcg/dose **Syrup:** 2 mg/5 ml **Tablet, immediate release:** 2 mg, 4 mg **Tablet, extended release:** 4 mg, 8 mg
	Airomir, Sandoz Salbutamol, Ventolin Diskus	
fenoterol	Not available	**inhalant solution:** 1 mg/ml **Inhaler MDI (Berotec AEM):** 100 mcg/dose
	Berotec, Berotec AEM	
levalbuterol	Xopenex, Xopenex HFA	**Inhaler (Xopenex HFA):** 45 mcg/actuation **Inhalant solution (Xopenex):** 0.31 mg/3 ml, 0.63 mg/3 ml, 1.25 mg/3 ml, 1.25 mg/0.5 ml
	Not available	
metaproterenol*	Alupent	**Inhaler (Alupent):** 0.65 mg/actuation **Inhalant solution:** 0.4%, 0.6% **Syrup:** 10 mg/5 ml **Tablet:** 10 mg, 20 mg
	not available	
pirbuterol	Maxair	**Inhaler MDI:** 0.2 mg/actuation
	Not available	
terbutaline*	Generics	**Inhalant powder (Bricanyl):** 0.5 mg/actuation **Solution, injection:** 1 mg/ml **Tablet:** 2.5 mg, 5 mg
	Bricanyl Turbuhaler	
Combinations		
albuterol + ipratropium bromide	Combivent, DuoNeb	**Inhaler MDI (Combivent):** albuterol 103 mcg/actuation + ipratropium bromide 18 mcg/actuation **Inhalant solution (DuoNeb):** albuterol 3 mg/3 ml + ipratropium bromide 0.5 mg/3 ml
	Combivent	
fenoterol hydrobromide + ipratropium bromide	not available	**Inhaler (MDI):** fenoterol hydrobromide 0.3125 mg + ipratropium bromide 0.125 mg
	DuoVent	

*Generic available.

TECH ALERT!
The following drugs have look-alike/ sound-alike issues: albuterol and atenolol; metoproterenol and metoprolol; Combivent and Combivir; terbutaline and terbinafine

Drugs Used to Prevent Asthma Flare-ups

Drugs that are intended for long-term use and are taken daily to prevent asthma symptoms are called "controllers." The five classes of drugs for prophylaxis of asthma are long-acting β₂ agonists, inhaled corticosteroids, leukotriene modifiers, mast cell stabilizers, and xanthine derivatives.

LONG-ACTING β₂-ADRENERGIC AGONISTS

The Food and Drug Administration (FDA) issued an advisory in 2005 to reduce the risk of asthma-related death by long-acting β₂-adrenergic agonists. According to the FDA, the World Health Organization (WHO), and National Heart, Lung, and Blood Institute (NHLBI), salmeterol and formoterol should not be administered as primary therapy and should only be administered as an optional add-on therapy when inhaled corticosteroids have not adequately controlled the patient's asthma.

Long-Acting β₂-Adrenergic Agonists

Generic name	U.S. brand name(s) / Canadian brand(s)	Dosage forms and strengths
formoterol	Foradil Aerolizer	**Capsule, for inhalation (Foradil):** 12 mcg **Inhaler (Oxeze):** 6 mcg, 12 mcg
	Foradil, Oxeze Turbuhaler	
salmeterol	Serevent Diskus	**Inhaler:** 50 mcg (Canada only) **Inhalation, powder:** 50 mcg
	Serevent Diskhaler, Serevent Diskus	

TECH NOTE!

The FDA advises that "long-acting β₂-adrenergic agonists, such as salmeterol, the active ingredient in Serevent Diskus, have been associated with an increased risk of severe asthma exacerbations and asthma-related death."

GLUCOCORTICOSTEROIDS

Glucocorticosteroids are antiinflammatory drugs. They reduce infiltration cells into the airway that mediate the inflammatory response, and they produce mucus and swelling that makes breathing difficult (see Figure 28-1). Glucocorticosteroids decrease the synthesis of proinflammatory substances—prostaglandins, leukotrienes, cytokines, arachidonic acid, and macrophages—that are released as part of the inflammatory response (see Figure 15-6).

MECHANISM OF ACTION AND PHARMACOKINETICS

The mechanism of action and pharmacokinetics of glucocorticosteroids are discussed in detail in Chapter 15. The primary route of administration for corticosteroids used for the treatment of asthma is inhalation; however, they may be administered orally for more severe symptoms. Inhaled corticosteroids include fluticasone (Flovent), budesonide (Pulmicort), triamcinolone (Azmacort), flunisolide (Aerobid), and beclomethasone (Qvar).

ADVERSE REACTIONS

Adverse reactions to inhaled corticosteriods are primarily local and include coughing, hoarseness, throat irritation, dry mouth, flushing, loss of taste, or unpleasant taste. Some patients may develop an infection in the mouth or throat called thrush. Risks can be minimized by gargling or rinsing the mouth after administering the prescribed dose of medicine. Systemic effects are dose dependent, and more likely to occur at higher doses. Flovent HFA is contraindicated in children less than 4 years, and budesonide, beclomethasone, and triamcinolone inhalers are contraindicated in children under 6 years old. Symbicort and Advair HFA are contraindicated in children less than 12 years old.

Inhaled Corticosteroids

Generic name	U.S. brand name(s) / Canadian brand(s)	Dosage forms and strengths
beclomethasone	Qvar	**Inhaler:** 40 mcg/actuation
	Qvar	
budesonide	Pulmicort, Pulmicort Respules	**Inhalant powder (Pulmicort):** 90 mcg, 180 mcg/actuation **Inhalant suspension (Pulmicort Respules):** 0.25 mg/2 ml, 0.5 mg/2 ml
	Pulmicort, Pulmicort Turbuhaler	
flunisolide	Aerobid	**Inhaler:** 250 mcg/actuation
	Not available	
fluticasone	Flovent Diskus, Flovent HFA	**Inhalant powder (Flovent Diskus):** 50 mcg/actuation **Inhaler:** 44 mcg, 110 mcg, 220 mcg/actuation
	Flovent Diskus	
triamcinolone	Azmacort	**Inhaler:** 100 mcg/actuation
	Not available	

Continued

Inhaled Corticosteroids—cont'd

Generic name	U.S. brand name(s)	Dosage forms and strengths
	Canadian brand(s)	
Long-acting β₂-adrenergic agonist + corticosteroid		
formoterol + budesonide	Symbicort	**Inhaler:**
	Symbicort	6 mcg formoterol + 100 mcg budesonide, 6 mcg formoterol + 200 mcg budesonide
salmeterol + fluticasone	Advair Diskus, Advair HFA	**Inhalant, powder (Advair Diskus):** 25 mcg salmeterol + 125 mcg fluticasone*, 25 mcg salmeterol + 250 mcg fluticasone*, 50 mcg salmeterol + 100 mcg fluticasone, 50 mcg salmeterol + 250 mcg fluticasone, 50 mcg salmeterol + 500 mcg fluticasone
	Advair Diskus	**Inhaler (Advair HFA):** 21 mcg salmeterol + 45 mcg fluticasone, 21 mcg salmeterol + 115 mcg fluticasone, 21 mcg salmeterol + 230 mcg fluticasone

*Strength available in Canada only.

TECH ALERT!
The following drugs have look-alike/sound-alike issues: Foradil and Toradol; salmeterol and salbutamol; Serevent and Serentil

TECH NOTE!
A common ending for leukotriene modifiers is "-lukast."

LEUKOTRIENE MODIFIERS

Leukotrienes are proinflammatory substances that are released as part of the inflammatory response. Leukotriene modifiers are administered to patients with mild asthma to reduce inflammation.

MECHANISM OF ACTION

Figure 28-2 shows the leukotriene pathway.

PHARMACOKINETICS

Montelukast is readily absorbed when administered orally. The maximum concentration of oral tablets is reached within 3 to 4 hours. Chewable tablets work faster, reaching maximum concentrations within approximately 2½ hours. Food does not decrease bioavailabilty of montelukast, unlike zafirlukast, which must be taken on an empty stomach. Montelukast,

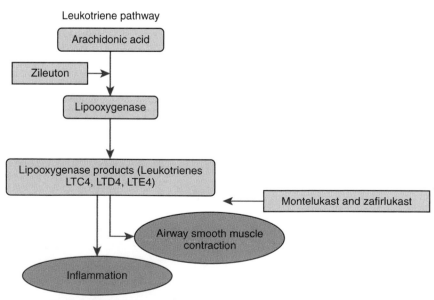

FIGURE 28-2 Leukotriene pathway.

zafirlukast, and zileutin are metabolized in the liver by CYP450 isozymes and can interfere with the metabolism of other drugs using the same metabolic pathway.

ADVERSE REACTIONS

Montelukast and zafirlukast may produce cough, hoarseness or sore throat, headache, indigestion, heartburn or stomach upset, and runny nose. Montelukast may also produce difficulty sleeping, dizziness, drowsiness, muscle aches or cramps, or unusual dreams. Zileuton extended release tablets may produce abdominal pain in addition to the adverse reactions listed for montelukast and zafirlukast.

PRECAUTIONS

The packet of montelukast granules should not be opened until ready for use. Once opened, packet contents (with or without mixing with food) must be administered within 15 minutes. Zileuton may produce abnormal liver function and jaundice, so liver function tests should be conducted every 2 to 3 months.

TECH ALERT!

The following drugs have look-alike/sound-alike: Singulair and Sinequan; Accolate, Accutane, and Aclovate

Leukotriene Modifiers

Generic name	U.S. brand name(s) / Canadian brand(s)	Dosage forms and strengths
montelukast	Singulair	**Chewable:** 4 mg, 5 mg **Oral granules:** 4 mg
	Singulair	**Tablet:** 5 mg, 10 mg
zafirlukast	Accolate	**Tablet:** 10 mg (U.S. only), 20 mg
	Accolate	
zileuton	Zyflo	**Tablet, controlled release:** 600 mg
	Not available	

MAST CELL STABILIZERS

Mast cells are released as part of the immune system response to allergens. Mast cell degranulation results in the release of histamine and mediators of inflammation (e.g., leukotrienes, eosinophils, basophils, cytokines, and prostaglandins). Cromolyn sodium and nedocromil are mast cell stabilizers. By making mast cells less reactive to antigens, they reduce the release of inflammatory substances responsible for producing the symptoms of asthma. Both drugs are administered for prophylaxis and do not control acute symptoms.

PHARMACOKINETICS

Cromolyn sodium may be administered by metered-dose inhaler (MDI) or nebulizer. Nedocromil is administered by MDI only. Cromolyn and nedocromil are similar in effectiveness; however, nedocromil prevents bronchoconstriction secondary to nonantigenic stimuli at much lower doses than cromolyn.

ADVERSE REACTIONS

Systemic absorption of cromolyn sodium is minimal, so side effects are generally localized. The most common adverse reactions are bad taste in the mouth, irritated dry throat, and cough or wheezing.

Mast Cell Stabilizers

	Generic name	U.S. brand name(s)	Dosage forms and strengths
		Canadian brand(s)	
	cromolyn sodium*	Intal	**Inhaler:** 0.8 mg/actuation
			Inhalant solution: 20 mg/2 ml
		Generics	
	nedocromil	Tilade	**Inhaler:** 1.75 mg/actuation
		Not available	

*Generic available.

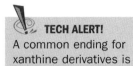

TECH ALERT!

A common ending for xanthine derivatives is *"-phylline."*

XANTHINE DERIVATIVES

The xanthines are one of the oldest classes of drug used in the treatment of asthma. Theophylline occurs naturally in tea and is chemically similar to caffeine. Xanthines have both bronchodilator and antiinflammatory properties.

MECHANISM OF ACTION

The exact mechanism of action of xanthines is unknown. They are believed to have a number of possible mechanisms of action: (1) prostaglandin antagonism, (2) inhibition of calcium ion influx into smooth muscle, (3) stimulation of endogenous catecholamines, (4) inhibition of release of mediators from mast cells and leukocytes, and (5) adenosine receptor antagonism. These actions are responsible for reducing airway inflammation (1, 4), reducing bronchospasm (2), and producing bronchodilation (3, 5).

PHARMACOKINETICS

The half-life ($T\frac{1}{2}$) of theophylline and aminophylline varies with patient age, liver function, smoking status, and use of concurrent drugs. Smoking decreases the $T\frac{1}{2}$ by nearly 50%. The $T\frac{1}{2}$ in children ages 1 to 9 years can be as much as 50% shorter than that in adults. Liver disease and pulmonary edema can prolong the $T\frac{1}{2}$ up to 24 hours. Theophylline is extensively metabolized by the CYP450 enzyme system and is involved in numerous drug interactions (Box 28-4). The bioavailability of theophylline varies between manufacturers. It is recommended that patients receive the same manufacturer's product each time their prescription is refilled.

ADVERSE REACTIONS

Xanthine derivatives (e.g., theophylline) may produce insomnia, dizziness, headache, irritability, decreased appetite, stomach cramps, and urinary retention.

BOX 28-4 DRUGS AND FOOD THAT MODIFY SERUM BLOOD LEVELS OF THEOPHYLLINE

Drugs and foods that increase levels	Oral contraceptives
	Erythromycin
	Calcium channel blockers
	Cimetidine
	Caffeine
	Chocolate
Drugs that decrease levels	Phenobarbital
	Phenytoin
	Carbamazepine
	Cigarette smoking

Xanthine Derivatives

Generic name	U.S. brand name(s)	Dosage forms and strengths
	Canadian brand(s)	
aminophylline*	Generics	**Injection, solution:** 25 mg/ml
		Tablet: 100 mg, 200 mg
	Phyllocontin	**Tablet, extended release (Phyllocontin):** 225 mg, 350 mg
theophylline*	Elixophyllin, Theo-24, TheoCap, Theochron, Uniphyl	**Elixir (Elixophyllin, Theolair liquid):** 80 mg/15 ml
		Capsule, extend release: 125 mg, 200 mg, 300 mg
	Theolair liquid, Uniphyl SRT	**Tablet, extended release (Theo-24):** 100 mg, 200 mg, 300 mg, 400 mg; (Theochron): 100 mg, 200 mg, 300 mg, 450 mg; (Uniphyl): 400 mg, 600 mg

*Generic available.

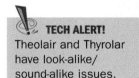

TECH ALERT!
Theolair and Thyrolar have look-alike/sound-alike issues.

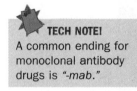

TECH NOTE!
A common ending for monoclonal antibody drugs is "-mab."

MONOCLONAL ANTIBODIES

Omalizumab (also called rhuMAb-E25) is recombinant human monoclonal antibody (anti-IgE) and is indicated for the treatment of moderate to severe allergic asthma. In patients with *allergic asthma,* symptoms occur as a result of a hypersensitivity reaction due to overexpression of immunoglobulin E (IgE) antibodies upon exposure to environmental allergens. Omalizumab is indicated as "add-on" therapy for patients whose asthma is not controlled with inhaled corticosteroids and β_2-adrenergic agonists.

MECHANISM OF ACTION AND PHARMACOKINETICS

The action of omalizumab is specifically directed toward IgE. Omalizumab prohibits IgE's binding to mast cells and prevents binding of the IgE-anti-IgE complex to $Fc_{epsilon}RI$ receptors on monocytes, eosinophils, dendritic cells, epithelial cells, and platelets. The result is prevention of early- and late-stage allergic response and the release of inflammatory mediators (e.g., cytokines).

Omalizumab is administered by subcutaneous injection. Maximum serum concentration is reached within 7 to 8 hours of the administered dose; however, maximum effects from omalizumab are not achieved for several weeks of administration.

ADVERSE REACTIONS

Adverse reactions due to omalizumab injections include mild redness, itching, swelling, or bruising at the injection site; headache; and nausea. Difficulty breathing, hives or skin rash, and unusual bleeding are more serious adverse effects and may be a prelude to anaphylaxis.

PRECAUTIONS

The package insert for omalizumab carries a Black Box warning that patients should be instructed to watch for signs and symptoms of anaphylaxis and be provided with instructions for self-treatment in the event of an emergency.

Monoclonal Antibodies

Generic name	U.S. brand name(s)	Dosage forms and strengths
	Canadian brand(s)	
omalizumab	Xolair	**Powder, injection:** 150 mg
	Xolair	

Drug Delivery Devices for Use With Asthma Medicines

Delivery of the prescribed dose of medication using an MDI is fast but may be challenging for some individuals and is inappropriate for small children. It is not uncommon for a substantial amount of the drug to be delivered to the back of the throat rather than into the lungs when an MDI is used. A nebulizer is a device that converts a liquid dose of medicine into an aerosolized mist that can be inhaled by normal breathing, when used with a mask (Figure 28-3). A mouthpiece may also be attached to the end of the nebulizer and the mist inhaled using slow deep breaths.

A spacer is a device that is attached to the end of the metered dose inhaler (Figure 28-4). The drug is sprayed into the device's chamber and then slowly inhaled into the lungs. Some devices produce a whistling sound to alert the patient when inhalation is too rapid or not controlled.

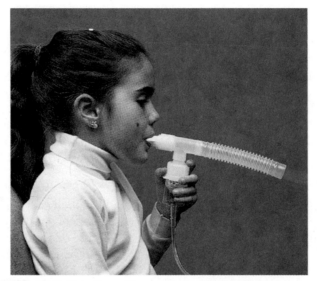

FIGURE 28-3 Nebulizer. *(From Hopper T:* Mosby's pharmacy technician, *ed 2, St. Louis, 2007, WB Saunders.)*

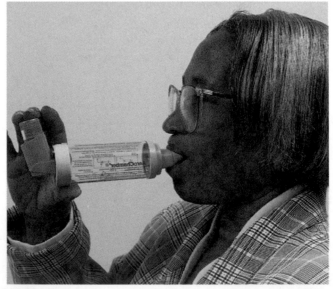

FIGURE 28-4 Spacer. *(From Hopper T:* Mosby's pharmacy technician, *ed 2, St. Louis, 2007, WB Saunders.)*

Summary of Drugs Used in the Treatment of Asthma and COPD

Generic name	U.S. brand name	Usual adult oral dose and dosing schedule*	Warning labels
Short-acting β₂-adrenergic agonists			
albuterol	Ventolin	**Asthma:** **Inhaler:** 1 to 2 puffs every 4 to 6 hours as needed **Inhalant solution:** 2.5 mg every 6 to 8 hours prn delivered over 5 to 15 minutes; *or* AccuNeb: 0.63 to 1.25 mg 3 to 4 times per day, deliver over 5 to 15 minutes as needed **Solution or tablet, immediate release:** 2 mg to 4 mg every 6 to 8 hrs (max: 32 mg/day) **Tablet, extended release:** 4 mg to 8 mg every 12 hours (max: 32 mg/day)	SHAKE WELL—Inhaler
levalbuterol	Xopenex	**Asthma:** **Inhalant solution:** 0.63 to 1.25 mg every 6 to 8 hours **Inhaler:** 2 puffs every 4 to 6 hours	
fenoterol	Berotec (Canada)	**COPD:** **Inhaler:** 100 to 200 mcg 3 to 4 times a day	
metoproteronol	Alupent	**Asthma/COPD:** **Syrup or tablets:** 20 mg 3 to 4 times per day. **Inhaler:** 2 to 3 puffs every 3 to 4 hours (max: 12 puffs/day) **Inhalant solution:** 0.2 to 0.3 ml of 5% solution, diluted in 2.5 to 3 ml NS, 3 to 4 times per day	
pirbuterol	Maxair	**Asthma/COPD:** **Inhaler:** 1 to 2 puffs every 4 to 6 hours (max: 12 puffs/day)	
terbutaline	generics	**Asthma/COPD:** **Injection:** 0.25 mg SC. Repeat in 15 to 30 minutes if needed **Tablet:** 2.5 to 5 mg 3 times a day **Asthma:** **Inhaler:** 2 puffs (400 mcg) every 4 hours	
Long-acting β₂-adrenergic agonists			
formoterol	Foradil Aerolizer	**Asthma/COPD:** Inhale contents of 1 capsule every 12 hours	
salmeterol	Serevent Diskus	**Asthma/COPD:** 1 inhalation every 12 hours	
β₂-Adrenergic agonists + anticholinergics			
albuterol + ipratropium bromide	Combivent, DuoNeb	**COPD:** Inhale 2 puffs 4 times a day (Combivent) or 3 ml 4 times a day (DuoNeb)	SHAKE WELL—Inhaler
fenoterol hydrobromide + ipratropium bromide	DuoVent	**COPD:** Inhale 4 ml every 4 to 6 hours	

Continued

Summary of Drugs Used in the Treatment of Asthma and COPD—cont'd

	Generic name	U.S. brand name	Usual adult oral dose and dosing schedule*	Warning labels
	Inhaled corticosteroids			
	beclomethasone	Q-Var	**Asthma:** 1 to 4 puffs twice daily (max: 320 mcg/day)	SHAKE WELL—Inhaler
	budesonide	Pulmicort	**Asthma:** 1 to 2 puffs twice a day	
	flunisolide	Aerobid	**Asthma:** 2 sprays twice daily	
	fluticasone	Flovent HFA	**Asthma:** 2 sprays up to 2 times a day (max: 440 mcg/day)	
	triamcinolone	Azmacort	**Asthma:** 2 puffs 3 to 4 times a day	
	β₂-Adrenergic agonists + inhaled corticosteroids			
	formoterol + budesonide	Symbicort	**Asthma:** 2 puffs twice daily	SHAKE WELL—Inhaler
	salmeterol + fluticasone	Advair HFA	**Asthma:** 2 puffs every 12 hours	
		Advair Diskus	**Asthma/COPD:** 1 puffs every 12 hours	
	Leukotriene modifiers			
	montelukast	Singulair	**Asthma:** 1 tablet daily	TAKE WITH A LARGE GLASS OF WATER— chewable tab DISCARD UNUSED PORTION OF GRANULES WITHIN 15 MINUTES
	zafirlukast	Accolate	**Asthma:** 20 mg (1 to 2 tablets) twice daily	TAKE ON AN EMPTY STOMACH (1 to 2 HOURS AFTER EATING)
	zileuton	Zyflo	**Asthma:** 2 tablets twice daily	TAKE WITH FOOD SWALLOW WHOLE DON'T CRUSH OR CHEW
	Mast cell stabilizers			
	cromolyn sodium	Intal	**Asthma:** **Inhaler:** 2 sprays 4 times a day **Nebulizer:** 20 mg (2 ml) 4 times a day	SHAKE WELL—Inhaler
	nedocromil	Tilade	**Asthma:** 2 sprays 4 times a day	

Summary of Drugs Used in the Treatment of Asthma and COPD—cont'd

	Generic name	U.S. brand name	Usual adult oral dose and dosing schedule*	Warning labels
Xanthine derivatives				
	aminophylline	generics	**Asthma/COPD:** 10 mg/kg/day PO/IV in divided doses every 6-8 hrs (max: 800 mg/day)	SWALLOW WHOLE; DON'T CRUSH OR CHEW—extended release
	theophylline	Theo-24	***Asthma/COPD:*** **Immediate release:** 10 mg/kg/day (max: 300 to 800 mg/day) PO/IV in divided doses every 6 to 8 hours **Extended release:** 10 mg/kg/day (max: 300 to 800 mg/day) PO/IV in divided doses every 12 to 24 hours (Theo-24)	TAKE 30-60 MINUTES BEFORE MEALS WITH A FULL GLASS OF WATER
Monoclonal antibody				
	omalizumab	Xolair	**Asthma:** 150 mg to 375 mg administered SC every 2 or 4 weeks (based on baseline IgE levels)	REFRIGERATE POWDER AND RECONSTITUTED SOLUTION BETWEEN 2°C AND 8°C DISCARD RECONSTITUTED SOLUTION AFTER 24 HOURS

*Adult dose for asthma and COPD unless specified.
aminophylline dose expressed as theophylline

CHAPTER SUMMARY

- Asthma is a chronic disease that affects the airways producing irritation, inflammation, and difficulty breathing.
- Asthma is classified according to frequency and severity of symptoms. The four classifications for asthma are mild intermittent, mild persistent, moderate persistent, and severe persistent asthma.
- Family history of asthma, smoking including exposure to second-hand smoke, chronic exposure to air pollution, exposure to some allergens, and infections early in life are risk factors for developing asthma.
- Symptoms of asthma are caused by airway irritation that causes bronchial constriction and impedes the passage of air. Airways also become inflamed, which produces swelling and further restricts the flow of air. Mucus production is increased, which further obstructs breathing passages.
- Symptoms of asthma include coughing, wheezing, shortness of breath, and chest tightness.
- Nocturnal asthma is a condition that is characterized by decreased FEV_1 and increased airway inflammation and hyperresponsiveness occurring in the middle of the night.
- Asthma triggers can precipitate an asthma attack. Examples of triggers are animal dander, cockroach droppings, environmental pollutants, cleaning fluids, mold, tobacco smoke, air pollution, upper respiratory infection, vigorous exercise, and even cold air.
- Asthma symptoms can be managed with a combination of medication, lifestyle modification, and home monitoring of breathing using a peak flow meter and medication.
- Chronic obstructive pulmonary disease (COPD) is a progressive disease of the airways that produces gradual loss of pulmonary function.
- Cigarette smoking or exposure to second-hand smoke, occupational irritants, industrial chemicals, or dust can increase the risk of developing COPD.
- Air pollution and viral infections may contribute and worsen existing COPD.

- Shortness of breath, chronic persistent cough, wheezing, and increased sputum production are symptoms of COPD.
- A peak flow meter permits self-management of asthma similar to how monitoring blood glucose levels enables self-management of diabetes.
- Low peak flow numbers signal that asthma is not controlled.
- Pharmacological treatment of COPD involves the administration of bronchodilators, glucocorticosteroids, and antibiotics, when infections are present.
- Nonpharmacological treatments include oxygen therapy and mechanical ventilation.
- Drugs used for the treatment and management of asthma are divided into two classes. Drugs for treatment of acute symptoms are classified as "rescue" or "reliever" medicines. Drugs administered to prevent asthma episodes are classified as "controllers."
- Short-acting β_2-adrenergic agonists provide short-term relief of acute symptoms. "Reliever" medicines currently prescribed for the treatment of asthma include levalbuterol, metaproteronol, and terbutaline.
- Inhaled anticholinergics such as ipratropium bromide may also be administered for relief of acute symptoms.
- Bronchial airways are comprised of smooth muscle, which is innervated by $\beta_2, \alpha_1, \alpha_2,$ and muscarinic (M1 and M3) receptors.
- Stimulation of β_2 receptors produces bronchodilation.
- Levalbuterol is an isomer of albuterol and is a moderately selective β_2-receptor agonist.
- Anticholinergics (e.g., ipratropium bromide) bind to muscarinic receptors and block the effects of acetylcholine, resulting in relaxation of bronchial smooth muscle.
- Drugs like albuterol can produce nervousness, difficulty sleeping, dry mouth, mild headache, and throat irritation (inhalants). Ipratropium bromide can additionally cause difficulty urinating and blurred vision.
- Drugs that are intended for long-term use and are taken daily to prevent asthma symptoms are called "controllers."
- The five classes of drugs for prophylaxis of asthma are long-acting β_2-agonists, inhaled corticosteroids, leukotriene modifiers, mast cell stabilizers, and xanthine derivatives.
- Salmeterol and formoterol should not be administered as primary therapy.
- "Long-acting β_2-adrenergic agonists have been associated with an increased risk of severe asthma exacerbations and asthma-related death."
- Glucocorticosteroids decrease the synthesis of proinflammatory substances: prostaglandins, leukotrienes, cytokines, arachidonic acid, and macrophages.
- Inhaled corticosteroids include fluticasone (Flovent), budesonide (Pulmicort), triamcinolone (Azmacort), flunisolide (Aerobid), and beclomethasone (Qvar).
- Adverse reactions to inhaled corticosteriods are primarily local and include coughing, hoarseness, throat irritation, dry mouth, flushing, loss of taste, or unpleasant taste.
- Risks for thrush can be minimized by gargling or rinsing the mouth after administering the prescribed dose of glucocorticosteroids.
- Leukotriene modifiers are administered to patients with mild asthma to reduce inflammation.
- Leukotriene modifiers inhibit the release of proinflammatory leukotrienes, substances that are released as part of the inflammatory response.
- The packet of montelukast granules should not be opened until ready for use. Once opened, packet contents (with or without mixing with food) must be administered within 15 minutes.
- Cromolyn sodium and nedocromil are mast cell stabilizers.
- They make mast cells less reactive to antigens and reduce the release of inflammatory substances responsible for producing the symptoms of asthma.
- Xanthines have both bronchodilator and antiinflammatory properties.
- Smoking cigarettes decreases the $T\frac{1}{2}$ of theophylline by nearly 50%.
- It is recommended that patients receive the same manufacturer's product each time their prescription for theophylline is refilled.
- Omalizumab is recombinant human monoclonal antibody (anti-IgE) and is indicated for the treatment of moderate to severe allergic asthma.

- Omalizumab is indicated as "add-on" therapy for patients whose asthma is not controlled with inhaled corticosteroids and β_2-adrenergic agonists.
- Omalizumab carries a Black Box warning that patients should be instructed to watch for signs and symptoms of anaphylaxis.
- A nebulizer is a device that converts a liquid dose of medicine into an aerosolized mist.
- A spacer is a device that is attached to the end of the metered-dose inhaler and used to control the delivery of an inhaled medicine.

REVIEW QUESTIONS

Multiple Choice

1. A drug that relaxes tightened airway muscles and improves airflow through the airways is known as a _____.
    a. bronchodilator
    b. bronchoconstrictor

2. Asthma is classified according to _____ and _____ of symptoms:
    a. frequency & duration
    b. duration & presentation
    c. frequency & severity
    d. timing & duration

3. Coughing, wheezing, shortness of breath, and chest tightness are symptoms of which of the following diseases?
    a. COPD
    b. bronchitis
    c. asthma
    d. pneumonia

4. A peak flow meter is a device _____.
    a. that is attached to the end of the metered-dose inhaler
    b. that aids in self-management of asthma
    c. used to administer asthma medication
    d. used to diagnose and treat COPD

5. Emphysema, chronic bronchitis, and chronic obstructive bronchitis are all classified under the heading of "_____."
    a. asthma
    b. COPD
    c. cystic Fibrosis
    d. RSV

6. Persons with _____ may also exhibit a chronic persistent cough, wheezing, and increased sputum production.
    a. smoking habit
    b. COPD
    c. bronchitis
    d. none of the above

7. Nonpharmacological treatments for COPD include which of the following?
    a. oxygen therapy
    b. mechanical ventilation.
    c. inhalers
    d. a and b

8. Pharmacological treatment of COPD, when infections are present, involves the administration of _____.
    a. bronchodilators
    b. glucocorticosteroids
    c. antiinfectives
    d. all of the above

9. **Ipratropium bromide is administered by the _____ route.**
   a. oral
   b. inhalation
   c. transdermal
   d. intravenous

10. **A _____ is a device that converts a liquid dose of medicine into an aerosolized mist that can be inhaled by normal breathing, when used with a mask.**
    a. aerosolizer
    b. nebulizer
    c. spacer
    d. inhaler

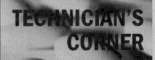

TECHNICIAN'S CORNER

1. Can lung damage be reversed when a smoker stops smoking?
2. What are some lifestyle modifications that can be implemented to manage asthma?

BIBLIOGRAPHY

National Center for Health Statistics: NCHS Health E-Stats. Atlanta, GA, Centers for Disease Control and Prevention, US Department of Health and Human Services, 2007. Available at: http://www.cdc.gov/nchs/products/pubs/pubd/hestats/ashtma03-05/asthma03-05.htm.

National Heart, Lung, and Blood Institute: Chronic obstructive pulmonary disease: data fact sheet. Bethesda, MD, National Heart, Lung, and Blood Institute, National Institutes of Health, US Department of Health and Human Services. NIH publication No. 03-5229, March 2003. Available at: http://www.nhlbi.nih.gov/.

National Heart, Lung, and Blood Institute: Asthma. Bethesda, MD, National Heart, Lung, and Blood Institute, National Institutes of Health, US Department of Health and Human Services, May 2006. Available at: http://www.nhlbi.nih.gov/health/dci/Diseases/Asthma/Asthma_WhatIs.html.

National Institute of Environmental Health Sciences: Asthma and its environmental triggers. Bethesda, MD, US Department of Health and Human Services, May 2006. Available at: http://www.niehs.nih.gov/.

National Institute of Occupational Safety and Health: Preventing allergic reactions to natural rubber latex in the workplace, NIOSH alert No. 97-135. Available at: http://www.cdc.gov/niosh/latexalt.html.

National Institute for Occupational Safety and Health: Latex allergy, prevention guide (2nd printing), NIOSH publication No. 98-113. Available at: http://www.cdc.gov/niosh/pubs/all_date_desc_nopubnumbers.html.

Page C, Curtis M, Sutter M, Walker M, Hoffman B: *Integrated pharmacology* (pp 415-423), Philadelphia, 2005, Mosby.

Papi A, Contoli M, Gaetano C, Mallia P, Johnston S: Models of infection and exacerbations in COPD, Curr Opin Pharmacol, 7:259-265, 2007.

Pleis JR, Lethbridge-Çejku M: Summary health statistics for U.S. adults: National health interview survey, 2005. National Center for Health Statistics. *Vital Health Stat,* 10(232), 2006. Available at: http://www.cdc.gov/nchs/data/series/sr_10/sr10_232.pdf.

Shigemitsu H, Afshar K: Nocturnal asthma, *Curr Opin Pulm Med,* 13:49-55, 2007.

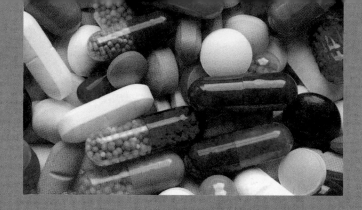

CHAPTER 29

Treatment of Allergies

LEARNING OBJECTIVES

- Learn the terminology associated with allergies.
- Describe the etiology of allergic reactions.
- List symptoms of an allergic reaction.
- List and categorize medications used in the treatment of allergies.
- Describe mechanism of action for drugs used to treat allergies.
- Identify warning labels and precautionary messages associated with medications used for the treatment allergies.
- Identify significant drug look-alike/sound-alike issues.
- List common endings for drug classes used for the treatment of allergies.

KEY TERMS

Allergen: Substance that produces an allergic reaction.

Allergic rhinitis: Seasonal condition that is characterized by inflammation and swelling of the nasal passageways (rhinitis) accompanied by runny nose (rhinorrhea).

Allergy: Hypersensitivity reaction by the immune system upon exposure to an allergen.

Anaphylaxis: Life-threatening allergic reaction.

Angioedema: Allergic skin disease characterized by patches of circumscribed swelling involving the skin and its subcutaneous layers, the mucous membranes, and sometimes the viscera.

Mast cells: Granule-containing cells found in tissue.

Urticaria: Hives.

Wheal: Raised blister-like area on the skin.

Overview

An allergy is a hypersensitivity reaction by the immune system upon exposure to an allergen. It is not known why some individuals are more likely than others to develop allergies; however, exposure to allergens in the environment is a major determinant for the development of allergies. Allergic conditions affect between 40 and 50 million people in the United States and are a public health issue. Allergic conditions affect the quality of life, productivity, and performance of sensitive individuals. Seasonal allergic rhinitis (SAR) occurs upon exposure to seasonal pollens. Up to 10% of the total U.S. population is sensitized to ragweed, and symptoms of seasonal allergic rhinitis are greatest between the months of August and October, when ragweed pollen levels are high.

What Triggers an Allergic Response?

The immune system functions to defend the body against invading germs and other substances it believes are harmful. When an allergic person first comes into contact with an allergen, the immune system treats the allergen as an invader and produces antibodies to the substance. An ***allergen*** is a substance that produces an allergic reaction. Human allergic response is engineered by T lymphocytes. There are different types of T lymphocytes (e.g., CD4$^+$, CD8$^+$, and natural killer T [NKT] cells). Their capacity to respond to allergens varies. CD4$^+$ T cells are the predominant T lymphocytes responsible for producing allergies, although CD8$^+$ is involved in allergic asthma. CD4$^+$ T cells exert their effects through production of interleukins (e.g., IL-4, IL-5, and IL-13) and secretion of cytokines, when activated by allergens (Figure 29-1). IL-4 is involved in immunoglobulin E (IgE) synthesis, a major risk factor for the development of allergic asthma (see Chapter 28). IL-5 orchestrates eosinophil recruitment. Eosinophils are cells that produce inflammation.

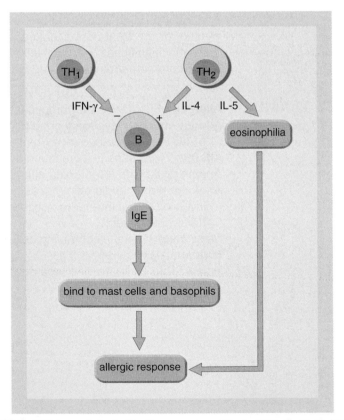

FIGURE 29-1 CD4$^+$ mediated allergic response. *(From Page C, et al.* Integrated pharmacology, *ed 3. Philadelphia, 2006, Mosby.)*
TH$_\epsilon$ = T helper cells
IFN-γ = interferon gamma
IL = interleukin

The production of allergen-specific IgE antibodies and T-cell responses directed against allergens develops within the first few years of life. It is now known that exposure early in life to high levels of multiple endotoxins, as occurs when children live with multiple pets, may reduce the risks for development of asthma and allergies. The degree of IgE antibody response varies and allergens from some sources (e.g., dust mite and cat) are more potent than others.

ALLERGIC RHINITIS

Allergic rhinitis is a condition characterized by nasal itching (rhinitis), runny nose (rhinorrhea), nasal congestion (stuffiness), and sneezing. Symptoms are caused by inflammation and swelling of the nasal passageways. The condition may be perennial, occurring throughout the year, or seasonal. With seasonal allergic rhinitis, allergy symptoms appear after a period of absence from allergen exposure. Symptoms are produced by T lymphocytes and eosinophils infiltration of the nasal epithelium, which occurs as a result of stimulation of mast cells by allergens. The reoccurrence of allergic symptoms seasonally is believed to be caused by the presence of memory $CD4^+$ T cells. There are two types of memory $CD4^+$ T cells. Central memory T cells (TCMs) multiply upon exposure to antigens. Effector memory T cells (TEMs) travel to inflamed tissues secreting cytokines, mediators of immune system response (and inflammation). Memory $CD4^+$ T cells are allergen specific (e.g., tree, grass, and weed pollen).

URTICARIA

Urticaria (also known as hives) is a condition that is characterized by itching and ***angioedema*** (swelling). Redness, swelling, and ***wheals*** (blister-like vesicles) appear on the skin. Itching is also present. Urticaria may be caused by an insect bite, drug or food allergy, or injection of allergen extracts ("allergy shots"). The condition usually subsides within a few days, but if it is severe it may need to be managed by administration of H_1-receptor antagonists and glucocorticosteroids. Acute pharyngeal or laryngeal angioedema must be managed by the administration of drugs that rapidly reduce swelling in the throat and restore breathing capacity (e.g., short-acting β_2-adrenergic agonists).

OCCUPATIONAL ALLERGENS

Pharmacy technicians are at risk for developing latex allergy. Allergic reactions occur when latex sensitive individuals breathe in or come in physical contact with latex proteins. Latex proteins in disposable gloves may form a complex with the lubricant powder used in some gloves. When the pharmacy technician changes gloves, the protein–powder particle complex may become airborne and then inhaled.

Latex allergy may produce mild reactions like skin redness, rash, hives, or itching. Respiratory symptoms such as runny nose, sneezing, itchy eyes, and scratchy throat may occur. More severe reactions involve asthma (difficult breathing, coughing spells, and wheezing) and, rarely, anaphylaxis, which is life threatening.

The National Institute for Occupational Safety and Health recommends taking the following steps to protect oneself from latex exposure and allergy in the workplace.

1. Avoid contact with latex gloves and products. Select non-latex gloves when possible. Appropriate barrier protection is necessary when handling infectious materials.
2. If you choose latex gloves, use powder-free gloves with reduced protein content.
3. Use appropriate work practices to reduce the chance of reactions to latex.
4. Do not use oil-based hand creams or lotions when wearing latex gloves as they can cause glove deterioration.
5. After removing latex gloves, wash hands with a mild soap and dry thoroughly.
6. Practice good housekeeping by frequently cleaning areas and equipment contaminated with latex-containing dust.
7. Avoid areas where you might inhale the powder from latex gloves worn by other workers.
8. Tell your employer and health care providers (physicians, nurses, dentists, etc.) that you have latex allergy.

BOX 29-1 EXAMPLES OF PRODUCTS CONTAINING LATEX

- Disposable gloves
- Intravenous tubing
- Intravenous bag ports
- Syringes

- Catheters
- Injection ports
- Rubber tops of multidose vials

BOX 29-2 COMMON ALLERGY SYMPTOMS

Dermal	Redness
	Swelling
	Urticaria
	Wheal
Respiratory	Itchy eyes, nose, and throat
	Runny nose
	Stuffy nose
	Sneezing
	Coughing and postnasal drip
	Watery eyes
	Conjuctivitis
	"Allergic shiners"
	"Allergic salute"

Pharmacy technicians may come in contact with a wide variety of products containing latex in the workplace. Box 29-1 provides examples of products that may contain latex.

Symptoms of Allergies

Symptoms associated with an allergic reaction may be localized to a specific area of contact as with contact dermatitis, or may be more generalized. Persons with chronic airborne allergies may develop "allergic shiners" (dark circles under the eyes caused by increased blood flow near the sinuses) and an "allergic salute" (a crease across the bridge of the nose caused by persistent upward rubbing of the nose). Common allergy symptoms are listed in Box 29-2.

Drugs Used in the Treatment of Allergies

Pharmacological treatment of allergies is aimed at reducing swelling and inflammation and at suppression of the release of cells that mediate immune system and inflammatory response, as well as blocking receptor sites of the mediators. Drugs used to treat allergic symptoms include antihistamines, inhaled corticosteroids and mast cell stabilizers, leukotriene modifiers, and vasoconstrictors.

H_1-RECEPTOR ANTAGONISTS

Allergic reactions that are associated with binding of histamine to H_1-receptor sites can be reduced by the administration of antihistamines. Recall that when allergens bind to specific IgE antibodies on mast cells, mast cell degranulation occurs, resulting in the release of histamine, prostaglandins, and leukotrienes. Histamine release causes vasodilation and swelling, itchiness, runny nose, watery eyes, and other allergic symptoms. It also produces smooth muscle contraction in the bronchial airways and gastrointestinal tract.

There are several classes of antihistamines: ethylendiamines, ethanolamines, alkylamines, piperazines, phenothiazines, and piperadines. Most are available without prescription. An additional use for piperazine antihistamines (e.g., meclizine and cyclizine) is the treatment of nausea and vomiting. Phenothiazines are also administered for their antiemetic properties and for the treatment of schizophrenia (see Chapter 7).

TECH NOTE!

Symptoms of allergy and a cold are similar; however, cold symptoms rarely last longer than 1 to 2 weeks.

TECH NOTE!

The CDC (2007) and FDA (2008) have issued public health warnings recommending cold and cough products containing antihistamines*, decongestants, and expectorants not to be used in children less than 2 years. The FDA nonprescription Drug Advisory Committee and Pediatric Advisory Committee recommendations extend to children less than 6 years (2007) *Chlorpheniramine, diphenhydramine, brompheniramine, clemastine

MECHANISM OF ACTION AND PHARMACOKINETICS

Administration of antihistamines prevents histamine binding to H_1-receptor sites. The drugs compete with free histamine for binding at H_1-receptor sites. All H_1-receptor antagonists have good oral absorption and reach maximum serum levels within 1 to 2 hours. The half-life ($T\frac{1}{2}$) of the antihistamines varies, ranging from as short as 4 to 6 hours (e.g., diphenhydramine) to 24 hours (fexofenadine). Hydroxyzine is metabolized to the active metabolite cetirizine (Zyrtec). Desloratadine and loratadine are formulated as disintegrating tablets for rapid dissolution and onset of action. The Food and Drug Administration approved the drug levocetirizine in May 2007.

ADVERSE REACTIONS

Antihistamines that cross the blood-brain barrier decrease alertness and/or produce sedation. Sedation, dizziness, decreased alertness, dry mouth, blurred vision, lack of coordination, and urinary retention are the most common adverse reactions of antihistamines. Antihistamines that are classified as ethanolamines (e.g., diphenhydramine) and phenothiazines (e.g., promethazine) produce the most sedation and have the greatest anticholinergic effects. Ethylenediamines (e.g., pyrilamine) and piperazines (e.g., cetirizine) produce fewer sedative effects and the newer agents produce least sedation. Piperadines (e.g., loratadine, fexofenadine) are relatively nonsedating.

PRECAUTIONS

Antihistamines should be used cautiously in men with prostate disease, persons with asthma, and women who are breastfeeding. Antihistamine use children less than 2 years is not recommended (CDC, 2007; FDA). The drugs can decrease urination, thicken bronchial secretions, and decrease milk supply.

TECH NOTE!
Due to its sedating effects, diphenhydramine is also administered for the treatment of insomnia.

TECH ALERT!
The following drugs have look-alike/sound-alike issues: diphenhydramine and dimenhydrinate; Allegra and Viagra; Zyrtec, Zantac, Xanax, and Serax; Claritin and Clarinex

Selected Antihistamines (H_1-Receptor Antagonists)

Generic name	U.S. brand name(s) / Canadian brand(s)	Dosage forms and strengths	Prescription status
Alkylamines			
brompheniramine*	Generics	**Suspension:** 12 mg/5 ml	OTC
	Generics	**Tablet, chewable:** 12 mg **Tablet:** 12 mg	
chlorpheniramine*	Chlor-Trimeton, Chlor-Trimeton Allergy 12 Hour, Teldrin HBP	**Syrup (Chlor-Tripolon):** 2.5 mg/5 ml	OTC
	Chlor-Tripolon, Chlor-Tripolon 12 mg Long Acting	**Tablet:** 4 mg **Tablet, extended release:** 12 mg	
Ethanolamines			
diphenhydramine*	Aler-Dryl, Benadryl Allergy, Complete Allergy, PediaCare Nighttime Cough	**Capsule:** 25 mg, 50 mg **Liquid:** 12.5 mg/5 ml **Tablet:** 25 mg, 50 mg	OTC
	Allerdryl, Benadryl, Benadry Elixir		
clemastine*	Allerhist-1, Tavist Allergy	**Tablet:** 1.34 mg, 1 mg (Canada)	OTC
	Tavist		
Piperazines			
cetirizine	Zyrtec	**Syrup:** 1 mg/ml **Tablet, chewable:** 5 mg **Tablet:** 5 mg, 10 mg, 20 mg (Canada)	OTC
	Reactine		

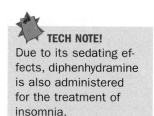

Continued

Selected Antihistamines (H₁-Receptor Antagonists)—cont'd

Generic name	U.S. brand name(s) / Canadian brand(s)	Dosage forms and strengths	Prescription status
levocetrizine	Xyzal	**Tablet:** 5 mg	Rx
Piperidines			
desloratadine	Clarinex, Clarinex RediTab / Aerius, Aerius Kids	**Syrup:** 0.5 mg/ml **Tablet:** 5 mg **Tablet, disintegrating (Clarinex RediTab):** 2.5 mg, 5 mg	Prescription (US) OTC (Canada)
loratadine	Claritin, Claritin Hives Relief, Claritin RediTab, Equate Allergy 24 Hour / Claritin, Claritin Kids, Claritin Rapid Dissolve	**Syrup:** 0.5 mg/ml, 1 mg/ml (Canada only) **Tablet:** 5 mg, 1 mg (Claritin Kids) **Tablet, disintegrating (Claritin RediTab):** 2.5 mg, 5 mg, 10 mg (Claritin Rapid Dissolve)	OTC
fexofenadine*	Allegra / Allegra 12 Hour, Allegra 24 Hour	**Suspension:** 30 mg/5 ml **Tablet:** 30 mg, 60 mg, 180 mg, 120 mg (Allegra 24 hour)	Prescription (OTC Canada)

*Generic available.

GLUCOCORTICOSTEROIDS

Glucocorticosteroids are antiinflammatory drugs. They are administered intranasally to control symptoms of rhinitis. When administered intranasally, they inhibit the onset of the inflammatory response by reducing the permeability of the nasal mucosa cells to T-lymphocytes and eosinophils, thereby decreasing the release of mediators of the inflammatory response (e.g., cytokines). They also reduce the number of inflammatory cells. The result is a reduction in mucus and swelling that makes breathing difficult. Additional mechanisms of action and pharmacokinetics of glucocorticosteroids are discussed in detail in Chapters 15 and 28. Glucocorticosteroids for intranasal use include fluticasone (Flonase), budesonide (Rhinocort), triamcinolone (Nasacort), flunisolide (Nasarel), and beclomethasone (Vancenase AQ).

ADVERSE REACTIONS

Adverse reactions to corticosteriods administered intranasally are primarily local and include nasal irritation, throat irritation, and nose bleed. Some patients may develop a *Candida* infection in the nostril that may present as burning or stinging in the nostril(s).

Mast Cell Stabilizers

Cromolyn sodium is the only mast cell stabilizers available for intranasal use. It is administered to reduce nasal reactivity upon exposure to allergens; therefore, decrease mast cell degranulation and release of inflammatory substances.

Cromolyn sodium is not used to treat acute symptoms. Therapy with cromolyn sodium should be initiated 1 full week before coming into contact with allergens and continued for the duration of allergen exposure. Mechanisms of action and pharmacokinetics and adverse reactions for cromolyn sodium are described in Chapter 28. Adverse effects include bad taste in the mouth; cough, dry throat, or difficulty breathing; headache; nose bleeds, runny nose; sneezing; and stinging, burning, or irritation inside the nose. Cromolyn sodium (Nasalcrom) is available without prescription.

Inhaled Corticosteroids

Generic name	U.S. brand name(s)	Dosage forms and strengths	Prescription status
	Canadian brand(s)		
beclomethasone	Beconase AQ, QVAR	**Pump Spray (Beconase AQ):** 42 mcg/actuation **Inhaler, aerosolized (QVAR):** 4 mcg/actuation	Prescription only
	Generics		
budesonide	Rhinocort Aqua	**Inhaler:** 32 mcg/actuation	Prescription only
	Rhinocort Aqua, Rhinocort Turbuhaler		
flunisolide*	Nasarel	**Pump spray (Rhinalar):** 25 mcg/actuation **Pump spray (Nasarel):** 29 mcg/actuation	Prescription only
	Rhinalar		
fluticasone propionate	Flonase	**Pump spray:** 50 mcg/actuation	Prescription only
	Flonase		
fluticasone furoate	Veramyst	**Spray Mist:** 27.5 mcg/actuation	Prescription only
	Not available		
triamcinolone	Nasacort AQ	**Pump spray:** 55 mcg/actuation, 100 mcg (Nasacort)	Prescription only
	Nasacort, Nasacort AQ		

*Generic available.

Mast Cell Stabilizer

Generic name	U.S. brand name(s)	Dosage forms and strengths	Prescription status
	Canadian brand(s)		
cromolyn sodium	Nasalcrom	**Pump Spray:** 5.2 mg/actuation	OTC
	Generics		

Summary of Drugs Used in the Treatment of Asthma and COPD

Generic name	U.S. brand name	Usual adult oral dose and dosing schedule*	Warning labels
Antihistamine (H$_1$-receptor antagonist)			
brompheniramine	Generic	**Allergic rhinitis, pruritus, and urticaria:** **Immediate release:** 4 to 8 mg every 6 to 8 hours **Extended release:** 1 to 2 tablets every 12 hours	MAY CAUSE DROWSINESS; ALCOHOL MAY INCREASE THIS EFFECT SWALLOW WHOLE; DON'T CRUSH OR CHEW—extended release
chlorpheniramine	Chlor-Trimeton	**Allergic rhinitis:** **Immediate release:** 4 mg every 4 to 6 hours up to 24 mg/day **Extended release:** 8 mg to 12 mg 2 to 3 times a day	
diphenhydramine	Benadryl	**Allergic rhinitis, pruritus, and urticaria:** 25 mg to 50 mg 3 to 4 times a day	

Continued

Summary of Drugs Used in the Treatment of Asthma and COPD—cont'd

	Generic name	U.S. brand name	Usual adult oral dose and dosing schedule*	Warning labels
	clemastine	Tavist	**Allergic rhinitis and urticaria:** 1.34 to 2.68 mg 2 to 3 times a day **Pruritus and angioedema:** 2.68 mg 1 to 3 times a day	
	cetirizine	Zyrtec	**Allergic rhinitis and urticaria:** 5 to 10 mg once daily	
	desloratadine	Clarinex	**Allergic rhinitis, pruritus, and urticaria:** 5 mg once daily	PROTECT FROM MOISTURE; LEAVE IN FOIL PACKET UNTIL READY FOR USE—disintegrating tablets
	fexofenadine	Allegra	**Allergic rhinitis and urticaria:** 60 mg twice daily or 180 mg once daily	DISSOLVE REDITAB UNDER THE TONGUE MAY CAUSE DIZZINESS OR DROWSINESS AVOID ORANGE, GRAPEFRUIT, and APPLE JUICE—fexofenadine
	levocetirizine	Xyzal	**Allergic rhinitis and urticaria:** 5 mg once daily in the evening	MAY CAUSE DIZZINESS OR DROWSINESS AVOID ALCHOLIC DRINKS
	loratadine	Alavert, Claritin	**Allergic rhinitis and urticaria:** 10 mg once daily	DO NOT DRIVE
Intranasal corticosteroids				
	beclomethasone	Beconase AQ	**Allergic rhinitis:** 1 to 2 sprays each nostril twice daily	SHAKE WELL
	budesonide	Rhinocort Aqua	**Allergic rhinitis:** 1 to 2 sprays each nostril once daily	
	flunisolide	Nasarel	**Allergic rhinitis:** 2 to 3 sprays each nostril twice daily	
	fluticasone propionate	Flonase	**Allergic rhinitis:** 1 spray each nostril twice daily or 2 sprays in each nostril daily	
	fluticasone furoate	Veramyst	**Allergic rhinitis:** 2 sprays once daily	
	triamcinolone	Nasacort	**Allergic rhinitis:** 1 to 2 sprays each nostril twice daily	
Mast cell stabilzers				
	cromolyn sodium	Nasalcrom	**Allergic rhinitis:** 1 spray each nostril 3 to 4 times daily (up to 6 times daily)	RINSE AND DRY TIP AFTER EACH USE

Immunotherapy

Allergy shots represent a form of immunotherapy. They may be administered to persons with perennial or seasonal allergies. The rationale for immunotherapy is to reduce the level of IgE antibodies in the blood while at the same time stimulating the production of IgG, a protective antibody. Allergy shots are administered by subcutaneous injection. They are administered as a series of shots; each injection has an increased concentration of the allergen that produces sensitivity. Allergy shots can reduce allergy symptoms over a longer period of time than all other treatments.

CHAPTER SUMMARY

- An allergy is a hypersensitivity reaction by the immune system upon exposure to an allergen.
- Allergic conditions affect the quality of life, productivity, and performance of sensitive individuals.
- Seasonal allergic rhinitis (SAR) occurs upon exposure to seasonal pollens.
- When an allergic person first comes into contact with an allergen, the immune system treats the allergen as an invader and produces antibodies to the substance.
- $CD4^+$ T cells are the predominant T lymphocytes responsible for producing allergies, although $CD8^+$ is involved in allergic asthma. $CD4^+$ T cells exert their effects through production of interleukins (e.g., IL-4, IL-5, and IL-13) and secretion of cytokines, when activated by allergens.
- IL-4 is involved in immunoglobulin E (IgE) synthesis.
- The production of allergen-specific IgE antibodies and T-cell responses directed against allergens develop within the first few years of life.
- The degree of IgE antibody response varies and allergens from some sources (e.g., dust mite and cat) are more potent than others.
- Allergic rhinitis is a condition characterized by nasal itching (rhinitis), runny nose (rhinorrhea), nasal congestion (stuffiness), and sneezing.
- The reoccurrence of allergic symptoms seasonally is believed to be caused by the presence of memory CD4+ T cells. There are two types of memory $CD4^+$ T cells. Central memory T cells multiply upon exposure to antigens. Effector memory T cells travel to inflamed tissues secreting cytokines, mediators of immune system response (and inflammation).
- Urticaria (also known as hives) is condition that is characterized by itching and angiodemia (swelling).
- Pharmacy technicians are at risk for developing latex allergy. Allergic reactions occur when latex-sensitive individuals breathe in or come in physical contact with latex proteins.
- Latex allergy may produce mild reactions like skin redness, rash, hives, or itching. Respiratory symptoms such as runny nose, sneezing, itchy eyes, and scratchy throat may occur.
- Pharmacological treatment of allergies is aimed at reducing swelling and inflammation and suppression of the release of cells that mediate immune system and inflammatory response, as well as blocking receptor sites of the mediators.
- Drugs used to treat allergic symptoms include antihistamines, inhaled corticosteroids and mast cell stabilizers, leukotriene modifiers, and vasoconstrictors.
- Antihistamines compete with free histamine for binding at $histamine_1$ (H_1)-receptor sites.
- There are six classes of antihistamine: ethylendiamines, ethanolamines, alkylamines, piperazines, phenothiazines, and piperadines.
- Sedation, dizziness, decreased alertness, dry mouth, blurred vision, lack of coordination, and urinary retention are the most common adverse reactions of antihistamines.
- Antihistamines that are classified as ethanolamines (e.g., diphenyhydramine) and phenothiazines (e.g., promethazine) produce the most sedation and have the greatest anticholinergic effects.
- Piperadines (e.g., loratadine, desloratadine, and fexofenadine) are relatively nonsedating.
- Antihistamines should be used cautiously in men with prostate disease, persons with asthma, and women who are breastfeeding. They are not recommended for use in children less than 2 years old.
- Glucocorticosteroids are administered intranasally to control symptoms of rhinitis.
- Glucocorticosteroids for intranasal use include fluticasone (Flonase), budesonide (Rhinocort), triamcinolone (Nasacort), flunisolide (Nasalide), and beclomethasone (Vancenase AQ).
- Adverse reactions to corticosteriods administered intranasally are primarily local and include: nasal irritation, throat irritation, and nose bleed.

- Cromolyn sodium is the only mast cell stabilizers available for intranasal use.
- Therapy with cromolyn sodium should be initiated 1 full week before coming into contact with allergens and continued for the duration of allergen exposure.
- Allergy shots are a form of immunotherapy.
- Allergy shots are administered as a series of subcutaneous injections and can reduce allergy symptoms over a longer period of time than all other treatments.

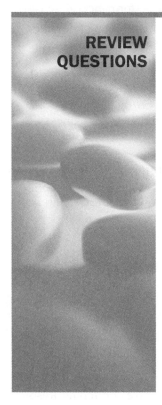

REVIEW QUESTIONS

Multiple Choice

1. **Which of the following is a life-threatening allergic reaction?**
   a. urticaria
   b. pruritus
   c. anaphylaxis
   d. wheal

2. **An allergy is a hypersensitivity reaction by the endocrine system upon exposure to an allergen.**
   a. true
   b. false

3. **A condition characterized by nasal itching (rhinitis), runny nose (rhinorhhea), nasal congestion (stuffiness), and sneezing is called _____.**
   a. urticaria
   b. allergic rhinitis
   c. wheals
   d. angioedema

4. **Symptoms associated with an allergic reaction are always localized.**
   a. true
   b. false

5. **Not all antihistamines are available without a prescription.**
   a. true
   b. false

6. **Glucocorticosteroids are administered intraorally to control symptoms of rhinitis.**
   a. true
   b. false

7. **Cromolyn sodium is the only _____ available for intranasal use.**
   a. mast cell stabilizer
   b. glucocorticoid
   c. antihistamine
   d. antiinflammatory

8. **Diphenhydramine has a side effect of _____.**
   a. hyperactivity
   b. sedation
   c. burning
   d. none of the above

9. **Loratadine is the generic name for Clarinex.**
   a. true
   b. false

10. **Cetirizine is available in which of the following dosage forms?**
    a. tablet
    b. chewable tablet
    c. syrup
    d. all of the above

TECHNICIAN'S CORNER

1. What is the best way to identify what is causing an allergy?
2. Should all antihistamines be available as OTC drugs?

BIBLIOGRAPHY

Kaiser H, Naclerio R, Given J, Toler T, Ellsworth A, Philpot E: Fluticasone furoate nasal spray: A single treatment option for the symptoms of seasonal allergic rhinitis, *J Allergy Clin Immunol,* 119, 2007.

Kalant H, Grant D, Mitchell J: *Principles of medical pharmacology* (pp 22-27, 397-400, 451, 453-454), ed 7. Toronto, 2007, Elsevier Canada, A Division of Reed Elsevier Canada.

National Institute of Allergy and Infectious Disease: *Airborne allergens: Something in the air,* Bethesda, MD, NIAID Health Info, National Institutes of Health, US Department of Health and Human Services. NIH publication No. 03-7045, April 2003 Available at: http://www.niaid.nih.gov/.

Page C, Curtis M, Sutter M, Walker M, Hoffman B: *Integrated pharmacology* (pp 330-336, 428-430), Philadelphia, 2005, Mosby.

Woodfolk J: T-cell responses to allergens, molecular mechanisms in allergy and clinical immunology, *J Allergy Clin Immunol,* 119, 2007.

UNIT VIII

Drugs Affecting the Urinary System

LEARNING OBJECTIVES

- Identify the organs of the urinary system.
- Understand the function of each part of the urinary system.
- Explain the process of the formation and elimination of urine.
- Understand the importance of the kidney in maintaining homeostasis.

Overview of the Urinary System

The principal organs of the urinary system are the **kidneys**, which process blood and form urine as a waste to be excreted. The excreted urine travels from the kidneys to the outside of the body via accessory organs: the **ureters, urinary bladder,** and **urethra**.

The urinary system is primarily thought of as a "urine producer" but a better image of it is that of "blood plasma balancer." The water content is adjusted to maintain constancy of the internal environment. Likewise, the blood content of sodium and potassium and the pH of blood can be altered to match the normal levels.

Anatomy of the Urinary System

KIDNEY

The kidneys lie in a retroperitoneal position against the posterior wall of the abdomen and located on either side of the vertebral column. Each kidney is roughly oval with a medial indentation. The medial surface has a concave notch called the **hilum** and it is here that the ureters and blood vessels enter and leave the kidney. The main internal structures of the kidney are the renal cortex (outer region), and the renal medulla (inner region), and renal pyramids (medullary tissue). Each point of a pyramid (papilla) juts into a cuplike structure called a **calyx.** Urine leaving the renal papilla is collected for transport out of the body. The calyces join together to form a large collection reservoir called the renal pelvis, which narrows as it exits the hilum to become the ureter.

BLOOD VESSELS OF THE KIDNEY

The renal artery, a branch of the aorta, brings blood to each kidney. The renal artery branches into smaller arteries, then into the afferent arteriole, which branches into a tuft-like grouping of five to eight capillaries (glomerular capillaries) called the **glomerulus.** Blood leaving the glomerular capillaries flows from efferent arterioles into the peritubular capillaries, then into venules and finally into the renal vein.

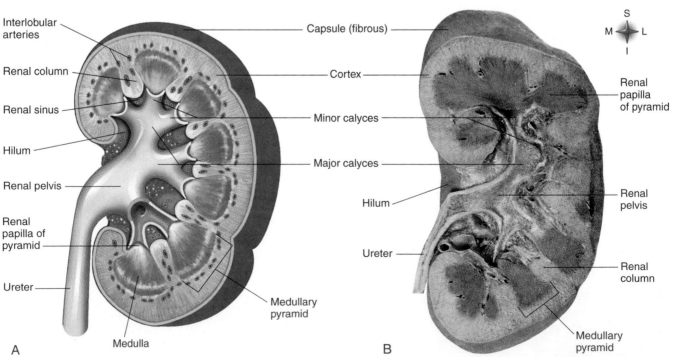

(**A,** from Brundage DJ: Renal disorders. St. Louis, Mosby, 1992. **B,** from Abrahams P, Hutchings RT, Marks SC: McMinn's color atlas of human anatomy, 4th ed. St. Louis, Mosby, 1999.)

THE NEPHRON

The microscopic functional units and working unit of the kidney are named **nephrons** and number 1.25 million per kidney. Each nephron contains the following structures: renal corpuscle, Bowman's capsule, proximal convoluted tubule, loop of Henle, distal convoluted tubule, and collecting duct.

Bowman's Capsule

Bowman's capsule is the cup-shaped mouth of the nephron and is formed by two layers of epithelial cells with a space, called *Bowman's space*. Fluids, waste products, and electrolytes constitute the glomerular filtrate, which will be processed in the nephron to form urine. The **glomerulus** is made up of a fine network of capillaries that fits neatly into the Bowman's capsule. The **proximal tubule, loop of Henle,** and the **distal tubule** extend out from the glomerulus and it is here that secretion of waste products, and re-absorption of nutrients take place. The **juxtaglomerular apparatus** is found at the point where the afferent arteriole brushes past the distal tubule. This structure is important in maintaining homeostasis of blood flow because it secretes renin when blood pressure in the afferent arteriole drops. The **collecting duct** is a straight tubule joined by the distal tubules of several nephrons. Collecting ducts join larger ducts, and converge to form one tube that opens at a renal papilla into one of the small calyces. See Figure 22-2 for the anatomy of the nephron.

URETERS

The ureters are the two tubes that actively transport urine from the kidneys to the urinary bladder. Each ureter is composed of three layers of tissue, a mucus lining, a muscular middle layer, and fibrous outer layer. The muscular layer is composed of smooth muscle and propels the urine by peristalsis.

URINARY BLADDER

The urinary bladder is located directly behind the symphysis pubis and in front of the rectum. In women it is anterior of the vagina and in front of the uterus, whereas in men, it rests on the prostate. The wall of the bladder is made of mostly smooth muscle tissue often called the detrusor muscle. The bladder is lined with mucus transitional epithelium that forms folds that are called **rugae**; and which enable it to distend considerably when full. There are three openings on the floor of the bladder—two from the ureters and one into the urethra. The bladder performs two major functions: a reservoir for urine and expelling urine from the body aided by the urethra.

URETHRA

The urethra is a small tube that leads from the floor of the bladder (trigone) to the exterior of the body. In females, it lies directly behind the symphysis pubis and anterior to the vagina as it passes through the muscular floor of the pelvis. It then extends down from the bladder and ends at the **external urinary meatus**. The male urethra passes through the center of the prostate gland just after leaving the bladder. Within the prostate, it is joined by two ejaculatory ducts. After leaving the prostate, the urethra extends down into the penis and ends as a urinary meatus at the tip of the penis.

Overview of Kidney Function

The chief functions of the kidney are to process blood plasma and excrete urine. These functions are vital because they maintain the homeostatic balance of the body, such as electrolyte and acid-balance. The following is a list of blood constituents that need to be held within their normal concentration ranges to prevent kidney failure: sodium, potassium, chloride, nitrogenous wastes (especially urea). Nitrogenous wastes from protein metabolism, notably urea, leave the blood by way of the kidneys.

The kidney also performs other functions such as influencing the rate of secretion of antidiuretic hormone (ADH) and aldosterone. The nephrons of the kidney function to reabsorb fluids and electrolytes, filter blood, and eliminate waste in urine.

1. *Filtration* is the movement of water and protein-free solutes from plasma in the glomerulus, across the glomerular membrane, and into the capsular space of Bowman's capsule. The result is about 180 liters of glomerular filtrate being formed each day.
2. *Tubular reabsorption* is the process of movement of molecules like water, sodium, and electrolytes out of the various segments of the tubule and into the blood.
3. *Tubular secretion* is the process of movement of molecules out of blood and into the tubule for excretion. The distal tubules and collecting tubules secrete potassium, hydrogen, and ammonium ions. Tubule cells also secrete certain drugs like penicillin.

REGULATION OF URINE VOLUME

Antidiuretic hormone (ADH) has a central role in the regulation of urine volume by reducing water loss by the body. Another hormone that tends to decrease urine volume and conserves water is *aldosterone*. It reabsorbs sodium, which in turn causes an osmotic imbalance that drives the re-absorption of water from the tubule. *Atrial natriuretic hormone (ANH)* also influences water re-absorption in the kidneys. ANH is secreted by specialized muscle fibers in the atrial wall of the heart. ANH promotes natriuresis (loss of sodium in urine).

MICTURITION

The mechanism of voiding urine begins with voluntary relaxation of the external sphincter muscle of the bladder. Injury to any of these nerves, by a cerebral hemorrhage or a spinal cord injury, for example, results in involuntary micturition or *incontinence*.

Urine Composition

Urine is approximately 95% water, in which are dissolved several different kinds of substances such as:

- **Nitrogenous wastes:** urea, uric acid, ammonia, and creatinine.
- **Electrolytes:** Sodium, potassium, ammonium, chloride, bicarbonate, phosphate, and sulfate (amounts vary with diet and other factors).
- **Toxins:** During disease, bacterial poisons leave the body in urine.
- **Pigments:** Yellowish pigments (urochromes) from the breakdown of old red blood cells in the liver and elsewhere (foods and drugs).
- **Hormones:** High hormone levels sometimes result in significant amounts of hormones in the filtrate (and therefore in the urine).
- **Abnormal constituents:** Blood, glucose, albumin (a plasma protein or calculi [kidney stones]) are substances that if found in the urine could signal disease or an infection.

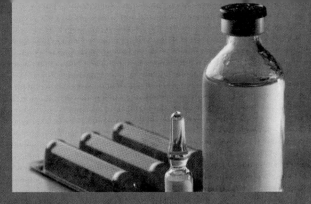

Treatment of Prostate Disease and Erectile Dysfunction

LEARNING OBJECTIVES

- Learn the terminology associated with prostate disease and erectile dysfunction.
- List symptoms of prostate disease.
- List symptoms of erectile dysfunction.
- List and categorize medications used for the treatment of prostate disease and erectile dysfunction.
- Describe mechanism of action for drugs used for the treatment of prostate disease and erectile dysfunction.
- Identify warning labels and precautionary messages associated with medications used for the treatment of prostate disease and erectile dysfunction.
- Identify significant drug look-alike/sound-alike issues.
- List common endings for drug classes used in the treatment of prostate disease and erectile dysfunction.

KEY TERMS

α-Blockers: Drugs used in the treatment of benign prostatic hyperplasia to relax muscles in the prostate and increase urine flow.

α-Reductase inhibitor: Drug that shrinks the prostate gland; used to treat BPH.

Benign prostatic hyperplasia (BPH): Noncancerous growth of cells in the prostate gland.

Digital rectal exam (DRE): Screening exam involving palpation of the prostate gland and conducted by insertion of a gloved, lubricated finger into the rectum.

Ejaculation: Release of semen from the penis during orgasm.

Erectile dysfunction (ED): Persistent inability to achieve and/or maintain an erection sufficient for satisfactory sexual intercourse.

Frequency: Need to urinate more often than is normal.

Hyperplasia: Abnormal increase in the number of cells in an organ or tissue.

Incontinence: Loss of bladder or bowel control.

Prostate: Gland in the male reproductive system just below the bladder and surrounding the urethra.

Prostate-specific antigen (PSA): Protein produced by the prostate gland. Levels are elevated in men that have prostate cancer, infection, or inflammation of the prostate gland and BPH.

Prostate-specific antigen test: Blood test to measure PSA, a substance produced by prostate gland cells. A free PSA test reports the percentage of PSA that is not attached to another chemical, compared to total PSA in a man's blood. Free PSA is linked to BPH but not to cancer.

Prostatitis: Inflammation of the prostate gland.

Semen: Fluid containing sperm and secretions from glands of the male reproductive tract.

Tumor: Abnormal mass of tissue that results from excessive cell division. Tumors may be benign (not cancerous) or malignant (cancerous).

Urgency: Feeling of needing to urinate immediately.

Urinanalysis: Microscopic and chemical examination of a fresh urine sample.

Benign Prostatic Hyperplasia

The *prostate gland* is a part of the male reproductive system. The gland produces *semen,* the fluid that contains sperm. The prostate gland in located just below the bladder and it surrounds the urethra. *Prostatitis* is an inflamed or infected prostate gland. Symptoms may be burning upon urination; fever; body ache; groin, rectal, or low back pain; difficulty urinating; painful ejaculation; and decreased libido. While some of the symptoms are similar, prostatitis is usually an acute condition, unlike benign prostatic hyperplasia. *Benign prostatic hyperplasia (BPH)* is a condition where noncancerous cells in the prostate grow and increase the size of the prostate gland (Figure 30-1). It may increase from the size of a walnut to the size of a small lemon. As the gland grows, it begins to obstruct the flow of urine through the urethra. The urethra is a small tube that carries urine and semen through the penis.

The risk for developing BPH increases with age. More than 50% of adult males will have BPH by age 60 years, and by age 85, approximately 90% will have BPH. Not all men with BPH have symptoms. Nearly 70% are asymptomatic.

DIAGNOSIS

Several tests are available to check the health of prostate. A *digital rectal exam (DRE)* is the first step for examining the prostate. The exam involves insertion of a gloved finger into the rectum and palpating the prostate to determine if it is enlarged. A *prostate*

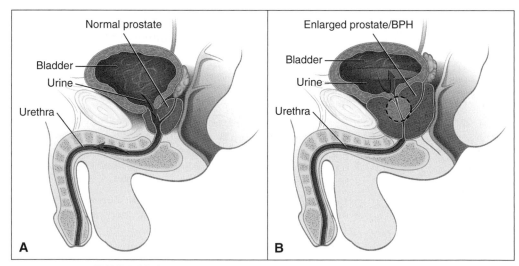

FIGURE 30-1 A, Normal prostate. **B,** Enlarged prostate. *(Courtesy National Institutes of Health, Bethesda, MD.)*

BOX 30-1 SYMPTOMS OF BENIGN PROSTATIC HYPERPLASIA

- Weak or slow stream of urine
- Delay in starting urination
- Urinary stream that starts and stops
- Frequent urination

- Urinary urgency
- Nighttime awakening to urinate
- Need to strain to urinate
- Incomplete bladder emptying

specific antigen (PSA) test may be performed to determine if levels of the PSA protein are elevated. Higher than normal levels are a sign of BPH, infection, inflammation, or prostate cancer. A free PSA test, the percentage of PSA that is not attached to another chemical, may be conducted to differentiate between BPH and cancer. Free PSA is linked to BPH but not to cancer. A biopsy of prostate tissue may also be taken.

SYMPTOMS OF BENIGN PROSTATIC HYPERPLASIA

The first symptoms of an enlarged prostate gland are a weak or slow stream (Box 30-1). There may also be a delayed start in the flow or urine or straining to urinate. As the disease progresses, the bladder becomes hypersensitive and the need to urinate becomes more frequent. Some men may develop urinary infection(s) from the condition. BPH may also produce bladder stones, sudden inability to urinate, or kidney damage.

Treatment of Benign Prostatic Hyperplasia

Pharmacotherapy for BPH is initiated when symptoms are uncomfortable enough to warrant treatment. *Watchful waiting* is recommended when patients are asymptomatic or symptoms do not produce much discomfort. Two classes of drugs are administered to manage symptoms: α-blockers and 5α-reductase inhibitors.

α-BLOCKERS

α_1-Adrenergic antagonists relax prostate and bladder smooth muscle, which reduces urethral resistance and improves the flow of urine. Some α-Blockers are also prescribed for the treatment of hypertension (see Chapter 22).

MECHANISM OF ACTION AND PHARMACOKINETICS

Alfuzosin, doxazosin, terazosin, and tamsulosin bind to α_1-receptor sites. Prostate muscle tone is primarily controlled through binding to α_{1A}-receptor sites. The drugs also have varying affinity for α_{1B} and α_{1D} subtypes. Binding to α_1-receptors blocks adrenergic mediated vasoconstriction.

Alfuzosin is available in immediate release and extended release dosage forms. The immediate release has a half-life ($T\frac{1}{2}$) of 3 hours, whereas the extended release $T\frac{1}{2}$ is approximately 11 hours. The other agents possess a long half-life ranging from 16 to 22 hours and are dosed once daily. Urine flow rates are usually improved within the first 2 weeks of therapy.

ADVERSE REACTIONS

Adverse drug effects linked to the administration of α-adrenergic antagonists are postural hypotension, dizziness, reflex tachycardia, headache, stuffy nose, weakness, and fatigue.

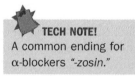

TECH NOTE!
A common ending for α-blockers *"-zosin."*

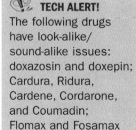

TECH ALERT!
The following drugs have look-alike/sound-alike issues: doxazosin and doxepin; Cardura, Ridura, Cardene, Cordarone, and Coumadin; Flomax and Fosamax

α₁-Adrenergic Antagonists

	Generic name	U.S. brand name(s) / Canadian brand(s)	Dosage forms and strengths
	alfuzosin	Uroxatral	**Tablet, immediate release:** 10 mg
		Xatral	**Tablet, extended release:** 10 mg
	doxazosin*	Cardura	**Tablet:** 1 mg, 2 mg, 4 mg, 8 mg (8 mg not available in Canada)
		Cardura	**Tablet, extended release (Cardura XL):** 4 mg, 8 mg
	terazosin*	Hytrin	**Capsule (Hytrin) and Tablet:** 1 mg, 2 mg, 5 mg, 10 mg
		Hytrin	
	tamsulosin	Flomax	**Capsule:** 0.4 mg
		Flomax, Flomax CR	**Capsule, extended release:** 0.4 mg

*Generic available.

5α-REDUCTASE INHIBITORS

Excess growth of prostate tissue in BPH is dependent on testosterone levels. High levels result in growth, whereas deprivation results in reduction in glandular size. Finasteride and dutasteride are antiandrogens, capable of reducing testosterone levels.

MECHANISM OF ACTION AND PHARMACOKINETICS

Prostate growth and size is reduced by the administration of 5α-reductase inhibitors. They inhibit 5α-reductase, an enzyme that controls the production of dihydrotestosterone (DHT) from testosterone. The effects of 5α-reductase inhibitors accumulate over time. It may take 6 to 12 months for therapeutic effects to be achieved.

ADVERSE REACTIONS

Adverse effects of dutasteride and finasteride are decreased desire for sex, erectile dysfunction (ED), and reduced semen. Dutasteride and finasteride are also harmful to the developing fetus. Pregnant women and women of child-bearing age should be advised to avoid contact with broken or crushed tablets. The use of barrier contraceptive, such as condoms, is recommended.

5α-reductase inhibitors

	Generic name	U.S. brand name(s) / Canadian brand(s)	Dosage forms and strengths
	dutasteride	Avodart	**Capsule:** 0.5 mg
		Avodart	
	finasteride*	Proscar, Propecia	**Tablet (Proscar):** 5 mg
		Proscar, Propecia	**Tablet (Propecia):** 1 mg

*Generic available.

Nonpharmacological Treatment Options

When symptoms of BPH are severe, surgery is indicated. There are several surgical options. Some procedures are more invasive than others. Surgical procedures are briefly described.

HoELP (holium laser enucleation of prostate): Excess prostate tissue is vaporized using a laser (holium).

TURP (transurethral resection of the prostate): Excess prostate tissue is trimmed away.

TUIP (transurethral incision of the prostate): One or two slits are made in the prostate to relieve the pressure and improve urine flow.

TUMT (transurethral microwave thermal therapy of the prostate): Computer-regulated microwaves are sent through a catheter to heat portions of the prostate.

TUNA (transurethral needle ablation): Excess prostate tissue is burned using radio waves.

Prostatic stent: A stent (scaffolding) is inserted into the urethra to open passage and improve urine flow.

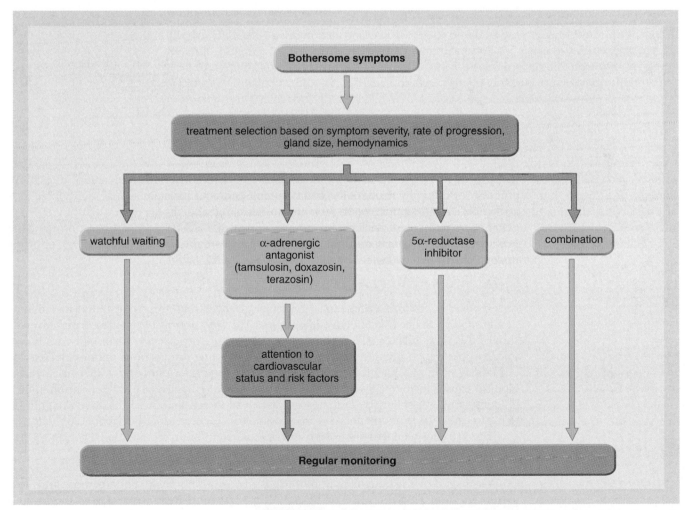

FIGURE 30-2 Summary of treatment options for BPH. *(From Page C, et al.: Integrated pharmacology, ed 3. Philadelphia, 2006, Mosby.)*

Summary of Drugs Used in the Treatment of Benign Prostatic Hyperplasia (BPH)

	Generic name	U.S. brand name	Usual adult oral dose and dosing schedule	Warning labels
α₁-Adrenergic antagonist				
	alfuzosin	Uroxatrol	10 mg once daily	DO NOT DISCONTINUE WITHOUT MEDICAL SUPERVISION
	doxazosin	Cardura	4 mg to 8 mg once daily	
	terazosin	Hytrin	10 mg at bedtime	MAY CAUSE DIZZINESS OR LIGHTHEADNESS
	tamsulosin	Flomax	0.4 mg once daily	AVOID DRIVING OR OPERATING HAZARDOUS MACHINERY
				SWALLOW WHOLE; DO NOT CRUSH OR CHEW—tamsulosin
				TAKE 30 MINUTES AFTER THE SAME MEAL EACH DAY—tamsulosin
5α-Reductase inhibitors				
	dutasteride	Avodart	0.5 mg once daily	SWALLOW CAPSULES WHOLE; DO NOT CHEW—dutasteride
	finasteride	Proscar	5 mg once daily	SWALLOW THE TABLETS WITH A DRINK OF WATER—finasteride
				PREGNANT WOMEN SHOULD AVOID CONTACT WITH BROKEN OR CRUSHED TABLETS

Erectile Dysfunction

ED is defined as a total inability to achieve erection, an inconsistent ability to achieve erection, or difficulty maintaining erection long enough to sustain sexual intercourse. It is also known as impotence. Up to 30 million American males have reported symptoms of ED. ED appears to increase with increasing age; however, it is not an evitable part of the aging process. By age 40 years, approximately 5% of males experience ED. By age 65, approximately 15% to 25% of males have ED.

WHAT CAUSES ERECTILE DYSFUNCTION?

An erection is produced pursuant to vascular changes that are orchestrated to enhance penile rigidity and enable effective intercourse. The smooth muscle of the corpus cavernosum of the penis relaxes. Arteries and sinusoids in the corpus cavernosum fill with blood. Intracorporal blood pressure increases, while at the same time venous outflow decreases.

ED may have physiological, psychological, neurological, or endocrinology causes. Physiological causes include age-related changes and chronic disease (e.g., hypertension, hyperlipidemia, multiple sclerosis). Diabetes is a disease of the endocrine system (see Chapter 33) that can cause vascular and nerve changes that affect erectile function. Depression may also produce ED. Lifestyle factors, smoking, obesity, and alcoholism are additional causes of ED.

Drugs Used in the Treatment of Erectile Dysfunction

ED is managed by the administration of drugs that promote penile engorgement and slow loss of erection. This control is orchestrated by relaxation and contraction of the smooth muscle in the corpus cavernosum. Neurotransmitters of the autonomic nervous system and the nonadrenergic noncholinergic system control relaxation and contractions. Neurotransmitters that promote relaxation produce an erection. They are listed in Box 30-2.

Nitric oxide is a mediator of smooth muscle relaxation and is released by the nonadrenergic noncholinergic system as a response to sexual stimulation. It activates several intracellular

BOX 30-2 NEUROTRANSMITTERS THAT RELAX SMOOTH MUSCLE IN THE PENIS

- Acetylcholine (ACh)
- Nitric oxide (NO)
- Prostaglandin E1 (PGE1)
- Vasoactive intestinal polypeptide (VIP)
- Calcitonin gene–related peptide (CGRP)

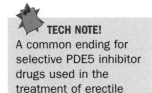

TECH NOTE!

A common ending for selective PDE5 inhibitor drugs used in the treatment of erectile dysfunction is *"-afil."*

enzymes, of which phosphodiesterase type 5 (PDE5), an enzyme that is involved in reversal of an erection, is one. Drugs currently marketed for the treatment of ED are PDE inhibitors and prostaglandin E analogs.

PHOSPHODIESTERASE INHIBITORS

MECHANISM OF ACTION

Sildenafil, tadalafil, and verdenafil are selective inhibitors of cyclic guanosine monophosphate (cGMP)-specific PDE5. They relax smooth muscle and blood vessels that supply the corpus cavernosum and control penile engorgement (Figure 30-3). At the cellular level, the drugs increase levels of nitric oxide (NO) in the corpus cavernosum, which blocks the opening of calcium voltage-gated channels and reduces calcium-mediated vascular contractions.

PHARMACOKINETICS

The oral absorption of sildenafil, vardenafil, and tadalafil is good, and maximum concentration (C_{max}) and onset of action of vardenafil are reached between 30 minutes and 2 hours after a dose of drug is administered. C_{max} for tadalafil and sildenafil is similar, averaging about 2 hours. The C_{max} may be reduced if the drugs are taken with a meal that is high in fat. Bioavailability can be reduced by up to 50%. Protein binding is approximately 94% to 95% for all PDEs.

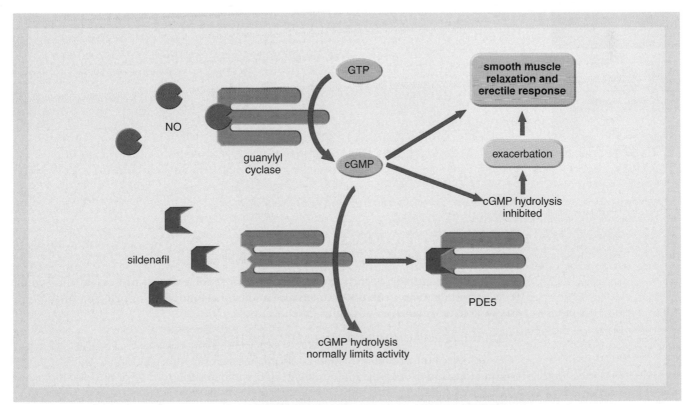

FIGURE 30-3 Mechanism of action for sildenafil. *(From Page C, et al.: Integrated pharmacology, ed 3. Philadelphia, 2006, Mosby.)* Sildenafil binds to receptors which blocks the degradation of cGMP and increases the effects of nitric oxide (No) on the corpus cavernosum (relaxation and increased erectile response).

ADVERSE REACTIONS

Many of the adverse reactions associated with the use of phosphodiesterase inhibitors are a result of vasodilatation. These side effects include dizziness, flushing, headache, and nasal congestion. Gastrointestinal side effects are diarrhea and indigestion. Sildenafil, tadalafil, and vardenafil may also produce visual effects that range from light sensitivity and difficulty distinguishing between green and blue, to loss of vision. The incidence of visual disturbances is greater with sildenafil than with vardenafil and tadalafil.

PRECAUTIONS

PDE inhibitors are involved in numerous drug interactions. A life-threatening drop in blood pressure has occurred in males who have taken nitrates such as nitroglycerin (for angina), so the use of nitrates, in all dosage forms, is contraindicated while taking PDE inhibitors. Concurrent administration of α-adrenergic agonists (e.g., alfuzosin, terazosin, doxazosin) used for the treatment of BPH requires caution. Other important drug interactions to avoid are concurrent administration of PDE inhibitors with antifungals (-*azoles*), cimetidine, grapefruit juice, and macrolide antiinfectives (e.g., erythromycin and clarithromycin). Drug interactions also occur with co-administration of selective serotonin reuptake inhibitor and monoamine oxidase inhibitor antidepressants.

Phosphodiesterase Inhibitors

	Generic name	U.S. brand name(s) Canadian brand(s)	Dosage forms and strengths
	sildenafil	Revatio,* Viagra	**Tablet:** 25 mg, 50 mg, 100 mg
		Revatio,* Viagra	
	tadalafil	Cialis	**Tablet:** 10 mg, 20 mg
		Cialis	
	verdenafil	Levitra	**Tablet:** 5 mg, 10 mg, 20 mg, 2.5 mg (U.S. only)
		Levitra	

*Used for the treatment of pulmonary hypertension.

PROSTAGLANDINS

Alprostadil is naturally occurring prostaglandin E_1 (PGE_1) that is present in the seminal vesicles and cavernous tissues of males. It can also be found in the placenta of the fetus. PGE_1 mediates relaxation of penile smooth muscle.

MECHANISM OF ACTION AND PHARMACOKINETICS

PGE_1 mobilizes intracellular calcium in the corpus cavernosum, resulting in smooth muscle contraction; however, in the endothelium, PGE_1 mediates the release of nitric oxide, which relaxes cavernosal smooth muscle, causing an erection.

Oral absorption of alprostadil is poor; therefore, the drug is formulated for intraurethral insertion and intracavernosal injection. The intracavernosal route of administration is more effective than the intraurethral route but has a higher incidence of pain and discomfort with administration of each dose.

ADVERSE REACTIONS

Adverse reactions are specific to the route of administration. Side effects caused by intra-cavernosal administration include hypotension, dizziness, bleeding, bruising, or pain at site of injection and painful erection. Adverse effects associated with intraurethral administration of alprostadil are itching in the penis, testicles, legs, and perineum; redness of the penis, warmth or burning sensation in the urethra, and leg swelling. Urethral bleeding or spotting may occur when the drug is administered improperly. Both dosage forms may produce prolonged erection (lasting longer than 4 hours).

INSTRUCTIONS FOR ADMINISTRATION OF INTRAURETHRAL PELLETS

1. Urinate prior to insertion and gently shake the penis.
2. Gently and slowly stretch the penis upward to its full length.
3. Slowly insert the stem of the applicator into the urethra up to the collar; then gently and completely push down the button at the top of the applicator until it stops (and medicated pellet is released).
4. Hold the applicator in this position for 5 seconds; then remove applicator while keeping the penis upright. Roll the penis firmly between the hands for at least 10 seconds to ensure that the medication is adequately distributed along the walls of the urethra.
5. An erection should begin to form within 10 minutes of application.

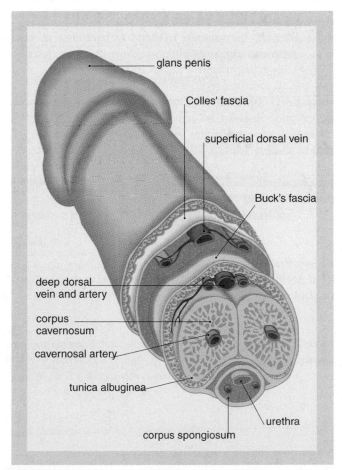

FIGURE 30-4 Structure of the penis. *(From Page C, et al.: Integrated pharmacology, ed 3. Philadelphia, 2006, Mosby.)*

INSTRUCTIONS FOR ADMINISTRATION OF INTRACAVERNOSAL INJECTION

1. Gently and slowly stretch the penis upward to its full length.
2. Insert the needle into the corpus cavernosum until the metal portion of the needle is almost completely into the penis. Avoid visible veins, urethra, and corpus spongiosum.
3. Slowly inject the contents of the syringe over 5 to 10 seconds.
4. Withdraw syringe and apply pressure to injection site for 5 minutes or until bleeding stops.

Prostaglandins

Generic name	U.S. brand name(s) / Canadian brand(s)	Dosage forms and strengths
alprostadil	Caverject, Muse, Prostin VR	**Injection, powder (Caverject):** 10 mcg, 20 mcg, 40 mcg
	Caverject, Muse, Prostin VR*	**Urethral insert (Muse):** 125 mcg, 250 mcg, 500 mcg, 1000 mcg
		Injection, solution (Prostin VR): 500 mcg/ml

*Prostin VR is administered as a continuous infusion to neonates with congenital heart disease such as ductus arteriosus, pumonary stenosis, or interruption of the aortic arch, until corrective surgery can be performed.

NONPHARMACOTHERAPEUTIC MANAGEMENT OF ERECTILE DYSFUNCTION

ED may also be treated by attaching a mechanical vacuum device to the penis, which uses suction to produce engorgement. An alternative approach is to surgically implant a device with inflatable tubes that can cause the penis to become erect. Vascular surgery may be performed to reconstruct arteries that supply the penis and to block off veins that allow blood to leak from penile tissue.

Summary of Drugs Used in the Treatment of Erectile Dysfunction

Generic name	U.S. brand name	Usual adult oral dose and dosing schedule	Warning labels
Phosphodiesterase inhibitors			
sildenafil	Viagra	25 to 100 mg ½ to 4 hours prior to sexual intercourse, not more than once daily	DO NOT DRINK ALCOHOL TO EXCESS (e.g., 5 glasses wine or 5 shots of whiskey)
tadalafil	Cialis	5 to 20 mg prior to sexual intercourse, not more than once daily or 2.5 to 5 mg once daily	MAY CAUSE DIZZINESS DO NOT TAKE WITHIN 4 HOURS OF TAKING α BLOCKERS (alfuzosin, doxazosin, or terazosin)
vardenafil	Levitra	5 to 20 mg up to 60 minutes prior to sexual intercourse, not more than once daily	AVOID GRAPEFRUIT JUICE
Prostaglandins			
alprostadil	Muse	Insert 1 pellet 30 to 60 minutes prior to sexual intercourse, not more than once daily	REFRIGERATE (may be stored at room temperature for 14 days)
	Caverject	Inject individualized dose not more than once in 24 hours or greater than 3 times per week	ROTATE SITE OF INJECTION MAY STORE AT ROOM TEMPERATURE FOR UP TO 3 MONTHS AVOID EXPOSURE TO EXTREMES IN HEAT OR COLD

CHAPTER SUMMARY

- The prostate gland is a part of the male reproductive system.
- Prostatitis is an inflamed or infected prostate gland.
- Benign prostatic hyperplasia (BPH) is a condition where noncancerous cells in the prostate grow and increase the size of the prostate gland.
- The risk for developing benign prostatic hyperplasia increases with age, and by age 85, approximately 90% of males will have BPH.
- A prostate specific antigen (PSA) test may be performed to determine if levels of the PSA protein are elevated. Higher than normal levels are a sign of BPH, infection, inflammation, or prostate cancer.
- Pharmacotherapy for BPH is initiated only when symptoms are uncomfortable enough to warrant treatment.
- Watchful waiting is recommended when patients are asymptomatic or symptoms do not produce much discomfort.
- Two classes of drugs are administered to manage symptoms: α-blockers and 5α-reductase inhibitors.
- A common ending for α-blockers *"-zosin."*
- α_1-Adrenergic antagonists relax prostate and bladder smooth muscle, which reduces urethral resistance and improves the flow of urine.
- Alfuzosin, doxazosin, terazosin, and tamsulosin bind to α_1-receptor sites. Prostate muscle tone is primarily controlled by binding to α_{1A}-receptor sites.
- Alfuzosin is available in immediate release and extended release dosage forms.
- Adverse drug effects linked to the administration of α-adrenergic antagonists are postural hypotension, dizziness, reflex tachycardia, headache, stuffy nose, weakness, and fatigue.
- A common ending for 5α-reductase inhibitors is *"-steride."*
- Finasteride and dutasteride are antiandrogens, capable of reducing testosterone levels.
- The effects of 5α-reductase inhibitors accumulate over time. It may take 6 to 12 months for therapeutic effects to be achieved.
- Dutasteride and finasteride are also harmful to the developing fetus. Pregnant women and women of child-bearing age should be advised to avoid contact with broken or crushed tablets. The use of barrier contraceptive is also recommended.
- Several surgical procedures are available for the management of prostate disease.
- Erectile dysfunction is defined as a total inability to achieve erection, an inconsistent ability to achieve erection, or difficulty maintaining erection long enough to sustain sexual intercourse.
- By age 65, approximately 15% to 25% of males have erectile dysfunction.
- Erectile dysfunction may have physiological, psychological, neurological, or endocrinology causes.
- Lifestyle factors, smoking, obesity, and alcoholism may cause erectile dysfunction.
- Erectile dysfunction is managed by the administration of drugs that promote penile engorgement and slow loss of erection.
- Drugs currently marketed for the treatment of erectile dysfunction are phosphodiesterase inhibitors and prostaglandin E analogs.
- A common ending for selective phosphodiesterase type 5 (PDE5) inhibitor drugs used in the treatment of erectile dysfunction is *"-afil."*
- Sildenafil, tadalafil, and verdenafil are selective inhibitors of cyclic guanosine monophosphate (cGMP)-specific PDE5.
- PDE5 inhibitors relax smooth muscle and blood vessels that supply the corpus cavernosum and control penile engorgement by increasing levels of nitric oxide.
- Side effects of PDE5 inhibitors are dizziness, flushing, headache, nasal congestion, diarrhea, indigestion, and visual disturbances.
- The administration of nitrates, such as nitroglycerin, in all dosage forms, is contraindicated in patients taking PDE inhibitors.
- Concurrent administration of α-adrenergic agonists (e.g., alfuzosin, terazosin, doxazosin) used for the treatment of BHP in patients taking PDE5 inhibitors should be done with caution.

- Alprostadil is a naturally occurring prostaglandin E_1 that is present in the seminal vesicles and cavernous tissues of males.
- Prostaglandin E_1 mediates relaxation of penile smooth muscle.
- Oral absorption of alprostadil is poor; therefore, the drug is formulated for intraurethral insertion and intracavernosal injection.
- Both dosage forms may produce prolonged erection (lasting longer than 4 hours).
- Erectile dysfunction may also be treated by attaching a mechanical vacuum device to the penis, which uses suction to produce engorgement.
- An alternative approach to treatment of erectile dysfunction is to surgically implant an inflatable device that can produce an erection.

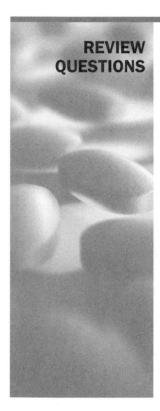

REVIEW QUESTIONS

Multiple Choice

1. Benign prostatic hyperplasia is a condition that is cancerous.
   a. true
   b. false
2. The first symptom(s) of an enlarged prostate gland is(are) _____.
   a. a weak or slow stream
   b. a delayed start in the flow or urine
   c. straining to urinate
   d. all of the above
3. Class(es) of drugs that are administered to manage symptoms of benign prostatic hyperplasia are _____.
   a. α-blockers and β-blockers
   b. α-reductase inhibitors and β-blockers
   c. α-blockers and α-reductase inhibitors
   d. all of the above
4. A common ending for α-blockers "-*zosin.*"
   a. true
   b. false
5. The generic name for Hytrin is _____.
   a. doxazosin
   b. tamulosin
   c. alfuzosin
   d. terazosin
6. Which of the following is *not* an adverse effect of dutasteride and finasteride?
   a. decreased desire for sex
   b. erectile dysfunction
   c. increased desire for sex
   d. reduced semen
7. Which of the following drugs is *not* used for erectile dysfunction?
   a. sildenafil
   b. penadafil
   c. tadalafil
   d. verdenafil

8. **Higher than normal levels of PSA are a sign of _____.**
   a. BPH
   b. infection, inflammation
   c. prostate cancer
   d. all of the above

9. **Finasteride and dutasteride are androgens, capable of reducing testosterone levels.**
   a. true
   b. false

10. **_____ are currently marketed for the treatment of erectile dysfunction.**
    a. phosphodiesterase inhibitors
    b. prostaglandin E analogs
    c. testosterone therapy
    d. all of the above

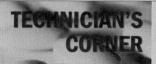

TECHNICIAN'S CORNER

1. What is the active ingredient in "saw palmetto" that promotes a healthy prostate gland?
2. What lifestyle changes can be made to prevent erectile dysfunction?

BIBLIOGRAPHY

American Urological Foundation: *Benign prostatic hyperplasia: Treatment choices*, 2005. Available at: www.AUAFoundation.org.

Lance L, Lacy C, Armstrong L, Goldman M: *Drug information handbook for the allied health professional,* ed 12. Hudson, OH, 2005, APhA Lexi-Comp.

National Information Clearinghouse: *Understanding prostate changes: A health guide for men.* Bethesda, MD, National Cancer Institute, National Institutes of Health, US Department of Health and Human Services, August 2004. NIH publication No. 02-5199. Available at: http://www.niddk.nih.gov.

National Kidney and Urological Diseases Information Clearinghouse: *Erectile dysfunction.* Bethesda, MD, National Institute of Diabetes and Digestive and Kidney Diseases, National Institutes of Health, US Department of Health and Human Services, December 2005. NIH publication No. 06-3923. Available at: http://www.kidney.niddk.nih.gov.

Page C, Curtis M, Sutter M, Walker M, Hoffman B: *Integrated pharmacology* (pp 495-500), Philadelphia, 2005, Mosby.

USP Center for Advancement of Patient Safety: *Use caution–avoid confusion,* USP Quality Review No. 79, Rockville, MD, April 2004, USP Center for Advancement of Patient Safety.

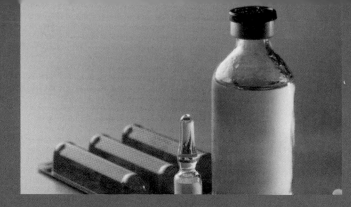

Treatment of Fluid and Electrolyte Disorders

LEARNING OBJECTIVES

- Learn the properties of electrolytes.
- Know the symptoms of electrolyte imbalances.
- Identify treatments for electrolyte imbalances.
- Describe mechanism of action for drugs used for the treatment of fluid and electrolyte disorders.
- Identify warning and precautionary messages associated with medications used for the treatment of fluid and electrolyte disorders.
- Identify significant drug look-alike/sound-alike issues.
- List common endings for drug classes used in the treatment of fluid and electrolyte imbalances.
- Learn terminology associated with fluid and electrolyte imbalances.

KEY TERMS

Anion: Negatively-charged particle.

Bicarbonate: Substance used as a buffer to maintain the normal levels of acidity (pH) in blood and other fluids in the body.

Cation: Positively charged electrolyte.

Chloride: Major anion (negatively-charged ion) found in the fluid outside of cells and in blood.

Colloids: Proteins or other large molecules that remain suspended in the blood for a long period of time and are too large to cross membranes.

Crystalloids: Intravenous solutions that contain electrolytes in concentrations resembling those of plasma.

Dehydration: Term used to describe the condition that results from excessive loss of body water.

Edema: Presence of abnormally large amounts of fluid in the intercellular tissue spaces of the body.

Electrolytes: Small, charged molecules essential for homeostasis that play an important role in body chemistry.

Extracellular fluid: Type of fluid that surrounds the cells and consists mainly of the plasma found in blood vessels.

Homeostasis: Constancy or balance that is maintained by the body despite constant changes.

Hyperchloremia: Condition in which the serum chloride level is higher than 107 mEq/L.

Hypernatremia: Elevation of the serum sodium concentration higher than 145 mEq/L.

Hyperkalemia: Condition in which the serum potassium level is above 5.5 mEq/L.

Hypertonic: Fluids with a higher osmolarity than serum.

Hypocalcemia: Condition in which the serum calcium level drops below 4.5 mEq/L.

Hypochloremia: Condition in which the serum chloride level is lower than 97 mEq/L.

Hypokalemia: Condition in which potassium is lost from the body, resulting in a serum potassium level below 3.5 mEq/L.

Hypomagnesemia: Condition in which the serum level of magnesium is below 1.5 mEq/L.

Hyponatremia: Condition of decreased serum sodium concentration below the normal range (less than 136 mEq/L).

Hypophosphatemia: Condition in which the serum phosphate level is defined as mild (2 to 2.5 mg/dl, or 0.65 to 0.81 mmol/L), moderate (1 to 2 mg/dl, or 0.32 to 0.65 mmol/L), or severe (<1 mg/dl, or 0.32 mmol/L).

Hypotonic: Fluid with less osmolarity than serum.

Intracellular fluid: Fluid inside cells.

Ions: Charged particles.

Isotonic fluids: Fluids close to the same osmolarity as serum.

Magnesium: Fourth most common cation in the body.

Millequivalents (mEq): Units used to measure the number of ionic charges or electro-valent bonds (electrolytes) in a solution.

Osmolarity: Osmotic pressure of a solution expressed as osmoles or millimoles per liter (mmol/L) of the solution.

Potassium: Main electrolyte in extracellular fluid.

Sodium: Chief electrolyte in interstitial fluid.

Overview of Fluid and Electrolyte Disorders

A *fluid and electrolyte disorder* is defined as an imbalance of electrolytes or fluids above or below the normal levels of serum concentrations in the body. The phrase "fluid and electrolyte balance" implies **homeostasis,** or constancy of body fluid and electrolyte levels. The volume of fluid and the electrolyte levels inside the cells, in the interstitial spaces, and in the blood vessels all remain relatively constant. For homeostasis to be maintained, body "input" of water and electrolytes must be balanced by "output." Fluid and electrolyte imbalance, then, means that both the total volume of water and the level of electrolytes in the body or the amounts in one or more of the compartments have increased or decreased beyond normal limits.

Electrolytes

Chemical bonds between molecules of certain chemical compounds break-up or disassociate when in solution. For example, sodium chloride (NaCl) disassociates into separate charged particles (Na^+ and Cl^-) that are called **electrolytes**. Positively-charged electrolytes are called **cations**. Examples of cations are calcium (Ca^{2+}), magnesium (Mg^{2+}), potassium (K^+), and sodium (Na^+). Negatively-charged ions are called **anions**. Examples of anions are bicarbonate (HCO_3^-), chloride (Cl^-), phosphate (PO_4^-), and sulfate (SO_4^{-2}).

The number of ionic charges or electrovalent bonds (electrolytes) in a solution is measured in **milliequivalents** (mEq). Common electrolytes that are measured by clinicians with blood testing include sodium, potassium, chloride, and bicarbonate. The normal range values for these electrolytes are described in Table 31-1.

Electrolytes are essential for homeostasis and play an important part in body chemistry. They circulate in the blood at specific levels where they are available when needed by the cells. An imbalance of electrolytes such as when levels are too high or too low can cause serious disease that requires treatment to restore balance in the body. Electrolytes are essential to many body functions such as nerve conduction, muscle contraction, and bone growth.

TABLE 31-1   Electrolyte Values

Electrolyte	Normal Adult Values
Calcium:	4.5 to 5.5 mEq/L
Chloride:	97 to 107 mEq/L
Potassium:	3.5 to 5.3 mEq/L
Magnesium:	1.5 to 2.5 mEq/L
Sodium:	135 to 145 mEq/L

Sodium is the major positive ion (cation) in fluid outside of cells. Sodium regulates the total amount of water in the body, and the transmission of sodium into and out of individual cells also plays a role in critical body functions. Many processes in the body, especially in the brain, nervous system, and muscles, require electrical signals for communication. The movement of sodium is critical in generation of these electrical signals. Too much or too little sodium therefore can cause cells to malfunction, and extremes (too much or too little) can be fatal. Excess sodium (such as from eating fast-food hamburgers and French fries) is excreted in the urine.

Potassium is the other major positive ion (cation) found inside of cells. The proper level of potassium is essential for normal cell function. Among the many functions of potassium in the body are regulation of the heartbeat and function of the muscles. A seriously abnormal increase of potassium (hyperkalemia) or decrease of potassium (hypokalemia) can profoundly affect the nervous system and increases the chance of irregular heartbeats (arrhythmias), which, when extreme, can be fatal.

Chloride is the major anion (negatively-charged ion) found in the fluid outside of cells and in blood. Seawater has almost the same concentration of chloride ion as human fluids. The balance of the chloride ion (Cl^-) is closely regulated by the body. Significant increases or decreases in chloride can have deleterious or even fatal consequences. Chloride plays a role in helping the body maintain a normal balance of fluids.

The bicarbonate ion acts as a buffer to maintain the normal levels of acidity (pH) in blood and other fluids in the body. The acidity is affected by foods or medications that we ingest and the function of the kidneys and lungs. The chemical notation for bicarbonate on most lab reports is HCO_3^- but may be represented as the concentration of carbon dioxide (CO_2). The normal serum range for bicarbonate is 22 to 30 mmol/L.

Magnesium, the fourth most common cation in the body, has been the recent focus of much clinical and scholarly interest. Previously underappreciated, this ion is now established as a central electrolyte in a large number of cellular metabolic reactions, including DNA and protein synthesis, neurotransmission, and hormone-receptor binding. It is a component of GTPase and a cofactor for Na^+,K^+-ATPase, adenylate cyclase, and phosphofructokinase. Magnesium also is necessary for the production of parathyroid hormone. Accordingly, magnesium deficiency has an effect on multiple body functions. Magnesium is present in greatest concentration within the cell and is the second most abundant intracellular cation after potassium. The total body content of magnesium is 2000 mEq. The intracellular concentration of magnesium is 40 mEq/L, while the serum concentration is 1.5 to 2 mEq/L. Most of the body's magnesium is found in bone. Only 1% of the total body magnesium is extracellular. Of this amount, one half is ionized, and 25% to 30% is protein bound.

Phosphorus is essential for membrane structure, energy storage, and transport in all cells. In particular, phosphate is necessary to produce ATP, which provides energy for nearly all cell functions. Phosphate is an essential component of DNA and RNA and is also necessary in red blood cells for the production of 2,3-diphosphoglycerate (2,3-DPG), which facilitates release of oxygen from hemoglobin. Approximately 85% of the body's phosphorus is in bone as hydroxyapatite, while most of the remainder (15%) is present in soft tissue. Only 0.1% of phosphorus is present in extracellular fluid, and it is this fraction that is measured with a serum phosphorus level.

Body Fluid Compartments

Functionally, the total body water can be divided into two major fluid compartments, called the extracellular and the intracellular fluid compartments. ***Extracellular fluid*** consists mainly of the plasma found in the blood vessels and the interstitial fluid that surrounds the cells. ***Intracellular fluid*** refers to the water inside the cells. When compared according to all sources of fluid volume in the body, intracellular fluid is the largest amount (25 L), plasma is the smallest amount (3 L), and interstitial fluid in between (12 L). The cardinal principal about fluid balance is this: Fluid balance can be maintained only if intake equals output.

Regulation of Water and Electrolyte Levels in Intracellular Fluid

It is the plasma membrane that separates the intracellular and extracellular fluid compartments. Most of the body sodium is outside of the cells. Sodium is the chief electrolyte by far in interstitial fluid. The main electrolyte of intracellular fluid is potassium. A change in the sodium or potassium concentration of either of these fluids causes the exchange of fluid between them to be unbalanced. Fluid balance depends on electrolyte balance. Conversely, electrolyte balance depends on fluid balance.

Types of Fluid and Electrolyte Disorders

Fluids and electrolytes are generally in equilibrium in the body. Internal body fluids, which are not leaked or excreted to the outside world, include those identified in Table 31-2. When fluid levels drop lower or go higher than normal, disorders result. This chapter will center on intracellular, interstitial, and plasma fluids.

DEHYDRATION

The term ***dehydration*** is used to describe a condition that results from excessive loss of body fluids. Water deprivation or loss triggers a complex series of protective responses designed to maintain homeostasis of water and electrolytes levels. If water intake is reduced to the point of dehydration, a corresponding quantity of electrolytes must be removed to maintain the normal ionic content of the body fluids. The same is true in the case of electrolyte loss when an accompanying loss of water must occur to maintain homeostasis of both fluid and electrolyte levels. Understanding the close interrelationships of water and electrolyte loss in dehydration provides the rationale for effective treatment. Signs and symptoms of dehydration include thirst, dry mucous membranes, weakness, dizziness, fever, low urine output, and poor skin turgor. Skin that is well hydrated will be elastic and quickly return to shape after being gently pinched.

Management of dehydration requires appropriate replacement therapy with oral electrolyte solutions, intravenous fluids with added electrolytes such as 0.9% sodium chloride, or normal saline. Water alone is inadequate (Box 31-1).

TABLE 31-2   Location of Body-Fluids

Body Fluid Types	Location in Body
Cerebrospinal fluid	Surrounding the brain and spinal cord
Synovial fluid	Surrounding bone joints
Intracellular fluid	Fluids inside cells
Blood	Connective tissue found all through the body mainly in blood vessels
Aqueous humor and vitreous humor	Fluids found in the eyeballs

BOX 31-1 MANAGEMENT AND TREATMENT OF DEHYDRATION

- Oral electrolyte solutions (mild diarrhea or vomiting)
- 2.0% to 2.5% glucose
- 0.9% Sodium chloride 75 to 90 mEq/L (parenteral)
- Sodium chloride 40 to 60 mEq/L (for rehydration and maintenance)

EDEMA

Edema is a classic example of fluid imbalance and may be described as the presence of abnormally large amounts of fluid in the intercellular tissue spaces of the body. Edema may occur in any organ or tissue of the body; however, the lungs, brain, and dependent body areas such as the legs and the lower part of the back are affected most often. One of the most common areas for swelling to occur is in the subcutaneous tissue of the ankle and foot. The following are causes of edema:

- Retention of electrolytes (especially Na^+) in the extracellular fluid
- An increase in capillary blood pressure. The general venous congestion of heart failure is the most common cause of widespread edema.
- A decrease in the concentration of plasma proteins normally retained in the blood. This can be caused by burns, infection, or shock.

HYPONATREMIA

Hyponatremia is a condition where serum sodium concentrations fall below the normal range (less than 136 mEq/L). Causes of hyponatremia include profuse perspiration (sweating), overzealous use of salt-wasting diuretics, adrenal insufficiency, renal or liver failure, low salt intake, or excessive water intake. Signs and symptoms of hyponatremia include muscle cramps, nausea and vomiting, cold and clammy skin, postural blood pressure changes, poor skin turgor, fatigue, and difficulty breathing, hypotension, irritability, and tachycardia. Cerebral swelling can occur in severe cases, causing confusion, hemiparesis (motor weakness on one side of the body), seizures, and coma.

Pseudohyponatremia occurs when too much water is drawn into the blood; it is commonly seen in people with hypoglycemia (low blood sugar).

Psychogenic polydipsia occurs in people who compulsively drink more than 4 gallons of water a day.

Hypovolemic hyponatremia (with low blood volume due to fluid loss) occurs in dehydrated people who rehydrate (drink a lot of water) too quickly, in patients taking thiazide diuretics, and after severe vomiting or diarrhea.

Hypervolemic hyponatremia (high blood volume due to fluid retention) occurs in people with live cirrhosis, heart disease, or nephrotic syndrome. Edema (swelling) often develops with fluid retention.

Euvolemic hyponatremia (decrease in total body water) occurs in people with hypothyroidism, adrenal gland disorder, and disorders that increase the release of the antidiuretic hormone (ADH), such as tuberculosis, pneumonia, and brain trauma.

CAN YOU REALLY DRINK TOO MUCH WATER?

In a word, yes. Drinking too much water can lead to a condition known as water intoxication and to a related problem resulting from the dilution of sodium in the body, hyponatremia. Water intoxication is most commonly seen in infants under 6 months of age and sometimes

BOX 31-2 MANAGEMENT AND TREATMENT OF EDEMA

- Treat underlying disease
- Decrease sodium and water intake
- Administer loop diuretics* (see Chapters 22 and 23)

*Loop diuretics (furosemide, bumetanide, and torsemide).

in athletes. A baby can get water intoxication as a result of drinking several bottles of water a day or from drinking infant formula that has been diluted too much. Athletes can also suffer from water intoxication. Athletes sweat heavily, losing both water and electrolytes.

WHAT HAPPENS DURING WATER INTOXICATION?

When too much water enters the body's cells, the tissues swell with the excess fluid. Your cells maintain a specific concentration gradient, so excess water outside the cells (the serum) draws sodium from within the cells out into the serum in an attempt to re-establish the necessary concentration. As more water accumulates, the serum sodium concentration drops—a condition known as hyponatremia. The other way cells try to regain the electrolyte balance is for water outside the cells to rush into the cells via osmosis. The movement of water across a semipermeable membrane from higher to lower concentration is called osmosis. Although electrolytes are more concentrated inside the cells than outside, the water outside the cells is 'more concentrated' or 'less dilute' because it contains fewer electrolytes. Both electrolytes and water move across the cell membrane in an effort to balance concentration. Theoretically, cells could swell to the point of bursting.

From the cell's point of view, water intoxication produces the same effects as would result from drowning in fresh water. Electrolyte imbalance and tissue swelling can cause an irregular heartbeat, allow fluid to enter the lungs, and may cause fluttering eyelids. Swelling puts pressure on the brain and nerves, which can cause behaviors resembling alcohol intoxication. Swelling of brain tissues can cause seizures, coma, and ultimately death unless water intake is restricted and a hypertonic saline (salt) solution is administered. If treatment is given before tissue swelling causes too much cellular damage, then a complete recovery can be expected within a few days.

HYPERNATREMIA

Hypernatremia is elevation of the serum sodium concentration to greater than 145 mEq/L. Causes of hypernatremia include lack of fluid intake, diarrhea, diabetes insipidus, loss of water via respiratory tract, heart disease or congestive heart failure, renal failure, and ingestion of salt in abnormal amounts. Signs and symptoms are similar to those of dehydration and include thirst, disorientation, lethargy, and seizures. The neurological symptoms are thought to be due to cerebral cellular dehydration. Administration of hypotonic solution helps lower the sodium level slowly, thereby reducing the risk of cerebral edema (Box 31-3).

HYPOKALEMIA

Hypokalemia is a condition in which potassium is lost from the body, resulting in a serum potassium level below 3.5 mEq/L. Causes of hypokalemia are overuse of potassium-wasting diuretics, increased urine output with loss of potassium, and vomiting or gastric suctioning without potassium replacement. Signs and symptoms include manifestations of anorexia, nausea, vomiting, depression, confusion, impaired thought processes, drowsiness, muscle weakness, decreased reflexes, low blood pressure, and cardiac arrhythmias.

HYPERKALEMIA

Hyperkalemia is a condition in which the serum potassium level is above 5.5 mEq/L. This can be even more dangerous than hypokalemia because myocardial muscle can be profoundly affected. Hyperkalemia can induce ventricular dysrhythmias, thereby possible

TECH NOTE!
Water "follows" sodium ions when they are moved through the cell membrane. Lots of sodium in the body means water stays inside (instead of leaving through kidney cells and then the bladder), which means there is more blood volume and blood pressure is higher.

BOX 31-3 MANAGEMENT OF HYPERNATREMIA AND HYPONATREMIA

HYPERNATREMIA
- Administration of hypotonic solution such as 0.45% NaCl (or ½ NS)

HYPONATREMIA
- Administration of sodium orally (salt tablets)
- Intravenous saline solution 3% sodium
- Water restriction

BOX 31-4 MANAGEMENT OF HYPERKALEMIA

- Restricting dietary intake of potassium in mild cases
- Emergency intravenous administration of calcium gluconate may be required to correct cardiac symptoms
- Dialysis to remove the excess potassium can be instituted to correct severe hyperkalemia

leading to cardiac arrest. Causes of hyperkalemia are kidney disease (most common), vomiting, diarrhea, potassium-conserving diuretics, extensive tissue damage as in burn or trauma victims, severe infections, and Cushing's syndrome. Signs and symptoms can include muscle weakness or failure of the respiratory muscles, intermittent diarrhea, nausea, vomiting, intestinal colic, irritability, anxiety, confusion, abdominal distress, and cardiac arrhythmias (Box 31-4).

HYPERCHLOREMIA

Elevations in chloride (*hyperchloremia*) may be associated with diarrhea, certain kidney diseases, and overactivity of the parathyroid glands. Hyperchloremia is often comorbid with diabetes or hyponatremia. Certain drugs, especially diuretics such as carbonic anhydrase inhibitors, hormonal treatments, and polypharmacy, may contribute to this disorder.

HYPOCHLOREMIA

Chloride is normally lost in the urine, sweat, and stomach secretions. Excessive loss can occur from heavy sweating, vomiting, and adrenal gland and kidney disease. Symptoms include dehydration, fluid loss, or high levels of blood sodium.

HYPOCALCEMIA

Hypocalcemia is a condition in which the serum calcium level falls below 4.5 mEq/L. Causes of hypocalcemia can be dietary deficiency, parathyroid disease, or accidental removal of the parathyroid glands during surgery of the thyroid gland. Signs and symptoms include tetany, muscle spasms, lethargy, and seizures.

HYPOMAGNESEMIA

Hypomagnesemia is a condition in which the serum level of magnesium is below 1.5 mEq/L. Hypomagnesemia may be caused by pregnancy-induced hypertension. Signs and symptoms include confusion, leg and foot cramps, hypertension, tachycardia, arrhythmias, weakness, nystagmus, neuromuscular irritability, tremor, hyperactive deep tendon reflexes, visual and auditory hallucinations, paresthesias, and seizures. Magnesium sulfate is used as replacement therapy in prevention and control of seizures in obstetric patients with pregnancy-induced hypertension.

HYPOPHOSPHATEMIA

Hypophosphatemia is a condition in which the serum phosphorus or phosphate level in adults is defined as mild (2 to 2.5 mg/dl, or 0.65 to 0.81 mmol/L), moderate (1 to 2 mg/dl, or 0.32 to 0.65 mmol/L), or severe (<1 mg/dl, or 0.32 mmol/L). Decreased dietary intake is a rare cause of hypophosphatemia because of the ubiquity of phosphate in foods. Certain conditions such as anorexia nervosa or chronic alcoholism may lead to hypophosphatemia. Signs and symptoms of hypophosphatemia are anorexia, bone or muscle weakness, respiratory failure, congestive heart failure, hemolysis, and rhabdomyolysis. Respiratory insufficiency may occur in some patients with severe hypophosphatemia, particularly when the underlying cause is malnourishment. Reducing available phosphate may compromise any organ system, alone or in combination. The critical role phosphate plays in every cell, tissue, and organ explains the systemic nature of injury caused by phosphate deficiency. As in the case of other intracellular ions (e.g., potassium, magnesium), a decrease in the level of serum

TECH NOTE!

0.9% Sodium chloride (NaCl) is also known as normal saline (NS) because it is the same concentration (isotonic) as in the body.

TECH ALERT!

The following drugs have look-alike/ sound-alike issues: Os-cal and Asacol; Citracal and Citrucel; calcium gluconate and calcium glubionate

TECH NOTE!

Many athletes consume oral electrolyte solutions e.g., Gatorade or Powerade

phosphate (hypophosphatemia) should be distinguished from a decrease in total body storage of phosphate (phosphate deficiency).

An electrolyte imbalance is diagnosed based on information gained from the following:
- History of symptoms
- Physical examination
- Urine and blood test results
- Electrocardiogram
- Ultrasound or radiography (if imbalance is caused by kidney problems)

Pharmaceuticals Used in the Treatment of Electrolyte Imbalances

The goal of treatment is to restore electrolyte balance for proper hydration and use of total body fluid. Electrolyte imbalances may be treated by the following means:
- Identifying the underlying problem
- Intravenous fluids
- Electrolyte replacement (many athletes consume Gatorade)
- Diet changes
- Restriction of water
- Fluid replacement

Electrolytes may be replaced via dietary or pharmaceutical therapy (Box 31-5).

BOX 31-5 MANAGEMENT OF ELECTROLYTE DEPLETION

• Diet rich in depleted electrolyte(s) • Dietary supplements	• Parenteral administration of depleted electrolyte(s), as necessary

Electrolyte Replacement Therapy—Sodium

Generic name	U.S. brand name(s) Canadian brand(s)	Dosage forms and strengths
sodium chloride*	Generics	**Intravenous solution:** 0.9% NaCl (NS), 0.45% NaCl (½ NS)
	Generics	**Solution for injection:** 2.5 mEq/ml, 4 mEq/ml, **Tablet:** 1 g

*Generic available.

Electrolyte Replacement Therapy—Chloride

Generic name	U.S. brand name(s) Canadian brand(s)	Dosage forms and strengths
ammonium chloride*	Generics	**Solution, injection:** 5 mEq/ml, 0.4 mEq/ml
	Generics	

*Generic available.

Electrolyte Replacement Therapy—Calcium

| Generic name | U.S. brand name(s) | Dosage forms and strengths |
	Canadian brand(s)	
calcium carbonate* (oyster shell calcium)	Calcium-600, Caltrate, Os Cal 500, Os Cal 1250, Tums, Tums Ex, Tums Ultra	**Tablets:** 500 mg, 600 mg, 750 mg, 1250 mg **Suspension:** 500 mg/5 ml, 1250 mg/5 ml
	Caltrate-600, Tums	
calcium citrate*	Cal-Citrate,	**Tablet (Cal-Citrate):** 250 mg
	—	
calcium gluconate†*	Generics	**Injection:** 100/ml **Tablet:** 500 mg, 648 mg, 650 mg, 972 mg
	Generics	
calcium chloride‡*	Generics	**Injection:** 1 g/10 ml
	—	
calcium lactate*	Ridactate	**Tablet:** 650 mg
	Generics	

*Generic available.
†Calcium is also used as an adjunct therapy for insect bites and stings to reduce muscle cramping (black widow spider bites).
‡Calcium chloride should not be given IM or SC because severe tissue necrosis can occur.

Electrolyte Replacement Therapy—Potassium

| Generic name | U.S. brand name(s) | Dosage forms and strengths |
	Canadian brand(s)	
potassium chloride*	Effer-K, Kaon, Kay Ciel, Klor Con M10, Klor Con M15, Klor Con M20, K-Lyte, Klotrix, K-Tab, Micro-K	**Capsule (Micro-K):** 8 mEq, 10 mEq **Tablet (K-Tab, Kaon Cl-10, Klor Con M10, Klotrix):** 600 mg (8 mEq), 750 mg (10 mEq), 1125 mg, 1500 mg **Liquid (Kaon):** 20 mEq/15 ml **Effervescent powder (K-Lyte, Kay Ciel):** 25 mEq, 1.5 g **Effervescent tablet (Effer K):** 25 mEq **IV (in D$_5$W):** 20 mEq/mL, 30 mEq, 40 mEq
	K-10, Kaochlor-10, Kaochlor-20, Roychlor, K-Lor, K-Lyte/Cl	
potassium gluconate*	Generics	**Oral liquid (Kaon):** 1.33 mEq/ml **Tablet:** 595 mg
	Kaon	
potassium acetate*	Generics	**Solution, injection:** 2 mg/ml
	Not available	

*Generic available.

Electrolyte Replacement Therapy—Phosphorus

Generic name	U.S. brand name(s)	Dosage forms and strengths
phosphorous salts*	K-Phos Original, Neutra Phos K	**Tablet (K-Phos Original):** 500 mg **Powder for solution (Neutra Phos K):** 14.25 mEq phosphate + 14.25 mEq potassium **Solution, injection (potassium phosphate):** 236 mg potassium phosphate (dibasic) + 224 mg potassium phosphate (monobasic) **Solution, injection (sodium phosphate):** 268 mg/ml sodium phosphate (dibasic) + 276 mg/ml sodium phosphate (konobasic); 142 mg sodium phosphate (dibasic) + 276 mg sodium phosphate (monobasic)

*Generic available.

Table 31-3 shows the phosphate, sodium, and potassium content of selected preparations of sodium phosphate and potassium phosphate.

TABLE 31-3 Phosphate, Sodium, and Potassium Content of Selected Preparations of Sodium Phosphate and Potassium Phosphate

Preparations of Sodium Phosphate and Potassium Phosphate	Dosage Forms and Strengths	Sodium Phosphate Content	Potassium Phosphate Content
Oral Preparations			
Skim cow's milk	1 g/L	28 mEq/L	38 mEq/L
Neutra-Phos	250 mg/packet	7.1 mEq/packet	7.1 mEq/packet
Neutra-Phos K	250 mg/capsule	0	14.25 mEq/capsule
K-Phos Original	150 mg/capsule	0	3.65 mEq/capsule
K-Phos Neutral	250 mg/tablet	13 mEq/tablet	1.1 mEq/tablet
Intravenous Preparations			
Neutral sodium potassium PO_4	1.1 mmol/ml	0.2 mEq/ml	0.02 mEq/ml
Neutral sodium potassium PO_4	0.09 mmol/L	0.2 mEq/ml	0
Sodium PO_4	3.0 mmol/ml	4.0 mEq/ml	0
Potassium PO_4	3.0 mmol/ml	0	4.4 mEq/ml

Electrolyte Replacement Therapy—Magnesium

Generic name	U.S. brand name(s)	Dosage forms and strengths
magnesium sulfate*	Mag-200	**Solution, injection:** 50%, 40 mg/ml, 80 mg/ml **Tablet (Mag-200):** 200 mg, 400 mg
magnesium oxide*	Mag-Ox 400, Mag-gel 600, Uro-Mag	**Tablet (Mag-Ox):** 400 mg **Capsule:** 140 mg (Uro-Mag); 600 mg (Mag-gel)
magnesium gluconate*	Mag-G, Magonate, Magtrate	**Liquid, oral (Magonate):** 54 mg/5 ml **Tablet (Mag-G, Magtrate):** 500 mg
magnesium chloride*	Chloromag	**Solution, injection:** 200 mg/ml
magnesium lactate*	Mag-Tab	**Tablet, extended release:** 84 mg

*Generic available.

Loop Diuretics

Generic name	U.S. brand name(s) Canadian brand(s)	Dosage forms and strengths
bumetanide*	Bumex	**Injection, solution:** 0.25 mg/ml **Tablet:** 0.5 mg, 1 mg, 2 mg (1 mg, 5 mg Canada)
	Burinex	
furosemide*	Lasix	**Injection, solution:** 10 mg/ml **Solution, oral:** 10 mg/ml; 40 mg/5 ml **Tablet:** 20 mg, 40 mg, 80 mg
	Lasix, Lasix Special	
torsemide*	Demadex	**Injection, solution:** 10 mg/ml **Tablet:** 5 mg, 10 mg, 20 mg, 100 mg
	Not available	

*Generic available.

TECH NOTE!
[*Lactated Ringer's
solution contains
28 mmol/L lactate,
4 mmol/L
potassium (K^+), and
3 mmol/L calcium
(Ca^{2+}).]

TECH ALERT!
K-Phos-Neutral and
Neutra-Phos-K have
look-alike and
sound-alike issues.

TECH ALERT!
The following drugs
have look-alike/
sound-alike issues:
magnesium sulfate,
morphine sulfate, and
manganese sulfate;
Magonate and Magtrate

Treatment of Fluid and Electrolyte Disorders with Intravenous Fluids

More than 200 types of commercially-prepared IV fluids are available to treat fluid and electrolyte imbalances. IV solutions are used to replace fluids and electrolytes that have been lost or provide volume replacement that has been lost through hemorrhage, severe burns, diarrhea, vomiting, or inadequate fluid intake; to administer medication; to provide electrolyte balance; for amino acid utilization; and to monitor cardiac functions.

IV electrolyte solutions may be classified as isotonic, hypotonic, or hypertonic according to their osmolality (tonicity)—the concentration of ions in a solution (Figure 31-1). The osmolality of blood plasma is approximately 290 mOsm/L. Fluids in the range of 240 to 340 mOsm/L are considered isotonic. Fluids with tonicities above 340 mOsm/L are hypertonic, and those with tonicities below 240 mOsm/L are hypotonic.

Isotonic fluids are close to the same osmolarity as serum. They remain inside the intravascular compartment, thus expanding it. They can be helpful in hypotensive or hypovolemic patients; however, their use may cause overloading, especially in patients with congestive heart failure (CHF) and hypertension.

Hypotonic fluids have less osmolarity than serum. They dilute the serum and pull fluids into cells; decreasing serum osmolarity. Water is then pulled from the vascular compartment into the interstitial fluid compartment. As the interstitial compartment is diluted, its osmolarity decreases, which draws water into adjacent cells. Hypotonic solutions can be helpful when cells are dehydrated, such as in a dialysis patient who is on diuretic therapy. They may also be used for hyperglycemic conditions such as diabetic ketoacidosis, in which high serum glucose levels draw fluid out of the cells and into the vascular and interstitial compartments. Hypotonic solutions are not given to patients who are hypotensive, as they can further increase the lowered blood pressure. They can cause a dangerous shift

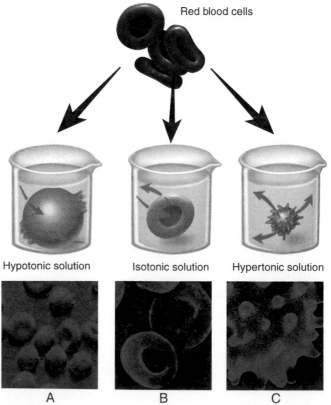

FIGURE 31-1 Beakers filled with Hypotonic/Isotonic/Hypertonic solutions. *(From Thibodeau GA, Patton KT:* Anatomy and physiology, *ed 6. St. Louis, 2007, Mosby.)*

in fluid from the intravascular space to the cells resulting in cardiovascular collapse and increased intracranial pressure.

Hypertonic fluids have a higher osmolarity than serum. They pull fluid and electrolytes from the intracellular and interstitial compartments into the intravascular compartment and can help stabilize blood pressure, increase urine output, and reduce edema.

IV fluids may be grouped into categories called colloids and crystalloids.

Colloids are proteins or other large molecules that remain suspended in the blood for a long period of time because they are too large to cross membranes. While circulating, they draw water molecules from the cells to the tissues into blood vessels through their ability to increase osmotic pressure. These agents are sometimes called plasma or volume expanders. Examples of colloids include plasma protein fraction, albumin, dextran 40, and hetastarch. Blood itself is a colloid.

Crystalloids are IV solutions that contain electrolytes in concentrations resembling those of plasma. Unlike colloids, crystalloids solutions leave the blood and enter cells. They are used to replace fluids that have been lost and promote urine output. Common crystalloids include normal saline (NS), lactated Ringer's, plasmalyte, hypertonic saline (3% sodium chloride), and 5% dextrose in water (D_5W) (Table 31-4).

If additional medications are required to be administered to a patient placed on an IV electrolyte solution, the piggyback method provides an intermittent IV drip of a second solution through the venipuncture site of an established primary IV system (Figure 31-2). The piggyback technique eliminates the need for another venipuncture and dilutes the medication to reduce irritation.

TABLE 31-4 Common Crystalloid Solutions Used for Intravenous Administration

Type of solution	Solution	Uses	Adverse effects
Isotonic	Dextrose 5% in sterile water (D_5W)	Fluid loss Dehydration Hypernatremia	Can cause fluid overload Use cautiously in renal and cardiac patients.
Isotonic	0.9% Sodium chloride (normal saline [NS])	Hyponatermia Blood transfusion Shock Resuscitation	Can lead to fluid overload Use cautiously In patients with heart failure (HF) or edema.
Isotonic crystalloid	Lactated Ringer's solution (LR)	Burns Dehydration Acute hemorrhage	Use cautiously in renal patients because of potassium content. Use cautiously in liver patients—cannot metabolize lactate.
Hypotonic crystalloid	0.45% Sodium chloride (½ NS)	Fluid (water) replacement Fluid loss from vomiting	May cause cardiovascular collapse or increase intracranial pressure Do not use in patients with liver disease, burns, or trauma.
Hypertonic	Dextrose 5% and 0.9% sodium chloride (D_5 NS)	Temporary treatment for shock, Addison's disease crisis	Do not use in cardiac or renal patients.
Hypertonic	Dextrose 10% in sterile water or $D_{10}W$	Water replacement Malnutrition	Monitor blood glucose levels.
Hypertonic	Dextrose 5% and 0.45% NaCl (D_5 and ½ NS)	Use when blood glucose levels fall below 250 mg/dl	Use cautiously in surgical patients and those with circulatory insufficiency and in pregnancy.

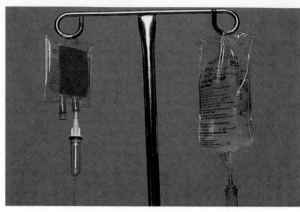

FIGURE 31-2 Piggyback method. *(From Hopper T: Mosby's pharmacy technician, ed 2. St. Louis, 2007, WB Saunders.)*

Summary of Drugs Used in the Treatment of Fluid and Electrolyte Disorders

Drug name	Usual dose and dosing schedule	Warning label(s)
Loop diuretics		
bumetanide	0.5 mg to 2 mg twice daily	MAY BE ADVISABLE TO EAT BANANAS OR DRINK ORANGE JUICE
furosemide	20 mg to 80 mg twice a day	MAY CAUSE DIZZINESS OR LIGHTHEADNESS
torsemide	2.5 mg to 10 mg daily	AVOID PROLONGED EXPOSURE TO SUNLIGHT
		SOME OTC DRUGS CAN AGGRAVATE YOUR CONDITION
Electrolyte replacement		
sodium chloride	**Hyponatremia and dehydration:** **IV:** individualized **Oral:** 650 mg to 2.25 g as directed for specific product (max: 4.8 g/day)	TAKE WITH A FULL GLASS OF WATER (Oral)
calcium carbonate	**Hypocalcemia:** 2 g to 4 g/day of elemental calcium (5 g to 10 g calcium carbonate), given in 3 to 4 divided doses	TAKE WITH FOOD—calcium carbonate AVOID FERROUS PRODUCERS WITHIN 1 TO 2 HOURS OF DOSE (May decrease iron absorption) TAKE 1-3 HOURS AFTER MEALS—calcium glubionate
calcium chloride	500 mg to 1 g in 1- to 3-day intervals	DO NOT INJECT CACLIUM CHLORIDE IM Or SEVERE SLOUGHING OR NECROSIS MAY OCCUR
potassium chloride	20 mEq/day given in 1 to 2 divided doses	TAKE WITH WATER SWALLOW WHOLE; DON'T CRUSH OR CHEW—extended release DILUTE EFFERVESCENT POWDERS AND TABS IN WATER OR JUICE

Summary of Drugs Used in the Treatment of Fluid and Electrolyte Disorders—cont'd

Drug name	Usual dose and dosing schedule	Warning label(s)
magnesium sulfate	25 mg/kg to 50 mg/kg/dose every 4 to 6 hours	MONITOR ARRHYTHMIAS, HYPOTENSION MAY CAUSE RESPIRATORY AND CNS DEPRESSION
magnesium oxide	250 mg to 1.5 g four times a day	
potassium phosphate K-Phos Neutral	**Hypophosphatemia:** **IV:** 0.5mmol/kg to 0.25 mmol/kg IV over 4 to 6 hours **Oral:** 700 mg per day	MONITOR FOR DIARRHEA OR SIGNS OF HYPERMAGNESEMIA

CHAPTER SUMMARY

- The phrase "fluid and electrolyte balance" implies homeostasis, or constancy, of body fluid and electrolyte levels. For homeostasis to be maintained, body "input" of water and electrolytes must be balanced by "output."
- Electrolytes are essential to many body functions such as nerve conduction, muscle contraction, and bone growth.
- Functionally, the total body water can be divided into two major fluid compartments, called the extracellular and the intracellular fluid compartments. *Extracellular fluid* consists mainly of the plasma found in the blood vessels and the interstitial fluid that surrounds the cells. *Intracellular fluid* refers to the water inside the cells.
- There are many causes of electrolyte imbalances, such as hormonal or endocrine disorders, kidney disease, dehydration, an inadequate diet, lack of dietary vitamins, malabsorption, and medications.
- The goal of treatment is to restore electrolyte balance and restore for proper hydration.
- An electrolyte imbalance is diagnosed based on information gained from the history of symptoms, physical examination, urine and blood test results, electrocardiography, ultrasonography, or radiography (if imbalance is caused by kidney problems).
- The term "dehydration" is used to describe the condition that results from excessive loss of body water.
- Edema is a classic example of fluid imbalance and may be described as the presence of abnormally large amounts of fluid in the intercellular tissue spaces of the body.
- Intravenous solutions are used to replace fluids and electrolytes that have been lost and to provide calories through their carbonate content.
- There are three main types of IV fluids: isotonic, hypotonic, and hypertonic.
- There are two main groups of fluids: crystalloid and colloid.

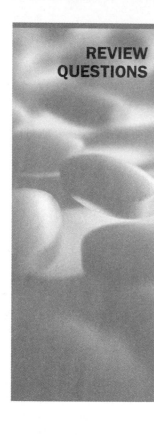

REVIEW QUESTIONS

Multiple Choice

1. A cation is a negatively-charged electrolyte and an anion is a positively-charged particle.
   a. true
   b. false

2. Fluids close to the same osmolarity as serum are called _____.
   a. hypotonic
   b. isotonic
   c. hypertonic
   d. serotonic

3. Which of the following is *not* an example of an electrolyte?
   a. calcium
   b. magnesium
   c. selenium
   d. sodium

4. Electrolytes are essential to many body functions such as _____.
   a. nerve conduction
   b. muscle contraction
   c. bone growth
   d. all of the above

5. Which of the following electrolytes is important for the regulation of the heartbeat and function of the muscles?
   a. calcium
   b. potassium
   c. sodium
   d. magnesium

6. The _____ ion acts as a buffer to maintain the normal levels of acidity (pH) in blood and other fluids in the body.
   a. chlorine
   b. magnesium
   c. bicarbonate
   d. phosphate

7. Which of the following is necessary to produce ATP, which provides energy for nearly all cell functions?
   a. phosphate
   b. bicarbonate
   c. citrate
   d. all of the above

8. Two types of fluid disorders are _____ and _____.
   a. edema and hydration
   b. dehydration and shock
   c. hyponatremia and hypomagnesmia
   d. water intoxication and diarrhea

9. What are two types of intravenous (IV) fluids used to treat fluid imbalances?
   a. crystalloids and osmoloids
   b. osmoloids and colloids
   c. colloids and crystalloids
   d. all of the above

10. Furosemide is the generic name for Bumex.
    a. true
    b. false

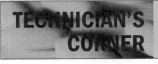

1. Why is the intake of water so important for proper cell function?
2. What types of food provide potassium?

BIBLIOGRAPHY

Fulcher EM, Fulcher RM, Soto CD: *Pharmacology: Principles and applications,* ed 2 (Appendix XI: Intravenous administration basics,). Philadelphia, 2005 Saunders.

Harris P, Nagy S, Vardaxis N: *Mosby's dictionary of medicine, nursing, and health professions* (pp 625, 626, 1008-1011), ed 7. Philadelphia, 2005, Elsevier Mosby.

http://en.wikipedia.org/wiki/IntravenousTherapy.

http://www.ncbi.nlm.nih.gov/sites/entrez?cmd=retrieveanddb=PubMedandlist_uids-3587116.

Martin S: *Intravenous therapy, business briefing, long term healthcare strategies* (pp 1-4). Fort Lauderdale, FL, 2003, College of Allied Health and Nursing, Nova Southeastern University.

Phillips B: *Critical care medicine: Electrolyte replacement, a review.* Boston, Boston Medical Center, Boston University of Medicine. Available at: http://www.ispub.com/ostia/index.php?xmlFilePath=journals/ijim/vol5n1/electrolytes.xml.

www.drugs.com.

www.rxlist.com.

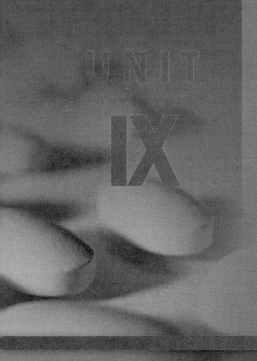

Drugs Affecting the Endocrine System

LEARNING
OBJECTIVES

- Identify the target organs and understand the functions of the endocrine system.
- Explain the process of the negative feedback system.
- Understand the importance of hormones in maintaining homeostasis.

Organization of the Endocrine System

The endocrine system and nervous system both function in a regulatory way to achieve and maintain stability of the internal environment. In the endocrine system, these regulatory functions are performed by chemical messengers called hormones. Unlike neurotransmitters, which are sent over short distances across synapse and rapidly produce effects,

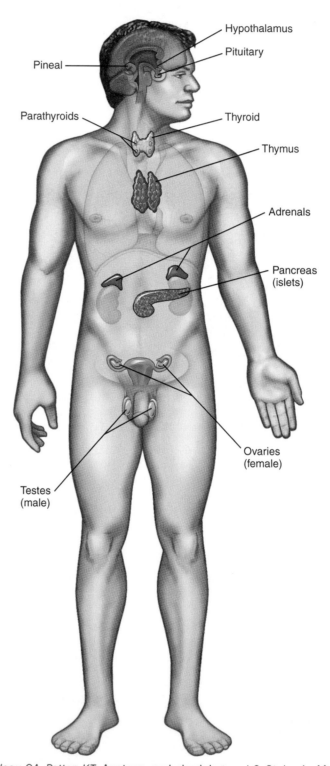

(From Thibodeau GA, Patton KT: Anatomy and physiology, ed 6, St. Louis, Mosby, 2007.)

hormones diffuse into the blood to be carried to nearly every point in the body and their effects appear more slowly and last longer. Endocrine glands are known as "ductless glands" because they secrete hormones directly into the blood.

Hormones

CLASSIFICATION OF HORMONES

Hormones are classified by their target site, their chemical composition (steroid or non-steroid), and whether they are hydrophilic or hydrophobic. *Tropic* hormones target other endocrine glands and stimulate their growth and secretion. Sex hormones target reproductive tissues. Anabolic hormones stimulate anabolism in their target cells.

STEROID HORMONES

Hormones secreted by endocrine tissues can be classified simply as steroid or non-steroid. Examples of important steroid hormones include cortisol, aldosterone, estrogen, progesterone, and testosterone. Estrogen, progesterone, and testosterone are sex hormones.

NONSTEROID HORMONES

Most nonsteroid hormones are proteins and are synthesized primarily from amino acids rather than from cholesterol. Insulin, parathyroid hormone (PTH), growth hormone (GH), prolactin (PRL), calcitonin (CT), glucagon, and adrenocorticotropic hormone (ACTH) are protein hormones. Protein hormones that have carbohydrates groups attached to the amino acids chains are classified as *glycoprotein hormones* and include follicle-stimulating hormone (FSH), leutinizing hormone (LH), thyroid-stimulating hormone (TSH), and human chorionic gonadotropin (hCG). Another category of nonsteroid hormones are *peptide hormones*. Examples of peptide hormones are oxytocin (OT), antidiuretic hormone (ADH), melatonin-stimulating hormone (MSH), somastatin (SS), thyrotropin-releasing hormone (TRH), gonadotropin-releasing hormone (GnRH), and atrial natriuretic hormone (ANH). Yet another category of nonsteroid hormones consists of amino acid derivative hormones derived from a single amino acid molecule. There are two subgroups within this category— *amine hormones* (epinephrine and norepinephrine) and those produced by the thyroid gland thyroxine (T_4) and triiodothyroinine (T_3).

How Hormones Work

Hormones signal a cell by binding to a specific receptor on or in the cell. In a "lock-and-key" mechanism, hormones will only bind to receptor molecules that "fit" them exactly. Any cell with more than one receptor for a particular hormone is said to be a target for that hormone. Hormones travel to their target cells by way of the circulating bloodstream. Because they only affect their target cells, the effects of a particular hormone may be limited to specific tissues in the body.

MECHANISM OF ACTION FOR STEROID HORMONES

Steroid hormones are lipids and are not very soluble in blood plasma. They attach to soluble plasma proteins and dissociate before approaching the target cell. After a steroid hormone diffuses into the cell, it passes into the nucleus where it binds to a hormone-receptor complex. Steroid hormones regulate cells by regulating their production of certain critical proteins, such as enzymes.

MECHANISM OF ACTION FOR NONSTEROID HORMONES

THE SECOND MESSENGER ACTION

Nonsteroid hormones typically operate according to a mechanism called the second messenger model. A nonsteroid hormone acts as the "first messenger" delivering its chemical messenger to fixed receptors on target cell's plasma membrane. The "messenger" is then passed into the cell where a "second messenger" triggers the appropriate cellular changes. In short, the first messenger hormone binds to a membrane receptor, triggering formation of an intracellular second messenger, which activates a cascade of chemical reactions that produce the target's cell response.

THE NUCLEAR-RECEPTOR MECHANISM

Not all nonsteroid hormones operate according to the second-messenger model. The iodinated amino acids thyroxine (T_4) and triiodothyronine (T_3) enter the target cells and bind to receptors already associated with a DNA molecule within the nucleus of the target cell.

Regulation of Hormone Secretion

The control of hormonal secretion is usually part of a ***negative feedback loop***. Secretion by many endocrine glands is regulated by a hormone produced by another gland. Secretion of hormones by the anterior pituitary gland is regulated by releasing hormones or inhibiting hormones secreted by the hypothalamus. Another mechanism that may influence the secretion of hormones by a gland is input from the nervous system. For example, secretion from the posterior pituitary gland is not regulated by releasing hormones but by direct nervous system input from the hypothalamus. Likewise, sympathetic nerve impulses that reach the medulla of the adrenal glands trigger the secretion of epinephrine and norepinephrine. Many other glands, including the pancreas, are also influenced to some degree by nervous system input.

Regulation of Target Cell Sensitivity

The sensitivity of a target cell to any particular hormone partly depends on how many receptors for that hormone it has. Production of too much hormone by a diseased gland is called ***hypersecretion***. If too little hormone is produced, the condition is called ***hyposecretion***.

Prostaglandins

The ***prostaglandins*** are a unique group of lipid molecules but do not meet the usual definition of a hormone. The term "tissue hormone" is appropriate because their secretion is produced in a tissue and diffuses only a short distance to other cells within the same tissue, thus integrating the activities of neighboring cells.

Secretory Glands

PITUITARY GLAND (HYPOPHYSIS)

The pituitary gland has been known as the "master gland." This gland has a stemlike stalk, the ***infundibulum***, which connects to the hypothalamus of the brain. The pituitary gland is divided into two parts: the ***adenohypophysis*** or anterior pituitary gland and the ***neurohypophysis*** or posterior pituitary gland. The release of hormones from the adenohypophysis is controlled by chemicals made in the hypothalamus called releasing hormones. The hypothalamus, through its releasing hormones, integrates the endocrine system and the nervous system particularly in times of stress. When survival is threatened, the hypothalamus can take over the adenohypophysis and thus gain control of every cell in the body. The neurohypophysis serves as a storage and release site for two hormones—antidiuretic hormone (ADH) and oxytocin, which are made by the hypothalamus and controlled by nervous stimulation.

THYROID GLAND

The thyroid gland is located in the neck on the anterior and lateral surfaces of the trachea, just below the larynx. Thyroid hormones are tetraiodothyronine (T_4) or thyronine, triiodothyronine (T_3), and calcitonin. Calcitonin helps control calcium levels in the body by increasing bone formation of osteoblasts and inhibiting bone breakdown by osteoclasts. It may slightly decrease blood calcium levels and promote conservation of hard bone matrix.

PARATHYROID GLANDS

There are four to five **parathyroid glands** embedded in the posterior surface of the thyroid's lateral lobes. They secrete parathyroid hormone (PTH), which, along with calcitonin, maintains calcium homeostasis. PTH acts on bone and kidney cells to increase the

Hormones of the Pituitary Gland

Hormone	Source	Principal Action	Target Organ
Growth hormone (somatotropin)	Adenohypophysis	Promotes body growth by stimulating protein anabolism and fat mobilization	Bone, muscle, other tissues
Prolactin	Adenohypophysis	Initiates milk secretion (lactation)	Mammary glands
Thyroid-stimulating hormone (thyrotropin)	Adenohypophysis	Promotes and maintains the growth and development	Thyroid gland
Adrenocorticotropic hormone (adrenocorticotropin)	Adenohypophysis	Promotes and maintains normal growth of the adrenal cortex	Adrenal gland (Cortex)
Follicle-stimulating hormone (FSH)	Adenohypophysis	**Female:** promotes development of ovarian follicles; stimulates estrogen secretion **Male:** promotes development of testes; stimulates sperm production	Ovaries, Testes (gonads)
Luteinizing hormone (LH)	Adenohypophysis	**Female:** Triggers ovulation; promotes development of corpus luteum **Male:** stimulates production of testosterone	Ovaries, Testes (gonads)
Antidiuretic Hormone	Neurohypophysis	Promotes water retention by kidney tubules; raises blood pressure by contraction of muscles in arterial walls	Kidney, small arteries
Oxytocin	Neurohypophysis	Stimulates the contractions of uterine muscles; stimulates ejection of milk into the ducts of lactating women	Uterus, mammary glands

release of calcium into the blood causing less new bone to be formed and more old bone to be dissolved. PTH increases the body's absorption of calcium from food by activating Vitamin D in the kidney, which then can be transported through the intestinal cells and into the blood.

ADRENAL GLANDS

The *adrenal glands* are located atop the kidneys, fitting like a cap over these organs. The outer portion of the gland is called the *adrenal cortex* and secretes three sets of hormones: mineralcorticoids, glucocorticocoids, and sex hormones. The inner portion is called the *adrenal medulla* and secretes two important hormones—epinephrine and norepinephrine. Both are in the class of nonsteroid hormones called catecholamines. Epinephrine or adrenaline, accounts for about 80% of the medulla's secretion. The other 20% is norepinephrine.

Hormones of the Adrenal Glands

	Hormone	Source	Principal Action	Target Organ
	Aldosterone (mineralcorticoids)	Adrenal Cortex	Stimulates kidney tubules to conserve sodium, which triggers the release of ADH, which then causes the conservation of water by the kidney	Kidney
	Cortisol (glucocorticoid)	Adrenal Cortex	Influences metabolism of food molecules; in large amounts, it has an antiinflammatory effect	General body
	Adrenal androgens (sex hormone)	Adrenal Cortex	Exact role uncertain but may support sexual function	Sex organs
	Adrenal estrogens (sex hormone)	Adrenal Cortex	Thought to be physiologically insignificant	Sex organs
	Epinephrine	Adrenal Medulla	Enhances and prolongs the effect of the sympathetic division of the autonomic nervous system	Sympathetic nervous system
	Norepinephrine	Adrenal Medulla	Enhances and prolongs the effects of the sympathetic division of the autonomic nervous system	Sympathetic nervous system

PANCREATIC HORMONES

The *pancreas* is an elongated gland lying at the beginning of the small intestine behind the stomach and touching the spleen. The tissue of the pancreas is made up of both endocrine and exocrine tissue. The endocrine portion is made up of scattered islands of cells called pancreatic islets (*islets of Langerhans*). These hormone-producing cells are surrounded by cells called *acini*, which secrete a serous fluid containing digestive enzymes that drain into the small intestine. The pancreatic islets cells are the *alpha* (α) *cells* which secrete the hormone glucagon, *beta* (β) *cells*, which secrete the hormone insulin, *delta cells*, which secrete the hormone somatostatin, and pancreatic polypeptide cells, which secrete pancreatic polypeptide.

Hormones of the Pancreatic Islets

	Hormone	Source	Principal Action	Target Organ
	Glucagon	Alpha (α) cells	Promotes increase of blood glucose levels by stimulating conversion of glycogen to glucose in liver cells	General tissues in the body
	Insulin	Beta (β) cells	Promotes movement of glucose, amino acids, and fatty acids out of the blood into tissue cells	General tissues in the body
	Somatostatin	Delta (δ) cells	Can have general effects on the body but primary role is to regulate pancreatic hormones	Pancreatic cells and other effectors
	Pancreatic Polypeptide	Pancreatic islets	Exact function uncertain but seems to influence absorption in the digestive tract	Intestinal cells and effectors

GONADS

Gonads are the primary sex organs in the male (testes) and female (ovaries). Each is structured differently and each produces its own set of hormones. The testes are composed mainly of coils of sperm-producing seminiferous tubules with a scattering of endocrine interstitial cells found in the area between the tubules. These interstitial cells produce *androgens* (male sex hormones); the principal androgen is testosterone. The ovaries are a set of paired glands in the pelvis that produce several types of sex hormones including estrogen and progesterone. Regulation of ovarian hormone secretion basically depends on changing levels of follicle-stimulating hormone (FSH) and leutinizing hormone (LH) from the adenohyophysis.

Hormones of the Gonads

Hormone	Source	Principal Action	Target Organ
Testosterone	Testes	Stimulates sperm production; stimulates growth and maintenance of male sexual characteristics, promotes muscle growth	Sperm-producing tissues of the testes, muscles and other tissues
Estrogen	Ovaries	Stimulates the development of female sexual characteristics, breast development, bone and nervous system maintenance	Uterus, breasts, and other tissues
Progesterone	Ovaries	Maintains the lining of the uterus necessary for successful pregnancy	Uterus, mammary glands, other tissues

Additional Hormones of the Body

Additional Hormones

Hormone	Source	Principal Action	Target Organ
Melatonin	Pineal gland	Helps "set" the biological clock by signaling light changes during the day, month, seasons; may help to induce sleep	Nervous system
Human chorionic gonadotropin (hCG)	Placenta	Stimulates secretion of estrogen and progesterone during pregnancy	Ovary
Thymosins and thymopoietins	Thymus gland	Stimulate development of T lymphocytes, which are involved in immunity	Certain lymphocytes (white blood cells)
Gastrin	Stomach mucosa	Triggers increased gastric juice secretion	Exocrine glands of stomach
Secretin	Intestinal mucosa	Increase alkaline secretions of the pancreas and slows emptying of the stomach	Stomach and pancreas
Cholecystokinin (CCK)	Intestinal mucosa	Triggers the release of bile from gallbladder and enzymes from the pancreas	Gallbladder and pancreas
Ghrelin	Stomach mucosa	Stimulates hypothalamus to boost appetite; affects energy balance in various tissues	Hypothalamus; other diverse tissues
Atrial natriuretic hormone (ANH)	Heart muscle	Promotes loss of sodium from the body into urine, thus promoting water loss and a decrease in blood volume and pressure	Kidney

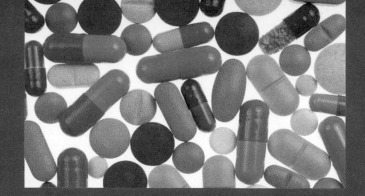

CHAPTER 32

Treatment of Thyroid Disorders

LEARNING OBJECTIVES

- Learn the terminology associated with thyroid disorders.
- List symptoms of hyperthyroidism and hypothyroidism.
- Describe the pathophysiology of hyperthyroidism and hypothyroidism.
- List and categorize medications used to treat hyperthyroidism and hypothyroidism.
- Describe mechanism of action for each class of drugs used to treat hyperthyroidism and hypothyroidism.
- Identify warning labels and precautionary messages associated with medications used to treat hyperthyroidism and hypothyroidism.
- Identify significant drug look-alike/sound-alike issues.
- List common endings for drug classes used in the treatment of hyperthyroidism and hypothyroidism.

KEY TERMS

Antithyroid drugs: Group of drugs administered to treat hyperthyroidism.

Graves' disease: Autoimmune disorder that causes hyperthyroidism.

Hashimoto's disease: Autoimmune disorder that causes hypothyroidism.

Hyperthyroidism: Condition in which there is an excessive production of thyroid hormones.

Hypothyroidism: Condition in which there is insufficient production of thyroid hormones.

Radioactive iodine uptake (RAIU): Test, using radioactive iodine, to screen for thyroid disease.

T_4 test: Measure of "free" circulating thyroid hormone.

Thyroid antibody test: Diagnostic test used to measure levels of thyroid antibodies that are diagnostic for autoimmune thyroid disease.

Thyroid releasing factor (TRF): Hormone released by the hypothalamus that stimulates the pituitary gland to release thyroid-stimulating hormone.

Thyroid stimulating hormone (TSH): Hormone released by the pituitary gland that stimulates the thyroid gland to produce and release thyroid hormones.

Tetraiodothyronine (T_4): Most abundant thyroid hormone. It contains 4 atoms of iodine and is also known as thyroxine.

Triiodothyronine (T_3): Hormone secreted by the thyroid gland. It contains 3 atoms of iodine.

TSH test: Diagnostic test to measure the level of thyroid-stimulating hormone in the blood.

Overview

More than 27 million Americans and 1 in 20 Canadians have abnormally active thyroid glands and half of the cases are undiagnosed. The disease affects greater than 200 million persons worldwide. Thyroid disorders result in overactivity of the thyroid gland or underactivity of the thyroid gland causing hypersecretion or hyposecretion of thyroid hormones, respectively. Risk factors of thyroid disease are gender, disease (e.g., diabetes and glycogen storage disease), aging, and pregnancy. Hyperthyroidism and hypothyroidism are more prevalent in women than in men and represent approximately 80% of patients diagnosed with thyroid disease. Women have a 5 to 8 times greater prevalence of hypothyroidism than do men, and hyperthyroidism is most common in women between the ages of 20 and 40 years. Diabetes is also a risk factor for thyroid disease; and diabetics as well as their parents and siblings are at increased risk. The incidence of hypothyroidism increases with age, and by age 60, up to 17% of women and 9% of men will have an underactive thyroid. Cigarette smoking increases the risk for developing thyroid-related eye disease. Smokers with Graves' disease are 5 times more likely than nonsmokers to develop thyroid-associated ophthalmopathy (TAO).

The thyroid gland secretes hormones that have an affect on nearly all cells in the body. ***Tetraiodothyronine (T$_4$)*** and ***triiodothyronine (T$_3$)*** are thyroid hormones and they function to regulate growth and metabolism. The physiologic actions of thyroid hormone are listed in Box 32-1. Calcitonin, another hormone secreted by the thyroid gland, helps to maintain calcium homeostasis.

THYROID HORMONE CONTROL

Thyroid levels are tightly controlled by the negative feedback loop. When an increased need for thyroid hormones is required, the hypothalamus secretes ***thyroid-releasing factor (TRF)***, a hormone that signals the pituitary to release ***thyroid-stimulating hormone (TSH)***. The target site of TSH is the thyroid gland, which produces and secretes T$_4$ and T$_3$. Once desired levels are achieved, TSH release in turned off (Figure 32-1).

SYNTHESIS OF THYROID HORMONES

The thyroid gland is one of the few glands that produces and stores its hormones. Thyroid hormones (T$_4$, T$_3$) are synthesized by a coupling process in which atoms of iodine are bound to the thyroid protein thyroglobulin. The process is activated by the oxidation of the enzyme peroxidase. When one atom of iodide is bound to thyroglobulin, the resultant product is monoiodotyrosine (MIT). When two atoms bind to thyroglobulin, the product formed is diiodotyrosine (DIT). Monoiodotyrosine (MIT) combines with diiodotyrosine (DIT) to form triiodothyronine (T$_3$). When two DIT molecules combine, tetraiodothyronine (T$_4$) is formed. Tetraiodothyronine is more commonly called thyroxine. In the body, T$_4$ is converted to T$_3$ by the process of deiodination.

Diagnosis of Thyroid Disorders

Diagnostic tests are available to determine the cause for excess or deficient thyroid hormone levels. The ***TSH test*** measures the level of thyroid-stimulating hormone in the blood. A low TSH level signals hyperthyroidism. This is to be expected because TSH levels are regulated by

BOX 32-1 PHYSIOLOGIC ACTIONS OF THYROID HORMONES

- Growth of skeletal tissues
- Fetal growth and development (cognitive and physical)
- Growth and development of the central nervous system
- Regulation of protein, lipid, and carbohydrate metabolism
- Regulation of hepatic metabolic enzymes
- Regulation of body temperature
- Cardiac functions (heart rate and contractility)
- Circulatory volume
- Respiratory functions
- Peripheral vasodilation
- Bone turnover
- Skin and soft tissue effects

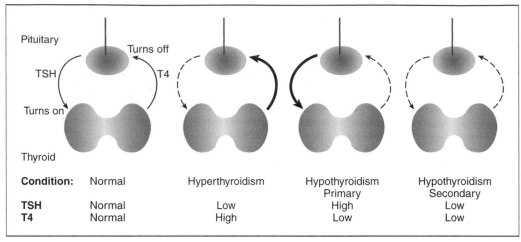

FIGURE 32-1 Comparison of TSH and T_4 levels for normal, hyperthyroidism, and hypothyroidism. *(Courtesy of the American Thyroid Association, www.thyroid.org.)*

the negative feedback loop. TSH release is "turned off" because the body recognizes the T_4 levels are high and is attempting to stop its further production and release. A high TSH level is a signal for hypothyroidism. A **T_4 test** measures "free" T_4 (FT4) and the free T_4 index (FT4I). FT4 and FT4I levels are high when hyperthyroidism is present and low when a person has hypothyroidism. The FT4 and FT4I test measures circulating thyroid hormone. In hyperthyroidism, FT4 levels are elevated and TSH levels are depressed. The reverse is true in the case of hypothyroidism. The presence of thyroid stimulating antibodies can be measured by administering a **thyroid antibody test**. When thyroid antibodies are present, autoimmune thyroid disease is diagnosed. A **radioactive iodine uptake (RAIU)** test may also be conducted to test for thyroid disease. Iodine is selectively taken up by the thyroid gland in the process of synthesizing thyroid hormones, T_4 and T_3 (Figure 32-2); thus, when a low dose of

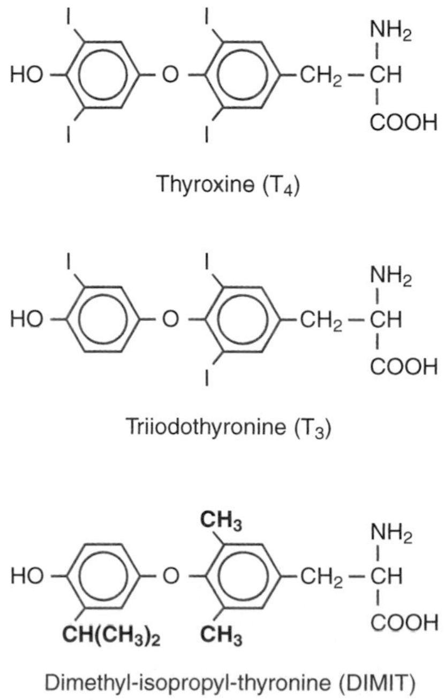

Thyroxine (T_4)

Triiodothyronine (T_3)

Dimethyl-isopropyl-thyronine (DIMIT)

FIGURE 32-2 Structural formula of thyroid hormones. *(From Kalant H, Grant DM, Mitchell J:* Principles of medical pharmacology, *ed 7, Philadelphia, 2007, WB Saunders.)*

radioactive iodine (^{131}I) is administered, the amount of radioactivity in the thyroid gland can be measured. The RAIU is very high when a person has hyperthyroidism and low when the person has hypothyroidism.

Types of Thyroid Disorders

HYPERTHYROIDISM

Hyperthyroidism is a condition in which the thyroid gland secretes excessive amounts of thyroid hormones. Conditions known to cause hyperthyroidism are (1) thyroid nodules (lumps on the thyroid gland that secrete thyroid hormone) and (2) inflammation of the thyroid gland (e.g., subacute thyroiditis, postpartum thyroiditis, and lymphatic thyroiditis). Graves' disease is autoimmune disease and a primary cause of thyroid hyperactivity. Thyroid-stimulating antibodies called thyroid-stimulating immunoglobulins (TSIs) mimic thyroid-stimulating hormone. When TSA binds to receptors on the thyroid gland, the gland releases hormones (see Figure 32-1). Circulating TSA is not sensitive to the negative feedback loop that turns off thyroid hormone release when levels are elevated.

SYMPTOMS OF HYPERTHYROIDISM

Given that thyroid hormones have an effect on numerous cells throughout the body, it is not surprising that symptoms of thyroid disease are widespread.

Symptoms of hyperthyroidism are listed in Box 32-2.

TREATMENT OF HYPERTHYROIDISM

Treatment of hyperthyroidism involves the administration of antithyroid drugs or radioactive iodine or surgery. Despite the knowledge that Graves' disease is an autoimmune disorder selectively affecting the thyroid gland, there are currently no effective therapies that block autoantibodies.

Radioactive Iodine

TECH NOTE!
Radioactive iodine ^{131}I is made in nuclear pharmacies and is regulated by the Nuclear Regulatory Commission (NRC). The limit for radioactive iodine (^{131}I) in workplace air is 2×10^{-8} microcurie per milliliter (μCi/ml).

Low-dose radioactive iodine is used for diagnosis, and higher-dose radioactive iodine is administered for the treatment of hyperthyroidism. It is selectively taken up by the thyroid gland, where it causes glandular destruction without producing damage to other tissues. The rate of cure is approximately 66%. Pretreatment with an antithyroid drug is recommended for about 2 weeks to block synthesis of thyroid hormone prior to the administration of iodine-131 (^{131}I). The full effects of ^{131}I therapy are achieved after 2 to 3 months in most people, but sometimes a second or third course of therapy is required. β-blockers may be administered concurrently with ^{131}I until tachycardia and tremors, symptoms of hyperthyroidism, subside. Radioactive iodine that is not retained by the thyroid is eliminated into the urine within 2 or 3 days.

Adverse Reactions. Treatment with ^{131}I produces few adverse effects. The most common side effect is temporary inflammation of the salivary glands. Most patients also develop an underactive thyroid gland after treatment, requiring lifelong therapy for hypothyroidism.

Precautions. Radioactive iodide therapy is contraindicated in pregnant women because

BOX 32-2 SYMPTOMS OF HYPERTHYROIDISM

- Palpitations or fluttering in the chest
- Rapid heart rate
- Muscle weakness
- Muscle wasting
- Tremor
- Shortness of breath
- Nervousness
- Excitability
- Restlessness
- Enlarged thyroid (goiter)
- Amenorrhea
- Breast enlargement
- Bulging eyes
- Rapid speech
- Sweating
- Facial flushing
- Heat intolerance, warm skin
- Weight loss

the drug can cross the placenta and cause thyroid damage in the developing fetus. Nursing mothers should also avoid breastfeeding until radioactive iodine can no longer be detected in their breast milk. Nonpregnant women and men treated with radioactive iodide should avoid close physical contact with pregnant women and young children for a few days after the dose is administered.

Radioactive Iodine (^{131}I)

Generic name	U.S. brand name(s)	Dosage forms and strengths
	Canadian brand(s)	
radioactive iodine (^{131}I)*	No commercial preparations	Individualized
	No commercial preparations	

*Generic available.

Thioamides

Thioamides are thiourea derivatives and are classified as antithyroid drugs. They are used for the primary treatment of hyperthyroidism or to deplete excess thyroid hormone in patients awaiting treatment with radioactive iodine or thyroid surgery.

Mechanism of Action and Pharmacokinetics. Propylthiouracil (PTU) and methimazole block the synthesis of T_4 and T_3. They bind thyroid peroxidase enzyme, which is the enzyme that activates the coupling of iodine and thyroglobulin and inhibits coupling of iodinated tyrosine (MIT and DIT). Only propylthiouracil is capable of blocking the deiodination process that converts T_4 to T_3. It takes 2 to 4 months of therapy with propylthiouracil before maximum effects are achieved, because thioamides do not antagonize the activity of thyroid hormones stored in the follicles of the thyroid gland. They only stop the synthesis of new thyroid hormone.

Adverse Reactions. Methimazole and PTU may cause nausea or vomiting, muscle aches and pains, or minor rash or itching. Side effects requiring medical attention are fever accompanied by sore throat and hoarseness, goiter, severe redness or itching, hepatitis, arthritis, and unusual bleeding, bruising, or red spots. Methimazole and PTU may also produce a dangerous drop in white blood cells (agranulocytosis), which increases the risk for serious infections. Dosages greater than 40 mg/day of methimazole may increase the risk for agranulocytosis.

Like radioactive thryoid therapy, treatment with antithyroid drugs typically induces hypothyroidism. Hypothyroidism may appear as soon as 6 months after the onset of therapy or as many as 25 years after disease remission and discontinuation of drug therapy.

Thioamides

Generic name	U.S. brand name(s)	Dosage forms and strengths
	Canadian brand(s)	
methimazole*	Tapazole	**Tablet:** 5 mg, 10 mg
	Tapazole	
propylthiouracil*	Generics	**Tablet:** 50 mg, 100 mg (Canada only)
	Propyl-Thyracil	

*Generic available.

HYPOTHYROIDISM

Hypothyroidism is a condition in which the thyroid gland secretes deficient amounts of thyroid hormones. Conditions known to cause hypothyroidism are (1) treatment for hyperthyroidism with radioactive iodine and antithyroid drugs; (2) treatment with medications for non–thyroid-related conditions (e.g., lithium, amiodarone); (3) thyroidectomy (removal of all or a portion of the thyroid gland); (4) pituitary gland damage that affects TSH secretion; (5) congenital conditions (birth defects); and (6) thyroiditis. Autoimmune thyroiditis occurs when the body produces antibodies to its own thyroid cells. The antibodies and white blood cells attack and damage the thyroid. Hashimoto's disease is an autoimmune disorder that causes hypothyroidism. Note that postpartum thyroiditis and subacute thyroiditis are also listed as a cause of hyperthyroidism. This is because both conditions may be followed by a period of temporary hypothyroidism.

SYMPTOMS OF HYPOTHYROIDISM

The effects of insufficient thyroid hormones can be felt throughout the body. Symptoms of hypothyroidism are listed in Box 32-3.

TREATMENT OF HYPOTHYROIDISM

TECH NOTE!

With the exception of liotrix, the generic name of thyroid replacement hormones contains the name of the naturally occurring hormone(s) they replace. For example, levothyroxine in the replacement for naturally occurring thyroxine.

Thyroid replacement therapy is the principal treatment for hypothyroidism. Replacement can be achieved by the administration of dessicated (dried, powdered) whole gland animal thyroid or synthetic T_4, synthetic T_3, or a ratio of the two hormones. The most prescribed treatment for hypothyroidism is synthetic T_4, which is converted in the body to T_3.

Mechanism of Action

Exogenously administered thyroid hormones, animal gland and synthetic, bind to the same receptor sites and produce the same actions as thyroid hormones produced by the body. Synthetic T_4, known as levothyroxine or L-thyroxin, is commonly the only thyroid hormone prescribed for the treatment of hypothyroidism. Additional administration of liothyronine is typically unnecessary because levothyroxine is converted to liothyronine in the body, just as naturally occurring T_4 is metabolized to T_3.

Pharmacokinetics

Liothyroinine (T_3) and levothyroxine are dissimilar in their onset and duration of action. They also differ in potency and dosing frequency. A comparison of the two drugs is shown in Table 32-1.

BOX 32-3 SYMPTOMS OF HYPOTHYROIDISM

- Slowed heart rate
- Slowed pulse
- Lethargy
- Dry, coarse hair
- Deep, coarse voice
- Slow speech, thick tongue
- Enlarged heart
- Hypertension
- Cold intolerance
- Facial swelling

TABLE 32-1 Comparison Between Liothyronine and Levothyroxine

Liothyronine	Levothyroxine
T_3	Synthetic T_4
Rapid onset	Longer onset
Short duration	Longer duration
Half-life (T½) up to 24 hours	T½ greater than 7 days
3 to 4 times more potent	Less potent
Administered in divided doses	Once daily dosing

BOX 32-4 MEDICATIONS THAT INTERACT WITH THYROID HORMONES

- Ferrous products (iron supplements)
- Calcium supplements and dairy products
- Soy isoflavones
- Food
- Raloxifene
- Cholestyramine

- Colestipol
- Oral contraceptives
- Phenytoin
- Carbamazepine
- Didanosine

 TECH NOTE!
Pharmacy technicians should attempt to dispense the same manufacturer's product each time the patient's prescription is refilled.

Bioavailability issues exist between different manufacturer's formulations of synthetic and naturally occurring thyroid preparations.

Numerous medications interact with thyroid hormones (Box 32-4). Ferrous products, calcium supplements, cholesterol-lowering agents (colestipol and cholestyramine), and didanosine interfere with the absorption of thyroid hormones. Food delays absorption. Antiseizure medicines, such as phenytoin and carbamazepine, accelerate the rate of metabolism of thyroid hormones. Soy isoflavones, oral contraceptives, and raloxifene reduce the clinical response to administered thyroid hormone by altering TSH, thyroglobulin, and T_4 and T_3 levels.

Adverse Reactions
Given that thyroid replacement therapy is achieved by administering naturally occurring or synthetic thyroid hormone, adverse effects produced are the same as symptoms of hypothyroidism (subtherapeutic doses) or symptoms of hyperthyroidism (taking too much thyroid hormone).

Precautions
Diabetic patients may require an adjustment in their dose of diabetes medicine once thyroid replacement therapy is initiated. Thyroid hormones can affect blood sugar levels.

Thyroid Replacements

	Generic name	U.S. brand name(s) / Canadian brand(s)	Dosage forms and strengths
	levothyroxine* (T_4)	Levothroid, Levoxyl, Synthroid, Unithroid Eltroxin, Euthrox,	**Powder, injection:** 0.2 mg, 0.5 mg **Tablet:** 0.025 mg, 0.05 mg, 0.075 mg, 0.88 mg, 0.1 mg, 0.112 mg, 0.125 mg, 0.137 mg, 0.15 mg, 0.175 mg, 0.2 mg, 0.3 mg
	liothyronine* (T_3)	Cytomel, Triostat Cytomel	**Solution, injection (Triostat):** 10 mcg/ml **Tablet:** 25 mcg, 50 mcg, 5 mcg (US only)
	liotrix* ($T_4:T_3$)	Thyrolar Not available	**Tablet:** levothyroxine 12.5 mcg + liothyronine 3.1 mcg levothyroxine 25 mcg + liothyronine 6.25 mcg levothyroxine 50 mcg + liothyronine 12.5 mcg levothyroxine 100 mcg + liothyronine 25 mcg levothyroxine 150 mcg + liothyronine 37.5 mcg
	dessicated thyroid*	Armour Generics	**Tablet:** 15 mg, 30 mg, 60 mg, 90 mg, 120 mg, 180 mg, 240 mg, 300 mg **Capsule:** 15 mg, 30 mg, 60 mg, 90 mg, 120 mg, 180 mg, 240 mg

*Generic available.

Summary of Drugs Used in the Treatment of Thyroid Disorders

Generic name	Brand name	Usual dose and dosing schedule	Warning labels
Hyperthyroidism			
methimazole	Tapazole	15 mg to 60 mg in 1 to 3 divided doses/day	TAKE ON AN EMPTY STOMACH OR WITH FOOD, BUT ALWAYS TAKE IT THE SAME WAY
propylthiouracil	Generics	Begin 300 mg to 1200 mg divided in 3 doses/day, maintenance 100 mg to 150 mg every 8 to 12 hours	AVOID PREGNANCY
radioactive iodine ^{131}I	Manufactured in pharmacy	6 to 15 mCi [microcuries (μCi)] as a single dose	AVOID PREGNANCY
Hypothyroidism			
levothyroxine	Synthroid, Levothroid	25 mcg to 150 mcg once daily	AVOID ANTACIDS, DAIRY, AND FE^{++} WITHIN 4 HOURS OF DOSE
liothyronine	Cytomel	25 mcg to 75 mcg once daily	TAKE ON AN EMPTY STOMACH
liotrix	Thyrolar	50 mcg to 100 mcg T$_4$ + 12.5 mcg to 25 mcg T$_3$ once daily	TAKE WITH A FULL GLASS OF WATER
desiccated thyroid	Generics	60 mg once daily	DON'T SKIP DOSES

TECH ALERT!

The following drugs have look-alike/ sound-alike issues: levothyroxine and liothyronine; Levoxyl, Luvox, and Lanoxin; Synthroid and Symmetrel

TECH NOTE!

The various strengths of levothyroxine are color-coded to help avoid dispensing errors.

TECH NOTE!

Sometimes the strength of dessicated thyroid is written as the grain strength. For example, 60 mg thyroid is equivalent to gr 1 thyroid.

CHAPTER SUMMARY

- Thyroid disorders result in overactivity of the thyroid gland or underactivity of the thyroid gland causing hypersecretion or hyposecretion of thyroid hormones, respectively.
- Hyperthyroidism and hypothyroidism are more prevalent in women than in men. Women have a 5 to 8 times greater prevalence of hypothyroidism than do men.
- Hyperthyroidism is most common in women between the ages of 20 and 40 years.
- Diabetics as well as their parents and siblings are at increased risk for developing thyroid disease.
- The incidence of hypothyroidism increases with age, and by age 60, up to 17% of women and 9% of men will have an underactive thyroid.
- Cigarette smoking increases the risk for developing thyroid-related eye disease.
- The thyroid gland secretes hormones that have an affect on nearly all cells in the body. Tetraiodothyronine (T$_4$) and triiodothyronine (T$_3$) are thyroid hormones, and they function to regulate growth and metabolism.
- The thyroid gland is one of the few glands that produces and stores its hormones.
- Thyroid hormones (T$_4$, T$_3$) are synthesized by a coupling process in which atoms of iodine are bound to the thyroid protein thyroglobulin. The process is activated by the oxidation of the enzyme peroxidase.
- Monoiodotyrosine (MIT) combines with diiodotyrosine (DIT) to form triiodothyronine (T$_3$). When two DIT molecules combine, tetraiodothyronine (T$_4$) is formed.
- The TSH test measures the level of thyroid-stimulating hormone in the blood. A low TSH level signals hyperthyroidism.
- Free T$_4$ index (FT4I) or FT4 levels are high when hyperthyroidism is present and low when a person has hypothyroidism.
- When thyroid antibodies are present, autoimmune thyroid disease is diagnosed.
- Low-dose radioactive iodine (^{131}I) is administered to measure the amount of radioactivity take up by the thyroid gland.
- High-dose ^{131}I is administered to treat hyperthyroidism.

- The RAIU is very high when a person has hyperthyroidism and low when the person has hypothyroidism.
- Hyperthyroidism is a condition in which the thyroid gland secretes excessive amounts of thyroid hormones.
- Thyroid-stimulating antibodies (TSAs) called thyroid-stimulating immunoglobulins mimic TSH. When TSA binds to receptors on the thyroid gland, the gland releases hormones.
- Graves' disease is an autoimmune disease that causes hyperthyroidism.
- Treatment of hyperthyroidism involves the administration of antithyroid drugs or radioactive iodine or surgery.
- Radioactive iodine is selectively taken up by the thyroid gland, where it causes glandular destruction without producing damage to other tissues. The rate of cure is approximately 66%. Pretreatment with an antithyroid drug is recommended.
- The full effects of ^{131}I therapy are achieved after 2 to 3 months in most people.
- Most patients treated with ^{131}I develop an underactive thyroid gland after treatment, requiring lifelong therapy for hypothyroidism.
- Radioactive iodide therapy is contraindicated in pregnant women because the drug can cross the placenta and cause thyroid damage in the developing fetus.
- Radioactive iodine ^{131}I is made in nuclear pharmacies and is regulated by the Nuclear Regulatory Commission (NRC).
- Propylthiouracil (PTU) and methimazole block the synthesis of T_4 and T_3. They bind thyroid peroxidase enzyme, which is the enzyme that activates the coupling of iodine and thyroglobulin and inhibits coupling of iodinated tyrosine (MIT and DIT).
- PTU is capable of blocking the process that converts T_4 to T_3.
- It takes 2 to 4 months of therapy with PTU before maximum effects are achieved.
- Treatment with antithyroid drugs typically induces hypothyroidism.
- Hypothyroidism is a condition in which the thyroid gland secretes deficient amounts of thyroid hormones.
- Hashimoto's disease is an autoimmune disorder that causes hypothyroidism.
- Thyroid replacement therapy is the principal treatment for hypothyroidism. Replacement can be achieved by the administration of dessicated (dried, powdered) whole gland animal thyroid or synthetic T_4, synthetic T_3, or a ratio of the two hormones.
- Synthetic T_4, known as levothyroxine or L-thyroxin, is most commonly prescribed for the treatment of hypothyroidism.
- Levothyroxine is converted to liothyronine in the body, just as naturally occurring T_4 is metabolized to T_3.
- Liothyroinine (T_3) and levothyroxine differ in their onset of action, duration of action, potency, and dosing frequency.
- Pharmacy technicians should attempt to dispense the same manufacturer's product each time the patient's prescription is refilled.
- Ferrous products, calcium supplements, and food decrease the absorption of thyroid hormones.
- Sometimes the strength of dessicated thyroid is written as the grain strength. For example, 60 mg thyroid is equivalent to gr 1 thyroid.
- The various strengths of levothyroxine are color-coded to help avoid dispensing errors.

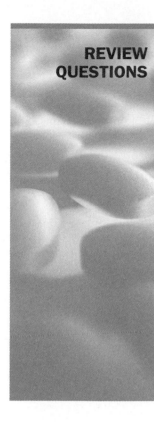

REVIEW QUESTIONS

Multiple Choice

1. Tetraiodothyronine is the most abundant thyroid hormone. It contains _____ atoms of iodine and is also known as thyroxine.
   a. 3
   b. 4
   c. 2
   d. 1

2. Hyperthyroidism and hypothyroidism are more prevalent in women than in men.
   a. true
   b. false

3. _____ is an autoimmune disease and the primary cause of thyroid hyperactivity.
   a. Hashimoto's disease
   b. TSH disease
   c. Graves' disease
   d. all of the above

4. Treatment of hyperthyroidism involves the administration of _____.
   a. antithyroid drugs
   b. radioactive iodine
   c. surgery
   d. all of the above

5. Which thyroid drug may produce a dangerous drop in white blood cells (agranulocytosis), which increases the risk for serious infection?
   a. Propylthiouracil
   b. Cytomel
   c. Synthroid
   d. Thyrolar

6. It takes _____ of therapy with propylthiouracil before maximum effects are achieved.
   a. 1 to 2 months
   b. 2 to 4 months
   c. 5 to 6 months
   d. 6 to 8 months

7. A brand name for levothyroxine is _____.
   a. Cytomel
   b. Thyrolar
   c. Proloid
   d. Synthroid

8. Ferrous products, calcium supplements, and food increase the absorption of thyroid hormones.
   a. true
   b. false

9. Hashimoto's disease is an autoimmune disorder that causes _____.
   a. hypothyroidism
   b. hyperthyroidism

10. Diabetes is not a risk factor for thyroid disease.
    a. true
    b. false

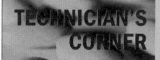

TECHNICIAN'S CORNER

1. What is an autoimmune disease, and what are the effects of an autoimmune disease like Graves' disease?
2. What types of food provide iodine?

BIBLIOGRAPHY

Agency for Toxic Substances and Disease Registry: *ToxFAQs for iodine.* Available at: http://www.atsdr. cdc.gov/tfacts158.html.

American Thyroid Association: Thyroid function tests, 2005. Available at: www.thyroid.org.

American Thyroid Association: Thyroid hormone treatment, 2005. Available at: www.thyroid.org.

Becker D, Hurley J, Detres R, Thyroid Foundation of Canada/La Fondation Canadienne de la Thyroïde: Radioactive iodine treatment of hyperthyroidism, *Bridge,* 7, 1992. Available at: www.thyroid.ca.

Cawood T, Moriarty P, O'Farrelly C, O'Shea D: Smoking and thyroid-associated ophthalmopathy: A novel explanation of the biological link, *J Clin Endocrinol Metab,* 92:59-64, 2007.

De Moraes A, Pedro A, Romaldini J: Spontaneous hypothyroidism in the follow-up of Graves hyperthyroid patients treated with antithyroid drugs, *South Med J,* 99, 2006.

Hormones and You Patient Information Page: Hyperthyroidism, The Hormone Foundation, May 2006. Available at: www.hormone.org.

Kalant H, Grant D, Mitchell J: *Principles of medical pharmacology* (pp 613-619), ed 7, Toronto, 2007, Elsevier Canada, A Division of Reed Elsevier Canada.

Lance L, Lacy C, Armstrong L, Goldman M: *Drug information handbook for the allied health professional,* ed 12. Hudson, OH, 2005, APhA Lexi-Comp.

Raffa R, Rawls S, Beyzarov E: *Netter's illustrated pharmacology* (pp 10-11, 136-142), Philadelphia, 2005, Saunders Elsevier.

Otto M: Class 1C antiarrhythmics, *Clin Pharmacol,* 2003. Available at: http://www.clinicalpharmacology. com/apps/default.asp?entry=11andrNum=96.

Page C, Curtis M, Sutter M, Walker M, Hoffman B: *Integrated pharmacology* (pp 288-291), Philadelphia, 2005, Mosby.

Wang S, Baker J Jr: Targeting B cells in Graves' disease, *Endocrinology,* 147:4559-4560, 2006.

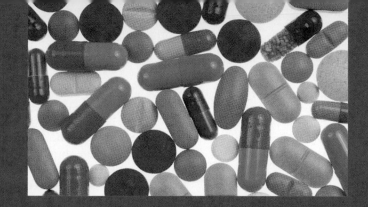

Treatment of Diabetes Mellitus

- Learn the terminology associated with diabetes mellitus.
- List the symptoms of diabetes mellitus.
- Describe the etiology of diabetes mellitus.
- Identify risk factors for diabetes mellitus.
- List and categorize medications used to treat diabetes mellitus.
- Describe mechanism of action for each class of drugs used to treat diabetes mellitus.
- Identify warning labels and precautionary messages associated with medications used to treat diabetes mellitus.
- Identify significant drug look-alike/sound-alike issues.
- List common endings for drug classes used in the treatment of diabetes mellitus.

Diabetes mellitus: Chronic condition in which the body is unable to properly convert food into energy.

Diabetic neuropathy: Nerve disorder caused by diabetes. This disorder leads to pain or loss of feeling in the toes, feet, legs, hands, or arms.

Fasting blood glucose: Blood glucose level after a person has not eaten for 8 to 12 hours (usually overnight).

Gestational diabetes: Diabetes that may be caused by the hormones of pregnancy or a shortage of insulin.

Hemoglobin A1c (Hb$_{A1c}$): Blood test that measures a person's average blood glucose level over a period of weeks or months.

Hyperglycemia: Elevated blood glucose levels.

Hypoglycemia: Decreased blood glucose levels.

Insulin resistance: Condition in which the body does not respond to insulin; is a precursor to type 2 diabetes.

Postprandial: After eating.

Prediabetes: Condition of impaired fasting glucose (IFG) and impaired glucose tolerance (IGT) in which the body consistently has high normal glucose levels.

Triglyceride: Form in which fat is stored in the body. High triglyceride levels in the blood may raise the risks for heart attack or stroke.

Type 1 diabetes: Autoimmune disease in which β cells are destroyed and insufficient amounts of insulin are produced.

Type 2 diabetes: Condition where the pancreas produces a sufficient amount of insulin, but insulin receptors lack sensitivity to the insulin produced. The body is unable to use the insulin effectively.

Overview

Diabetes mellitus is a disorder of metabolism that involves glucose utilization. It is a chronic condition in which the body cannot properly convert food into energy. Glucose is the body's primary energy source. Under normal conditions, as glucose levels in the blood rise, hormones are released that move the glucose out of the bloodstream and into cells, where it is needed for growth and energy. In diabetes, glucose accumulates in the blood. Much like a person with sticky hands walking through a room, glucose in the bloodstream leaves a sticky residue over all the body's organs and cells in which it comes in contact and causes damage.

As much as 7% of the U.S. population (20.8 million) and 5% (1.3 million) of the Canadian population over the age of 12 years is estimated to have diabetes mellitus, and its prevalence is growing. According to the Centers for Disease Control and Prevention (CDC), it is estimated that by 2050 the number of people diagnosed with diabetes will jump 165% above current levels. Strikingly, nearly half of the cases of diabetes are undiagnosed, accounting for about 6.2 million people. The number of people diagnosed with prediabetes is also alarmingly high at 54 million.

Diabetes mellitus is one of the leading causes of disability in the United States. It is the leading cause of non–war-related amputations. In the United States, diabetes was the sixth leading cause of death in 2002, and according to the 2005 Canadian Community Health Survey, diabetes is the seventh leading cause of death in Canada. In the United States, $1 of $8 federal health care dollars is spent treating people with diabetes. More than $9.88 billion was spent on diabetes drugs in the United States in 2005. According to Medco's 2007 Drug Trend Report, 2009 expenditures for diabetes drugs is predicted to be up to 68% above 2006 levels.

HORMONE REGULATION OF BLOOD GLUCOSE LEVELS

Insulin is a hormone that is essential for the regulation of carbohydrates, fat, and protein metabolism. When blood glucose levels rise, as occurs after a meal, β cells in the islets of Langerhans secrete insulin. The control of glucose levels occurs by a second messenger reaction. Insulin binds to receptors on the cell membrane. This stimulates the docking of intracellular glucose transporters that carry glucose out of the bloodstream and into cells where it is needed. Insulin, along with glucagon, is released by the pancreas in response to the rise and fall of blood glucose levels, amino acids, and gut-derived hormones (Figure 33-1).

When glucose levels drop, glucagon is secreted by α cells in the islets of Langerhans. The physiological effects of insulin are primarily anabolic; for example, glucose that is not needed for energy immediately is stored in the liver as glycogen, a reservoir for future energy needs (Figure 33-2). The physiological effects of glucagon are primarily catabolic. It releases energy stores. The physiological effects of insulin are listed in Box 33-1.

Types of Diabetes Mellitus

Prediabetes, type 1 diabetes, type 2 diabetes, and gestational diabetes all produce elevated blood glucose levels.

PREDIABETES

Prediabetes causes impaired fasting glucose (IFG) and impaired glucose tolerance (IGT). When blood glucose levels range between 100 and 125 mg/dL after an overnight fast fasting, glucose levels are said to be impaired. With IGT, blood glucose level is high, ranging between 140 to 199 mg/dL after a 2-hour oral glucose tolerance test. Prediabetes increases risks for cardiovascular disease.

TYPE 1 DIABETES

Type 1 diabetes is an autoimmune disease. The immune system attacks and destroys the insulin-producing β cells in the pancreas. Hypotheses for the cause of this autoimmune disorder are exposure to environmental factors, viruses, or possibly genetics. Only 5% to 10% of all persons with diabetes have type 1 diabetes. Type 1 diabetes is also known as

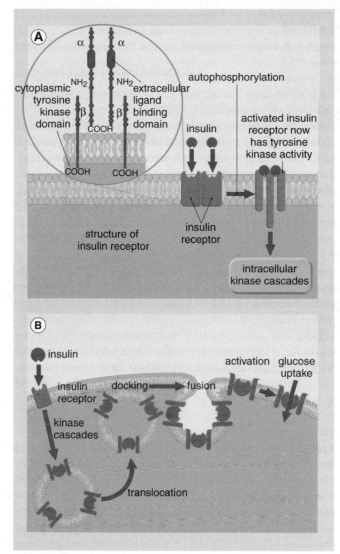

FIGURE 33-1 Insulin action. *(From Page C, et al.* Integrated pharmacology, *ed 3. Philadelphia, 2006, Mosby).*

insulin-dependent diabetes mellitus (IDDM) or juvenile-onset diabetes mellitus. This is because persons with this type of diabetes must inject insulin daily. Their body can no longer produce sufficient amounts of the hormone insulin. The onset of type 1 diabetes is typically in childhood, although it can occur later in life—hence, the name *juvenile-onset diabetes mellitus.* Type 1 diabetes occurs equally among males and females but is more common in whites than in nonwhites.

TYPE 2 DIABETES

Type 2 diabetes is most common, accounting for 90% to 95% of all cases of diabetes. It is also known as non–insulin-dependent diabetes mellitus (NIDDM) because administration of insulin is not the only treatment options for this type of diabetes. This is because in type 2 diabetes, the pancreas is usually producing sufficient amounts of insulin, but for unknown reasons the body is unable to use the insulin effectively. This condition is called *insulin resistance.* Insulin production eventually decreases; however, this may not occur for several years. Risk factors of type 2 diabetes are obesity, lack of physical activity, family history of diabetes, prior gestational diabetes, and increasing age. Approximately 80% of persons diagnosed with type 2 diabetes are overweight.

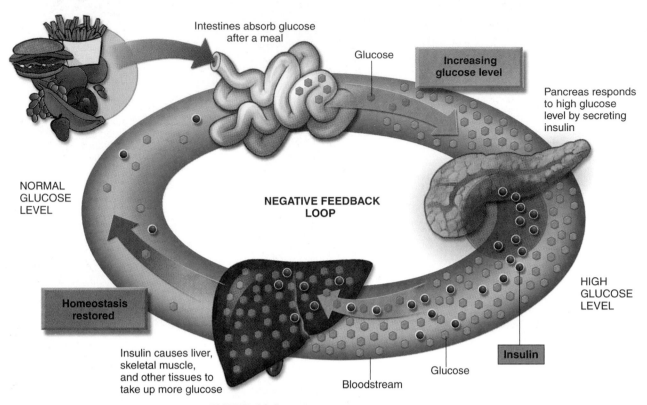

Intestines absorb glucose after a meal

Glucose

Increasing glucose level

Pancreas responds to high glucose level by secreting insulin

NORMAL GLUCOSE LEVEL

NEGATIVE FEEDBACK LOOP

HIGH GLUCOSE LEVEL

Homeostasis restored

Insulin

Insulin causes liver, skeletal muscle, and other tissues to take up more glucose

Glucose

Bloodstream

FIGURE 33-2 Role of insulin. *(From Thibodeau GA, Patton KT:* Anatomy and physiology, *ed 6, St. Louis, 2007, Mosby.)*

The prevalence of type 2 diabetes is high in Aborginals and Native Americans, African Americans, and Mexican Americans. It is believed that this may be linked to exposure to racism, chronic stress, and consumption of a "diabetes" diet that is high in fat and carbohydrates.

GESTATIONAL DIABETES

Gestational diabetes occurs in about 3% to 8% of all pregnant women. It occurs late in pregnancy. Because it may have no symptoms, pregnant women are routinely tested for gestational diabetes. Blood glucose levels are normally lower than normal during pregnancy so an elevated blood glucose level is a sign of gestational diabetes. Gestational diabetes may be caused by the hormones of pregnancy or by a shortage of insulin. Symptoms often disappear after delivery; however, women that have had gestational diabetes have a 20% to 50% increased risk for the development of type 2 diabetes within 5 to 10 years.

BOX 33-1 THE PHYSIOLOGICAL EFFECTS OF INSULIN

CARBOHYDRATE METABOLISM
- Increased glycogen synthesis (liver)
- Decreased gluconeogenesis (liver)
- Increased glucose transport (muscle and fat cells)

LIPID METABOLISM
- Sets the level of triglyceride production from "free fatty acids"
- Decreased lipolysis

PROTEIN METABOLISM
- Increased amino acid synthesis
- Increased amino acid transport (precursors for protein synthesis)

What Causes Diabetes?

INSULIN RESISTANCE

Insulin resistance is a condition in which the body does not respond to insulin. It is a precursor to type 2 diabetes. Insulin resistance is a syndrome that is associated with genetic factors, inactivity, diet, and obesity that leads to a set of metabolic dysregulatory conditions that increase the risk for cardiovascular disease, hypertension, dyslipidemia, elevated triglycerides and LDLs, decreased HDLs, microalbuminuria, and diabetes. It may also increase risk for obesity (a risk factor for type 2 diabetes) because one role of the hormone insulin is to signal the need to increase food intake. Feedback signals are proportionate to body fat (Table 33-1).

Symptoms of Diabetes Mellitus

Symptoms of diabetes mellitus are listed in Box 33-2.

Diagnostic Tests for Diabetes Mellitus

Blood glucose testing for elevated levels is the principle method used to diagnose diabetes. Typically, blood glucose levels are measured after fasting however an oral glucose tolerance test may be administered. The **hemaglobin A1c (Hb$_{A1c}$)** test is the only test that provides information about blood glucose levels over a 2- to 3-month period.

- **Fasting blood glucose test:** Blood glucose level of 126 milligrams per deciliter (mg/dL) or more after an 8-hour fast.
- **Oral glucose tolerance test (OGTT):** Blood glucose level of 200 mg/dL or more 2 hours after drinking a beverage containing 75 grams of glucose dissolved in water.
- **Random blood glucose:** Blood glucose level of 200 mg/dL or more, along with the presence of diabetes symptoms.
- **Hemoglobin A1c (Hb$_{A1c}$) test:** Reflects average blood glucose over a 2- to 3-month period.

Diabetes Complications

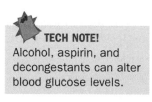

TECH NOTE!
Alcohol, aspirin, and decongestants can alter blood glucose levels.

Complications of untreated or poorly controlled diabetes mellitus occur throughout the body (Box 33-3). Diabetes mellitus causes microvascular damage and macrovascular damage. Microvascular damage may lead to weakened blood vessels in the eye that leak contents into

---

TABLE 33-1   Risk Factors for Diabetes Mellitus

Nonmodifiable	Age (≥45 years), family history of diabetes
Modifiable	Obesity (body mass index ≥ 25 kg/m2)
	Physical inactivity
	Smoking
Disease	Hypertension, angina, myocardial infarction, stroke, metabolic syndrome, insulin resistance, hyperlipidemia

---

BOX 33-2 SYMPTOMS OF DIABETES MELLITUS

TYPE 1	TYPE 2
Increased thirst (polydipsia)	Fatigue
Frequent urination (polyuria)	Frequent urination
Constant hunger (polyphagia)	Hunger
Weight loss	Weight loss
Blurred vision	Blurred vision
Extreme fatigue	Increased thirst
Diabetic ketoacidosis	Slow healing of wounds or sores
Hyperglycemia	Hyperglycemia

BOX 33-3 DIABETES COMPLICATIONS

Retinopathy	Hyperlipidemia
Blindness	Peripheral neuropathy
Blurred vision	Infections
Nephropathy	Amputations
Stroke	Pregnancy complications
Heart attack	Increased birth defects
Hypertension	Ketoacidosis
Angina	

the retina (retinopathy) leading to blurred vision and blindness. Nephropathy (kidney damage) also occurs. Macrovascular changes can lead to hypertension, angina, and myocardial infarction. Diabetes can also cause hyperlipidemia and peripheral neuropathy (nerve damage and numbness in the lower limbs). In fact, patients with diabetes must frequently inspect their feet because, should they develop a foot injury, they may not feel it. Diabetes causes poor wound healing, so foot infections sometimes become serious enough to require limb amputations. Individuals with untreated or poorly controlled type 1 diabetes may develop ketoacidosis, a condition in which the body breaks down fats to obtain its energy needs. Ketones are a byproduct of lipid metabolism, and their accumulation can lead to coma and death.

Nonpharmacological Management of Diabetes

Diabetes mellitus is sometimes classified as a disease of lifestyle because lifestyle factors can increase the risk for type 2 diabetes, and all types diabetes can be improved by weight loss, engaging in physical activity, consuming foods with a low glycemic index, quitting smoking, and other lifestyle changes. Physical activity lowers the risk of type 2 diabetes by up to 30%. For those with diabetes, increased physical activity decrease risks of mortality from the disease. A minimum of 150 minutes of exercise per week is recommended to maintain glycemic control, of which at least 90 minutes is vigorous aerobic exercise. Loss of 5% to 7% of body weight through diet and increased physical activity can lower the risks of diabetes (Box 33-4).

BLOOD GLUCOSE MONITORING

TECH ALERT!
Pharmacy technicians knowledgeable about the various blood glucose monitors can help patients select the monitor that best suits their needs.

Blood glucose monitoring is an essential component of diabetes management (Figure 33-3). Measurement of blood glucose levels may be recommended 2 to 4 times a day depending on whether the individual has type 1, type 2, or gestational diabetes. Knowledge of blood glucose levels enables individuals with diabetes to take "control" of their disease and adjust their level of diet, exercise, and insulin.

Treatment of Diabetes Mellitus

Maintenance of blood glucose level within normal ranges has been shown to minimize the risk of diabetic complications. According to the Diabetes Control and Complications Trial (DCCT), a 10-year study sponsored by the National Institute of Diabetes and Digestive and Kidney Diseases (NIDDK) and the United Kingdom Prospective Diabetes Study, intensive control of blood glucose and blood pressure reduces complications in type 1 and type 2 diabetes.

BOX 33-4 RECOMMENDED LIFESTYLE MODIFICATIONS

Weight loss	Stop smoking
Engage in physical activity	Eat low glycemic index foods

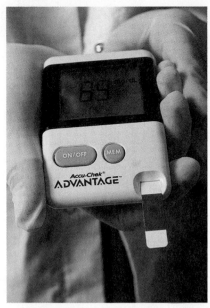

FIGURE 33-3 Blood glucose monitor. *(From Bonewit-West K:* Clinical Procedures for Medical Assistants, *ed 7, St. Louis, Saunders, 2008)*

TECH NOTE!
Remember when mixing insulin that if one is cloudy, it gets drawn up second. Lantus should not be mixed together in a syringe with any other form of insulin.

TECH NOTE!
Regular insulin solutions that appear cloudy should be discarded.

TECH NOTE!
Individuals with diabetes must eat scheduled meals. A combination of rapid-acting and intermediate-acting insulin is typically administered to mimic normal fluctuations of insulin levels throughout the day in response to preprandial and postprandial glucose levels.

At present, type 1 diabetes may be treated only with insulin. Type 2 diabetes may be treated with oral agents. Oral hypoglycemic agents and oral antidiabetic agents are only indicated as an adjunct to diet and exercise in the treatment of type 2 diabetes mellitus.

INSULIN

Insulin is administered for the management of all types of diabetes. It helps the body metabolize carbohydrates, fats, and proteins from the diet. It may be the sole drug administered as in the case of type 1 diabetes or may be added to oral therapy or replace oral therapy, as in type 2 diabetes. Insulin is manufactured from animal sources (pig and cow) and genetically engineered using recombinant DNA technology (see Chapter 1), to match human insulin. Animal source insulin is no longer marketed in the United States or Canada but is still available in other parts of the world.

MECHANISM OF ACTION AND PHARMACOKINETICS

Insulin is a protein, so it cannot be taken orally, as it would be digested in the stomach by gastric acids. Insulin is administered parenterally. The insulin that is administered for the treatment of diabetes has the identical mechanism of action as naturally occurring human insulin. It is formulated in ultra-rapid-acting, short-acting, intermediate-acting, and long-acting form. The onset of action for ultra-rapid-acting insulin (lispro insulin) begins within 15 minutes, whereas the onset of action for long acting insulin is 4 to 6 hours (Table 33-2). Ultra-rapid-acting insulin (e.g., insulin aspart) must be injected 5 to 15 minutes before eating.

Regular insulin is a clear solution that may be administered intravenously; however, other parenteral forms of insulin are suspensions for subcutaneous injection. Dosage delivery systems for the administration of insulin are the insulin pump, autoinjector, and pen cartridges.

ADVERSE REACTIONS

Adverse reactions to insulin administration are associated with hypersecretion (hypergylcemia) or hyposecretion (hypoglycemia) of the hormone from pancreatic β cells. Symptoms of hyperglycemia and hypoglycemia are listed in Box 33-5. Adverse effects due to inhaled insulin are cough, mild shortness of breath, sore throat, hoarseness, runny nose, and nose bleeds.

TECH NOTE!

Insulin must be protected from extremes in heat and cold. Refrigerate unopened vials; do not freeze. Opened vials of insulin may be stored at room temperature, but this will shorten the expiry date for most insulins. Check manufacturer's insert (see Table 33-3).

TABLE 33-2   Onset and Duration of Action of Insulin

Insulin	Onset of Action	Duration of Action
Ultra-Rapid-Acting		
insulin lispro	15 minutes	6 to 8 hours
insulin aspart	15 minutes	3 to 5 hours
insulin glulisine	20 minutes	5 to 6 hours
Short-Acting		
insulin regular	15 minutes (IV)	30 to 60 minutes (IV)
	30 minutes (SC)	8 to 12 hours (SC)
Intermediate-Acting		
insulin isophane "NPH"	1 to 4 hours	10 to 24 hours
Long-Acting		
isuline glargine	1.5 hours	24 hours
insulin detemir	4 to 12 hours	24 hours

BOX 33-5 SYMPTOMS OF HYPERGLYCEMIA AND HYPOGLYCEMIA

HYPERGLYCEMIA	HYPOGLYCEMIA
Elevated blood glucose	Low blood glucose
Extreme thirst	Anxiety, nervousness, irritability
Frequent urination	Confusion
Extreme hunger	Difficulty concentrating
Weakness	Hunger
Blurred vision	Pale skin
Dry mouth	Nausea
Upset stomach and vomiting	Fatigue, uncontrolled yawning
Shortness of breath	Sweating
Breath that smells fruity	Headache
Decreased consciousness	Palpitations, rapid heartbeat
	Numbness of the mouth
	Tingling in the fingers
	Tremors
	Muscle weakness
	Blurred vision
	Cold sensations
	Shallow breathing
	Loss of consciousness

TABLE 33-3   Recommended Storage for Opened Vials and Cartridges of Insulin

insulin aspart and insulin glulisine	Vials: ROOM TEMP OR FRIDGE; DISCARD AFTER 28 DAYS Cartridges: STORE AT ROOM TEMP; DISCARD AFTER 28 DAYS
insulin detemir	Vials: ROOM TEMP OR FRIDGE; DISCARD AFTER 42 DAYS Cartridges: STORE AT ROOM TEMP; DISCARD AFTER 42 DAYS
insulin glargine	ROOM TEMP: DISCARD AFTER 14 DAYS (5 ml) or 28 DAYS (10 ml) REFRIGERATED: DISCARD AFTER 28 DAYS (5 ml and 10 ml)

Insulin

	Generic name	U.S. brand name(s) Canadian brand(s)	Dosage forms and strengths
	insulin aspart (rDNA origin)	Novolog, Novolog FlexPen, Novolog Penfill	**Injection, suspension (vial, pen, cartridge):** 100 units/ml
		Novorapid	
	insulin lispro	Humalog	**Injection, suspension (vial, pen, cartridge):** 100 units/ml
		Humalog, Humalog Pen, Humalog cartridge	
	insulin glulisine	Apidra	**Injection, solution (vial):** 100 units/ml
		Not available	
	insulin regular (rDNA origin)	Humulin R, Novolin R, Novolin R Innolet	**Injection, solution (vial, pen, cartridge):** 100 units/ml
		Humulin R	
	insulin isophane (rDNA origin)	Humulin N, Humulin N Pen, Novolin N, Novolin N Innolet	**Injection, suspension (vial, pen, cartridge):** 100 units/ml
		Humulin N, Novolin GE NPH	
	insulin detemir (rDNA origin)	Levemir, Levemir FlexPen	**Injection, solution (vial, pen):** 100 units/ml
		Levemir	
	Insulin glargine (rDNA origin)	Lantus	**Injection, solution:** 100 units/ml
		Lantus	
Insulin mixtures			
	insulin regular + insulin isophane	Humulin 50/50, Humulin 70/30, Novolin 70/30, Mixtard 70/30	**Injection, suspension:** 30 units/ml insulin + 70 units/ml insulin isophane 50 units/ml insulin + 50 units/ml insulin isophane 10 units/ml insulin +90 units/ml insulin isophane* 20 units/ml insulin + 80 units/ml insulin isophane* 40 units/ml insulin + 60 units/ml insulin isophane*
		Humulin 30/70 Novolin GE Penfill 10/90 Novolin GE Penfill 20/80 Novolin GE Penfill 30/70 Novolin GE Penfill 40/60	
	lispro insulin + lispro protamine suspension	Humalog Mix 50/50, Humalog Mix 75/25	**Injection, suspension (cartridge):** 25 units lispro insulin + 75 units lispro protamine suspension 50 units lispro insulin + 50 units lispro protamine suspension
		Humalog Mix 25, Humalog Mix 50	
	insulin aspart + insulin aspart protamine	Novolog Mix	**Injection, suspension:** 30 units insulin aspart + 70 units insulin aspart protamine
		Novomix-30	

*Strength available in Canada only.

SULFONYLUREAS

Sulfonylureas are also called oral hypoglycemic agents (OHAs). They are only effective for the treatment of type 2 diabetes.

MECHANISM OF ACTION AND PHARMACOKINETICS

Sulfonylureas stimulate insulin release from pancreatic β cells and increase insulin binding and insulin receptor sensitivity. Sulfonylureas also decrease glycogenolysis, the process of converting glycogen (storage form of glucose) to glucose.

Sulfonylureas differ in pharmacokinetics, pharmacodynamics, and incidence of hypoglycemic reactions. For example, glyburide (or dibenclamide) has a long T½ and active metabolites. The second-generation agents, glipizide and glyburide, are more potent than first-generation agents.

ADVERSE REACTIONS

Sulfonylureas can produce hypoglycemia, a serious side effect. Other side effects include abdominal pain, diarrhea, dyspepsia, nausea and vomiting, headache, and dizziness. Infrequently, sulfonylureas may produce bone marrow toxicity and cholestatic jaundice.

Sulfonylureas

	Generic name	U.S. brand name(s) / Canadian brand(s)	Dosage forms and strengths
	First generation		
	tolazamide*	Generics	**Tablet:** 100 mg, 250 mg, 500 mg
		Not available	
	tolbutamide*	Generics	**Tablet:** 500 mg
		Generics	
	Second generation		
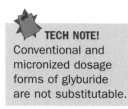	glyburide* (glibenclamide)	Diabeta, Glynase PresTab, Micronase	**Tablet, conventional (Diabeta, Micronase):** 1.25 mg, 2.5 mg, 5 mg **Tablet, micronized:** 1.5 mg, 3 mg, 6 mg
		Diabeta, Euglucon	
	glipizide*	Glucotrol, Glucotrol XL	**Tablet, immediate release (Glucotrol):** 5 mg, 10 mg **Tablet, extended release (Glucotrol XL):** 2.5 mg, 5 mg, 10 mg
		Not available	
	glimepiride*	Amaryl	**Tablet:** 1 mg, 2 mg, 4 mg
		Amaryl	

*Generic available.

BIGUANIDES

Metformin is classified as a biguanide antidiabetic agent. It is only effective in individuals who have some pancreatic islet cell function. Metformin acts to control fasting blood glucose.

MECHANISM OF ACTION

Metformin improves glucose tolerance and insulin resistance; lowers postprandial plasma glucose; decreases hepatic gluconeogenesis (new glucose) production; decreases intestinal absorption of glucose; and improves insulin sensitivity by increasing peripheral glucose uptake and utilization.

PHARMACOKINETICS

Metformin may be administered in immediate-release (tablets and solution) and extended-release dosage forms. Peak blood levels are achieved in 2.5 hours for immediate-release tablets, 2.2 hours for oral solution, and 7 hours for extended-release tablets. Food decreases the absorption of immediate release tablets but increases the absorption of metformin solution and extended release tablets. Glumetza, Glucophage XR, and Fortamet are extended-release dosage forms of metformin but not substitutable. Different processes are used to make the extended-release dosage form release drug content over time.

ADVERSE REACTIONS

Gastrointestinal adverse events are common. They include gas, heartburn, metallic taste in the mouth, mild stomachache, nausea, and weight loss.

Biguanides

		U.S. brand name(s)	
	Generic name	Canadian brand(s)	Dosage forms and strengths
	metformin*	Fortamet, Glucophage, Glucophage XR, Glumetza, Riomet	**Solution, oral (Riomet):** 100 mg/ml **Tablet, immediate release:** 500 mg, 850 mg, 1000 mg (1000 mg U.S. only) **Tablet, extended release:** **(Glumetza):** 500 mg **(Fortamet):** 500 mg, 1000 mg **(Glucophage XR):** 500 mg, 750 mg
		Glucophage, Glumetza	
	Combination biguanide + sulfonylureas		
	metformin + glyburide*	Glucovance	**Tablet:** 250 mg metformin + 1.25 mg glyburide 500 mg metformin + 2.5 mg glyburide 500 mg metformin + 5 mg glyburide
		Not available	
	metformin + glipizide*	Metaglip	**Tablet:** 250 mg metformin + 2.5 mg glipizide 500 mg metformin + 2.5 mg glipizide 500 mg metformin + 5 mg glipizide
		Not available	

*Generic available.

α-GLUCOSIDASE INHIBITORS

α-Glucosidase inhibitors prolong the digestion of carbohydrates and delay their absorption in the small intestine. They reduce peak plasma glucose levels. Acarbose does not promote insulin secretion like other antidiabetic agents, nor does it cause hypoglycemia.

MECHANISM OF ACTION AND PHARMACOKINETICS

Acarbose is an inhibitor of several α-glucosidases (e.g., glycoamylase, sucrase, maltase, and dextranase). The antidiabetic agent miglitol also inhibits the α-glucosidases maltase and sucrase. α-Glucosidases are enzymes that break down carbohydrates. Acarbose and miglitol must be administered with the first bite of each meal because the drug is an oral oligosaccharide that competes for binding sites with oligosaccharides and disaccharides in foods. It is important to eat a diet rich in complex carbohydrates while taking acarbose.

ADVERSE REACTIONS

α-Glucosidase inhibitors most commonly produce gastrointestinal side effects. Adverse reactions include bloated feeling, diarrhea, stomach or intestinal gas, or rumbling stomach and stomach pain or discomfort.

Alpha glucosidase Inhibitors

Generic name	U.S. brand name(s)	Dosage forms and strengths
	Canadian brand(s)	
acarbose	Precose	**Tablet:** 25 mg (U.S. only), 50 mg, 100 mg
	Glucobay	
miglitol	Glyset	**Tablet:** 25 mg, 50 mg, 100 mg
	Not available	

MEGLITINIDES

Meglitinides are oral antidiabetic agents used in the treatment and management of type 2 diabetes. Meglitinides, like other classes of antidiabetic agents, are only effective in individuals that have a functioning pancreas.

MECHANISM OF ACTION AND PHARMACOKINETICS

Meglitinides stimulate insulin secretion from pancreatic β cells, similar to sulfonylureas. Repaglinide is rapidly and completely absorbed from the intestinal tract; however, it is highly protein bound and metabolized via the CYP450 system, so it is subject to many drug interactions. Peak effects of repaglinide and nateglinide are achieved in about 1 to 1.5 hours, and elimination is equally as rapid. Their short half-life may account for the multiple daily dosing. Repaglinide and nateglinide both lower postprandial blood glucose levels. The drugs differ in that postprandial insulin levels peak earlier with nateglinide than with repaglinide.

ADVERSE REACTIONS

Meglitinide administration may cause hypoglycemia; however, the risk is lower than with sulfonylureas. Other side effects are headache, nausea, and vomiting. Repaglinide should be used with caution in patients with liver dysfunction.

Meglitinides

Generic name	U.S. brand name(s)	Dosage forms and strengths
	Canadian brand(s)	
nateglinide	Starlix	**Tablet:** 60 mg, 120 mg, 180 mg (Canada only)
	Starlix	
repaglinide	Prandin	**Tablet:** 0.5 mg, 1 mg, 2 mg
	Gluconorm	

THIAZOLIDINEDIONES

Thiazolidinediones are also called "insulin sensitizers" and are used in the treatment of type 2 diabetes. They are especially useful in the treatment of insulin resistance. Two agents are currently marketed in the United States and Canada. They are pioglitazone and rosiglitazone. Both drugs reduce fasting plasma glucose (FPG) and hemoglobin A1c (Hb$_{A1c}$).

MECHANISM OF ACTION

Thiazolidinediones increase tissue sensitivity to insulin. They do not increase insulin secretion. Increased receptor sensitivity is more prominent in adipose tissue, skeletal muscle, and the liver. Pioglitazone and rosiglitazone also increase uptake of glucose in the liver and muscles. Pioglitazone lowers free fatty acid and trigylcerides, too. Plasma glucose concentrations, insulin concentrations, and glycosylated hemoglobin are all reduced.

PHARMACOKINETICS

Pioglitazone and rosiglitazone are both administered orally. The time to reach peak plasma concentration is within 1 hour for rosiglitazone and 2 hours for pioglitazine. Food doubles the time needed to reach the maximum concentration for pioglitazone but has no effect on rosiglitazone. Food does not reduce the bioavailability of either drug.

ADVERSE REACTIONS

The most common adverse reactions of therapy with pioglitazone and rosiglitazone are headache, weight gain, diarrhea, nausea, and vomiting. Patients should be instructed to report signs of muscle pain, jaundice, blurred vision, and signs of hypoglycemia or hyperglycemia. Serious side effects linked to proglitazone and rosiglitazone are heart failure, heart attack, and liver failure.

Thiazolidinediones

	Generic name	U.S. brand name(s) Canadian brand(s)	Dosage forms and strengths
	pioglitazone	Actos	**Tablet:** 13 mg, 30 mg, 45 mg
		Actos	
	rosiglitazone	Ava ndia	**Tablet:** 2 mg, 4 mg, 8 mg
		Avandia	

Thiazolidinediones + biguanides

	pioglitazone + metformin	Actosplus Met	**Tablet:** pioglitazone 15 mg + metformin 500 mg
		Not available	pioglitazone 15 mg + metformin 850 mg
	rosiglitazone + metformin	Avandamet	**Tablet:** rosiglitazine 1 mg + metformin 500 mg (Canada only)
		Avandamet	rosiglitazone 2 mg + metformin 500 mg
			rosiglitazone 4 mg + metformin 500 mg
			rosiglitazone 2 mg + metformin 1000 mg
			rosiglitazone 4 mg + metformin 1000 mg

Thiazolidinediones + sulfonylureas

	pioglitazone + glimepiride	Duetact	**Tablet:** pioglitazone 30 mg + glimepiride 2 mg
		Not available	pioglitazone 30 mg + glimepiride 4 mg
	rosiglitazone + glimepiride	Avandaryl	**Tablet:** rosiglitazone 4 mg + glimepiride 1 mg
		Avandaryl	rosiglitazone 4 mg + glimepiride 2 mg
			rosiglitazone 4 mg + glimepiride 4 mg
			rosiglitazone 8 mg + glimepiride 2 mg
			rosiglitazone 8 mg + glimepiride 4 mg

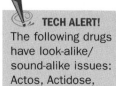

DIPEPTIDYL PEPTIDASE-4 INHIBITOR

Sitagliptin is an oral agent that is administered for the treatment of type 2 diabetes. It increases insulin release and decreases glucagon levels by potentiating the activity of peptide hormones that are released in response to eating a meal. Sitagliptin decreases fasting plasma glucose, *postprandial* glucose, and hemoglobin A1c.

MECHANISM OF ACTION AND PHARMACOKINETICS

Sitagliptin is a dipeptidyl peptidase-4 inhibitor. It inhibits the activity of dipeptidyl peptidase-4 (DPP-4), the enzyme that is responsible for the degradation of circulating glucagon-like peptide-1 (GLP-1) and glucose-dependent insulinotropic peptide (GIP). These peptide hormones are key agents in glucose homeostasis. The action of the hormones is prolonged by sitagliptin. Sitagliptin also increases β cells responsive to glucose in the islets of Langerhans.

Oral absorption and bioavailability of sitagliptin are good, and peak effects are reached 1 to 4 hours after administration. It is primarily eliminated in the urine, so some dosage adjustments may be required in individuals with kidney disease.

ADVERSE REACTIONS

The most common adverse reactions linked to the use of sitagliptin are intestinal upset, gas, heartburn, stomach pain, decreased appetite and weight loss, metallic taste, and stuffy or runny nose. The drug may also cause hypoglycemia especially in patients taking sulfonylureas.

Dipeptidyl Peptidase-4 Inhibitor

Generic name	U.S. brand name(s)	Dosage forms and strengths
	Canadian brand(s)	
sitagliptin	Januvia	**Tablet:** 50 mg
	Not available	
Combination dipeptidyl peptidase-4 inhibitor + biguanide		
sitagliptin + metformin	Janumet	**Tablet:**
	Not available	sitagliptin 50 mg + metformin 500 mg sitagliptin 50 mg + metformin 1000 mg

INCRETIN MIMETIC

Exenatide (Byetta) is parenterally administered adjunct to insulin therapy that may only be administered for type 2 diabetes mellitus.

MECHANISM OF ACTION AND PHARMACOKINETICS

Exenatide mimics the effect of the hormone incretin. Incretin stimulates the pancreas to secrete insulin when blood sugar levels are high, slows the emptying of the stomach, and causes decreased appetite. Exenatide is administered subcutaneously within 60 minutes *before* the morning and evening meals.

ADVERSE EFFECTS

Side effects of exenatide include hypoglycemia, heartburn, itching, burning, swelling, or rash at the injection site, diarrhea, reduced appetite, or a slight weight loss. Exenatide may cause mild dizziness, weakness or headaches, or nausea (these are also signs of hypoglycemia and hyperglycemia).

Incretin Mimetic

Generic name	U.S. brand name(s)	Dosage forms and strengths
	Canadian brand(s)	
exenatide	Byetta	Injection solution: 250 mcg/ml
	Not available	

TECH NOTE!
Pramlintide may cause hypoglycemia. The risk may be greater during the first 3 hours after pramlintide is injected.

TECH NOTE!
Do not mix pramlintide with any other injection, including insulin.

AMYLIN ANALOG

Pramlintide (Symlin) is a synthetic analog of the hormone amylin. Amylin levels are absent in type 1 diabetes and decreased in type 2 diabetes. Pramlintide is used with mealtime insulin to control blood sugar levels in people who have type 1 or type 2 diabetes mellitus.

MECHANISM OF ACTION AND PHARMACOKINETICS

Like amylin, pramlintide slows gastric emptying, reduces postprandial glucagon secretion, and reduces appetite. The maximum concentration of pramlintide is reached within 20 minutes of administration, and the therapeutic effects last approximately 3 hours.

ADVERSE REACTIONS

Adverse reactions associated with pramlintide are redness, swelling, bruising, itching at the injection site, loss of appetite, stomach pain, indigestion, upset stomach, excessive tiredness, dizziness, coughing, sore throat, or joint pain.

Amylin Analog

Generic name	U.S. brand name(s)	Dosage forms and strengths
	Canadian brand(s)	
pramlintide	Symlin, Symlin Pen 60, Symlin Pen 120	injection solution: 0.6 mg/ml
	Not available	

Complementary and Alternative Medicine and Diabetes

Six dietary supplements have been of interest as adjunct therapy for people with diabetes. They are alpha-lipoic acid (ALA), chromium, coenzyme Q10, garlic, magnesium, and omega-3 fatty acids. None have been extensively studied using randomized, double-blind studies. Of the six dietary supplements alpha-lipoic acid, magnesium, omega-3 fatty acids, and garlic show the greatest evidence of possible usefulness.

ALPHA-LIPOIC ACID

Alpha-lipoic acid is an antioxidant. Antioxidants prevent cell damage caused by oxidative stress by substances called free radicals. Elevated blood glucose can cause oxidative stress. ALA might lower blood sugar too much, so blood glucose levels must be monitored closely when it is used.

MAGNESIUM

Magnesium is a mineral that is found in green leafy vegetables, nuts, seeds, and some whole grains. Magnesium levels are depressed in people with diabetes. Low magnesium levels may worsen glucose control in type 2 diabetes by interrupting insulin secretion and increasing insulin resistance.

OMEGA-3 FATTY ACIDS

Omega-3 fatty acids are naturally found in fish, fish oil, canola and soybean oil, walnuts, and wheat germ. Studies have shown that supplementation with omega-3 fatty acids can reduce the incidence of cardiovascular disease (CVD) and slow the progression of atherosclerosis. Omega-3 fatty acids have been of interest for diabetes because diabetes can increase the risk of CVD.

GARLIC

Evidence about the value of garlic is mixed. It is believed that garlic may be involved in some biological activities associated with type 2 diabetes.

Summary of Drugs Used in the Treatment of Diabetes

	Generic name	Brand name	Usual dose and dosing schedule	Warning labels
Insulin				
	insulin	Humulin, Novolin	Individualized	STORE IN THE REFRIGERATOR; DO NOT FREEZE
Sulfonylureas				
	tolazamide	Generics	100 mg to 250 mg once daily (maximum 500 mg twice a day)	AVOID ALCOHOL TAKE BEFORE BREAKFAST
	tolbutamide	Generics	250 mg to 2000 mg daily	
	glipizide	Glucotrol	10 mg to 15 mg once daily	TAKE 30 MINUTES BEFORE BREAKFAST
		Glucotrol XL	5 mg to 10 mg once daily	TAKE WITH BREAKFAST
	glyburide	Diabeta, Micronase	1.25 mg/day to 20 mg/day given in single or divided doses	
		Glynase PresTab	0.75 mg/day to 12 mg/day, given in single or divided dose	
	glimepiride	Amaryl	1 mg to 4 mg once daily, with a maximum of 8 mg/day	
Biguanides				
	metformin	Glucophage	500 mg twice daily or 850 mg PO once daily (maximum 2000 mg/day)	TAKE WITH THE EVENING MEAL
		Glumetza	1000 mg 1 to 2 times a day	
		Fortamet	500 mg to 1000 mg once daily	
α-Glucosidase inhibitors				
	acarbose	Precose	25 mg to 100 mg 3 times a day	TAKE WITH THE FIRST BITE OF A MEAL
	miglitol	Glyset	25 mg to 100 mg 3 times a day	PROTECT FROM MOISTURE
Dipeptidyl Peptidase-4 Inhibitor				
	sitagliptin	Januvia	100 mg once daily	TAKE AT THE SAME TIME EACH DAY WITH OR WITHOUT FOOD

Summary of Drugs Used in the Treatment of Diabetes—cont'd

	Generic name	Brand name	Usual dose and dosing schedule	Warning labels
	Meglitinides			
	nateglinide	Starlix	120 mg 3 times a day	TAKE IMMEDIATELY PRIOR TO A MEAL
	repaglinide	Prandin	1 mg to 4 mg up to 4 times a day	SWALLOW TABLETS WITH WATER; DO NOT CHEW
	Thiazolidinediones			
	pioglitazone	Actos	15 mg to 45 mg once daily	AVOID ALCOHOL
	rosiglitazone	Avandia	4 mg daily in single or divided doses	TAKE WITH A FULL GLASS OF WATER
	Combinations			
	metformin + glipizide	Metaglip	1 to 2 tablet 1 to 2 times/day (maximum 2000 mg metformin + 20 mg glipizide per day)	TAKE WITH FOOD AVOID ALCOHOL DON'T SKIP DOSES
	metformin + glyburide	Glucovance	1 to 2 tablet 1 to 2 times/day (maximum 2500 mg metformin + 20 mg glyburide per day)	
	metformin + pioglitazone	Actoplus Met	1 tablet 1 to 2 times/day (maximum 2250 mg metformin + 45 mg pioglitazone per day)	
	metformin + rosiglitazone	Avandamet	1 tablet 1 to 2 times/day	
	metformin + sitagliptin	Janumet	1 tablet twice a day	
	pioglitazone + glimepiride	Duetact	1 tablet daily with the first meal of the day	TAKE WITH FOOD
	rosiglitazone + glimepiride	Avandaryl	1 tablet daily with the first meal of the day	

CHAPTER SUMMARY

- Diabetes mellitus is a disorder of metabolism that involves glucose utilization.
- In diabetes, glucose accumulates in the blood. Much like a person with sticky hands walking through a room, glucose in the bloodstream leaves a sticky residue over all the body's organs and cells in which it comes in contact and causes damage.
- Diabetes mellitus is one of the leading causes of disability in the United States. It is the leading cause of non–war-related amputations.
- Diabetes is the seventh leading cause of death in Canada.
- Insulin is released by the β cells in the islets of Langerhans of the pancreas in response to the rise of blood glucose levels, amino acids, and gut-derived hormones.
- When glucose levels drop, glucagon is secreted by α cells in the islets of Langerhans.
- Prediabetes causes impaired fasting glucose and impaired glucose tolerance.
- Type 1 diabetes is an autoimmune disease. The immune system attacks and destroys the insulin-producing β cells in the pancreas.

- Type 1 diabetes is also known as insulin-dependent diabetes mellitus because the body can no longer produce sufficient amounts of the hormone insulin.
- Type 2 diabetes is most common, accounting for 90% to 95% of all diabetes. It is also known as non–insulin-dependent diabetes mellitus.
- In type 2 diabetes, the pancreas usually produces sufficient amounts of insulin, but for unknown reasons the body is unable to use the insulin effectively.
- Gestational diabetes may be caused by the hormones of pregnancy or a shortage of insulin.
- Insulin resistance is a condition in which the body does not respond to insulin. It is a precursor to type 2 diabetes.
- The hemoglobin A1c (HbA1c) test is the only test that provides information about blood glucose levels over a 2- to 3-month period.
- Blood glucose testing is the principle method used to diagnose diabetes.
- Individuals with type 1 or type 2 diabetes will reduce risks for complications by weight loss, engaging in physical activity, consuming foods with a low glycemic index, quitting smoking, and other lifestyle changes.
- Insulin is administered for the management of all types of diabetes. It is available in dosage forms to be administered by intravenous infusion, insulin pump, and subcutaneous injection.
- It is formulated in ultra-rapid-acting, short-acting, intermediate-acting, and long-acting form.
- Ultra-rapid-acting insulin (e.g., insulin aspart) must be injected 5 to 15 minutes before eating.
- Regular insulin solutions that appear cloudy should be discarded.
- Sulfonylureas are also called oral hypoglycemic agents. They are only effective for the treatment of type 2 diabetes.
- Sulfonylureas stimulate insulin release from pancreatic β cells, increase insulin binding and insulin receptor sensitivity, and decrease glycogenolysis.
- Metformin is classified as a biguanide antidiabetic agent. Metformin improves glucose tolerance and insulin resistance, lowers postprandial plasma glucose, decreases hepatic gluconeogenesis, decreases intestinal absorption of glucose, and improves insulin sensitivity.
- α-Glucosidase inhibitors prolong the digestion of carbohydrates and delay their absorption in the small intestine. They reduce peak plasma glucose levels.
- Acarbose and miglitol must be administered with the first bite of each meal.
- Meglitinides (nateglinide and repaglinide) stimulate insulin secretion from pancreatic β cells, similar to sulfonylureas.
- A common ending for thiazolidinediones is *"-glitazone."*
- Thiazolidinediones are also called "insulin sensitizers" and are used in the treatment of type 2 diabetes.
- Sitagliptin is a dipeptidyl peptidase-4 inhibitor. It decreases fasting plasma glucose, postprandial glucose, and hemoglobin A1c.
- Alpha-lipoic acid, magnesium, omega-3 fatty acids, and garlic are nutritional supplements that show some evidence of usefulness in the treatment of diabetes mellitus.

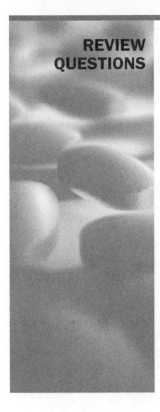

REVIEW QUESTIONS

Multiple Choice

1. The condition of elevated blood glucose levels is termed _____.
   a. hypoglycemia
   b. hyperglycemia

2. An autoimmune disease in which β cells are destroyed and insufficient amounts of insulin are produced is _____.
   a. type 1 diabetes
   b. type 2 diabetes
   c. gestational diabetes
   d. all of the above

3. In diabetes, _____ accumulates in the blood.
   a. calcium
   b. glucose
   c. magnesium
   d. insulin

4. A hormone that is essential for the regulation of carbohydrate, fat, and protein metabolism is _____.
   a. aldosterone
   b. serotonin
   c. dopamine
   d. insulin

5. Type 2 diabetes is most common, accounting for 90% to 95% of all cases of diabetes.
   a. true
   b. false

6. Select the common symptoms of diabetes _____.
   a. polyphagia
   b. polydipsia
   c. polyuria
   d. all of the above

7. The risk for diabetes mellitus cannot be lowered by making lifestyle changes.
   a. true
   b. false

8. Insulin is only administered for the management of type 1 diabetes.
   a. true
   b. false

9. Glipizide and glyburide are examples of _____.
   a. sulfonylureas
   b. dipeptidyl peptidase-4 inhibitors
   c. thiazolidinediones
   d. nutritional supplements

10. Pioglitazone and rosiglitazone are both administered parenterally.
    a. true
    b. false

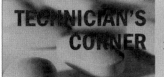

TECHNICIAN'S CORNER

1. If your family has a history of type 2 diabetes, what lifestyle precautions should you take to reduce your risk for developing the disease?
2. What are some basic changes in diet that can be implemented to avoid developing type 2 diabetes?

BIBLIOGRAPHY

Berkrot B: Study finds staggering cost of treating diabetes, June 19, 2007, Rueters, Copyright © 2007 Reuters Limited. Available at: http://www.nlm.nih.gov/medlineplus/news/fullstory_51076.html.

Bloomgarden Z: Insulin resistance concepts, *Diabetes Care,* 30:1320-1326, 2007.

Bosi E, Camisasca R, Collober C, Rochette E, Garber A: Effects of vildagliptin on glucose control over 24 weeks in patients with type 2 diabetes inadequately controlled with metformin, *Diabetes Care,* 30:890-895, 2007.

Gangji A, Cukierman T, Gerstein H, Goldsmith C, Clase C: A systemic review and met-analysis of hypoglycemia and cardiovascular events, *Diabetes Care,* 30:389-394, 2007.

Kalant H, Grant D, Mitchell J: *Principles of medical pharmacology* (pp 635-642), ed 7, Toronto, 2007, Elsevier Canada, A Division of Reed Elsevier Canada.

Lance L, Lacy C, Armstrong L, Goldman M: *Drug information handbook for the allied health professional,* ed 12, Hudson, OH, 2005, APhA Lexi-Comp.

Morrato E, Hill J, Wyatt H, Ghushchyan V, Sullivan P: Physical activity in US adults with diabetes and at risk for developing diabetes, *Diabetes Care,* 30:203-209, 2007.

National Diabetes Information Clearinghouse: *Diabetes overview,* Bethesda, August 2006, National Institute of Diabetes and Digestive and Kidney Diseases (NIDDK), National Institutes of Health, US Department of Health and Human Services, NIH publication No. 06-3873. Available at: www.diabetes. niddk.nih.gov.

NCCAM Clearinghouse: *Treating type 2 diabetes with dietary supplements: Research report,* Bethesda, June 2005, National Center for Complimentary and Alternative Medicine (NCCAM), National Institutes of Health, US Department of Health and Human Services.

Ottawa Health Statistics Division: *Your community, your health: Findings from the 3.1 smoking and diabetes care: Results from the Canadian Community Health Survey (CCHS) cycle,* Ottawa, 2005, Health Statistics Division, catalog No. 82-621-XIE, No. 002, pp 49-59.

Page C, Curtis M, Sutter M, Walker M, Hoffman B: *Integrated pharmacology* (pp 293-299), Philadelphia, 2005, Mosby.

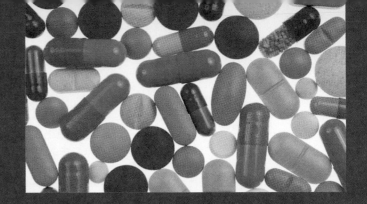

CHAPTER 34

Drugs That Affect the Reproductive System

LEARNING OBJECTIVES

- Learn the terminology associated with the reproductive system.
- Describe the pathophysiology of reproductive system disorders.
- Describe the physiology of pregnancy and methods of pregnancy prevention.
- List and categorize medications that affect the reproductive system.
- Describe mechanism of action for each class of drugs used that affects the reproductive system.
- Identify warning labels and precautionary messages associated with medications that affect the reproductive system.
- Identify significant drug look-alike/sound-alike issues.
- List common endings for drug classes that affect the reproductive system.

KEY TERMS

Amenorrhea: Absence of normal menstruation.

Atrophic vaginitis: Postmenopausal thinning and dryness of the vaginal epithelium related to decreased estrogen levels.

Condom: Thin flexible penile sheath made of synthetic or natural materials.

Craniopharyngioma: Pituitary tumor that causes hormonal deficiencies.

Diaphragm: Rubber or plastic cup that fits over the cervix and used for contraceptive purposes.

Dysfunctional uterine bleeding: Irregular or excessive uterine bleeding that results either from a structural problem or hormonal imbalance.

Dysmenorrhea: Difficult or painful menstruation.

Endometriosis: Presence of functioning endometrial tissue outside the uterus.

Fertility: Quality of being productive or fertile.

Hypogonadism: Inadequate production of sex hormones.

Hysterectomy: Surgical removal of the uterus.

Infertility: Inability to achieve pregnancy during a year or more of unprotected intercourse.

Intrauterine device: Contraceptive device inserted in the uterus usually made of cooper coils.

Kallman's syndrome: Congenital disorder that causes hypogonadism and loss of the sense of smell.

Klinefelter's syndrome: A chromosome disorder in males. People with the condition are born with at least one extra X chromosome.

Menopause: Termination of menstrual cycles and is an event that is usually marked by the passage of at least 1 full year without menstruation.

Menorrhagia: Excessive menstrual bleeding.

Osteoporosis: Loss of bone mass that occurs throughout the skeleton, predisposing patients to fractures.

Pelvic inflammatory disease: Infection of the uterus, fallopian tubes, and adjacent pelvic structures that is not associated with pregnancy or surgery.

Polycystic ovary disease: Condition that is characterized by ovaries twice the normal size that are studded with fluid-filled cysts.

Pregnancy: Condition of having a developing embryo or fetus in the body after successful conception.

Premenstrual dysphoric disorder: Disorder characterized by symptoms such as depression, anxiety, hopelessness, sad feelings, self-depreciation.

Premenstrual syndrome: Condition involving a set of symptoms (headache, irritability, depression, fatigue, sleep changes, weight gain) that occur before the start of the menstrual cycle.

Prolactinoma: Pituitary tumor that produces excessive amount of prolactin.

Salpingitis: Inflammation of the fallopian tube, usually as a result of an STI.

Supraovulation: Simultaneous rupture of multiple mature follicles.

Toxic shock syndrome (TSS): Rare disorder caused by certain *Staphyococcus aureus* strains seen in women using tampons.

Turner's syndrome: Congenital endocrine disorder caused by a failure of the ovaries to respond to pituitary hormone (gonadotropin) stimulation.

Vaginitis: Inflammation of the vagina.

Types of Reproductive System Conditions

PREGNANCY

Pregnancy is the condition of having a developing embryo or fetus in the body after successful conception. The average gestational period is 280 days or 40 weeks. About 7 million Americans become pregnant each year, and about two-thirds of those pregnancies result in live births. Common symptoms include *amenorrhea*, nausea and vomiting, breast tenderness, urinary frequency, fatigue, and changes in skin pigmentation (chloasma). Physiological changes and disorders that affect body systems are outlined in Table 34-1.

PREGNANCY PREVENTION

A variety of methods exist to prevent pregnancy (Box 34-1). *Hormonal* methods of contraception began with the establishment of the relationship between sex hormone levels and ovulation. This led to the development of oral contraceptives. In addition to oral contraceptives taken as a pill, other types of hormonal birth control "delivery mechanisms" are also available. They include hormone-impregnated vaginal inserts, hormone injections, skin "patches," and surgical implants. Many other methods of contraception exist. They have differing rates of effectiveness and unique advantages and disadvantages. For example, *spermicidal methods* involve use of preparations (foams, jellies, and creams) that act to kill sperm, and *mechanical barrier methods* use devices such as condoms, diaphragms, and cervical cap to block sperm from entering the uterus. *Surgical methods* such as tubal ligation and male vasectomy result in permanent sterility. *Behavioral methods* involve abstaining from sexual intercourse for a specified number of days before, during, and after ovulation. The rhythm method is a natural method that is based on calculating the fertile period by the use of a calendar, on which the supposed infertile days are marked. The ovulation method includes keeping a temperature chart to detect a minute change in temperature at the time of ovulation or judging the time of ovulation by observing changes in cervical mucus.

TABLE 34-1   Physiological Changes During Pregnancy

Body systems affected by pregnancy	Physiological changes	Disorders
Mammary	Enlarged, tender, and more nodular	
	Aerolae darken; nipples become more sensitive and erectile	
	Colostrum may leak out during the last trimester as the breasts prepare for lactation	
Reproductive: uterine, cervix	Softening	Vaginal bleeding
	Change in size, shape, and consistency	
	Increase in muscle mass	
Vagina	Increase in secretions	
	Lowering of pH levels	
	Elongation, increase in vascularity, elasticity	
	Thickening of mucus	
	Discharge	
Endocrine system	Elevated levels of estrogen and progesterone	*Placenta*
	Increased size and activity of thyroid gland	Abruptio placentae
	Increased level of triiodothyronine and globulin	Placenta previa
	Placental hormones prevent ovulation; development of corpus luteum	Placentitis
		Gestational diabetes
Cardiovascular	Increase in circulation blood volume	*Preeclampsia*
	Increase in RBC count	Hypertension
	Rising levels of clotting factors (VII, VIII, IX, X)	Edema
	Increase in pulse rate and stroke volume	Proteinuria
		Eclampsia
		Severe hypertension
		Convulsions
		Coma
		Varicose veins
		Hemorrhoids
Musculoskeletal	Softening, increased mobility of pelvic articulations	Cramping "charley horse"
		Back pain
	Increase in lumbar curve	Pedal edema
Respiratory	Decreased airway resistance	Edema
	Shortness of breath	Congestion of nasal mucosa (nosebleeds and stuffiness)
Gastrointestinal		Nausea and vomiting (first trimester)
		Heartburn
		Constipation
Skin	Chloasma	Prutritus
	Areolar darkening	
	Linea negra (pigmented line vertically bisecting abdomen)	
Urinary	Increase in urinary frequency	
	Increase in bladder capacity	
	Increased voiding	
Weight	Weight gain of 25 to 39 lb (11.4 to 17.7 kg)	

BOX 34-1   METHODS OF CONTRACEPTION

- Hormonal
- Spermicidal
- Mechanical barriers
- Behavioral
- Natural

CONDOMS

A **condom** is a device, usually made of latex or polyurethane, that is used during sexual intercourse. It is put on a man's erect penis and physically blocks ejaculated semen from entering the body of the sexual partner. Condoms are used to prevent pregnancy and transmission of sexually transmitted infections (STIs) such as gonorrhea, syphilis, and HIV. Condoms are easy to use and inexpensive, have few side effects, and offer protection against STIs. Condom use is typically combined with as spermicide for greater protection. Condoms come in various sizes, from magnum to snug. Mass-produced condoms do not vary much in width but do vary significantly in length.

Latex condoms are the most distributed type of condom in the world, and there are thousands of variants in regard to thickness, size, and texture.

Polyurethane condoms are thinner than latex condoms (0.02 mm). They conduct heat better than latex, are not as sensitive to temperature and ultraviolet light, can be used with oil-based lubricants, are less allergenic than latex, and do not have an odor. They are more likely to slip or break than is latex and are more expensive.

Lambskin condoms made from lamb intestines are the oldest form of condom available. They have a greater availability to transmit body warmth and tactile sensation compared to synthetic condoms and are less allergenic than latex. Because the pores of the lambskin condoms are larger, they are considered ineffective in preventing the transmission of STIs.

The "**Invisible Condom**," developed in Quebec, Canada, is a gel that hardens upon increased temperature after insertion into the vagina or rectum. In the laboratory, it has been shown to effectively block HIV and herpes simplex virus. The barrier breaks down and liquefies after several hours. The invisible condom is in the clinical trial phase and has not yet been approved for use.

The "**female condom**" or "**femidom**" is larger and wider than male condoms but equivalent in length. It has a flexible ring-shaped opening and is designed to be inserted into the vagina. It contains an inner ring that aids insertion and helps keep the condom from sliding out of the vagina during sexual intercourse. This condom is made from polyurethane or nitrile.

DIAPHRAGMS AND IUD

The **diaphragm** is a cervical barrier type of birth control. It is a soft latex or silicone dome with a spring molded rim. The spring creates a seal against the wall of the vagina. The rim of the diaphragm is squeezed into an oval or arc shape for insertion. A water-based lubricant (usually spermicide) may be applied to the rim of the diaphragm to aid insertion. One teaspoon (5 ml) of spermicide is placed in the dome of the diaphragm before insertion or with an applicator after insertion. The diaphragm must be inserted sometime before sexual intercourse and remain in the vagina for 6 to 8 hours after a man's last ejaculation. Upon removal, a diaphragm should be cleaned with warm soapy water before storage. The diaphragm must be removed for cleaning at least once every 24 hours. Oil-based products should not be used with latex diaphragms. Lubricants or vaginal medications that contain oil will cause the latex to rapidly degrade and greatly increases the chances of the diaphragm breaking or tearing. A latex diaphragm should be replaced every 1 to 3 years. Silicone diaphragms may last much longer—up to 10 years. Diaphragms come in different sizes. A correctly fitting diaphragm will cover the cervix and rest snugly against the pubic bone. A diaphragm that is too small might fit inside the vagina without covering the cervix or might become dislodged from the cervix during intercourse or bowel movements. Diaphragms should be refitted after a weight change of 4.5 kg (10 lb) or more. Diaphragms should also be refitted after any pregnancy of 14 weeks or longer. In the United States, diaphragms are available by prescription only. Many European countries do not require prescriptions.

Adverse Reactions

Diaphragms are associated with an increased risk of urinary tract infection. ***Toxic shock syndrome (TSS)*** occurs at a rate of 2.4 cases/100,000 women using diaphragms, almost exclusively when the device is left in place longer than 24 hours.

Types of Diaphragms

Generic name	U.S. brand name(s) / Canadian brand(s)	Dosage forms and strengths
flat spring	Reflexions	50 mm to 105 mm (2 to 4 inches)
coil spring	Ortho Coil	50 mm to 150 mm (2 to 4 inches)
	Milex Wide-Seal Omniflex Semina	
arcing spring	Ortho All-Flex	50 mm to 105 mm (2 to 4 inches)
	Milex Wide-Seal Arcing	

LEA'S SHIELD

Lea's Shield (Canada) and Lea Contraceptive (United States) is a female barrier method of contraception. It is a reusable barrier made of medical-grade silicone, inserted in the vagina over the cervix with the intention to block sperm. It is used in conjunction with spermicide. Like the cervical cap, Lea's Shield stays in place by suction. It differs from the other female barrier methods, such as the cervical cap and the diaphragm, in that it comes in one size (does not need to be specifically fitted to each woman) and it has a one-way valve to aid in creation of suction. This valve also allows for passage of cervical mucus. The shield also has a loop to assist in removal. It is available by prescription in the United States, although it is obtainable over the counter in Europe and Canada.

INTRAUTERINE DEVICE

An **intrauterine device** is a birth control device also known as an IUD or a coil (based on the coil-shaped design of early IUDs). It is a device placed in the uterus and is the world's most widely used method of reversible birth control currently used by 160 million women. The device has to be fitted inside or removed from the uterus by a physician or qualified medical practitioner. Depending on the type, a single IUD is approved for 5 to 10 years' use (the copper T380A is effective for at least 12 years). There are two broad categories of intrauterine contraceptive devices: copper-based devices and those that work by releasing a progestogen. In the United States, there are two types of intrauterine devices available: the copper Paraguard and the hormonal Mirena. Most nonhormonal IUDs have a plastic T-shaped frame that is wrapped with copper and/or has copper bands. In some IUDs, such as the Nova T 380, the pure copper wire has a silver core, which has been shown to prevent breaking of the wire. The arms of the frame hold the IUD in place near the top of the uterus. The GyneFix does not have a T-shape but rather a loop that holds several copper tubes. The GyneFix is held in place by a suture to the fundus of the uterus.

Mechanism of Action

The presence of an object in the uterus prompts the release of leukocytes and prostaglandins by the endometrium. These substances are hostile to both sperm and eggs; the presence of the copper increases the spermicidal effect. While the primary mechanism of the IUD is spermicidal/ovicidal, postfertilization mechanisms are believed to contribute significantly to their effectiveness. IUDs do not protect against STDs or PID.

Some physicians prefer to insert the IUD during menstruation to verify that the woman is not pregnant at the time of insertion. However, IUDs may be safely inserted at anytime during the menstrual cycle. The pregnancy rate for IUDs is less than 1% per year. If pregnancy does occur, presence of the IUD increases the risk of miscarriage, particularly during the second trimester. Hormonal uterine devices reduce menstrual bleeding or prevent menstruation all together and can be used as a treatment for **menorrhagia** (heavy periods). Mirena is the only intrauterine system available and releases levonorgestrel (a progestogen) and may be used for 5 years.

Adverse Reaction

Insertion of an IUD may introduce bacteria into the uterus. The insertion carries a small transient risk of PID in the first 20 days after insertion.

Intrauterine Devices

Generic name	Brand name(s)
copper based IUD	Paraguard Copper T 380A, Nova T 380A, GyneFix
levonorgestrel	LNG-20 IUS (US), Mirena (Canada)

ORAL CONTRACEPTIVES

Oral contraceptives (OCs) are collectively called "the pill." Numerous OC products are available containing different types, combinations, and dosages of estrogen and progesterone (Table 34-2). The so-called "mini-pill" contains only progestin. The pill can be used to regulate menstruation and to prevent pregnancy. If used correctly and consistently, the pill is an extremely effective contraceptive with an unintended pregnancy rate estimated at between 0.1% and 3%. Only total abstinence is 100% in preventing pregnancy.

Mechanism of action

Most hormonal contraceptives were developed to prevent pregnancy by initiating negative feedback inhibition of follicle-stimulating hormone (FSH) and luteinizing hormone (LH) secretion. As a result, mature follicles do not develop, and LH levels required to initiate ovulation do not occur. The next menses does take place, however, if the progesterone and estrogen dosage is stopped in time to allow blood levels to decrease as they normally do near the end of the cycle to bring on menstruation.

Adverse Reactions

Smoking increases risk of adverse reactions, including increased risk of thromboembolic events and heart attacks. Loss of appetite and constipation can also be experienced. Women taking OCs should immediately report pain or muscle soreness, swelling, heat, or redness in calves; shortness of breath; sudden loss of vision; unresolved leg or foot swelling or weight gain (>5 lb); change in menstrual pattern; breast tenderness, that does not go away; acute abdominal cramping; signs of vaginal infection; blurred vision; and changes in central nervous system (confusion, acute anxiety, or unresolved depression).

OTHER CONTRACEPTIVE DOSAGE FORMS

Depo-Provera injection is a synthetic derivative of progesterone that induces and maintains the endometrium; prevents ovulation; and produces a thick cervical mucus that prevents the passage of sperm. An advantage is that the injection is administered every 3 months, but there are many disadvantages such as sensitivity to sunlight, dizziness, anxiety, depression, changes in appetite, decreased libido, hot flashes, and increased body hair (reversible when drug is discontinued), and osteoporosis, among others.

TABLE 34-2   Types of Oral Contraceptives

Monophasic estrogen/ progestin combinations	Provide a fixed dose of estrogen and progestin throughout the cycle of 21 or 28 days' package
Biphasic estrogen/ progestin combinations	Amount of estrogen remains the same throughout cycle, less progestin in first half of cycle and increased progestin in second half of cycle
Triphasic estrogen/ progestin combinations	Amount of estrogen is the same or varies throughout cycle; progestin amount varies

Ortho-Evra is a transdermal patch containing a combination of estrogen and progestin. One patch is applied each week for 3 weeks followed by 1 patch-free week. Each patch should be applied on the same day each week and only one patch should be worn at a time. No more than 7 days should pass during the patch-free interval. An advantage over other methods of contraception is that it is a weekly dose, noninvasive, and easy to use. Disadvantages are that the patch can become partially or completed detached and can irritate the skin.

Nuva-Ring is a hormonal vaginal ring inserted for 3 weeks and then removed for 1 week. A new ring is inserted 7 days after the last one was removed and should be inserted the same time as the insertion of the previous ring. Advantages are that it is easy to use and it is a once-per-month dosing. Although rare, it is possible for the ring to slip outside of the vagina, and then it must be replaced within 3 hours.

Adverse Reactions

Adverse reactions include increased blood pressure; loss of appetite, constipation; pain or muscle soreness, swelling, heat, redness in calves; shortness of breath, sudden loss of vision, weight gain; breast tenderness, acute abdominal cramping; signs of vaginal infection; and changes in the CNS. Smoking increases the risk of thromboembolic events and heart attacks.

Types of Oral Contraceptives

Generic name	U.S. brand name(s) Canadian brand(s)	Dosage forms and strengths
Estrogen and progestin combinations		
ethinyl estradiol + desogestrel	Apri, Cyclessa, Desogen, Kariva, Mircette, Ortho-Cept, Solia, Velivet Marvelon	**Tablet:** ethinyl estradiol 0.02 mg/desogstrel 0.15 mg (low-dose formulation) **Monophasic formulation:** ethinyl estradiol 0.03 mg/desonorgestrel 0.15 mg (21days) **Triphasic formulation:** Days 1 to 7 (ethinyl estradiol 0.025 mg/desonorgestrel 0.1 mg); Days 8 to 14 (ethinyl estradiol 0.025 mg/desonorgestrel 0.125 mg); Days 14 to 21(ethinyl estradiol 0.025 mg/desonorgestrel 0.15 mg)
ethinyl estradiol + drospirenone	Yasmin, Yaz Yasmin, Angeliq	**Tablet:** ethinyl estradiol 0.03 mg/drospirenone 3 mg
ethinyl estradiol + etonogestrel	Nuva-Ring Nuva-Ring	**Intravaginal ring:** ethinyl estradiol 0.015 mg/day/etonoethinylenonorgestrel 0.12 mg/day
ethinyl estradiol + levonorgestrel	Alesse, Aviane, Enpresse, Lessina, Levlen, Levlite, Levora, Lutera, Nordette, Portia, Seasonale, Tr-Levlen, Triphasil, Trivora Min-Ovral, Triquilar	**Tablet** **Low-dose formulation:** ethinyl estradiol 0.02 mg/levonorgestrel 0.1 mg **Monophasic formulation:** ethinyl estradiol 0.03 mg/levonorgestrel 0.15 mg **Triphasic formulation:** Days 1 to 6 ethinyl estradiol 0.03 mg/levonorgetrel 0.05 mg; Days 7 to 11 ethinyl estradiol 0.04 mg/levonorgestrel 0.075 mg Days 12 to 21 ethinyl estradiol 0.03 mg/levonorgestrel 0.125 mg

Continued

Types of Oral Contraceptives—cont'd

	Generic name	U.S. brand name(s) / Canadian brand(s)	Dosage forms and strengths
	ethinyl estradiol + norethindrone*	Aranelle, Brevicon, Estrostep Fe, femHRT, Junel, Junel 0.5/35, Necon 1/35, Necon 7/7/7, Necon 7/11, Norinyl 1+35, Nortrel, Nortrel 7/7/7, Ortho-Novum, Ovcon, Tri-Norinyl	**Tablet** **Monophasic formulation:** varied dosages **Biphasic formulation:** varied dosages **Triphasic formulation:** varied dosages
		Minestrin 1/20, Select 1/35, Symphasic	
	ethinyl estradiol + norgestimate*	MonoNessa, Ortho-Cyclen, Ortho Tri-Cyclen, Previfem, Sprintec, TriNessa, Tri-Prevofem, Tri-Sprintec	**Tablet** **Monophasic formulation:** ethinyl estradiol 0.035 mg/ norgestimate 0.25 mg **Triphasic formulation:** Days 1 to 7 ethinyl estradiol 0.035 mg/norgestimate 0.18 mg Days 8 to 14 ethinyl estradiol 0.035 mg/norgestimate 0.215 mg Days 15 to 21 ethinyl estradiol 0.035 mg/ norgestimate 0.25 mg
Progesterone			
	progesterone, progestin*	Crinone, Prochieve, Progestasert, Prometrium	**Capsule (Prometrium):** 100 mg, 200 mg **Vaginal gel (Crinone, Prochieve):** 4%, 8% **Injection:** 50 mg/ml **Intrauterine system:** 38 mg
		Crinone, Prometrium	

*Generic available.

EMERGENCY CONTRACEPTION

Emergency use of OC pills containing levonorgestrel alone reduces the risk for pregnancy after unprotected intercourse by 89%. Pills containing a combination of ethinyl estradiol and either norgestrel or levonorgestrel can be used and reduce the risk for pregnancy by 75%. Emergency contraception with oral contraceptive pills (levonorgestrel—Plan B) should be initiated as soon as possible after unprotected intercourse. Plan B should be used within 72 hours of unprotected sexual intercourse; a second tablet should be taken 12 hours after first dose. It may be used anytime during the menstrual cycle. The only medical contraindication to provision of emergency contraception is current pregnancy.

Emergency insertion of a copper IUD also is highly effective, reducing the risk by as much as 99%.

Emergency Contraceptives

	Generic name	U.S. brand name(s) / Canadian brand(s)	Dosage forms and strengths
	levonorgestrel	Plan B	Tablet 0.75 mg
		Plan B	

MENOPAUSE AND ATROPHIC VAGINITIS

Unlike other body systems, the female reproductive system does not begin to perform its functions until puberty, and unlike the male reproductive system, the female reproductive system ceases its principal function in middle adulthood around 35 to 58 years of age. *Menopause* is the termination of menstrual cycles and is an event that is usually marked by the passage of at least 1 full year without menstruation. Natural menopause will occur in 25% of women by age 47, 50% by age 50, 75% by age 52, and 95% by age 55. After that time, a woman may continue to enjoy normal sexual activity, but she cannot produce more offspring. Menopause due to surgical removal of the ovaries (*hysterectomy*) has occurred in almost 30% of U.S. women who are 50 years or older.

Symptoms of menopause may last from a few months to years and vary from hardly noticeable to severe. Symptoms include vasomotor instability, nervousness, hot flashes (flushes), chills, excitability, fatigue, apathy, mental depression, crying episodes, insomnia, palpitation, vertigo, headache, numbness, tingling, myalgia, urinary disturbances (such as incontinence), atrophic vaginitis, and various disorders of the gastrointestinal system. The long-range effects of lower estrogen levels are osteoporosis and atherosclerosis.

Atrophic vaginitis is the postmenopausal thinning and dryness of the vaginal epithelium related to decreased estrogen levels. Symptoms include burning and pain during intercourse. Hormone replacement therapy or application of topical estrogen restores the integrity of the vaginal epithelium and supporting tissues and relieves symptoms.

HORMONE REPLACEMENT THERAPY

Hormone replacement therapy (HRT) is medication containing one or more female hormones, commonly estrogen plus progestin (synthetic progesterone). Some women receive estrogen-only therapy (usually women who have had their uterus removed). HRT is most often used to treat symptoms of menopause such as "hot flashes," vaginal dryness, mood swings, sleep disorders, and decreased sexual desire. This medication may be taken in the form of a pill, a patch, or vaginal cream. Based on earlier studies, many physicians used to believe that HRT might be beneficial for reducing the risk of heart disease and bone fractures caused by osteoporosis (thinning of the bones) in addition to treating menopausal symptoms. The results of a new study by the Women's Health Initiative (WHI) have led physicians to revise their recommendation regarding HRT. Part of the study was intended to examine the health benefits and the risks of HRT including the risk of developing breast cancer, heart attacks, strokes, and blood clots. One component of the WHI, which studied the use of estrogen and progestin in women who had a uterus, was stopped early because the health risks exceeded the health benefits. The estrogen-progestin study showed there was a 26% increase in breast cancer. A second component of the WHI, which studies estrogen-only therapy in women who no longer had a uterus, was also stopped early because it showed an increase in the risk of strokes.

Hormone replacement typically involves administration of oral or vaginal estrogens with or without progestins (synthetic progesterone). Table 34-3 shows examples of oral estrogen and estrogen/progestin products.

TABLE 34-3   Examples of Oral Estrogen and Estrogen/Progestin Products

Estrogen Pills		Progestin Pills		Estrogen-Plus-Progestin Pills	
Brand	Generic	Brand	Generic	Brand	Generic
Premarin	conjugated equine estrogens	Cycrin	medroxyprogesterone acetate	Premphase	conjugated equine estrogens and medroxyprogesterone acetate
Cenestin	synthetic conjugated estrogens	Provera	medroxyprogesterone acetate	Prempro	conjugated equine estrogens and medroxyprogesterone acetate
Estratab	esterified estrogens	Aygestin	norethindrone acetate	Femhrt	ethinylestradiol and norethindrone acetate
Menest	esterified estrogens		norethindrone acetate		
Ortho-Est	estropipate (piperazine estrone sulfate)	Norlutate	progesterone USP (in peanut oil)	Activella	17-β-estradiol and norethindrone acetate
Ogen	estropipate (piperazine estrone sulfate)	Prometrium		Ortho-Prefest	17-β-estradiol and norgestimate
Estrace	micronized 17-β-estradiol				
Estinyl	ethinyl estradiol				

Courtesy of National Library of Medicine, NIH publication No. 05-5200.

BOX 34-2 EXAMPLES OF TYPICAL HORMONAL REPLACEMENT THERAPY REGIMENS

- Cyclic or sequential
  - Estrogen every day
  - Progesterone or progestin added for 10 to 14 days out of every 4 weeks
- Continuous-combined
  - Estrogen and progestin daily without a break

Courtesy of the National Library of Medicine, NIH publication No. 05-5200.

TABLE 34-4   Examples of Gels, Creams, Patches, and Other Hormone Products

Type	Brand	Generic
Estrogen Products		
Vaginal Cream	Estrace	micronized 17-β-estradiol
	Ortho Dienestrol	dienestrol
	Ogen	estropipate (piperazine estrone sulfate)
	Premarin	conjugated equine estrogens
Vaginal Tablet	Vagifem	estradiol hemihydrate
Vaginal Ring	Estring	micronized 17-β-estradiol
	Femring	estradiol acetate
Skin Patch	Alora	micronized 17-β-estradiol
	Climara	micronized 17-β-estradiol
	Esclim	micronized 17-β-estradiol
	Estraderm	micronized 17-β-estradiol
	Vivelle	micronized 17-β-estradiol
	Vivelle-Dot	micronized 17-β-estradiol
Skin Gel	Estrogel	estradiol gel
Skin Cream	Estrasorb	estradiol topical emulsion
Progestin Products		
Vaginal Gel	Crinone	progesterone
IUD	Mirena	levonorgestrel
Estrogen Plus Progestin Products		
Skin Patch	Combipatch	17-β-estradiol and norethindrone acetate
		17-β-estradiol and norgestimate
	Ortho-Prefest	

Courtesy of the National Library of Medicine, NIH publication No. 05-5200.

Treatment protocols vary according to whether or not the woman has a uterus or has had a hysterectomy.

The dosage form may vary according to symptoms to be treated. For example, a vaginal estrogen ring or cream can ease vaginal dryness, urinary leakage, or vaginal or urinary infections but does not relieve hot flashes.

Adverse Reactions

HRT may increase risk of heart disease, pulmonary embolism, and breast and endometrial cancers. Other adverse effects are nausea, vomiting, bloating, cramping, breast tenderness, return of menstruation or spotting, migraine headaches, and weight gain.

Hormone Replacement Therapy

	Generic name	U.S. brand name(s)	Dosage forms and strengths
	Estrogen		
	estradiol*	Climara-25, -50, -75, -100, Delesterogen, Estrace, Estraderm-25, -50, -100, Estradot-25, -37.5, -100, Estring, Estrogel, Oesclim, Vagifem, Vivelle	**Vaginal cream (Estrace):** 0.1 mg/g **Topical gel (Estrogel):** 0.06% **Injection (Delesterogen):** 10 mg/ml **Vaginal ring (Estring):** 0.05 mg **Tablet:** (Estrace): 0.5 mg, 1 mg, 2 mg **Vaginal tablet (Vagifem):** 25 mcg **Transdermal patch:** 2 mg, 3.8 mg, 5.7 mg, 7.6 mg (Climara) 2 mg, 4 mg, 8 mg (Estraderm) 0.39 mg, 0.585 mg, 1.56 mg (Estradot) 50 mcg (Vivelle)
	conjugated estrogens* (equine)	C.E.S.; Congest Premarin	**Vaginal cream:** 0.625 mg/g **Injection:** 25 mg **Tablet:** 0.3 mg, 0.45 mg, 0.625 mg, 0.9 mg, 1.25 mg, 2.5 mg
	estrogen (esterified)	Neo Estrone	**Tablet:** 0.3 mg, 0.625 mg, 1.25 mg, 2.5 mg
	estropipate*	Ogen	**Tablet:** 0.625 mg, 1.25 mg, 2.5 mg
	Estrogen and progesterone combinations		
	estradiol + norethindrone	Estalis 140/50, 250/50, Estalis-Sequi	0.62 mg estradiol + 2.7 mg norethindrone (Estalis) 0.51 mg estradiol + 4.8 mg norethindrone (Estalis) 0.62 mg estradiol + 4.33 mg estradiol + 2.7 mg norethindrone (Estalis Sequi) 0.51 mg estradiol + 4.33 mg estradiol + 4.8 mg norethindrone (Estalis Sequi)
	estrogens + medroxyprogesterones	Premplus	**Tablet:** conjugated estrogens 0.625 mg + medroxyprogesterone 5 mg (Premplus)
	ethinyl estradiol + etonorgestrel	Nuvaring	2.6 mg ethinyl estradiol + 11.4 mg etonorgestrel
	ethinyl estradiol + norethindrone	FemHRT	5 mcg ethinyl estradiol + 1 mg norethindrone

*Generic available.

Hormonal and Menstrual Disorders

PREMENSTRUAL SYNDROME

Premenstrual syndrome (PMS) is a condition that involves a collection of symptoms that regularly occur in women during the premenstrual phase of their reproductive cycles. Symptoms include headache, irritability fatigue, nervousness, weight gain, sleep changes, depression, and other problems that are distressing enough to limit activity and affect personal

TECH ALERT!

The following drugs have look-alike/ sound-alike issues: fluoxetine and fluvastatin; Prozac, Prilosec, Proscar, Prosom, and Prostep; Sarafem and Serophene; Paroxetine and pyridoxine; Paxil, Plavix, and Taxol; sertraline, selegiline, and Serentil; Zoloft and Zocor

relationships. Because the causes of PMS are still unclear, current treatments focus on relieving the symptoms. A more severe form of PMS is premenstrual dysphoric disorder (PMDD). It is characterized by more pronounced characteristics of PMS and occurs during the last week of the luteal phase in most menstrual cycles during the year preceding diagnosis. These symptoms begin to remit within a few days of the onset of the menses (follicular phase) and are always absent the week following menses. Five or more of the following symptoms must be present to be diagnosed with PMDD: feeling sad, hopeless, or self-depreciating; feeling tense, anxious, or "on edge"; marked lability of mood interspersed with frequent tearfulness; persistent irritability, anger, and increased interpersonal conflicts; decreased interest in usual activities, difficulty concentrating, feeling fatigue, lethargic, or lacking in energy; marked changes in appetite such as binge eating and cravings; hypersomnia or insomnia; a subjective feeling of being out of control; and physical symptoms such as "bloating," weight gain, breast tenderness, and joint or muscle pain. The symptoms may be accompanied by suicidal thoughts. Women commonly report that their symptoms worsen with age until relieved by the onset of menopause. PMDD is treated with antidepressants such as SSRIs.

Selective Serotonin Reuptake Inhibitors for Treatment of PMDD

Generic name	U.S. brand name(s)	Dosage forms and strengths
	Canadian brand(s)	
fluoxetine*	Prozac, Prozac Weekly, Sarafem	**Capsule (Prozac):** 10 mg, 20 mg, 40 mg; (Serafem) 10 mg, 40 mg **Capsule, delayed release (Prozac Weekly):** 90 mg
	Prozac	**Solution, oral (Prozac): 20 mg/5 ml Tablet (Prozac):** 10 mg, 20 mg
sertraline*	Zoloft	**Solution, oral concentrate:** 20 mg/ml
	Zoloft	**Tablet:** 25 mg, 50 mg, 100 mg
paroxetine*	Paxil, Paxil CR, Prexeva	**Suspension, oral:** 10 mg/5 ml (250 ml) **Tablet, as hydrochloride (Paxil):** 10 mg, 20 mg, 30 mg, 40 mg
	Paxil, Paxil CR	**Tablet, as mesylate (Pexeva):** 10 mg, 20 mg, 30 mg, 40 mg **Tablet, as controlled release (Paxil CR):** 12.5 mg, 25 mg, 37.5 mg

*Generic available.

TECH ALERT!

The following drugs have look-alike/ sound-alike issues: Aleve and Alesse Anaprox, Anaspaz, and Avapro Naprelan and Naprosyn Naprosyn, naproxen, Natacyn, and Nebcin Oruvail, Clinoril, and Elavil

DYSMENORRHEA

Dysmenorrhea, or "painful menstruation," is the term used to describe *menstrual cramps*. As many as 75% to 85% of women will have painful periods sometime during their reproductive years. Severe lower abdominal cramping and back pain accompanied by headache, nausea, and vomiting will disrupt their school, work, athletic, or other activities. *Primary dysmenorrhea* is the most common type, occurring primarily in adolescents and young women. Symptoms, which can last from hours to days and vary in severity from cycle to cycle, are caused by an abnormally increased concentration of certain prostaglandins produced by the uterine lining. High concentrations of prostaglandin E_2 (PGE_2) and prostaglandin F_2 (PGF_2) cause painful spasms by decreasing blood flow and oxygen delivery to the uterine muscle. Fortunately, primary dysmenorrhea is not associated with pelvic disease, such as an infection or a tumor. In more severe cases, antiinflammatory drugs or certain hormones, including OCs, are administered to alter menstrual cycle activity or reduce the level of cyclical uterine contractions. *Secondary dysmenorrhea* refers to menstrual-related pain caused by some pelvis pathological condition, including inflammatory conditions and cervical stenosis. Treatment involves treating the underlying disorder. Primary dysmenorrhea can generally be treated effectively with over-the-counter (OTC) drugs such as nonsteroidal antiinflammatory drugs (NSAIDS) as discussed in Chapter 10.

Nonsteroidal Antiinflammatory Drug (NSAID) Treatment for Dysmenorrhea

Generic name	U.S. brand name(s)	Dosage forms and strengths
	Canadian brand(s)	
ibuprofen*	Advil, Motrin, Midol	**Caplet, tablet:** 200 mg
	Advil, Motrin	
naproxen*	Aleve, Anaprox, Anaprox DS, Naprelan, Naprosyn, Pamprin	**Caplet:** 220 mg **Tablet:** 250 mg, 375 mg, 500 mg (Anaprox DS: 550 mg) **Tablet CR, ER:** 375 mg, 500 mg
	Anaprox, Anaprox DS, Naprelan, Naprosyn, Naprosyn E	
ketoprofen*	Orudis KT, Oruvail	**Caplet:** 50 mg, 75 mg **Capsule (Oruvail ER):** 100 mg, 150 mg, 200 mg **Tablet (Orudis KT):** 12.5 mg
	generics	
meclofamate*	Generics	**Capsule:** 50 mg, 100 mg
	not available	

*Generic available.

AMENORRHEA

Amenorrhea is the absence of normal menstruation. *Primary amenorrhea* is the failure of the menstrual cycles to begin, and it may be caused by various factors, such as hormone imbalances, genetic disorders, brain lesions, or structural deformities of the reproductive organs. *Secondary amenorrhea* occurs when a woman who has previously menstruated slows to three or fewer cycles per year. Amenorrhea may be a symptom of excessive weight loss, pregnancy, lactation, menopause, or disease of the reproductive system. If amenorrhea occurs because of sports training, then treatment may become part of extensive long-term strategy to address a number of complex nutritional, hormonal, and self-image issues.

Pharmaceutical Treatment of Amenorrhea

Generic name	U.S. brand name(s)	Dosage forms and strengths
	Canadian brand(s)	
bromocriptine*	Parlodel	**Tablet:** 2.5 mg **Capsule:** 5 mg
	Parlodel	
oral contraceptives	See mini-drug monograph "types of oral contraceptives"	See mini-drug monograph "types of oral contraceptives"

*Generic available.

DYSFUNCTIONAL UTERINE BLEEDING

Dysfunctional uterine bleeding (DUB) is defined as irregular or excessive uterine bleeding resulting from a structural problem or hormonal imbalance that causes a disruption of blood supply. Excessive uterine bleeding from any cause can result in life-threatening anemia. DUB is a significant medical problem, one that affects nearly 2 million women in the United States every year. To diagnose the cause, a physician may use specialized ultrasound or x-ray studies, look directly inside the uterus, or examine tissue obtained by biopsy to exclude cancer. Symptoms may include excessive bleeding and cramping for an abnormal period of time beyond the normal menstrual cycle.

If hormonal imbalance is the cause of DUB, it is the excessive growth (hyperplasia) and breakdown of delicate endometrial tissue that results in heavy bleeding. In these cases, treatment begins with NSAIDs and hormonal manipulation using low-dose birth control pills. If conservative treatment fails to stop the endometrial lining from hemorrhaging, hysterectomy remains one of the most curative options.

Disorders Caused by Infection or Inflammation of the Reproductive System

Pelvic inflammatory disease (PID) may be an acute or chronic inflammatory condition and is caused by several different pathogens, which usually spread upward from the vagina. PID is a major cause of infertility and sterility and affects more than 800,000 women each year in the United States and Canada. It is a common complication following an STI by chlamydial and gonoccoccal STI organisms. Infection involving the uterus, uterine tubes, ovaries, and other pelvic organs and often results in development of scar tissue and adhesions.

Salpingitis is a uterine tube inflammatory condition characterized by obstruction of the lumen and marked by dilation at the end of the tube. Fluids accumulate that cannot escape.

Vaginitis is inflammation or infection of the vaginal lining. Vaginitis most often results from STIs or from a "yeast infection." So-called yeast infections are opportunistic infections of the fungus *Candidiasis albicans,* producing candidiasis. Candidiasis infections are characterized by a whitish discharge (leukorrhea).

Sexually transmitted infections (STIs) and venereal diseases are infections caused by communicable pathogens such as viruses, bacteria, fungi, and protozoa. They can all be transmitted by sexual contact. Diseases classified as STIs can be transmitted sexually but do not have to be. For example, acquired immunodeficiency syndrome (AIDS) is a viral condition that can be spread through sexual contact but is also spread by transfusion of infected blood and the use of contaminated medical instruments such as intravenous needles and syringes.

> **TECH ALERT!**
>
> The following drugs have look-alike/ sound-alike issues: Azithromycin and erythromycin
> Rocephin and Roferon
> Floxin and Flexeril
> doxycyline, doxepin, doxylamine, and dicyclomine
> Monodox and Maalox
> Trobicin and tobramycin
> Zinacef and Zithromax

Treatment of Selected Sexually Transmitted Infections

Generic name	U.S. brand name(s)	Dosage forms and strengths
	Canadian brand(s)	
Chancroid		
azithromycin	Zithromax	1 g single dose
ceftriaxone	Rocephin	250 mg IM single dose
ciprofloxacin	Cipro	500 mg twice daily for 3 days
erythromycin	E-Mycin, Eryc E.E.S., Ery-tab, Erythrocin, PCE, Romycin	500 mg three times daily for 7 days
	ERYC, PCE, EES	
Chlamydia		
azithromycin	Zithromax	1 g single dose
doxyclycline*	Adoxa, Doryx, Doryx-100, Monodox, Periostat, Vibramycin, Vibra-Tabs	100 mg twice daily for 7 days
	Vibramycin, Vibra-Tabs	

Treatment of Selected Sexually Transmitted Infections—cont'd

Generic name	U.S. brand name(s) Canadian brand(s)	Dosage forms and strengths
Gonnorhea		
ceftriaxone*	Rocephin	125 mg IM in single dose
ciprofloxacin*	Cipro, Cipro XR, Ciloxan	500 mg single dose
cefixime*	Suprax	400 mg single dose
cefoxitin	Mefoxin	1 to 2 g every 6 hours
cefuroxime*	Generic	1 g single dose
	Ceftin, Kefurox,	
spiramycin (Canada only)	Rovamycine	12 million to 13.9 million units (8 to 9 capsules) as a single dose
spectinomycin	Trobicin	2 g IM single dose
gatafloxacin	Tequin	400 mg single dose
	Zymar	
ofloxacin*	Generics	400 mg as a single dose
	Generics	
doxycycline*	Adoxa, Doryx, Doryx-100, Monodox, Periostat, Vibramycin, Vibra-Tabs	100 mg twice daily × 14 days
	Vibramycin, Vibra-Tabs	
tetracycline*	Sumycin,	Tablet 200 mg to 500 mg every 6 hours
	Generics	

*Generic available.

INFERTILITY AND HYPOGONADISM

Infertility is often defined as a failure to conceive after 1 year of regular unprotected intercourse. Infertility may be caused by a wide variety of medical, environmental, and even lifestyle factors, such as smoking or alcohol abuse. Ninety percent of the causal factors may be traced to various problems in either the male or the female partner. For the remaining 10%, the reason is never determined. Approximately 25% of women in the overall population will experience some period of infertility during their reproductive years. In many cases, infertility results from an inability to ovulate—often caused by a medical condition such as *polycystic ovary disease,* a condition that is characterized by ovaries twice the normal size that are studded with fluid-filled cysts. Significant numbers of infertile women experiencing ovulatory dysfunction desire to become pregnant and, after a sometimes long and complex medical "workup" and selection process, become candidates to receive so-called fertility drugs, either alone or in combination with other "assisted reproductive procedures" such as artificial insemination.

Hypogonadism is when the sex glands produce little or no hormones. In men, these glands (gonads) are the testes; in women, they are the ovaries. The cause of hypogonadism may be "primary" or "central." In primary hypogonadism, the ovaries or testes themselves do not function properly. Some causes of primary hypogonadism include surgery, radiation, genetic or developmental disorders, liver or kidney disease, infection, and certain autoimmune disorders. The most common genetic disorders that cause primary hypogonadism are *Turner syndrome* (in women) and *Klinefelter syndrome* (in men). In central hypogonadism, the centers in the brain that control the gonads (hypothalamus and pituitary) do not function properly. Some causes of central hypogonadism include tumors, surgery, radiation, infections, trauma, bleeding, genetic problems, nutritional deficiencies, and iron excess (hemochromatosis). A genetic cause of central hypogonadism that also produces an inability to smell is *Kallman syndrome* (males). In girls, hypogonadism during childhood will result in lack of menstruation and breast development and short height. If hypogonadism occurs after puberty, symptoms include loss of menstruation, low libido, hot flashes, and loss of body hair. In boys, hypogonadism in childhood results in a lack of muscle and beard development and growth problems. In men, the usual complaints are sexual dysfunction, decreased beard and body hair, breast enlargement, and muscle loss. If a brain tumor is present, there may be headaches or visual loss or symptoms of other hormonal deficiencies (hypothyroidism). In *prolactinoma,* there may be a milky breast discharge. Anorexia nervosa (excessive dieting to the point of starvation) may produce central hypogonadism.

TREATMENT OF INFERTILITY

Pharmaceutical treatment of infertility may involve the administration of antiestrogens, menotropins, human chorionic gonadotropin, and recombinant human FSH.

ANTIESTROGENS

Clomiphene is an antiestrogen agent that competes with estrogen for estrogen-receptor binding sites. By blocking estrogen it acts as an ovulatory stimulant. This medication works by effectively "tricking" the pituitary gland into producing FSH and LH.

GONADOTROPINS

Supraovulation, or simultaneous rupture of multiple mature follicles, is an infertility treatment option that may be used if clomiphene use proves ineffective or if multiple ova are deemed desirable in assisted reproductive procedures such as in vitro fertilization. It most frequently involves self-administered injections of either (1) menotropins or (2) genetically developed (recombinant) gonadotropins. Menotropins are purified combination preparations of the human pituitary gonadotropins, FSH, and LH. Menotropins contain a small amount of human chorionic gonadotropin (hCG). Menotropins are derived from the urine of postmenopausal women. hCG may be derived from natural or synthetic sources. The synthetic, recombinant formulation is called choriogonadotropin alfa (rhCG). The natural source comes from the urine of pregnant females.

Follitropin, rFSH, is a recombinant version of human FSH. It mimics the actions of naturally released FSH and is required for normal follicular growth, maturation, and gonadal steroid production.

MECHANISM OF ACTION AND PHARMACOKINETICS

The production of FSH and LH (gonadotropins) causes normal follicle growth and subsequent ovulation. Clomiphene is given starting on day 5 of the menstrual cycle and, if treatment is successful, ovulation begins 5 to 10 days after a course of the drug.

The action of hCG on adult females is essentially identical to those of LH. hCG and human menotropins (hMG) are peptides and therefore are quickly destroyed in the gastrointestinal tract, so they must be administered parenterally either as intramuscular (IM) injections or, for select products, as subcutaneous (SC) injections. Urine-derived hCG is administered IM and recombinant hCG is administered SC. The action of hMG is to mimic the action of naturally released FSH. Administration usually results in follicular growth and maturation. It is immediately followed by administration of hCG to produce ovulation.

ADVERSE REACTIONS

Clomiphene may cause visual disturbances, dizziness, and lightheadedness. It should not be used during pregnancy. Side effects of gonadotripin administration include headache lightheadedness, nausea, abdominal discomfort, flushing, and local inflammation at injection site.

TECH ALERT!
The following drugs have look-alike/sound-alike isssues: clomiphene, clomipramine, and clonidine; serophene and Sarafem

The incidence of multiple births when clomiphene is administered is about 5% to 7% (mostly twins). This percentage is much lower than what is observed following direct administration (injection) of FSH and LH, where the intent is to produce multiple follicles before inducing ovulation.

Infertility Therapy

Generic name	U.S. brand name(s) / Canadian brand(s)	Dosage forms and strengths
clomiphene	Clomid, Serophene Clomid, Serophene	Tablet 50 mg
follitropin-alpha	Follistim AQ, Gonal-f, Gonal-f RFF Gonal-f, Gonal-f RFF	**Gonal-f powder for injection (Gonal-f):** 75 international units/(Gonal-f RFF), 450 international units/vial, 1050 international units/vial **Solution, injection (Follistim AQ):** 75 international units **Cartridge for injection (Follistim AQ):** 300 international units, 900 international units - (Gonal-f RFF, Follistim AQ) 600 international units (Follistim AQ only)
human chorionic gonadotropin (hCG)* (choriogonadotropin)	Novarel, Ovidrel, Pregnyl Ovidrel, Pregnyl, Profasi HP	**Powder for injection (Novarel, Profasi HP, Pregnyl):** 10,000 units/vial **Solution prefilled syringe, injection (Ovidrel):** 250 mcg/0.5 ml
human menopausal gonadotropin (hMG)	Menopur, Repronex Menopur, Repronex	**Powder for injection:** 75 international units, 150 international units (U.S. only)

*Generic available.

Treatment of Hypogonadism

Treatment of hypogonadism involves the administration of synthetic LH, estrogens, and androgens. Gonadotropin therapy works by stimulating the anterior pituitary to release the gonadotropin LH. The effect that LH produces in males is differs from the effect in females. In females, recombinant human LH (rhLH) is indicated for the stimulation of follicular development in infertile hypogonadotropic, hypogonadal women with profound LH deficiency. In males, androgens (e.g., testosterone) play a critical role in sexual maturation throughout life.

Gonadotropin therapy is also used to evaluate functional capacity and response of the gonadotropes of the anterior pituitary and in suspected gonadotropin deficiency. It is also used to evaluate residual gonadotropic function of the pituitary gland following surgical or radiologic removal of a pituitary tumor. Unlabeled uses are treatment of delayed puberty, amenorrhea, and infertility in males.

ADVERSE REACTIONS

Common adverse effects produced by rhLH are abdominal bloating, breast tenderness, diarrhea, and gas. Less common adverse reactions are fast heartbeat, itching of skin, lightheadedness, headache, stomach, painful menstrual periods and heavy bleeding, and redness, pain, or swelling at the injection site.

Treatment for Hypogonadism

	Generic name	U.S. brand name(s) Canadian brand(s)	Dosage forms and strengths
Female			
	lutropin alfa	Luveris	**Injection:** 75 international units
		Luveris	
	estrogens	See mini-drug monograph "types of oral contraceptives" and "Hormone Replacement Therapy"	See mini-drug monograph "types of oral contraceptives" and "Hormone Replacement Therapy"
Male			
	methyltestosterone	See mini-drug monograph "Androgen Agonists"	See mini-drug monograph "Androgen Agonists"
	testosterone	See mini-drug monograph "Androgen Agonists"	See mini-drug monograph "Androgen Agonists"

TECH ALERT!
A common ending of androgen agonists is "-sterone."

TECH ALERT!
Testosterone and other anabolic steroids are schedule C-III controlled substances in the united states.

TECH ALERT!
Testosterone patches are NOT substitutable.

TECH ALERT!
The following drugs have look-alike/ sound-alike issues: Testoderm (scrotal patch) and Testoderm TTS (transdermal patch) Testoderm and Estraderm methylTESTOSTERone and medroxy PROGESTERone Testosterone and testolactone

Treatment of Androgen Deficiency in Men

ANDROGEN AGONISTS

The male hormone testosterone and its derivatives are collectively called *androgens*. They are secreted by the anterior pituitary gland and are responsible for masculinization (development of male secondary sexual characteristics). Small amounts are produced by the adrenal gland. Anabolic steroids closely resemble the androgen testosterone. Androgen therapy is used as replacement therapy for testosterone deficiency such as hypogonadism, selected cases of delayed puberty, and postpuberty testosterone deficiency. Anabolic steroids are synthetic drugs chemically related to androgens. They promote the tissue-building process and in normal dosages can have a minimal effect on accessory sex organs and secondary sex characteristics.

MECHANISM OF ACTION AND PHARMACOKINETICS

Androgens aid in the development and maintenance of secondary sexual characteristics in adolescent boys such as facial hair, deepening of voice, growth of body hair, fat distribution, and muscle development. Testosterone also stimulates the growth of accessory sex organs (penis, testes, vas deferens, prostate). Androgens also promote tissue-building processes (anabolism) and tissue-depleting processes (catabolism).

They are available in different dosage forms such as patches, gels, tablets, capsules, mucoadhesive (buccal), injections, transdermal patches, and pellets. The mucoadhesive form produces twice the androgen activity of oral tablets; the transdermal patch is applied daily to the scrotum or other parts of the body; and the gel is applied to the shoulder, upper arm, and abdomen—it should not be applied to the genitals.

ADVERSE REACTIONS

Androgens may produce gyneomastia (breast enlargement), testicular atrophy, impotence, inhibition of testicular function, penis enlargement, nausea, jaundice, headache, anxiety, male pattern baldness, acne, and depression. Fluid electrolyte imbalances (sodium, chloride, potassium, calcium, phosphate, water retention) may also occur. Prolonged usage of anabolic steroids can cause many of the same serious adverse effects as androgens, as well as testicular atrophy, blood-filled cysts in liver or spleen, malignant and benign liver tumors, increased risk of atherosclerosis, and mental changes (e.g., rage). These adverse effects are the reason why androgens (anabolic steroids) are regulated as Class III controlled substances.

Androgen Agonists

	Generic name	U.S. brand name(s)	Dosage forms and strengths
		Canadian brand(s)	
	fluoxymesterone	Halotestin	**Tablet:** 2 mg, 5 mg, 10 mg
		Not available	
	methyltestosterone	Android, Methitest, Testred	**Capsule:** 10 mg
		Not available	**Tablet (Methitest):** 10 mg
	oxandrolone	Oxandrin	**Tablet:** 2.5 mg, 10 mg
		Not available	
	testosterone*	Androderm, Delatestryl, Striant, Testim Depo-Testoderm, Testoderm TTS	**Capsule (Andriol):** 40 mg **Topical gel (Striant, Testim):** 25 mg/2.5 g, 1% unit-dose packet
		Andriol, Androderm, Androgel, Delatestryl, Testim	**Solution, injection:** 200 mg/ml **Oil, injection:** 100 mg/ml, 200 mg/ml **Mucoadhesive (buccal):** 30 mg **Pellet:** 75 mg **Patch (Androderm):** 2.5 mg/hr, 5 mg/24 hr

*Generic available.

Endometriosis

Endometriosis is the benign but painful condition that commonly affects the female reproductive tract. It is characterized by the presence of functioning endometrial tissue outside of the uterus. The displaced endometrial tissue is most often attached to an ovary or to the pelvic or abdominal organs and is occasionally found in other places throughout the body. The development of endometriosis is an important clinical condition, often causing infertility, dysmenorrhea, and severe pain. Symptoms reflect that fact that displaced endometrial tissue reacts to ovarian hormones in the same way as the normal endometrium—exhibiting a cycle of growth and sloughing off. The disorder affects approximately 10% of women, a majority aged 30 to 45 years.

TREATMENT OF ENDOMETRIOSIS

DANAZOL

Danazol, an androgen steroid derivative of testosterone, is used to treat endometriosis and fibrocystic breast disease to reduce breast pain, tenderness, and nodules. It is also used to prevent attacks of angioedema in both males and females.

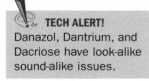

TECH ALERT!
Danazol, Dantrium, and Dacriose have look-alike sound-alike issues.

Mechanism of Action and Pharmacokinetics

Danazol works by suppressing pituitary output of FSH and LH, resulting in anovulation and associated amenorrhea. It interrupts the progression and pain of endometriosis by causing atrophy of both normal and ectopic endometrial tissue.

Adverse Reactions

Adverse reactions include masculinity effects; gastrointestinal distress, diarrhea, or jaundice; and menstrual irregularities.

Treatment for Endometriosis

	Generic name	U.S. brand name(s) / Canadian brand(s)	Dosage forms and strengths
	danazol*	Generics	**Capsule:** 50 mg, 100 mg, 200 mg
		Cyclomen	

*Generic available.

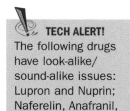

TECH ALERT!
The following drugs have look-alike/sound-alike issues: Lupron and Nuprin; Naferelin, Anafranil, and enalapril

GONADOTROPIN-RELEASING HORMONE ANALOGS

Gonadotropin-releasing hormone analogs are synthetic agonists and used to treat prostate cancer, endometriosis, advanced breast cancer, and endometrial thinning. It is a synthetic form of LH-releasing hormone (LHRH or GNRH) that inhibits pituitary gonadotropin secretion. With chronic administration, serum testosterone levels fall into the range of normally seen with castrated males.

Mechanism of Action and Pharmacokinetics
Goserelin acetate works by inhibiting gonadotropin secretion.

Adverse Reactions
Adverse reactions for goserelin acetate are headache, tumor flare, gyneomastia, breast swelling and tenderness, postmenopausal symptoms, vaginal spotting, breakthrough bleeding, decreased libido, impotence, bone pain, and bone loss.

Gonadotropin-Releasing Hormone and Its Analogs

	Generic name	U.S. brand name(s) / Canadian brand(s)	Dosage forms and strengths
	buserelin	Not available	**Implant (Suprefact Depot):** 6.3 mg, 9.45 mg
		Suprefact, Suprefact Depot	**Solution, injection:** 1 mg/ml
	goserelin	Zoladex	**Injection (1-month implant):** 3.6 mg
		Zoladex LA	**Injection (3-month implant):** 10.8 mg
	leuprolide*	Eligard, Lupron, Lupron Depot, Viadur	**Implant (Viadur):** 65 mg
		Eligard, Lupron, Lupron Depot	**Injection:** 5 mg/ml
			Lupron Depot (1 month): 3.75 mg, 7.5 mg
			Lupron Depot (3 months): 11.25 mg, 22.5 mg
			Lupron Depot (4 months): 30 mg
	nafarelin	Synarel	**Solution, nasal spray:** (200 mcg, 60 metered doses)
		Synarel	
	histrelin	Vantas	**Implant:** 50 mg
		Vantas	

*Generic available.

Summary of Drugs That Affect the Reproductive System

Generic name	Brand name	Usual dose and dosing schedule	Warning labels
Treatment of PMDD—selective serotonin reuptake inhibitors			
fluoxetine	Prozac, Sarafem	20 mg/day starting 14 days prior to menstruation through the first full day of menses	MAY CAUSE DIZZINESS MAY IMPAIR ABILITY TO DRIVE
sertraline	Zoloft	50 mg/day through luteal phase; can increase to 100 mg/day in 3-day increments	AVOID ALCOHOL SWALLOW WHOLE; DON'T CRUSH OR CHEW (delayed release)
paroxetine	Paxil, Paxil CR, Prexeva	12.5 mg/day to 25 mg/day through luteal phase; increase dose at 1-week intervals if needed	
Nonsteroidal antiinflammatory drugs (NSAIDs) used for dysmenorrhea			
ibuprofen	Advil, Motrin, Midol	200 mg/dose to 400 mg/dose every 4 to 6 hours Maximum daily dose 1200 mg/24 hr period	TAKE WITH FOOD AVOID ASPIRIN WHILE TAKING THIS PRODUCT
naproxen	Aleve, Anaprox, Naprelan, Naprosyn, Pamprin	Initial dose 500 mg; then 250 mg every 6 to 8 hours Maximum daily dose 1250 mg	MAY CAUSE DROWSINESS
ketoprofen	Orudis KT, Oruvail	25 mg to 50 mg every 6 to 8 hours Maximum daily dose 300 mg	
meclofamate	Generic	50 mg every 6 to 8 hours Maximum daily dose 400 mg	
Treatment of amenorrhea			
bromocriptine	Parlodel	1.25 mg/day to 2.5 mg/day Maximum daily dose 2.5 mg 2 to 3 times/day	TAKE WITH FOOD OR MILK MAY CAUSE DROWSINESS LIMIT ALCOHOL USE
oral contraceptives	See mini-drug monograph "types of oral contraceptives"	See mini-drug monograph "types of oral contraceptives"	See mini-drug monograph "types of oral contraceptives"
Oral contraceptives			
Estrogen and progestin combinations			
ethinyl estradiol + desogestrel	Apri, Cyclessa, Desogen, Kariva, Mircette, Ortho-Cept, Solia, Velivet, Marvelon	Take 1 tablet daily at same time every day	DO NOT BREASTFEED WHILE ON THIS DRUG REPORT ANY OF THE FOLLOWING: SEVERE HEADACHES, VOMITING, DISTURBED VISION OR SPEECH, NUMBNESS OR WEEKENSS IN EXTREMITIES, DEPRESSION OR UNUSUAL BLEEDING
ethinyl estradiol + drospirenone	Yasmin		
ethinyl estradiol + etonogestrel	Nuva-Ring	Insert ring vaginally and leave in place for 3 weeks. Remove for 1 week. Insert new ring 7 days after last one was removed	

Continued

Summary of Drugs That Affect the Reproductive System—cont'd

	Generic name	Brand name	Usual dose and dosing schedule	Warning labels
	ethinyl estradiol + levonorgestrel	Alesse, Aviane, Enpresse, Lessina, Levlen, Levlite, Levora, Lutera, Nordette, Portia, Seasonale, Tr-Levlen, Triphasil, Trivora Min-Ovral, Triquilar	Take 1 tablet at same time every day	USE EXACTLY AS PRESCRIBED AVOID SMOKING
	ethinyl estradiol + norethindrone	Aranelle, Brevicon, Estrostep Fe, Junel, Junel 0.5/35, Necon 1/35, Necon 7/7/7, Necon 7/11, Norinyl 1+35, Nortrel, Nortrel 7/7/7, Ortho-Novum, Ovcon, Tri-Norinyl, Minestrin 1/20, Select 1/35, Symphasic		
	ethinyl estradiol + norgestimate	MonoNessa, Ortho-Cyclen, Ortho Tri-Cyclen, Previfem, Sprintec, Tri-Nessa, Tri-Prevofem, Tri-Sprintec	Take 1 tablet at same time every day	
Intrauterine devices				
	progesterone, progestin	Progestasert	**Intrauterine system (IUD):** Insert IUD into uterine cavity and replace 1 year after insertion	REPORT SUDDEN LOSS OF VISION OR MIGRAINE HEADACHE
	levonorgestrel	Mirena	**Intrauterine system (IUD):** Insert IUD into uterine cavity and replace 5 years after insertion	REPORT SUDDEN LOSS OF VISION OR MIGRAINE HEADACHE
Emergency contraceptives				
	levonorgestrel	Plan B	Take 1 tablet within 72 hours of unprotected sexual intercourse; taken another tablet 12 hours later	AVOID SMOKING REPORT SUDDEN LOSS OF VISION OR SUDDEN ACUTE HEADACHE
Hormone replacement therapy				
Estrogen				
	Estradiol	Alora, Climara, Delestrogen, Depo-estradiol, Esclim, Estrace, Estraderm, Estrasorb, Estring, EstroGel, Femring, Gynodiol, Menostar, Vagifem, Vivelle, Vivelle-Dot, Estradot, Oesclim	**Vaginal cream:** Insert 2 g/day to 4 g/day intravaginally for 2 weeks; then reduce to ½ initial dose for 2 weeks, followed by maintenance dose of 1 g 2 to 3 times/week **Topical emulsion:** Apply 3.84 g once daily in the morning **Topical gel:** 1.25 g/day applied at same time daily **Patch:** Apply 0.025 mg once/week; 0.05 mg twice/week **Vaginal ring:** Insert 0.05 mg ring Intravaginally: leave in for 3 months **Vaginal tablet:** **Insert 1 tablet daily for 2 weeks; maintenance:** insert 1 tablet twice weekly	REPORT SUDDEN SEVERE HEADACHE, VOMITING, VISON OR SPEECH DISTURBANCE, LOSS OF VISION, NUMBNESS OR WEAKNESS IN EXTREMITIES, SHARP OR CRUSHING CHEST PAIN, SHORTNESS OF BREATH, SEVERE ABDOMINAL PAIN OR MASS, DEPRESSION, UNUSUAL BLEEDING

Summary of Drugs That Affect the Reproductive System—cont'd

Generic name	Brand name	Usual dose and dosing schedule	Warning labels
estrogens (conjugated)	Cenestin	0.45 mg/day to 1.25 mg/day **Vulvular atrophy:** 0.3 mg daily	TAKE WITH FOOD
estrogens (equine)	Premarin C.E.S. Congest	**Vaginal cream:** Insert ½ g/day to 2 g/day intravaginally for 3 weeks, then 1 week off (cyclically) **Tablet:** 0.3 mg/day cyclically or daily	TAKE WITH FOOD—tablet
estrogen (esterified)	Menest Estratab	**Tablet:** 0.3 mg/day to 1.25 mg/day cyclically	TAKE WITH FOOD
estropipate	Ogen, Ortho-est	**Tablet:** 0.75 mg to 6 mg daily	
Estrogen and progesterone combinations			
estradiol + levonoregestrel	ClimaraPro	**Transdermal:** apply 1 patch weekly	DO NOT EXPOSE PATCH TO SUNLIGHT FOR LONG PERIODS OF TIME
estradiol + norethindrone	Activella, CombiPatch Estalis, Estalis-Sequi	**Transdermal patch:** apply new patch twice weekly during 28-day cycle **Combo:** apply estradiol patch only for 14 days, followed by Estalis patch twice weekly for 14 days for 28-day cycle **Tablet:** 1 daily	
estradiol + norgestimate	Prefest	**Tablet:** 1 mg pink tablet daily for 3 days followed by 0.09 mg white tablet for 3 days: repeat sequence	
estrogens + medroxypro-gesterones	Premphase, Premplus, Prempro Premplus	**Premphase:** 1 maroon tablet days 1 to 14 followed by 1 light blue tablet days 15 to 28 **Prempro:** one 0.3 mg to 0.625 mg/MPA 1.5 mg to 5 mg tablet daily	TAKE WITH FOOD
estrogen + methyl testosterone	Estratest, Estratest H.S., Syntest D.S., Syntest H.S.	**Tablet:** 1 daily 3 weeks on, 1 week off	TAKE WITH FOOD
Infertility therapy			
clomiphene	Clomid, Serophene	**Male:** 25 mg/day for 25 days with 5 days rest OR 100 mg every M, W, F **Female:** 50 mg/day for 5 days	TAKE EXACTLY AS DIRECTED; DON'T SKIP DOSES
menotropins	Pergonal	**Pergonal:** Male: IM injection 75 international units to 150 international units 3 times/week **Female:** 75 international units to 150 international units for 7 to 12 days **Repronex:** Female: 150 international units to 450 international units daily for 5 to 12 days	REFRIGERATE DILUTED POWDER; DO NOT FREEZE PROTECT FROM LIGHT

Continued

Summary of Drugs That Affect the Reproductive System—cont'd

Generic name	Brand name	Usual dose and dosing schedule	Warning labels
follitropin-alpha	Gonal-f	**Infertility:** 75 international units/day SC; if no response in 5 to 7 days may increase by 37.5 international units weekly until maximum 300 international units **Hypogonadism (men):** 150 international units SC 3 times per week with hCG 1000 units	USE IMMEDIATELY AFTER RECONSTITUTION
human chorionic gonadotropin (recombinant)	Profasi	**Injection:** Female: 5000 to 10,000 units 1 day **Male:** 1500 to 3000 units 2 times/week	DISCARD ANY UNUSED RECONSTITUTED SOLUTION
Endometriosis			
danazol	Danocrine Cyclomen	**Capsule:** 200 mg/day to 400 mg/day in 2 divided doses (individualized dosage) **Maintenance dose:** 800 mg/day in 2 divided doses	TAKE WITH FOOD
Gonadotropin-releasing hormone and its analogs			
goserelin	Zoladex Zoladex LA	**Injection:** Inject dose every 28 days **Implant:** Insert every 1 to 3 months (1-month implant 3.6 mg; 3-month implant 10.8 mg)	STORE AT ROOM TEMPERATURE UNTIL READY FOR USE. DO NOT FREEZE INJECT ACCORDING TO PRESCRIBED SCHEDULE
leuprolide	Eligard, Lupron, Lupron Depot,	**Precocious puberty:** **Injection:** 7.5 mg, 11.25 mg, or 15 mg as a single dose monthly **Anemia due to uterine fibroids:** Lupron Depot: 3.5 mg monthly or 11.25 mg every 3 months)	RE-SHAKE SUSPENSION IF SETTLING OCCURS. DISCARD ANY UNUSED SUSPENSION—DEPOT SUSPENSION STORE AT ROOM TEMP—SOLUTION ROTATE INJECTION SITE
nafarelin	Synarel	**Endometriosis:** 2 sprays in one nostril in the morning and 1 spray in the other nostril in the evening: **Precocious puberty:** 2 sprays in each nostril every morning and evening	DO NOT USE NASAL DECONGESTANTS FOR 30 MINUTES AFTER USING NAFARELIN SPRAY
Treatment for hypogonadism			
lutropin alfa	Luveris	75 international units to 150 international units SC once daily	DISCARD ANY UNUSED PORTION OF VIAL
Androgen agonists			
fluoxymesterone	Halotestin	**Tablet:** 5 mg/day to 20 mg/day	TAKE AS DIRECTED

Summary of Drugs That Affect the Reproductive System—cont'd

Generic name	Brand name	Usual dose and dosing schedule	Warning labels
methyltestosterone	Android	**Oral:** 10 mg/day to 50 mg/day **Buccal:** 5 mg/day to 25 mg/day	TAKE WITH FOOD DISSOLVE BUCCAL TABLETS IN CHEEK: do not eat, drink, chew, or smoke while buccal tablet is in place
oxandrolone	Oxandrin	**Cachexia:** 2.5 mg to 20 mg daily in 2 to 4 divided doses for 2 to 4 weeks	TAKE AS DIRECTED
testosterone	Androderm, Delatestryl, Striant Testoderm	**Pellet:** SC implantation 150 mg to 450 mg every 3 to 6 months **Scrotal patch (Testoderm):** 6 mg daily to scrotum **Transdermal patch (Androderm, Testoderm TTS):** Apply daily to back, abdomen, thigh, or arm **Injection:** 50 mg to 400 mg every 2 to 4 weeks **Gel:** 5 g daily **Oral, buccal (Striant):** 30 mg every 12 hours	ROTATE SITE OF APPLICATION—patch, injection APPLY TO THE UPPER GUM ABOVE THE INCISOR TOOTH—buccal tab APPLY TO ARM, ABDOMEN, BACK, OR THIGH—Androderm APPLY TO SCROTUM—Testoderm

CHAPTER SUMMARY

- The average gestational period for pregnancy is 280 days, or 40 weeks. About 7 million American women become pregnant each year, and about two thirds of those pregnancies result in live births.
- Infertility may be caused by a wide variety of medical, environmental, and even lifestyle factors, such as smoking or alcohol abuse.
- Symptoms of premenstrual syndrome include headache, irritability fatigue, nervousness, weight gain, sleep changes, depression, and other problems that are distressing enough to limit activity and affect personal relationships.
- Amenorrhea may be a symptom of weight loss, pregnancy, lactation, menopause, or disease of the reproductive system.
- Dysfunctional uterine bleeding is irregular or excessive uterine bleeding that most often results from either a structural problem or some type of hormonal imbalance.
- Pelvic inflammatory disease occurs either as an acute or chronic inflammatory condition and is caused by several different pathogens, which usually spread upward from the vagina.
- Sexually transmitted infections or venereal diseases are infections caused by communicable pathogens such as viruses, bacteria, fungi, and protozoa. They can all be transmitted by sexual contact.
- Menopause is the termination of menstrual cycles and is an event that is usually marked by the passage of at least 1 full year without menstruation.
- Endometriosis is a benign but painful condition that commonly affects the female reproductive tract and is characterized by the presence of functioning endometrial tissue outside of the uterus.

- Condoms are used to prevent pregnancy and transmission of sexually transmitted infections such as gonorrhea, syphilis, and HIV.
- Most hormonal contraceptives were developed to prevent pregnancy by initiating negative feedback inhibition of follicle-stimulating hormone and luteinizing hormone secretion.
- The diaphragm must be inserted sometime before sexual intercourse and remain in the vagina for 6 to 8 hours after a man's last ejaculation.
- The presence of an intrauterine device in the uterus prompts the release of leukocytes and prostaglandins by the endometrium. These substances are hostile to both sperm and eggs. The presence of the copper increases the spermicidal effect.
- If used correctly and consistently, the pill is an extremely effective contraceptive with an unintended pregnancy rate estimated at between 0.1% and 3%.
- Emergency use of oral contraceptive pills containing levonorgestrel alone reduces the risk for pregnancy after unprotected intercourse by 89%.
- Hormone replacement therapy is most often used to treat symptoms of menopause such as "hot flashes," vaginal dryness, mood swings, sleep disorders, and decreased sexual desire.
- The results of a new study called the Women's Health Initiative have led physicians to revise their recommendation regarding hormone replacement therapy.
- Gonadotropin-releasing hormone analogs are used to treat prostate cancer, endometriosis, advanced breast cancer, and endometrial thinning.
- The male hormone testosterone and its derivatives are collectively called androgens, are secreted by the anterior pituitary gland, and are responsible for masculinization (development of male secondary sexual characteristics).

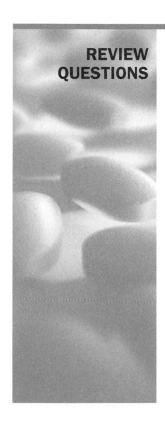

REVIEW QUESTIONS

Multiple Choice

1. **The average human gestational period is _____.**
   a. 280 days or 40 weeks
   b. 294 days or 42 weeks
   c. 290 days or 42 weeks
   d. 273 days or 39 weeks

2. **Menorrhagia is a term used for _____ menstrual bleeding.**
   a. diminished
   b. excessive
   c. absence of
   d. painful

3. **Bromocriptine is a drug used to treat _____.**
   a. premenstrual dysphoric disorder
   b. dysmenorrhea
   c. amenorrhea
   d. all of the above

4. **Pelvic inflammatory disease is a common complication following infection by _____.**
   a. human immunodeficiency virus (HIV)
   b. chlamydial organism
   c. gonoccoccal organism
   d. b and c

5. **Menopause is the termination of menstrual cycles and is an event that is usually marked by the passage of at least 2 full years without menstruation.**
   a. true
   b. false

6. **Oral contraceptives ("the pill") are 100% effective in preventing pregnancy.**
   a. true
   b. false

7. **The WHI study on hormonal replacement therapy concludes that hormonal replacement therapy may increase the risk for _____ .**
   a. heart disease and breast cancer
   b. heart attack and blood clots
   c. strokes
   d. all of the above

8. **Clomiphene is a drug used to treat _____ .**
   a. contraception
   b. infertility
   c. hypogonadism
   d. amenorrhea

9. **Gonadotropin therapy works by stimulating the _____ pituitary to release the gonadotropin LH.**
   a. anterior
   b. posterior
   c. interior
   d. exterior

10. **Testosterone and anabolic steroids are _____ controlled substances.**
    a. Class I
    b. Class II
    c. Class III
    d. Class IV

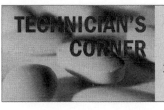

TECHNICIAN'S CORNER

1. Since the WHI study, many women have turned to herbal preparations to combat menopausal symptoms. How effective are these preparations in improving these symptoms?
2. Many athletes are using anabolic steroids to gain an "edge" in their sport. What are some long-term effects of these steroids on the body and mind?

BIBLIOGRAPHY

Amenorrhea. Available at: http://www.nlm.nih.gov/health/topics/Amenorrhea.cfm.

Condom. Available at: http://en.wikiperdia.org/wiki/Condom.

Diaphragm. Available at: http://en.wikiperdia.org/wiki/Diaphragm_28%Contraceptive%29.

Hormone replacement therapy. Available at: http://www.nlm.nih.gov/medlineplus/ency/article/007111.htm.

Hypogonadism. Available at: http://www.nlm.nih.gov/medlineplus/ency/article/001195.htm.

Intrauterine devices. Available at: http://en.wikiperdia.org/wiki/Intrauterine_device.

Lance L, Lacy C, Armstrong L, Goldman M: *Drug information handbook for the allied health professional,* ed 12. Hudson, OH, 2005, APhA Lexi-Comp.

MBC 3320 androgens. Available at: http://www.neurosci.pharm.utoledo.edu/MBC3320/androgens.htm.

National Heart, Lung, and Blood Institute: *Facts about menopausal hormone therapy.* Bethesda, MD, 2002, revised June 2005, National Institutes of Health, U.S. Department of Health and Human Services. NIH Publication No. 05-5200. Available at: http://www.nhlbi.nih.gov/health/women/pht_facts.pdf.

Roach S: *Pharmacology for health professionals.* Baltimore, 2005, Lippincott, Williams and Wilkins.

Sexually transmitted diseases treatment and guidelines, *Morb Mortal Wkly Rep,* 55:August 4, RR-11, 2006. Available at: www.cdc.gov.

Shannon M, Wilson B, Stang C: *Health professionals drug guide 2005-2006.* Upper Saddle River, NJ, 2006, Prentice-Hall.

Taber's cyclopedic medical dictionary, ed 20, Philadelphia, 2005, FA Davis.

Thibodeau G, Patton K: *Anatomy and physiology,* ed 6, St. Louis, 2007, Mosby.

Drugs Affecting the Immunological System

- Identify the organs and vessels and understand the functions of the lymphatic system.
- Understand the function of cells of the immune system.
- Explain the process of adaptive and innate immunity.

Overview of the Lymphatic System

The lymphatic system serves various functions in the body. The two most important functions of this system is maintenance of fluid balance in the internal environment and immunity. A third function is that of the absorption of fats from the small intestines by lymphatic vessels located in the intestinal wall with transportation to the bloodstream. The lymphatic system consists of moving fluid (**lymph**) derived from the blood and tissue fluid through a group of vessels (**lymphatics**) that return the lymph to the blood. In addition to lymph and the lymphatic vessels, the system includes lymphoid tissue containing lymphocytes and other specialized cells. Lymph nodes are located along the paths of collecting lymphatic vessels. Peyer's patches are in the intestinal wall. Additional lymphoid structures include the tonsils, thymus, spleen, and bone marrow.

LYMPH VESSELS

Lymph capillaries are thin-walled tubes that form complex networks transporting lymph from tissue spaces to larger lymphatic vessels. The larger lymphatic vessels lead to specialized masses of tissue called *lymph nodes* located along the paths of the lymph vessels. After leaving the nodes, the vessels merge to form even larger vessels called lymphatic trunks that join one of two collecting ducts, the right lymphatic duct or the thoracic duct. After leaving the collecting ducts, lymph enters the venous system through the left subclavian vein.

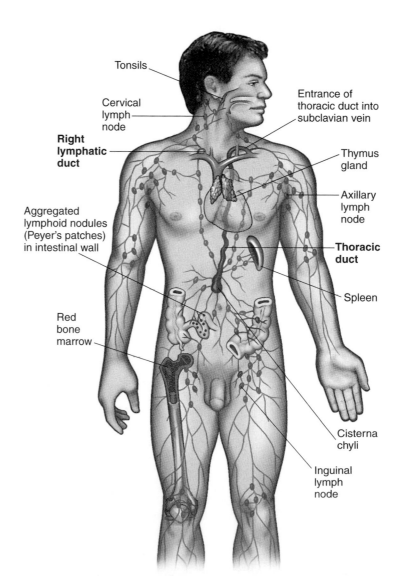

(From Thibodeau GA, Patton KT: Anatomy and physiology, *ed 6, St. Louis, 2007, Mosby.)*

LYMPH NODES

Lymph nodes not only produce lymphocytes but also filter and trap substances from inflammatory and cancerous lesions. They contain specialized cells called **macrophages** located in the lymph nodes (as well as in the spleen, liver, lungs, brain, and spinal cord) that engulf and destroy antigens (substances not recognized as "self"). This process is called phagocytosis. Specialized lymphocytes (**B cells**) present in the nodes produce antibodies. **T-cell** lymphocytes attack bacteria and foreign cells by accurately recognizing a cell surface protein as "non-self," attaching to them and destroying them.

SPLEEN AND THYMUS GLAND

The **spleen** is located in the upper left quadrant of the abdomen, adjacent to the stomach, and has several important functions—destruction of old erythrocytes by macrophages, filtration of microorganisms and other harmful substances from the blood, activation of lymphocytes as it filters antigens from the blood, and storage of blood, especially erythrocytes and platelets. The **thymus gland** is a lymphatic organ located in the upper mediastinum between the lungs. During fetal life and childhood it is quite large, but it becomes smaller with age. The thymus gland is composed of nests of lymphoid cells and plays an important role in the body's ability to protect itself from disease, especially in the early years of growth.

Organization of the Immune System

The components and mechanisms of the immune system are continually patrolling the body for harmful or internal enemies. To do this the immune system must recognize unique molecules and groups of molecules on the surface of cells, viruses, and other particles that can be used to identify them. Likewise, our own cells have unique cell markers (**antigens**) embedded in our plasma membrane that identify our cells as **self**. Foreign cells or particles have **non-self** molecules that serve as recognition markers for our immune system. The ability of our immune system to attack abnormal cells but spare our own normal cells is called **self-tolerance**. All of these defensive mechanisms can be categorized into major categories: innate immunity and adaptive immunity.

INNATE IMMUNITY

The primary types of cells involved in innate immunity are epithelial barrier cells, phagocytic cells (neutrophils, macrophages), and natural killer (NK) cells. **Cytokines**, which are chemicals released from cells to trigger or release innate and adaptive immune responses, also participate in innate immunity. Examples of cytokines include interleukins, leukotreines, and interferons. In addition to cytokines, other chemicals play a regulatory role in immunity, such as complements, other enzymes, and the amine histamine.

Mechanisms of Innate Defense

Mechanism	Description
Species resistance	Refers to a phenomenon in which the genetic characteristics common to a particular kind of organisms, or species, provide defense against certain pathogens (disease-causing agents).
Mechanical and chemical barriers	Physical impediments to the entry of foreign cells or substances. The skin and mucosa form a continuous wall that separates the internal environment from the external environment, preventing the entry of pathogens. Secretions such as sebum, mucus, and enzymes, and hydrochloric acid chemically inhibit the activity of pathogens.
Inflammatory response	Isolates the pathogens and stimulates the speedy arrival of a large numbers of immune cells. The inflammation mediators include histamine, kinins, prostaglandins, leukotrines, interleukins, and related compounds. Many of these mediators are chemotactic factors. They attract white blood cells to the area in the process called chemotaxis.

Continued

Mechanisms of Innate Defense—cont'd

Mechanism	Description
Phagocytosis	Ingestion and destruction of pathogens by phagocytic cells such as neutrophils and macrophages (monocytes). The movement of phagocytes from blood vessel to inflammation sites is called *diapedesis*. Phagocytes have a very short life span, and thus dead cells tend to "pile up" at the inflammations site, forming a white substance called *pus*.
Natural killer (NK) cells	Group of lymphocytes that kill many different types of cancer cells and virus-infected cells. They are produced in red bone marrow and are neither T cells nor B cells.
Interferon	Protein produced by cells after they become infected by a virus; inhibits the spread or further development of a viral infection.
Complement	Group of plasma proteins (about 20 inactive enzymes) that produce a cascade of chemical reactions that ultimately causes lysis (rupture) of a foreign cell.

ADAPTIVE IMMUNITY

Adaptive immunity is also called *specific immunity* and involves mechanisms that recognize specific threatening agents and then adapts, or responds, by targeting their activity against these agents—and these agents only. The primary types of cells involved in adaptive immunity are T-cell lymphocytes and B-cell lymphocytes. B-cell lymphocytes do not attack pathogens themselves but instead produce molecules called *antibodies* that attack the pathogens or direct other cells, such as phagocytes, to attack them. B-cell mechanisms are classified as antibody-mediated immunity or *humoral immunity*. Because T cells attack pathogens more directly, T-cell mechanisms are classified as *cell-mediated immunity* or cellular immunity. The densest populations of lymphocytes occur in the bone marrow, thymus gland, lymph nodes, and spleen

Types of Adaptive Immunity

Type	Description or example
Natural immunity	**Exposure to a causative agent that is not deliberate**
Active (exposure)	A child develops measles and acquires an immunity to a subsequent infection.
Passive (exposure)	A fetus received protection from the mother through the placenta, or an infant receives protection through the mother's milk.
Artificial immunity	**Exposure to a causative agent that is deliberate**
Active (exposure)	Injection of the causative agent, such as a vaccination against polio, confers immunity.
Passive (exposure)	Injection of a protective material (antibodies) that was developed by another individual's immune system.

ANTIBODIES (IMMUNOGLOBULINS)

Antibodies are proteins called *immunoglobulins (Igs)*. There are five classes of antibodies, identified by letter names as immunoglobulins M, G, A, E, and D. *IgM* is the antibody that immature B cells synthesize and insert into their plasma membranes. It is also the predominant class of antibody produced after initial contact with an antigen. The most abundant circulating antibody is *IgG*. The *IgG* antibodies cross the placental barrier during pregnancy to impart natural passive immunity to the offspring. *IgA* is present in the mucous membranes of the body, in saliva, and in tears. *IgE* can produce major harmful effects, such as those associated with allergies. *IgD's* precise function is unknown. The function of antibody molecules is to produce antibody-mediated immunity. They fight disease first by recognizing substances that are foreign or abnormal.

Complement

Complement is a component of blood plasma that consists of about 20 protein compounds. They are inactive enzymes and are triggered by either adaptive or innate immunity mechanisms. Ultimately they cause the lysis (rupture) of the cell that triggered it. Complement also marks microbes for destruction by phagocytic cells in a process called *opsonization*, and it promotes the inflammatory response.

T Cells and Cell-Mediated Immunity

DEVELOPMENT OF T CELLS

T cells, by definition, are lymphocytes that have made a detour through the thymus gland before migrating to the lymph nodes and spleen. Each T cell, like each B cell, displays antigen receptors on its surface membrane. Thus, T cells react to cells that are already infected, or otherwise engulfed, the antigen. B cells, on the other hand, react mainly to antigens that are in plasma. When an antigen is present, the T cells are activated or sensitized. The T cells then divide repeatedly to form identical clones: *effector T cells* and *memory T cells*. Effector T cells include cytotoxic T cells, which are also called *killer T cells* because they kill the target cell. Besides cytotoxic T cells, there are two types of effector T cells found in the body: *helper T cells* and *suppressor T cells*. Both types of cells help regulate adaptive immune function by regulating B-cell and T-cell function. Helper T cells help other lymphocytes by secreting cytokines that stimulate B cells and cytotoxic T cells. Suppressor T cells act to suppress B-cell differentiation into plasma cells. The antagonistic action allows the immune system to fine tune its antibody-mediated response. Suppressor T cells also regulate other T cells, helping to "turn off" an immune response to restore homeostasis.

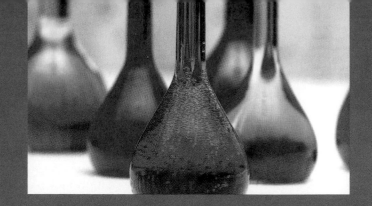

Treatment of Bacterial Infection

LEARNING OBJECTIVES

- Learn the terminology associated with treatments for infection.
- Describe the morphology of bacterial cells.
- List and categorize antiinfective agents.
- Describe mechanism of action for antiinfective agents.
- Compare "bacteriostatic" to "bactericidal."
- Explain antimicrobial resistance and list several reasons for its development.
- Identify warning labels and precautionary messages associated with antiinfective agents.
- Identify significant drug look-alike/sound-alike issues.
- List common endings for antiinfective agents.

KEY TERMS

Antibiotic: Natural substance produced by one organism that is capable of destroying or inhibiting the growth of bacteria.

Antiinfective: Natural or synthetic substance capable of destroying or inhibiting the growth of bacteria.

Bactericidal: Able to destroy bacteria.

Bacteriostatic: Able to inhibit bacterial proliferation; host defense mechanisms destroy the bacteria.

β-Lactamase: Enzyme secreted by some microbes that has the ability to destroy β-lactam antibiotics.

Microbial resistance: Ability of bacteria to overcome the bactericidal effects of an antiinfective. Resistance traits are encoded on bacterial genes and can be transferred to other bacteria.

OVERVIEW

While chronic, noninfectious disease is a leading cause of disability and death in developed, industrialized countries, infectious disease is still one the leading causes of morbidity and mortality globally. In developing countries, infectious diarrhea is a major cause for infant mortality. The incidence of infectious diseases such as malaria and tuberculosis is also high. Poverty, malnutrition, lack of clean water, poor sanitation, and inadequate housing increase the risk for infectious disease and decrease the likelihood for adequate treatment.

Antibiotics and their synthetic analogs (***antiinfectives***) have played a key role in improving the survival of individuals with bacterial infections. An ***antibiotic*** is a naturally occurring substance produced by one organism that is capable of destroying of inhibiting the growth of bacteria.

Mechanisms of Antimicrobial Action

Effective treatment of bacterial infections is dependent upon host factors, bacterial factors, and drug factors (Figure 35-1).

BACTERICIDAL VERSUS BACTERIOSTATIC

Antiinfective agents may be classified as bactericidal or bacteriostatic. ***Bactericidal*** agents are able to destroy rapidly proliferating, pathogenic bacteria. ***Bacteriostatic*** agents slow the growth of bacteria enough for the host (our bodies) defense mechanism to destroy the invading bacteria. Whether an antiinfective agent is bactericidal or bacteriostatic is dependent on the concentration administered or the length of time the bacteria is exposed to toxic concentrations.

INHIBIT BACTERIAL CELL WALL SYNTHESIS

Many bacteria have a cell wall, and this is the target of a variety of antiinfective agents. Because human cells lack cell walls, antiinfective agents that target the cell wall harm the bacteria without damaging the host. β-Lactam antibiotics target the bacterial cell wall (Figure 35-2). Penicillins, cephalosporins, cabapenems, and monobactams are β-lactam antibiotics that inhibit cell wall synthesis. Glycopeptides also target the bacterial cell wall. Vancomycin is the only glycopeptide antibiotic available in the United States and Canada.

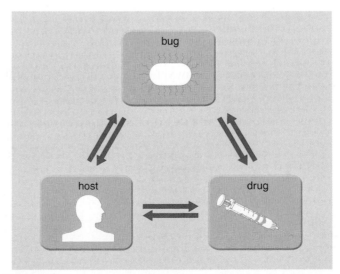

FIGURE 35-1 Factors that influence successful antimicrobial therapy. *(From Page C, et al.: Integrated pharmacology, ed 3, Philadelphia, 2006, Mosby.)*

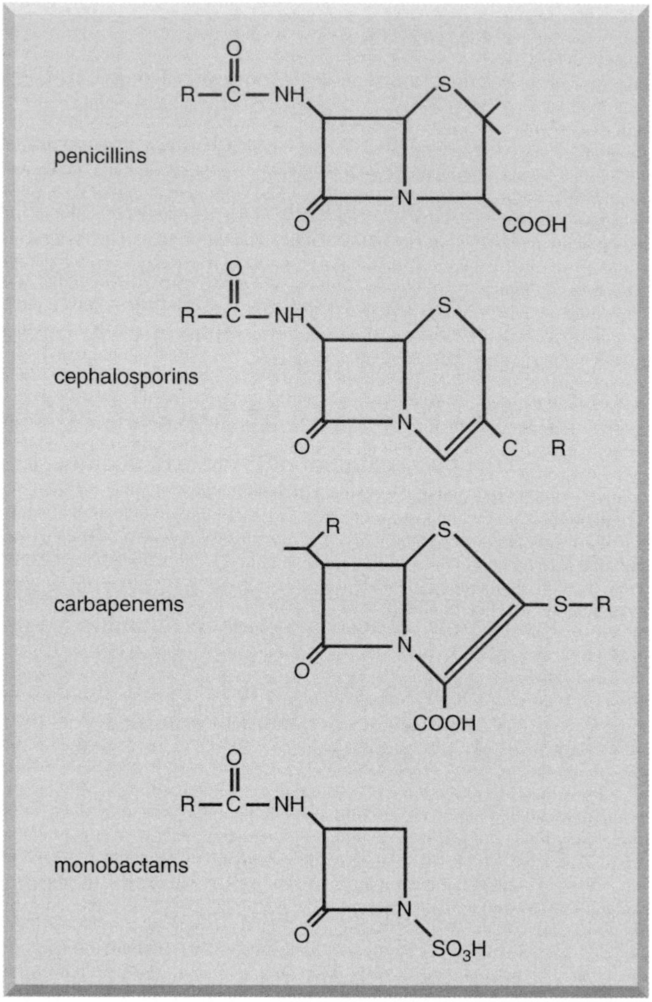

FIGURE 35-2 Basic structure of β-lactam antibiotics. *(From Page C, et al.:* Integrated pharmacology, *ed 3, Philadelphia, 2006, Mosby.)*

INHIBIT BACTERIAL CELL WALL FUNCTION

Antibiotics that inhibit the function of the bacterial cell wall work by binding to bacterial membranes, where the antibiotic produces a detergent-like action that increases cell membrane permeability. This causes essential cell contents to leak out of the cell and destroys the bacteria. Polymyxin B is an example of an antibiotic that interferes with cell wall function.

INHIBIT PROTEIN SYNTHESIS

There are five classes of antiinfective agents that act to inhibit bacterial protein synthesis. They are the aminoglycosides, macrolides, tetracyclines, amphenicols, and oxazolidiones. These antiinfective agents reduce the number of disease-causing bacteria by interfering with the bacteria's ability to replicate (Figure 35-3).

INHIBIT BACTERIAL DNA AND RNA SYNTHESIS

Genetic code is stored in DNA. In the replication process, a strand of RNA forms along a strand of DNA. The job of transfer RNA (tRNA) is to get the base pairs in the correct sequence. The job of messenger RNA (mRNA) is to carry the code message to the ribosome. RNA also regulates specific cell functions such as editing strands of code. Editing occurs on the ribosome by the RNA enzyme (ribozyme). Without the ability to transfer genetic codes for the synthesis of bacteria cell constituents, bacteria are unable to replicate and spread.

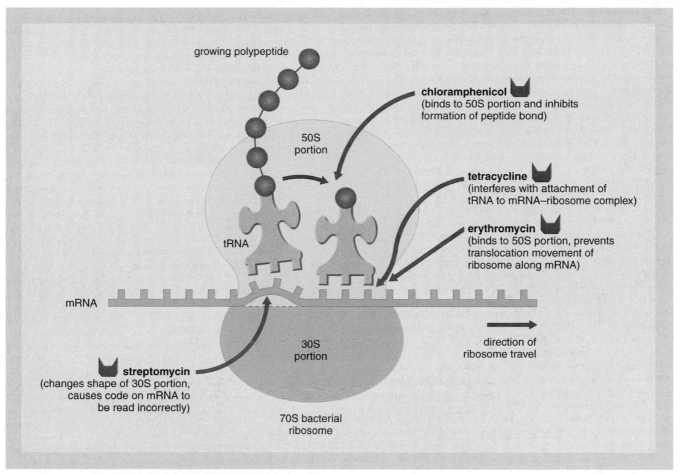

FIGURE 35-3 Antibiotics that inhibit bacterial protein synthesis. *(From Page C, et al.:* Integrated pharmacology, *ed 3, Philadelphia, 2006, Mosby.)*

Fluoroquinolones and nitroimidazoles are classes of antiinfectives capable of inhibiting DNA synthesis. The action of fluoroquinolones (e.g., ciprofloxacin) and nitroimidazoles (e.g., metronidazole) is predominantly bactericidal.

Rifampin inhibits bacterial RNA synthesis.

ANTIFOLATES

Folic acid is needed for bacterial synthesis of DNA, and unlike humans, bacteria must synthesize its own folic acid. It cannot get it from external sources. Bacteria synthesize folic acid from *para*-aminobenzoic acid (PABA). Antifolate antiinfective agents and dihydrofolate reductase inhibitors block bacterial synthesis of folic acid. Sulfonamides are antifolate drugs and trimethoprim is a dihydrofolate reductase inhibitor (Figure 35-4).

What Is Microbial Resistance?

Microbes proliferate rapidly, mutate frequently, and adapt with relative ease to new environments and hosts. Unfortunately, microbes can learn how to withstand the effects of antibiotics and now new "superbugs" exist that are resistant to currently available antiinfective agents. Multidrug resistance is a serious problem, and while previously only a risk for hospitalized patients, multidrug-resistant tuberculosis (MDR-TB), vancomycin-resistant enterococci (VRE), and methicillin-resistant *Staphylococcus aureus* (MRSA) are spreading outside of hospitals. *Microbial resistance* is the ability of bacteria to overcome the bactericidal effects of an antibiotic. Resistance traits are encoded on bacterial genes on chromosomal or plasmid DNA and can be transferred to other bacteria. Bacteria resistant to one penicillin antibiotic may also be resistant to most penicillins and other β-lactams including cephalosporins.

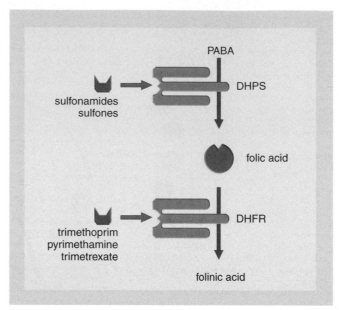

FIGURE 35-4 The folate biosynthetic pathway. *(From Page C, et al.:* Integrated Pharmacology, *ed 3, Philadelphia, Mosby, 2006.)*

Misuse of antimicrobial agents is a major cause for the development and spread of microbial resistance. Misuse includes (1) inappropriate prescribing, (2) failure to complete the full course of therapy, (3) administration of antibacterial agents for viral infections (e.g., the common cold), (4) antibiotics in the food chain (agriculture, animal husbandry, fish farms), and (5) lack of guidelines for preventing spread of infections in institutional care settings.

Mechanisms of Microbial Resistance

SECRETION OF ENZYMES THAT INACTIVATE THE ANTIBIOTIC

β-*Lactamase* is an enzyme produced by some microbes that have the ability to destroy β-lactam antibiotics. It breaks the bonds of the β-lactam ring. β-Lactamase inhibitors have no antimicrobial activity of their own. They are added to some β-lactam antibiotics (e.g., amoxicillin + clavulanic acid) to increase the antibiotic's resistance to microbial destruction. There are three β-lactamase inhibitors. They are clavulanic acid (clavulanate), sulbactam, and tazobactam. Macrolides are inactivated by bacterial production of the esterases e.g., phosphodiesterase enzymes.

MODIFICATION OF THE RIBOSOMAL TARGET

Microbial resistance develops when bacteria mutate to modify the site on the ribosome that the antibiotic normally binds to. This is a mechanism of microbial resistance to macrolide antibiotics.

PRODUCTION OF ANTIBIOTIC-MODIFYING ENZYMES

Bacteria previously sensitive to the effects of aminoglycosides can become resistant by adding an acetyl group or phosphoryl group to the antibiotic that inhibits the antibiotic's ability to reach the bacterial binding site.

MUTATIONS THAT CHANGE BACTERIAL TRANSPORT MECHANISMS

Bacteria that are resistant to tetracyclines have mutated to change the transport mechanism that causes the antibiotic to accumulate in the bacterial cell. Bacteria resistant to macrolides are capable of lowering the concentration of the antibiotic by transporting the antibiotic out of the cell.

Classification of Antiinfective Agents

AMINOGLYCOSIDES

Aminoglycoside antibiotics are effective for treating aerobic gram-negative bacilli, staphylococci, and mycobacterium. They are used in the treatment of serious infections of the bone, abdomen, heart, brain, urinary tract, reproductive system, skin, and kidneys. Examples are lower respiratory infections, peritonitis, septicemia, meningitis, pelvic inflammatory disease, endocarditis, and osteomylitis. Ophthalmic dosage forms may also be administered to sterilize the bowel prior to bowel surgery. The topical forms are also prescribed for the treatment of blepharitis and conjunctivitis (see Chapter 20).

MECHANISM OF ACTION AND PHARMACOKINETICS

Aminoglycosides inhibit bacterial protein synthesis. They enter the bacterial cell via an oxygen dependent transport system, which explains why they are effective against *aerobic* bacteria and not *anaerobic* bacteria. They bind on a site on the bacterial ribosome that causes the genetic code carried by mRNA to be read incorrectly.

Aminogylcosides are not absorbed systemically when administered by mouth. The only aminoglycoside that is administered orally is used to reduce the bacteria in the bowel prior to colorectal surgery. Other nonparenteral use occurs when they are administered topically for skin, eye, and ear infections.

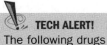
ADVERSE REACTIONS

Serious adverse reactions are linked to aminoglyoside use including hearing loss (ototoxicity) and kidney damage (nephrotoxicity). These effects limit their use to serious infections.

Aminoglycosides

Generic name	U.S. brand name(s) / Canadian brand(s)	Dosage forms and strengths
amikacin*	Amikin	**Solution for injection:** 50 mg/ml, 250 mg/ml
	Generic	
gentamicin*	Genoptic S.O.P, Gentak	**Powder for injection:** 60 mg, 80 mg, 100 mg/vial
	Garamycin, Garasone	**Solution for injection:** 0.6 mg/ml, 0.8 mg/ml, 1 mg/ml, 1.2 mg/ml, 1.6 mg/ml, 2 mg/ml, 10 mg/ml, 40 mg/ml **Ophthalmic ointment and solution (Genoptic, Gentak, Garasone):** 0.3% **Topical cream and ointment (Garamycin):** 0.1%
kanamycin*	Generic	**Solution for injection:** 333 mg/ml
	not available	
neomycin*	Generic	**Tablet:** 500 mg
	not available	
streptomycin*	Generics	**Powder for injection:** 1 g
	Generics	
tobramycin*	Tobi, Tobrex OS	**Powder for injection:** 1.2 g **Inhalation solution (Tobi):** 500 mg/5 ml **Solution for injection:** 10 mg/ml; 40 mg/ml **Solution for injection in NS:** 0.8 mg/ml; 60 mg/50 ml **Ophthalmic solution (Tobrex):** 0.3%
	Tobi, Tobrex OS	

*Generic available.

TECH ALERT!

A common beginning for cephalosporin drugs is "-ceph" or "-cef."

TECH ALERT!

The following drugs have look-alike/ sound-alike issues: Kefzol and Cefzil; Ceftin and Cefzil; cefoxitin and Cytoxan; Mefoxin and Lanoxin; Vantin and Ventolin; Rocephin and Roferon; ceftizoxime, cefotaxime, ceftazidime, and cefuroxime; Suprax and Sporanox

CEPHALOSPORINS

Cephalosporins also have a β-lactam ring structure. Like penicillins, the different side chains added to the basic β-lactam ring structure can affect antiinfective spectrum of activity. Cephalosporins are classified as first generation, second generation, and third generation. First-generation cephalosporins are most effective against gram-positive (+), aerobic bacteria. Second-generation cephalosporins have effectiveness against gram-positive and gram-negative (−) bacteria, but third-generation cephalosporins are the most effective against gram-negative, anaerobic bacteria. For example, first-generation cephalosporins are effective in the treatment of staphlococcal infections and streptococcal infections of the skin and soft tissue. Second-generation cephalosporins are effective for treating upper respiratory infections such as *Haemophilus influenzae.* Third-generation cephalosporins are effective for treating bacterial meningitis, gonorrhea, intraabdominal infections (e.g., peritonitis), and bone and joint infections.

MECHANISM OF ACTION

Cephalosporins inhibit the third and final stage of bacterial cell wall synthesis by binding to specific penicillin-binding proteins (PBPs) that are located inside the bacterial cell wall. Because PBPs vary among different bacterial species, cephalosporin spectrum of activity is dependent on the drug's ability to bind to a specified bacterial PBP.

PHARMACOKINETICS

Cephalosporins are formulated for oral, intramuscular, and intravenous use. All except one third-generation cephalosporin (cefixime) is administered parenterally, and only two second-generation cephalosporins are available for oral use (cefaclor and cefuroxime). First-generation cephalosporins do not penetrate the cerebrospinal fluid (CSF) in adequate concentrations to treat meningitis, whereas most third-generation agents do.

ADVERSE REACTIONS

Adverse reactions produced by cephalosporins include diarrhea, headache, dizziness, nausea, vomiting, gas, abdominal pain, dry mouth, and heartburn.

Cephalosporins

Generic name	U.S. brand name(s) Canadian brand(s)	Dosage forms and strengths
First generation		
cefazolin	Generics	**Powder for injection:** 0.5 g, 1 g, 10 g
	Generics	**Solution for injection:** 10 mg/ml, 20 mg/ml (U.S. only)
cefadroxil*	Duricef	**Capsule:** 500 mg
	Duricef	**Powder for oral suspension:** 250 mg/5 ml, 500 mg/5 ml **Tablet:** 1 g (U.S. only)
cephalexin*	Keflex	**Capsule:** 250 mg, 500 mg
	Keflex	**Powder for oral suspension:** 125 mg/5 ml, 250 mg/5 ml
cephalothin	Not available	**Powder for injection:** 1 g (Canada only)
	Ceporacin	
Second generation		
cefaclor*	Generics	**Capsule:** 250 mg, 500 mg
	Ceclor	**Powder for oral suspension:** 125 mg/5 ml, 187 mg/5 ml (U.S. only), 250 mg/5 ml, 375 mg/5 ml **Tablet, extended release:** 500 mg

Cephalosporins—cont'd

	Generic name	U.S. brand name(s) / Canadian brand(s)	Dosage forms and strengths
	cefotetan	Cefotan	**Powder for injection:** 1 g, 2 g, 10 g
		Not available	**Solution for injection:** 1 g/50 ml
	cefoxitin*	Mefoxin	**Powder for injection:** 1 g, 2 g, 10 g
		generic	**Solution for injection:** 1 g/50 ml, 2 g/50 ml, 20 mg/50 ml
	cefuroxime*	Ceftin, Zinacef	**Add-Vantage powder for injection (Zinacef):** 750 mg, 1.5 g
		Ceftin, Zinacef	**Powder for injection (Zinacef):** 750 mg, 1.5 g **Powder for oral suspension (Ceftin):** 125 mg/5 ml, 250 mg/5 ml **Tablet:** 250 mg, 500 mg
Third generation			
	cefotaxime	Claforan	**Add-Vantage powder for injection:** 1 g, 2 g
		Claforan	**Powder for injection:** 500 mg, 1 g, 2 g, 10 g **Solution for injection:** 20 mg/ml, 40 mg/ml
	ceftazidime*	Fortaz, Tazicef	**Add-Vantage powder for injection (Fortaz only):** 1 g, 2 g
		Fortaz	**Powder for injection:** 500 mg, 1 g, 2 g, 6 g
	ceftizoxime	Cefizox	**Powder for injection:** 2 g
		Not available	**Solution for injection:** 1 g, 2 g
	ceftriaxone*	Rocephin	**Powder for injection:** 250 mg, 500 mg, 1 g, 2 g, 10 g
		Rocephin	
	cefixime*	Suprax	**Powder for oral suspension:** 100 mg/5 ml, 200 mg/5 ml
		Suprax	**Tablet:** 400 mg
	cefpodoxime*	Vantin	**Powder for oral suspension:** 50 mg/5 ml, 100 mg/5 ml **Tablet:** 100 mg, 200 mg
	ceftibuten	Cedax	**Capsule:** 400 mg **Powder for oral suspension:** 90 mg/5 ml

*Generic available.

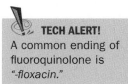

TECH ALERT!
A common ending of fluoroquinolone is "-floxacin."

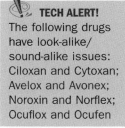

TECH ALERT!
The following drugs have look-alike/sound-alike issues: Ciloxan and Cytoxan; Avelox and Avonex; Noroxin and Norflex; Ocuflox and Ocufen

FLUOROQUINOLONES

Fluoroquinolones are indicated for the treatment of urinary tract infections, sinusitis, sexually transmitted infections (see Chapter 34), bacterial conjunctivitis (see Chapter 20), infectious diarrhea, anthrax, and numerous other infections.

MECHANISM OF ACTION

The process of DNA replication and transcription begins with the separation of the two strands of DNA. Excessive coiling (supercoiling) occurs when the strands separate. An enzyme, DNA gyrase, is responsible for blocking the supercoiling. Fluoroquinolones inhibit the enzyme DNA gyrase. This results in inhibition of bacterial DNA synthesis.

TECH ALERT!
Oral and parenteral fluoroquinolones are contraindicated in pregnant women and children less than 16 to 18 years old because of the risk for cartilage malformations.

PHARMACOKINETICS

Fluoroquinolones are formulated for oral, ophthalmic, and parenteral use. Oral absorption is good. The half-life ($T\frac{1}{2}$) of the newer agents such as moxifloxacin is long, permitting once-daily dosing, whereas ciprofloxacin ($T\frac{1}{2}$ approximately 4 hours) is dosed every 12 hours.

ADVERSE REACTIONS

Common adverse reactions are diarrhea, crystalluria, photosensitivity, dizziness, drowsiness, headache, nausea, and stomach upset. Oral gatafloxacin, grepafloxacin, and sparfloxacin have been discontinued due to risk of fatal adverse effects.

Fluoroquinolones

	Generic name	U.S. brand name(s) / Canadian brand(s)	Dosage forms and strengths
	ciprofloxacin*	Cipro, Cipro XR, Ciloxan, ProQuin XR Ciloxan, Cipro, Cipro XL	**Tablet:** 250 mg, 500 mg, 750 mg **Tablet, extended release:** 500 mg, 1000 mg **Ophthalmic ointment and solution:** 0.3% **Powder for suspension:** 25 mg/5 ml, 500 mg/5 ml **Solution for injection:** 10 mg/ml **Solution for injection in 5% dextrose:** 2 mg/ml **Mini-bags for IV:** 2 mg/ml (Canada only) **Oral suspension:** 10 g/100 ml (Canada only)
	gatifloxacin	Zymar Zymar	**Ophthalmic solution:** 0.3%
	levofloxacin	Iquix, Levaquin, Quixin Levaquin	**Ophthalmic solution:** 0.5% (Quixin), 1.5% (Iquix) **Solution for injection:** 25 mg/ml (U.S. only) **Solution for injection in 5% dextrose:** 5 mg/ml **Solution, oral:** 25 mg/ml (U.S. only) **Tablet:** 250 mg, 500 mg, 750 mg
	moxifloxacin	Avelox, Vigamox Avelox, Vigamox	**Ophthalmic solution (Vigamox):** 0.5% **Tablet:** 400 mg **Solution for IV:** 400 mg/250 ml 0.8% NaCl
	ofloxacin*	Floxin Otic, Ocuflox Ocuflox	**Ophthalmic solution (Ocuflox):** 0.3% **Otic solution (Floxin Otic):** 0.3% **Tablet (generics):** 200 mg, 300 mg, 400 mg
	norfloxacin*	Noroxin generics	**Tablet:** 400 mg

*Generic available.

TECH ALERT!
A common ending for macrolides is "-thromycin."

TECH ALERT!
Clarithromycin, erythromycin, and telithromycin have look-alike/ sound-alike issues.

MACROLIDES AND RELATED ANTIINFECTIVES

Macrolide antiinfectives are primarily used for the treatment of upper respiratory infections (URIs). The newer macrolides—azithromycin and clarithromycin—are more active against the bacteria *H. influenzae* than is erythromycin. Clarithromycin is a key ingredient in treatment regimens for peptic ulcer disease caused by the bacteria *H. pylori* (see Chapter 26). Erythromycin, the prototype for the macrolides, is used for the prevention of neonatal eye infections and acne in addition to URI treatment. Ketolides are structurally similar to macrolides but have greater antiinfective effects and a lower incidence of antimicrobial resistance. Telithromycin is currently the only marketed ketolide. Due to its risk for serious side effects, telithromycin is only indicated for community-acquired pneumonia.

MECHANISM OF ACTION

Macrolides inhibit bacterial protein synthesis by binding to the 50S ribosomal unit and blocking the translocation movement along mRNA.

PHARMACOKINETICS

Macrolides are formulated for oral, parenteral, and ophthalmic use. Several salts of erythromycin are in use and include erythromycin base, erythromycin ethylsuccinate, erythromycin stearate, and erythromycin lactobionate. Erythromycin base is formulated for immediate release and delayed release. Delayed-release tablets have a lower incidence of gastrointestinal side effects than do immediate-release tablets.

The expiration date of powder for oral suspension of erythromycin, clarithromycin, and azithromycin is shortened once the drug is reconstituted. Refrigeration is recommended for oral suspensions of erythromycin, whereas storage at room temperature is recommended for clarithromycin and azithromycin.

ADVERSE REACTIONS

Gastrointestinal upset is common with the use of macrolides. It occurs in up to 21% of individuals who take erythromycin. Gastrointestinal upset is less with clarithromycin (10%) and azithromycin (5%). Erythromycin and clarithromycin can cause arrhythmias by prolongation of the QT interval. Other adverse reactions include headache and tinnitus. Macrolides may decrease the effectiveness of oral contraceptives.

In 2007, the Food and Drug Administration required the package label for telithromycin to indicate that the drug is contraindicated in individuals with myasthenia gravis due to risk of fatal respiratory failure. The drug may also cause liver toxicity.

Macrolides and Related Antiinfectives

	Generic name	U.S. brand name(s) / Canadian brand(s)	Dosage forms and strengths
	azithromycin*	Azasite, Zithromax Z-pak, Zithromax, Zmax Zithromax	**Capsule:** 250 mg **Ophthalmic solution (Azasite):** 1% **Powder for injection:** 500 mg **Powder for oral suspension:** 100 mg/5 ml, 200 mg/5 ml **Powder of oral suspension, extended-release (Zmax):** 2 g **Tablet:** 250 mg, 500 mg, 600 mg
	clarithromycin*	Biaxin, Biaxin XL Biaxin, Biaxin BID, Biaxin XL	**Powder for suspension:** 125 mg/5 ml, 250 mg/5 ml **Tablet:** 250 mg, 500 mg **Tablet, extended release:** 500 mg
	erythromycin base* (immediate release)	Ery Pads, Ery gel Erysol	**Tablet (generics):** 250 mg, 500 mg **Topical solution (Ery pads, Ery gel, Erysol):** 2%
	erythromycin base* (delayed release)	Ery-tab, ERYC, PCE ERYC, PCE	**Tablet:** 250 mg, 333 mg, 500 mg
	erythromycin stearate*	Erythrocin Generic	**Tablet:** 250 mg, 500 mg

Continued

Macrolides and Related Antiinfectives—cont'd

Generic name	U.S. brand name(s) Canadian brand(s)	Dosage forms and strengths
erythromycin ethylsuccinate*	EES, Eryped	**Granules for oral suspension:** 200 mg/5 ml **Suspension:** 200 mg/5 ml, 400 mg/5 ml **Tablet:** 400 mg, 600 mg (Canada)
	EES	
erythromycin lactobionate*	Erythrocin	**Powder for injection:** 500 mg, 1 g
	Generic	
Ketolides		
telithromycin	Ketek	**Tablet:** 300 mg, 400 mg
	Ketek	

*Generic available.

OXAZOLIDINONES

Linezolid is a new antiinfective agent that is indicated for the treatment of gram-positive bacterial pneumonia and skin structure infections. Its use is limited due to side effects and in order to limit the development of bacterial resistance.

MECHANISM OF ACTION AND PHARMACOKINETICS

Linezolid inhibits bacterial protein synthesis. Its action on the bacterial ribosome blocks a key step in the translation process, which inhibits bacterial replication.

ADVERSE REACTIONS

Linezolid inhibits monoamine oxidase, the enzyme that is responsible for the breakdown of monoamine neurotransmitters (e.g., norepinephrine). Drug or drug-food interactions may cause a rise in blood pressure. More common side effects are skin rash, itching, change in taste, headache, mild diarrhea, dizziness, mild stomach upset, nausea, vomiting, and temporary tongue discoloration.

Oxazolidinones

Generic name	U.S. brand name(s) Canadian brand(s)	Dosage forms and strengths
linezolid	Zyvox	**Powder for suspension:** 100 mg/5 ml (U.S. only) **Solution for injection:** 2 mg/ml **Tablet:** 600 mg
	Zyvoxam	

TECH ALERT!
A common ending of penicillin-family drugs is "-cillin."

TECH ALERT!
Persons who are allergic to penicillin may also be allergic to cephalosporins.

PENICILLINS AND CARBAPENEMS

Penicillin is a true antibiotic. An antibiotic is a naturally occurring substance produced by one organism that is capable of destroying another organism. Oral penicillins are used to treat many infections including upper respiratory infections, otitis media, skin infections, and strep throat. It is also prescribed to prevent recurrent rheumatic fever. Penicillins may also be administered before dental and other medical procedures, to prevent bacterial endocarditis in individuals with prosthetic heart valves. Ampicillin may be prescribed for pelvic inflammatory disease (see Chapter 34). Parenteral penicillins are also used for the treatment of numerous infections including bone and joint infections, diabetic foot ulcers, infectious arthritis, sexually transmitted infections, meningitis, and septicemia.

MECHANISM OF ACTION

Penicillins are β-lactam antibiotics. Penicillins inhibit the synthesis of the cell wall of sensitive microbes. They do this by inhibiting the cross-linkage of peptide side chains of the bacterial cell wall. All penicillins are similar in structure. They each have a sulfur-containing ring-like structure. Side chains on this structure alter the antibacterial and pharmacological properties of basic penicillin molecule. The side chains can extend the antimicrobial spectrum. For example, amoxicillin and ticarcillin are effective against more types of bacteria than penicillin. Staphylococci are bacteria that have developed resistance to penicillin-type antiinfectives. Antistaphylococcal penicillins are penicillinase resistant. They are not inactivated by penicillinase (staphylococcal β-lactamase), a substance produced by the bacteria that destroys the antibiotic's β-lactam ring.

Carbapenems have a β-lactam ring fused with a penem ring. Carbapenems inhibit the third step in bacterial cell wall synthesis. Their spectrum of activity is broad and they resist inactivation by microbial enzymes (e.g., β-lactamase). Carbapenems are more effective against gram-negative bacteria than are other β-lactam antiinfective agents because they have a greater ability to penetrate the outer membrane of the bacteria.

PHARMACOKINETICS

Standard penicillins lack stability in gastric acids, which is why most are administered intramuscularly or must be taken on an empty stomach. The exception is penicillin VK, which is relatively acid stable.

Procaine penicillin G and benzathine penicillin G are formulated to delay absorption and achieve prolonged blood levels. Levels of benzathine penicillin G can be detected in the blood up to 1 month after an intramuscular injection of the drug is given.

Penicillins that are formulated as powders for reconstitution have shortened expiry dates once mixed with water. Expiration dates range between 10 and 14 days depending on the drug. Must suspensions should be refrigerated once they are reconstituted.

ADVERSE REACTIONS

Gastrointestinal side effects are the most common adverse reactions to penicillins. Examples are diarrhea, loss of appetite, nausea, vomiting, sore mouth, and stomach gas or heartburn. Other adverse effects include superinfection and hypersensitivity, hematological, and neurological reactions. Penicillins may decrease the effectiveness of oral contraceptives.

Penicillins

Generic name	U.S. brand name(s) / Canadian brand(s)	Dosage forms and strengths
Standard penicillins		
penicillin G potassium*	Pfizerpen	**Powder for injection:** 2 million units, 5 million units
	not available for human use	
phenoxymethyl penicillin potassium* (penicillin VK)	Veetids	**Powder for oral suspension:** 125 mg/5 ml, 250 mg/5 ml (Veetids), 180 mg/5 ml, 300 mg/5 ml (Pen Vee)
	Pen Vee	**Tablets:** 250 mg, 500 mg
procaine penicillin G*	Generics	**Suspension for IM injection:** 600,000 units/ml, 1,200,000 units/2 ml
	Not available for human use	
benzathine penicillin G*	Bicillin L-A	**Suspension for IM injection:** 600,000 units/ml
	Not available	

Continued

Penicillins—cont'd

	Generic name	U.S. brand name(s) / Canadian brand(s)	Dosage forms and strengths
	benzylpenicillin (penicillin G sodium)	Crystapen	**Powder for injection:** 1,000,000 units/ml, 5,000,000 units/ml (Canada only)

Aminopenicillins: extended spectrum

	Generic name	U.S. brand name(s) / Canadian brand(s)	Dosage forms and strengths
	amoxicillin*	Amoxil Generics	**Capsule:** 250 mg, 500 mg **Powder for oral suspension:** 50 mg/ml, 125 mg/5 ml, 200 mg/5 ml, 250 mg/5 ml, 400 mg/5 ml **Tablet:** 500 mg, 875 mg **Tablet, chewable:** 125 mg, 200 mg, 250 mg, 400 mg
	ampicillin*	Generics Generics	**Capsule:** 250 mg, 500 mg **Powder for injection:** 125 mg 250 mg, 500 mg, 1 g, 2 g, 10 g **Powder for oral suspension:** 125 mg/5 ml, 250 mg/5 ml

Antistaphyloccocal penicillins: penicillinase resistant

	Generic name	U.S. brand name(s) / Canadian brand(s)	Dosage forms and strengths
	cloxacillin*	Not available in U.S. Generics	**Capsule:** 250 mg, 500 mg **Powder for oral suspension:** 125 mg/5 ml **Powder for injection:** 0.5 g, 1 g, 2 g
	dicloxacillin*	Generics Not available	**Capsule:** 250 mg, 500 mg
	nafcillin*	Generics Not available	**Powder for injection:** 1 g, 2 g, 10 g **Solution for injection:** 20 mg/ml
	oxacillin*	Generics Not available	**Powder for injection:** 1 g, 2 g, 10 g **solution for injection:** 20 mg/ml

Antipseudomonal penicillins

	Generic name	U.S. brand name(s) / Canadian brand(s)	Dosage forms and strengths
	carbenicillin	Geocillin Not available	**Tablet:** 382 mg
	piperacillin*	Generics Generics	**Powder for injection:** 2 g, 3 g, 4 g, 40 g

Penicillin combinations

	Generic name	U.S. brand name(s) / Canadian brand(s)	Dosage forms and strengths
	amoxicillin + clavulanic acid*	Amoclan, Augmentin, Augmentin ES, Augmentin XR Clavulin	**Powder for oral suspension:** amoxicillin 125 mg + clavulanic acid 31.25 mg amoxicillin 200 mg + clavulanic acid 28.5 mg amoxicillin 250 mg + clavulanic acid 62.5 mg amoxicillin 400 mg + clavulanic acid 57 mg amoxicillin 600 mg + clavulanic acid 42.9 mg (Augmentin ES) **Tablet:** amoxicillin 250 mg + clavulanic acid 125 mg amoxicillin 500 mg + clavulanic acid 125 mg amoxicillin 875 mg + clavulanic acid 125 mg **Tablet, chewable:** amoxicillin + clavulanic acid amoxicillin 200 mg + clavulanic acid 28.5 mg amoxicillin 250 mg + clavulanic acid 62.5 mg amoxicillin 400 mg + clavulanic acid 57 mg amoxicillin 500 mg + clavulanic acid 125 mg Tablet extended release (Augmentin XR) amoxicillin 1000 mg + clavulanic acid 62.5 mg

Penicillins—cont'd

	Generic name	U.S. brand name(s) / Canadian brand(s)	Dosage forms and strengths
	ampicillin + sulbactam	Unasyn	**Powder for injection:**
		Not available	ampicillin 1 g + sulbactam 0.5 g ampicillin 2 g + sulbactam 1 g
	piperacillin + tazobactam	Zosyn	**Powder for injection:**
		Tazocin	piperacillin 2 g + tazobactam 0.25 g piperacillin 3 g + tazobactam 0.375 g piperacillin 4 g + tazobactam 0.5 g piperacillin 36 g + tazobactam 4.5 g **Solution for injection:** piperacillin 2 g + tazobactam 0.25 g/50 ml piperacillin 3 g + tazobactam 0.375 g/50 mg piperacillin 4 g + tazobactam 0.5 g/100 ml
	ticarcillin + clavulanic acid	Timentin	**Powder for injection:**
		Timentin	ticarcillin 3 g + clavulanic acid 100 mg ticarcillin 30 g + clavulanic acid 1 g **Solution for injection:** ticarcillin 3 g + clavulanic acid 100 mg/100 ml

*Generic available.

Carbapenems

	Generic name	U.S. brand name(s) / Canadian brand(s)	Dosage forms and strengths
	Imlpenem + cilastatin	Primaxin	**Powder for injection:**
		Primaxin	imipenem 500 mg + cilastatin 500 mg imipenem 250 mg + cilastatin 250 mg (Canada)
	meropenem	Merrem	**Powder for injection:**
		Merrem	500 mg, 1 g

TECH ALERT!
The warning label TAKE WITH LOTS OF WATER is applied to prescription vials for sulfonamides. This reduces the risk of kidney damage due to crystalluria.

SULFONAMIDES

Sulfonamides are the oldest antiinfective agents. They were developed in the 1930s, but their use did not spread until the 1940s in World War II. Sulfonamides are commonly called "sulfa" drugs because the generic name of all agents begins with *"sulf."* Sulfonamides and trimethoprim are used in the treatment of various upper respiratory, urinary tract, and skin infections. They are also indicated for the treatment of AIDS-related pneumonia (*Pneumocystis carinii*).

MECHANISM OF ACTION AND PHARMACOKINETICS

Sulfonamides and trimethoprim are antifolate drugs. They interfere with microbial synthesis of folic acid at separate steps in the biosynthetic pathway that ultimately leads to bacterial DNA synthesis (see Figure 35-4). Food may slightly decrease the absorption of sulfonamides; however, the drug may be taken with small amounts of food to reduce gastric upset.

ADVERSE REACTIONS

Adverse reactions that are common with the use of sulfonamides are nausea, vomiting, abdominal pain, headache, drowsiness, dizziness, diarrhea, and photosensitivity. Sulfonamides may produce the formation of crystals in the urine (crystalluria), especially if taken with acidic foods or beverages.

Sulfonamides

Generic name	U.S. brand name(s) / Canadian brand(s)	Dosage forms and strengths
Sulfonamides		
sulfadiazine*	Silvadene	**Cream (Silvadene):** 1%
	Dermazin, Flumazine	**Tablet:** 500 mg
sulfamethoxazole*	Not available	**Tablet:** 500 mg
	Generics	
sulfisoxazole*	Gantrisin	**Suspension:** 500 mg/5 ml
	Generics	**Tablet (generics):** 500 mg
Combination Sulfonamides		
sulfisoxizole + erythromycin ethylsuccinate*	Pediazole	**Granules for suspension:** sulfisoxizole 600 mg/5 ml + erythromycin ethylsuccinate 200 mg/5 ml
	Pediazole	
sulfamethoxazole + trimethoprim* (SMX-TMP) (COTRIMOX)	Bactrim, Bactrim DS, Septra, Septra DS	**Solution for injection:** Sulfamethoxazole 80 mg/ml + trimethoprim 16 mg/ml **Tablet:** sulfamethoxazole 400 mg + trimethoprim 80 mg, sulfamethoxazole 800 mg + trimethoprim 160 mg **Suspension:** sulfamethoxazole 200 mg/5 ml + trimethoprim 40 mg/5 ml
	Septra, Sulfatrim	

*Generic available.

TETRACYCLINES

Tetracylines are broad-spectrum antiinfective agents. They may be bactericidal or bacteriostatic. They are used for the treatment of acne, sexually transmitted infections such as *Chlamydia*, Lyme's disease, and Rocky Mountain spotted fever.

MECHANISM OF ACTION AND PHARMACOKINETICS

Tetracyclines inhibit protein synthesis. Their site of action is the 30S ribosomal unit (Figure 35-3). They block the binding of tRNA to the mRNA-ribosome complex. Tetracycline interacts with dairy products, calcium, aluminum, and ferrous supplements to form a chelated complex. The complex significantly reduces the absorption of tetracycline.

Doxycycline and minocycline are more stable in the acidic stomach contents than tetracycline. They also have a longer duration of action. They are dosed 1 to 2 times a day compared to tetracycline, which is dosed 4 times a day.

ADVERSE REACTIONS

The tetracylines can cause nausea, vomiting, diarrhea, and photosensitivity. Serious, but less common, side effects include hepatotoxicity, pseudomembranous colitis, and kidney disease. Outdated tetracyline becomes toxic. Patients should be advised to discard old medicines. Tetracyclines man decrease the effectiveness of oral contraceptives.

Tetracyclines

	Generic name	U.S. brand name(s)	Dosage forms and strengths
		Canadian brand(s)	
	demeclocycline*	Declomycin	**Tablet:** 150 mg, 300 mg
		Declomycin	
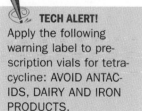	doxycycline hyclate*	Doryx, Periostat, Vibra-tabs, Vibramycin	**Capsule (Vibramycin):** 100 mg **Powder for suspension (Vibramycin):** 25 mg/5 ml **Syrup, oral (Vibramycin):** 50 mg/5 ml **Tablet:** 20 mg (Periostat), 100 mg (Vibra-tabs) **Tablet (delayed release):** 75 mg, 100 mg
	doxycycline monohydrate* (U.S. only)	Aldoxa, Aldoxa Pak, Monodox	**Tablet:** 50 mg, 75 mg, 150 mg
	minocycline*	Cleeravue-M Kit, Dynacin, Dynacin PAC, Minocin, Myrac, Soladyn	**Capsule:** (Dyacin, Minocin, Enca): 50 mg, 75 mg, 100 mg **Tablet:** 50 mg (Cleeravue, Dynacin, Myrac), 75 mg, 100 mg
		Enca, Minocin	**Tablet, extended release (Soladyn):** 45 mg, 90 mg, 135 mg
	tetracycline*	Emtet, Sumycin	**Capsule (Emtet):** 500 mg (U.S. only) **Ophthalmic oint:** 1%
		Generics	**Syrup: (Sumycin):** 125 mg/nl **Tablet (Sumycin):** 250 mg, 500 mg (U.S. only)

*Generic available.

TECH ALERT!
Apply the following warning label to prescription vials for tetracycline: AVOID ANTACIDS, DAIRY AND IRON PRODUCTS.

TECH ALERT!
Tetracyclines are contraindicated in pregnancy and small children as they can weaken fetal bone, retard bone growth, weaken tooth enamel, and stain teeth.

TECH ALERT!
The following drugs have look-alike/sound-alike issues: Bactroban, baclofen, and bacitracin; Cleocin and Clinoril

MISCELLANEOUS ANTIINFECTIVES

Isoniazid is used for the treatment of tuberculosis. It inhibits the synthesis of mycolic acid, an important constituent of the highly lipid cell wall of Mycobacteria. Isoniazid may cause liver disease and nerve damage. Concurrent administration of vitamin B_6 is recommended to prevent neurotoxicity. Isoniazid is abbreviated as INH, but the use of acronyms may cause medication errors.

Metronidazole is an amoebacide. It destroys the protozoa that cause giardiasis (traveler's diarrhea) and trichomoniasis (a sexually transmitted infection). It is the drug of choice for the treatment of *C. difficile* enteritis, a condition that may cause pseudomembranous colitis. Topical preparations are used for the treatment of acne rosacea. It is formulated for oral, parenteral, vaginal, and topical use. Alcohol beverages or medicines containing high levels of alcohol may produce nausea, vomiting, stomach pains, headache, and dizziness. The drug may also produce a metallic taste.

Mupirocin is a topically applied antiinfective used to treat staphylococcal infections of the skin such as impetigo.

Chloramphenicol is a broad-spectrum antiinfective agent that inhibits protein synthesis. Its use is limited and is indicated when alterative, less-toxic drugs cannot be used (e.g., drug allergy). It may be used for treatment of bacterial meningitis, brain abscess, and Rocky Mountain spotted fever. Neonates are unable to fully metabolize the drug and may accumulate toxic levels. Its use in children may produce "gray baby syndrome" or cyanosis.

Clindamycin is an antiinfective agent that is commonly used topically for the treatment of acne and vaginosis. Systemic use of clindamycin is associated with the development of *C. difficile*, a bacteria that causes diarrhea and pseudomembranous colitis. Drinking lots of fluids can lower the risk for the development of this condition.

Miscellaneous

	Generic name	U.S. brand name(s) Canadian brand(s)	Dosage forms and strengths
	isoniazid*	Nydrazide	**Solution for injection (Nydrazide):** 100 mg/ml **Syrup (generics):** 50 mg/5 ml **Tablet:** 100 mg, 300 mg
		Isotamine-100, Isotamine-300, Isotamine B-300	
	metronidazole*	Flagyl, Flagyl ER, Metrocreme, Metrogel, Metrolotion, Noritate, Vandazole	**Capsule:** 375 mg **Cream:** 0.75% (Metrocreme), 1% (Noritate) **Gel, topical (Metrogel, Rosasol):** 1% **Gel, vaginal (Metrogel, Nidagel, Vandazole):** 0.75% **Lotion:** 0.75% **Powder for injection:** 500 mg **Solution for injection:** 5 mg/ml **Tablet:** 250 mg, 500 mg **Tablet, extended release (Flagyl ER, Flurozole ER):** 750 mg
		Flagyl 500 S-Pak, Flurozole ER, Metrocreme, Metrogel, Metrolotion, Nidagel, Noritate, Rosasol Cream	
	mupirocin*	Bactroban Cream, Centany	**Cream:** 2% **Ointment, topical:** 2% **Ointment, nasal:** 2%
		Bactoban, Bactoban Cream	
	chloramphenicol*	Generics	**Powder for injection:** 1GM **Ophthalmic solution:** 0.5% (Chloroptic), 0.25% (Pentamycetin) **Ophthalmic ointment:** 1%
		Chloroptic, Pentamycetin	
	clindamycin*	Cleocin, Cleocin Pediatric, Cleocin T, Clindagel, Clindamax, Clindets pledgets, Evoclin	**Capsule:** 75 mg, 150 mg, 300 mg **Foam (Evolclin):** 1% **Pledgets (Clindets):** 1% **Powder for injection:** 150 mg/ml (Dalacin C, Cleocin), 900 mg/6ml, 900 mg/50 ml **Powder for oral solution:** 75 mg/5 ml **Topical gel, lotion, solution:** 1% **Vaginal cream:** 2% **Vaginal suppositories (Cleocin Ovules):** 100 mg
		Clindasol, Clindets, Dalacin C-150, Dalacin C-300, Dalacin C phosphate, Dalacin T 1%, Dalacin Vaginal Cream	

*Generic available.

Summary of Drugs Used for the Treatment of Bacterial Infections

	Generic name	Brand name	Usual dose and dosing schedule	Warning labels
	Cephalosporins			
	cefadroxil*	Duricef	1 g to 2 g orally per day given in 1 to 2 daily doses (maximum 4 g per day)	COMPLETE FULL COURSE OF THERAPY TAKE WITH FOOD—cefadroxil
	cephalexin*	Keflex	Varies (maximum 4 g per day)	REFRIGERATE, SHAKE WELL AND DISCARD AFTER 14 DAYS
	cefaclor*	Ceclor Ceclor CD	250 mg to 500 mg orally every 8 hours. (maximum dose is 2 g/day)	COMPLETE FULL COURSE OF THERAPY STORE AT ROOM TEMPERATURE, SHAKE WELL AND DISCARD AFTER 14 DAYS SWALLOW WHOLE, DON'T CRUSH OR CHEW—extended release TAKE WITH FOOD—extended release

Summary of Drugs Used for the Treatment of Bacterial Infections—cont'd

	Generic name	Brand name	Usual dose and dosing schedule	Warning labels
	cefuroxime	Ceftin	250 mg to 500 mg orally every 12 hours (maximum dose is 1 g/day)	COMPLETE FULL COURSE OF THERAPY REFRIGERATE, SHAKE WELL AND DISCARD AFTER 10 DAYS
	cefixime	Suprax	400 mg orally divided every 12 to 24 hours (maximum dose is 800 mg/day)	COMPLETE FULL COURSE OF THERAPY STORE AT ROOM TEMPERATURE, SHAKE WELL AND DISCARD AFTER 14 DAYS
Fluoroquinolones				
	ciprofloxacin*	Cipro Cipro XR	500 mg to 750 mg orally every 12 hours (maximum 1.5 g/day)	COMPLETE FULL COURSE OF THERAPY TAKE WITH LOTS OF WATER AVOID PROLONGED SUNLIGHT
	levofloxacin	Levaquin	250 mg to 500 mg every 24 hours (maximum 750 mg/day)	MAY CAUSE DIZZINESS OR DROWSINESS, DO NOT DRIVE, USE MACHINERY
	moxifloxacin	Avelox	400 mg orally or IV once daily	AVOID ANTACIDS AND VITAMINS CONTAINING IRON AND ZINC
	norfloxacin	Noroxin	400 mg orally twice daily	REFRIGERATE, SHAKE WELL AND DISCARD AFTER 14 DAYS— suspension SWALLOW WHOLE, DON'T CRUSH OR CHEW—extended release TAKE ON AN EMPTY STOMACH
Macrolides				
	azithromycin	Zithromax	500 mg the first 1 to 3 days of therapy, followed by 250 mg once daily for 4 days	COMPLETE FULL COURSE OF THERAPY STORE AT ROOM TEMPERATURE, DISCARD IN 14 DAYS—clarithromycin and azithromycin extended release suspension
	clarithromycin	Biaxin, Biaxin XL	250 mg to 500 mg every 12 hours up to 1000 mg once daily	SHAKE WELL—suspension
	erythromycin base-delayed release	Ery-Tab, ERYC, PCE	250 mg to 500 mg every 6 to 8 hours (maximum 4 g/day)	REFRIGERATE, DISCARD IN 10 DAYS— azithromycin suspension (immed. release)
	erythromycin ethylsuccinate	EES	400 mg to 800 mg every 6 to 8 hours (maximum 4 g/day)	TAKE ON AN EMPTY STOMACH— azithromycin suspension MAY DECREASE THE EFFECTIVENESS OF ORAL CONTRACEPTIVES TAKE WITH FOOD—delayed release

Continued

Summary of Drugs Used for the Treatment of Bacterial Infections—cont'd

	Generic name	Brand name	Usual dose and dosing schedule	Warning labels
Ketolides				
	telithromycin	Ketek	800 mg once daily	COMPLETE FULL COURSE OF THERAPY
Sulfonamides and sulfonamide combinations				
	sulfisoxazole	Gantrisin	Varies 2 g to 4 g initially then 4 g/day to 8 g/day in 4 to 6 equally divided doses (maximum dose is 12 g/day)	COMPLETE FULL COURSE OF THERAPY TAKE WITH LOTS OF WATER AVOID PROLONGED EXPOSURE TO SUNLIGHT SHAKE WELL—suspension
	sulfisoxizole + erythromycin ethylsuccinate	Pediazole	400 mg erythromycin + 1200 mg sulfisoxazole every 6 hours (maximum 4 g per day erythromycin base or 12 g per day sulfisoxazole)	
	sulfamethoxazole + trimethoprim	Septra, Bactrim	160 mg trimethoprim + 800 mg sulfamethoxazole every 12 hours	
Penicillins				
	ampicillin	Generics	250 mg to 1000 mg orally every 6 hours (maximum 4 g/day)	COMPLETE FULL COURSE OF THERAPY TAKE ON AN EMPTY STOMACH—ampicillin, dicloxacillin
	amoxicillin	Amoxil	Varies 500 mg to 875 mg every 12 hours or 250 mg to 500 mg PO every 8 hours (maximum 1750 mg/day)	REFRIGERATE, SHAKE WELL AND DISCARD AFTER 14 DAYS—suspension (ampicillin, dicloxacillin, pen VK)
	carbenacillin	Geocillin	1 to 2 tablets 4 times a day	MAY DECREASE EFFECTIVENESS OF ORAL CONTRACEPTIVES
	dicloxacillin	Generics	125 mg to 500 mg orally every 6 hours (maximum 4 g/day)	REFRIGERATE, SHAKE WELL AND DISCARD AFTER 10 DAYS—suspension (amoxicillin + clavulanic acid)
	penicillin VK	Veetids	125 mg to 500 mg orally every 6 hours (maximum 3 g/day)	
	amoxicillin + clavulanic acid	Augmentin	Varies 250 mg to 500 mg every 8 hours or 500 mg to 875 mg every 12 hours—maximum Augmentin tablets, chewable tablets, or suspension 1750 mg/day (amoxicillin component), Augmentin XR tablets 4 g/day (amoxicillin component)	
	penicillin G benzathine	Bicillin L-A	Varies	REFRIGERATE, DO NOT FREEZE

Summary of Drugs Used for the Treatment of Bacterial Infections—cont'd

Generic name	Brand name	Usual dose and dosing schedule	Warning labels
Tetracyclines			
doxycycline	Vibramycin, Monodox	600 mg/day for 5 days in acute gonococcal infections, 300 mg/day for all other infections	COMPLETE FULL COURSE OF THERAPY TAKE WITH LOTS OF WATER AVOID PROLONGED SUNLIGHT AVOID ANTACIDS AND VITAMINS CONTAINING IRON AND ZINC
minocycline	Minocin	Varies (maximum 350 mg on day 1, then 200 mg/day)	MAY DECREASE EFFECTIVENESS OF ORAL CONTRACEPTIVES
tetracycline	Sumycin	Varies (maximum 4 g/day)	SHAKE WELL—tetracycline suspension TAKE ON AN EMPTY STOMACH—tetracycline
Miscellaneous			
metronidazole	Metrogel, Metrocreme Noritate Metrogel Flagyl	**Acne rosecea:** Apply a thin film 1 to 2 times daily **Bacterial vaginosis:** 1 applicatorful once daily at bedtime **Other infections:** 500 mg to 750 mg PO twice daily or 250 mg PO three times per day (maximum 4 g per day)	COMPLETE FULL COURSE OF THERAPY TAKE WITH A FULL GLASS OF WATER AVOID ALCOHOL MAY CAUSE DIZZINESS OR DROWSINESS, DO NOT DRIVE, USE MACHINERY
isoniazid	Generics	**TB prophylaxis:** 300 mg orally once daily or 900 mg/day twice weekly with pyridoxine (50 mg once daily or 100 mg twice weekly) for 9 months	COMPLETE FULL COURSE OF THERAPY AVOID ANTACIDS AVOID ALCOHOL
clindamycin	Cleocin	150 mg to 450 mg orally every 6 hours (maximum 2700 mg/day)	COMPLETE FULL COURSE OF THERAPY TAKE WITH A FULL GLASS OF WATER
mupirocin	Bactroban	Apply 3 times daily or apply 2 times daily for intranasal infections	COMPLETE FULL COURSE OF THERAPY

 TECH ALERT!
The following drugs have look-alike/sound-alike issues: doxycycline hyclate and doxycycline monohydrate; doxycycline and dicyclomine; Monodox and Maalox; Dynacin, Dynabac, Dyazide, and Dynapen; Minocin and Minizide

CHAPTER SUMMARY

- Chronic, noninfectious disease is a leading cause of disability and death in developed, industrialized countries; however, infectious disease is still one the leading causes of morbidity and mortality globally.
- Poverty, malnutrition, lack of clean water, poor sanitation, and inadequate housing increase the risk for infectious disease and decrease the likelihood for adequate treatment.
- Antibiotics have played a key role in improving the survival of individuals with bacterial infections.
- Microbes can "learn" how to withstand the effects of antibiotics, and new "superbugs" exist that are resistant to currently available antiinfective agents. Multidrug resistance is a serious problem.

- Microbial resistance is the ability of bacteria to overcome the bactericidal effects of an antibiotic. Resistance traits are encoded on bacterial genes on chromosomal or plasmid DNA and can be transferred to other bacteria.
- Causes of microbial resistance are (1) inappropriate prescribing, (2) failure to complete the full course of therapy, (3) administration of antibacterial agents for viral infections (e.g., the common cold), (4) antibiotics in the food chain (agriculture, animal husbandry, fish farms), and (5) lack of guidelines for preventing spread of infections in institutional care settings.
- Examples of mechanisms of antimicrobial resistance are (1) secretion of enzymes that inactivate the antibiotic, (2) modification of the target site for antibiotic binding, (3) production of antibiotic-modifying enzymes, and (4) mutations that affect antibiotic transport into the cell.
- Bactericidal agents are able to destroy rapidly proliferating, pathogenic bacteria.
- Bacteriostatic agents slow the growth of bacteria enough for the host (our bodies) defense mechanism to destroy the invading bacteria.
- β-Lactam antibiotics target the bacterial cell wall. Penicillins, cephalosporins, cabapenems, and monobactams are β-lactam antibiotics that inhibit cell wall synthesis.
- Vancomycin is a glycopeptide antibiotic that inhibits cell wall synthesis.
- Antibiotics that inhibit the function of the bacterial cell wall work by binding to bacterial membranes and producing a detergent-like action that increases cell membrane permeability. Polymyxin B is an example.
- There are five classes of antiinfective agents that act to inhibit bacterial protein synthesis. They are the aminoglycosides, macrolides, tetracyclines, amphenicols, and oxazolidiones.
- Fluoroquinolones and nitroimidazoles are classes of antiinfectives capable of inhibiting DNA synthesis.
- Rifampin inhibits bacterial RNA synthesis.
- Bacteria must synthesize folic acid.
- Sulfonamides are antifolate drugs and trimethoprim is a dihydrofolate reductase inhibitor and interfere with bacterial folic acid synthesis.
- Aminoglycosides are not absorbed, systemically when administered by mouth but may be given orally to reduce bacteria of the bowel prior to colonorectal surgery.
- The most serious adverse reactions linked to aminoglyoside use are hearing loss (ototoxicity) and kidney damage (nephrotoxicity).
- A common beginning for cephalosporin drugs is *"-ceph"* or *"cef."*
- Cephalosporins are classified as first, second, and third generation.
- First-generation cephalosporins are most effective against gram-positive, aerobic bacteria. Second-generation cephalosporins have effectiveness against gram-positive and gram-negative bacteria, but third-generation cephalosporins are the most effective against gram-negative, anaerobic bacteria.
- A common ending of fluoroquinolones is *"-floxacin."*
- Oral and parenteral fluoroquinolones are contraindicated in pregnant women and children less than 16 to 18 years old because of the risk for cartilage malformations.
- A common ending for macrolides is *"-thromycin."*
- Clarithromycin is a key ingredient in treatment regimens for peptic ulcer disease caused by the bacteria *H. pylori.*
- Gastrointestinal upset is common with the use of macrolides. It occurs in up to 21% of individuals who take erythromycin.
- Macrolides and penicillins may decrease the effectiveness of oral contraceptives (OC). Tetracyclines also decrease OC effectiveness.
- Penicillins may also be administered before dental and other medical procedures, to prevent bacterial endocarditis in individuals with prosthetic heart valves.
- Antistaphlococcal penicillins are penicillinase resistant.
- Standard penicillins lack stability in gastric acids, which is why most are administered intramuscularly or must be taken on an empty stomach.
- A common beginning for sulfonamides *"-sulf."*
- Sulfonamides are indicated for the treatment of AIDS-related pneumonia (*Pneumocystis carinii*), urinary tract infections, and upper respiratory infections.

- Sulfonamides may produce the formation of crystals in the urine (crystalluria), especially if taken with acidic foods or beverages.
- Tetracyclines are used for the treatment of acne, sexually transmitted infections such as *Chlamydia,* Lyme's disease, and Rocky Mountain spotted fever.
- Tetracyclines are contraindicated in pregnancy and small children as they can weaken fetal bone, retard bone growth, weaken tooth enamel, and stain teeth.
- Isoniazid is used for the treatment of tuberculosis. Vitamin B_6 should be taken with isoniazid to reduce neurotoxicity.
- Metronidazole is the drug of choice for treatment of *C. difficile* enteritis, a condition that may cause pseudomembranous colitis.
- Individuals taking metronidazole should avoid drinking alcoholic beverages or taking medicines containing alcohol.
- Mupirocin is a topically applied antiinfective used to treat staphylococcal infections of the skin such as impetigo.
- Systemic use of clindamycin is associated with the development of *C. difficile,* a bacteria that causes diarrhea and pseudomembranous colitis. Drinking lots of fluids can lower the risk for the development of this condition.

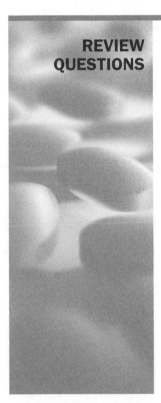

REVIEW QUESTIONS

Multiple Choice

1. Antibiotics are _____ substances produced by one organism that is capable of destroying or inhibiting the growth of bacteria.
   a. natural
   b. synthetic

2. Misuse of antimicrobial agents is a major cause for the development and spread of microbial resistance.
   a. true
   b. false

3. Antiinfective agents may be classified as _____ .
   a. bactericidal
   b. bacteriolytic
   c. bacteriostatic
   d. a and c

4. Fluoroquinolones and nitroimidazoles are classes of antiinfectives capable of inhibiting _____ synthesis.
   a. RNA
   b. DNA
   c. tPA
   d. GABA

5. Second-generation cephalosporins have effectiveness only against gram-positive bacteria.
   a. true
   b. false

6. Fluoroquinolones are formulated for oral, ophthalmic, and parenteral use.
   a. true
   b. false

7. Macrolide antiinfectives are primarily used for the treatment of upper respiratory infections (URIs) and lower respiratory infections (LRIs).
   a. true
   b. false

8. Oral penicillins are used to treat many infections including _____.
   a. upper respiratory infections
   b. otitis media, skin infections
   c. strep throat
   d. all of the above

9. **Outdated tetracyline becomes toxic and should be discarded.**
   a. true
   b. false

10. **Isoniazid is used for the treatment of _____.**
    a. upper respiratory infections
    b. AIDS
    c. tuberculosis
    d. peptic ulcers

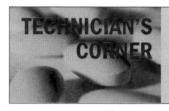

1. With microbial resistance developing against antibiotics, what steps should be taken by the pharmaceutical industry, patients, health care providers, and the food industry to combat this problem?
2. Can the practice of universal precautions (handwashing, etc.) reduce the incidences of nosocomial infections?

BIBLIOGRAPHY

Kalant H, Grant D, Mitchell J: *Principles of medical pharmacology* (pp 671-686, 702-707, 713-722), ed 7. Toronto, 2007, Elsevier Canada, A Division of Reed Elsevier Canada.

Lance L, Lacy C, Armstrong L, Goldman M: *Drug information handbook for the allied health professional,* ed 12, Hudson, OH, 2005, APhA Lexi-Comp.

Page C, Curtis M, Sutter M, Walker M, Hoffman B, et al: *Integrated pharmacology* (pp 111-134), Philadelphia, 2005, Elsevier Mosby.

Prosser T, Gold Standard Inc, Clinical Pharmacology: *Quinolones,* revised April 18, 2007. Available at: http://www.clinicalpharmacology.com/.

Reents S, Prosser T, Gold Standard Inc, Clinical Pharmacology: *Cephalosporins,* revised July 31, 2002. Available at: http://www.clinicalpharmacology.com/.

Reents S, Prosser T, Gold Standard Inc, Clinical Pharmacology: *Macrolides,* revised December 16, 2005. Available at: http://www.clinicalpharmacology.com/.

USP Center for Advancement of Patient Safety: *Use caution–avoid confusion,* USP Quality Review No. 79, Rockville, MD, April 2004, USP Center for Advancement of Patient Safety.

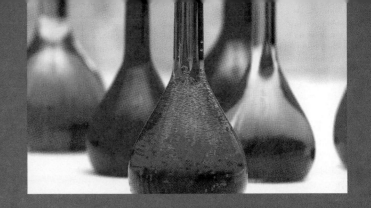

CHAPTER

36

Treatment of Viral Infections

LEARNING OBJECTIVES

- Learn the terminology associated with treatments for viral infections.
- Describe the mechanism of virus entry into cells.
- Describe antiviral resistance.
- List and categorize antiviral agents.
- Describe mechanism of action for antiviral agents.
- Identify warning labels and precautionary messages associated with antiinfective agents.
- Identify significant drug look-alike/sound-alike issues.
- List common endings for antiviral agents.

KEY TERMS

Adherence: Closely following or adhering to the treatment regimen.

AIDS (acquired immune deficiency syndrome): AIDS is the most severe form of HIV infection. HIV-infected patients are diagnosed with AIDS when their CD4 cell count falls below 200 cells/mm^3 or if they develop an AIDS-defining illness (an illness that is very unusual in someone who is not HIV positive).

Antiretroviral: Medication that interferes with the replication of retroviruses. HIV is a retrovirus.

Antiviral: Medication that is able to inhibit viral replication.

Antiviral resistance: Ability of a virus to overcome the suppressive action of antiviral agents.

CD4 count: Number of CD4 cells in a sample of blood.

CD4 T lymphocyte: White blood cells that fight infection.

Cross-resistance: Development of resistance to one drug in a particular class that results in resistance to the other drugs in that class.

Drug resistance testing: Laboratory test to determine if an individual's HIV strain is resistant to any anti-HIV medications.

Highly active antiretroviral therapy (HAART): Combination of three or more antiretroviral medications taken in a regimen.

Host: Individual infected with a virus.

Viral load: Amount of materials from the virus that get released into the blood when the HIV reproduces.

Mother-to-child transmission (also called perinatal transmission): Transmission of the HIV from an HIV-infected mother to her baby during pregnancy or delivery or through breast milk.

Virion: Infectious particles of a virus.

Virostatic: Able to suppress viral proliferation.

Virus: Intracellular parasite that consists of a DNA and RNA core surrounded by a protein coat and sometimes an outer covering of lipoprotein.

OVERVIEW

A *virus* is an intracellular parasite that consists of a DNA or RNA core surrounded by a protein coat and sometimes an outer covering of lipoprotein. The infectious particles (*virions*) do not have the cellular components necessary for reproduction so they use their host's cellular machinery to replicate (Figure 36-1). The virus attaches itself to the host cell and then releases viral genetic material (RNA and DNA) into the host cell. The viral material takes control of the host cell machinery for replication. The host cell eventually dies because the virus keeps it from performing its normal functions. When it dies, the cell releases replicated viruses that proliferate and attack more and more host cells.

Viruses may cause minor illness such as the common cold and warts, as well as serious infections such as human immunodeficiency virus (HIV), smallpox, and hepatitis C. Some viral infections are linked to cancers. For example, human papillomavirus (HPV) is linked to cervical cancer. Epstein-Barr virus (EBV) is associated with nose and throat cancers, and hepatitis C virus is associated with liver cancer.

An *antiviral* is a medication that is able to inhibit viral replication. All antiviral agents work best when the host (the individual with the infection) has a healthy immune system. This is because antivirals do not destroy viruses; they are virustatic. When the rate of virus proliferation is slowed, the macrophages, immunoglobulins, T cells, interleukins, interferons, and other cells released by the host in response to attack ultimately are responsible for recovery from the infection (see Unit Introduction). Like bacterial infections, effective treatment of viral infections is dependent upon host factors, virus factors, and drug factors. Figure 35-1 shows factors that influence successful therapy.

Factors that influence the outcome of antiviral therapy are (1) stage of illness at the time of initiation of therapy, (2) dosage of antiviral agent used, (3) ability of the virus to penetrate the central nervous system, (4) ability of the virus to remain latent within its host, and

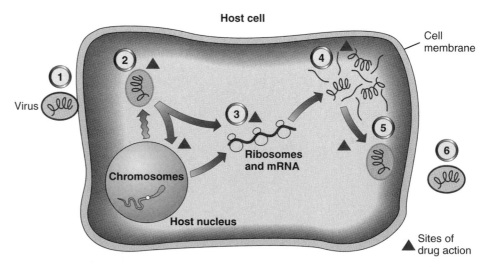

1. Attachment to host cell
2. Uncoating of virus, and entry of viral nucleic acid into host cell nucleus
3. Control of DNA, RNA, and/or protein production
4. Production of viral subunits
5. Assembly of virions
6. Release of virions

FIGURE 36-1 Virus invasion of a host cell, viral replication, and release of virions. *(Modified from Brody TM, Larner J, Minneman KP:* Human pharmacology: molecular to clinical, *ed 3, St. Louis, 1998, Mosby.)*

(5) development of antiviral resistance. Herpes simplex (HSV-1, HSV-2) is an example of a virus that demonstrates the importance of timing as related to initiation of drug therapy. Severity of the infection and symptoms are reduced only when antiviral therapy is initiated within the first 24 to 48 hours of exposure to the virus or onset of symptoms. Other viral infections that are improved by early initiation of antiviral therapy are influenza (type A and type B) and varicella zoster virus (VZV). HSV-1, HSV-2, and VZV are examples of viruses that lay dormant in host cells and periodically awaken to cause recurrent disease.

Unlike antibiotics, antivirals are only effective against a specific virus. For example, antiviral agents indicated for the treatment of influenza are not effective for the treatment of HIV, HPV, or HSV. Antibiotics are not effective against viral infections.

What Causes Viral Resistance?

The growth of viral colonies involves viral replication. In the process of replication, the virus may mutate. While mutations may result in a virus that is not able to reproduce, frequently, mutations result in adaptations that make it easier for the virus to exist in new environments and hosts. *Antiviral resistance* is the ability of a virus to overcome the suppressive action of antiviral agents. Antiviral resistance may occur when an individual taking an antiviral drug skips doses or takes them irregularly. Vomiting is an additional cause for subtherapeutic levels. Rather than having drug levels in the body high enough to suppress viral replication, low levels of residual drug are sufficient to allow the virus to reproduce. The virus may accidentally mutate into a form that is resistant to the antiviral drug(s) taken.

Because viruses continually mutate, it is difficult to develop a vaccine to prevent virus infection. For example, each year a new flu vaccine must be developed to the latest virulent strain of influenza. A triple "cocktail" of drugs is administered for HAART therapy to decrease mutations and improve antiretroviral therapy for the treatment of HIV/AIDS.

Mechanisms of Antiviral Action

Antivirals inhibit virus-specific steps in the replication cycle. Specific steps that are blocked by antiviral agents aim to:
- Interfere with the virus attachment to the host cell receptors, cell penetration, and viral uncoating
- Inhibit reverse transcriptase, transamidase, and other virion-associated enzymes
- Inhibit viral transcription
- Inhibit viral mRNA
- Interfere with virus regulatory proteins
- Interfere with virus cleavage
- Interfere with viral assembly
- Interfere with release of virus

INHIBITORS OF VIRAL UNCOATING

Amantadine and rimantidine are used for the prevention and treatment of influenza A. They are not effective against influenza B. Due to antiviral resistance, amantadine and rimantidine were not Food and Drug Administration (FDA) recommended for use during the 2006–2007 flu season.

MECHANISM OF ACTION AND PHARMACOKINETICS

Both drugs interfere with the uncoating of the influenza A virus, a necessary step in the virus replication process. More specifically, they inhibit the activity of the influenza virus M2 protein, which forms a channel in the virus membrane and enables replication after the virus enters the host cell.

ADVERSE REACTIONS

Amantadine and rimantadine may produce anxiety, irritability, nervousness, drowsiness, confusion, and headache. They can also cause diarrhea or constipation, difficulty sleeping, or nightmares, dry mouth, loss of appetite, nausea or vomiting, unusual tiredness, and, rarely, kidney damage.

TECH ALERT!
A common ending for antivirals that inhibit viral uncoating is "-mantidine."

TECH ALERT!
The following drugs have look-alike/ sound-alike issues: Amantadine and rimantadine; Flumadine, fludarabine, and flutamide

Inhibitors of Viral Uncoating

	Generic name	U.S. brand name(s)	Dosage forms and strengths
		Canadian brand(s)	
	amantidine	Symmetrel	**Capsule (generics):** 100 mg
		Symmetrel	**Syrup (Symmetrel):** 50 mg/ml
			Tablet (generics): 100 mg
	rimantadine	Flumadine	**Syrup (Flumadine):** 50 mg/5 ml
		Not available	**Tablet (generics):** 100 mg

*Generic available.

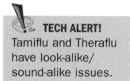

TECH ALERT!
Tamiflu and Theraflu have look-alike/sound-alike issues.

NEURAMINIDASE INHIBITORS

Oseltamivir and zanamivir are indicated for the treatment of influenza A and influenza B. They inhibit virus proliferation by blocking virus release from the host cell.

MECHANISM OF ACTION AND PHARMACOKINETICS

The surfaces of influenza viruses are dotted with neuraminidase proteins. Neuraminidase inhibitors inhibit viral release by inhibiting the enzyme that breaks the bonds that hold the virus particle to the outside of the infected cell. This limits the spread of the virus. Oseltamivir (Tamiflu) is formulated for oral use, and zanamivir (Relenza) is formulated as a powder for oral inhalation.

ADVERSE REACTIONS

Side effects common to the use of oseltamivir and zanamivir are coughing, difficulty, sleeping, dizziness, headache, nausea, and vomiting. Psychosis and other emotional changes have been reported with the use of neuraminidase inhibitors. Zanamivir may precipitate bronchospasm in individuals who have asthma.

Neuraminadase Inhibitors

	Generic name	U.S. brand name(s)	Dosage forms and strengths
		Canadian brand(s)	
	oseltamivir	Tamiflu	**Capsule:** 75 mg
		Tamiflu	**Powder for suspension:** 12 mg/ml
	zanamivir	Relenza	**Powder for inhalation:** 5 mg
		Relenza	

*Generic available.

INHIBITORS OF TRANSCRIPTION

INTERFERONS

There are approximately 2000 interferon receptors on each normal and malignant cell. These receptors recognize and bind interferons that are released as part of the body's normal immune response. Interferons may also be produced by recombinant DNA technology. They are not technically antiviral agents. Instead, they protect uninfected cells by promoting a resistance to virus infection.

Interferon alfa-2a, interferon alfa-2b, interferon alfacon-1, peginterferon alfa-2a, and peginterferon alfa-2b are administered to treat viral infections. Interferon alfa-2a, interferon alfacon-1, and peginterferon alfa-2b are indicated for the treatment of hepatitis C virus. Interferon alfa-2b and peginterferon alfa-2a may be used for the treatment of hepatitis B and hepatitis C.

MECHANISM OF ACTION AND PHARMACOKINETICS

Interferons inhibit viral transcription by activating enzymes that cleave single-stranded viral RNA. Depending on the virus and cell type they also may inhibit viral uncoating, inhibit the synthesis of mRNA, and interfere with the translation, assembly, and release of viral proteins.

ADVERSE REACTIONS

The most common adverse reactions associated with interferons are flu-like symptoms: fever, chills, headache, fatigue, muscle aches, and joint pain. They may also cause nausea, vomiting, diarrhea, dizziness, and depression. More serious adverse affects are a drop in white blood cell count (neutropenia) and platelets (thrombocytopenia).

Interferons

Generic name	U.S. brand name(s) Canadian brand(s)	Dosage forms and strengths
interferon alfa-2a	Roferon A	**Solution for injection, prefilled syringe:** 3 mIU/0.5 ml
	Not available	**Solution for injection, prefilled syringe:** 6 mIU/0.5 ml **Solution for injection, prefilled syringe:** 9 mIU/0.5 ml
interferon alfa-2b	Intron-A	**Solution for injection, prefilled syringe:** 6 mIU/0.5 ml **Solution for injection, prefilled syringe:** 10 mIU/0.5 ml
	Intron-A	**Solution for injection, prefilled syringe:** 18 mIU/0.5 ml **Solution for injection, prefilled syringe:** 25 mIU/0.5 ml **Solution for injection, prefilled syringe:** 50 mIU/0.5 ml
interferon alfacon-1	Infergen	**Solution for injection:** 9 mcg/ml **Solution for injection:** 15 mcg/ml
	Infergen	
peginterferon alfa-2a	Pegasys	**Solution for injection:** 180 mcg/ml **Solution for injection, prefilled syringe:** 180 mcg/0.5 ml
	Pegasys	
peginterferon alfa-2b	PEG-intron	**Powder for injection:** 50 mcg, 80 mcg, 120 mcg, 150 mcg **Powder for injection, Redipen:** 50 mcg, 80 mcg, 120 mcg, 150 mcg
	Pegetron	

*Generic available.

INHIBITION OF DNA AND RNA REPLICATION

Antivirals that inhibit DNA and RNA replication are used for the treatment of herpes simplex type 1 and type 2, herpes zoster, and cytomeglovirus (CMV).

MECHANISM OF ACTION AND PHARMACOKINETICS

Genetic code is stored in DNA. RNA regulates specific cell functions such as editing strands of code, carrying the code message (mRNA), and accurately transferring the code. These are essential steps in the process of viral replication.

Acyclovir inhibits viral DNA synthesis. It is used for the treatment of herpes simplex virus (HSV-1), the virus that causes cold sores; herpes genitalis (HSV-2), one of the viruses that cause genital warts; and varicella zoster virus (VZV), the virus that causes chickenpox and shingles. Acyclovir is approximately 10 times more potent against HSV-1 and -2 than against VZV. So higher doses are required for the treatment of chickenpox and shingles. Acyclovir may be administered topically, orally, or parenterally. GI absorption is poor and bioavailability of orally administered acyclovir is much lower than parenterally administered acyclovir. Systemic effects from topical administration are limited.

Valacyclovir is an ester of acyclovir. It has greater oral absorption. It is also for the treatment of the same conditions as acyclovir but requires less frequent dosing.

Cidofovir is an acyclic phosphonate *nucleotide* analog. Nucleotides are the individual units that make up RNA and DNA. Cidofovir inhibits viral DNA polymerase, the enzyme responsible for replication of new viral RNA and DNA. Cidofovir is indicated for the treatment of cytomegalovirus retinitis. It is used for the treatment of herpes infections, although it is not FDA approved for this condition.

Foscarnet inhibits the viral-specific DNA polymerases and reverse transcriptases. It inhibits HIV reverse transcriptase and hepatitis B DNA polymerase. It also inhibits replication of the herpes simplex virus, varicella-zoster, EBV, human herpevirus 6, and CMV. It is indicated for the treatment of CMV retinitis in individuals with AIDS. It is also indicated for the treatment of acyclovir-resistant HSV-1, HSV-2, and herpes labialis.

Ganciclovir is also used for the treatment of CMV. It is similar in structure to acyclovir. Ganciclovir is a competitive inhibitor of viral DNA polymerases that results in inhibition of viral DNA synthesis.

Famciclovir is metabolized to penciclovir. It has a similar spectrum of activity to acyclovir and is also indicated for the treatment of HSV-1, HSV-2, and acute herpes zoster infections. It has a longer duration of action than acyclovir.

Penciclovir is an active metabolite of famciclovir. It is indicated for the treatment of herpes labialis, commonly known as cold sores. It is administered topically.

Trifluridine (trifluorothymidine) is indicated for the treatment of keratoconjunctivitis of the eye caused by HSV-1 and HSV-2 (see Chapter 20).

TECH ALERT!

The following drugs have look-alike/ sound-alike issues: Zovirax and Zostrix; Denavir and indinavir; Virotic and Timoptic

ADVERSE REACTIONS

Adverse reactions that are common to acyclovir, famciclovir, ganciclovir, penciclovir, valacyclovir, and cidofovir are diarrhea, nausea, vomiting, headache, fatigue, dizziness, and confusion. Penciclovir may also cause irritation and discoloration of the skin. Cidofovir may produce neutropenia, hair loss, tinnitus, and hearing loss. Foscarnet has a side effect profile similar to that of cidofovir but can additionally cause arrhythmias, heart failure, and peripheral neuropathy.

Treatment of Herpes and CMV—Inhibition of DNA and RNA Replication

	Generic name	U.S. brand name(s) Canadian brand(s)	Dosage forms and strengths
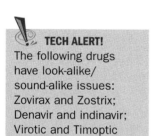	acyclovir*	Zovirax	**Capsule:** 200 mg
		Zovirax	**Cream:** 5% **Ointment:** 5% **Powder for injection:** 500 mg, 1000 mg/vial **Solution, injection:** 50 mg/ml **Suspension:** 200 mg/5 ml **Tablet:** 400 mg, 800 mg
	cidofovir	Vistide	**Solution for injection:** 75 mg/ml
		Not available	
	famciclovir*	Famvir	**Tablet:** 125 mg, 250 mg, 500 mg
		Famvir	
	foscarnet*	Foscavir	**Solution for injection:** 24 mg/ml
		Not available	
	ganciclovir	Cytovene	**Capsules:** 250 mg, 500 mg **Powder for injection:** 500 mg/vial **Invitreal implant (Vitrasert):** 4.5 mg/implant (Canada only)
		Cytovene, Vitrasert	
	penciclovir	Denavir	**Cream:** 1%
		Denavir	

Treatment of Herpes and CMV—Inhibition of DNA and RNA Replication—cont'd

Generic name	U.S. brand name(s) / Canadian brand(s)	Dosage forms and strengths
trifluridine (trifluorothymidine)	Viroptic / Viroptic	**Ophthalmic solution:** 1%
valacyclovir	Valtrex / Valtrex	**Tablet:** 500 mg, 1 g
valganciclovir	Valcyte / Valcyte	**Tablet:** 450 mg

Ribavirin is indicated for the treatment of respiratory syncytial virus (RSV). It is also indicated for the treatment of hepatitis C when combined with interferon alfa. It is effective against RNA and DNA viruses. The mechanism of action is not completely understood, but it is believed that the drug increases the mutation rate of the virus leading to a growing number of viruses unable to replicate. Ribavirin is formulated as a tablet, capsule, and solution for oral use. It is also formulated for intranasal and oral inhalation.

Treatment of Respiratory Syncytial Virus—Inhibition of DNA and RNA Replication

Generic name	U.S. brand name(s) / Canadian brand	Dosage forms and strengths
ribavirin*	Copegus, Rebetol, Ribapak, RibaTab, Virazole / Virazole	**Capsule (Rebetol):** 200 mg **Oral solution (Rebetol):** 40 mg/ml **Powder for inhalation (Virazole):** 6 g **Tablet (Copegus, RibaTab):** 200 mg **Tablet (Ribapak), compliance pack (1200 mg/day):** ribavirin 600 mg **Tablet, compliance pack (1000 mg/day):** ribavirin 600 mg and 400 mg **Tablet, compliance pack (800 mg/day):** ribavirin 400 mg

*Generic available.

Summary of Drugs Used for the Treatment of Influenza, Herpes, Hepatitis, RSV, and CMV Viral Infections

Generic name	Brand name	Usual dose and dosing schedule	Warning labels
Influenza A or B treatment			
amantidine	Symmetrel	**Influenza A treatment and prophylaxis:** 200 mg/day as 1 or 2 divided doses. Begin 24 to 48 hours of onset of signs/symptoms and continue for 24 to 48 hours after symptoms resolve or for prophylaxis at least 10 days.	MAY CAUSE DIZZINESS OR DROWSINESS COMPLETE FULL COURSE OF THERAPY
rimantidine	Flumadine	**Influenza A treatment and prophylaxis:** 100 mg twice daily. Begin 24 to 48 hours of onset of signs/symptoms and continue for 5 to 7 days.	

Continued

Summary of Drugs Used for the Treatment of Influenza, Herpes, Hepatitis, RSV, and CMV Viral Infections—cont'd

Generic name	Brand name	Usual dose and dosing schedule	Warning labels
oseltamivir	Tamiflu	**Influenza A or B treatment and prophylaxis:** 75 mg twice daily for 5 days for acute infection and once daily for 10 days—prophylaxis	REFRIGERATE; SHAKE WELL; DISCARD AFTER 10 DAYS COMPLETE FULL COURSE OF THERAPY
zanamivir	Relenza	**Influenza A treatment:** 2 doses to start; then 2 oral inhalations twice daily for 5 days. Begin within 48 hours of onset of signs/symptoms. **Influenza A prophylaxis:** 2 oral inhalations daily for 28 days.	COMPLETE FULL COURSE OF THERAPY
Herpes infections			
acyclovir	Zovirax	**Varies according to type of infection (HSV-1, HSV-2, VZV) and acute versus recurrent infection. Dosage range:** **IV:** 5 to 10 mg/kg every 8 hours for 5 to 10 days **Oral:** 200 mg 5 times a day or 400 mg 3 times a day for 5 to 10 days **Topical:** Apply every 3 hours for 7 days	SHAKE WELL—suspension COMPLETE FULL COURSE OF THERAPY (Begin therapy within 72 hours of the onset of symptoms) PROTECT FROM LIGHT AND MOISTURE SWALLOW WHOLE; DON'T CRUSH OR CHEW—ganciclovir AVOID PREGNANCY—ganciclovir TAKE WITH FOOD—ganciclovir
famciclovir	Famvir	**Varies according to type of infection (HSV-1, HSV-2, VZV) and acute versus recurrent infection. Dosage range:** 125 mg to 500 mg 2 to 3 times daily for 5 to 10 days or 1000 to 1500 mg twice daily for 1 day	
ganciclovir	Cytovene	**Varies according acute or recurrent CMV infection. Dosage range:** **IV:** 5 mg/kg IV every 12 to 24 hours for 7 to 21 days. **Oral:** 1000 mg 3 times daily or 500 mg 6 times daily	
penciclovir	Denavir	**Cold sores:** Apply every 2 hours while awake for 4 days. Start within 1 hour of onset of symptoms.	
valacyclovir	Valtrex	**Varies according to type of infection (HSV-1, HSV-2, VZV) and acute versus recurrent infection. Dosage range:** 500 mg to 2 g 2 to 3 times a day for 5 to 10 days	
foscarnet	Foscavir	**Varies according to type of infection (HSV-1, HSV-2, VZV, CMV) and acute versus recurrent infection. Dosage range:** 40 to 90 mg/kg IV every 8 to 12 hours for 2 to 3 weeks	STORE AT ROOM TEMPERATURE DISCARD DISCOLORED SOLUTION
trifluridine	Viroptic	1 drop in affected eye(s) every 2 hours while awake (maximum 9 drops/day)	REMOVE CONTACT LENSES BEFORE USE
Hepatitis B or C virus			
interferon alfa-2a	Roferon A	**Hepatitis C:** 3 million international units SC 3 times weekly for 12 months or 6 mIU SC 3 times per week for 3 months followed by 3 mIU SC 3 times per week for 9 months	REFRIGERATE; DO NOT FREEZE

Summary of Drugs Used for the Treatment of Influenza, Herpes, Hepatitis, RSV, and CMV Viral Infections—cont'd

Generic name	Brand name	Usual dose and dosing schedule	Warning labels
interferon alfa-2b	Intron A	**Hepatitis B:** 30 to 35 mIU weekly SC/IM for 16 weeks **Hepatitis C:** 3 mIU SC/IM 3 times weekly for up to 18 to 24 months	
interferon alfacon-1	Infergen	**Hepatitis C:** 9 to 15 mcg SC three times per week for 24 weeks At least 48 hours should elapse between doses	
peginterferon alfa-2a	Pegasys	**Hepatitis B and hepatitis C:** 180 mcg SC once weekly for 48 weeks	
peginterferon alfa-2b	PEG-Intron	**Hepatitis C:** 1mcg/kg once weekly for 1 year	
ribavirin	Copegus	**Hepatitis C:** 600 mg twice daily plus interferon alfa-2b for 24 to 48 weeks **RSV:** not established	
Cytomeglovirus			
cidofovir	Vistide	**CMV retinitis:** 5 mg/kg IV once per week for 2 weeks with probenecid; prophylaxis 5 mg/kg IV once every other week	USE WITHIN 24 HOURS OF PREPARATION REFRIGERATE OR STORE AT ROOM TEMPERATURE

HIV/AIDS Overview

HIV/AIDS is a global public health issue. According to 2007 estimates, nearly 33 million people are infected with HIV (UNAIDS, 2007). Millions more are affected by the disease. Women accounted for 46% of all adults living with HIV worldwide, and youth under 15 years old account for nearly 17 percent of all new HIV infections. HIV/AIDS is worsened by poverty. Poverty creates conditions in which individuals knowingly engage in risky sexual behaviors such as the sex trade; it increases malnutrition, which can weaken the immune system; it decreases access to health care and HIV medicines and this can increase drug resistance; and many HIV medicines should be taken with food and access to regular meals may be limited.

HIV is the virus that causes acquired immune deficiency syndrome (AIDS). The virus attacks CD4 T lymphocytes and weakens the immune system. As the **CD4 count** declines below 200 cells/mm^3 and the **viral load** increases, HIV-infected individuals are at increasing risk for developing opportunistic infections like tuberculosis (TB), candidiasis, and CMV and other AIDS-defining conditions. The viral load is commonly believed to be the amount of HIV in the blood, but actually it is the amount of materials from the virus that are released into the blood when the HIV reproduces.

The HIV Life Cycle

The HIV, like other viruses, lacks the cellular machinery to reproduce itself. It incorporates its DNA into the DNA of the host cell and then, when the host cell tries to make new proteins, it accidentally makes new HIV as well. The steps in the HIV life cycle are briefly described below.

Step 1: Binding

The HIV binds to CD4 surface receptors.

Step 2: Fusion

The HIV is activated by proteins on the cell's surface, allowing the HIV envelope to fuse to the outside of the cell.

Step 3: Uncoating

The virus is uncoated, permitting the contents of the viral capsid (viral RNA and enzymes) to be released into the infected host cell.

Step 4: Reverse transcription

A viral enzyme called reverse transcriptase makes a DNA copy of the viral RNA.

Step 5: Integration

Viral DNA is incorporated into the host cellular DNA.

Step 6: Genome replication

The strands of viral DNA in the nucleus separate, and mRNA provides instructions for making new virus (genome). This process is called transcription.

Step 7: Protein synthesis

The HIV mRNA genome acts as a template for synthesizing viral proteins needed to make a new virus in a process called translation.

Step 8: Protein cleavage and viral assembly

Protease is an enzyme that cuts the long chain of viral protein into smaller individual proteins. Some of the cleaved proteins become structural elements of new HIV, while others become enzymes, such as reverse transcriptase. The new particles are assembled into new HIV.

Step 9: Virus release

New virus buds off from the host cell.

Pharmacotherapy for HIV/AIDS

Antiretrovirals are medicines that interfere with replication of retroviruses. HIV is a retrovirus. Antiretrovirals are administered to reduce viral load; increase CD4 counts; delay the development of AIDS-related conditions and opportunistic infections; and improve survival. Antiretrovirals fall into four classes:

- Nucleoside reverse transcriptase inhibitors (NRTIs)
- Non-nucleoside reverse transcriptase inhibitors (NNRTIs)
- Protease inhibitors (PIs)
- Fusion inhibitors

Initiation of drug therapy with antiretrovirals is in accordance with international guidelines. Therapy is initiated in adults when CD4 counts fall below 200 cells/mm^3 and the individual has symptoms. Antiretroviral therapy should be offered or considered in asymptomatic or mildly symptomatic HIV-infected adults when the CD4 count range is between 200 and 350 cells/mm^3. Antiretroviral therapy is generally not necessary if the individual is asymptomatic and the CD4 count exceeds 350 cells/mm^3. Different guidelines exist for children. Antiretroviral therapy is a life-long commitment and requires strict adherence to treatment regimens.

To reduce antiviral resistance, *highly active antiretroviral therapy (HAART)*—a combination of three or more medications in a regimen also known as an AIDS "cocktail"—is prescribed. The medications administered for HAART therapy fall into two or more antiretroviral classes. Combination therapy increases adverse reactions, yet *adherence* to antiviral therapy is essential to decrease the risk of developing resistance. Antiretroviral *drug resistance testing* is recommended prior to initiation of therapy with antiretrovirals and prior to changing therapy for treatment failure.

Nucleoside and Nucleotide Reverse Transcriptase Inhibitors

Nucleoside and nucleotide reverse transcriptase inhibitors (NRTIs) are prodrugs. They are activated by intracellular phosphorylation by host cell enzymes. They competitively inhibit reverse transcriptase, the enzyme that makes a DNA copy of the viral RNA.

ABACAVIR

Abacavir is an NRTI. It is an ingredient in the triple antiretroviral therapy that combines abacavir with zidovudine and lamivudine. It is also formulated with lamivudine as a duo-combination therapy. It is linked to a fatal hypersensitivity reaction that necessitates discontinuation of the drug. Symptoms include fever and chills, muscle and joint pain, fatigue and feeling rundown, nausea and vomiting, skin rash, or shortness of breath.

DIDANOSINE (ddI)

Didanosine is an NRTI. It is metabolized to an active metabolite that has an intracellular half-life of 25 to 40 hours; therefore, the drug can be dosed once daily. It is acid labile, so it must be buffered to prevent inactivation by gastric acids. Didanosine is formulated for pediatric use as a powder for solution and as delayed release capsules. Side effects such as pancreatitis and peripheral neuropathy limit the use of didanosine.

EMTRICITABINE (FTC)

Emtricitabine is an NRTI similar to lamivudine. *Cross-resistance* occurs between lamivudine and emtricitabine. Cross-resistance refers to the development of resistance to one drug in a particular class that results in resistance to the other drugs in that class. Emtricitabine is formulated as an oral capsule and oral solution. Refrigeration is recommended for the oral solution; however, the solution is stable at room temperature for 3 months should refrigeration not be available.

LAMIVUDINE (3TC)

Lamivudine is an NRTI that is effective against HIV, including zidovudine-resistant strains of HIV. Lamivudine also inhibits replication of hepatitis B virus (HBV). It is a good choice of therapy for individuals who have HIV and HBV coinfections. Lamivudine is an ingredient in HIV combination therapies. (All antiretrovirals should be used in combination.) The drug has good oral absorption, and the relatively long intracellular half-life (12 hours) permits once-daily dosing.

STAVUDINE (d4T)

Stavudine is an NRTI. It is similar to zidovudine; however, a drug interaction occurs between stavudine and zidovudine that reduces the effectiveness of stavudine because zidovudine inhibits the activation of stavudine. Stavudine has a short half-life and must be administered more frequently than some of the other NRTIs. It is formulated for oral administration and food does not interfere with absorption.

TENOFOVIR (TDF)

Tenofovir is an NRTI. It is administered orally. Food increases bioavailablity of the drug. Tenofovir has a long intracellular half-life ($T\frac{1}{2}$) of up to 50 hours.

ZIDOVUDINE (AZT)

Zidovudine was the first available antiretroviral. It was introduced in 1987. It is an NRTI. It is formulated for oral and parenteral administration. The drug may be administered orally to pregnant women and intravenously during delivery and as a suspension to neonates. It has been shown to decrease perinatal mother-to-child transmission (PMTCT) of HIV from 25% to 8%. Current PMTCT guidelines are shown in Table 36-1.

TABLE 36-1 WHO 2006 PMTCT Guidelines*

Mother	
Antepartum	zidovudine starting at 28 weeks of pregnancy or as soon as feasible thereafter
Intrapartum	Sd-NVP + zidovudine/3TC
Postpartum	zidovudine/3TC × 7 days
Infant	Sd-NVP + zidovudine × 7 days

*WHO 2006 PMTCT guidelines.
Sd-NVP, single-dose nevirapine; 3TC, lamivudine.

An alternative regimen is as follows:

MOTHER

- Oral zidovudine starting at 14 to 34 weeks of pregnancy
- Intravenous zidovudine during labor and delivery

INFANT

- Zidovudine (in liquid form) every 6 hours for 6 weeks after birth

ADVERSE REACTIONS

Possible side effects from NRTI therapy are liver problems, muscle inflammation and weakness, diabetes, abnormal fat distribution (lipodystrophy syndrome), high cholesterol, decreased bone density due to osteonecrosis and osteopenia, skin rash, pancreatitis (inflammation of the pancreas), peripheral neuropathy (especially with the "d" drugs—ddI [didadosine] and d4T [stavudine]), leukopenia (a drop in white blood cell count), and increased bleeding in patients with hemophilia. Side effects that are associated with nearly all NRTIs are headache, stomach upset, fatigue or insomnia, muscle ache, and diarrhea. Additionally, zidovudine may cause nail discoloration, and zalcitabine may cause dry mouth and mouth ulcers.

Nucleoside Reverse Transcriptase Inhibitors (NRTI)

Generic name	U.S. brand name(s) Canadian brand(s)	Dosage forms and strengths
abacavir (ABC)	Ziagen Ziagen	**Tablet:** 300 mg **Solution:** 20 mg/ml
didanosine* (ddI)	Videx, Videx EC Videx, Videx EC	**Powder for pediatric solution:** 10 mg/ml **Tablet:** 125 mg, 200 mg, 250 mg, 400 mg
emtricitabine (FTC)	Emtriva Emtriva	**Capsule:** 200 mg **Solution:** 10 mg/ml
lamivudine (3TC)	Epivir, Epivir HBV Epivir, Heptovir	**Solution:** 5 mg/ml (Epivir HBV), 10 mg/ml (Epivir) **Tablet:** 100 mg (Epivir HBV, Heptovir); 150 mg, 300 mg (Epivir)
stavudine (d4T)	Zerit Zerit	**Capsule, immediate release:** 15 mg, 20 mg, 30 mg, 40 mg **Powder for oral solution:** 1 mg/ml
tenofovir DF (TDF)	Viread Viread	**Tablet:** 300 mg
zidovudine* (AZT)	Retrovir Retrovir	**Capsule:** 100 mg **Solution, injection:** 10 mg/ml **Syrup:** 50 mg/5 ml **Tablet:** 300 mg (U.S. only)
FIXED DOSE COMBINATIONS		
abacavir + lamivudine	Epzicom Kivexa	**Tablet:** 600 mg abacavir + 300 mg lamivudine
emtricitabine + tenofovir	Truvada Truvada	**Tablet:** 200 mg emtricitabine + 300 mg tenofovir

Nucleoside Reverse Transcriptase Inhibitors (NRTI)—cont'd

Generic name	U.S. brand name(s) Canadian brand(s)	Dosage forms and strengths
lamivudine + zidovudine	Combivir	**Tablet:** 150 mg lamivudine + 300 mg zidovudine
	Combivir	
efavirenz + emtricitabine + tenofovir	Atripla	**Tablet:** 600 mg efavirenz + 200 mg emtricitabine + 300 mg tenofovir
	not available	
abacavir + lamivudine + zidovudine	Trizivir	**Tablet:** 300 mg abacavir + 150 mg lamivudine + 300 mg zidovudine
	Trizivir	

*Generic available.

Non-Nucleoside Reverse Transcriptase Inhibitors

Non-nucleoside reverse transcriptase inhibitors (NNRTIs) bind to viral transcriptase. They differ from NRTIs in three important ways. (1) NNRTIs are noncompetitive inhibitors of reverse transcriptase. (2) They do not need to be activated by host enzymes. (3) They are not effective against HIV-2. With the exception of nevirapine, NNRTIs are only used in combination therapy with NRTIs and PIs because resistance develops rapidly. All NNRTIs are metabolized by CYP450 hepatic enzymes and reduce their own half-life as well as the T½ of other drugs coadministered with them that are metabolized by the same enzymes. Numerous drug interactions are seen when NNRTIs are administered concurrently with benzodiazepines, HMG-CoA inhibitors ("*-statins*"), and proton pump inhibitors ("*-prazoles*").

DELAVIRDINE

Delavirdine has a short half-life and must be given in multiple daily doses. It is administered 3 times a day compared to nevirapine and efavirenz, which are dosed once daily. Cross-resistance, frequency of dosing, and the number of tablets per dose (4 tablets) have limited the use of delavirdine.

EFAVIRENZ

Efavirenz is an ingredient in the fixed dose combination medicine Atripla used for the treatment of HIV-1 infection. It is also available as a single ingredient product; however, monotherapy is not recommended, due to the rapid development of resistance. The drug is administered by mouth and due to its long half-life (40 to 55 hours) may be given once daily.

Efavirenz is teratogenic and classified in pregnancy category D. The drug should not be administered in the first trimester of pregnancy and women taking the drug should be advised to avoid pregnancy.

NEVIRAPINE

Nevirapine is the one NNRTI that may be administered as monotherapy for the PMTCT of HIV. It is administered as a single dose. Controversy exists about use of single-dose nevirapine therapy because of the risk of development of drug resistance. Treatment of mothers with triple antiretroviral therapy reduces the risk of antiretroviral resistance.

Nevirapine is associated with fatal liver toxicity, and the FDA has required changes in the package labeling to warn of this adverse effect. Risk for development of liver toxicity with the use of single doses of nevirapine to the mother and to the child for prevention of perinatal HIV infection is minimal.

ADVERSE REACTIONS

Rash is a common side effect of all NNRTIs. Nevirapine is associated with fatal hepatotoxicity. The risk is greatest in the first 6 to 18 weeks of therapy and is more common in women than in men. Efavirenz may cause dizziness, drowsiness or insomnia, abnormal dreams, confusion, abnormal thinking, impaired concentration, amnesia, agitation, hallucinations, depersonalization, and euphoria.

Non-Nucleoside Reverse Transcriptase Inhibitors (NNRTIs)

Generic name	U.S. brand name(s)	Dosage forms and strengths
	Canadian brand(s)	
delavirdine (DLV)	Rescriptor	**Tablet:** 100 mg, 200 mg
	Rescriptor	
efavirenz (EFV)	Sustiva	**Capsule:** 50 mg, 100 mg, 200 mg **Tablet:** 600 mg
	Sustiva	
nevirapine	Viramune	**Suspension:** 50 mg/5 ml **Tablet:** 200 mg
	Viramune	

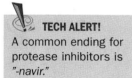

TECH ALERT!
A common ending for protease inhibitors is "-navir."

Protease Inhibitors

PIs interfere with Step 8 of the HIV life cycle. They block cleavage of long-chain viral proteins into individual proteins that are assembled to make new virus. PIs are administered as combination therapy, and most are recommended to be dosed along with ritonavir.

AMPRENAVIR AND FOSMAMPRENAVIR

Fosamprenavir and amprenavir are indicated for the treatment of HIV-1 infection. Fosamprenavir is a prodrug that is metabolized to the active drug amprenavir. The therapeutic dose of fosamprenavir (700 mg twice daily) is lower than the therapeutic dose of amprenavir (1200 mg twice daily). The effects of both drugs are boosted with coadministration of ritonavir.

ATAZANAVIR

Atazanavir is another PI that is effective against HIV-1. Its effectiveness is increased when the drug is coadministered with ritonavir. Concurrent administration with the NNRTI efavirenz can decrease its bioavailability. Atazanavir may be given orally once daily. Administration with a light meal increases bioavailability compared to a heavy meal or fasting. Atazanavir does not produce hyperlipidemia like other proteases, although it can increase cholesterol levels and blood glucose levels. The drug may produce jaundice but does not cause liver toxicity.

DARUNAVIR

Darunavir was approved by the FDA in 2006. It has advantages over other PIs in that cross-resistance is low and it produces greater reduction in viral load after 24 weeks of treatment. Like other PIs, it must be administered along with ritonavir.

INDINAVIR

Indinavir must be administered in three daily doses. Absorption is affected by food so the drug is taken on an empty stomach. To avoid the formation of kidney stones, indinavir should be taken with at least 1.5 liters of water daily. The effects of indinavir are boosted by coadministration of ritonavir.

NELFINAVIR

Nelfinavir is a competitive inhibitor of HIV protease. Current Centers for Disease Control and Prevention (CDC) recommendations advise that nelfinavir be administered as part of a three-drug regimen that typically also includes indinavir, efavirenz, and/or abacavir. Unlike indinavir and atazanavir, absorption of nelfinavir is enhanced by a fatty meal. Nelfinavir should be taken with food. Nelfinavir oral powder is stable for 6 hours, once mixed with food or liquid, if refrigerated.

RITONAVIR

Ritonavir is a competitive inhibitor of HIV protease. It differs from other PIs in that it is effective against HIV-1 and HIV-2 proteases. Ritonavir boost the effects of other PIs by inhibiting their metabolism. Ritonavir inhibits the metabolic enzyme CYP 3A4. Most PIs must be coadministered with ritonavir. Ritonavir is also formulated as a fixed-dose combination with lopinavir (Kaletra). Resistance to ritonavir appears to occur more slowly than with other PIs. The drug has excellent oral bioavailability and is dosed twice daily. A disadvantage is that adverse effects are common and occur in more than 85% of individuals taking the drug.

SAQUINAVIR

Saquinavir is formulated as a hard gelatin capsule and a film-coated tablet. Bioavailability following oral administration is low for both formulations. Extensive first-pass metabolism further reduces the actions of the drug. Similar to other PIs, saquinavir's effects are boosted by coadministration with ritonavir. Saquinavir should be taken with food.

TIPRANAVIR

Tipranavir is a sulfonamide that selectively binds to HIV-1 protease. It was approved in 2005 and currently has a lower rate for the development of resistance than some other PIs. The drug should be taken with food to increase absorption.

The FDA requires the manufacturer of tipranavir to provide a black box warning in the package labeling regarding reports of fatal and nonfatal intracranial hemorrhage. Like other PIs, tipranavir is not used for monotherapy but instead is administered with other antiretrovirals.

ADVERSE REACTIONS

PIs can elevate triglyceride levels, cholesterol levels (see Chapter 24), and blood glucose levels and can produce insulin resistance (see Chapter 33). They also cause redistribution of fat, causing accumulation in the abdomen and loss in the face and limbs. All PIs produce nausea, vomiting, and diarrhea.

Protease Inhibitors

Generic name	U.S. brand name(s) Canadian brand(s)	Dosage forms and strengths
amprenavir (APV)	Agenerase Agenerase	**Capsule:** 50 mg, 150 mg (Canada only) **Solution:** 15 mg/ml
atazanavir (ATV)	Reyataz Reyataz	**Capsule:** 150 mg, 200 mg, 300 mg
darunavir (TMC114)	Prezista Prezista	**Tablet:** 300 mg
fosamprenavir (FPV)	Lexiva Telzir	**Suspension:** 50 mg/5 ml **Tablet:** 700 mg
indinavir (IDV)	Crixivan Crixivan	**Capsule:** 200 mg, 400 mg

Continued

Protease Inhibitors—cont'd

Generic name	U.S. brand name(s) Canadian brand(s)	Dosage forms and strengths
nelfinavir (NFV)	Viracept ———— Viracept	**Powder for oral suspension:** 50 mg/g **Tablet:** 250 mg, 625 mg
ritonavir (RTV)	Norvir ———— Norvir	**Capsule:** 100 mg **Solution, Oral:** 80 mg/ml
saquinavir mesylate (SQV)	Invirase ———— Invirase	**Capsule:** 200 mg **Tablet:** 500 mg
tipranavir	Aptivus ———— Aptivus	**Capsule:** 250 mg
Combination		
lopinavir + ritonavir	Keletra ———— Keletra	**Capsule:** 133.3 mg lopinavir + 33.3 mg ritonavir **Solution, oral:** 80 mg/ml lopinavir + 20 mg/ml ritonavir **Tablet:** 200 mg lopinavir + 50 mg ritonavir

FUSION INHIBITORS

Fusion inhibitors are the latest medicines in the arsenal of antiretrovirals to treat HIV infection. Enfuvirtide is currently the only drug in this class. It interferes with Step 2 in the HIV life cycle attachment of the HIV to the host cell membrane. Fusion is required in order for the virus capsid to release its contents (genetic material) into the host cell. As with other HIV medicines, enfuvirtide is intended to be administered in combination with other antiretrovirals.

Enfuvirtide must be administered by subcutaneous injection in the thigh, arm, or abdomen. It is formulated as a powder that is reconstituted prior to administration. Once reconstituted, the solution is stable for only 24 hours, if refrigerated.

ADVERSE REACTIONS

Irritation, pain, redness, itchiness, and formation of nodules and cysts at the site of injection are common adverse reactions. Allergic reactions also occur and produce rash, chills, fever, stiffness, hypotension, nausea, and vomiting.

Fusion Inhibitors

Generic name	U.S. brand name(s) Canadian brand	Dosage forms and strengths
enfuvirtide (T-20)	Fuzeon ———— Fuzeon	**Powder for solution:** 90 mg/vial (U.S.); 108 mg/vial (Canada)

Summary of Drugs Used for the Treatment of HIV/AIDS

Generic name	Brand name	Usual dose and dosing schedule	Warning labels
Nucleoside Reverse Transcriptase Inhibitors (NRTIs)			
abacavir	Ziagen	300 mg twice daily or 600 mg once daily	TAKE EXACTLY AS DIRECTED; DON'T SKIP DOSES AVOID ALCOHOL PROTECT FROM MOISTURE
didanosine	Videx	Varies according to body weight and dosage form **Extended release cap:** 400 mg once daily (>60 kg) **Oral solution:** (>60 kg) 250 mg twice daily	SWALLOW WHOLE; DON'T CRUSH OR CHEW TAKE ON AN EMPTY STOMACH REFRIGERATE; DISCARD 30 DAYS AFTER RECONSTITUTION TAKE EXACTLY AS DIRECTED; DON'T SKIP DOSES
emtricitabine	Emtriva, Coviracil	Varies according to body weight and dosage form **Capsule:** 200 mg once daily (>33 kg) **Oral solution:** 6 mg/kg up to 240 mg once daily	TAKE EXACTLY AS DIRECTED; DON'T SKIP DOSES REFRIGERATE; DO NOT FREEZE—solution
lamivudine	Epivir	**HIV:** 300 mg once daily or 150 mg twice daily **Hepatitis B:** 100 mg once daily for up to 1 year if HIV (−) 300 mg twice daily for 1 year if HIV (+)	TAKE EXACTLY AS DIRECTED; DON'T SKIP DOSES AVOID EXCESSIVE ALCOHOL
stavudine	Zerit	Varies according to body weight and dosage form **Capsule, extend release:** 100 mg once daily (>60 kg) or 75 mg once daily (<60 kg) **Oral solution/capsule:** 40 mg every 12 hours (>60 kg) or 30 mg every 12 hours (<60 kg)	TAKE EXACTLY AS DIRECTED; DON'T SKIP DOSES PROTECT FROM MOISTURE—capsules REFRIGERATE; DISCARD 30 DAYS AFTER RECONSTITUTION
tenofovir DF	Viread	300 mg once daily	TAKE EXACTLY AS DIRECTED; DON'T SKIP DOSES TAKE WITH FOOD
zidovudine	Retrovir	**Oral:** 300 mg PO twice daily or 200 mg PO three times daily **IV:** 1 mg/kg IV given 5 to 6 times per day around the clock	TAKE EXACTLY AS DIRECTED; DON'T SKIP DOSES TAKE WITH LOTS OF WATER REFRIGERATE DILUTED IV SOLUTION; DISCARD AFTER 48 HOURS (stable for 24 hours at room temperature)
lamivudine + zidovudine	Combivir	1 tablet twice daily	TAKE EXACTLY AS DIRECTED; DON'T SKIP DOSES AVOID EXCESSIVE ALCOHOL
abacavir + lamivudine	Epzicom	1 tablet once daily	TAKE EXACTLY AS DIRECTED; DON'T SKIP DOSES
emtricitabine + tenofovir	Truvada	1 tablet once daily	TAKE EXACTLY AS DIRECTED; DON'T SKIP DOSES
efavirenz + emtricitabine + tenofovir	Atripla	1 tablet daily at bedtime	TAKE EXACTLY AS DIRECTED; DON'T SKIP DOSES TAKE ON AN EMPTY STOMACH

Continued

Summary of Drugs Used for the Treatment of HIV/AIDS—cont'd

	Generic name	Brand name	Usual dose and dosing schedule	Warning labels
	abacavir + lamivudine + zidovudine	Trizivir	1 tablet twice daily	TAKE EXACTLY AS DIRECTED; DON'T SKIP DOSES
Non-Nucleoside Reverse Transcriptase Inhibitors (NNRTIs)				
	delavirdine	Rescriptor	400 mg 3 times a day	TAKE EXACTLY AS DIRECTED; DON'T SKIP DOSES AVOID ANTACIDS WITHIN 1 HOUR OF DOSE
	efavirenz	Sustiva	600 mg once daily at bedtime	TAKE EXACTLY AS DIRECTED; DON'T SKIP DOSES TAKE ON AN EMPTY STOMACH MAY CAUSE DIZZINESS OR DROWSINESS; ALCOHOL INTENSIFIES THIS EFFECT AVOID PREGNANCY
	nevirapine	Viramune	200 mg once daily for the first 14 days, then 200 mg twice daily	TAKE EXACTLY AS DIRECTED; DON'T SKIP DOSES SHAKE GENTLY—suspension
Protease Inhibitors				
	amprenavir	Agenerase	1200 mg twice daily or 1200 mg once daily with ritonavir	TAKE EXACTLY AS DIRECTED; DON'T SKIP DOSES AVOID ANTACIDS WITHIN 1 HOUR OF DOSE AVOID VIT E SUPPLEMENTS
	atazanavir	Reyataz	300 mg once daily (taken with ritonavir)	TAKE EXACTLY AS DIRECTED; DON'T SKIP DOSES TAKE WITH LIGHT MEAL AVOID ANTACIDS WITHIN 1 HOURS OF DOSE SWALLOW WHOLE; DON'T CRUSH OR CHEW
	darunavir	Prezista	600 mg twice daily (taken with ritonavir)	TAKE EXACTLY AS DIRECTED; DON'T SKIP DOSES TAKE WITH FOOD
	fosamprenavir	Lexiva	700 mg twice daily (taken with ritonavir)	TAKE EXACTLY AS DIRECTED; DON'T SKIP DOSES TAKE WITH FOOD—oral suspension (children) TAKE WITHOUT FOOD—oral suspension (adults)
	indinavir	Crixivan	800 mg every 8 hours or 400 mg twice daily with ritonavir	TAKE EXACTLY AS DIRECTED; DON'T SKIP DOSES TAKE ON AN EMPTY STOMACH MAINTAIN ADEQUATE HYDRATION PROTECT FROM MOISTURE
	nelfinavir	Viracept	1250 mg twice daily or 750 mg 3 times a day	TAKE EXACTLY AS DIRECTED; DON'T SKIP DOSES TAKE WITH FOOD MIX ORAL POWDER WITH SMALL AMOUNT OF FOOD OR NON-ACIDIC LIQUID. CONSUME ENTIRE DOSE— mixture stable for 6 hours if refrigerated

Summary of Drugs Used for the Treatment of HIV/AIDS—cont'd

Generic name	Brand name	Usual dose and dosing schedule	Warning labels
ritonavir	Norvir	600 mg twice daily	TAKE EXACTLY AS DIRECTED; DON'T SKIP DOSES TAKE WITH FOOD REFRIGERATE; DON'T FREEZE—capsule stable for 30 days at room temperature SHAKE WELL—suspension STORE AT ROOM TEMPERATURE—suspension DISPENSE IN MANUFACTURER'S ORIGINAL CONTAINER
saquinavir	Invirase	1000 mg twice daily (taken with ritonavir)	TAKE EXACTLY AS DIRECTED; DON'T SKIP DOSES TAKE WITH FOOD
tipranavir	Aptivus	500 mg twice daily (taken with ritonavir)	TAKE EXACTLY AS DIRECTED; DON'T SKIP DOSES TAKE WITH FOOD REFRIGERATE; DON'T FREEZE—capsule stable for 60 days at room temperature
lopinavir + ritonavir	Keletra	3 capsules, 5 ml, or 2 tablets twice daily (400 mg lopinavir + 100 mg ritonavir) or 6 capsules, 10 ml, or 4 tablets once daily (800 mg lopinavir + 200 mg ritonavir)	TAKE EXACTLY AS DIRECTED; DON'T SKIP DOSES SWALLOW WHOLE; DON'T CRUSH OR CHEW- tablets TAKE WITH FOOD REFRIGERATE; DON'T FREEZE—solution stable for 60 days at room temperature DISPENSE TABLETS IN MANUFACTURER'S ORIGINAL CONTAINER
enfuvirtide	Fuzeon	90 mg SC twice daily	TAKE EXACTLY AS DIRECTED; DON'T SKIP DOSES REFRIGERATE DILUTED SOLUTION; DON'T FREEZE; DISCARD AFTER 24 HOURS

CHAPTER SUMMARY

- A virus is an intracellular parasite that consists of a DNA or RNA core surrounded by a protein coat and sometimes an outer covering of lipoprotein.
- The infectious particles (virions) do not have the cellular components necessary for reproduction, so they use their host's cellular machinery to replicate.
- Viruses may cause minor illness such as the common cold and warts or serious infections such as human immunodeficiency virus (HIV), smallpox, and hepatitis C.
- Some viruses are linked to cancer; for example, human papillomavirus (HPV) is associated with cervical cancer.
- An antiviral is a medication that is able to inhibit viral replication.
- All antiviral agents work best when the host (the individual with the infection) has a healthy immune system.
- Effective treatment of viral infections is dependent upon host factors, virus factors, and drug factors.

- Severity of influenza, herpes, and varicella viral infection and severity of symptoms are reduced when antiviral therapy is initiated within the first 24 to 72 hours of exposure to the virus or onset of symptoms.
- Some viruses can lay dormant in host cells and periodically awaken to cause recurrent disease.
- Antivirals are only effective against a specific virus.
- Antibiotics are not effective against viral infections.
- Antiviral resistance is the ability of a virus to overcome the suppressive action of antiviral agents.
- Because viruses continually mutate, it is difficult to develop a vaccine to prevent virus infection.
- Antivirals inhibit virus-specific steps in the replication cycle.
- A common ending for antivirals that inhibit viral uncoating and are administered to prevent influenza A infection is *"-mantidine."* Amantidine and rimantidine inhibit viral uncoating.
- Uncoating of the influenza A virus is a necessary step in the virus replication process.
- Oseltamivir and zanamivir are indicated for the treatment of influenza A and influenza B. They are neuraminidase inhibitors.
- Neuraminidase inhibitors inhibit viral release.
- Zanamivir (Relenza) is formulated as a powder for oral inhalation.
- Inteferons protect uninfected cells by promoting a resistance to virus infection.
- Interferon alfa-2a, interferon alfacon-1, and peginterferon alfa-2b are indicated for the treatment of hepatitis C virus.
- Interferon alfa-2b and peginterferon alfa-2a may be used for the treatment of hepatitis B and hepatitis C.
- A common ending for antivirals used for the treatment of herpes virus infections in *"cyclovir"* and *"ciclovir."*
- Acyclovir, famciclovir, and valacyclovir are used for the treatment of herpes simplex virus (HSV-1), the virus that causes cold sores; herpes genitalis (HSV-2), one of the viruses that cause genital warts; and varicella zoster virus (VZV), the virus that causes chickenpox and shingles.
- Cidofovir is indicated for the treatment of cytomeglovirus (CMV) retinitis.
- Foscarnet is indicated for the treatment of CMV retinitis in individuals with acquired immune deficiency syndrome (AIDS). It is also indicated for the treatment of acyclovir-resistant HSV-1, HSV-2, and herpes labialis infections.
- Ganciclovir is indicated for the treatment of CMV.
- Penciclovir is a metabolite of famciclovir that is used for the treatment of cold sores.
- Trifluridine is indicated for the treatment of keratoconjunctivitis of the eye caused by herpes virus.
- Ribavirin is indicated for the treatment of respiratory syncytial virus and hepatitis C when combined with interferon alfa.
- HIV/AIDS is a global public health issue. According to 2007estimates, nearly 33 million people are infected with the HIV.
- HIV is the virus that causes AIDS. The virus attacks CD4 T lymphocytes and weakens the immune system.
- The steps in the HIV life cycle are (1) binding, (2) fusion, (3) uncoating, (4) reverse transcription, (5) integration, (6) genome replication, (7) protein synthesis, (8) protein cleavage and assembly, and (9) virus release.
- Antiretrovirals are medicines that interfere with replication of retroviruses. HIV is a retrovirus.
- Antiretrovirals fall into four classes: (1) nucleoside reverse transcriptase inhibitors (NRTIs), (2) non-nucleoside reverse transcriptase inhibitors (NNRTIs), (3) protease inhibitors (PIs), and (4) fusion inhibitors.
- To reduce antiviral resistance, highly active antiretroviral therapy (HAART), a combination of three or more medications in a regimen known as AIDS "cocktail" is prescribed.

- Nucleoside and nucleotide reverse transcriptase inhibitors (NRTIs) are prodrugs.
- NRTIs competitively inhibit reverse transcriptase, the enzyme that makes a DNA copy of the viral RNA.
- Abacavir, didanosine, emtricitabine, lamivudine, stavudine, tenofovir, and zidovudine are NRTIs.
- Zidovudine may be administered to pregnant women and neonates and is used to prevent mother-to-child transmission (PMTCT) of HIV.
- NNRTIs differ from NRTIs in three important ways: (1) NNRTIs are noncompetitive inhibitors of reverse transcriptase; (2) they do not need to be activated by host enzymes; and (3) they are not effective against HIV-2.
- With the exception of nevirapine, NNRTIs are only used in combination therapy with NRTIs and protease inhibitors because resistance develops rapidly.
- Delavirdine, efavirenz, and nevirapine are NNRTIs.
- Nevirapine is administered as a single dose for the PMTCT of HIV. Controversy exists about use of single-dose nevirapine therapy because of the risk of development of drug resistance.
- Nevirapine is associated with fatal liver toxicity and the FDA has required changes in the package labeling to warn of this adverse effect.
- A common ending for protease inhibitors is *"-navir."*
- PIs interfere with Step 8 of the HIV life cycle. They block to cleavage of long chain viral proteins into individual proteins that are assembled to make new virus.
- PIs are administered as combination therapy.
- Fosamprenavir, amprenavir, atazanavir, darunavir, indinavir, nelfinavir, ritonavir, saquinavir, and tipranavir are PIs.
- Ritonavir is effective against HIV-1 and HIV-2 proteases.
- Tipranivir is a sulfonamide that selectively binds to HIV-1 protease.
- The FDA requires the manufacturer of tipranavir to provide a black box warning in the package labeling regarding reports of fatal and nonfatal intracranial hemorrhage.
- Fusion inhibitors are the latest medicines in the arsenal of antiretrovirals to treat HIV infection. Enfuvirtide is currently the only drug in this class.
- Fusion inhibitors interfere with Step 2 in the HIV life cycle attachment of the HIV to the host cell membrane.

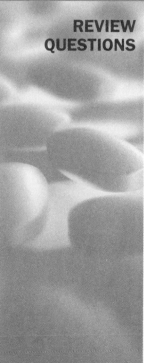

REVIEW QUESTIONS

Multiple Choice

1. _____ is the most severe form of HIV infection.
   a. CMV
   b. AIDS
   c. HPV
   d. HSV

2. The individual who infects another with a virus is a host.
   a. true
   b. false

3. An antiviral is a medication that is able to _____ viral replication.
   a. stop
   b. inhibit
   c. proliferate
   d. induce

4. Interferons are not technically antiviral agents.
   a. true
   b. false

5. **Which of the following is(are) indicated for the treatment of cytomegalovirus?**
    a. acyclovir
    b. ganciclovir
    c. cidofovir
    d. b and c

6. **Human immunodeficiency virus (HIV) is the virus that causes acquired immune deficiency syndrome (AIDS). The virus attacks _____ and weakens the immune system.**
    a. CD4 monocytes
    b. CD4 T lymphocytes
    c. CD2 T lymphocytes
    d. none of the above

7. **Antiretroviral therapy for HIV/AIDS is a short-term commitment and requires strict adherence to treatment regimens.**
    a. true
    b. false

8. **Lamivudine is an NRTI that is effective against _____.**
    a. HIV
    b. HBV
    c. CMV
    d. a and b

9. **Which of the following drugs does the FDA require the manufacturer to provide a black box warning in the package labeling regarding reports of fatal and nonfatal intracranial hemorrhage?**
    a. acyclovir
    b. famciclovir
    c. tipranavir
    d. foscarnet

10. **Enfuvirtide is currently the only drug in class of fusion inhibitors to treat HIV infection.**
    a. true
    b. false

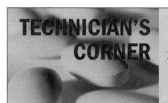

TECHNICIAN'S CORNER

1. We have yet to find a cure for the common cold. Why is it to difficult to find that cure?
2. We have publicized and educated worldwide about preventing the spread of AIDS, yet more and more cases are seen every year. What else can be done to stop the spread of this deadly disease?

BIBLIOGRAPHY

Canadian AIDS Treatment Information Exchange: *Plain and simple fact sheet: HIV viral load,* 2001. Available at: www.catie.ca.

Kalant H, Grant D, Mitchell J: *Principles of medical pharmacology* (pp 739-759), ed 7. Toronto, 2007, Elsevier Canada, A Division of Reed Elsevier Canada.

Lance L, Lacy C, Armstrong L, Goldman M: *Drug information handbook for the allied health professional,* ed 12. Hudson, OH, 2005, APhA Lexi-Comp.

National Institute of Allergy and Infectious Disease: *Flu drugs,* Besthesda, MD, November 2006, National Institutes of Health, U.S. Department of Health and Human Services. Available at: http://www.niaid.nih.gov/factsheets/fludrugs.htm.

Page C, Curtis M, Sutter M, Walker M, Hoffman B, et al: *Integrated pharmacology* (pp 91-109), Philadelphia, 2005, Elsevier Mosby.

US Food and Drug Administration, Center for Drug Evaluation and Research: *FDA public health advisory for nevirapine (Viramune),* revised July 19, 2005. Available at: http://www.fda.gov/Cder/drug/advisory/nevirapine.htm.

US Department of Health and Human Services, AIDSinfo: HIV and its treatment—HIV and .regnancy. Available at: http://aidsinfo.nih.gov/contentfiles/HIVandItsTreatment_cbrochure_en.pdf. Accessed August 2006.

USP Center for Advancement of Patient Safety: *Use caution–avoid confusion,* USP Quality Review No. 79, Rockville, MD, April 2004, USP Center for Advancement of Patient Safety.

Vieson K, Dawson J, Gold Standard Inc, Clinical Pharmacology: *Overview: anti-retroviral non-nucleoside reverse transcriptase inhibitors (NNRTIs).* Available at: http://www.clinicalpharmacology.com/apps/default.asp?entry=11andrNum=431.

World Health Organization: *Antiretroviral drugs for treating pregnant women and preventing HIV infection in infants: towards universal access—recommendations for a public health approach,* 2006 version (pp 27-28, 45), Geneva, Switzerland, WHO Press.

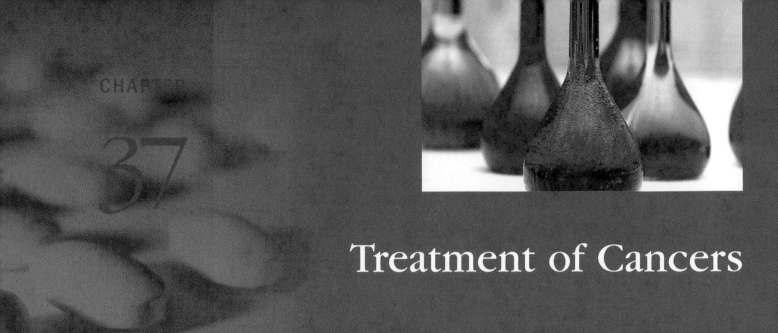

Treatment of Cancers

LEARNING OBJECTIVES

- Learn the terminology associated with cancer.
- Identify causes for specific cancers.
- List methods for screening for specific cancers.
- Identify risk factors for specific cancers.
- List and categorize medications used for the treatment of specific cancers.
- Describe mechanism of action for drugs used for the treatment of specific cancers.
- Identify warning labels and precautionary messages associated with medications used for the treatment of specific cancers.
- Identify significant drug look-alike/sound-alike issues.
- List common endings and/or beginnings for drug classes used in the treatment of for the treatment of specific cancers.

KEY TERMS

Benign: Tumor that is not cancerous and does not spread to surrounding tissues or other parts of the body.

Biopsy: Removal of cells or tissues for examination by a pathologist. The three types of biopsy are (1) incisional, (2) excisional, and (3) fine-needle aspiration.

Cancer: Term for diseases in which abnormal cells divide without control. Specific cancers are named according to the site where the cancerous growth begins.

Chemotherapy: Treatment with drugs that kill cancer.

Complementary and alternative medicine (CAM): Treatments that may include dietary supplements, herbal preparations, acupuncture, massage, magnet therapy, spiritual healing, and meditation.

Computed tomography (CT) scan: Diagnostic examination in which a series of detailed pictures taken of areas inside the body that are created by a computer that is linked to an x-ray machine.

Double-contrast barium enema: Diagnostic test to examine the colon and rectum in which an individual is administered a barium-containing enema and then radiographs are taken.

Excisional biopsy: Surgical procedure in which an entire lump or suspicious-looking tissue is removed for diagnosis.

External radiation: Radiation therapy that uses a machine to aim high-energy rays at the cancer.

Fecal occult blood test (FOBT): Test to check for blood in stool.

Implant radiation: Procedure, also known as brachytherapy, in which radioactive material sealed in needles, seeds, wires, or catheters is placed directly into or near a tumor.

Ionizing radiation: Type of high-frequency radiation produced by x-ray procedures, radioactive substances, and UV light that can lead to health risks, including cancer, at certain doses.

Leukemia: Cancer that starts in blood-forming tissue such as the bone marrow.

Lymphoma: Cancer that begins in cells of the immune system.

Malignant: Cancerous tumors that can invade and destroy nearby tissue and spread to other parts of the body.

Mammogram: Screening examination to detect breast cancer in which a radiograph is taken of the breast.

Melanoma: Form of skin cancer that arises in melanocytes, the cells that produce pigment.

Metastasis: Spread of cancer from one part of the body to another.

Neoplasm: Tumor.

Pap test or Pap smear: Screening test in which cells from the cervix are examined to detect cancer and changes that may lead to cancer.

Polyp: Growth that protrudes from a mucous membrane.

Positron emission tomography (PET) scan: Diagnostic examination used to detect cancer cells in the body in which a small amount of radioactive glucose (sugar) is injected into a vein and then a scanner is used to make detailed, computerized pictures of areas inside the body where the glucose is used.

Primary tumor: Original tumor or initial tumor.

Prostate-specific antigen (PSA) test: Test that measures level of free PSA, a protein produced by the prostate gland. Levels are elevated in men who have prostate cancer, infection, or inflammation of the prostate gland and BPH.

Radiation therapy: Use of high-energy radiation from x-rays, gamma rays, neutrons, and other sources to kill cancer cells and shrink tumors.

Radionuclide scan: Diagnostic test in which an individual is administered a small amount of radioactive material. A scanner is used to take pictures of the internal parts of the body to detect where the radiation concentrates.

Radon: Radioactive gas that if inhaled in sufficient quantity can lead to lung cancer.

Sonogram: Computer image of internal organs and tissues produced by ultrasound.

Stage: Extent of a cancer within the body. Staging is based on the size of the tumor, whether lymph nodes contain cancer, and whether the disease has spread from the original site to other parts of the body.

Stem cell: Type of cell from which other types of cells develop; for example, blood cells develop from blood-forming stem cells.

Stem cell transplantation: Procedure used to replace cells that were destroyed by cancer treatment.

Tumor: Mass of excess tissue that results from abnormal cell division. Tumors may be benign or malignant.

Tumor marker: Substance sometimes found in the blood, other body fluids, or tissues that may signal the presence of a certain type of cancer; for example, a high level of PSA is a signal for possible prostate cancer.

What Is Cancer?

Cancer is a disease that occurs when the normal cell renewal process fails. When old cells fail to die and new cells form more rapidly than needed, the cells may accumulate and form a mass called a *tumor*. Tumors are caused by abnormal cell division. They may be benign or malignant. A *malignant tumor* is cancerous and can invade and destroy nearby tissue and spread (*metastasize*) to other parts of the body, whereas a *benign tumor* is not cancerous and does not spread. Specific cancers are named according to the site where the cancerous growth began. This is the site of the *primary tumor*. For example, carcinoma begins in skin or tissues covering internal organs; leukemia begins in blood-forming tissues; and lymphoma begins in cells of the immune system.

Risk Factors for Cancer

There are many risk factors for cancer, including age, tobacco use, and many others discussed in this section (Box 37-1).

AGE

The risk for developing cancer increases with age. Cancers are more prevalent in persons over the age of 65.

TOBACCO

Inhalation of cigarette, cigar, and pipe tobacco smoke may increase the risk for developing cancer of the lungs, larynx, mouth, esophagus, bladder, kidney, throat, stomach, pancreas, and cervix and acute myeloid leukemia. Smokers as well as nonsmokers exposed to "second-hand" tobacco smoke are at increased risk. Chewing tobacco may increase risk for mouth cancer.

IONIZING RADIATION AND SUNLIGHT

X-rays, nuclear fallout (from atomic weapons testing or leaks from nuclear power plants), and radon gas are examples of ionizing radiation. Radon is a radioactive gas that is odorless, colorless, and tasteless. High levels may be found in mine shafts and in some homes. Exposure to radioactive fallout increases risk for the development of leukemia, thyroid cancer, and breast cancer. Exposure to radon gas may increase the risk for developing lung cancer.

Ultraviolet (UV) radiation comes from the sun. The ozone layer of the atmosphere provides protection from excessive exposure to UV radiation prompting concerns over depletion of the earth's ozone layer. UV radiation is classified as UVA and UVB. UVA levels are highest during midday, whereas UVB levels occur throughout the day. Exposure to both UVA and UVB can increase the risk for skin cancer (melanoma). Exposure to UV light from sunlamps and tanning booths also increases cancer risk. While protection from excess exposure to UV radiation is important, some exposure to sunlight is necessary in order for the skin to make the hormone vitamin D.

HAZARDOUS CHEMICALS AND ENVIRONMENTAL POLLUTANTS

Cancer-causing chemicals (carcinogens) are found in the workplace, home, and the environment through pollution. Industrial solvents, cleaning fluids, pesticides, and used engine oil are examples of hazardous chemicals. Known workplace carcinogens include benzene,

BOX 37-1 RISK FACTORS FOR CANCER

- Increasing age
- Tobacco
- Environmental pollutants
- Ionizing radiation
- Sunlight and tanning salons (UV light)
- Carcinogenic chemicals (e.g., benzene)
- Viruses (e.g., HPV, Epstein-Barr)

- Bacteria (e.g., *H. pylori*)
- Hormone therapy (e.g., diethylstilbesterol [DES])
- Family history
- Alcohol
- Poor diet, lack of physical activity, and overweight

vinyl chloride, polychlorinated biphenyls (PCBs), asbestos, cadmium, and nickel. These carcinogens may get into the environment through improper disposal or chemical spills or are released into the air in the process of incineration.

BACTERIAL AND VIRAL INFECTION

Heliocobacter pylori is a bacteria that is known to cause peptic ulcer disease (PUD). It is also associated with stomach cancer. Exposure to certain virus may increase the risk of developing certain cancers. *Epstein-Barr virus (EBV)* is a common virus that remains dormant in most people; however, it has been associated with the certain lymphomas such as Burkitt's lymphoma and immunoblastic lymphoma. The virus is also linked to nasopharyngeal carcinoma. *Hepatitis B virus (HBV)* and *hepatitis C virus (HBC)* are linked to liver cancer. *Human papillomavirus (HPV)* is a virus that causes genital warts and cancer of the cervix. *Human immunodeficiency virus (HIV)* and *human herpesvirus 8 (HHV8)* can cause Kaposi's sarcoma. *Human T-cell leukemia virus type 1* is another retrovirus; it can cause leukemia and lymphoma.

HORMONE THERAPY

The use of hormone replacement therapy (HRT), once the principal treatment for menopausal symptoms and also prescribed to reduce osteoporosis and heart disease, is now limited due to risk for the development of breast cancer, heart attack, stroke, and blood clots. Diethystilbesterol (DES) is an estrogen-type drug that was taken by pregnant women between 1940 and 1971. Girls born to women who took DES have a higher risk for cancer of the cervix than do girls born to women who did not take the drug. Women who took DES have a higher incidence of breast cancer.

FAMILY HISTORY

In the absence of contact with tobacco, carcinogenic chemicals and drugs, aging, and exposure to certain viruses and bacteria, it is not known why one individual will develop cancer while another does not. With the exception of cancers of the breast, ovary, prostate, skin, and colon, most cancers do not run in families. For example, if a father develops stomach cancer, his children have no greater risk for stomach cancer than would a non–family member.

ALCOHOL

Chronic alcohol consumption (up to two drinks daily over a period of years) may increase the risk for cancer of the liver, mouth, throat, esophagus, larynx, and breast.

DIET, PHYSICAL INACTIVITY, AND OBESITY

A diet is that is high in fat may increase the risk of cancers of the colon, uterus, and prostate. Cancers of the breast, colon, esophagus, kidney, and uterus are higher in individuals who have little physical activity and are overweight.

Types of Cancers

BREAST CANCER

In 2007, there were 178,480 new cases of breast cancer diagnosed. Approximately 128 of every 100,000 women will be diagnosed with the disease. The median age at the time of diagnosis is 61 years old. One or both breasts may be involved. The mortality rate is about 25 per 100,000 women, accounting for 40,460 deaths in 2007. Risk factors for breast cancer are (1) family history, (2) nulliparity (no pregnancies), (3) early onset of menses ("periods"), (4) advanced age, (5) a personal history of breast cancer, and (6) history of HRT. Signs and symptoms of breast cancer are listed in Box 37-2.

CANCER OF THE CERVIX, ENDOMETRIUM, AND OVARIES

Cancer of the cervix is linked to human papillomavirus (HPV) and exposure to the drug DES while in still in the uterus. Approximately 8.7 of 100,000 women are diagnosed annually with cancer of the cervix, and it is estimated that in 2007, nearly 11,150 women will

BOX 37-2 SIGNS AND SYMPTOMS OF BREAST CANCER

- Nipple tenderness
- Lump or mass in the breast of near the underarm area
- Fluid coming out of nipples
- Nipple that has turned inward

- Changes in size of shape of the breast
- Changes in appearance of skin of the breast, areola, or nipple (scaly, red, swollen, ridged, pitting, or pock-marked)

be diagnosed and 3,670 women will die from the disease. Ovarian cancer is more common than cervical cancer, with an incidence rate of 13.5 of 100,000 women annually. It is expected that nearly twice as many new cases of ovarian cancer will be diagnosed in 2007 compared with new cases of cervical cancer. The endometrium is the lining of the uterus. Endometrial cancer most commonly affects postmenopausal women.

SKIN CANCER

Skin cancer is one of the most common types of cancer. It is estimated that 65,050 men and women (37,070 men and 27,980 women) will be diagnosed with the disease in 2007 and 10,850 men and women will die of cancer of the skin. Skin cancer is divided into two categories: melanoma and nonmelanoma. The most treatable form is nonmelanoma.

Skin cancer is associated with excessive exposure to ultraviolet light, from either the sun or UV lights used in tanning salons. UV light and ionizing radiation are described earlier in "Risk Factors for Cancer." Protection from harmful UV light is the best way to prevent skin cancer. This can be achieved by wearing protective clothing when outdoors or by using sunscreens. Warning signs for skin cancer are shown in Box 37-3.

LUNG CANCER

Lung cancer is the most common form of cancer. It is estimated that 81 of each 100,000 men and 52 of each 100,000 women will be diagnosed with cancer of the lung and bronchus in 2007. That is nearly 213,380 men and women! Nearly 160,390 men and women are anticipated to die of cancer of the lung and bronchus in 2007!

There are two types of lung cancer. They are small cell lung cancer (SCLC) and non-small cell lung cancer (NSCLC). Antineoplastic agents used in the treatment of lung cancer are typically effective against one but not both forms of the disease. A history of smoking tobacco is nearly always the cause of small cell lung cancer.

COLORECTAL CANCER

Cancer of the colon and rectum affects an estimated 51.6 per 100,000 men and women annually. That is a total of 153,760 new cases each year. The first signs of colon cancer may be the appearance of a small polyp and blood in the stool. Early detection through the administration of screening examinations helps to reduce death from the disease. Colonoscopy and fecal occult blood test (FOBT) are screening tests for colorectal cancer.

BOX 37-3 SIGNS OF SKIN CANCER

Asymmetry: A mole that looks different on one half than the other half.
Border: The edges of the mole are blurry or jagged.
Color: The color of a mole changes (e.g., darkens, spreads, loses color, or appears as multiple colors (blue, red, white, pink, purple, or gray).

Diameter: The mole is larger than 1/4 inch in diameter.
Elevation: The mole is raised above the skin and has an uneven surface.

PROSTATE CANCER

The incidence of prostrate cancer increases as men grow older. Approximately 0.5% of men will be diagnosed with prostate cancer between age of 35 to 44 years, and this increases to 36.7% between 65 and 74 years of age. Levels begin to slowly decline again after the age of 75. It is estimated that approximately 218,890 men will be diagnosed with prostate cancer in 2007. Prostate disease, diagnosis, and treatment were described in Chapter 30.

Cancer Screening Tests

Early diagnosis is critical to successful treatment. Screening tests are recommended for early diagnosis of breast cancer, colorectal cancer, cancer of the cervix, and prostate cancer. A mammogram is a screening examination that is used to detect breast cancer. A radiograph is taken of the breast and inspected for evidence of tumors. A sonogram is an alternative method for screening for breast cancers. If a lump is found, a biopsy is performed. A *biopsy* is a procedure whereby the cells or tissue is removed for examination by a pathologist. The three types of biopsy are (1) incisional, (2) excisional, and (3) fine-needle aspiration. Regular self-examination of the breast is another important method for screening for breast cancer.

Several tests exist to screen for colorectal cancer. They are the FOBT, colonoscopy, sigmoidoscopy, double contrast barium enema, and a digital rectal examination (DRE). The FOBT is a test that screens for blood in stool. Bleeding may indicate the presence of polyps or cancer. A *polyp* is a growth that protrudes from a mucous membrane. A colonoscopy and sigmoidoscopy involve insertion of a lighted tube into the colon to inspect for abnormal growths. Radiographs may be taken of the colon. With this screening procedure, the individual is administered a *double contrast barium enema* to permit greater visualization of the bowel. A DRE is a screening test for colon cancer and prostate cancer (see Chapter 30). Another test that is performed to screen for prostate cancer is a PSA test. Prostate-specific antigen (PSA) is a protein produced by the prostate gland. Levels are elevated in men who have prostate cancer, infection, or inflammation of the prostate gland and BPH (see Chapter 30). A *Pap smear* is a screening test for cancer of the cervix. The Pap smear, also known as a Pap test, is a simple procedure in which cells from the cervix are removed and examined to detect cancer and changes that may lead to cancer.

The results of the screening test may indicate that more diagnostic examinations are warranted. Before a diagnosis of cancer is made, the individual may undergo additional radiographs, *CT scans*, biopsy, *sonogram, radionuclide scan, MRI,* or *PET scan*.

Staging

Staging is a method used to describe how far the cancer has progressed within the body. Staging is based on the size of the tumor, whether lymph nodes contain cancer, and whether the cancer has spread from the original site to other parts of the body.

Treatment of Cancer

Cancer may be treated with chemotherapy, biological therapy, radiation therapy, and surgery. Chemotherapy is the use of drugs to kill or slow the growth of cancerous cells. Biological therapy is the administration of immune system modulators to boost the body's natural defense against abnormal, invasive and cancerous cells. Factors influencing the selection of treatment options are (1) type of cancer, (2) the stage of cancer, (3) individual tolerance for adverse effects of treatment, (4) patient's age, (5) histologic and nuclear grade of the primary tumor, and (6) the capacity of the cancer to metastasize. This chapter focuses on antineoplastic agents and biological therapy.

Chemotherapeutic or antineoplastic agents may be administered parenterally or by mouth. They work by various mechanisms to interrupt the cell replication cycle. Some agents are cell cycle specific. They interrupt a specific stage of the cell cycle (Table 37-1); examples are mitotic inhibitors and DNA synthesis inhibitors. Other antineoplastic agents are nonspecific. The site of action of chemotherapeutic agents is shown in Figure 37-1.

TECH ALERT!

All chemotherapy agents are prepared in a Class II biohazard safety cabinet or using a vertical flow hood containing a high-efficiency particulate air (HEPA) filter with a vertical downward flow of air. The pharmacy technician is protected by a glass front and wears a fluid-proof gown, double gloves, mask, and goggles. USP 797 requires the use of a bonnet and shoe covers, also.

TABLE 37-1   Summary of the Cell Life Cycle

Phase of Cell Life Cycle	Description
Cell growth	**Interphase**
Protein synthesis	Proteins are manufactured according to the cell's genetic code; functional proteins, the enzymes, direct the synthesis of other molecules in the cells and thus the production of more and larger organelles and plasma membrane; sometimes called the *first growth phase or G1, phase* of interphase.
DNA replication	Nucleotides, influenced by newly synthesized enzymes, arrange themselves along the open sides of an "unzippered" DNA molecule, thereby creating two identical daughters DNA molecules; produces two identical sets of the cell's genetic code, which enables the cell to later split into two different cells, each with its own complete set of DNA; sometimes called the *[DNA] synthesis stage or S phase* of interphase.
Protein synthesis	After DNA is replicated, the cell continues to grow by means of protein synthesis and the resulting synthesis of other molecules and various organelles; this *second growth phase* is also called the *G2 phase.*
Cell reproduction	**M phase**
Mitosis or meiosis	The parent cell's replicated set of DNA is divided into two sets of separated by an orderly process into distinct cell nuclei; mitosis is subdivided into at least four phases: *prophase, metaphase, anaphase,* and *telophase.*
Cytokinesis	The plasma membrane of the parent cell "pinches in" and eventually separates the cytoplasm and two daughter nuclei into two genetically identical daughter cells.

From Thibodeau G, Patton K: *Anatomy and physiology,* ed 6, St. Louis, 2007, Mosby.

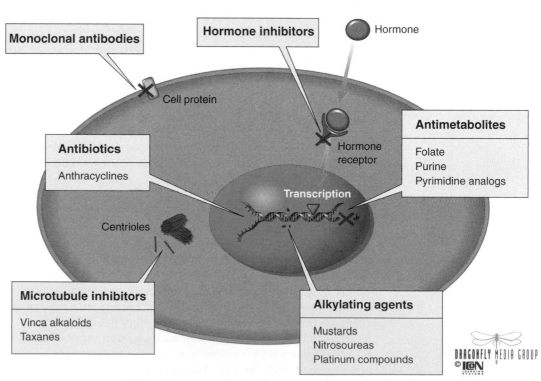

FIGURE 37-1   Site of action of chemotherapeutic agents. *(From Raffa RB, Rawls SM, Beyzarov EP:* Netter's illustrated pharmacology, *Philadelphia, 2005, WB Saunders.)*

Antineoplastic Agents

HORMONE THERAPY

Hormone therapy is a treatment of choice for breast cancer. Treatment choice is influenced by the woman's menopausal status, the affinity of the tumor for estrogen receptors and progesterone receptors, and human epidermal growth factor receptor 2 (*HER2/neu*) gene amplification, in addition to the other factors listed earlier.

The hormones estrogen and progesterone can promote the growth of estrogen-receptor positive (ER-positive) and/or progesterone-receptor positive (PR-positive) breast cancer. The administration of the estrogen receptor antagonist (antiestrogens) can reduce the risk of breast cancer reoccurrence for up to 5 years after the treatment of the primary tumor.

SELECTIVE ESTROGEN RECEPTOR MODULATORS (ANTIESTROGENS)

Tamoxifen is indicated for the treatment of ER-positive breast cancer that is noninvasive or invasive (metastatic). It is approved for the treatment of metastatic breast cancer in premenopausal and postmenopausal women. It is also approved for the treatment of metastatic breast cancer in men. Toremifene is a derivative of tamoxifen that is indicated for the treatment of metastatic breast cancer in postmenopausal women.

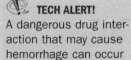

TECH ALERT!
Tamoxifen is classified in Food and Drug Administration pregnancy risk category D, so the warning label AVOID PREGNANCY should be applied to the prescription vial.

Mechanism of Action and Pharmacokinetics

Tamoxifen and torimefene are antiestrogens. Tamoxifen is a selective ER modulator (SERM) that has both antiestrogenic and estrogenic activity. Tamoxifen is an estrogen antagonist in breast tissue. It induces maspin, a tumor suppression gene that is abundant in normal breast cells and lacking in cancerous breast tissue. This may prevent the tumor from becoming invasive. Tamoxifen acts as a partial agonist in the endometrium (lining of the uterus). Its agonist effects on bone cells increase bone turnover (remodeling) and can decrease postmenopausal bone loss. Tamoxifen also has agonist effects on cholesterol metabolism and genitourinary epithelium. Tamoxifen has an active metabolite and long half-life and accumulates with continued administration. It may be dosed once or twice a day. The action of torimefene is primarily antiestrogenic.

TECH ALERT!
A dangerous drug interaction that may cause hemorrhage can occur when tamoxifen is taken with the anticoagulant warfarin.

Adverse Reactions

Tamoxifen and torimefene commonly produce menopause-like symptoms such as hot flashes, sweating, vaginal itchiness, discharge or dryness, nausea, and vomiting. Tamoxifen may additionally cause menstrual changes, and its agonist effects on the endometrium may result in endometrial cancer. Women taking tamoxifen have a 2 to 7 times increased risk for endometrial cancer compared with women who did not take tamoxifen. Other adverse effects produced by tamoxifen include hair loss, impotence, bone or muscle pain, deep vein thrombosis (DVT), lowered platelets and white blood cell count, pulmonary embolism, and visual changes (cataracts). Torimefene may produce ocular, vascular, and heart problems.

Selective Estrogen Receptor Modulators

Generic name	U.S. brand name(s) Canadian brand(s)	Dosage forms and strengths
tamoxifen	Soltamox	**Solution, oral (Soltamox):** 10 mg/5 ml
	Tamofen, Tamone	**Tablet (Tamofen, Tamone):** 10 mg, 20 mg
torimefene	Fareston	**Tablet:** 60 mg
	not available	

ESTROGEN RECEPTOR DOWNREGULATORS

Fulvestrant is an ER downregulator. It is indicated for the treatment of ER-positive metastatic breast cancer in postmenopausal women with disease progression, following antiestrogen therapy.

Mechanism of Action and Pharmacokinetics

Fulvestrant is an analog of estradiol. It acts as a competitive antagonist. When fulvestrant binds to ERs, it inhibits estrogen activity, causes changes in the ER function, and triggers ER degradation. Fulvestrant is administered intramuscularly. Plasma concentrations are maintained at therapeutic levels for up to 1 month.

Adverse Reactions

Adverse effects caused by fulvestrant include pain at the injection site, generalized bone and back pain, hot flashes, headache, nausea and vomiting, diarrhea or constipation, and weakness.

Estrogen Receptor Downregulators

| Generic name | U.S. brand name(s) | Dosage forms and strengths |
	Canadian brand name	
fulvestrant	Faslodex	Solution, injection: 50 mg/ml
	Faslodex	

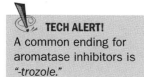

TECH ALERT!
A common ending for aromatase inhibitors is "-trozole."

AROMATASE INHIBITORS

Anastrozole, exemestane, and letrozole are aromatase inhibitors. They may be prescribed alone or in combination with tamoxifen. They are Food and Drug Administration (FDA) approved for the first-line treatment of postmenopausal women with advanced or metastatic ER-positive breast cancer. They are additionally approved for adjuvant treatment of early-stage breast cancer.

Mechanism of Action and Pharmacokinetics

The adrenal gland is the primary source of estrogen after menopause. Aromatase is an enzyme that is responsible for converting androgens produced by the adrenal gland into the estrogens estrone and estradiol in the peripheral tissues. Aromatase inhibitors block this process. Anastrozole and letrozole are nonsteroidal aromatase inhibitors and are potent inhibitors of serum estradiol levels. Exemestane is a steroidial aromatase inhibitor. It is a more potent inhibitor of estrogen than the other aromatase inhibitors.

TECH ALERT!
Femara and FemHRT have look-alike/sound-alike issues.

Adverse Reactions

Like tamoxifen, aromatase inhibitors produce menopause-like symptoms, nausea, and vomiting. Additional adverse effects include dizziness, cough, headache, hair loss, constipation, mood changes, and bone pain. Administration of steroid aromatase inhibitors requires adrenal hormone replacement therapy to replenish depleted glucocorticoids (cortisol) and mineralcorticoids (aldosterone). Symptoms may be fatigue, weight gain, and swelling.

Aromatase Inhibitors

Generic name	U.S. brand name(s)	Dosage forms and strengths
	Canadian brand(s)	
anastrozole	Arimidex	**Tablet:** 1 mg
	Arimidex	
exemestane	Aromasin	**Tablet:** 25 mg
	Aromasin	
letrozole	Femara	**Tablet:** 2.5 mg
	Femara	

GONADOTROPIN-RELEASING HORMONE AGONISTS AND LUTEINIZING HORMONE–RELEASING HORMONE AGONISTS

Gonadotropin-releasing hormone (GnRH) is also known as luteinizing hormone–releasing hormone (LHRH). Goserelin is a GnRH agonist that is indicated for the treatment of advanced breast cancer in premenopausal and perimenopausal women with ER-positive disease. The drug initially increases hormone levels and is followed by desensitization to the hormone's effects. GnRH and its analogs are described in depth in Chapter 34. GnRH agonists may be prescribed to treat premenopausal women, whereas SERMs and aromatase inhibitors are only indicated for use in postmenopausal women.

Luteinizing Hormone–Releasing Hormone and Gonadotropin-Releasing Hormone Agonists

Generic name	U.S. brand name(s)	Dosage forms and strengths
	Canadian brand(s)	
gosrelin	Zoladex	**Injection (1-month implant):** 3.6 mg
	Zoladex LA	**Injection (3-month Implant):** 10.8 mg

TECH ALERT!
Megesterol suspension is prescribed to increase appetite and combat wasting syndrome in patients with AIDS.

PROGESTINS

Megestrol acetate is a progestin that is approved for the treatment of breast cancer. It is indicated for the treatment of inoperable, advanced metastatic breast cancer following treatment with tamoxifen or aromatase inhibitors. It is also indicated for the treatment of endometrial cancer. Medroxyprogesterone acetate is approved for treatment of inoperable, metastatic endometrial cancer and renal cell cancer.

Mechanism of Action

It is not fully known how megestrol works to suppress estrogen-dependent breast tumors; however, suppression of LH release from the pituitary and increased metabolism of estrogen are believed to be involved.

Adverse Reactions

The most common adverse effects associated with megestrol use are hot flashes, breakthrough menstrual bleeding, and weight gain. Breast tenderness, hair loss, and hyperglycemia may also occur.

Progestins Used in the Treatment of Cancer

Generic name	U.S. brand name(s)	Dosage forms and strengths
	Canadian brand(s)	
megestrol acetate	Megace, Megace ES	**Suspension, oral:** 40 mg/ml; 125 mg/ml (concentrate)
	Megace, Megace OS	**Tablet:** 20 mg, 40 mg

AKYLATING AGENTS

Akylating agents are one of the oldest classes of antineoplastic agents. They are related to nitrogen mustard, a lethal gas that was used for chemical warfare in World War I. Cyclophosphamide (Cytoxan), busulfan (Busulfex, Myleran), ifosfamide (Ifex), melphalan (Alkeran), mechlorethamine (Mustargen), and chlorambucil (Leukeran) are all akylating agents. Only cyclophosphamide is approved for the treatment of breast cancer. It is also indicated for the treatment of Hodgkin's disease, non-Hodgkin's lymphoma, acute lymphocytic leukemia (ALL), ovarian cancer, multiple myeloma, chronic lymphocytic leukemia (CLL), mycosis fungoides, and retinoblastoma.

Mechanism of Action and Pharmacokinetics

The alkylating agents vary in their antitumor effects and in toxicity, but their mechanism of action is the same. All alkylating agents damage DNA when they substituting an alkyl group (saturated carbon atoms) on the amino acid guanine or, in some cases, cytosine. This changes the guanine-cytosine base-pair and impairs DNA replication and the growth phase of the cell life cycle (Table 37-1). Alkylating agents can cause cell mutations and are themselves carcinogenic. They are toxic to cancer cells and noncancerous cells.

Cyclophosphamide is a prodrug. It is available for oral and parenteral use. Resistance can develop to the effects of cyclophosphamide and other alkylating agents.

Adverse Reactions

Cylcophosphamide commonly causes hair loss, appetite and weight loss, skin discoloration, mouth sores, and fatigue.

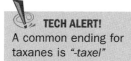

TECH ALERT!
The following drugs have look-alike/ sound-alike issues: cyclophosphamide and cyclosporine; Cytocin, Cytosar-U, Cytotec, Ciloxan, and cefoxitin

Alkylating Agents

Generic name	U.S. brand name(s)	Dosage forms and strengths
	Canadian brand(s)	
cyclophosphamide*	Cytoxan	**Powder for solution:** 500 mg/vial; 1000 mg/vial; 2000 mg/vial
	Cytoxan, Procytox	**Tablet:** 25 mg, 50 mg

*Generic available.

TECH ALERT!
A common ending for taxanes is "-taxel"

TECH ALERT!
The following drugs have look-alike/ sound-alike issues: paclitaxel and albumin-bound nanopaclitaxel; Taxotere and Taxol

TAXANES

Taxanes are cytotoxic drugs that are naturally derived from the Western Yew (paclitaxel) and the European Yew tree (docetaxel). They are approved for the treatment of breast cancer.

Mechanism of Action and Pharmacokinetics

Taxanes interfere with the process of mitosis. Mitosis is a key step in the process of cell division and is the stage where DNA is organized and distributed. Taxanes are microtubular inhibitors. They bind to tubulin subunits resulting in overly stable, nonfunctional microtubles that do not disassociate and disappear in the final phase of mitosis. Microtubles or spindles are normally formed during the prophase of mitosis and are supposed to disappear by the end of the telophase. The four phases of mitosis are shown in Table 37-2.

TABLE 37-2   The Major Events of Mitosis

Prophase	Metaphase	Anaphase	Telophase
1. Chromosomes shorten and thicken (from coiling of the DNA molecules that compose them); each chromosome consists of two chromatids attached at the centromere.	1. Chromosomes align across the equator of the spindle fiber at its centromere.	1. Each centromere splits, thereby detaching two chromatids that compose each chromosome from each other elongating (DNA molecules start uncoiling).	1. Changes occurring during telophase essentially reverse of those taking place during prophase; new chromosomes start elongating (DNA molecules start uncoiling).
2. Centrioles move to opposite poles of the cell; spindle fibers appear and begin to orient between opposing poles.		2. Sister chromatids (now called chromosomes) move to opposite poles; there are now twice as many chromosomes as there were before mitosis started.	2. A nuclear envelope forms again to enclose each new set of chromosomes.
3. Nucleoli and the nuclear membrane disappear.			3. Spindle fibers disappear.

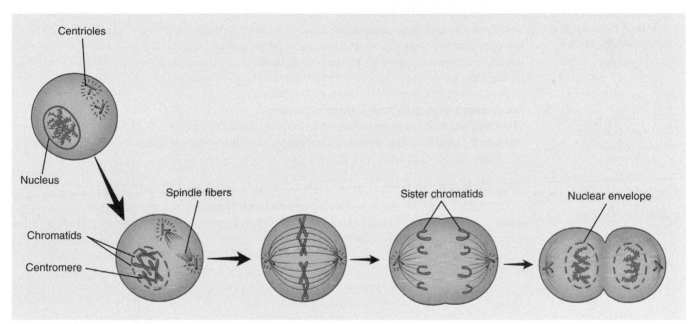

From Thibodeau G, Patton K: Anatomy and physiology, *ed 6, St. Louis, 2007, Mosby.*

 TECH ALERT!
Paclitaxel is insoluble in water, so it is prepared as an emulsion using cremophor. Allergic reactions to the cremophor emulsion are common.

Adverse Reactions

Common adverse reactions produced by taxanes are diarrhea, total body hair loss, nausea, muscle, joint and low back aches and pain, flushing, and sweating. They also decrease white blood cells, red blood cells, and platelets. When white blood cell levels drop, individuals may get infections more easily. Docetaxel may also cause discoloration of fingernails and loosening from the nail bed. Paclitaxel may cause mouth sores.

Taxanes

	Generic name	U.S. brand name(s) / Canadian brand(s)	Dosage forms and strengths
	docetaxel	Taxotere	Solution for injection: 40 mg/ml
		Taxotere	
	paclitaxel*	Onxol, Taxol	Solution: 6 mg/ml
		Taxol	
	albumin-bound nanoparticle paclitaxel	Abraxane	Powder for suspension: 100 mg/vial
		Abraxane	

*Generic available.

TECH ALERT!
A common beginning for Vinca Alkaloids is "vin-"

TECH ALERT!
Vinblastine and vincristine have look-alike/sound-alike issues

TECH ALERT!
Vincristine is usually stored in the refrigerator

VINCA ALKALOIDS

Vinorelbine, vincristine, and vinblastine are vinca alkaloids. They are naturally derived from the periwinkle plant. Vinca alkaloids are used for the treatment of non–small cell lung cancer, breast cancer, Kaposi's sarcoma, Hodgkin's disease, non-Hodgkin's lymphoma, and testicular cancer.

Mechanism of Action and Pharmacokinetics

The mechanism of action of vinca alkaloids is similar to taxanes. Both drugs act on microtubules to inhibit mitosis. Vinca alkaloids inhibit microtubule formation (taxanes inhibit microtubule degradation).

Adverse Reactions

Side effects linked to vinca alkaloids are similar to those for taxanes and include hair loss, nausea and vomiting, constipation, joint and muscle pain, mouth sores, increased risk for infections, and pain at the injection site.

Vinca Alkaloids

	Generic name	U.S. brand name(s) / Canadian brand(s)	Dosage forms and strengths
	vinorelbine*	Navelbine	Solution for injection: 10 mg/ml
		Navelbine	
	vinblastine*	Generics	Powder for injection: 10 mg/vial
		Generics	Solution for injection: 1 mg/ml
	vincristine*	Vincasar PFS	Solution for injection: 1 mg/ml
		Generics	

*Generic available.

TECH ALERT!
A common ending for anthracyclines is "-rubicin."

ANTHRACYCLINES

Doxorubicin, epirubicin, and idarubicin are anthracyclines. Mitoxantrone is a related compound and is classified as an anthracenedione. Only doxorubicin and epirubicin are indicated for the treatment of breast cancer, typically in combination with other antineoplastic agents. Doxorubicin is also approved for the treatment of numerous other cancers such as bladder cancer, lung cancer, Hodgkin's disease, leukemia, gastric cancer, ovarian cancer, soft tissue sarcoma, and thyroid cancer. Doxorubicin liposomal is approved for the treatment of ovarian cancer, Kaposi's sarcoma, and multiple myeloma. Idarubacin and mitxantrone are approved for the treatment of acute myelogenous leukemia (AML).

Mechanism of Action and Pharmacokinetics

Anthracyclines damage cellular DNA. They form a complex with DNA that changes the shape of the helix-shaped strand and results in inhibition of the DNA and RNA enzymes that cause protein synthesis (Figure 37-2). This impairs DNA replication and the growth phase of the cell life cycle (Table 37-1).

Anthracyclines also inhibit the activity of the enzyme topoisomerase (see "Topoisomerase Inhibitors"). Secondary mechanisms for cellular destruction involve the formation of free radicals and complexes with iron. Doxorubicin is a prodrug. It is metabolized to the active metabolite idarubicin (Idamycin PFS). It has a long half-life and may be administered as a weekly or monthly infusion. Mitoxantrone is a related compound that damages DNA by producing breaks in the strand.

Adverse Reactions

Doxorubicin is cardiotoxic and may cause heart failure. Mitoxanthrone produces less cardiotoxicity. Other side effects produced by the anthracyclines and anthracenediones include heart burn, mouth sores, hair loss, diarrhea, flushing, red or watery eyes, flu-like symptoms, and decreased red and white blood cells and platelets. The anthracyclines may turn urine and nails red, whereas mitoxantrone causes them to turn blue-green.

> **TECH ALERT!**
> Doxorubicin and doxorubicin lisosomal are not substitutable.

> **TECH ALERT!**
> The following drugs have look-alike/sound-alike issues: doxorubicin and doxorubicin liposomal; Ellence and Elase; Mitoxantrone and methotrexate

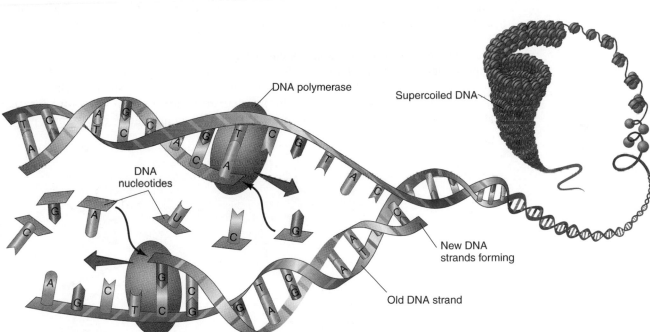

FIGURE 37-2 DNA Replication. *(From Thibodeau G, Patton K:* Anatomy and physiology, *ed 6, St. Louis, 2007, Mosby.)*

Anthracyclines

Generic name	U.S. brand name(s)	Dosage forms and strengths
	Canadian brand(s)	
doxorubicin*	Adriamycin, Rubex	**Powder for injection:** 10 mg, 20 mg, 50 mg, 100 mg (Rubex)
	Adriamycin PFS	**Solution for injection:** 2 mg/ml
doxorubicin liposomal	Doxil	**Solution for injection:** 2 mg/ml
	Caelyx, Myocet	

Continued

Anthracyclines—cont'd

Generic name	U.S. brand name(s)	Dosage forms and strengths
	Canadian brand(s)	
epirubicin*	Ellence	**Powder for injection:** 50 mg, 200 mg
		Solution for injection: 2 mg/ml
	Pharmorubicin PFS	
mitoxantrone*	Novantrone	**Solution for injection:** 2 mg/ml
	Generic	

*Generic available.

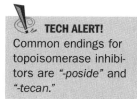

TECH ALERT!
Common endings for topoisomerase inhibitors are *"-poside"* and *"-tecan."*

TOPOISOMERASE INHIBITORS

Etoposide, teniposide, irinotecan, and topotecan are topoisomerase inhibitors. Topoisomerase inhibitors are derived from natural and semisynthetic sources. Etoposide and teniposide are semisynthetic derivatives of an extract from the mandrake plant. Irinotecan and topotecan are camptothecin derivatives and are extracted from *Camptotheca accuminata* (a Chinese tree). Irinotecan is a prodrug. Etoposide is approved for the treatment of testicular and small cell lung cancer. Teniposide is approved for the treatment of acute lymphocytic leukemia. Topotecan is indicated for the treatment of ovarian, cervical, and small cell lung cancer. Irinotecan is only indicated for the treatment of colorectal cancer.

Mechanism of Action and Pharmacokinetics

Topoisomerases are enzymes that cleave DNA strands; a step needed for DNA replication and RNA transcription (Figure 37-3). Topoisomerase I cleaves one strand of DNA, and topoisomerase II cleaves two strands. Topoisomerase II also plays a role in successful mitosis. Oral absorption of the drugs is good but penetration in the central nervous system is poor.

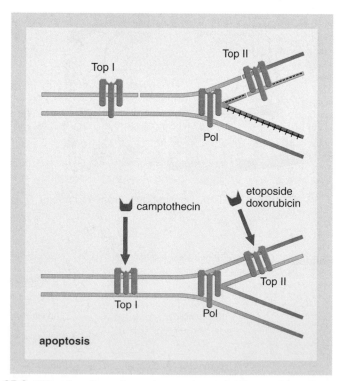

FIGURE 37-3 Site of action of topoisomerase inhibitors. *(From Page C, et al.: Integrated pharmacology, ed 3, Philadelphia, 2006, Mosby.)*

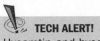

TECH ALERT!
Hycamtin and hycomine have look-alike/sound-alike issues.

Adverse Reactions

Etoposide and teniposide may cause diarrhea, hair loss, nausea, skin rash, fatigue, irritation at injection site, flu-like symptoms, bleeding, or bruising. Irinotecan and topotecan produce similar side effects plus headache, gas, and weight loss. Rarely, individuals on high-dose etoposide therapy may develop acute nonlymphocytic leukemia.

Topoisomerase Inhibitors

Generic name	U.S. brand name(s) Canadian brand(s)	Dosage forms and strengths
etoposide*	Etopophos, Toposar, VePesid	**Capsule (VePesid):** 50 mg
	VePesid	**Powder, injection (Etopophos):** 100 mg/vial **Solution, injection (Topsar, VePesid):** 20 mg/ml
teniposide	Vumon	**Solution, injection:** 10 mg/ml
	Vumon	
irinotecan	Camptosar	**Solution, injection:** 20 mg/ml
	Camptosar	
topotecan	Hycamtin	**Powder, injection:** 4 mg/vial
	Hycamtin	

*Generic available.

TECH ALERT!
Platinum compounds have the common ending "-platin."

TECH ALERT!
The following drugs have look-alike/sound-alike issues:
Carboplatin and cisplatin;
Eloxatin and Aloxi;
Platinol AQ, Plaquenil, Paraplatin AQ, and Patanol

PLATINUM COMPOUNDS

Carboplatin, cisplatin, and oxaliplatin are platinum compounds. Cisplatin is FDA approved for the treatment of testicular and ovarian cancer. Carboplatin is approved for the treatment of ovarian cancer, and oxalipatin is approved for the treatment of colorectal cancer.

Mechanism of Action and Pharmacokinetics

The action of platinum compounds on purine bases (adenine and guanine) results in the formation of faulty cross-linkages and defective DNA.

Adverse Reactions

Side effects of platinum compounds are fatigue, loss of appetite, loss of hair, metallic taste, pain at the site of injection, increased infections, bleeding, bruising, and nausea. Cisplatin may additionally cause irreversible hearing loss and neurotoxicity. Sensory neurotoxicity produced by oxaliplatin is reversible.

Platinum Compounds

Generic name	U.S. brand name(s) Canadian brand(s)	Dosage forms and strengths
carboplatin*	Generics	**Powder for injection:** 50 mg, 150 mg, 450 mg/vial
	Paraplatin AQ	**Solution for injection:** 10 mg/ml
cisplatin	Platinol AQ	**Solution for injection:** 1 mg/ml
	Generics	
oxaliplatin	Eloxatin	**Solution for injection:** 5 mg/5 ml, 50 mg/10 ml, 100 mg/20 ml; 200 mg/40 ml
	Eloxatin	

*Generic available.

FLUOROPYRIMIDINES

Capecitabine, cytarabine, gemcitabine, and 5-fluorouracil (5-FU) are fluoropyrimidines, also known as fluorinated pyrimidines. The drugs are indicated for the treatment of several cancers such as colorectal cancer (capecitabine, 5-FU), leukemia (cytarabine), gastric cancer (5-FU), basal cell carcinoma (5-FU), metastatic breast cancer (capecitabine, gemcitabine, 5-FU), lung cancer (gemcitabine), ovarian cancer (gemcitabine), and pancreatic cancer (gemcitabine, 5-FU).

Mechanism of Action and Pharmacokinetics

Capecitabine and 5-FU are prodrugs. Capecitabine is converted to 5-FU by an enzyme that is present in high levels in tumors. 5-FU must be activated, too. Once activated, 5-FU inhibits the enzyme responsible for making thymidine (a DNA nucleoside), inhibits RNA formation, and causes mismatched DNA base-pairs (see Figure 37-2).

Adverse Reactions

Adverse effects linked to capecitabine and 5-FU are stomach upset, loss of appetite, diarrhea or constipation, fatigue, muscle and bone pain, insomnia, headache, and dry, itchy skin. Additional adverse reactions include paresthesia (pricking or tingling sensation) in the hands and feet, jaundice, bone marrow suppression, fatal autoimmune anemias, increased opportunistic infections and cardiotoxicity (capecitabine, 5-FU, and fludarabine).

Fluoropyrimidines Used in the Treatment of Colorectal Cancer

Generic name	U.S. brand name(s) / Canadian brand(s)	Dosage forms and strengths
capecitabine	Xeloda	**Tablet:** 150 mg, 500 mg
	Xeloda	
5-fluorouracil (5-FU)*	Adrucil	**Solution for injection:** 50 mg/ml
	Generics	
cytarabine*	Generics	**Powder, injection:** 100 mg, 500 mg, 1 g, 2 g/vial
	Cytosar	**Solution for injection (Cytosar):** 20 mg/ml (U.S.); 100 mg/ml
cytarabine, liposomal	Depocyt	**Suspension, intrathecal:** 10 mg/ml
	Depocyt	
fludarabine	Fludara	**Powder for injection:** 50 mg/vial
	Fludara	**Solution for injection:** 25 mg/ml **Tablet:** 10 mg (Canada only)
gemcitabine	Gemzar	**Powder for injection:** 200 mg, 1 g/vial
	Gemzar	

*Generic available.

ANTIMETABOLITES

Methotrexate (MTX) is the principal drug in this class. Pemetrexed is a related compound. Methotrexate is indicated for the treatment of lung cancer, breast cancer, bladder cancer, acute lymphocytic leukemia (ALL), cutaneous T-cell lymphoma, lung cancer, non-Hodgkins lymphoma, and osteogenic sarcoma. It is also indicated for the treatment of rheumatoid arthritis (see Chapter 15). The purine antimetabolites 6-mercaptopurine and 6-thioguanine are primarily indicated for the treatment of acute lymphocytic leukemia. Pentostatin is a structural analog of the purine adenosine and is indicated for the treatment of hairy cell leukemia.

Mechanism of Action and Pharmacokinetics

Antimetabolites are chemotherapeutic agents that work most effectively against rapidly dividing cancerous cells. They inhibit normal DNA synthesis by forming abnormal nucleic acid base-pairs, resulting in abnormal DNA. Methotrexate is structurally similar to the vitamin folic acid and inhibits folate metabolism, which is essential to the formation of the purines. Pentostatin, 6-mercaptopurine, and 6-thioguanine are purine analogs. Purine bases, along with pyrimidine bases, make up the DNA strand. Methotrexate also causes the depletion of thymidine, a DNA nucleoside, so DNA synthesis ceases and cells die.

Adverse Reactions

Methotrexate and pemetrexed commonly cause hair loss, photosensitivity, loss of appetite, and nausea. They also decrease white and red blood cells and platelets. When white blood cell levels drop, individuals may get infections more easily. Similar adverse reactions are produced by 6-mercaptopurine and 6-thioguanine with the exception of photosensitivity.

> **TECH ALERT!**
> The warning label AVOID ASPIRIN AND NSAIDs should be applied to prescription vials for methotrexate because the drugs may decrease methotrexate clearance and cause toxicity.

Antimetabolites

Generic name	U.S. brand name(s) / Canadian brand(s)	Dosage forms and strengths
methotrexate* (MTX)	Rheumatrex, Trexall / Generics	**Powder for injection (generics):** 1 g/vial **Solution for injection (generics):** 25 mg/ml **Tablet:** 2.5 mg dosepak (Rheumatrex); 5 mg, 7.5 mg, 10 mg, 15 mg (Trexall)
pemetrexed	Alimta / Alimta	**Powder for injection:** 500 mg/vial
6-mercaptopurine*	Purinethol / Purinethol	**Tablet:** 50 mg
6-thioguanine	Tabloid / Lanvis	**Tablet:** 40 mg
pentostatin	Nipent / Not available	**Powder for injection:** 10 mg/vial

*Generic available.

> **TECH ALERT!**
> The following drugs have look-alike/sound-alike issues: methotrexate and Mitoxantrone; purinethol and propylthiouracil; pentostatin and Pentosan

MISCELLANEOUS

Bleomycin, dactinomycin, and mitomycin are antineoplastic agents that are approved for the treatment of various cancers. Bleomycin is indicated for the treatment of cervical, penile, testicular and vulvar cancers in addition to Hodgkin's disease and head and neck cancer. Dactinomycin is indicated for the treatment of testicular cancer, choriocarcinoma, and rhabdomyosarcoma. Mitomycin is approved for gastric and pancreatic cancer treatment. Hydroxyurea is indicated for the treatment of head and neck cancers, ovarian cancer, leukemia, and sickle cell anemia.

Mechanism of Action and Pharmacokinetics

The primary mechanism of action for bleomycin is to produce breaks in single and double DNA strands. The breaks result in chromosomal gaps and deletions that impair DNA replication. This group of drugs binds reduced iron (Fe^{2+}), which is a secondary mechanism of action. For example, a complex is formed between Fe^{2+}-bleomycin-oxygen (O_2) in the DNA

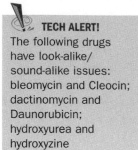

TECH ALERT!
The following drugs
have look-alike/
sound-alike issues:
bleomycin and Cleocin;
dactinomycin and
Daunorubicin;
hydroxyurea and
hydroxyzine

strand reducing the O_2 necessary for cleavage of the DNA strand. The action of dactinomycin on DNA causes the DNA helix to uncoil and inhibits DNA, RNA, and protein synthesis. Mitomycin therapy as results in DNA breaks. Mitomycin also binds to DNA to form abnormal cross-links.

Adverse Reactions

Bleomycin, dactinomycin, and mitomycin may produce pain at the injection site, fatigue, nausea, vomiting decreased appetite, hair loss, and darkened skin color. Mitomycin may discolor the urine and nails. Mitomycin and bleomycin therapy may result in pulmonary fibrosis and death. Bleomycin and mitomycin may also cause MI and stroke. Dactinomycin and hydroxyurea may cause bone marrow suppression and severe anemias increasing risk for infection. Bone marow suppression and severe anemias are also linked to hydroxyurea.

Miscellaneous Antineoplastic Agents

Generic name	U.S. brand name(s) / Canadian brand(s)	Dosage forms and strengths
bleomycin*	Blenoxane	**Powder for injection:** 15 units/vial (Blenoxane), 30 units/vial (generic)
	Blenoxane	
dactinomycin (actinomycin D)	Cosmegen	**Powder for injection:** 500 mcg/vial
	Cosmegen	
mitomycin C*	Mitozytrex	**Powder for injection:** 5 mg/vial
	Generics	
hydroxyurea*	Droxia, Hydrea	**Capsule:** 200 mg, 300 mg, 400 mg, 500 mg (Hydrea)
	Hydrea	

*Generic available.

MONOCLONAL ANTIBODIES

Trastuzumab (Herceptin) is a monoclonal antibody that is used in the treatment of metastatic breast cancer (when tumors overexpress the HER2 protein). The mechanism of action of monoclonal antibodies is described in Chapter 15.

Summary of Drugs Used in the Treatment of Selected Cancers

Generic name	U.S. brand name	Dose and dosing schedule*	Warning labels
Hormones			
Selective Estrogen Receptor Modulators			
tamoxifen	Soltamox	AVOID PREGNANCY DISCARD SOLUTION WITHIN 3 MONTHS OF OPENING—Soltamox STORE AT ROOM TEMPERATURE—solution	
torimefene	Fareston		
Estrogen-Receptor Downregulators			
fulvestrant	Faslodex	REFRIGERATE; DO NOT FREEZE STORE IN ORIGINAL CONTAINER	

Summary of Drugs Used in the Treatment of Selected Cancers—cont'd

Generic name	U.S. brand name	Dose and dosing schedule*	Warning labels
Aromatase Inhibitors			
anastrozole	Arimidex	TAKE AT THE SAME TIME EACH DAY WITH A DRINK OF WATER	
exemestane	Aromasin	TAKE WITH MEALS—exemestane	
letrozole	Femara		
Gonadotropin-Releasing Hormone Agonist			
gosrelin	Zoladex	STORE AT ROOM TEMPERATURE UNTIL READY FOR USE. DO NOT FREEZE INJECT ACCORDING TO PRESCRIBED SCHEDULE	
Progestins			
megestrol acetate*	Megace	SHAKE WELL—suspension	
Anthracyclines			
doxorubicin	Adriamycin	AVOID PREGNANCY	
epirubacin	Ellence	SHAKE WELL—powder for injection MAY STORE RECONSTITUTED SOLUTION FOR 24 HOURS AT ROOM TEMPERATURE PROTECT FROM LIGHT MAY CAUSE DISCOLORATION OF URINE EXERCISE PRECAUTIONS FOR HANDLING, PREPARING, AND ADMINISTERING CYTOTOXIC DRUGS	
Taxanes			
docetaxel	Taxotere	DO NOT SHAKE—docetaxel	
paclitaxel	Taxol, Onxol	REFRIGERATE; DON'T FREEZE—docetaxel RECONSTITUTED SOLUTION IS STABLE FOR _____ HOURS—docetaxel	
nanoparticle albumin bound paclitaxel	Abraxane	(4 hours); paclitaxel (27 hours), nanoparticle albumin-bound paclitaxel (8 hours) MAY STORE AT ROOM TEMPERATURE—paclitaxel DO NOT MIX IN PVC BAGS OR USE PVC SETS—docetaxel, paclitaxel EXERCISE PRECAUTIONS FOR HANDLING, PREPARING, AND ADMINISTERING CYTOTOXIC DRUGS—docetaxel, paclitaxel AVOID ASPIRIN AND NSAIDs	
Fluoropyrimidines			
5-fluorouracil	Adrucil	EXERCISE PRECAUTIONS FOR HANDLING, PREPARING, AND ADMINISTERING CYTOTOXIC DRUGS ONCE THE PHARMACY BULK VIAL IS OPENED, ANY UNUSED PORTION SHOULD BE DISCARDED AFTER 1 HOUR AVOID PREGNANCY AVOID PROLONGED EXPOSURE TO SUNLIGHT	
capecitabine	Xeloda	TAKE WITH FOOD AVOID PREGNANCY	
cytarabine, liposo-mal (ARA-C)	Depocyt	EXERCISE PRECAUTIONS FOR HANDLING, PREPARING, AND ADMINISTERING CYTOTOXIC DRUGS	
fludarabine	Fludara	REFRIGERATE; DO NOT FREEZE RECONSTITUTED SOLUTIONS ARE STABLE FOR 8 HOURS—fludarabine	
gemcitabine	Gemzar	EXERCISE PRECAUTIONS FOR HANDLING, PREPARING, AND ADMINISTERING CYTOTOXIC DRUGS IV SOLUTION IS STABLE FOR 24 HOURS STORE AT ROOM TEMPERATURE	

Continued

Summary of Drugs Used in the Treatment of Selected Cancers—cont'd

	Generic name	U.S. brand name	Dose and dosing schedule*	Warning labels
	Antimetabolites			
	methotrexate	generics	RECONSTITUTE POWDER IMMEDIATELY BEFORE USE AND DISCARD ANY UNUSED PORTION—methotrexate	
	pemetrexed	Alimta	DO NOT DRINK ALCOHOLIC BEVERAGES AVOID PROLONGED EXPOSURE TO SUNLIGHT AVOID PREGNANCY EXERCISE PRECAUTIONS FOR HANDLING, PREPARING, AND ADMINISTERING CYTOTOXIC DRUGS REFRIGERATE AND USE WITHIN 24 HOURS OF RECONSTITUTION; DISCARD ANY UNUSED PORTION—pemetrexed	
	6-mercaptopurine	Purinethol	AVOID ASPIRIN AND NSAIDs	
	6-thioguanine	Tabloid	AVOID PREGNANCY TAKE AS DIRECTED; DON'T SKIP DOSES	
	Vinca Alkaloids			
	vinorelbine	Navelbine	REFRIGERATE; DO NOT FREEZE—vinorelbine DILUTED SOLUTION IS STABLE FOR 24 HOURS	
	vinblastine	Generics	AVOID ASPIRIN AND NSAIDs—vinblastine, vinorelbine	
	vincristine	Vincasar PFS	EXERCISE PRECAUTIONS FOR HANDLING, PREPARING, AND ADMINISTERING CYTOTOXIC DRUGS Syringes must be labeled: "FATAL IF GIVEN INTRATHECALLY. FOR IV USE ONLY."	
	Platinum Compounds			
	carboplatin	Generics	RECONSTITUTED SOLUTION IS STABLE FOR 24 HOURS—(IV INFUSION IS STABLE FOR 8 HOURS) EXERCISE PRECAUTIONS FOR HANDLING, PREPARING, AND ADMINISTERING CYTOTOXIC DRUGS	
	cisplatin	Platinol AQ	STABLE FOR 28 DAYS ONCE VIAL IS PENETRATED PROTECT FROM LIGHT	
	oxaliplatin	Eloxatin	RECONSTITUTED SOLUTION AND IVs ARE STABLE FOR 24 HOURS IF REFRIGERATED	
	Topoisomerase Inhibitors			
	etoposide	VePesid	RECONSTITUTED SOLUTION IS STABLE FOR 24 HOURS	
	teniposide	Vumon	EXERCISE PRECAUTIONS FOR HANDLING, PREPARING, AND ADMINISTERING CYTOTOXIC DRUGS	
	irinotecan	Camptosar	RECONSTITUTED SOLUTION IS STABLE FOR 48 HOURS if refrigerated—(STABLE FOR 6 HOURS if not refrigerated)—irinotecan	
	topotecan	Hycamtin	RECONSTITUTED SOLUTION IS STABLE FOR 24 HOURS—(IV INFUSION IS STABLE FOR 8 HOURS)—topotecan EXERCISE PRECAUTIONS FOR HANDLING, PREPARING, AND ADMINISTERING CYTOTOXIC DRUGS	
	Miscellaneous			
	actinomycin D (dactinomycin)	Cosmegen	EXERCISE PRECAUTIONS FOR HANDLING, PREPARING, AND ADMINISTERING CYTOTOXIC DRUGS	
	bleomycin	Blenoxane	RECONSTITUTED SOLUTION IS STABLE FOR 24 HOURS	
	mitomycin C	Mitozytrex	REFRIGERATE; DO NOT FREEZE—bleomycin powder EXERCISE PRECAUTIONS FOR HANDLING, PREPARING, AND ADMINISTERING CYTOTOXIC DRUGS MAY DISCOLOR URINE—mitomycin C	
	hydroxyurea	Droxia	TAKE WITH LOTS OF WATER AVOID ASPIRIN AND NSAIDs	

*Protocols vary for Dose and Dosing Schedule depending on the site of the cancer; see manufacturer recommendations and institutional protocol.

CHAPTER SUMMARY

- Cancer is a disease that occurs when new cells form more rapidly than needed; the cells accumulate and form a mass called a tumor.
- A malignant tumor is cancerous and can invade and destroy nearby tissue and spread to other parts of the body, whereas a benign tumor is not cancerous and does not spread.
- Cancers are named according to the site where the cancerous growth began. This is the site of the primary tumor.
- Age; tobacco smoking or chewing; ionizing radiation and sunlight; hazardous chemicals; environmental pollutants; bacterial and viral infection; hormone therapy; family history; alcohol consumption; and diet, obesity, and lack of physical activity are all risk factors for cancer.
- Advancing age (>61 years) and a history of hormone replacement therapy increase the risk for breast cancer.
- The mortality rate for breast cancer is about 25 per 100,000 women accounting for 40,460 deaths in 2007.
- Mammogram and breast self-examination are important screening examinations used to detect breast cancer.
- Cancer of the cervix is linked to human papillomavirus and exposure to the drug diethystilbesterol.
- A Pap smear is a screening test for cancer of the cervix.
- Endometrial cancer most commonly affects postmenopausal women.
- Skin cancer is one of the most common types of cancer.
- Skin cancer is divided into two categories: melanoma and nonmelanoma. The most treatable form is nonmelanoma.
- Skin cancer is associated with excessive exposure to ultraviolet light, from either the sun or UV lights used in tanning salons. Wearing protective clothing or using sunscreens when outdoors is recommended.
- Lung cancer is the most common form of cancer with nearly 213,000 newly diagnosed individuals in 2007.
- There are two types of lung cancer. They are small cell lung cancer and non–small cell lung cancer.
- A history of smoking tobacco is nearly always the cause of small cell lung cancer.
- Colonoscopy and the fecal occult blood test are screening tests for colorectal cancer.
- The incidence of prostate cancer increases as men grow older.
- Screening tests are recommended for early diagnosis of breast cancer, colorectal cancer, cancer of the cervix, and prostate cancer.
- A digital rectal examination and a PSA test are screening tests for prostate cancer.
- Staging is a method used to describe how far the cancer has progressed within the body.
- Cancer may be treated with chemotherapy, biological therapy, radiation therapy, and surgery.
- Chemotherapy is the use of drugs to kill of slow the growth of cancerous cells.
- Biological therapy is the administration of immune system modulators to boost the body's natural defense against abnormal, invasive, and cancerous cells.
- Factors influencing the choice for treatment are (1) type of cancer, (2) the stage of cancer, (3) individual tolerance for adverse effects of treatment, (4) patient's age, (5) histologic and nuclear grade of the primary tumor, and (6) the capacity of the cancer to metastasize.
- The hormones estrogen and progesterone can promote the growth of estrogen-receptor positive (ER-positive) and/or progesterone-receptor positive (PR-positive) breast cancer.
- Antiestrogens are used in the treatment of ER-positive breast cancer.
- Tamoxifen and toremifene are selective estrogen-receptor modulators that are indicated for the treatment of estrogen-receptor positive breast cancer.
- Women taking tamoxifen have a 2 to 7 times increase risk for endometrial cancer than women who did not take tamoxifen.

- Tamoxifen and most other antineoplastic agents are classified in FDA pregnancy risk category D. The warning label AVOID PREGNANCY should be applied to the prescription vial.
- Fulvestrant is an ER downregulator that is approved for the treatment of breast cancer.
- A common ending for aromatase inhibitors is *"-trozole."*
- Anastrozole, exemestane, and letrozole are aromatase inhibitors approved for the treatment of breast cancer.
- Goserelin is a gonadotropin-releasing hormone agonist that is indicated for the treatment of advanced breast cancer in premenopausal and perimenopausal women with ER-positive disease.
- Megestrol acetate is a progestin that is approved for the treatment breast cancer.
- Medroxyprogesterone acetate is approved for treatment of inoperable, metastatic endometrial cancer, and renal cell cancer.
- Cyclophosphamide (Cytoxan), busulfan (Busulfex, Myleran), ifosfamide (Ifex), melphalan (Alkeran), mechlorethamine (Mustargen), and chlorambucil (Leukeran) are all akylating agents.
- A common ending for taxanes is *"-taxel."*
- Taxanes are cytotoxic drugs that are naturally derived from the Western Yew (paclitaxel) and the European Yew (docetaxel) trees.
- Vinorelbine, vincristine, and vinblastine are vinca alkaloids. They are naturally derived from the periwinkle plant. A common beginning for vinca alkaloids is "vin-".
- A common ending for anthracyclines is *"-rubicin."*
- Doxorubicin, epirubicin, and idarubicin are anthracyclines. Mitoxantrone is a related compound and is classified as an anthracenedione.
- Doxorubicin and epirubicin are indicated for the treatment of breast cancer.
- Doxorubicin liposomal and is approved for the treatment of ovarian cancer, Kaposi's sarcoma, and multiple myeloma.
- The anthracyclines may turn urine and nails red, whereas mitoxantrone causes them to turn blue-green.
- Common endings for topoisomerase inhibitors are *"-poside"* and *"-tecan."*
- Etoposide, teniposide, irinotecan, and topotecan are topoisomerase inhibitors.
- Teniposide is approved for the treatment of acute lymphocytic leukemia. Topotecan is indicated for the treatment of ovarian, cervical, and small cell lung cancer. Irinotecan is only indicated for the treatment of colorectal cancer.
- Platinum compounds have the common ending *"-platin."*
- Cisplatin is approved for the treatment of testicular and ovarian cancer, carboplatin is approved for the treatment of ovarian cancer, and oxalipatin is approved for the treatment of colorectal cancer.
- Capecitabine, cytarabine, gemcitabine, and 5-fluorouracil (5-FU) are fluoropyrimidines, also known as fluorinated pyrimidines.
- Antimetabolites are chemotherapeutic agents that work by inhibiting normal DNA synthesis by forming abnormal nucleic acid base-pairs, resulting in abnormal DNA.
- Pentostatin, 6-mercaptopurine, and 6-thioguanine are purine analogs. Purine bases, along with pyrimidine bases, make up the DNA strand.
- Bleomycin, dactinomycin, and mitomycin are antineoplastic agents that are approved for the treatment of various cancers. They interfere with DNA, RNA, and protein synthesis.
- Trastuzumab (Herceptin) is a monoclonal antibody that are used in the treatment of metastatic breast cancer.

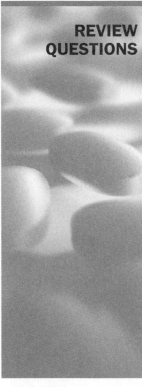

REVIEW QUESTIONS

Multiple Choice

1. Leukemia is cancer that starts in the _____.
    a. immune systems
    b. bones
    c. blood-forming tissues
    d. skin

2. Cancerous tumors that can invade and destroy nearby tissue and spread to other parts of the body are termed _____.
    a. benign
    b. malignant
    c. invasive
    d. tumors

3. Cancers are more prevalent in persons over the age of 65.
    a. true
    b. false

4. Cancer of the cervix is linked to the _____.
    a. herpes simples virus
    b. human immunodeficiency virus
    c. varicella zoster virus
    d. human papillomavirus

5. Early diagnosis is really not that critical for successful treatment of cancer.
    a. true
    b. false

6. Cancer may be treated with _____.
    a. chemotherapy
    b. biological therapy
    c. radiation therapy
    d. all of the above

7. Hormone therapy is a treatment of choice for _____ cancer.
    a. breast
    b. lung
    c. cervical
    d. skin

8. _____ are one of the oldest classes of antineoplastic agents. They are related to nitrogen mustard a lethal gas that was used for chemical warfare in World War I.
    a. Antimetabolites
    b. Antitumor antibiotics
    c. Akylating agents
    d. Hormones

9. Which one of the following is *not* a vinca alkaloid?
    a. vinorelbine
    b. vincristine
    c. vinblastine
    d. venlafaxine

10. These drugs commonly cause hair loss, photosensitivity, loss of appetite, and nausea. They also decrease white and red blood cells and platelets.
    a. methotrexate
    b. pemetrexed
    c. paclitaxel
    d. a and b

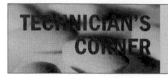

1. There have been many reports of the destruction of the rainforests and the possibility of losing potential cures for cancer. What can we do to prevent this from happening?
2. What are some new innovations being used to deliver chemotherapy doses that will not harm good cells?

BIBLIOGRAPHY

Gold Standard Inc., Clinical Pharmacology: Available at: http://www.clinicalpharmacology.com.

Health Canada Drug and Health Product Database. Available at: http://www.hc-sc.gc.ca/dhp-mps/prodpharma/databasdon/index_e.html.

Kalant H, Grant D, Mitchell J: *Principles of medical pharmacology* (pp 777-790), ed 7. Toronto, 2007, Elsevier Canada.

Lance L, Lacy C, Armstrong L, Goldman M: *Drug information handbook for the allied health professional,* ed 12. Hudson, OH, 2005, APhA Lexi-Comp.

National Cancer Institute: *Surveillance Epidemiology and End Results (SEER).* Available at: http://seer.cancer.gov/statfacts/html/lungb.html.

National Cancer Institute: *What you need to know about cancer,* Bethesda, MD, revised February 2005, National Institutes of Health, U.S. Department of Health and Human Services. NIH publication No. 06-1566. Available at: http://www.cancer.gov/publications.

Page C, Curtis M, Sutter M, Walker M, Hoffman B, et al.: *Integrated pharmacology* (pp 163-185), Philadelphia, 2005, Elsevier Mosby.

Thibodeau G, Patton K: *Anatomy and physiology,* ed 6 (pp 121-133), St. Louis, 2007, Mosby.

USP Center for Advancement of Patient Safety: *Use caution–avoid confusion,* USP Quality Review No. 79, Rockville, MD, April 2004, USP Center for Advancement of Patient Safety.

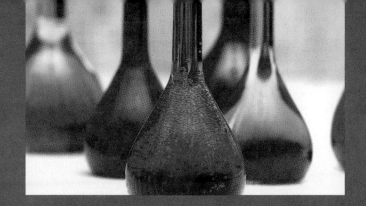

CHAPTER 38

Vaccines, Immunomodulators, and Immunosuppressants

LEARNING OBJECTIVES

- Learn the terminology associated with vaccines, immunomodulators, and immuno-suppressants.
- Describe how vaccines work.
- Describe types of vaccines.
- Discuss the importance of the "cold chain" and identify vaccines requiring cold storage.
- Provide examples of the pharmacy technician's role in maintaining the cold chain.
- List procedures that must be followed if the cold chain is broken.
- List and categorize immunosuppressants.
- Describe mechanism of action for immunosuppressants.
- Identify warning labels and precautionary messages associated with selected vaccines, immunomodulators, and immunosuppressants.
- Identify significant drug look-alike/sound-alike issues.
- List common endings for selected vaccines, immunomodulators, and immunosuppressants.

KEY TERMS

Cold chain: Set of safe handling practices that ensure vaccines and immunologicals requiring refrigeration are maintained at the required temperature from the time of manufacture until the time of administration to patients.

Conjugate vaccine: Vaccine that links antigens or toxoids to the polysaccharide or sugar molecules that certain bacteria use as a protective device to disguise themselves.

Immunosuppressants: Drugs that inhibit proliferation of the cells of the immune system; also known as immunopharmacologicals.

Immunization: Deliberate, artificial exposure to disease to produce acquired immunity.

Inactivated, killed vaccine: Killed vaccine. It provides less immunity than live vaccines but has fewer risks for vaccine-induced disease.

Live, attenuated vaccine: Living, but weakened, version of the invader that does not cause disease (nonvirulent).

Toxoid vaccine: Vaccine that stimulates the immune system to produce antibodies to a specific toxin that causes illness.

Vaccine: Substance that prevents disease by taking advantage of your body's ability to make antibodies and release "killer" cells to disease.

OVERVIEW

An *immunization* is defined as a deliberate, artificial exposure to disease to produce acquired immunity. Immunization is achieved by administering vaccines. Vaccines prevent disease by taking advantage of your body's ability to make antibodies and release "killer" cells to disease-causing microbes and viruses that attack it. Under normal circumstances, cells of your immune system can distinguish between the cells that are part of your body, harmless bacteria normally found in your body, and harmful invaders that need to be destroyed. The first time your body is exposed to a harmful virus, the immune system releases macrophages, cytotoxic T cells, and B cells. The macrophages digest most parts of the viruses but save the antigens. B cells secrete antibodies to the antigens and if the person is exposed to the virus again, the antibodies will attack. Cytotoxic T cells designed to destroy the virus are also released upon exposure to antigens. A vaccine is an altered antigen injected into your body that does not cause disease but stimulates your immune system's production of antibodies and cytotoxic T cells, and therefore provides protection against the disease should you be exposed to it again.

Types of Vaccines

Live, attenuated vaccines are a living, but weakened, version of the invader, so they do not cause disease (nonvirulent). They can mutate to a virulent strain of the virus. Polio, measles, mumps, and rubella vaccines are live vaccines. *Inactivated, killed vaccines* are advantageous because they cannot mutate but they produce less immunity than live vaccines. Booster shots are usually required to ensure continued immunity. Flu, hepatitis A, and polio vaccines are inactivated, killed vaccines. *Toxoid vaccines* stimulate the immune system to produce antibodies to the toxins that cause illness (e.g., tetanus and diphtheria). *Conjugate vaccines* link antigens or toxoids to the polysaccharide or sugar molecules that certain bacteria use as a protective device to disguise themselves. Conjugate vaccines allow the immune system to recognize and attack these "disguised" bacteria. *Haemophilus influenzae* type B (Hib) is a conjugate vaccine.

Special Handling Conditions for Vaccines

THE "COLD CHAIN"

Vaccines and immunologicals requiring refrigeration (Box 38-1) must be protected from extremes in temperature. Exposure to freezing temperatures or heat can destroy their integrity and make them unusable.

The cold chain refers to a set of safe handling practices that ensure vaccines and immunologicals requiring refrigeration are maintained at required temperature from the time of manufacture until the time of administration to patients. This means that they must be maintained at a constant temperature between 2°C to 8°C throughout the transport process and placed in appropriate store units once they are delivered to their final destination.

TECH ALERT!
Pharmacies, pharmacists, and pharmacy technicians play a key role in ensuring that breaches in the cold chain are avoided.

BOX 38-1 VACCINES REQUIRING REFRIGERATION (2°C TO 8°C)

- Diphtheria and tetanus toxoids (DT)
- Diphtheria and tetanus toxoids, and pertussis (adsorbed) (DPT)
- Diphtheria toxoid + hepatitis B surface antigen + pertussis vaccine (adsorbed) + poliovirus vaccine (inactivated) + tetanus toxoid
- Diphtheria and tetanus toxoids, adsorbed pertussis vaccine (adsorbed), inactivated polio vaccine and *Haemophilus influenzas* type b (Hib) conjugate vaccine
- Hepatitis A vaccine
- Hepatitis B vaccine

- Hib conjugate vaccine
- Inactivated polio vaccine
- Influenza vaccine
- Measles, mumps, and rubella (MMR) vaccine
- Meningicoccal A/C/Y/W vaccine
- Pneumococcal polysaccharide 7-polyvalent vaccine
- Pneumococcal polysaccharide 23-polvalent vaccine
- Rabies vaccine
- Tuberculosis testing solution
- Varicella vaccine

WHY COLD STORAGE IS IMPORTANT

Disruption of the cold chain is a public health threat. When the cold chain is disrupted, the effectiveness and shelf-life of vaccines are reduced. The stability of the vaccine decreases exponentially with each increase in temperature. Once the integrity of the vaccine is compromised, it cannot be restored by returning the vaccine to the refrigerator. Loss of potency and effectiveness are cumulative. Each time the cold chain is breached, the vaccine's effectiveness is further reduced. Ultimately, patients are placed at risk when suboptimal vaccines are administered. In addition to vaccine failure, patients may experience increased reactions at the injection site. The severity of problems linked to disruption of the cold chain is dependent on whether the vaccine is chemical or biological and whether the dosage form is aqueous solution, suspension, or dry powder. Dry powders and chemicals are least affected by breaches in the cold chain. Vaccines and other biological solutions and suspensions are most sensitive to breaches in the cold chain. They are more sensitive to degradation. Disruption of the cold chain is also very costly. Vaccines that expire or that have been stored improperly must be destroyed.

COLD CHAIN MAINTENANCE

Maintenance of the cold chain involves appropriate selection and maintenance of refrigeration units and transport containers capable of storing drug products at required temperatures.

REFRIGERATION UNITS

When feasible, the pharmacy should place vaccines in a refrigerator designated solely to vaccines. If a separate refrigerator is not feasible, vaccines should be segregated from other refrigerated pharmaceuticals. Pharmacies that handle a large volume of vaccines should purchase a walk-in refrigeration unit. If the refrigerator is overstocked, air circulation is insufficient to maintain constant temperatures. The refrigeration unit should be equipped with a minimum/maximum thermometer, to monitor temperature fluctuations and a continuous temperature-recording device. An alarm that signals when the refrigeration unit is out of range should be installed in the refrigerator. Monitors and thermometers should be calibrated routinely.

It is important to place the refrigerator in a location that is away for a heat source as this can affect the performance of the unit. The refrigerator cord should also be strategically placed to avoid accidental unplugging from the electrical outlet.

PROTOCOLS FOR RECEIVING, STOCKING, AND STORAGE

An important component of the cold chain is establishment and adherence to protocols for receiving, stocking, storage, and transport of drugs requiring refrigeration. The pharmacy team should develop these protocols in accordance with national guidelines. Protocols for receiving vaccines should include accurate assessment of the condition of vaccines received by the pharmacy. Pharmacy personnel should be alert for warning signs that the cold chain has been broken during shipment. This might be as simple as noticing that freezer packs have thawed or that dry ice placed in the transport container with polio vaccine has evaporated. Unfortunately, damage to the vaccines themselves, by exposure to heat or freezing, is not easy to detect. No changes in color or appearance occurs so visual indicators are unavailable. Shaking the vaccine may reveal clumps in the vaccine that indicate freezing; however, often no clumps are visible, making this method unreliable.

A procedure should be established to ensure that vaccines stocked are rotated to avoid wastage due to outdated supplies. Expiry dates should be checked and vaccines stocked so those that will expire soon are placed in front of vaccines that expire later. Vaccines should not be removed from the refrigerator until the time of dispensing or unless the vaccine must be transported. This is especially important for pneumococcal or influenza vaccines that are purchased in multidose vials.

TRANSPORT

Pharmacy personnel in charge of transporting vaccines are responsible for making sure that vaccines arrive at their destination at the proper temperature. The amount of time that the vaccine will be out of the refrigerator must be considered when determining the type of transport container. In most cases, vaccines should be transported in an insulated container. Protocols should be followed regarding the number of ice packs needed. Vaccines should always be positioned to avoid direct contact with the ice packs. Heat and cold monitors should also be included in the transport container if necessary.

Vaccines should be dispensed to patients with accurate advice for transport and storage. Extremes in heat and cold must be avoided so vaccines should never be placed in the hot glove compartment of a car. If the travel time between the pharmacy and the patient's destination, where a refrigerator is located, is less than 20 minutes, the vaccine should be dispensed in an insulated bag. If transport time is greater than 20 minutes, the vaccine should be transported with ice packs in an insulated container. See Figure 38-1 for a diagram explaining the importance of the pharmacy technician in cold chain management.

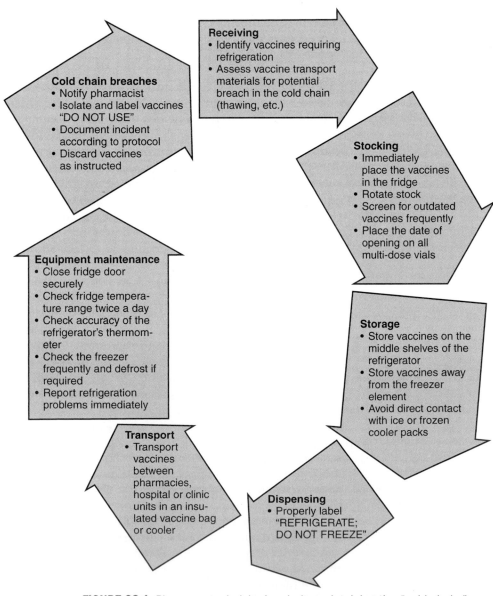

FIGURE 38-1 Pharmacy technician's role in maintaining the "cold chain."

Immunizations

Vaccines are administered to provide immunity to a wide variety of childhood diseases, such as influenza, hepatitis, pneumonia, viral meningitis, rabies, and other conditions. Sufficient immunity may be achieved after a single immunization; however, many vaccines must be administered as a series or require a "booster shot." Epidemiologists track flu infections from sentinel sites around the globe to determine which strains of the flu virus are most virulent. Vaccines are developed for the most infectious strains of the virus. Flu vaccines are must be reformulated each year. Please see Figures 38-2, 38-3, and 38-4 for age-specific immunization schedules recommended by the Centers for Disease Control and Prevention (CDC).

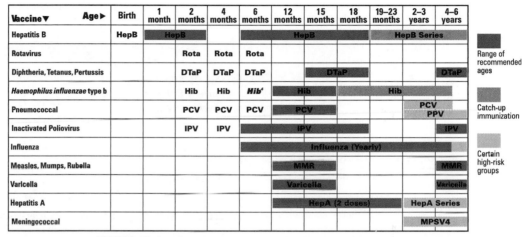

FIGURE 38-2 Recommended immunization schedule for persons aged 0-6 years. *(Courtesy Centers for Disease Control and Prevention, Atlanta, GA. Available at http://www.cdc.gov.)*

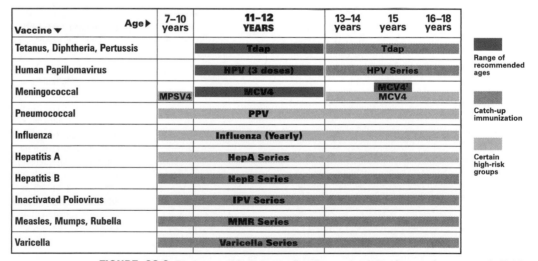

FIGURE 38-3 Recommended immunization schedule for persons aged 7-18 years. *(Courtesy Centers for Disease Control and Prevention, Atlanta, GA. Available at http://www.cdc.gov.)*

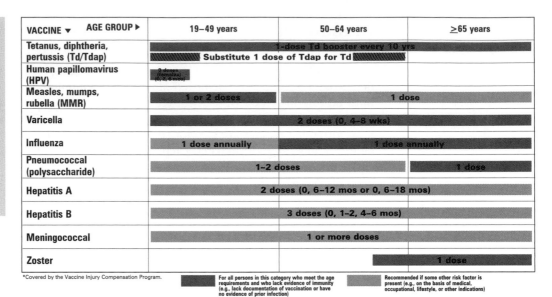

VACCINE ▼ AGE GROUP ►	19–49 years	50–64 years	≥65 years
Tetanus, diphtheria, pertussis (Td/Tdap)	1-dose Td booster every 10 yrs		
	Substitute 1 dose of Tdap for Td		
Human papillomavirus (HPV)	3 doses (females) (0, 2, 6 mos)		
Measles, mumps, rubella (MMR)	1 or 2 doses	1 dose	
Varicella	2 doses (0, 4–8 wks)		
Influenza	1 dose annually	1 dose annually	
Pneumococcal (polysaccharide)	1–2 doses		1 dose
Hepatitis A	2 doses (0, 6–12 mos or 0, 6–18 mos)		
Hepatitis B	3 doses (0, 1–2, 4–6 mos)		
Meningococcal	1 or more doses		
Zoster			1 dose

*Covered by the Vaccine Injury Compensation Program.

■ For all persons in this category who meet the age requirements and who lack evidence of immunity (e.g., lack documentation of vaccination or have no evidence of prior infection)

■ Recommended if some other risk factor is present (e.g., on the basis of medical, occupational, lifestyle, or other indications)

FIGURE 38-4 Recommended adult immunization schedule, by vaccine and age group. *(Courtesy Centers for Disease Control and Prevention, Atlanta, GA. Available at http://www.cdc.gov.)*

Selected Vaccines, Dosage Forms, and Strength

Generic name	U.S. brand name(s) / Canadian brand(s)	Dosage forms and strengths
diphtheria and tetanus toxoids (Td)	DECAVAC (Adult) / TD Adsorbed	**Suspension for injection (all):** **DECAVAC prefilled syringe:** diphtheria toxoid (adsorbed) 2 Lf/0.5 ml + tetanus toxoid (adsorbed) 5 Lf/0.5 ml **pediatric suspension:** diphtheria toxoid (adsorbed) 6.7 Lf/0.5 ml + tetanus toxoid (adsorbed) 5 Lf/0.5 ml
diphtheria and tetanus toxoids, and pertussis (acellular) (Tdap)	Infanrix, Adacel, Boostrix, Daptacel, Tripedia / Adacel, Boostrix	**Suspension for injection (all):** **Infanrix:** diphtheria toxoid (adsorbed) 25 Lf/0.5 ml + pertussis (adsorbed) 58 mcg/0.5 ml + tetanus toxoid (adsorbed) 10 Lf/0.5 ml **Adacel:** diphtheria toxoid (adsorbed) 2 Lf/0.5 ml + pertussis (adsorbed) 2.5 mcg/0.5 ml + tetanus toxoid (adsorbed) 5 Lf/0.5 ml **Boostrix:** diphtheria toxoid (adsorbed) 2.5 Lf/0.5 ml + pertussis (adsorbed) 18.5 mcg/0.5 ml + tetanus toxoid (adsorbed) 5 Lf/0.5 ml **Daptacel:** diphtheria toxoid (adsorbed) 15 Lf/0.5 ml + pertussis (adsorbed) 23 mcg/0.5 ml + tetanus toxoid (adsorbed) 5 Lf/0.5 ml **Tripedia:** diphtheria toxoid (adsorbed) 6.7 Lf/0.5 ml + pertussis (adsorbed) 46 mcg/0.5 ml + tetanus toxoid (adsorbed) 5 Lf/0.5 ml
diphtheria toxoid, + hepatitis B surface antigen + pertussis vaccine (adsorbed) + poliovirus vaccine (inactivated) + tetanus toxoid	Pediarix / Not available	**Pediarix:** diphtheria toxoid (adsorbed) 25 Lf/0.5 ml + hepatitis B surface antigen 10 mcg/0.5 ml + pertussis (adsorbed) 58 mcg/0.5 ml + poliovirus vaccine (inactivated) 80 DAgU/ 0.5 ml + tetanus toxoid (adsorbed) 10 Lf/0.5 ml

Selected Vaccines, Dosage Forms, and Strength—cont'd

Generic name	U.S. brand name(s) Canadian brand(s)	Dosage forms and strengths
diphtheria + tetanus toxoids, adsorbed + pertussis vaccine (acellular), 1 *Haemophilus influenzae* type b (Hib) conjugate vaccine	ActHIB with Tripedia Trihibit Not available	**Powder for injection:** Diphtheria toxoid adsorbed: 6.7 Lf/0.5 ml **Haemophilus B conjugate vaccine:** 10 mcg **Pertussis vaccine (adsorbed):** 46.8 mcg/0.5 ml **Tetanus toxoid (adsorbed):** 5 Lf/0.5 ml
Hib conjugate vaccine	PedvaxHIB PedvaxHIB	**Solution for injection:** **Haemophilus B conjugate vaccine:** 7.5 mcg/0.5 ml
inactivated polio vaccine	IPOL Imovax Polio	**Suspension for injection:** **Poliovirus vaccine (inactivated) (Mahoney):** 40 D antigen units/0.5 ml **Poliovirus vaccine (inactivated) (MEF-1):** 8 D antigen units/0.5 ml **Poliovirus vaccine (inactivated) (Saukett):** 32 D antigen units/0.5 ml
measles, mumps and rubella (MMR) vaccine	MMR II MMR II	**Powder for injection solution:** **Measles virus vaccine (live attenuated):** 1000 TCID **Mumps virus vaccine (live):** 20,000 TCID **Rubella virus vaccine (live):** 1000 TCID
hepatitis A vaccine (inactivated)	Havrix, VAQTA Avaxim, Havrix, VAQTA	**Suspension for injection (Havrix):** **Hepatitis A vaccine:** 720 ELU/0.5 ml (pediatric) **Hepatitis A vaccine:** 1440 ELU/ml **Solution for injection (VAQTA):** **Hepatitis A vaccine:** 50 units/ml **Hepatitis A vaccine:** 25 units/0.5 ml (pediatric) **Suspension for injection:** (Avaxim): **Hepatitis A vaccine:** 160 units/0.5 ml
hepatitis B vaccine	Energix-B, Recombivax Energix-B, Recombivax HB, Recombivax HB- Adult	**Suspension for injection (Energix-B):** **Hepatitis B virus vaccine (recombinant):** 10 mcg/0.5 ml (pediatric) **Hepatitis B surface antigen (recombivax):** 10 mcg/1 ml, 5 mcg/0.5 ml, 40 mcg/ml
influenza vaccine	Fluarix, Flulaval not available	**Suspension for injection:** **Influenza virus vaccine (avian):** 45 mcg/0.5 ml (Fluarix) **Influenza virus vaccine trivalent:** 45 mcg/0.5 ml (Flulaval, Fluzone)
meningicoccal vaccine	Menomune A/C/Y/W-135 Menomune A/C/Y/W-135	**Powder for injection:** **Meningococcal polysaccharide vaccine A:** 50 mcg **Meningococcal polysaccharide vaccine C:** 50 mcg **Meningococcal polysaccharide vaccine W135:** 50 mcg **Meningococcal polysaccharide vaccine Y:** 50 mcg
pneumococcal polysaccharide 7-polyvalent vaccine	Prevnar Prevnar	**Suspension for injection:** Pneumococcal polysaccharide-7 isolates 2 mcg of saccharide serotypes 4, 9V, 14, 18C, 19F, and 23F; 4 mcg of serotype 6B per dose; 20 mcg of CRM197.
pneumococcal polysaccharide 23-polyvalent vaccine	Pneumovax 23 Pneumovax 23	**Solution for Injection:** Pneumococcal polysaccharide-23 polyvalent 25 mcg /0.5mL

*D.C.O. = diploid cell origin

Continued

Selected Vaccines, Dosage Forms, and Strength—cont'd

	Generic name	U.S. brand name(s) Canadian brand(s)	Dosage forms and strengths
	rabies vaccine	Imovax, Rabavert	**Powder for injection:** **Rabies vaccine:** 2.5 units
		Imovax rabies, Rabavert	
	varicella vaccine (live)	Varivax	**Powder for injection:** **Varicella virus vaccine live:** 1350 units/0.5 ml
		Varivax III	
	varicella virus vaccine live + rubella virus vaccine (live) + mumps virus vaccine (live) + measles virus vaccine (live attenuated)	ProQuad	**Powder for injection:** **Measles virus vaccine (live attenuated):** 1000 TCID50 **Mumps virus vaccine (live):** 20,000 TCID50 **Rubella virus vaccine (live):** 1000 TCID50 **Varicella virus vaccine live:** 9772 units
		Not available	

Immunosupressants

Immunosuppressants inhibit proliferation of the cells of the immune system. They are also known as immunopharmacological drugs. Their actions may be cell specific or nonspecific. Antineoplastic and cytotoxic drugs, also called chemotherapeutic agents, generally act against any type of proliferating cell and are used in the treatment of a variety of cancers. Drugs that have their primary action on cells of the immune system are used in the treatment of autoimmune diseases, such as multiple sclerosis, rheumatoid arthritis, systemic lupus erythematosus (see Chapter 15), and Crohn's disease (see Chapter 27). They are also used to prevent tissue or organ rejection after transplant surgery. When drugs that are immune cell specific are used in the treatment of cancers, they are typically administered in high doses and 3- to 6-week intervals.

Corticosteroids, antineoplastics, cyclosporine, macrolides, mycophenolate mofetil, antithymocyte globulin (ATG), monoclonal antibodies, intravenous γ-globulin (IVIg), Rh_o [D] immunglobulin, and cytokine inhibitors are all categorized as immunopharmacologicals. Drugs that specifically target cells of the immune system are discussed in this chapter. Antineoplastic agents are described in Chapter 37.

CYCLOSPORINE

Cyclosporine is produced by a fungus (*Tolypocladium inflatum*) and is used to improve survival rates for individuals with organ transplants. It suppresses cell destruction in graft-versus-host reactions.

MECHANISM OF ACTION AND PHARMACOKINETICS

Cyclosporine acts on T-lymphocyte cells. It blocks cellular activation of mature immunocompetent T cells and suppresses immune interferon (IFN)γ and other macrophage growth factors. Cyclosporine is formulated as capsules, modified and nonmodified oral solutions, and solution for injection. Cyclosporine-modified solution has greater absorption than capsules. Cyclosporine inhibits CYP450 microsomal pathways, which are responsible for several drug interactions.

ADVERSE REACTIONS

Adverse reactions of cyclosporine include acne, bleeding or tender gums, overgrowth of gum tissue, diarrhea, hirsuitism, headache, leg cramps, anorexia, nausea and vomiting, and tremors. More serious adverse reactions are nephrotoxicity, neurotoxicity, and seizures. Because cyclosporine is an immunosuppressant, it can increase risk for infections.

TECH ALERT!
Cyclosporine oral liquid *nonmodified* (Sandimmune) is NOT substitutable with cyclosporine oral liquid *modified* (Neoral, Gengraf).

Cyclosporine

Generic name	U.S. brand name(s)	Dosage forms and strengths
	Canadian brand(s)	
cyclosporine*	Gengraf, Neoral, Pulminiq, Restasis, Sandimmune	**Capsule:** 25 mg, 100 mg **Solution, inhalation (Pulminiq):** 300 mg/4.8 ml **Solution, Injection:** 50 mg/ml, 250 mg/5 ml
	Neoral, Sandimune	**Solution, oral:** 100 mg/ml **Emulsion, ophthalamic (Restasis):** 0.05%

*Generic available.

TECH ALERT!
A common ending for macrolides used for immunosuppression is "-limus."

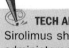

TECH ALERT!
Sirolimus should not be administered with 4 hours of cyclosporine.

MACROLIDES

Tacrolimus is another immunosuppressant that is derived from a fungus (*Streptomyces tsukubaensis*). Both tacrolimus and sirolimus are classified as macrolides. Like cyclosporine, they are used to prevent transplant rejections. Tacrolimus ointment is used for the treatment of eczema (see Chapter 42).

MECHANISM OF ACTION AND PHARMACOKINETICS

Tacrolimus inhibits the enzyme that is involved in gene transcription of interleukins (IL-2), interferons (INFγ), and cytokines. It interferes with the first phase of T-cell activation. Tacrolimus is more potent than cyclosporine. Sirolimus interferes with a key enzyme that regulates the second phase of T-cell activation and proliferation. It decreases levels of IgM, IgG, and IgA.

Sirolimus tablets and oral solution are not bioequivalent and so are not substitutable. A meal high in fats can reduce the absorption of tacrolimus and sirolimus.

ADVERSE REACTIONS

Tacrolimus and sirolimus may produce gastrointestinal adverse reactions such as diarrhea or constipation, loss of appetite, nausea, and vomiting. Other side effects are difficulty sleeping, nightmares, dizziness or drowsiness, hair loss or unusual hair growth, headache, mood changes, depression, confusion, muscle cramps, tremor, and unusual sensitivity to touch. More serious adverse reactions include seizures, hepatitis, and hemolytic anemias.

Macrolides

Generic name	U.S. brand name(s)	Dosage forms and strengths
	Canadian brand(s)	
sirolimus	Rapamune	**Solution, oral:** 1 mg/ml
	Rapamune	**Tablet:** 1 mg, 2 mg
tacrolimus	Prograf, Protopic	**Capsule:** 0.5 mg, 1 mg, 5 mg
	Prograf, Protopic	**Solution, injection:** 5 mg/ml **Ointment (Protopic):** 0.03%, 0.1%

ANTITHYMOCYTE GLOBULIN (ATG)

ATG is prepared by immunizing horses or rabbits with human thymocytes. The resulting horse immune globins (Atgam) or rabbit immune globulins (Thymoglobulin) that fight against human T cells are then collected and purified. ATG is primarily administered to reduce rejection associated with organ and bone marrow transplantation.

MECHANISM OF ACTION AND PHARMACOKINETICS

ATG reduces the number of T-cell lymphocytes. T-cell depletion persists for several days following a single dose of ATG and takes approximately 2 months before T-cell levels return to normal.

ADVERSE REACTIONS

Side effects associated with ATG administration are fever, chills, leukopenia, and skin rash. Additional adverse reactions are headache, dizziness, tiredness, and diarrhea.

Antithymocyte Globulin

Generic name	U.S. brand name(s)	Dosage forms and strengths
	Canadian brand(s)	
antithymocyte globulin	Atgam, Thymoglobulin	**Powder for injection:** 25 mg
	Atgam, Thymoglobulin	**Solution, injection:** 50 mg/ml

MYCOPHENOLATE MOFETIL

Mycophenolate is used in conjunction with corticosteroids and cyclosporine to decrease the rejection of transplanted organs.

MECHANISM OF ACTION AND PHARMACOKINETICS

Mycophenolate mofetil is a prodrug. It is metabolized to mycophenolic acid. Mycophenolic acid is an immunosuppressive agent that inhibits the enzyme required for synthesis of purines needed for T-cell and B-cell proliferation.

ADVERSE REACTIONS

Gastrointestinal side effects are common and include constipation, diarrhea or soft stools, gas, loss of appetite, nausea, vomiting, stomach pain, or indigestion. Mycophenolate mofetil, like other immunosuppressives, can increase the risk of bacterial and viral infections. Other serious adverse effects are leukopenia, infections, lymphomas, and other malignancies.

Mycophenolate Mofetil

Generic name	U.S. brand name(s)	Dosage forms and strengths
	Canadian brand(s)	
mycophenolate mofetil	CellCept, Myfortic	**Capsule:** 250 mg
	CellCept, Myfortic	**Powder for injection:** 500 mg
		Powder for oral suspension: 200 mg/ml
		Tablet: 500 mg
		Tablet, delayed release (Myfortic): 180 mg, 360 mg

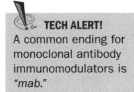

TECH ALERT!
A common ending for monoclonal antibody immunomodulators is *"mab."*

MONOCLONAL ANTIBODIES

Basiliximab, daclizumab, and muromonab are monoclonal antibody immunomodulators that are used to reduce transplant rejections and to prolong the life of transplanted organs. They are active against a variety of leukocyte surface antigens including CD3, CD4 (T-helper cells), and T-cell activation markers (IL-2, CD20, and CD25). Muromonab CD3 is administered with cyclosporine to reduce transplant rejections. Basiliximab is used to prolong the life of transplanted organs. Additional monoclonal antibody immunomodulators are described in Chapters 15 and 37.

MECHANISM OF ACTION

Basiliximab binds to and blocks the interleukin-2 receptor α-chain receptor (IL-2Rα), also known as CD25 antigen. *Daclizumab* blocks T-cell activation by binding to the α subunit of the interleukin (IL)-2 receptor (IL-2Rα) and inhibiting the binding of IL-2 to IL-2Rα. *Muromonab-CD3* blocks T-cell functions by binding to T lymphocytes that lead to cytokine release and T-cell activation.

ADVERSE REACTIONS

Administration of basiliximab, daclizumab, muromonab, and other monoclonal antibody immunomodulators may produce nausea, stomach pain, headache, redness, itching at the site of infusion, chest pain, hypertension, dyspnea, increased susceptibility to opportunistic infections, reactivation of dormant infections (e.g., TB), or worsening of existing infection.

Monoclonal Antibody Immunomodulators

Generic name	U.S. brand name(s) Canadian brand(s)	Dosage forms and strengths
basiliximab	Simulect	**Powder for injection:** 10 mg, 20 mg
	Simulect	
daclizumab	Zenapax	**Solution, injection:** 5 mg/ml
	Zenapax	
muromonab-CD3	Orthoclone OKT3	**Solution, injection:** 5 mg/5 ml
	Orthoclone OKT3	

INTRAVENOUS γ-IMMUNE GLOBULIN

Intravenous γ-immune globulin (IVIg) is collected from human plasma. It is classified as a biological response modifier. IVIg is used for the treatment of a variety of infections and chronic lymphatic leukemia. Immunoglobulins are described in the Unit 10 introduction.

Immunoglobulin IV

Generic name	U.S. brand name(s) Canadian brand(s)	Dosage forms and strengths
IV γ-immunoglobulin (IVIg)	Carimune NF, Gammagard, Iveegam, Panglobulin, Polygam S/D, Vigam	**Powder for injection (Carimune NF, Panglobulin):** 1 mg, 3 mg, 6 mg, 12 mg **Gammagard, Polygam, Vigam):** 5%, **(Iveegam):** 50 mg/ml
	Vivaglobulin	**Solution, injection (Gammagard):** 10%

RH₀ [D] IMMUNE GLOBULIN

Rh₀ [D] immune globulin is administered to pregnant women who are Rh negative who have been exposed to blood that is Rh negative. This may occur through exposure to fetal blood, amniocentesis, ectopic pregnancy, abdominal trauma during pregnancy, or whole blood transfusions. When an Rh incompatibility exists between the pregnant woman and the fetus, maternal antibodies are produced that act against fetal red blood cells. This condition is called erythroblastosis fetalis. It is a severe hemolytic disease of the fetus (see Unit 5 Introduction). Anti-D, administered within 72 hours of delivery, can prevent erythroblastosis fetalis in the fetus in a subsequent pregnancy.

MECHANISM OF ACTION AND PHARMACOKINETICS

Antibodies contained in Rh₀ [D] immune globulin interact directly with the Rh₀ [D] antigens, thereby preventing the interaction between the antigens and the maternal immune system. Rh₀ [D] immune globulin (Anti-D) opsonizes D+ red blood cells and blocks platelet destruction. It may cause immunosuppression by stimulating cytokines. It is formulated for intramuscular and intravenous administration.

ADVERSE REACTIONS

Side effects are headache, muscle aches and pains, pain and tenderness at the injection site chills, fever, and allergic reactions. Dizziness, weight gain, and difficulty breathing are additional side effects.

Rh₀ Immune Globulin

Generic name	U.S. brand name(s)	Dosage forms and strengths
	Canadian brand(s)	
Rh₀ immune globulin	HyperRHO S/D, MICRhoGAM, RhoGAM, WinRho SDF and Rhophylac	**Solution, IM injection only (HyperRHO S/D, MICRhoGAM, RhoGAM):** 50 mcg/ml **Powder for injection (WinRho SDF) for IM or IV:** 1500 international units per vial
	WinRho	**Solution for injection (Rhophylac):** 300 mcg/2 ml

CYTOKINE INHIBITORS

Enteracept is a genetically engineered inhibitor of tumor necrosis factor (TNF)-α. TNF-α inhibitors block the inflammatory process triggered by high concentrations of TNF. They prevent cell lysis (destruction) and release of the substances that cause inflammation. Anakinra is a genetically engineered interleukin 1 (IL-1) receptor antagonist. Anakinra interferes with the binding of interleukins that promote inflammatory responses. Drug-receptor binding results in fewer lymphocytes and macrophages in synovial fluid. Adverse reactions to anakinra include redness or irritation at injection site, infections, and bone or muscle weakness. Enteracept and ankinra are used in the treatment of rheumatoid arthritis and discussed in Chapter 15.

Interleukin Antagonists

Generic name	U.S. brand name(s)	Dosage forms and strengths
	Canadian brand(s)	
anakinra	Kineret	**Injection, solution:** 100 mg/0.67 ml (1 ml prefilled syringe)
	Kineret	

Tumor Necrosis Factor-α Inhibitors

Generic name	U.S. brand name(s)	Dosage forms and strengths
	Canadian brand(s)	
etanercept	Enbrel	**Injection, powder for reconstitution:** 25 mg **Injection, solution:** 50 mg/ml (0.98 ml prefilled syringe)
	Enbrel	

Summary of Immunosuppressant Drugs

Generic name	Brand name	Usual dose and dosing schedule	Warning labels
Cyclosporine			
cyclosporine	Neoral, Sandimmune	**Oral:** 15 mg/kg as a single dose 4 to 12 hours before transplantation. For maintenance therapy, continue initial daily in 2 divided doses or adjust dose downward. **IV:** 5 mg/kg to 6 mg/kg IV as a single dose 4 to 12 hours before transplantation as a slow infusion	AVOID PREGNANCY DILUTE ORAL SOLUTION IN LIQUID SWALLOW CAPSULES WHOLE, DON'T CRUSH OR CHEW AVOID GRAPEFRUIT JUICE DO NOT REFRIGERATE ORAL SOLUTION MUST BE USED WITHIN 2 MONTHS OF OPENING DISCARD DISCOLORED OR CLOUDY SOLUTION FOR INJECTION
Macrolides			
sirolimus	Rapamune	**Oral:** 6 mg as soon as possible following transplantation, then 2 mg PO once daily	AVOID GRAPEFRUIT JUICE DILUTE ORAL SOLUTION WITH WATER OR O.J. AVOID CONTACT WITH SKIN REFRIGERATE; DISCARD WITHIN 30 DAYS OF OPENING
tacrolimus	Prograf	**Oral:** 0.2 mg/kg/day in 2 divided doses, every 12 hours within 24 hours of transplantation **IV:** 0.03 mg/kg/day to 0.05 mg/kg/day continuous IV infusion within 24 hours of transplantation	AVOID GRAPEFRUIT JUICE TAKE ON AN EMPTY STOMACH
Antithymocyte Globulin			
antithymocyte globulin	Atgam	**Kidney transplantation:** 15 mg/kg/day IV given within 24 hours of the transplant, then once daily for the next 14 days **Bone marrow transplantation:** 10 mg/kg/day to 20 mg/kg/day IV infusion for 8 to 14 days, continuing with every-other-day dosing up to a total of 21 doses	GENTLY ROTATE SOLUTION; DO NOT SHAKE REFRIGERATE DILUTED SOLUTION
Mycophenolate Mofetil			
mycophenolate mofetil	CellCept	**Oral:** 1 g twice daily **IV:** 1 g IV over at least 2 hours twice daily given within 24 hours of the transplant	SHAKE WELL—suspension SWALLOW WHOLE; DON'T CRUSH OR CHEW TAKE ON AN EMPTY STOMACH STORE RECONSTITUTED SUSPENSION AT ROOM TEMPERATURE AND DISCARD IN 60 DAYS
Monoclonal Antibody Immunomodulators			
basiliximab	Simulect	20 mg IV 2 hours prior to transplantation, then 20 mg IV 4 days after transplantation	REFRIGERATE; DO NOT FREEZE PROTECT FROM LIGHT DO NOT SHAKE SOLUTION SHOULD BE USED WITHIN 4 HOURS OF PREPARATION—daclizumab, basiliximab
daclizumab	Zenapax	1 mg/kg IV up to 24 hours before transplantation, then 4 more doses of 1 mg/kg IV once every 2 weeks	
muromonab CD3	Orthoclone OKT3	5 mg IV once daily for 10 to 14 day	

Continued

Summary of Immunosuppressant Drugs—cont'd

	Generic name	Brand name	Usual dose and dosing schedule	Warning labels
Cytokines				
	ankinra	Kineret	**SC:** 100 mg once daily	PROTECT FROM LIGHT
	etanercept	Enbrel	25 mg twice weekly or 50 mg once weekly	REFRIGERATE; DON'T FREEZE
Rh$_0$ Immune Globulin				
	Rh$_0$ immune globulin		IM dosage (BayRho-D (HyperRHO S/D) Full dose, RhoGAM): 300 mcg IM at 28 weeks gestation. Repeat within 72 hours of delivery of a confirmed Rh$_0$ [D]-positive infant. IV /IM dossage (WinRho SDF, Rhophylac): 300 mcg IM or IV at 28 to 30 weeks' gestation. Repeat dose within 72 hours of delivery of a confirmed Rh$_0$ [D]-positive infant. (repeat dose for WinRho SDF is 120 mcg)	REFRIGERATE; DO NOT FREEZE PROTECT FROM LIGHT

CHAPTER SUMMARY

- An immunization is defined as a deliberate, artificial exposure to disease to produce acquired immunity.
- Vaccines prevent disease by taking advantage of your body's ability to make antibodies and release "killer" cells to disease-causing microbes and viruses that attack it.
- Live, attenuated vaccines are a living, but weakened, nonvirulent version of the invader microbe or virus.
- Inactivated, killed vaccines are advantageous because they cannot mutate but they produce less immunity than live vaccines.
- Toxoid vaccines stimulate the immune system to produce antibodies to the toxins that cause illness.
- Conjugate vaccines link antigens or toxoids to the polysaccharide or sugar molecules that certain bacteria use as a protective device to disguise themselves.
- The cold chain refers to a set of safe handling practices that ensure vaccines and immunologicals requiring refrigeration are maintained at required temperature from the time of manufacture until the time of administration to patients.
- When the cold chain is disrupted, the effectiveness and shelf-life of vaccines are reduced.
- Loss of potency and effectiveness are cumulative. Each time the cold chain is breached, the vaccine's effectiveness is further reduced.
- Patients are placed at risk when suboptimal vaccines are administered.
- Vaccines and other biological solutions and suspensions are most sensitive to breaches in the cold chain.
- Vaccines should be placed in a refrigerator designated solely to vaccines or, if a separate refrigerator is not feasible, vaccines should be segregated from other refrigerated pharmaceuticals.
- An important component of the cold chain is establishment and adherence to protocols for receiving, stocking, storage, and transport of drugs requiring refrigeration.
- Pharmacy personnel should be alert for warning signs that the cold chain has been broken during shipment. This might be as simple as noticing that freezer packs have thawed or that dry ice placed in the transport container with polio vaccine has evaporated.
- Vaccine stock should be rotated to avoid wastage due to outdated supplies. Expiry dates should be checked frequently.

- Vaccines should not be removed from the refrigerator until the time of dispensing or unless the vaccine must be transported.
- In most cases, vaccines should be transported in an insulated container.
- Extremes in heat and cold must be avoided so vaccines should never be placed in the hot glove compartment of a car.
- Vaccines are administered to provide immunity to a wide variety of childhood diseases, influenza, hepatitis, pneumonia, viral meningitis, rabies, and other conditions.
- Immunosuppressants inhibit proliferation of cells of the immune system.
- Drugs that have their primary action on cells of the immune system are used in the treatment of autoimmune diseases such as multiple sclerosis, rheumatoid arthritis, systemic lupus erythematosus, and Crohn's disease; to prevent tissue or organ rejection after transplant surgery; and in the treatment of cancer.
- Corticosteroids, antineoplastics, cyclosporine, macrolides, mycophenolate mofetil, antithymocyte globulin, monoclonal antibodies, intravenous γ-globulin (IVIg), Rh_o [D] immunoglobulin and cytokine inhibitors are all categorized as immunopharmacologicals.
- Cyclosporine is produced by a fungus (*Tolypocladium inflatum*), and it is used to improve survival rates for individuals with organ transplants.
- Cyclosporine acts on T-lymphocyte cells.
- Tacrolimus and sirolimus are classified as macrolides. Like cyclosporine, they are used to prevent transplant rejections.
- Tacrolimus interferes with the first phase of T-cell activation, and sirolimus interferes with a key enzyme that regulates the second phase of T-cell activation and proliferation.
- Antithymocyte globulin (ATG) is prepared by immunizing horses or rabbits with human thymocytes and then collecting the immunoglobulins.
- T-cell depletion persists for several days following a single dose of ATG and takes approximately 2 months before T-cell levels return to normal.
- Mycophenolate mofetil is a prodrug. It inhibits T-cell and B-cell proliferation.
- Basiliximab, daclizumab, and muromonab are monoclonal antibody immunomodulators that are used to reduce transplant rejections and to prolong the life of transplanted organs.
- They are active against a variety of leukocyte surface antigens.
- Intravenous γ-immunoglubulin (IVIg) is collected from human plasma. It is used for the treatment of a variety of infections and chronic lymphatic leukemia.
- Rh_o [D] immune globulin is administered to pregnant women who are Rh negative and have been exposed to blood that is Rh positive.
- When an Rh incompatibility exists between the pregnant woman and the fetus, maternal antibodies are produced that act against fetal red blood cells.
- Etanercept is genetically engineered inhibitor of tumor necrosis factor-α and blocks the inflammatory process triggered by high concentrations of tissue necrosis factor.
- Anakinra is a genetically engineered interleukin 1 receptor antagonist.
- Etanercept and ankinra are used in the treatment of rheumatoid arthritis.

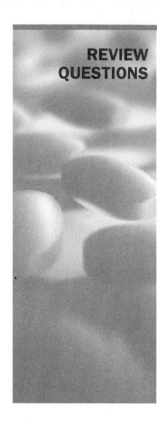

REVIEW QUESTIONS

Multiple Choice

1. **A living, but weakened version of the invader that does not cause disease (nonvirulent) is called a _____.**
   a. live, attenuated vaccine
   b. dead, attenuated vaccine
   c. live, encapsulated vaccine
   d. live, strengthened vaccine

2. **Drugs that inhibit proliferation of cells of the immune system; also known as immunopharmacologicals, are termed _____.**
   a. immunostimulants
   b. immunosuppressants
   c. immunologicals
   d. immunostablizers

3. **Immunization is not always achieved by administering vaccines.**
   a. true
   b. false

4. **Examples of inactivated, killed vaccines are _____.**
   a. flu
   b. hepatitis A
   c. polio
   d. all of the above

5. **These vaccines stimulate the immune system to produce antibodies to the toxins that cause illness such as tetanus and diphtheria.**
   a. conjugated vaccine
   b. live, attenuated vaccines
   c. toxoid vaccines
   d. inactivated, killed vaccines

6. **Disruption of the cold chain is NOT a public health threat.**
   a. true
   b. false

7. **Which of the following drugs are NOT categorized as immunopharmacologicals?**
   a. corticosteroids
   b. antineoplastics
   c. antivirals
   d. intravenous γ-globulin

8. **Cyclosporine is produced by a bacteria (*Tolypocladium inflatum*) and is used to improve survival rates for individuals with organ transplants.**
   a. true
   b. false

9. **A common ending for monoclonal antibody immunomodulators is _____.**
   a. "-tan"
   b. "-mab"
   c. "-ine"
   d. "-olol"

10. **Rh_0 [D] immune globulin is administered to pregnant women who are Rh _____ who have been exposed to blood that is Rh _____.**
    a. negative, positive
    b. positive, negative
    c. both a and b
    d. 0, negative

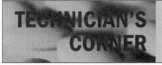

1. If a patient receives a vaccine, can that patient still become ill with the disease related to the vaccine?
2. Why does the body reject transplanted organs and not manufactured parts?

BIBLIOGRAPHY

Canada Communicable Disease Report: *Effects of freezing on DPT and DPT-IPV vaccines, adsorbed,* Vol. 21-11, June 15, 1995 F-6.

Canada Communicable Disease Report: *National guidelines for vaccine storage and transportation,* Vol. 21-11, June 15, 1995 F1-3.

Gold Standard Inc, Clinical Pharmacology: *Rh$_o$ [D] immune globulin,* revised April 3, 2007. Available at: http://www.clinicalpharmacology.com/apps/default.asp?entry=11&rNum=467.

Kalant H, Grant D, Mitchell J: *Principles of medical pharmacology* (pp 546-552), ed 7. Toronto, 2007, Elsevier Canada.

Lance L, Lacy C, Armstrong L, Goldman M: *Drug information handbook for the allied health professional,* ed 12. Hudson, OH, 2005, APhA Lexi-Comp.

Moscou K: *The vaccine cold chain,* Tech Talk CE. Available at: www.pharmacygateway.ca.

Murdoch J: Chill out: what pharmacists need to know about the room temperature stability of refrigerated pharmaceutical products, *Pharm Pract,* 22:32-42, 2006.

National Institute of Allergy and Infectious Disease: *Understanding vaccines: what they are, how they work,* Bethesda, MD, July 2003, NIAID, National Institutes of Health, U.S. Department of Health and Human Services. NIH publication No. 03-4219. Available at: http://www.niaid.nih.gov/.

Seto J, Marra F: *Keeping it cool: a pharmacist's guide, executive summary,* University of British Columbia, Continuing Pharmacy Professional Development, Home Study Program, February 2005, Rogers Publishing Ltd, pp 1-7.

Weir E, Hatch K: Preventing cold-chain failure: vaccine storage and handling, *JAMC,* 171(9), 2004.

Drugs Affecting the Integumentary System

- Identify the layers of the skin and its accessory structures.
- Understand the function of each part of the integumentary system.
- Identify the different types of cells of the integumentary system and their function.

Overview

Vital, diverse, complex, and *extensive* describe the largest, thinnest, and one of the most important organs of the body, the skin. It forms a self-repairing and protective boundary between the internal environment of the body and an often external hostile world. *Integument* is another name for skin, and ***integumentary system*** is a term used to denote the skin and its appendages (hair, nails, and skin glands).

Structure of the Skin

The skin is classified as a cutaneous membrane with two primary layers—the ***epidermis***, the superficial, thinner layer, and ***dermis***, the deep, thicker layer. The specialized area where the cells of the epidermis meet the connective cells of the dermis is called the ***dermal-epidermal junction***. Beneath the dermis lies a loose ***hypodermis*** (subcutaneous tissue), rich in fat and areolar tissue.

Sturcture of the Skin

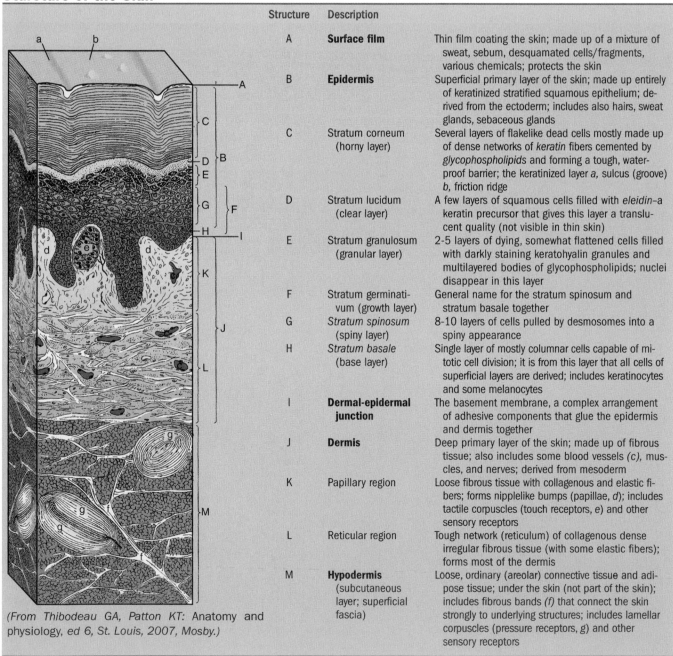

Structure		Description
A	**Surface film**	Thin film coating the skin; made up of a mixture of sweat, sebum, desquamated cells/fragments, various chemicals; protects the skin
B	**Epidermis**	Superficial primary layer of the skin; made up entirely of keratinized stratified squamous epithelium; derived from the ectoderm; includes also hairs, sweat glands, sebaceous glands
C	Stratum corneum (horny layer)	Several layers of flakelike dead cells mostly made up of dense networks of *keratin* fibers cemented by *glycophospholipids* and forming a tough, waterproof barrier; the keratinized layer *a,* sulcus (groove) *b,* friction ridge
D	Stratum lucidum (clear layer)	A few layers of squamous cells filled with *eleidin*–a keratin precursor that gives this layer a translucent quality (not visible in thin skin)
E	Stratum granulosum (granular layer)	2-5 layers of dying, somewhat flattened cells filled with darkly staining keratohyalin granules and multilayered bodies of glycophospholipids; nuclei disappear in this layer
F	Stratum germinativum (growth layer)	General name for the stratum spinosum and stratum basale together
G	*Stratum spinosum* (spiny layer)	8-10 layers of cells pulled by desmosomes into a spiny appearance
H	*Stratum basale* (base layer)	Single layer of mostly columnar cells capable of mitotic cell division; it is from this layer that all cells of superficial layers are derived; includes keratinocytes and some melanocytes
I	**Dermal-epidermal junction**	The basement membrane, a complex arrangement of adhesive components that glue the epidermis and dermis together
J	**Dermis**	Deep primary layer of the skin; made up of fibrous tissue; also includes some blood vessels (*c*), muscles, and nerves; derived from mesoderm
K	Papillary region	Loose fibrous tissue with collagenous and elastic fibers; forms nipplelike bumps (papillae, *d*); includes tactile corpuscles (touch receptors, *e*) and other sensory receptors
L	Reticular region	Tough network (reticulum) of collagenous dense irregular fibrous tissue (with some elastic fibers); forms most of the dermis
M	**Hypodermis** (subcutaneous layer; superficial fascia)	Loose, ordinary (areolar) connective tissue and adipose tissue; under the skin (not part of the skin); includes fibrous bands (*f*) that connect the skin strongly to underlying structures; includes lamellar corpuscles (pressure receptors, *g*) and other sensory receptors

(From Thibodeau GA, Patton KT: Anatomy and physiology, *ed 6, St. Louis, 2007, Mosby.)*

EPIDERMIS

The *epidermis* is the outermost layer of the skin that is composed of squamous epithelium. Epithelium is the covering for both the internal and external surfaces of the body. The outer layer of the skin is arranged in several layers (strata) and is therefore called stratified squamous epithelium. The epidermis lacks blood vessels, lymphatic vessels, and connective tissue (elastic fibers, cartilage, and fat) and is therefore dependent on the deeper dermis layer and its rich network of capillaries for nourishment.

EPIDERMAL CELLS

The epidermis is composed of several types of epithelial cells. *Keratinocytes* are filled with a tough, fibrous protein called *keratin*. *Melanocytes* contribute to the color of the skin and serve to decrease the amount of ultraviolet (UV) light that can penetrate into the deeper layers of the skin. *Langerhans cells* are branched cells that play a role in immunity. The cells of the epidermis are found in up to five distinct layers or strata.

Layer of the Epidermis

Layers of epidermis	Description
Stratum basale (base layer)	Single layer of mostly columnar cells capable of mitotic cell division; keratinocytes and melanocytes are derived from this layer
Stratum spinosum (spiny layer)	8 to 10 layers of irregularly shaped cells that are rich in ribonucleic acid (RNA) and well equipped to initiate the protein synthesis required for production of keratin
Stratum granulosum (granular layer)	2 to 5 layers of dying, somewhat flattened cells filled with intensely staining granules called *keratohyalin*, which is required for keratin formation
Stratum lucidum (clear layer)	A few layers of squamous cells filled with *eleidin*—a keratin precursor that gives this layer a translucent quality
Stratum corneum	Several layers of flake-like dead cells mostly made of keratin fibers cemented by *glycophospholipids* and forming a tough, waterproof barrier

EPIDERMAL GROWTH AND REPAIR

The epidermis has the ability to create new cells and repair itself after injury or disease. New cells must be formed at the same rate that old keratinized cells flake off from the stratus corneum to maintain a constant thickness of the epidermis. The regeneration time required for completion of mitosis, differentiation, and movement of new keratinocytes from stratum basale to the surface of the epidermis is about 35 days.

DERMAL-EPIDERMAL JUNCTION

This basement membrane is a complex arrangement of adhesive components that glue together the epidermis and dermis. It serves as a partial barrier to the passage of some cells and large molecules, preventing the passage of chemicals or disease-causing organisms through the skin from the external environment.

DERMIS

The *dermis*, or corium, is sometimes called the "true skin." In addition to serving as a protective function against mechanical injury and compression, this layer of skin provides a reservoir or storage area for water and important electrolytes. A specialized network of nerves and nerve endings in the dermis called somatic sensory receptors also process the sensory information such as pain, pressure, touch, and temperature. A variety of muscle fibers, hair follicles, sweat and sebaceous glands, and many blood vessels are embedded in the dermis.

Layers of the Dermis

Layers of dermis	Description
Papillary region	Loose fibrous tissue with collagenous and elastic fibers; form nipple-like bumps (papillae); Papillae include tactile corpuscles (touch receptors. etc.) and other sensory receptors
Reticular region	Tough network (reticulum) of collagenous dense irregular fibrous tissue (with some elastic fibers); forms most of the dermis

HYPODERMIS

The hypodermis is sometimes called the **subcutaneous layer**, or **superficial fascia**. It lies deep in the dermis and forms a connection between the skin and the underlying structures of the body. The hypodermis is mainly composed of loose fibrous and adipose (fat) tissue. Bands of fibers running through the hypodermis help hold the skin to underlying structures such as deep fascia and muscles.

SKIN COLOR

The main determinant of skin color is the quantity of melanin deposited in the cells of the epidermis. Prolonged exposure to the UV radiation in sunlight in light-skinned individuals causes melanocytes to increase melanin production and darken skin color. UV radiation can also reach into the DNA of the melanocyte and cause severe damage that can lead to skin cancer. Unless protected by melanin, UV radiation can also break down the vitamin folic acid. Other pigments like beta-carotene (or β-carotene) (found in vegetables and roots) also contribute to skin color. β-Carotene can be converted by the body to vitamin A, a critically important nutrient for skin growth that is stored in skin tissue.

Functions of the Skin

The major functions of the skin are protection, sensation, growth, synthesis of important chemicals and hormones (vitamin D), excretion, temperature regulation, and immunity.

Functions of the Skin

Function	Example	Mechanism
Protection from:	Microorganisms	Surface film/mechanical barrier
	Dehydration	Keratin
	UV radiation	Melanin
	Mechanical trauma	Tissue strength
Sensation	Pain	Somatic sensory receptors
	Heat and cold	
	Pressure	
	Touch	
Body growth and movement	Body growth and change in body contours during movement	Elastic and recoil properties of skin and subcutaneous tissue
Endocrine	Vitamin D production	Activation of precursor compound in skin cells by UV light
Excretion	Water	Regulation of sweat volume and content
	Urea	
	Ammonia	
	Uric acid	
Immunity	Destruction of microorganisms and interaction with immune cells (helper T cells)	Phagocytic cells and Langerhans' cells
Temperature regulation	Heat loss or retention	Regulation of blood flow to the skin and evaporation of sweat

Appendages of the Skin

Appendages of the skin consist of *hair, nails*, and *skin glands.*

HAIR

Only a few areas of the skin are hairless. They are the palms of the hands, the soles of the feet, the lips, nipples, and some areas of the genitalia. Hair growth begins when cells of the epidermis spread down into the dermis to form a small tube, the follicle part of the hair. The root lies hidden in the follicle and the visible part is called the shaft. Deposited in the cells of the hair are varying amounts of melanin, which is responsible for hair color. Two or more **sebaceous glands** secrete **sebum,** an oily substance into each hair follicle. The sebaceous gland secretions lubricate and condition the hair and surrounding skin to keep it from becoming dry, brittle, and easily damaged.

NAILS

Heavily keratinized epidermal cells compose fingernails and toenails. The visible part of each nail is called the **nail body.** The root of the nail lies in the flat sinus hidden by a fold of skin bordered by the **cuticle.** The nail body near the root has a crescent-shaped white area known as the **lunula**, or "little moon." Under the nail lies a layer of epithelium called the nail bed.

SKIN GLANDS

The skin glands include three kinds of microscopic glands: sweat, sebaceous, and ceruminous.

SWEAT GLANDS

Sweat or **sudoriferous glands** are the most numerous of the skin glands. They are classified as *eccrine* and *apocrine.* **Eccrine sweat glands** are distributed over the total body surface except the lips, ear canal, glans penis, and nail beds. They function throughout life to produce a transparent watery liquid (perspiration or sweat) rich in salts, ammonia, uric acid, urea, and other wastes. Sweat plays a critical role in maintaining a constant core temperature. Eccrine sweat glands are also numerous on the soles of the feet, forehead, and upper part of the torso. **Apocrine sweat glands** are located deep in the subcutaneous layer of the skin in the armpit (axilla), the areola of the breast, and the pigmented skin areas around the anus. Apocrine glands enlarge and begin to function at puberty.

SEBACEOUS GLANDS

Sebaceous glands secrete oil for the hair and skin. The oil, or sebum, keeps the hair supple and the skin soft and pliant. Sebaceous glands are found in the dermis, except in the skin of the palms and the soles. Some sebaceous glands open directly to the skin surface in such areas as the glans penis, lips, and eyelids. Sebum secretion increases during adolescence because it is stimulated by the increased blood levels of hormones.

CERUMINOUS GLANDS

Ceruminous glands are a special variety of apocrine sweat glands. They appear as excretory ducts that open onto the free surface of the skin in the external ear canal or with sebaceous glands into the necks of hair follicles in this area. The mixed secretions of sebaceous and ceruminous glands form a brown waxy substance called **cerumen.** It serves a useful purpose in protecting the skin of the ear canal from dehydration.

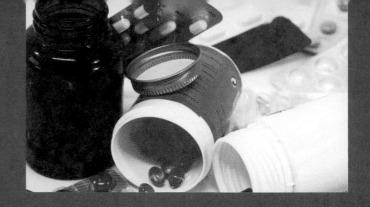

Treatment of Fungal Infections

CHAPTER 39

LEARNING OBJECTIVES

- Learn the terminology associated with fungal infections.
- Identify risk factors for fungal infections.
- List and categorize medications used for the treatment of fungal infections.
- Describe mechanism of action for drugs used for the treatment of fungal infections.
- Identify warning labels and precautionary messages associated with medications used for the treatment of fungal infections.
- Identify significant drug look-alike/sound-alike issues.
- List common endings for drug classes used for the treatment of specific fungal infections.

KEY TERMS

Antifungal: Drug used to treat a fungal infection.

Candida: Type of fungus. It is also called yeast.

Dermatophytes: Group of fungi responsible for most fungal infections of the skin, the hair, and the nails.

Fungus (*pl.* fungi): Primitive plant that reproduces by budding, releasing spores, or fusing hyphae (body of the fungus made of tiny filaments).

Mycoses: General term for fungal infections.

Onychomycosis: Fungal infection involving the fingernails or toenails, also known as tinea unguium.

Ringworm: Group of tinea infections involving the body or scalp that have a characteristic ring-like shape. Ringworm is spread person-person and animal-person.

Vulvovaginal candidiasis: Yeast vaginitis.

What Are Fungi and Yeast?

Fungi are primitive plants that reproduce by budding, releasing spores, or fusing hyphae (body of the fungus made of tiny filaments). Thousands of different fungi exist on earth. Mold, mildew, yeast, and mushrooms are all types of fungi. Many fungi are beneficial and do not cause disease. For example, mushrooms are fungi that we eat as food. The antibiotic penicillin is derived from a mold, and yeast causes bread to rise. Other fungi can cause severe illness. *Pneumocystis carinii* is a fungus that can cause pneumonia in individuals who have a decreased immune system response, and *Aspergillus fumigatus* is a mold that also causes serious respiratory infection.

Fungal Infections of the Skin and Nails

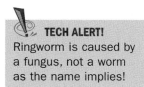

TECH ALERT!
Ringworm is caused by a fungus, not a worm as the name implies!

The general term used to describe a fungal infection is *mycoses*. Most fungal infections of the skin are caused by a group of fungi called dermatophytes. *Dermatophytes* thrive on dead keratin, a tough protein substance that is found in the top layer of skin, nails, and hair. They are not typically found in the mouth or vaginal mucosa. *Candida*, also called yeast, is a type of fungus that thrives in warm moist areas and is responsible for fungal infections in the vagina, groin, and mouth. To identify *Candida*, a potassium hydroxide (KOH) stain is applied to a sample of cells from the infected area. A *Candida* stain is shown in Figure 39-1.

Mycoses caused by the dermatophyte tinea are named for the site of the infection. For example, tinea manus is a fungal infection on the hands, tinea corporis is an infection on the body, and tinea capitis is located on the head ("cap"). Tinea infections are also called ringworm.

Dermatophyte infections are common and affect up to 20% of the population. This is because fungi are ubiquitous (found everywhere)! They are found in the air, soil, plants, and water. They are also found on surfaces in the home, office, schools, and gyms and even occur normally on our bodies. Fungi that are part of the normal body flora may become pathogenic (cause infection) only when the normal balance of flora is upset. For example, women who take broad-spectrum antibiotics may get a yeast infection because the bacteria and fungi that keep the yeast normally present in the vagina from overgrowing are killed by the antibiotic.

ATHLETE'S FOOT

Athlete's foot (tinea pedis) (Figure 39-2) is a common fungal infection that affects athletes and nonathletes. Symptoms are peeling, flaking skin between the toes, redness, itchiness, burning or stinging, and blisters and thickening of skin on the soles of the feet and heels. It may be accompanied by a foul odor. If severe, it may cause cracking of the skin, oozing, and secondary bacterial infection.

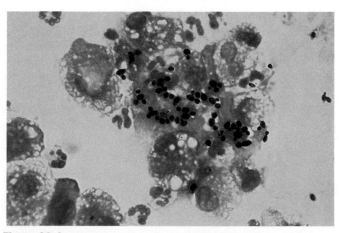

Figure 39-1 Candida stain. *(From Mahon CR, Lehman DC, Manuselis G: Textbook of diagnostic microbiology, ed 3, St. Louis, Saunders, 2007.)*

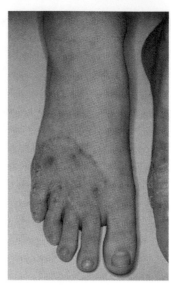

FIGURE 39-2 Athlete's foot. *(From Callen JP, Greer KE, Hood A, et al.:* Color atlas of dermatology, *Philadelphia, Saunders, 1993.)*

BOX 39-1 PREVENTION OF ATHLETE'S FOOT

- Keep feet clean and dry.
- Wear open sandals to permit feet to "breathe" if possible.
- Avoid walking barefoot across the floor of public facilities.

- Wear cotton socks and change socks daily.
- Use antifungal powders to prevent recurrent infections.

Individuals who have abrasions on the feet, as is caused by improperly fitted shoes that rub, are more susceptible to athlete's foot should they walk barefoot across an infected surface. Tips for prevention of athlete's foot are listed in Box 39-1.

Ringworm infections are caused by tinea fungi (*T. mentagrophytes*, T. rubrum, and *M. canis*) and may occur on the scalp, body, feet, fingernails, or toenails. Ringworm is contagious and is spread from person-person by physical contact with infected surfaces or lesions. Ringworm can also spread between humans and animals. Cats and dogs may be carriers of the fungus.

Ringworm of the body is also known as **tinea corporis**. Patches and plaques appear pink-to-red with raised scaly borders. They form in a distinctive circular pattern that gives the name of "ring" worm (Figure 39-3).

Tinea capitis is also called ringworm of the scalp. It occurs more frequently in children than in adults and is spread by sharing contaminated hats, combs, clothing, bedding, and linens. It may be spread animal-person, too. The fungus can cause bald patches on the scalp (Figure 39-4).

Tinea manus affects the hands, and **tinea unguium** affects the nails. Fungal infections of the nails are also called onychomycosis. Infected nails become discolored and thick and may crumble or fall off. Onychomycosis is hard to treat with topically applied antifungals because it is difficult for drugs to penetrate the nails and nail bed.

CANDIDIASIS

Candida is yeast that can cause infections of the skin and mucus membranes. Sites of infection are the groin, mouth, vagina, penis, skin folds, corners of the mouth, and nail beds. *Candida* is normally present in the gastrointestinal tract and vagina but only causes infection when conditions are favorable to the overgrowth of yeast.

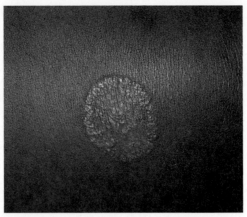

FIGURE 39-3 Tinea corporis. *(From Zitelli BJ, Davis HW:* Atlas of pediatric physical diagnosis, *ed 5, Philadelphia, Mosby, 2008.)*

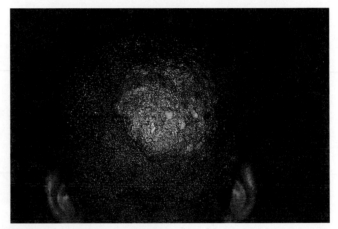

FIGURE 39-4 Ringworm of the scalp. *(From Callen JP, Greer KE, Paller LJ, et al.:* Color atlas of dermatology, *ed 2, Philadelphia, Saunders, 2000.)*

Vulvovaginal candidiasis is also known as yeast vaginitis or moniliasis. The risk for getting yeast vaginitis increases with age. Changes in hormone levels, such as occurs during pregnancy or when taking oral contraceptives or hormone replacement therapy, can also increase the risk of infection. When the body's ability to fight infection is suppressed because of infections like HIV or if taking immunosuppressive drugs (e.g., corticosteroids, antineoplastic agents), fungal infections may flourish. Risk factors of vulvovaginal candidiasis are listed in Box 39-2. Signs and symptoms of vulvovaginal candidiasis are shown in Box 39-3.

Candida can also cause infections in the oral cavity and in the area surrounding the mouth. A *Candida* infection in the oral cavity is called *thrush* (Figures 39-5 and 39-6). Thrush is most common in infants. A thrush infection in adults is a sign that the immune system is compromised. Thrush is an opportunistic infection that occurs in individuals with diseases that affect the immune system such as HIV, persons who take immunosuppressive medicines for cancer treatment or after stem cell and organ transplantation, and individuals taking broad-spectrum antiinfective agents.

Treatment of Fungal and Yeast Infections

Treatment of many fungal infections can be achieved with the use of nonprescription antifungal agents. Fungal infections that are cured using over-the-counter drugs are vulvovaginal candidiasis, jock itch, and athlete's foot.

There are three primary mechanisms of action for antifungal agents. Most antifungal agents act by destroying the fungus's cell membrane. The cell membrane of fungi differs from the cell membrane of human cells so destruction of the fungi does not destroy the

BOX 39-2 RISK FACTORS FOR VULVOVAGINAL CANDIDIASIS

- Age
- Decreased immune status
- Diabetes
- Drug therapy (hormone replacement therapy, oral contraceptives, antibiotics, immunosuppressives, corticosteroids)

- Pregnancy
- Sexual activity
- Poor hygiene

BOX 39-3 SIGNS OF VULVOVAGINAL CANDIDIASIS

- Itching
- "Cottage-cheese"–like vaginal discharge

- Burning
- Pain during intercourse

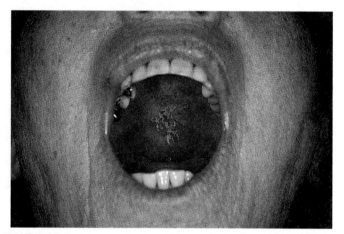

FIGURE 39-5 Thrush. *(From Callen JP, Greer KE, Paller LJ, et al.: Color atlas of dermatology, ed 2, Philadelphia, Saunders, 2000.)*

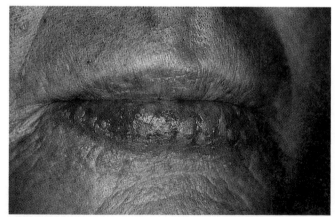

FIGURE 39-6 Oral candidiasis. *(From Callen JP, Greer KE, Paller LJ, et al.: Color atlas of dermatology, ed 2, Philadelphia, Saunders, 2000.)*

human cell. A second mechanism is interference with the synthesis of nucleic acids needed for replication. A third mechanism is to inhibit the synthesis of the fungal cell wall.

IMIDAZOLES AND TRIAZOLES

Imidazoles and triazoles are formulated for the treatment of cutaneous fungal infections (skin) and systemic infections. Several imidazoles are available for topical use, without prescription. They are butoconazole, clotrimazole, ketoconazole, miconazole, and tioconazole. These "-azoles" are used to treat athlete's foot, vulvovaginal candidiasis, jock itch, ringworm, and oral candidiasis. The remaining imidazoles (econazole, oxiconazole, and sulconazole) are restricted to prescription use only. Fluconazole, itraconazole, posaconazole, terconazole, and voriconazole are triazoles and require a prescription.

MECHANISM OF ACTION AND PHARMACOKINETICS

The imidazoles and triazoles interfere with ergosterol, an essential component needed for the synthesis of the fungal cell membrane. This causes cellular contents to leak out and the cell dies. Topical "-azoles" are formulated for application to the skin (creams, gel, lotion), mucous membranes (vaginal creams, suppositories), and scalp (shampoo).

ADVERSE REACTIONS

Adverse effects linked to topical use of imidazoles and triazoles are stinging or burning at the application site, redness, itchiness, or blistering. Nausea and vomiting, skin rash, liver toxicity, and photophobia are adverse reactions linked to oral use of ketoconazole.

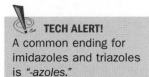

TECH ALERT!
A common ending for imidazoles and triazoles is "-azoles."

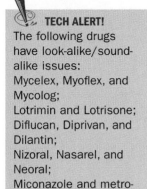

TECH ALERT!
The following drugs have look-alike/sound-alike issues:
Mycelex, Myoflex, and Mycolog;
Lotrimin and Lotrisone;
Diflucan, Diprivan, and Dilantin;
Nizoral, Nasarel, and Neoral;
Miconazole and metronidazole;
Terconazole and tioconazole

Imidazoles and Triazoles

Generic name	U.S. brand name / Canadian brand(s)	Dosage forms and strengths	Rx/OTC status
butoconazole	Gynezole-1, Mycelex-3	**Vaginal cream:** 2%	Rx (Gynezole-1) OTC (Mycelex-3)
	Gynezole-1		
clotrimazole*	Cruex, Desenex AF, Gyne-Lotrimin, Gyne-Lotrimin Combo Pak and 3 Day Combo Pak, Gyne-Lotrimin 3 Day Cr., Lotrimin, Lotrimin AF Jock Itch, Lotrimin AF, Mycelex, Mycelex-7, Mycelex Troche	**Cream:** 1% **Lozenge (Mycelex Troche):** 10 mg **Topical powder (Desenex AF):** 1% **Topical solution:** 1% **Vaginal cream (Gyne-Lotrimin):** 1%, 2% **Vaginal suppository (Gyne-Lotrimin, Mycelex-7):** 100 mg, 200 mg	OTC
	Canasten 1, Canasten Combo Pak, Clotrimaderm		
econazole*	Spectazole	**Cream:** 1%	Rx
	Not available		
fluconazole*	Diflucan	**Capsule:** 150 mg (Canada) **Powder for oral suspension:** 10 mg/ml; 40 mg/ml (U.S.) **Solution for injection:** 2 mg/ml in dextrose or normal saline **Tablet:** 50 mg, 100 mg, 150 mg; 200 mg (U.S.)	Rx
	Diflucan		
itraconazole*	Sporonox	**Capsule:** 100 mg **Solution, oral:** 10 mg/ml **Solution, injection:** 10 mg/ml (U.S. only)	Rx
	Sporonox		

Continued

Imidazoles and Triazoles—cont'd

Generic name	U.S. brand name / Canadian brand(s)	Dosage forms and strengths	Rx/OTC status
ketoconazole*	Extina, Kuric, Nizoral, Nizoral A-D, Xolegel Ketoderm, Nizoral	**Cream (Kuric):** 2% **Gel (Xolegel):** 2% **Shampoo (Nizoral):** 2% **Tablet:** 200 mg **Topical foam (Extina):** 2%	Rx OTC (Nizoral A-D)
miconazole*	Desenex, Dexenex Jock Itch, Fungoid Tincture, Lotrimin AF Deodorant Spray, Monistat, Micaderm, Micatin Jock Itch, Monistat, Monistat 1 Combo Pak, Neosporin AF, Zeasorb Micatin, Monistat 3 Dual Pak, Monistat 1, Monistat 7, Monistat Derm	**Cream (Micaderm, Micatin Athlete's Foot, Monistat Derm):** 2% **Lotion (Zeasorb):** 2% **Micatin Jock Itch, Neosporin AF:** 2% **Tincture (Fungoid):** 2% **Topical powder (Desenex):** 2% **Topical spray (Desenex Jock Itch, Lotrimin AF Deodorant, Micatin Jock Itch):** 2% **Vaginal cream (Monistat):** 2% Vaginal cream 2% + suppository 1200 mg (Monistat 1 Combo Pak, Monistat 3 Dual pak)	OTC
oxiconazole	Oxistat not available	**Cream:** 1% **Lotion:** 1%	Rx
posaconazole	Noxafil Spriafil	**Oral suspension:** 200 mg/5 ml	Rx
sulconazole	Exelderm not available	**Cream:** 1%	Rx
terconazole*	Terazol 3, Terazol 7, Zazole Terazol 3, Terazol 7	**Vaginal cream:** 0.8% (Terazol 3), 0.4% (Terazol 7) **Vaginal suppository:** 80 mg	Rx
tioconazole*	Monistat 1 Day, Tioconastat AF, Vagistat-1 Not available	**Vaginal ointment:** 6.5%	OTC
voriconazole	Vfend Vfend	**Powder of injection:** 200 mg **Powder of oral suspension:** 40 mg/ml (U.S.) **Tablet:** 50 mg, 200 mg	Rx

*Generic available.

ALLYLAMINE ANTIFUNGALS

Butenafine, naftifine, and terbinafine are classified as allylamine antifungals. Lamisil (terbinafine) is effective for treating fungal infections involving the nails.

MECHANISM OF ACTION AND PHARMACOKINETICS

Allylamines distort hyphae and stunt the growth of susceptible fungi by blocking an enzyme needed for the synthesis of ergosterol. Butenafine and naftifine are only available for topical application. Terbinafine is formulated for topical and oral use. When administered orally, therapeutic levels are reached within 3 to 18 weeks. Therapeutic levels persist in the skin for 2 to 3 weeks after terbinafine has been discontinued.

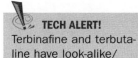

TECH ALERT!
Terbinafine and terbutaline have look-alike/ sound-alike issues.

ADVERSE REACTIONS

Orally administered terbinafine may produce nausea, vomiting, altered taste, headache, and tiredness. Topical application of terbinafine, butenafine, or naftifine may produce burning, stinging, redness, itchiness, and drying of the skin.

Allylamines

Generic name	U.S. brand name(s)	Dosage forms and strengths	Rx/OTC Status
	Canadian brand(s)		
butenafine	Mentax, Lotrimin Ultra Jock Itch	**Cream:** 1%	Rx (Mentax)
	Not available		OTC (Lotrimin Ultra Jock Itch)
naftifine	Naftin	**Cream:** 1%	Rx
	Naftin	**Gel:** 1%	
terbinafine*	Lamisil, Lamisil AT, Lamisil AT Athlete's Foot Cream, Lamisil AT for Women, Lamisil AT Jock Itch	**Cream:** 1% **Tablet:** 250 mg **Spray:** 1% **Topical solution:** 1%	Rx OTC (all Lamisil AT formulations)
	Lamisil		

*Generic available.

POLYENE CLASS OF ANTIFUNGALS

Nystatin, natamycin, and amphotericin B are all derived from the fungi-like bacteria streptomyces. They belong to the class of antifungals called polyenes. Nystatin is used for the treatment of *Candida* infections on the skin and mucous membranes. Nystatin suspension is commonly prescribed for the treatment of thrush. Amphotericin B is prescribed for systemic infections caused by various fungi including candidiasis, histoplasmosis, and aspergillosis. Natamycin is used to treat fungal infections in the eye (blepharitis, conjunctivitis, and keratitis). These infections are described in Chapter 20.

MECHANISM OF ACTION AND PHARMACOKINETICS

Nystatin, natamycin, and amphotericin B inhibit the synthesis of the fungal cell membrane by binding irreversibly to ergosterol. Nystatin is only available for oral and topical use. Oral absorption of amphotericin B is low so the drug is administered parenterally. Natamycin is formulated for ophthalmic use.

ADVERSE REACTIONS

Systemic absorption of nystatin is low when administered topically and orally, so adverse effects are minimal. Oral administration may produce nausea or diarrhea. Amphotericin B may produce nausea, vomiting, kidney damage, fever, chills, headache, and thrombophlebitis when administered intravenously. Amphotericin B may also cause potassium loss (hypokalemia).

Polyenes

Generic name	U.S. brand name(s)	Dosage forms and strengths	Rx/OTC status
	Canadian brand(s)		
amphotericin B*	Generic	**Powder for injection (Ambisome, Fungizone):** 50 mg/vial **IV suspension (Abelcet):** 5 mg/ml	Rx
	Abelcet, Ambisome Fungizone		
natamycin	Natacyn	**Ophthalmic suspension:** 5%	Rx
	Not available		

Continued

Polyenes—cont'd

Generic name	U.S. brand name(s)	Dosage forms and strengths	Rx/OTC status
	Canadian brand(s)		
nystatin*	BioStatin, Mycostatin, Nystop	**Cream:** 100,000 units **Capsule (BioStatin):** 500,000 units, 1,000,000 units **Lozenge (Mycostatin):** 200,000 units **Tablet, delayed release:** 500,000 units **Powder, topical (Candistatin, Mycostatin, Nystop):** 100,000 units **Suspension, oral:** 100,000 units **Vaginal cream:** 25,000 units/g **Vaginal insert:** 100,000 units/insert	Rx
	Candistatin, Mycostatin, Nyaderm		

*Generic available.

THIOCARBAMATES

Tolnaftate is the only antifungal belonging to the thiocarbamate class. It is approved for treatment and prevention of athlete's foot. It is also indicated for the treatment of ringworm and jock itch. Tolnaftate is available without prescription.

MECHANISM OF ACTION AND PHARMACOKINETICS

The mechanism of action for tolnaftate is similar to the terbinafine and naftifine. It stunts the growth of susceptible dermatophytes.

ADVERSE REACTIONS

Adverse reactions are mild and include irritation at the site of application, itching, or burning.

TECH ALERT!
The following drugs have look-alike/sound-alike issues:
tolnaftate and Tornalate
Tinactin and Talacen

Thiocarbamates

Generic name	U.S. brand name(s)	Dosage forms and strengths
	Canadian brand(s)	
tolnaftate*	Absorbine Jr Antifungal, Absorbine Jr Athlete's Foot, Fungi-Guard, Tinactin, Tinactin Jock Itch, Tinaderm, Ting	**Cream:** 1% **Gel:** 1% **Spray:** 1% **Topical powder:** 1% **Topical solution:** 1%
	Absorbine Jr Antifungal, Dr Scholl's Athlete's Foot, Fungicure, Pitrex, Tinactin, Zeasorb	

*Generic available.

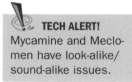

TECH ALERT!
A common ending for echinocandin antifungals is "-fungin."

TECH ALERT!
Mycamine and Meclomen have look-alike/sound-alike issues.

ECHINOCANDINS

Anidulafungin, caspofungin, and micafungin belong to a class of antifungal agents called echinocandins. They are effective for treating infections caused by *Candida* and *Aspergillus*.

MECHANISM OF ACTION AND PHARMACOKINETICS

Echinocandins interfere with the synthesis of the fungal cell wall. They are not toxic to human cells because their target is a cell wall component that does not exist in human cells. Oral absorption is poor so echinocandins are formulated for parenteral use.

ADVERSE REACTIONS

Echinocandins have fewer adverse effects and drug interactions than other oral or parenterally administered antifungals. They can cause elevated liver enzymes.

Echinocandins

	Generic name	U.S. brand name(s)	Dosage forms and strengths
		Canadian brand(s)	
	anidulafungin	Eraxis	**Powder for injection:** 50 mg
		Not available	
	caspofungin	Cancidas	**Powder for injection:** 50 mg, 70 mg
		Cancidas	
	micafungin	Mycamine	**Powder for injection:** 50 mg, 100 mg
		Not available	

MISCELLANEOUS

The remaining antifungal agents work by various mechanisms of action. Ciclopirox and undecylenic acid are effective in treating athlete's foot and jock itch. Ciclopirox is a broad-spectrum antifungal agent and is additionally approved for the treatment of ringworm and mild onychomycosis, a fungal infection of the nails. Griseofulvin is an orally administered drug used to treat onychomycosis.

MECHANISM OF ACTION AND PHARMACOKINETICS

Ciclopirox, povidone-iodine, and undecylenic acid are topical antifungal agents. Griseofulvin is administered orally. Ciclopirox interferes with DNA and RNA synthesis. Undecylenic acid and zinc undecylate are combined to produce a drug the decreases the spread of susceptible fungi. Formulations must contain not less than 10% undecylenate to be effective. The range falls between 10% and 27% undecylenate. Additionally, zinc undecylenate is an astringent and reduces irritation.

Griseofulvin is an orally administered antifungal agent. It interferes with fungal mitosis (see Table 37-2). This disrupts the ability of the fungus to replicate. Griseofulvin formulations made with ultramicronized crystals (Gris-PEG) offer the best absorption. Absorption is also increased when the drug is taken with a fatty meal.

Povidone-iodine is used to treat thrush and vulvovaginal candidiasis. It is also used as an antiseptic wash.

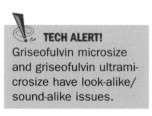

TECH ALERT!
Griseofulvin microsize and griseofulvin ultramicrosize have look-alike/sound-alike issues.

ADVERSE REACTIONS

Topically applied antifungals may produce mild burning, stinging, itching, swelling, or other signs of skin irritation. Common adverse effects due to the administration of griseofulvin are nausea, vomiting, headache, dizziness, gas, and heartburn.

Miscellaneous Antifungal Agents

	Generic name	U.S. brand name(s)	Dosage forms and strengths	Rx/OTC status
		Canadian brand(s)		
	ciclopirox*	Loprox, Penlac	**Cream:** 0.77%	Rx
		Loprox, Penlac, Steiprox	**Gel:** 0.77% **Nail lacquer (Penlac):** 8% **Shampoo:** 1% (Loprox), 1.5% (Steiprox) **Suspension, topical:** 0.77%	
	griseofulvin*	Grifulvin V, Gris-PEG	**Suspension:** 125 mg/5ml	Rx
		Not available for human use	**Tablet:** 125 mg, 250 mg (Gris-PEG); 500 mg (Grifulvin V)	

Continued

Miscellaneous Antifungal Agents—cont'd

Generic name	U.S. brand name(s) / Canadian brand(s)	Dosage forms and strengths	Rx/OTC status
povidone-iodine*	Betadine	**Ointment:** 10%	OTC
	Alphadine, Betadine, E-Z Scrub	**Scrub:** 7.5% (Alphadine, Betadine), 10%, 20% (E-Z Scrub) **Spray:** 5% **Solution:** 10% **Vaginal douche:** 10% **Vaginal suppository:** 200 mg	
undecylenic acid*	Desenex, Cruex Antifungal Cream	**Liquid, topical:** 12.5% **Powder:** undecylenic acid 2% + undecylenate 27.1%	OTC
	Desenex, Fungicure Professional Formula		

*Generic available.

Summary of Drugs Used for the Treatment of Fungal and Yeast Infections

Generic name	U.S. brand name	Usual dose and dosing schedule*	Warning labels
Imidazoles and triazoles			
butoconazole	Gynezole-1	**Vaginal:** 1 applicator full vaginally at bedtime for 3 to 7 days depending on product formulation	COMPLETE THE FULL COURSE OF THERAPY
clotrimazole	Lotrimin Canasten	**Vaginal:** 1 applicator full at bedtime for 3 to 14 days depending on product formulation **Topical:** Apply twice daily	
econazole	Spectazole	**Topical:** Apply twice daily	
fluconazole	Diflucan	**Oral or IV:** 200 mg on day 1, then 100 mg daily for 2 weeks (esophageal or oropharyngeal candidiasis) *Or* 150 mg to 200 mg as a single dose or for 3 doses of 3 days each (vulvovaginal candidiasis)	COMPLETE THE FULL COURSE OF THERAPY SHAKE WELL—suspension
itraconazole	Sporonox	**Oral:** 100 mg to 400 mg once daily	COMPLETE THE FULL COURSE OF THERAPY TAKE WITH FOOD AVOID GRAPEFRUIT JUICE
ketoconazole	Nizoral	**Oral:** 200 mg to 400 mg once daily **Topical:** apply daily for up to 6 weeks **For dandruff:** use every 3 to 4 days for up to 8 weeks	TAKE WITH FOOD—tablets AVOID ALCOHOL COMPLETE THE FULL COURSE OF THERAPY
miconazole	Monistat	**Vaginal:** 1 applicator full or 1 suppository at bedtime for 1 to 14 days depending on product formulation **Topical:** Apply twice daily	COMPLETE THE FULL COURSE OF THERAPY
oxiconazole	Oxistat	**Topical:** Apply 1 to 2 times daily	COMPLETE THE FULL COURSE OF THERAPY
posaconazole	Noxafil	**Oral:** 200 mg 3 times daily	COMPLETE THE FULL COURSE OF THERAPY SHAKE WELL TAKE WITH FOOD

Summary of Drugs Used for the Treatment of Fungal and Yeast Infections—cont'd

Generic name	U.S. brand name	Usual dose and dosing schedule*	Warning labels
sulconazole	Exelderm	**Topical:** Apply 1 to 2 times daily	COMPLETE THE FULL COURSE OF THERAPY
terconazole	Terazol 3, Terazol 7	**Vaginal:** 1 applicator full or 1 suppository at bedtime for 3 to 7 days depending on product formulation	
tioconazole	Vagistat	**Vaginal:** 1 applicator full as a single dose	
voriconazole	Vfend	**Parenteral:** 6 mg/kg IV every 12 hours **Oral:** 400 mg every 12 hours as loading dose on Day 1, followed by 200 mg every 12 hours	AVOID GRAPEFRUIT JUICE TAKE ON AN EMPTY STOMACH AVOID ALCOHOL
Allylamines			
butenafine	Mentax	**Topical:** Apply once daily for 2 to 4 weeks	COMPLETE THE FULL COURSE OF THERAPY
naftifine	Naftin	**Topical:** Apply cream once daily and apply gel twice daily	
terbinafine	Lamisil	**Topical:** Apply cream twice daily and apply gel once daily for 1 to 4 weeks **Oral:** 250 mg once daily for 6 to 12 weeks	COMPLETE THE FULL COURSE OF THERAPY TAKE WITH FOOD—tablets
Polyenes			
amphotericin B	Fungizone	**IV:** 0.25-1.5/kg/day (maximum 1.5 mg/day)	COMPLETE THE FULL COURSE OF THERAPY SHAKE WELL TAKE ON AN EMPTY STOMACH PROTECT FROM LIGHT—IV solution
natamycin	Natacyn	**Ophthalmic:** (see Chapter 20)	SHAKE WELL
nystatin	Generics	**Capsule:** 1 capsule 3 times daily **Suspension:** 4 ml to 6 ml swished in mouth 4 times a day **Topical:** Apply twice daily **Vaginal:** 1 insert nightly for 14 days	COMPLETE THE FULL COURSE OF THERAPY SHAKE WELL—suspension
Thiocarbamates			
tolnaftate	Tinactin	**Topical:** Apply twice daily for 2 to 4 weeks	COMPLETE THE FULL COURSE OF THERAPY
Echinocandins			
anidulafungin	Eraxis	100 mg IV loading dose on day 1, followed by 50 mg IV daily for 7 days after symptoms resolve	COMPLETE THE FULL COURSE OF THERAPY REFRIGERATE; DON'T FREEZE—caspofungin
caspofungin	Cancidas	70 mg IV infusion as a loading dose on Day 1, followed by 50 mg IV infusion once daily for at least 14 days	
micafungin	Mycamine	150 mg IV daily for 10 to 30 days	
Miscellaneous			
griseofulvin	Gris-PEG	**For tinea unguium:** **Oral:** 660 mg to 750 mg (ultramicrosize) or 750 mg to 1 g (microsize) once daily or in 2 to 4 divided doses	COMPLETE THE FULL COURSE OF THERAPY TAKE WITH FOOD SHAKE WELL
ciclopirox	Loprox	**Topical:** Apply twice daily	COMPLETE THE FULL COURSE OF THERAPY

*Usual dose for candidiasis or tinea.

CHAPTER SUMMARY

- Fungi are primitive plants, and thousands of species exist on earth.
- Some fungi are beneficial to humans, whereas other cause serious infections.
- The general term used to describe a fungal infection is *mycoses.*
- Most fungal infections of the skin are caused by a group of fungi called dermatophytes.
- Mycoses caused by the dermatophyte tinea are named for the site of the infection. For example, tinea manus is a fungal infection on the hands, tinea corporis is an infection on the body, and tinea capitis is located on the head ("cap").
- Women who take broad-spectrum antiinfectives may get a yeast infection because the bacteria and fungi that keep the yeast normally present in the vagina from overgrowing are killed by the antibiotic.
- Athlete's foot (tinea pedis) is a common fungal infection that affects athletes and nonathletes.
- Athlete's foot can be prevented by (1) keeping feet clean and dry, (2) wearing open sandals to permit feet to "breathe," (3) not walking barefoot across the floor of public facilities, (4) wearing cotton socks and changing socks daily, and (5) using antifungal powders to prevent recurrent infections.
- Tinea infections are also called ringworm. Ringworm has a characteristic "ring-like" shape and may affect the body, scalp, nails, or feet.
- Ringworm is contagious and is spread via person-person and animal-person.
- *Candida,* also called yeast, is a type of fungus that thrives in warm moist areas and is responsible for fungal infections in the vagina, groin, and mouth.
- Vulvovaginal candidiasis is also known as yeast vaginitis or moniliasis.
- A *Candida* infection in the oral cavity is called thrush.
- Treatment of many fungal infections can be achieved with the use of nonprescription antifungal agents.
- Fungal infections that are cured using over-the-counter drugs are vulvovaginal candidiasis, jock itch, and athlete's foot.
- There are three primary mechanisms of action for antifungal agents: (1) destroy the fungus' cell membrane, (2) interfere with the synthesis of nucleic acids needed for replication, and (3) inhibit the synthesis of the fungal cell wall.
- A common ending for imidazoles and triazoles is *"-azoles."*
- The imidazoles and triazoles interfere with ergosterol, an essential component needed for the synthesis of the fungal cell membrane.
- Topical "-azoles" are formulated for application to the skin (creams, gel, lotion), mucous membranes (vaginal creams, suppositories), and scalp (shampoo).
- Butenafine, naftifine, and terbinafine are classified as allylamine antifungals.
- Nystatin, natamycin, and amphotericin B are all derived for the fungi-like bacteria streptomyces and belong to the class of antifungals called polyenes.
- Nystatin, natamycin, and amphotericin B inhibit the synthesis of the fungal cell membrane.
- Tolnaftate is the only antifungal belonging to the thiocarbamate class. It is approved for treatment and prevention of athlete's foot.
- Anidulafungin, caspofungin, and micafungin belong to a class of antifungal agents called echinocandins.
- Echinocandins interfere with the synthesis of the fungal cell wall.
- The bioavailability of griseofulvin formulations varies. Formulations made with ultramicronized crystals (Gris-PEG) have better absorption than formulations made from micronized crystals. Absorption is also increased when the drug is taken with a fatty meal.

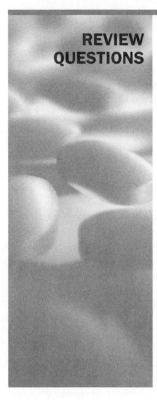

REVIEW QUESTIONS

Multiple Choice

1. *Candida* is a type of _____. It is also called yeast.
   a. virus
   b. bacteria
   c. fungus
   d. protozoan

2. The antibiotic _____ is derived from a mold.
   a. tetracycline
   b. penicillin
   c. doxycycline
   d. cephalosorin

3. Ringworm is caused by a worm.
   a. true
   b. false

4. Fungal infections of the _____ are called onychomycosis.
   a. hair
   b. skin
   c. scalp
   d. nails

5. Primary mechanisms of action for antifungal agents.
   a. destroying the fungus' cell membrane
   b. interfering with the synthesis of nucleic acids needed for replication
   c. inhibiting the synthesis of the fungal cell wall
   d. all of the above

6. _____ is effective for treating fungal infections involving the nails.
   a. Lamisil
   b. Tioconazole
   c. Nystatin
   d. Clotrimazole

7. Nystatin suspension is commonly prescribed for the treatment of thrush.
   a. true
   b. false

8. Natamycin is formulated for _____ use.
   a. topical
   b. ophthalmic
   c. otic
   d. oral

9. Echinocandins are formulated for oral use.
   a. true
   b. false

10. Griseofulvin is a(n) _____ administered antifungal agent.
    a. topically
    b. orally
    c. parenterally
    d. all of the above

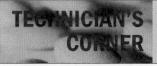

TECHNICIAN'S CORNER

1. There are many reports of onychomycosis due to artificial nails. What is causing these infections, and how can they be prevented?
2. How did the term "athlete's foot" come about?

BIBLIOGRAPHY

Aetna InteliHealth:*Candidiasis*.Available at:http://www.intelihealth.com/IH/ihtIH/WSIHW000/9339/31092.html.

Cappelletty D, Eiselstein-McKitrick K:The echinocandins, *Pharmacotherapy*, 27(3):369-388, 2007.

Gold Standard Inc., Clinical Pharmacology:Available at: http://www.clinicalpharmacology.com.

Health Canada Drug and Health Product Database. Available at: http://www.hc-sc.gc.ca/dhp-mps/prodpharma/databasdon/index_e.html.

Kalant H, Grant D, Mitchell J: *Principles of medical pharmacology* (pp 688, 691-695), ed 7.Toronto, 2007, Elsevier Canada.

Lance L, Lacy C,Armstrong L, Goldman M: *Drug information handbook for the allied health professional*, ed 12. Hudson, OH, 2005,APhA Lexi-Comp.

Merck Manual Online Professional Library: *Dermatophytoses: fungal infections of the skin*.Available at: http://www.merck.com/mmpe/sec10/ch120/ch120c.html?qt=ringwormandalt=sh.

National Institute of Allergy and Infectious Diseases: *Sexually transmitted infections: vaginitis: vaginal yeast infection*.Available at: http://www3.niaid.nih.gov/healthscience/healthtopics/vaginitis/yeast/cause.htm.

National Institute of Allergy and Infectious Diseases: *Understanding microbes in sickness and in health*. Bethesda, MD, January 2006, National Institutes of Health, U.S. Department of Health and Human Services. NIH publication No. 06-4914.Available at: www.niaid.nih.gov.

National Library of Medicine, National Institutes of Health: *Cutaneous candidiasis*. http://www.nlm.nih.gov/medlineplus/ency/article/000880.htm.

National Library of Medicine, National Institutes of Health: *Ringworm*.Available at: http://www.nlm.nih.gov/medlineplus/ency/article/001439.htm.

National Library of Medicine, National Institutes of Health: *Vaginal yeast infection*. Available at: http://www.nlm.nih.gov/medlineplus/ency/article/001511.htm.

Pray W: *Nonprescription product therapeutics* (pp 542-551), Baltimore, 1999, Lippincott, Williams and Wilkins.

USP Center for Advancement of Patient Safety: *Use caution–avoid confusion*, USP Quality Review No. 79, Rockville, MD,April 2004, USP Center for Advancement of Patient Safety.

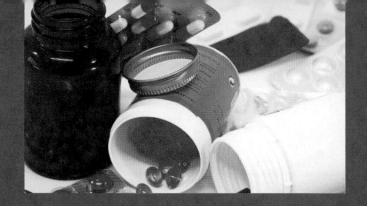

Treatment of Decubitus Ulcers and Burns

LEARNING OBJECTIVES

- Learn the terminology associated with decubitus ulcers.
- Learn the terminology associated with burns.
- Describe the stages of decubitus ulcers and degrees of burns.
- List and categorize medications used to treat decubitus ulcers and burns.
- Describe mechanism of action for each class of drugs used to treat decubitus ulcers and burns.
- Identify warning labels and precautionary messages associated with medications used to treat decubitus ulcers and burns.
- Identify significant drug look-alike/sound-alike issues.

KEY TERMS

Blister: Collection of fluid below or within the epidermis.

Decubitus ulcer: Pressure sore or "bedsore."

Eschar: Blackened necrotic tissue of a decubitus ulcer.

Escharotomy: Removal of necrotic skin and underlying tissue.

First-degree burn: Minor discomfort and reddening of the skin.

Fourth-degree burn: Burn that involves underlying muscles, fasciae, or bone.

Full-thickness burn: Third-degree burn where the epidermis and dermis are destroyed.

Partial-thickness burns: First- and second-degree burns.

Rules of palms: Rule for determining the extent of a burn surface area. A palm size of a burn victim is about 1% of total body surface area.

Rules of nines: Formula for estimating the percentage of adult body surface covered by burns by assigning 9% to the head and each arm, twice 9% (18%) to each leg and the anterior and posterior trunk, and 1% to the perineum. This is modified in infants and children because of the proportionately larger head size.

Second-degree burn: Burn that involves deep epidermal layers and causes damage to the upper layers of dermis.

Third-degree burn: Burn that is characterized by destruction of the epidermis and dermis.

Decubitus Ulcers

A *decubitus ulcer* is a pressure sore and is commonly called a "bedsore" (Figure 40-1). Decubitus means "lying down," a name that hints at a common cause and nature of pressure sores, lying in a prone position for long periods. Pressure sores typically occur in patients who are in bed or chair bound. Patients with sensory or mobility deficits like spinal cord injury, stroke, coma, and malnourished; patients with peripheral vascular disease; hospitalized elderly patients; and nursing home residents are all at risk. Decubitus ulcers can range from a very mild pink coloration of the skin, which disappears in a few hours after pressure is relieved on the area, to a very deep wound extending to and sometimes through a bone into internal organs. These ulcers, as well as other wound types, are classified in stages according to the severity of the wound.

All decubitus ulcers have a course of injury similar to a burn wound. This can be a mild redness of the skin and/or blistering, such as a first-degree burn, to a deep open wound with blackened tissue, as in a third-degree burn. This blackened tissue is called **eschar**.

MECHANISM OF FORMATION

The usual mechanism of forming a decubitus ulcer is from pressure. However, it can also occur from friction caused by rubbing against something such as a bed sheet, cast, brace, etc. or prolonged exposure to cold. The most common sites where decubitus ulcers are likely to form are over bony prominences. These areas include the spine, coccyx, hips, heels, and elbows, to name a few. The weight of a body presses on the bone, and the bone presses on the tissue and the skin that it covers. This tissue begins to decay from lack of blood circulation. This is the basic formation of decubitus ulcer development.

STAGES OF WOUNDS

Wounds are often categorized according to severity by the use of stages. This is similar to the staging system used to classify burn and decubitus ulcers.

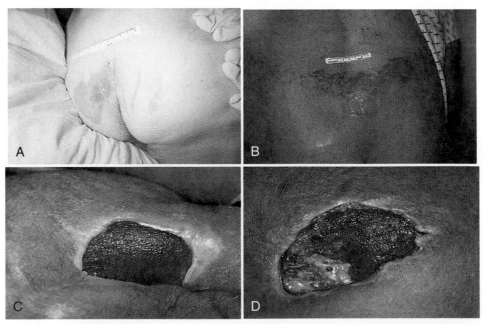

FIGURE 40-1 Decubitus ulcers. (**A**) Stage I, (**B**) stage II, (**C**) stage III, (**D**) stage IV. *(Courtesy Laurel Wiersma. From Potter PA, Perry AG:* Fundamentals of nursing, *ed 4, St. Louis, 1997, Mosby.)*

STAGE I

This stage is characterized by a surface reddening of the skin. The skin is unbroken and the wound is superficial. Examples of stage I wounds are a light sunburn; a first-degree burn, or a decubitus ulcer. The burn heals spontaneously or the decubitus ulcer quickly fades when pressure is relieved on that area. The key factor to consider in a stage I wound is what were the causes of the wound and how to alleviate the pressure on the area to prevent it from worsening. Improving the nutritional status of the individual should also be considered early to prevent wound worsening. The presence of a stage I wound is an indication or early warning of a problem and a signal to take preventative action.

STAGE II

This stage is characterized by a *blister* either broken or unbroken. A partial layer of the skin is injured. Involvement is no longer superficial. The goal of care is to cover, protect, and clean the area. Coverings designed to insulate and absorb as well as protect are used. Close attention to prevention, protection, nutrition, and hydration is important also. With quick attention, a stage II wound can heal very rapidly. Generally, decubitus ulcers or pressure wounds developing beyond stage II are from lack of aggressive intervention when first noted at stage I.

STAGE III

In stage III, the wound has extended through all layers of the skin. It is the primary site for a serious infection to occur. The goal of treatment is to alleviate pressure, cover and protect the wound, same as stage II, as well as an increased emphasis on nutrition and hydration is applied. Medical care is necessary to promote healing and to treat and prevent infection. This type of wound will progress rapidly if left unattended. Infection is of grave concern.

STAGE IV

Stage IV wounds extend through the skin and involve underlying muscle, tendons, and bone. The diameter of the wound is not as important as the depth. This is very serious and can produce a life-threatening infection, especially if not aggressively treated. All of the goals of protecting, cleaning, and alleviation of pressure on the area still apply. Nutrition and hydration are now critical. Without adequate nutrition, this wound will not heal.

Anyone with a stage IV wound requires medical care by someone skilled in wound care. Surgical removal of the necrotic or decayed tissue is often necessary for wounds of larger diameter. A skilled wound care physician, physical therapist, or nurse can sometimes successfully treat a smaller-diameter wound without the necessity of surgery. Surgery is the usual course of treatment for larger stage IV wounds. Amputation may be necessary in some situations.

STAGE V

This is an older classification and is not used in all areas. A stage V wound is a wound that is extremely deep, having gone through the muscle layers and now involves underlying organs and bones. It is difficult to heal. Surgical removal of the necrotic or decayed tissue is the usual treatment. Amputation may be necessary is some situations.

CARE, PREVENTION, AND TREATMENT OF DECUBITUS ULCERS

In at-risk patients, one method of determining the patient risk is with simple assessment tools such as the Norton or Braden scale (Table 40-1).

The most important principle of therapy is to prevent initial skin damage that promotes ulceration. In patients at risk, aggressive nursing practices, such as frequent turning of immobile patients, changing position every 2 hours or more frequently if needed, and the application of skin protection to bone body parts, frequently are effective. This 2-hour time frame is generally accepted as the maximum interval that the tissue can tolerate pressure without damage. Maintaining hydration, nutrition high in protein, and hygiene are also very important parts of prevention and treatment. Range-of-motion exercises and early ambulation are encouraged, and the use of low-pressure mattresses and special beds are also used.

TABLE 40-1   The Norton Scale

Physical condition	Mental state	Activity	Mobility	Incontinence	Total score
Good	Alert	Ambulatory	Full	Not	
4	4	4	4	4	
Fair	Apathetic	Walks with help	Slightly limited	Occasionally	
3	3	3	3	3	
Poor	Confused	Chair bound	Very limited	Usually urinary output	
2	2	2	2	2	
Very bad	Stuporous	Confined to bed	Immobile	Double urinary output	
1	1	1	1	1	

The patient is rated from 1 to 4 on the five risk factors listed. A score of ≤14 indicates risk for decubitus ulcers, or pressure sores.

BOX 40-1 TOPICAL TREATMENT OF DECUBITUS ULCERS

- Occlusive hydrocolloid dressings
- Polyurethane films
- Absorbable gelatin sponges
- Karaya gum patches
- Antiseptic irrigations
- Antibiotic ointments

- Air-permeable occlusive clear dressings (allows aspiration of collected fluids)
- Supportive adhesive-backed foam padding
- Absorptive dextranomer beads
- Proteolytic enzyme debriding agents

The treatment for a decubitus ulcer involves keeping the area clean and removing necrotic (dead) tissue, which can form a breeding ground for infection. There are many procedures and products available for this purpose. Topical treatments aid the healing of partial-thickness sores (Box 40-1). Some deep wounds even require surgical removal or debridement of necrotic tissue. In some situations, amputation may be necessary.

COLLAGENASE

Collagenase is used to promote debridement of necrotic tissue in dermal ulcers and severe burns. Collagenase is a water-soluble proteinase that specifically breaks down collagen into gelatin, allowing less specific enzymes to act. Collagenase is most effective within a narrow pH range of 6 to 8. The commercially available preparation of collagenase (Santyl) is derived from the bacterium *Clostridium histolyticum*. In addition, there is new evidence that elastin and fibrin are also degraded by collagenase but to a lesser degree.

PAPAIN AND UREA

Papain and urea is used as an enzymatic debridement ointment for treatment of chronic and acute wounds. Papain is purified from the carica papaya fruit. The most commonly used papain/urea–based product is Accuzyme. The mechanism of action is for papain to attach to and break down any proteins containing cysteine residues. This process is nonselective as most proteins, including growth factors, contain cysteine residues. Collagen contains no cysteine residues and is therefore unaffected by papain. The primary use of a papain-urea product is for nonspecific bulk debridement with a broad pH range (3 to 12).

TRYPSIN, BALSAM PERU, AND CASTOR OIL

Trypsin, balsam Peru, and castor oil are used in the treatment of decubitus ulcers, varicose ulcers, debridement of eschar, dehiscent wounds, and sunburns. Trypsin is used to debride necrotic tissue; balsam Peru stimulates circulation at the wound site and may be mildly bactericidal; and castor oil improves epithelialization and acts as a protectant covering and helps reduce pain. Local application may produce temporary stinging at the application site.

ANTIBACTERIALS

Antibacterial drugs may be used if the decubitus ulcer is not healing or it continues to ooze after 2 weeks of proper cleansing and bandage changes. Some antibacterial preparations can be applied directly to the skin. Antiinfectives given by mouth or injection are needed for those who have blood poisoning or infections in the skin or underlying bone. Antiinfectives are also given to prevent diseased heart valves from getting infected, or when the ulcer needs surgical repair.

Treatment of Decubitus Ulcers

Generic name	U.S. brand name(s) / Canadian brand(s)	Dosage forms and strengths
collagenase	Santyl	Ointment: 250 units/g
	Santyl	
papain and urea	Accuzyme, Ethezyme, Gladase, Accuzyme SE	Ointment: 650,000 units papain + 10% urea 830,000 units papain + 10% urea 1,100,000 units papain + 10% urea
	Not available	Spray (Accuzyme SE): 830,000 units papain + 10% urea
trypsin, balsam Peru, and castor oil	Optase Granul-Derm Allan Derm T	Aerosol: (Granul-Derm) trypsin 0.1 mg, balsam Peru 72.5 mg, caster oil 650 mg
	Not available	Gel (Optase): trypsin 0.12 mg, balsam peru 87 mg, caster oil 788 mg Ointment (Allan Derm T): trypsin 90 units, balsam peru 87 mg, caster oil 788 mg
Topical antibacterials		
bacitracin	Baciguent, BaciiM	Injection: 50,000 units
	Baciguent	Ointment: 500 units/g
gentamycin gentamicin	Gentak	Cream: 0.1%
	Garamycin	Ointment: 0.1% Injection (various): 40 mg/ml, 1 mg/ml, 1.2 mg/ml, 1.6 mg/ml
metronidazole	Metrocreme, Metrogel, Metrolotion, Noritate, Vandazole	Cream: 0.75% (Metrocreme), 1% (Noritate) Gel, topical (Metrogel, Rosasol): 1% Lotion: 0.75%
	Metrocreme, Metrogel, Metrolotion, Nidagel, Noritate Rosasol Cream	Powder for injection: 500 mg Solution for injection: 5 mg/ml
mupirocin	Bactroban Cream, Centany	Cream: 2%
	Bactroban, Bactroban Cream	Ointment: 2%
silver sulfadiazine	Silvadene, SSD, SSD AF	Cream: 1%
	Dermazin, Flamazine, SSD silver sulfadiazine	
Antiseptics		
aluminum acetate solution (Burow's solution)	Domeboro	Topical powder: 648 mg
	Not available	
povidone-iodine	Antisept Soap, Betadine, Clinidine Solution, Iodex Ointment, Minidyne, Pharmadine, Operand,	Gel: 10% Ointment: 10%, 4.7% (Iodex) Pad: 10%
	Alfadine Scrub, Betadine, E-Z Scrub sponge	Scrub: 7.5%, 20% Solution: 10% (Minidyne) Spray: 5% Swabsticks: 7.5%, 10%

Burns

Typically, we think of a burn as a thermal injury or lesion caused by contact of the skin with some hot object or fire. In addition, overexposure to ultraviolet light (sunburn) or contact with an electric current or corrosive chemicals and radioactive agents causes injury or death to skin cells. The injuries that result can be classified as burns and the effects may be local or systemic involving primary shock (which occurs immediately after injury and rarely fatal) or secondary shock (which develops insidiously following severe burns and is often fatal). In the United States and Canada, about 1.25 million persons receive medical treatment for burns annually. More than 50,000 of these burn victims are hospitalized as a result of a severe burn injury.

ESTIMATING BODY SURFACE AREA

When burns involve large areas of skin, treatment and the prognosis for recovery depend in large part on the total area involved and the severity of the burn. The severity of a burn is determined by the depth and extent (percentage of body surface area [BSA]) of the lesion. There are several ways to estimate the extent of BSA burned. One method is called the "*rules of palms*" and is based on the assumption that the palm size of a burn victim is about 1% of the total BSA. Therefore, estimating the number of "palms" that are burned approximates the percentage of BSA involved.

The "*rule of 9s*" (Figure 40-2) is another, more accurate method of determining the extent of a burn injury. In this technique, the body is divided into 11 areas of 9%, with the area around the genitals, called the perineum, representing the additional 1% of BSA. As Figure 40-2 shows, 9% of the skin covers the head and upper extremity, including the front and back surfaces. Twice as much, or 18%, of the total skin area covers the front and back of the trunk and each lower extremity, including the front and back surfaces. The rule of nines works well with adults but does not reflect the differences of BSA in small children. Special tables called *Lund-Browder* charts, which takes the large surface area of certain body areas (such as the head) in a growing child into account, are used by physicians to estimate burn percentages in children.

The depth of a burn injury depends on the tissue layers of the skin that are involved (Figure 40-3). A *first-degree burn* (typical sunburn) causes minor discomfort and some reddening of the skin. Although the surface layers of the burned area may peel in 1 or 2 days, no blistering occurs, and the actual tissue destruction is minimal. First- and second-degree burns are called *partial-thickness burns*.

Second-degree burns involve the deep epidermal layers and always cause injury to the upper layers of the dermis. In deep second-degree burns, damage to sweat glands, hair follicles, and sebaceous glands may occur, but tissue death is not complete. Blisters, severe pain, generalized swelling, and edema characterize this type of burn. Scarring is common.

Third-degree, or *full-thickness, burns* are characterized by destruction of both the epidermis and dermis. Tissue death extends below the follicles and sweat glands. If burning involves underlying muscles, fasciae, or bone, it may be called a *fourth-degree burn*. A distinction between second- and third- or fourth-degree burning is the fact that a third- or fourth-degree lesion is insensitive to pain immediately after injury because of the destruction of nerve endings. Scarring is a serious problem. Third- and fourth-degree burns are best managed in specialized burn centers.

COMPLICATIONS

Sloughing of skin, gangrene, scarring, erysipelas (skin infection caused by group A staphylococci), nephritis (kidney infection), pneumonia, immune system impairment, and intestinal disturbances are possible complications. The risk of complication is greatest when more than 25% of the body surface is burned. Two common complications of burns are infection and dehydration.

Signs of infection are:
- Change in color of the burned area or surrounding skin
- Purplish discoloration, particularly if swelling is also present

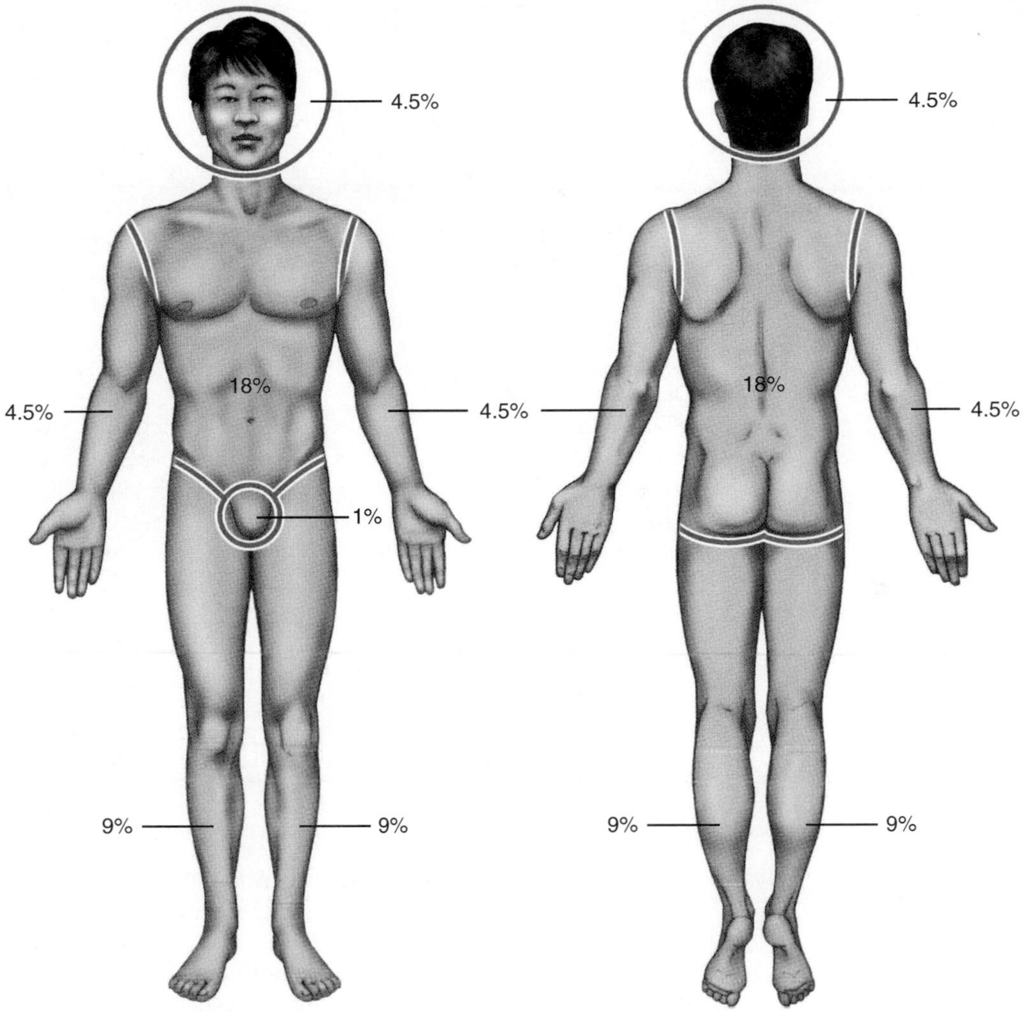

FIGURE 40-2 Rules of 9s. *(From Thibodeau GA, Patton KT: Anatomy and physiology, ed 6, St. Louis, 2007, Mosby.)*

- Change in thickness of the burn
- Greenish discharge or pus
- Fever
  Signs of dehydration are:
- Thirst
- Lightheadedness or dizziness (when moving from lying or sitting, standing)
- Weakness
- Dry skin
- Urinating less often than usual

PRECAUTIONS

"Stop," "drop," and "roll" should be the first actions if a person is experiencing burns due to a fire. A rug, a blanket, or anything within reach can be used to smother flames. Care must be taken so the individual does not inhale the smoke. Clothing must be carefully cut away so that skin is not pulled away. Blisters should not be opened, as this will increase the chance for infection. All burned patients must receive appropriate tetanus prophylaxis.

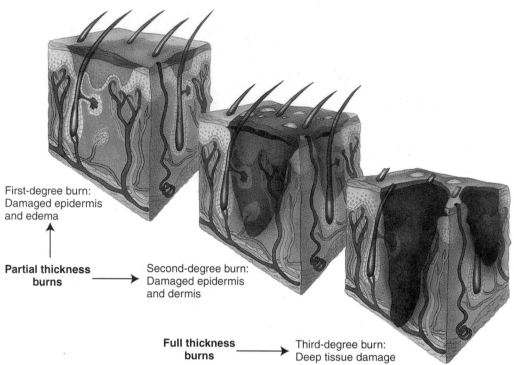

FIGURE 40-3 Classification of burns. *(From Thibodeau GA, Patton KT:* Anatomy and physiology, *ed 6, St. Louis, 2007, Mosby.)*

Partial thickness burns → First-degree burn: Damaged epidermis and edema

Partial thickness burns → Second-degree burn: Damaged epidermis and dermis

Full thickness burns → Third-degree burn: Deep tissue damage

TREATMENT

The *first step* in the care of the burn patient is to check for airway injury or impaired breathing. Airway injury is most likely to occur after facial burns or smoke inhalation in closed spaces. The *second* task in burn care is to ensure cardiac output and tissue perfusion. Volume replenishment with crystalloid intravenous fluids is given per standard protocols; at the same time urinary output, blood pressure and pulse, body weight, and renal function are closely monitored to ensure adequate hydration. The *third* task in burn care is the removal of overlying clothing and the irrigation of affected tissues, taking care to avoid excessively cooling the body. Gentle tissue debridement should be followed by application of nonadherent dressings, skin substitutes, topical antiseptics, or autografts, as dictated by circumstances. *Escharotomy* (removal of necrotic skin and underlying tissue) for circumferential burns (burns that extend right around the body), antibiotic therapy for infections, intravenous analgesics, pressor support for hypotension, or nutritional support may be needed. Fluid balance is carefully monitored as well as nutritional therapy. β-Blockers are given to reduce hypermetabolic state associated with large burns. Emotional support is offered to help patients cope with altered body image or lifestyle concerns. Burned tissues are positioned per protocols to minimize edema and contractures. Therapies are instituted to prevent venous thrombosis, pneumonia, and complications resulting from immobility.

DRUG TREATMENT

SILVER SULFADIAZINE

Silver sulfadiazine is the most frequently used topical agent for burns. It is thought to act via inhibition of DNA replication and modification of the cell membrane and cell wall. The drug is bactericidal against both gram-positive and gram-negative organisms, but resistance has occasionally been reported.

Adverse Effects

Local skin reactions, such as pain, burning, or itching and hypersensitivity, are occasionally reported. Transient leukopenia occurs in 5% to 15% of patients, but there is no increased incidence of infectious complications.

MAFENIDE

Mafenide appears to act on bacterial cellular mechanisms. It interferes with bacterial folic acid synthesis through competitive inhibition of *para*-aminobenzoic acid. In topical application, mafenide is bacteriostatic against gram-positive and gram-negative bacteria.

Adverse Reactions

Pain or burning sensation following mafenide application is the most frequently reported adverse effect. Mafenide is a strong carbonic anhydrase inhibitor, and its use leads to alkaline diuresis, which can cause acid-base abnormalities. Carbonic anhydrase inhibitors block carbonic anhdrase, an enzyme that affects acid-base balance by its ability to form carbonic acid from water and carbon dioxide. It also inhibits epithelial regeneration (growth of new tissue).

SILVER NITRATE

Silver nitrate is a broad-spectrum agent. It is bacteriostatic at a concentration of 5%. The effects of silver nitrate may result from silver ions readily combining with several biologically important chemical groups.

Adverse Effects

Silver nitrate is prepared with distilled water resulting in an extremely hypotonic solution leading to electrolyte imbalance.

POVIDONE-IODINE

Povidone-iodine acts by destroying microbial protein and DNA. This drug has excellent in vitro (a test that is done in glass or plastic vessels in the laboratory) antimicrobial activity but is inactivated by wound exudates.

Adverse Effects

Systemic absorption of iodine results in renal and thyroid dysfunction.

Topical Treatment of Burns

Generic name	U.S. brand name(s) Canadian brand(s)	Dosage forms and strengths
mafenide	Sulfamylon	**Cream:** 85 mg/g
	Sulfamylon	**Powder for topical solution:** 5%
silver sulfadiazine	Silvadene, SSD, SSD AF	**Cream:** 1%
	Dermazin, Flamazine	
silver nitrate	Generic	**Applicator sticks:** 75% silver nitrate, 25% potassium nitrate
	Not available	**Ointment, topical:** 10%
		Solution, topical: 0.5%, 10%, 25%, 50%

REHABILITATION

During rehabilitation, individually fitted elastic garments are applied to prevent hypertrophic scar formation, and joints are exercised to promote a full range of motion. Referrals for occupational therapy, psychological counseling, support groups, or social services are often necessary to assist the patient with life adjustments.

Summary of Drugs Used in the Treatment of Decubitus Ulcers and Burns

Generic name	Brand name	Usual dose and dosing schedule	Warning labels
Debriding Agents			
collagenase	Santyl	Apply once daily (more if dressing becomes soiled)	DO NOT TOUCH THE TIP OF THE TUBE TO ANY SURFACE, INCLUDING A FINGER, THE WOUND, OR STERILE GAUZE PAD
papain and urea	Accuzyme, Ethezyme, Gladase	Apply directly to wound; secure into place and reapply 1 to 2 times/day	
trypsin, balsam Peru, and castor oil	Granul-Derm	Apply a minimum of twice daily or as often as necessary	
Topical antibacterials			
bacitracin	Baciguent	Apply 1 to 5 times daily	NOT TO BE USED FOR LONGER THAN A WEEK UNLESS PRESCRIBED BY A PRESCRIBER
gentamicin	Garamycin	**Topical:** Apply 3 to 4 times/day to affected area	REPORT ANY DIZZINESS OR SENSATIONS OF RINGING OR FULLNESS IN EARS
mupirocin	Bactoban	Apply small amount to affected area 2 to 5 times/day for 5 to 14 days	FOR TOPICAL USE ONLY DISCONTINUE IF RASH, ITCHING, OR IRRITATION OCCURS
silver sulfadiazine	Silvadene	Apply 1 to 2 times/day with sterile-gloved hand; apply to thickness of $\frac{1}{16}$ inch	FOR EXTERNAL USE ONLY
mafenide	Sulfamylon	Apply 1 to 2 times/day with a sterile-gloved hand; apply to thickness of 16 mm; the burned area should be covered with cream at all times	DISCONTINUE AND REPORT IMMEDIATELY IF RASH, BLISTERS, OR SWELLING APPEAR WHILE USING CREAM FOR EXTERNAL USE ONLY
silver sulfadiazine	Silvidene, SSD, SSD AF, Thermazene, Dermazin, Flamazine	Apply 1 to 2 times/day with sterile-gloved hand; apply to thickness of $\frac{1}{16}$ inch	
silver nitrate	Generics	Apply a cotton applicator dipped in solution on the affected area 2 to 3 times/week for 2 to 3 weeks	DISCONTINUE IF REDNESS OR IRRITATION DEVELOPS
Antiseptics			
povidone-iodine	Betadine	Apply as needed for treatment and prevention of susceptible microbial infections	DO NOT SWALLOW FOR EXTERNAL USE AVOID CONTACT WITH THE EYES
aluminum acetate solution	Domeboro	Soak affected area in the solution 2 to 4 times/day for 15 to 30 minutes or apply wet dressing soaked in the solution	KEEP DRESSING MOIST

CHAPTER SUMMARY

- Decubitus ulcers can range from a very mild pink coloration of the skin, which disappears in a few hours after pressure is relieved on the area, to a very deep wound extending to and sometimes through a bone into internal organs.
- The usual mechanism of forming a decubitus ulcer is from pressure. However it can also occur from friction by rubbing against something such as a bed sheet, cast, brace, etc. or prolonged exposure to cold.
- Stage I of a decubitus ulcer is characterized by a surface reddening of the skin.
- Stage II is characterized by a blister either broken or unbroken.
- In stage III, the wound has extended through all layers of the skin.
- Stage IV wounds extends through the skin and involves underlying muscle, tendons, and bone.
- Stage V is an older classification and is not used in all areas. A stage V wound is a wound that is extremely deep, having gone through the muscle layers and now involving underlying organs and bones.
- The treatment for a decubitus ulcer involves keeping the area clean and removing necrotic (dead) tissue, which can form a breeding ground for infection.
- Collagenase is used to promote debridement of necrotic tissue in dermal ulcers and severe burns.
- Papain and urea is used as an enzymatic debridement ointment for treatment of chronic and acute wounds.
- Trypsin, balsam Peru, and castor oil are used in the treatment of decubitus ulcers, varicose ulcers, debridement of eschar, dehiscent wounds, and sunburns.
- Antibacterial drugs may be used if the decubitus ulcer is not healing or it continues to ooze after 2 weeks of proper cleansing and bandage changes.
- The injuries that result from electrical, chemical, or radioactive agents can be classified as burns and the effects maybe local or systemic involving primary shock (which occurs immediately after injury and rarely fatal) or secondary shock (which develops insidiously following severe burns and is often fatal).
- The severity of a burn is determined by the depth and extent (percentage of body surface area) of the lesion.
- There are several ways to estimate the extent of body surface area burned. One method is called the "rules of palms" and is based on the assumption that the palm size of a burn victim is about 1% of the total body surface area.
- The "rule of 9s" is another and more accurate method of determining the extent of a burn injury. In this technique the body is divided into 11 areas of 9%, with the area around the genitals, called the perineum, representing the additional 1% of body surface area.
- A first-degree burn (typical sunburn) causes minor discomfort and some reddening of the skin.
- Second-degree burns involve the deep epidermal layers and always cause injury to the upper layers of the dermis.
- Third-degree, or full-thickness, burns are characterized by destruction of both the epidermis and dermis.
- If burning involves underlying muscles, fasciae, or bone, it may be called a fourth-degree burn.
- Two common complications of burns are infection and dehydration.
- The procedures for the care of the burn patient include assessing the airway to ensure that breathing is unimpaired; ensure cardiac output and tissue perfusion; the removal of overlying clothing and the irrigation of affected tissues. Gentle tissue debridement should be followed by application of nonadherent dressings, skin substitutes, topical antiseptics, or autografts, as dictated by circumstances.
- Silver sulfadiazine is the most frequently used topical agent for burns. It is thought to act via inhibition of DNA replication and modification of the cell membrane and cell wall.
- Mafenide appears to act on bacterial cellular mechanism. It interferes with bacterial folic acid synthesis through competitive inhibition of *para*-aminobenzoic acid.
- Silver nitrate is a broad-spectrum agent. It is bacteriostatic at a concentration of 5%.

REVIEW QUESTIONS

Multiple Choice

1. Pressure sores typically occur in patients who are _____.
   a. confined to the bed
   b. chair bound
   c. ambulatory
   d. a and b

2. The usual mechanism of forming a decubitus ulcer is from _____.
   a. pressure
   b. infection
   c. inflammation
   d. laceration

3. In stage _____ of the decubitus ulcer, the wound has extended through all layers of the skin.
   a. I
   b. II
   c. III
   d. IV

4. Frequent turning is optional to alleviate pressure on the wound and to promote healing.
   a. true
   b. false

5. The severity of a burn is determined by the _____ (percentage of body surface area) of the lesion.
   a. depth
   b. width
   c. extent
   d. a and c

6. The "rule of 9s" is a more accurate method of determining the extent of a burn injury than the "rule of palms".
   a. true
   b. false

7. Third-degree, or _____ burns are characterized by destruction of both the epidermis and dermis.
   a. partial-thickness
   b. full-thickness
   c. total thickness
   d. all of the above

8. Common complications of burns are _____ and _____.
   a. infection
   b. dehydration
   c. stroke
   d. a and b

9. _____ is the most frequently used topical agent for burns.
   a. Gentamycin
   b. Silver sulfadiazine
   c. Silver nitrate
   d. Mupirocin

10. The removal of necrotic skin and underlying tissue from a burn or decubitus ulcer is termed _____.
    a. echarectomy
    b. escharotomy
    c. necrotomy
    d. ulcerectomy

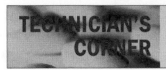

1. Aloe vera is widely used to treat minor burns. What active ingredient in the aloe vera promotes healing of burns?
2. Can decubitus ulcers be prevented from developing? If so, how?

BIBLIOGRAPHY

Burns: injuries, poisoning. Available at: http://www.merck.com/mmpe/sec21/ch315/ch315a.html.

Lance L, Lacy C, Armstrong L, Goldman M: *Drug information handbook for the allied health professional,* ed 12. Hudson, OH, 2005, APhA Lexi-Comp.

LDHP Medical Review Services Corporation: *Decubitus ulcer information and wound stages,* December 1999. Available at: http://www.expertlaw.com/library/malpractice/decubitus_ulcers.html.

Local burn treatments. Available at: http://www.medbc.com/annals/review/vol_13/num_4/text/vol13n4p216.htm.

Moore J, Jensen P: *Assessing the role and impact of enzymatic debridement.* Available at: http://www.podiatrytoday.com/article/2785.

Sussman C, Bates-Jensen B: *Wound care,* Gaithersburg, MD, 1998, Aspen Publishers.

Thibodeau G, Patton K: *Anatomy and physiology,* ed 6, St. Louis, 2007, Mosby.

http://www.edu/altmed/articles/burns-000021.htm.

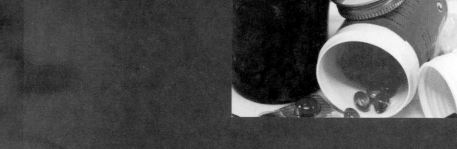

Treatment of Acne

- Learn the terminology associated with acne.
- Describe the causes of acne.
- Describe the types of acne.
- List and categorize medications used to treat acne.
- Describe mechanism of action for each class of drugs used to treat acne.
- Identify warning labels and precautionary messages associated with medications used to treat acne.
- Identify significant drug look-alike/sound-alike issues.

KEY TERMS

Acne: Disorder resulting from the action of hormones and other substances on the skin's oil glands (sebaceous glands) and hair follicles.

Acne vulgaris: Most common form of acne.

Blackhead (open comedone): Trapped sebum and bacteria partially open to the surface that turn black due to melanin, the skin's pigment; can last for a long time because the contents very slowly drain to the surface.

Comedone: Enlarged and plugged hair follicle and the most characteristic sign of acne.

Cysts: End products of pustules or nodules.

Keratolytic: Pertaining to keratolysis, the softening and shedding of the horny outer layer of the skin. A keratolytic agent is a peeling agent.

Milia: Tiny little bumps that occur when normally sloughed skin cells get trapped in small pockets on the surface of the skin.

Nodule: Ruptured pustules that form abscesses.

Papule: Obstructed follicle that becomes inflamed.

Pilosebaceous units (PSUs): PSUs consist of a sebaceous gland connected to a canal, called a follicle, and contain a fine hair.

Pustule: Larger lesions that are more inflamed than papules and can be superficial or deep.

Whitehead (closed comedo): Trapped sebum and bacteria that stay below the skin surface; may show up as tiny white spots, or they may be so small that they are invisible to the naked eye.

Acne

Acne is a disorder resulting from the action of hormones and other substances on the skin's oil glands (sebaceous glands) and hair follicles (Figure 41-1). These factors lead to plugged pores and outbreaks of lesions commonly called "pimples or zits." Acne lesions usually occur on the face, neck, back, chest, and shoulders. Although acne is usually not a serious health threat, it can be a source of significant emotional distress. Severe acne can lead to permanent scarring.

Physicians describe acne as a disease of the *pilosebaceous units* (PSUs). Found over most of the body, PSUs consist of a sebaceous gland connected to a canal, called a follicle, that contains a fine hair (Figure 41-2). These units are most numerous on the face, upper back, and chest. The sebaceous glands make an oily substance called sebum that normally empties onto the skin surface through the opening of the follicle, commonly called a pore. Cells called keratinocytes line the follicle.

The hair, sebum, and keratinocytes that fill the narrow follicle may produce a plug, which is an early sign of acne. The plug prevents sebum from reaching the surface of the skin through a pore. The mixture of oil and cells allows bacteria *Propionibacterium acnes*

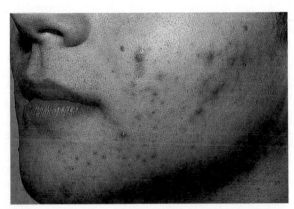

FIGURE 41-1 Adult acne. *(From Callen JP, Paller AS, Greer KE, Swinyer LF: Color atlas of dermatology, ed 2, Philadelphia, 2000, WB Saunders.)*

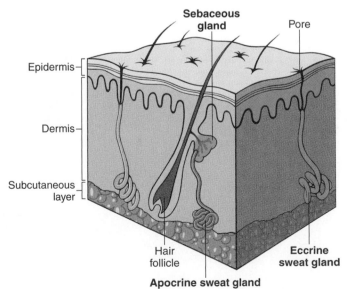

FIGURE 41-2 Normal pilosebaceous Unit. *(From Chabner DE: The language of medicine, ed 8, St. Louis, 2007, WB Saunders.)*

(P. acnes) that normally live on the skin to grow in the plugged follicles. These bacteria produce chemicals and enzymes and attract white blood cells that cause inflammation. Inflammation is a characteristic reaction of tissues to disease or injury and is marked by four signs: swelling, redness, heat, and pain. When the wall of the plugged follicle breaks down, it spills sebum, shedding skin cells and bacteria into the nearby skin, leading to lesions or pimples.

Common *acne*, or **acne vulgaris**, occurs most frequently in the adolescent years as a result of overactive secretion by the sebaceous glands, accompanied by blockages and inflammation of their ducts. People of all races and ages get acne. An estimated 80% of all people between the ages of 11 and 30 have acne outbreaks at some point. The rate of sebum secretion increases more than 5-fold between 10 and 19 years of age. For most people, acne tends to go away by the time they reach their 30s; however, some people in their 40s and 50s continue to have this skin problem.

People with acne frequently have a variety of lesions. The basic acne lesion, called the **comedone**, is simply an enlarged and plugged hair follicle and is the most characteristic sign of acne. If the plugged follicle, or comedone, stays beneath the skin, it is called a closed comedone and produces a white bump called a **whitehead**. A comedone that reaches the surface of the skin and opens up is called an open comedone or **blackhead** because it looks black on the skin's surface (Figure 41-3). This black discoloration is due to changes in sebum as it is exposed to air. It is not due to dirt. Both whiteheads and blackheads may stay in the skin for a long time and are considered to be noninflammatory acne.

Pus-filled pimples or pustules result from secondary infections within or beneath the epidermis, often in a hair follicle or sweat pore. Troublesome acne lesions can develop, including the following:

- **Papules**—inflamed lesions that usually appear as small, pink bumps on the skin and can be tender to the touch
- **Pustules (pimples)**—papules topped by white or yellow pus-filled lesions that may be red at the base
- **Nodules**—large, painful, solid lesions that are lodged deep within the skin
- **Cysts**—deep, painful, pus-filled lesions that can cause scarring

Blackheads and whiteheads normally release their contents at the surface of the skin then heal. If the follicle wall ruptures, inflammatory acne can ensue. This rupture can be caused by random occurrence or by picking or touching the skin. This is why it is important to leave acne-prone skin relatively untouched.

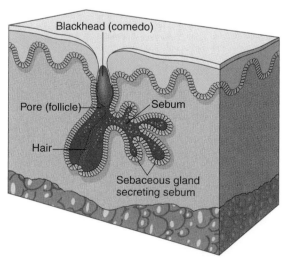

FIGURE 41-3 Open comedone. *(From Chabner DE:* The language of medicine, *ed 8, St. Louis, 2007, WB Saunders.)*

Milia are tiny little bumps that occur when normally sloughed skin cells get trapped in small pockets on the surface of the skin. They are common in newborns across the nose and upper cheeks and can also be seen on adult skin. The bumps disappear as the surface is worn away and the dead skin is sloughed. In newborns, the bumps usually disappear within the first few weeks of life. However, for adults milia may persist indefinitely. Treatment is not indicated in children. Adults can have them removed by a physician for cosmetic improvement.

What Causes Acne?

The exact cause of acne is unknown, but physicians believe it results from several related factors. One important factor is an increase in hormones called androgens (male sex hormones). These increase in both boys and girls during puberty and cause the sebaceous glands to enlarge and make more sebum. Hormonal changes related to pregnancy or starting or stopping birth control pills can also cause acne.

Another factor is heredity or genetics. Researchers believe that the tendency to develop acne can be inherited from parents. For example, studies have shown that many school-age boys with acne have a family history of the disorder. Other risk factors for acne are the use of certain drugs including androgens and lithium (Box 41-1) and the use of comedogenic, greasy cosmetics. They may alter the cells of the follicles and make them stick together, producing a plug.

FACTORS THAT CAN MAKE ACNE WORSE

Factors that can cause an acne flare include
- Changing hormone levels in adolescent girls and adult women 2 to 7 days before their menstrual period starts
- Oil from skin products (moisturizers or cosmetics) or grease encountered in the work environment (for example, a kitchen with fry vats)
- Pressure from sports helmets or equipment, backpacks, tight collars, or tight sports uniforms
- Environmental irritants, such as pollution and high humidity
- Squeezing or picking at blemishes
- Hard scrubbing of the skin
- Stress

MYTHS ABOUT THE CAUSES OF ACNE

There have been many theories concerning the causes of acne. Because adolescents commonly suffer from acne and indulge in "fast food," "junk food," and sweets, these food items are often blamed as the causes of acne. Not keeping one's skin clean is also blamed for the causes of blackheads but that also is a myth. Another stated cause of acne is stress. Stress in itself does not cause acne but can compound existing acne making it worse.

BOX 41-1 MEDICATIONS THAT TRIGGER OR EXACERBATE ACNE

MORE COMMON
- Anabolic steroids (e.g., danazol [Danocrine], testosterone)
- Bromides
- Corticosteroids (e.g., prednisone [Deltasone])
- Corticotropin (H.P. Acthar)
- Isoniazid (Nydrazid)
- Lithium
- Phenytoin (Dilantin)

LESS COMMON
- Azathioprine (Imuran)
- Cyclosporine (Sandimmune, Neoral)
- Disulfiram (Antabuse)
- Phenobarbital
- Quinidine
- Tetracycline
- Vitamins B_1, B_6, B_{12}, and D_2

Treatment of Acne

The goals of treatment are to heal existing lesions, stop new lesions from forming, prevent scarring, and minimize the psychological stress and embarrassment caused by this disease. Drug treatment is aimed at reducing several problems that play a part in causing acne:

- Abnormal clumping of cells in the follicles
- Increased oil production
- Bacteria
- Inflammation

All medicines can have side effects. Some side effects may be more severe than others. Pharmacy technicians should remind customers to review the package insert that comes with the medicine and ask the pharmacist if they have any questions about the possible side effects. Depending on the severity of the acne, the physician may recommend one of several over-the-counter (OTC) medicines and/or prescription medicines. Some of these medicines may be topical (applied to the skin), and others may be oral (taken by mouth). One or more topical medicines may be used or combined therapy with oral and topical medicines may be recommended.

Mild acne consists of small lesions, such as blackheads, whiteheads, or pustules, which appear at or near the surface of the skin. As such, mild cases of acne can sometimes be controlled at home by gently washing the affected area(s) with warm water and a mild soap twice a day to remove dead skin cells and excess oil and use of the following products:

TREATMENT OF MILD ACNE: OTC MEDICATIONS

Topical OTC medicines are available in many forms, such as gels, lotions, creams, soaps, or pads. At home treatment with OTC topical medicines may take up to 8 weeks before noticeable improvement can be seen. Once acne clears, treatment must be continued to prevent new lesions from forming. If the acne does not respond to at-home treatment, a dermatologist can assess the situation and determine an appropriate alternative therapy. In these cases, combination therapy of two or more treatments may be used. Combination therapy may include use of a prescription topical antimicrobial or topical retinoid. These prescription topicals can be very effective in clearing mild acne.

COMEDOLYTICS (KERATOLYTICS)

Salicyclic Acid

Salicyclic acid is a mild comedolytic agent that provides a milder, less effective alternative to the prescription agent tretinoin. In cleansing preparations, salicyclic acid is considered an adjunctive treatment.

Mechanism of Action. Salicyclic acid acts as a surface keratolytic (peeling agent) helping to break down blackheads and whiteheads. It also helps cut down the shedding of cells lining the hair follicles.

Adverse Effects. The adverse effects are burning, redness, and peeling of skin.

Sulfur-Resorcinol Combination

Combinations of sulfur 3% to 8% with resorcinol 2%, which enhances the effects of the sulfur, are available without prescription for the treatment of acne.

Mechanism of Action. Sulfur and resorcinol function as keratolytics, fostering cell turnover and desquamation helping to break down blackheads and whiteheads.

Adverse Effects. The adverse effects are redness and peeling of skin.

ANTIMICROBIALS

Sulfur and Sulfacetamide Combination

Sodium sulfacetamide is an antibacterial agent and is used in the treatment of acne, rosacea, and seborrheic dermatitis (a red, flaking skin rash).

Mechanism of Action. Sodium sulfacetamide interferes with the growth of bacteria on the skin. Sulfur may also inhibit the growth of bacteria on the skin, and it may cause drying of the skin.

Adverse Effects. The adverse effects are redness, warmth, swelling, itching, stinging, burning, or irritation of the treated area.

BENZOYL PEROXIDE

Benzoyl peroxide is the most effective and widely used nonprescription medication currently available for treatment of noninflammatory acne.

Mechanism of Action. Benzoyl peroxide causes irritation and desquamation that prevents closure of the pilosebaceous duct. Its irritant effects cause an increased turnover rate of epithelial cells lining the follicular duct, which then increases sloughing and promotes resolution of the comedones. When benzoyl peroxide combines with proteins in the comedones, oxygen is released. *P. acne* is anaerobic and is destroyed in the presence of oxygen.

Adverse Effects. The adverse effects are dryness and irritation of the skin. Benzoyl peroxide may also bleach clothing or hair that it comes in contact with.

Over-the-Counter Acne Products

Generic name	U.S. brand name(s) Canadian brand(s)	Dosage forms and strengths
benzoyl peroxide*	Clearplex, Exact Acne Medication, Fostex 10% BPO, Loroxide, Neutrogena Acne Mask, Neutrogena On The Spot Acne Medication, Oxy 10 Balanced Medicated Face Wash, Oxy 10 Balance Spot Treatment, Palmer's Skin Success Acne, PanOxyl Bar, Zapzyl	**Cream:** 5%, 10% **Gel:** 2.5%, 5%, 10%, 4% (Solugel) **Liquid:** 2.5%, 5%, 10% **Lotion:** 5%, 10%, 20% (Oxyderm) **Soap:** 5%, 10%
	Acetoxyl, Benoxyl, Benzac AC, Benzac W Wash, Desquam X, Oxyderm, Pan Oxyl, Oxy 5, PanOxyl-AQ, Solugel, Clear Pore on the Spot Acne Treatment	
resorcinol and sulfur*	Clearasil Adult Care, Acnomel	**Cream:** resorcinol 2%, sulfur 8% **Cake:** resoricnol 1%, sulfur 4% **Gel:** resoricinol 1.25%, sulfur 2.5% **Lotion:** resorcinol 2%, sulfur 5%, resorcinol 2%, sulfur 8% **Stick:** resorcinol 1%, sulfur 8%
	Acnomel	
salicylic acid*	NeoCeuticals Acne Spot Treatment, Neutrogena Acne Wash, Neutrogena Clean Pore, Neutrogena Maximum Strength T-Sal, Neutrogena On the Spot Acne Patch, Oxy Balance, Oxy Balance Deep Pore, Palmer's Skin Success Acne Cleanser, SalAc, Sal-Acid, Stri-Dex, Stridex Facewipes To Go, Zapzl Acne Wash, Zapzyl Pore Treatment	**Cream:** 2% **Cloths:** 2% **Foam:** 2% **Gel:** 2% **Liquid:** 2% **Pads:** 0.5% **Patch:** 2% **Soap:** 2%
	Neutrogena Acne Wash Foam Cleanser, Clean and Clear Blackhead Clearing Scrub	
sulfur and salicyclic acid*	Aveeno Cleansing Bar, Fostex, SAStid Plain Therapeutic Shampoo and Acne Wash	**Cake:** sulfur 2%, salicylic acid 2% **Cleanser:** sulfur 2%, salicylic acid 1.5% **Soap:** sulfur 2%, salicylic acid 2% **Wash:** sulfur 1.6%, salicylic acid 1.6%
	Meted, Sebulex	
sulfur and sulfacetamide*	AVAR, AVAR Cleanser, AVAR Green, Clenia, Nocosyn, Plexion, Plexion SCT, Plexion TS, Rosanil, Rosula, Sulfacet-R, Zetacet	**Cream:** sulfur 5%, sulfacetamide sodium 10% **Gel:** sulfur 5%, sulfacetanide sodium 10% **Liquid soap:** sulfur 5%, sulfacetamide 10% **Lotion:** sulfur 5%, sulfacetamide 10% **Suspension:** sulfur 5%, sulfacetamide 10%
	Sulfacet-R	

*Generic available.

TREATMENT OF MODERATE TO MODERATELY SEVERE ACNE

In moderate to moderately severe acne, numerous whiteheads, blackheads, papules, and pustules appear to cover from one-fourth to three-fourths of the face and/or other affected area(s). Moderate to moderately severe acne usually requires the help of a dermatologist and combination therapy. Treatment used to treat moderate to moderately severe acne are

- Physical methods, such as comedone, extraction or UV light therapy
- Oral antibiotics—help stop or slow the growth of bacteria and reduce inflammation
- Vitamin A derivatives (retinoids)—unplug existing comedones (plural of comedo), allowing other topical medicines, such as antibiotics, to enter the follicles. Some may also help decrease the formation of comedones. These drugs contain an altered form of vitamin A.
- Prescription-strength topical keratolytics
- Oral contraceptives

ANTIBIOTICS

Oral and topical antibiotics may be prescribed for the treatment of acne. Oral antibiotics commonly are initial therapy in patients with moderate to severe inflammatory acne. Systemic antibiotics decrease *P. acne*s colonization and have intrinsic antiinflammatory effects. First-line oral antibiotics have included **tetracycline, erythromycin, doxycycline,** and **minocyline**. Because *P. acne*'s resistance to erythromycin is increasing, this antibiotic is becoming a second-line agent that is used when treatment with tetracycline or other macrolide antibiotics fails or is not tolerated. The mechanism of action and adverse effects produced by these antibiotics is described in Chapter 35.

Oral antibiotics must be taken for 6 to 8 weeks before results are evident, and treatment should be given for 6 months to prevent the development of microbial resistance. Oral antibiotics may be discontinued after inflammation has resolved. Topical antibiotics may be continued for prophylaxis. Some patients may require long-term oral antibiotic therapy to control their acne and prevent scarring.

Other oral medicines less commonly used are clindamycin (Cleocin) and sulfonamides (Bactrim).

Dermatologists recommend early treatment for moderate to moderately severe acne because if not treated early, scars can develop. Acne scars can take two forms—as raised thickened tissue or as a depression, such as pits or pock marks. The only reliable method of preventing or limiting the extent of these scars is to treat acne early in its course, and for as long as necessary.

Topical antiinfective agents are used in the treatment of acne to reduce inflammation caused by bacteria rather than by a direct bactericidal effect. Topical antiinfectives used for the treatment of acne are clindamycin, erythromycin, metronidazole, and sulfacetamide.

RETINOIDS

Retinoids include vitamin A and its derivatives. Adapalene, tretinoin, and tazarotene are retinoids.

Adapalene

Adapalene is a retinoid-type drug. It affects the growth of skin cells and thereby reduces the formation of pimples. It is available for topical use only.

Mechanism of Action. Adapalene modulates cell differentiation and keratinization that are responsible for the drug's ability to break down comedones. It is also a potent antiinflammatory.

Adverse Effects. The adverse effects are irritation, redness, dryness, itching, and flares of acne.

Tretinoin

Tretinoin is a retinoid. It is used for the treatment of mild to moderate acne.

Mechanism of Action. Tretinoin increases cell turnover in the follicular wall and decreases the cohesiveness of cells, leading to the extrusion of comedones and inhibition of the formation of new comedones. In patients with acne, new cells replace the cells of existing pimples, and the rapid turnover of cells prevents new pimples from forming.

Adverse Effects. The adverse effects are dry skin, peeling, itching, burning, stinging, and redness.

Clindamycin/Tretinoin

Mechanism of Action. Clindamycin binds to the 50S ribosomal subunits of susceptible bacteria and prevents elongation of the peptide chains by interfering with the peptidyl transfer, thereby suppressing bacterial protein synthesis. Tretinoin increases cell turnover in the follicular wall and decreases the cohesiveness of cells, leading to the extrusion of comedones and inhibition of the formation of new comedones.

Adverse Effects. The adverse effects are inflammation of the nose and throat, throat pain, dry skin, cough, and sinus inflammation.

Tazarotene

Tazarotene is a retinoid prodrug.

Mechanism of Action. Tazarotene modulates the differentiation and proliferation of epithelial tissue and exerts to some degree some antiinflammatory and immunological activity.

Adverse Effects. The adverse effects are itching burning, stinging, redness, irritation, swelling, dryness of the skin, and pain.

Azelaic Acid

Mechanism of Action. Azelaic acid works by killing the bacteria that infect pores and by decreasing the production of keratin, a natural substance that could lead to the development of acne.

Adverse Effects. The adverse effects are slight stinging or burning, tingling, redness, or drying of the skin may occur.

TECH ALERT!

The following drugs have look-alike/sound-alike issues:

Benoxyl, Brevoxyl, and Peroxyl;

Fostex and pHisohex;

Akne-Mycin and AK-Mycin;

doxycycline, dicyclomine, doxepin, and doxylamine;

Doxy-100 and Doxil;

Monodox and Maalox;

Dynacin, Dyazide, Dynabac, DynaCirc, and Dynapen;

Minocin, Indocin, Minizide, Mithracln, and niacin;

tretinoln and trientine

Drug Treatment for Moderate to Moderately Severe Acne

Generic name	U.S. brand name(s) / Canadian brand(s)	Dosage forms and strengths
adapalene	Differin	**Cream:** 0.1%
	Differin	**Gel:** 0.1% **Pledget:** 0.1% **Solution:** 0.1%
azelaic acid	Azelex, Finacea	**Cream:** 20%
	Finacea	**Gel:** 15%
benzoyl peroxide*	Zenzac AC, Brevoxyl, Triaz,	**Gel:** 2.5%
	Acetoxyl, Benoxyl, Benzac, Benzac AC, Benzac W GEL, Benzac W Wash, Desquam-X, Oxyderm, Pan Oxyl, Solugel	
erythromycin base* USP	Akne-Mycin, A/T/S, E mgel, Erycette, Eryderm, Erygel, Erymax, Ery-sol, Erythra-derm, ETS, Staticin Theramycin Z	**Gel:** 2% **Ointment:** 2% **Solution:** 2% (60 ml)
	Staticin, Sans-Acne	
benzoyl peroxide and erythromycin*	Benzamycin, Benzamycin Pak	**Gel:** benzoyl peroxide 5%, erythromycin 3%
	Benzamycin	

Continued

Drug Treatment for Moderate to Moderately Severe Acne—cont'd

Generic name	U.S. brand name(s) Canadian brand(s)	Dosage forms and strengths
doxycycline*	Vibramycin, Adoxa, Doryx, Doxy-100, Monodox, Periostat, Vibra-Tabs	**Capsule:** 50 mg. 100 mg **Capsule (coated pellets [Doryx]):** 75 mg, 100 mg **Tablet:** 50 mg, 75 mg, 100 mg
	Doxycin, Vibra-Tabs, Vibramycin	
benzoyl peroxide and clindamycin*	Benzaclin Duac	**Gel:** benzoyl peroxide 5% + clindamycin phosphate 1%
	Benzaclin	
minocylcine*	Minocin, Dynacin	**Capsule:** 50 mg, 75 mg, 100 mg **Capsule pellet-filled:** 50 mg, 100 mg **Tablet:** 50 mg, 75 mg, 100 mg
	Enca, Minocin	
tetracycline*	Sumycin, Wesmycin	**Capsule:** 250 mg, 500 mg **Tablet:** 250 mg, 500 mg
	Generics	
tazarotene	Avage, Tazorac	**Cream:** 0.05%, 0.1% **Gel:** 0.05%, 0.1%
	Tazarac	
tretinoin*	Altinac, Avita, Renova, Retin-A, Retin-A Micro	**Cream:** 0.025%, 0.05%, 0.1% **Gel:** 0.025% **Liquid:** 0.05%
	Rejuva-A, Retin-A, Retin-A Micro, Renova	
clindamycin + tretinoin	Ziana	**Gel:** clindamycin phosphate 1.2%, tretinoin 0.025%
	Not available	

*Generic available.

TREATMENT OF SEVERE ACNE

Severe acne is characterized by deep cysts, inflammation, extensive damage to the skin, and scarring. It requires an aggressive treatment regimen and should be treated by a dermatologist. Severe, disfiguring forms of acne can require years of treatment and individuals may experience one or more treatment failures. Almost every case of acne can be successfully treated. People with nodules or cysts should be treated by a dermatologist. Physical methods and medications that dermatologists use to treat severe acne include

- Drainage and surgical excision
- Inter-lesional corticoid injection
- Isotretinoin
- Oral antibiotics
- Oral contraceptives

ISOTRETINOIN

For patients with severe inflammatory acne that does not improve with medicines previously described, a physician may prescribe isotretinoin (Accutane), a retinoid (vitamin A derivative). Isotretinoin is an oral drug that is usually taken once or twice a day with food for 15 to 20 weeks. It markedly reduces the size of the oil glands so that much less oil is produced. As a result, the growth of bacteria is decreased.

Mechanism of Action. Isotretinoin noticeably reduces the production of sebum and shrinks the sebaceous glands. It stabilizes keratinization and prevents comedones from forming. Isotretinoin works by altering DNA transcription. This effect decreases the size and output of sebaceous glands, makes the cells that are sloughed off into the sebaceous glands less sticky, and therefore less able to form comedones.

Adverse Reactions. Treatment with isotretinoin can help prevent scarring; however, the drug must be used cautiously in women of childbearing age because it can produce fetal abnormalities. Isotretinoin is classified in FDA pregnancy category D. Women must use two separate effective forms of birth control at the same time for 1 month before treatment begins, during the entire course of treatment, and for 1 full month after stopping the drug.

Other possible side effects of isotretinoin include dry eyes, mouth, lips, nose, or skin (very common); itching; nosebleeds; muscle aches; sensitivity to the sun; poor night vision; changes in mood, depression, and suicidal thoughts; changes in the blood, such as an increase in fats in the blood (triglycerides and cholesterol); and change in liver function. To be able to determine if isotretinoin should be stopped if side effects occur, your physician may test your blood before you start treatment and periodically during treatment. Side effects usually go away after the medicine is stopped.

FDA iPLEDGE Program for Accutane and Generic Isotretinoin. The Food and Drug Administration (FDA) announced the approval of a strengthened risk management program, called iPLEDGE, for Accutane and generic isotretinoin. The sponsors have implemented a program that requires registration in the iPLEDGE program of wholesalers, prescribers, pharmacies, and patients who agree to accept specific responsibilities designed to minimize pregnancy exposures in order to distribute, prescribe, dispense, and use Accutane. The FDA approved a strengthened risk management plan for Accutane and generic isotretinoin on August 12, 2005, to make sure females do not become pregnant while taking this medicine. Isotretinoin causes birth defects. FDA approved this program under its regulations at 21 CFR 314, Subpart H. The starting date that began patient registration and qualification in iPLEDGE was December 30, 2005. Since March 1, 2006, only prescribers registered and activated in iPLEDGE can able to prescribe isotretinoin and only patients registered and qualified in iPLEDGE are able to be dispensed isotretinoin.

Isotretinoin is approved to treat the most severe form of acne (nodular acne) that has not responded to other acne treatments and that can leave permanent scars. However, isotretinoin can cause birth defects. Previous programs to reduce the risk of fetal exposure to isotretinoin were assessed in February 2004 by the FDA and the results of the assessment were presented at a joint meeting of the Drug Safety and Risk Management and Dermatologic and Ophthalmic Drugs Advisory Committees. Those committees strongly recommended the need for improvements in the isotretinoin risk management program to strengthen processes to ensure pregnancy testing and counseling of patients before and during treatment to reduce the risk of fetal exposure. The iPLEDGE program is a technology-based, closed system of registered wholesalers, prescribers, pharmacies, and patients. See the following Web sites for more details on the iPLEDGE program.

http://69.20.19.211/Cder/drug/infopage/accutane/default.htm
http://69.20.19.211/Cder/drug/advisory/isotretinoin2005.htm
https://www.ipledgeprogram.com/

Treatment for Severe Acne

Generic name	U.S. brand name(s) / Canadian brand(s)	Dosage forms and strengths
isotretinoin	Accutane, Amnesteem, Claravis, Sotret,	**Capsule:** 10 mg, 20 mg, 40 mg
	Accutane, Clarus	
oral antibiotics	See "Topical corticosteroid," mini drug monograph in Chapter 42 and Chapter 35	See "Topical corticosteroid," mini drug monograph in Chapter 42
oral contraceptives	See Chapter 34	See Chapter 34

TREATMENTS FOR HORMONALLY INFLUENCED ACNE IN WOMEN

In some women, acne is caused by an excess of androgen (male) hormones. Clues that this may be the case include hirsutism (excessive growth of hair on the face or body), premenstrual acne flares, irregular menstrual cycles, and elevated blood levels of certain androgens. The physician may prescribe one of several drugs to treat women with this type of acne.

Oral contraceptives (OCPs) help suppress the androgen produced by the ovaries. Side effects are nausea, weight gain, menstrual spotting, and breast tenderness. When an OCP is used to treat acne, the physician should prescribe a formulation that contains progestins with low androgenic possibility. Appropriate progestins include norethindrone (Norlutin), norethindrone acetate (Aygestin), ethynodiol diacetate (Zovia), and norgestimate (Ortho-Cyclen). Ultimately, the choice of OCP should be based on tolerability and compliance.

Treatments for Hormonally Induced Acne in Women

Generic name	U.S. brand name(s) Canadian brand(s)	Dosage forms and strengths
oral contraceptives*	See Chapter 34	See Chapter 34

*A complete listing of oral contraceptives is located in Chapter 34.

OTHER TREATMENTS FOR ACNE

Physicians may use other types of procedures in addition to drug therapy to treat patients with acne. For example, the physician may remove the patient's comedones during office visits. Sometimes, the physician will inject corticosteroids directly into lesions to help reduce the size and pain of inflamed cysts and nodules.

If scarring has occurred, dermabrasion (or microdermabrasion), which is a form of "sanding down" scars, is sometimes used. Another treatment option for deep scars caused by cystic acne is the transfer of fat from another part of the body to the scar. Alternatively, a synthetic filling material may be injected under the scar to improve its appearance.

Summary of Drugs Used for the Treatment of Acne

Generic name	Brand name	Usual dose and dosing schedule	Warning labels
benzoyl peroxide	Various brands and generics (see "Over the Counter Acne" products mini-drug monograph	**Cleansers:** Wash once or twice daily **Topical:** Apply sparingly once daily; increase to 2 to 3 times/day if needed	BLEACHING AGENT—AVOID CONTACT WITH FABRIC AND HAIR
resorcinol and sulfur	Clearasil Adult Care	Apply a small amount to affected area as directed by physician	FOR EXTERNAL USE ONLY
salicylic acid	Various brands and generics (see "Over the Counter Acne" products mini-drug monograph	**Cream, cloth, foam, liquid, gel:** Apply to skin once or twice daily and rinse thoroughly **Pads:** Apply to affected area 1 to 3 times a day **Patch:** apply over affected area at night; remove in the morning Bath gels or soap—wash once daily	AVOID THE EYES, MOUTH, LIPS, INSIDE THE NOSE, GENITALS, AND ANAL AREA

Summary of Drugs Used for the Treatment of Acne—cont'd

Generic name	Brand name	Usual dose and dosing schedule	Warning labels
sulfur and salicyclic acid	SAStid	**Soap:** Use every day or every other day	AVOID CONTACT WITH EYES FOR EXTERNAL USE ONLY
sulfur and sulfacetamide	Sulfacet-R	Apply a thin film 1 to 3 times/day Cleansing products should be used 1 to 2 times/day	FOR EXTERNAL USE ONLY AVOID CONTACT WITH EYES, EYELIDS, LIPS, MOUTH
adapalene	Differin	Apply once daily at bedtime	FOR EXTERNAL USE ONLY
azelaic acid	Azelex	Apply and massage a thin film into affected area twice daily	FOR EXTERNAL UE ONLY KEEP AWAY FROM EYES, EARS AND MUCOUS MEMBRANES
erythromycin	Various brands and generics	**Oral:** 250 mg to 500 mg twice daily **Topical:** Apply over affected area twice daily	FOR EXTERNAL USE ONLY
benzoyl peroxide and erythromycin	Benzamycin, Benzamycin Pak	Apply twice daily, morning and evening	FOR EXTERNAL USE ONLY
doxycycline	Vibramycin	50 mg to 100 mg twice daily	AVOID SUNLIGHT AVOID TAKING ANTACIDS, IRON, OR DAIRY PRODUCTS
benzoyl peroxide and clindamycin	Benzaclin, Duac	**BenzaClin:** Apply twice daily **Duac:** Apply once daily in the evening	MAY BLEACH HAIR AND FABRIC FOR EXTERNAL USE ONLY AVOID CONTACT WITH EYES, NOSE, MOUTH, AND ALL MUCOUS MEMBRANES
minocylcine	Minocin	50 mg to 100 mg once or twice daily	AVOID SUNLIGHT AVOID TAKING ANTACIDS, IRON, OR DAIRY PRODUCTS
tetracycline	Generics	250 mg to 500 mg/dose every 6 hours	AVOID SUNLIGHT AVOID TAKING ANTACIDS, IRON, OR DAIRY PRODUCTS
tazarotene	Avage, Tazorac Tazarac	Apply thin film once daily, in the evening to the affected area	DO NOT USE IF PREGNANT FOR EXTERNAL USE ONLY
tretinoin	Renova, Retin-A	Apply once daily to acne lesions once daily before bedtime or on alternate days	MAY CAUSE SENSITIVITY TO SUNLIGHT
clindamycin + tretinoin	Ziana	Apply to entire face every night at bedtime	AVOID EXCESSIVE EXPOSURE TO THE SUN, COLD AND WIND FOR EXTERNAL USE ONLY
isotretenoin	Accutane	0.5 mg/kg/day to 2 mg/kg/day for 15 to 20 weeks	TAKE WITH FOOD AVOID PREGNANCY AVOID USE OF VITAMIN A PRODUCTS

CHAPTER SUMMARY

- Acne is a disorder resulting from the action of hormones and other substances on the skin's oil glands (sebaceous glands) and hair follicles.
- Doctors describe acne as a disease of the pilosebaceous units (PSUs). Found over most of the body, PSUs consist of a sebaceous gland connected to a canal, called a follicle, that contains a fine hair.
- Common acne, or acne vulgaris, occurs most frequently in the adolescent years as a result of overactive secretion by the sebaceous glands accompanied by blockages and inflammation of their ducts.
- Pus-filled pimples or pustules result from secondary infections within or beneath the epidermis, often in a hair follicle or sweat pore.
- Milia are tiny bumps that occur when normally sloughed skin cells get trapped in small pockets on the surface of the skin.
- The goals of treatment for acne are to heal existing lesions, stop new lesions from forming, prevent scarring, and minimize the psychological stress and embarrassment caused by this disease.
- Benzoyl peroxide is the most effective and widely used nonprescription medication currently available for treatment of noninflammatory acne.
- Salicyclic acid is a mild comedolytic (keratolytic) agent that provides a milder, less effective alternative to the prescription agent tretinoin.
- Topical OTC medicines are available in many forms, such as gels, lotions, creams, soaps, or pads. In some people, OTC acne medicines may cause side effects such as skin irritation, burning, or redness, which often get better or go away with continued use of the medicine.
- Adapalene is believed to affect the growth of skin cells and thereby reduce the formation of pimples.
- Azelaic acid works by killing the bacteria that infect pores and by decreasing the production of keratin, a natural substance that could lead to the development of acne.
- Tazarotene modulates the differentiation and proliferation of epithelial tissue and exerts to some degree some antiinflammatory and immunological activity.
- Tretinoin increases cell turnover in the follicular wall and decreases the cohesiveness of cells, leading to the extrusion of comedones and inhibition of the formation of new comedones.
- Severe acne is characterized by deep cysts, inflammation, extensive damage to the skin, and scarring. It requires an aggressive treatment regimen and should be treated by a dermatologist.
- For patients with severe inflammatory acne a physician may prescribe isotretinoin, a retinoid (vitamin A derivative).
- Early treatment is the best way to prevent acne scars. Once scarring has occurred, dermabrasion may be used to treat irregular scars.
- Medical researchers are working on new drugs to treat acne, particularly topical antibiotics to replace some of those in current use.

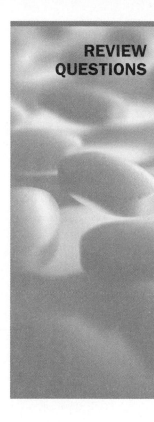

REVIEW QUESTIONS

Multiple Choice

1. **An enlarged and plugged hair follicle, the most characteristic sign of acne, is termed a _____.**
   a. milia
   b. pustule
   c. comedone
   d. papule

2. **Physicians know the exact cause of acne.**
   a. true
   b. false

3. **_____ is the most effective and widely used nonprescription medication currently available for the treatment of noninflammatory acne.**
   a. Salicylic acid
   b. Benzoyl peroxide
   c. Sulfur
   d. Doxycycline

4. **At-home treatment for acne requires _____ to see improvement.**
   a. 2 to 4 weeks
   b. 4 to 8 weeks
   c. 6 to 10 weeks
   d. 8 to 10 weeks

5. **When acne is resistant to topical therapies, intravenous antibiotics may be used.**
   a. true
   b. false

6. **Which of the following oral antibiotics is LESS commonly used for the treatment of moderate to severe acne?**
   a. doxycycline
   b. tetracycline
   c. clindamycin
   d. minocycline

7. **_____ works by killing the bacteria that infect pores and by decreasing the production of keratin, a natural substance that could lead to the development of acne.**
   a. Azelaic acid
   b. Adapalene
   c. Benzoyl peroxide
   d. A and c

8. **_____ is a very effective medicine that can help prevent scarring.**
   a. Tretinoin
   b. Isotretinoin
   c. Retinoin
   d. All of the above

9. **Oral contraceptives are used to treat what type of acne?**
   a. mild
   b. moderate
   c. severe
   d. hormonally induced

10. **Which of the following drugs are used for treating hormonally influenced acne?**
    a. corticosteroids
    b. antiandrogens
    c. progestins
    d. all of the above

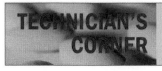

TECHNICIAN'S CORNER

1. There are many OTC and prescription medications available for the treatment of acne. Are there any natural/herbal remedies available?
2. What advice can one give to a teenager experiencing acne?

BIBLIOGRAPHY

Acne vulgaris. Available at: http://en.wikipedia.org/wiki/Acne_vulgaris.

American Academy of Dermatology. Available at: www.aad.org.

Berardi RR, et al., American Pharmacists Association (APhA): *Handbook of nonprescription drugs,* ed 15, Washington DC, 2006.

Diagnosis and treatment of acne. Available at: http://www.aafp.org/afp/20040501/2123.html.

National Institute of Arthritis and Musculoskeletal and Skin Diseases (NIAMS): Available at: www.niams.nih.gov.

Lance L, Lacy C, Armstrong L, Goldman M: *Drug information handbook for the allied health professional,* ed 12. Hudson, OH, 2005, APhA Lexi-Comp.

Thibodeau G, Patton K: *Anatomy and physiology,* ed 6, St. Louis, 2007, Mosby.

Treating severe acne. Available at: www.skincarephysicians.com/acnenet/treatsevereacne.html.

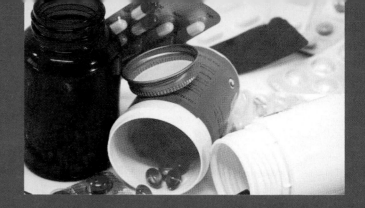

Treatment of Eczema and Psoriasis

LEARNING OBJECTIVES

- Learn the terminology associated with eczema and psoriasis.
- Describe the etiology of eczema and psoriasis.
- List the symptoms of eczema and psoriasis.
- List and categorize medications used to treat eczema and psoriasis.
- Describe mechanism of action for drugs used to treat eczema and psoriasis.
- Identify warning labels and precautionary messages associated with medications used to treat eczema and psoriasis.
- Identify significant drug look-alike/sound-alike issues.
- List common endings for drug classes used in the treatment of eczema and psoriasis.

KEY TERMS

Atopic: Group of diseases where there is an inherited tendency to develop other allergic conditions.

Atopic dermatitis: Chronic disease of the skin.

Cutaneous: Pertaining to the skin.

Dermatitis: Inflammation of the skin.

Eczema: General term used to describe several types of inflammation of the skin.

Exacerbation: Aggravation of symptoms or increases in the severity of the disease.

Phototherapy: Treatment for atopic dermatitis that involves exposing the skin to ultraviolet A or B light waves.

Psoriasis: Chronic disease of the skin that is characterized by itchy red patches covered with silvery scales.

Remission: Lessening in severity or an abatement of symptoms.

OVERVIEW

Eczema is a general term used to describe several types of inflammation of the skin. It is a common condition affecting millions of Americans and Canadians. There are several types of eczema. They are atopic dermatitis, allergic contact eczema, contact eczema, dyshidrotic eczema, neurodermatitis, nummular eczema, seborrheic eczema, and stasis dermatitis. These types of eczema are described in Box 42-1.

Atopic dermatitis is the most common from of eczema, affecting more than 15 million Americans. It is a chronic disease of the skin that often develops in infancy and may continue throughout adulthood. *Atopic* is defined as a group of diseases where there is an inherited tendency to develop other allergic conditions. Up to 75% of children with eczema (atopic dermatitis) are prone to developing asthma and hay fever.

Unlike contact dermatitis, where symptoms appear after exposure to an allergen, the cause for eczema (atopic dermatitis) is unknown. People who live in dry climates and in large cities seem to have a higher incidence of the condition. Perhaps it is because atopic dermatitis appears to be linked to environmental factors. Heredity and a malfunction of the body's immune system are other important factors that are associated with the condition. Atopic diseases are autoimmune disorders and persons with atopic dermatitis have a hyperactive dermal response to irritants.

Common irritants are listed in Box 42-2.

Langerhans cells in the skin are potent activators of T cells (see Unit 10), and levels are increased in the skin of individuals with atopic diseases. Psoriasis is also caused by hyperactivity of the T cells. *Psoriasis* is a condition associated with rapid turnover of skin cells. Whereas the normal rate of cell turnover is approximately 30 days, with psoriasis the cell turnover rate may be as short as a few days. Individuals with psoriasis have thick, silvery, scaly patches. They may also have some redness and swelling. Itchy psoriatic

BOX 42-1 TYPES OF ECZEMA

- Allergic contact eczema (dermatitis): a red, itchy, weepy reaction where the skin has come into contact with a substance that the immune system recognizes as foreign, such as poison ivy or certain preservatives in creams and lotions
- Atopic dermatitis: a chronic skin disease characterized by itchy, inflamed skin
- Contact eczema: a localized reaction that includes redness, itching, and burning where the skin has come into contact with an allergen (an allergy-causing substance) or with an irritant such as an acid, a cleaning agent, or other chemical
- Dyshidrotic eczema: irritation of the skin on the palms of hands and soles of the feet characterized by clear, deep blisters that itch and burn
- Neurodermatitis: scaly patches of the skin on the head, lower legs, wrists, or forearms caused by localized itch (such as an insect bite) that become intensely irritated when scratched
- Nummular eczema: coin-shaped patches of irritated skin—most common on the arms, back, buttocks, and lower legs—that may be crusted, scaling, and extremely itchy
- Seborrhic eczema: yellowish, oily, scaly patches of skin on the scalp, face, and occasionally other parts of the body
- Statis dermatitis: a skin irritation on the lower legs, generally related to circulatory problems

(From National Institute of Arthritis and Musculoskeletal and Skin Diseases, Bethesda, MD.)

BOX 42-2 COMMON IRRITANTS

- Wool or synthetic fibers
- Soaps and detergents
- Perfumes and cosmetics
- Cleaning solvents, mineral oil and chlorine
- Dust
- Sand
- Cigarette smoke

patches may be found on the neck, elbows, genitals, scalp, hands, and feet. Factors that aggravate psoriasis are

- Stress
- Dry skin
- Environmental factors that produce dry skin (e.g., heating systems and weather)
- Infections
- Some medicines

Symptoms of Atopic Dermatitis (Eczema)

Atopic *dermatitis* commonly produces symptoms of intense itching, redness (from scratching), skin irritation, and inflammation. Eczematous patches may form that are flaky and crusting and may even ooze a clear fluid (Figure 42-1).

Individuals with eczema (atopic dermatitis) (Box 42-3) and psoriasis may experience periods when their symptoms worsen (*exacerbation*) and periods when they get better or go away completely (*remission*). It is not uncommon for eczema that has gone into remission in childhood to return with the onset of puberty. Factors that exacerbate symptoms of eczema are

- Stress
- Contact with environmental pollutants and household cleaning products
- Food allergy (eggs, peanuts, milk, fish, soy products, and wheat)
- Wearing wool or clothing that rubs and irritates skin
- Factors that cause dry skin (low humidity environments, not applying moisturizers, and hot baths)
- Scratching

Scratching can break down the protective layer of the skin and increase the risk of developing secondary bacterial or viral infections.

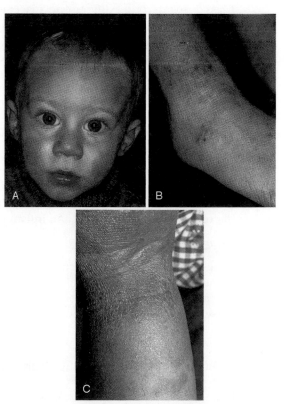

FIGURE 42-1 Eczema. **A,** infantile phase. **B,** childhood phase. **C,** Adolescent phase. *(From Fitzpatrick JE, Morelli JG: Dermatology secrets in color, ed 3, Philadelphia, Mosby, 2007 C, Courtesy James E. Fitzpatrick, MD.)*

BOX 42-3 SIGNS AND SYMPTOMS OF ECZEMA

- Dry, rectangular scales on the skin
- Small rough bumps and papules on arms, legs, face
- Thickened, leathery patches of skin
- Inflammation around the corners of the mouth and face rash
- Darkened eyelids and skin around the eyes

- Extra skin fold under the eye
- Excess creases in the palms of the hands
- Hives (urticaria)
- Intense itching
- Redness
- Rashes in creases of elbows and knees

Nonpharmaceutical Treatment of Eczema and Psoriasis

Nonpharmaceutical treatment for eczema involves using skin care regimens (Box 42-4) that reduce irritation and avoiding allergens and irritants and may include the use of phototherapy. *Phototherapy* involves exposing the skin to ultraviolet (UV) A or B light waves. It may be used alone or in combination with drug therapy. Phototherapy is only recommended for individuals older than 12 years. Adverse reactions to the use of UV light therapy are premature aging of the skin and increased risk for skin cancer.

Pharmaceutical Treatment of Eczema and Psoriasis

CORTICOSTEROIDS

The use of topical corticosteroids continues to be a mainstay of therapy for the treatment of eczema. Corticosteroids are also used for the treatment of psoriasis, seborrhea, and other skin conditions where inflammation is present. The use of oral corticosteroids is reserved for severe symptoms.

Topical corticosteroids are categorized into seven groups based on potency (Box 42-5). Class I agents (e.g., diflorasone diacetate [Psorcon]) are super-high potency. Class VII agents include hydrocortisone, which is mild enough for OTC use. The vehicle (base) in which the corticosteroid is suspended may influence the potency. For example, betamethasone dipropionate in an optimized vehicle is super potent (Class II), whereas the same drug in a regular vehicle is classified as potent (Class IV). Higher potency corticosteroids have more adverse reactions. Only the mildest potency agents, like hydrocortisone, should be used on the face.

MECHANISM OF ACTION AND PHARMACOKINETICS

Topical corticosteroids possess antiinflammatory and immunosuppressive properties and produce vasoconstriction. They reduce the permeability of the cells T-lymphocytes and eosinophils, thereby decreasing the release of mediators of the inflammatory response (e.g., cytokines). They also reduce the number of inflammatory cells, which decreases redness, swelling, and inflammation.

ADVERSE REACTIONS

Long-term use of topical corticosteroids can result in thinning of the skin, stretch marks (striae), spider veins, acne, milia, rosacea (enlarged blood vessel especially on nose), bruising, atrophy, lacerations, poor wound healing, and growth suppression (in children). Adverse reactions are more extensive when high-potency corticosteroids are used.

TECH ALERT!
The following drugs have look-alike/sound-alike issues: flucinolone and flucinonide; hydrocortisone acetate, hydrocortisone butyrate, and hydrocortisone valerate; betamethasone dipropionate and betamethasone valerate; betamethasone dipropionate augmented formula and betamethasone dipropionate regular

BOX 42-4 RECOMMENDED SKIN CARE FOR PERSONS WITH ECZEMA

- Avoid hot bathes or showers
- Air-dry or gently pat dry skin after bathing (Avoid vigorous rubbing)

- Apply moisturizing cream or ointment after bathing (lotions may be drying)

BOX 42-5 POTENCY CLASSIFICATION OF SELECTED TOPICAL CORTICOSTEROIDS (GENERIC NAMES)

CLASS I SUPER-HIGH POTENCY
- clobetasol propionate
- diflorasone diacetate

CLASS II SUPER POTENT
- betamethasone dipropionate (optimized vehicle)
- halobetasol propionate

CLASS III VERY POTENT
- amcinonide
- desoximetasone
- halcinonide
- fluocinonide
- mometasone furoate
- diflorasone diacetate (cream)
- triamcinolone > 0.5%

CLASS IV POTENT
- betamethasone dipropionate (regular vehicle)
- flurandrenolide (ointment)
- mometasone furoate

CLASS V MEDIUM POTENCY
- beclomethasone
- betamethasone valerate
- diflucortolone valerate
- fluocinolone acetonide
- flurandrenolide (cream)
- fluticasone propionate (cream)
- hydrocortisone butyrate (cream)
- hydrocortisone valerate (cream)
- triamcinolone acetonide < 0.5%

CLASS VI MILD POTENCY
- alclometasone dipropionate (cream, ointment)
- desonide (cream)
- prednicarbate

CLASS VII MILDEST POTENCY
- dexamethasone
- hydrocortisone base

Adapted from Clinical Pharmacology, Gold Standard, Inc. http://www.clinicalpharmacology.com and Raymond, G. and Houle, M.-C., A Review of Corticosteroids for the Treatment of Psoriasis, *Dermatology Service, Centre Hospitalier Université de Montréal, Montréal, QC, Canada.*

Topical Corticosteroids

Generic name	U.S. brand name(s) / Canadian brand(s)	Dosage forms and strengths
alclometasone dipropionate*	Aclovate / Not available	**Cream:** 0.05% **Ointment:** 0.05%
amcinonide*	Generics / Cyclort	**Cream:** 0.1% **Lotion:** 0.1% **Ointment:** 0.1%
betamethasone dipropionate*	Diprolene, Diprolene AF / Diprolene, Diprosone	**Cream, augmented:** 0.05% **Cream:** 0.05%, 0.064% (Diprosone) **Gel, augmented:** 0.05% **Lotion, augmented:** 0.05% **Lotion:** 0.05% **Ointment:** 0.05%
betamethasone valerate*	Luxiq / Betaderm, Valisone	**Cream:** 0.1% **Lotion:** 0.1% **Ointment:** 0.1% **Topical foam (Luxiq):** 0.12%
clobetasol propionate*	Clobevate, Clobex, Cormax, Olux, Olux-E, Temovate, Temovate-E / Clobex, Dermovate	**Cream:** 0.05% **Gel:** 0.05% **Lotion:** 0.05% **Ointment:** 0.05% **Shampoo:** 0.05% **Spray:** 0.05% **Solution:** 0.05% **Topical foam (Olux):** 0.05%

Continued

Topical Corticosteroids—cont'd

Generic name	U.S. brand name(s) Canadian brand(s)	Dosage forms and strengths
desonide*	Desowen, LoKara, Verdeso	**Cream:** 0.05% **Lotion:** 0.05% **Ointment:** 0.05% **Topical foam (Verdeso):** 0.05%
	Desocort	
desoximetasone*	Topicort, Topicort LP	**Cream:** 0.25% (Topicort), 0.05% (Topicort LP, Topicort Mild) **Gel (Topicort):** 0.05% **Ointment (Topicort):** 0.25%
	Topicort, Topicort Mild	
diflucortolone valerate	Not available	**Cream:** 0.1% **Oily cream:** 0.1% **Ointment:** 0.1%
	Nerisone, Nerisone Oily	
diflorasone diacetate*	Apexicon, Apexicon-E, Psorcon-E	**Cream:** 0.05% **Ointment (Apexicon):** 0.05%
	Not available	
fluocinolone acetonide*	Capex, DermaSmoothe FS Eczema	**Cream:** 0.01%, 0.025% **Ointment:** 0.025% **Shampoo (Capex):** 0.01% **Solution:** 0.01% **Topical oil (DermaSmoothe FS):** 0.01%
	Capex, DermaSmoothe FS Eczema, Synalar	
fluocinonide*	Lidex, Vanos	**Cream (Lidex, Vanos):** 0.05% **Cream, emulsified (Lidex, Lidemol):** 0.05% **Gel:** 0.05% **Ointment:** 0.05% **Solution:** 0.05%
	Lidex, Lidemol, Lyderm, Tiamol, Topactin	
flurandrenolide	Cordran, Cordran SP, Cordran Tape	**Cream (Cordran SP):** 0.05% **Lotion (Cordran):** 0.05% **Tape:** 4 µg
	Not available	
fluticasone propionate	Cutivate	**Cream:** 0.05% **Lotion:** 0.05% (U.S. only) **Ointment:** 0.005% (U.S. only)
	Cutivate	
halcinonide	Halog	**Cream:** 0.1% **Ointment:** 0.1% **Solution:** 0.1% (U.S. only)
	Halog	
halobetasol propionate*	Ultravate	**Cream:** 0.05% **Ointment:** 0.05%
	Ultravate	
hydrocortisone base* (only Rx trade names listed)	Hytone, Instacort, Keratol, Nutracort	**Cream:** 1%; 2.5% (Hytone) **Gel (Instacort):** 1%
	Dermaflex HC, Emo Cort, Hyderm	
hydrocortisone butyrate*	Locoid	**Cream:** 0.1% **Cream, lipocream:** 0.1% **Ointment:** 0.1% **Solution:** 0.1%
	Not available	
hydrocortisone valerate*	Westcort	**Cream:** 0.2% **Ointment:** 0.2%
	Westcort	
mometasone furoate*	Elocon	**Cream:** 0.1% **Ointment:** 0.1% **Solution:** 0.1%
	Elocom	

Topical Corticosteroids—cont'd

Generic name	U.S. brand name(s) Canadian brand(s)	Dosage forms and strengths
prednicarbate*	Dermatop-E	**Cream:** 0.1% **Ointment:** 0.1%
	Dermatop, Dermatop-E	
triamcinolone acetonide*	Cinalog, Delta Tritex, Kenalog, Triderm	**Cream:** 0.025%, 0.1%, 0.5% (Cinalog) **Lotion:** 0.025%, 0.1%
	Aristocort, Kenalog, Triaderm	**Ointment:** 0.025%, 0.1%, 0.5% **Topical spray (Kenalog):** 0.147 mg/g

*Generic available.

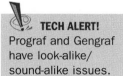

TECH ALERT!
Prograf and Gengraf have look-alike/sound-alike issues.

IMMUNOMODULATORS: CALCINEURIN INHIBITORS

Calcineurin inhibitors are immunomodulators. They control inflammation and reduce immune system response to allergens. Pimecrolimus is indicated for the treatment of mild-to-moderate eczema. It is approved for short-term and intermittent long-term therapy. Tacrolimus is approved for the treatment of moderate-to-severe atopic dermatitis that has failed to respond to corticosteroid treatment.

MECHANISM OF ACTION AND PHARMACOKINETICS

Pimecrolimus and tacrolimus inhibits T-cell activation and the production of cytokines, interleukins, and interferons; mediators of the inflammatory response.

ADVERSE REACTIONS

Common adverse reactions associated with topical application are local burning and stinging of the skin. The U.S. Food and Drug Administration and Health Canada require manufacturers to include a Black Box warning in the package insert, advising health care providers that pimecrolimus and tacrolimus may increase the risk for development of lymphoma. The risk for lymphoma is minimal with topical application compared to parenteral use according to the Canadian Dermatology Association.

Calcineurin Inhibitors

Generic name	U.S. brand name(s) Canadian brand(s)	Dosage forms and strengths
pimecrolimus	Elidel	**Cream:** 1%
	Elidel	
tacrolimus	Prograf, Protopic	**Capsule:** 0.5 mg, 1 mg, 5 mg **Ointment:** 0.03%, 0.1%
	Prograf, Protopic	**Solution for injection:** 5 mg/ml

VITAMIN D ANALOGS

Calcipotriene is a synthetic analog of vitamin D. The generic name is calcipotriol in Canada. The drug is approved for the treatment of psoriasis. Signs of improvement can be seen in about 2 weeks; however, maximum effects may take 4 to 8 weeks.

MECHANISM OF ACTION AND PHARMACOKINETICS

Calcipotriene (calcipotriol) inhibits the rapid and repeated production of new skin cells (proliferation). It inhibits the proliferation of T cells and inhibits the release of mediators of inflammation (e.g., cytokines, interleukins, and interferons).

ADVERSE REACTIONS

Most adverse reactions are localized to the site of application. Irritation and redness are common. When large areas of the body are covered with the drug, some systemic absorption may occur. Vitamin D plays an important role in calcium absorption. Systemic effects produced by calcipotriene (calcipotriol) are increased calcium in the blood and urine.

Vitamin D Analogs

Generic name	U.S. brand name(s)	Dosage forms and strengths
	Canadian brand(s)	
calcipotriene (calcipotriol–Canada)	Dovonex	**Cream:** 0.005%
	Dovonex	**Solution, scalp:** 0.005% **Solution, topical:** 0.005%
calcipotriene + betamethasone dipropionate	Taclonex	**Ointment:** 0.005% calcipotriene + 0.064% betamethasone dipropionate
	Dovobet	

FURANOCOUMARINS

Psoralens are a class of drugs that increase photosensitivity and are classified as furanocoumarins. Methoxsalen is the only drug in this class. It is approved for the treatment of atopic dermatitis and psoriasis along with UV light therapy. Methoxsalen and UV light work synergistically. Methoxalen increases the skins sensitivity to UV light and UV light activates methoxsalen. Psoralens plus UV light A therapy is also known as PUVA.

MECHANISM OF ACTION AND PHARMACOKINETICS

The action of methosoxalen on pyramidine bases of the DNA molecule results in suppression of DNA synthesis. This decreases cell replication and proliferation. DNA photodamage produces *cutaneous* immunosuppression by affecting leukocyte regulatory mechanisms. Psoralens may be administered orally, topically, or parenterally. The bioavailability of methoxsalen hard gelatin capsules (8-MOP) and soft gelatin capsules (Oxsoralen-Ultra) is not equivalent so product substitution is not permitted. 8-MOP should be taken with food or milk, whereas Oxsorelan-Ultra should be taken with low-fat food or milk.

ADVERSE REACTIONS

Adverse reactions produced by oral methoxsalen therapy are photosensitivity, insomnia, headache, dizziness, leg cramps, itching, dry skin, nausea, and vomiting. Topical application can cause burning, blistering, and swelling at the site of application.

Furanocoumarins

Generic name	U.S. brand name(s)	Dosage forms and strengths
	Canadian brand(s)	
methoxsalen	8-MOP, Oxsoralen, Oxsoralen Ultra, UVADEX	**Capsule (Oxsoralen Ultra, 8-MOP):** 10 mg **Lotion (Oxsoralen):** 1%
	Oxsoralen, Oxsoralen Ultra, UltraMOP	**Solution, injection (UVADEX):** 20 mcg/ml

IMMUNOSUPPRESSANTS AND ANTIMETABOLITES

Atopic dermatitis is believed to be an autoimmune disease; therefore, immune system modulation and immunosuppression can downregulate the body's response to allergens and other irritants. Cyclosporine and azathioprine are immunosuppressants (see Chapter 15). Cyclosporine is FDA approved for the short-term treatment of severe atopic dermatitis and psoriasis. Azathioprine is used for the treatment of severe psoriasis, although not FDA approved. Methotrexate is an antimetabolite (see Chapter 37 and 15) that is indicated for the treatment of moderate to severe chronic psoriasis and psoriatic arthritis.

MECHANISM OF ACTION

Cyclosporine selectively interferes with T-cell proliferation and interleukin production. The result is a decreased immune system response. Azathioprine also suppresses T-cell–mediated immune system response. Additionally, azathioprine blocks the synthesis of RNA and DNA needed for cell replication. Methotrexate also interferes with normal DNA synthesis. Azathioprine and methotrexate slow the rapid rate of skin cell turnover that occurs with eczema and psoriasis.

ADVERSE REACTIONS

Cyclosporine, azathioprine, and methotrexate may produce nausea and vomiting. They also may increase the risk for infections. Azathioprine and methotrexate use may cause a dangerous drop in red and white blood cells. Cyclosporine can cause kidney toxicity, whereas azathioprine can cause liver toxicity. Weight gain and hypertension are other side effects of cyclosporine therapy. See Chapter 15 for a complete list of adverse reactions.

Immunosuppressants

Generic name	U.S. brand name(s) / Canadian brand(s)	Dosage forms and strengths
azathioprine*	Azasan, Imuran / Imuran	**Injection, powder for reconstitution:** 100 mg **Tablet:** 25 mg, 50 mg, 75 mg, 100 mg (Imuran only available as 50 mg)
cyclosporine*	Gengraf, Neoral, / Neoral	**Capsule, modified (Gengraf, Neoral):** 25 mg, 100 mg **Solution, oral, modified (Gengraf, Neoral):** 100 mg/ml (See Chapter 15 for additional dosage forms and brand names)
methotrexate* (MTX)	Rheumatrex, Trexall / generics	**Powder for injection (generics):** 1 g/vial **Solution for injection (generics):** 25 mg/ml **Tablet:** 2.5 mg dosepak (Rheumatrex); 5 mg, 7.5 mg, 10 mg, 15 mg (Trexall)

*Generic available.

TUMOR NECROSIS FACTOR-α INHIBITORS

Etanercept is a tumor necrosis factor (TNF)-α inhibitor indicated for the treatment of psoriasis.

TNF-α inhibitors are genetically engineered drugs that block the inflammatory process triggered by high concentrations of TNF. Psoriasis is a condition that is linked to high levels of TNF. TNF-α inhibitors prevent cell lysis (destruction) and release of the substances that cause inflammation. Adverse reactions of etanercept are nausea, stomach pain, headache, opportunistic infections, redness, and itching at the injection site.

Tumor Necrosis Factor-α inhibitors

Generic name	U.S. brand name / Canadian brand	Dosage forms and strengths
etanercept	Enbrel / Enbrel	**Injection, powder for reconstitution:** 25 mg **Injection, solution:** 50 mg/ml (0.98 ml prefilled syringe)

MISCELLANEOUS

Anthralin is one of the oldest drugs approved for the treatment of psoriasis. It was approved in 1939.

MECHANISM OF ACTION

Anthralin reduces cell turnover by inhibiting mitosis in skin cells. Mitosis is the part of the cell replication process in which DNA is replicated, divided, and split between the old cell and a new cell.

ADVERSE REACTIONS

Anthralin causes skin discoloration and may cause discoloration of hair and nails.

Miscellaneous

Generic name	U.S. brand name(s) Canadian brand(s)	Dosage forms and strengths
anthralin	Drithro-Scalp, Psoriatec	**Cream:** 0.5% (Dritho-Scalp); 1% (Psoriatec)
	Not available	

Summary of Drugs Used for the Treatment of Eczema

	Generic name	Brand name	Usual dose and dosing schedule	Warning labels
	Topical corticosteroids			
	alclometasone dipropionate*	Aclovate	**Cream or ointment:** Apply a thin film 2 to 3 times/day	FOR EXTERNAL USE
	amcinonide*	Generics	**All dosage forms:** Apply a thin film 2 to 3 times/day	
	betamethasone dipropionate*	Diprolene AF Diprosone	**Cream, lotion, ointment:** Apply a thin film 2 to 4 times/day	
	betamethasone valerate*	Betaderm, Luxiq, Valisone	**Foam:** Apply twice daily Cream, lotion, ointment: Apply a thin film 2 to 4 times/day	FOR EXTERNAL USE SHAKE WELL—foam, lotion
	clobetasol propionate*	Clobex	**All dosage forms:** Apply twice daily	
	desonide*	Desowen Desocort	**Foam:** Apply twice daily **Cream, lotion, ointment:** Apply a thin film 2 to 4 times/day	
	desoximetasone*	Topiocort	**Cream, gel, ointment:** Apply a thin film 2 times/day	FOR EXTERNAL USE
	diflucortolone valerate	Nerisone	Apply 3 times/day	FOR EXTERNAL USE
	diflorasone* diacetate	Psorcon-E	**Nonemollient dosage forms:** Apply a thin film 1 to 4 times/day **Emollient dosage forms:** Apply a thin film 1 to 3 times/day	FOR EXTERNAL USE
	fluocinolone acetonide*	Synalar Derma Smoothe FS	**Cream, ointment, solution:** Apply a thin film 2 to 4 times/day **Oil:** Apply a thin film 3 times/day	FOR EXTERNAL USE

Summary of Drugs Used for the Treatment of Eczema—cont'd

	Generic name	Brand name	Usual dose and dosing schedule	Warning labels
	halcinonide	Halog	**Cream, ointment, solution:** Apply a thin film 2 to 4 times/day	FOR EXTERNAL USE
	halobetasol propionate*	Ultravate	**Cream or ointment:** Apply a thin film 1 to 2 times/day	FOR EXTERNAL USE
	hydrocortisone, acetate*	Keratol HC	**All dosage forms:** Apply 3 to 4 times/day	FOR EXTERNAL USE
	hydrocortisone butyrate*	Locoid	**All dosage forms:** Apply 1 to 2 times/day	FOR EXTERNAL USE
	hydrocortisone valerate*	Westcort	**All dosage forms:** Apply 2 to 4 times/day	FOR EXTERNAL USE
	mometasone furoate*	Elocon	**Topical dosage forms:** Apply once daily	FOR EXTERNAL USE
	prednicarbate*	Dermatop	**Cream or ointment:** Apply a thin film 2 times/day	FOR EXTERNAL USE
	triamcinolone acetonide*	Kenalog	**Cream, lotion, ointment:** Apply a thin film 2 to 4 times/day	FOR EXTERNAL USE
Calcineurin Inhibitors				
	pimecrolimus	Elidel	Apply a thin layer twice daily	AVOID EXCESS EXPOSURE TO SUNLIGHT
	tacrilimus	Protopic	Apply a thin layer twice daily	AVOID GRAPEFRUIT JUICE—capsule
Immunosuppressives				
	cyclosporine	Neoral	1.25 mg/kg orally twice daily up to 4 mg/kg daily	TAKE WITH FOOD AVOID PREGNANCY AVOID ALCOHOL SWALLOW WHOLE, DON'T CRUSH OR CHEW
	methotrexate	generics	10 mg to 25 mg oral/IV/IM given as a single weekly dose or 2.5 mg to 5 mg orally every 12 hours for 3 doses every week	DO NOT DRINK ALCOHOLIC BEVERAGES AVOID PROLONGED EXPOSURE TO SUNLIGHT AVOID PREGNANCY EXERCISE PRECAUTIONS FOR HANDLING, PREPARING, AND ADMINISTERING CYTOTOXIC DRUGS
Vitamin D Analogs				
	calcipotriene	Dovonex	Apply a thin layer 2 times/day	FOR EXTERNAL USE AVOID EXCESS EXPOSURE TO SUNLIGHT AVOID FACE
	calcipotriene + betamethasone	Taclonex	Apply thin layer once daily	

Continued

Summary of Drugs Used for the Treatment of Eczema—cont'd

	Generic name	Brand name	Usual dose and dosing schedule	Warning labels
Furanocoumarins				
	methoxsalen	Oxsoralen Ultra	**Capsule:** 1 capsule 1½ to 2 hours before UVA therapy	TAKE WITH FOOD OR MILK AVOID SUN EXPOSURE FOR 24 HOURS BEFORE AND 48 HOURS AFTER TREATMENT
Tumor Necrosis Factor-α Inhibitors				
	etanercept	Enbrel	**Psoriasis:** 50 mg SC weekly given as one 50 mg SC injection or as two 25 mg SC injections 3 to 4 days apart	PROTECT FROM LIGHT REFRIGERATE; DON'T FREEZE
Miscellaneous				
	anthralin	Psoriatec	Apply once daily at bedtime	MAY STAIN SKIN, FABRIC, OR HAIR

*generic available

CHAPTER SUMMARY

- *Eczema* is a general term used to describe several types of inflammation of the skin.
- Atopic dermatitis, allergic contact eczema, contact eczema, dyshidrotic eczema, neurodermatitis, nummular eczema, seborrheic eczema, and stasis dermatitis are all types of eczema.
- Atopic dermatitis is the most common from of eczema.
- Atopic dermatitis is a chronic disease of the skin that often develops in infancy and may continue throughout adulthood.
- People who live in dry climates and in large cities seem to have a higher incidence of atopic dermatitis.
- Atopic diseases are an autoimmune disorder.
- Psoriasis is also caused by hyperactivity of the T cells.
- Psoriasis is a condition associated with rapid turnover of skin cells.
- Individuals with psoriasis have thick, silvery, scaly patches. They may also have some redness and swelling.
- Atopic dermatitis commonly produces symptoms of intense itching, redness (from scratching), skin irritation, and inflammation. Eczematous patches may form that are flaky and crusting and may even ooze a clear fluid.
- Individuals with eczema (atopic dermatitis) and psoriasis may experience periods when their symptoms worsen (exacerbation) and periods when they get better or go away completely (remission).
- Nonpharmaceutical treatment for eczema involves using skin care regimens that reduce irritation and avoiding allergens and irritants and may include the use of phototherapy.
- Phototherapy involves exposing the skin to ultraviolet A or B light waves.
- Adverse reactions to the use of UV light therapy are premature aging of the skin and increased risk for skin cancer.
- The use of topical corticosteroids continues to be a mainstay of therapy for the treatment of eczema.
- Corticosteroids are also used for the treatment of psoriasis, seborrhea, and other skin conditions where inflammation is present.
- Topical corticosteroids are categorized into seven groups based on potency.
- The vehicle (base) in which the corticosteroid is suspended may influence the potency.
- Higher-potency corticosteroids have more adverse reactions.

- Only the mildest potency agents, like hydrocortisone, should be used on the face.
- Long-term use of topical corticosteroids can result in thinning of the skin, stretch marks (striae), spider veins, acne, milia, rosacea (enlarged blood vessel especially on nose), bruising, atrophy, lacerations, poor wound healing, and growth suppression (in children).
- Calcineurin inhibitors are immunomodulators that control inflammation and reduce immune system response to allergens.
- Pimecrolimus is indicated for the treatment of mild-to-moderate eczema.
- Tacrolimus is approved for the treatment of moderate-to-severe atopic dermatitis that has failed to respond to corticosteroid treatment.
- The U.S. Food and Drug Administration and Health Canada require manufacturers to include a Black Box warning in the package insert, advising health care providers that tacrolimus and pimecrolimus may increase the risk for development of lymphoma.
- Calcipotriene is a synthetic analog of vitamin D. It is known as calcipotriol in Canada.
- Calcipotriene (calcipotriol) inhibits the rapid and repeated production of new skin cells.
- Psoralens are a class of drugs that increase photosensitivity and are classified as furanocoumarins. Methoxsalen is the only drug in this class.
- Psoralens plus ultraviolet light A therapy is also known as PUVA.
- The bioavailability of methoxsalen hard gelatin capsules (8-MOP) and soft gelatin capsules (Oxsoralen-Ultra) is not equivalent, so product substitution is not permitted.
- Cylcosporine is FDA approved for the short-term treatment of severe atopic dermatitis and psoriasis. It decreases immune system hyperactivity.
- Methotrexate is an antimetabolite that is indicated for the treatment of moderate to severe chronic psoriasis and psoriatic arthritis.
- Azathioprine and methotrexate slow the rapid rate of skin cell turnover that occurs with eczema and psoriasis.
- Anthralin is one of the oldest drugs approved for treatment of psoriasis.
- Anthralin causes skin discoloration and may cause discoloration of hair and nails.

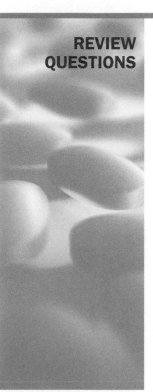

REVIEW QUESTIONS

Multiple Choice

1. A chronic disease of the skin that is characterized by itchy red patches covered with silvery scales is termed _____.
   - a. eczema
   - b. psoriasis
   - c. dermatitis
   - d. rosacea

2. _____ is defined as a group of diseases where there is an inherited tendency to develop other allergic conditions.
   - a. Atopic
   - b. Ectopic
   - c. Dermatopic
   - d. Allergic

3. When symptoms worsen, it is called _____, and periods when they get better or go away completely are called _____.
   - a. exacerbation and metastasis
   - b. exacerbation and remission
   - c. metastasis and inflammation
   - d. allergic and nonallergic

4. Phototherapy reduces the risk for skin cancer.
   - a. true
   - b. false

5. A mainstay of therapy for the treatment of eczema is _____.
   a. antibiotics
   b. corticosteroids
   c. antihistamines
   d. none of the above
6. Pimecrolimus is indicated for the treatment of moderate-to-severe eczema.
   a. true
   b. false
7. For which two drugs is it required to place a Black Box warning in the package insert advising health care providers that the drugs may increase the risk for development of lymphoma?
   a. desonide
   b. pimecrolimus
   c. tacrolimus
   d. b and c
8. Methoxsalen is the only drug in this class.
   a. immunomodulators
   b. furanocumarins
   c. calcineurin inhibitors
   d. immunosuppressants
9. _____ is an antimetabolite that is indicated for the treatment of moderate to severe chronic psoriasis and psoriatic arthritis.
   a. Anthralin
   b. Cyclosporine
   c. Methotrexate
   d. Calcipotreine
10. Anthralin is one of the oldest drugs approved for treatment of psoriasis.
    a. true
    b. false

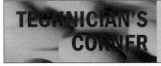

TECHNICIAN'S CORNER

1. Because eczema is allergy related, how can one prevent "flareups" from occurring?
2. How well do calamine lotion and oatmeal soap (both OTC products) work in decreasing the symptoms of atopic dermatitis?

BIBLIOGRAPHY

Gold Standard Inc., Clinical Pharmacology: Available at: http://www.clinicalpharmacology.com/apps/default.asp?entry=11andrNum=897.

Health Canada Drug and Health Product Database. Available at: http://www.hc-sc.gc.ca/dhp-mps/prodpharma/databasdon/index_e.html.

Kalant H, Grant D, Mitchell J: *Principles of medical pharmacology* (pp 891-898), ed 7. Toronto, 2007, Elsevier Canada.

Lance L, Lacy C, Armstrong L, Goldman M: *Drug information handbook for the allied health professional*, ed 12. Hudson, OH, 2005, APhA Lexi-Comp.

National Institute of Arthritis and Musculoskeletal and Skin Diseases: *Atopic aermatitis (a type of eczema)*, Bethesda, MD, January 1999, U.S. Department of Health and Human Services, National Institutes of Health. NIH publication No. 03-4272, revised April 2003. Available at: http://www.niams.nih.gov/hi/topics/dermatitis/index.html.

National Institute of Arthritis and Musculoskeletal and Skin Diseases: *What is psoriasis? Fast facts*, Bethesda, MD, May 2005, U.S. Department of Health and Human Services, National Institutes of Health. Available at: http://www.niams.nih.gov/hi/topics/psoriasis/ffpsoriasis.pdf.

Page C, Curtis M, Sutter M, Walker M, Hoffman B, et al.: *Integrated pharmacology* (pp 506-508, 512-514), Philadelphia, 2005, Elsevier Mosby.

Raymond G, Houle M-C: A review of corticosteroids for the treatment of psoriasis, *Skin Ther Lett Pharmacist Ed*, 1(3), March 2007. Available at: http://www.skinpharmacies.ca/2_1_2.html.

USP Center for Advancement of Patient Safety: *Use caution–avoid confusion*, USP Quality Review No. 79, Rockville, MD, April 2004, USP Center for Advancement of Patient Safety.

Vender R: Management of eczema, *Skin Ther Lett Pharmacist Ed*, 1(2, September-October), 2006. Available at: http://www.skinpharmacies.ca/2_1_2.html.

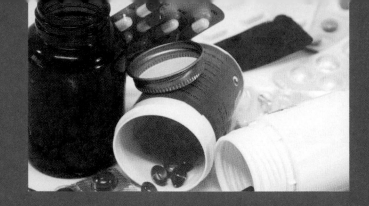

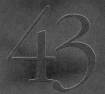

Treatment of Lice and Scabies

Treatment of Lice and Scabies

LEARNING OBJECTIVES	• Learn the terminology associated with lice and scabies. • Describe the epidemiology of lice and scabies infestation. • List the symptoms of lice and scabies infestation. • List and categorize medications used to treat lice and scabies. • Describe mechanism of action for drugs used to lice and scabies. • Identify warning labels and precautionary messages associated with medications used to treat lice and scabies. • Identify significant drug look-alike/sound-alike issues. • List common endings for drug classes used in the treatment of lice and scabies. • List prevention strategies.
KEY TERMS	**Lice:** Group of parasites (*Pediculus humanus capitis, Pediculus humanus corporis, Phthirus pubis*) that can live on the body, scalp, or genital area of humans. **Nits:** Head lice eggs. **Nymph:** Baby louse. **Ovicidal:** Kills eggs. **Parasite:** Organism that benefits by living in, with, or on another organism. **Pediculicide:** Drug that kills lice. **Scabicide:** Drug that kills the scabies mite. **Scabies:** Parasitic infection caused by the mite *Sarcoptes scabei.*

Epidemiology of Lice and Scabies Infestation

Lice and scabies infestations affect people around the globe without regard for social status or race. They are caused by parasites and are readily spread person-person. A *parasite* is an organism that benefits by living in, with, or on another organism (host), usually to the detriment of the host.

LICE

HEAD LICE

Head lice most commonly infests children aged 3 to 11 years and their families, but anyone can become infested (Figure 43-1, *A, B*). Infestation is caused by the parasite *Pediculus humanus capitis*. Head lice is spread between individuals through head-head contact as occurs during

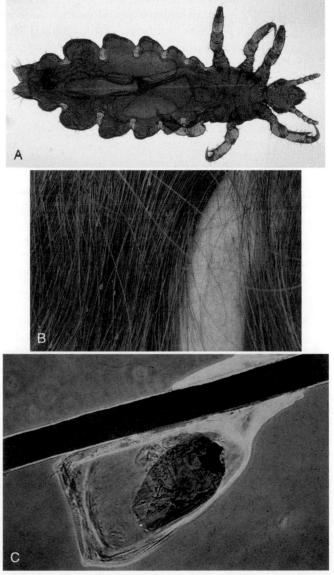

FIGURE 43-1 (A) Adult head louse. *(Photograph by Dr. Dennis D. Juranek, Courtesy of the Centers for Disease Control and Prevention.)* **(B)** Head lice infestation. *(From Callen J, Greer K, Hood A, et al: Color atlas of dermatology, Philadelphia, 1993, WB Saunders.)* **(C)** Nit attached to hair shaft. *(From Kumar V, Abbas AK, Fausto M: Robbins and Cotran pathologic basis of disease, ed 7, Philadelphia, 2005, WB Saunders.)*

children's play and sports. Less commonly, transmission occurs by sharing personal items such as combs, brushes, hats, towels, scarves, and coats with someone who has head lice.

The life cycle of a head louse is about 4 to 6 weeks. Adults lay eggs, also called *nits*, at the base of the hair shaft (Figure 43-1, *C*). In about 7 days, the nits hatch and a nymph emerges. A *nymph* is a baby louse. The nymph becomes an adult in about 7 days; and the adult lives for approximately 30 days.

Lice are parasites that feed on blood. This is the reason why eggs are laid within ¼ inch of the scalp—so newly hatched nymphs can be close to a blood source. If nit shells are found farther from the base of the scalp, they are remains of an earlier infestation and treatment is not necessary. An adult louse can live for only 2 days away from a human host.

BODY LICE

Body lice infestations are caused by the parasite *Pediculus humanus corporis*. Infestations are a serious public health concern because body lice may cause epidemics of typhus and louse-borne relapsing fever. Body lice thrive in crowded environments where chronic poverty and unsanitary conditions exist such as refugee camps, temporary housing from natural disasters, and prisons. In the United States and Canada, body lice infestations rarely occur except in homeless populations without access to bathing facilities.

Like head lice, body lice infestation is spread person-person through direct contact with a person who has body lice. An alternate mode of transmission is through shared bedding or clothes. In fact, body lice live in the seams of the clothing of infested individuals.

The life cycle of body lice is similar to head lice and begins with laying eggs. The nits hatch and nymphs mature to adults in 7 days. Adults can only survive away from a human host for 10 days.

PUBIC LICE

Pubic lice, or "crabs," is sometimes classified as a sexually transmitted infection (STI) because it is most commonly spread through sexual contact (Figure 43-2). It is rare for lice to be spread through contact with bedding, linens, or clothes. Although the life cycle of pubic lice is the same as the life cycle of head lice, pubic lice and head lice are different species of lice. Head lice do not inhabit the genitalia and pubic lice do not live in the hair. Lice infestation in the pubic region is caused by the parasite *Phthirus pubis*.

SCABIES

Scabies infestations are common and affect individuals of all social classes and race. Infestations are caused by a parasitic mite called *Saroptes scabei*. The mite flourishes and spreads person-person in environments where the population density is high, such as hospitals, nursing homes, child care facilities, and schools. Transmission occurs through close contact and sharing bedding, linen, clothing, or sexual relations.

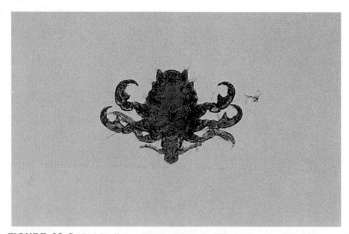

FIGURE 43-2 Pubic lice. *(From Mahon CR, Lehman DC, Manuselis G: Textbook of diagnostic microbiology, ed 3, St. Louis, 2007, WB Saunders.)*

The scabies mite burrows beneath the skin. Sites of the infestation can be seen in the webbing between fingers and toes; skin folds of the breast, penis, and shoulder blades; and in the bend of elbows, knees, and wrist. Like lice, *S. scabei* feeds on blood and dies if away from a human host for greater than 48 to 72 hours. The adult mite can live for approximately 30 days.

Symptoms of Lice and Scabies Infestation

Symptoms of lice and scabies infestation are listed in Box 43-1.

Prevention of Lice Reinfestation

Ways to prevent lice reinfestation are listed in Box 43-2.

Treatment of Head Lice, Pubic Lice, and Scabies

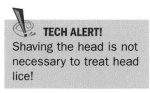
TECH ALERT!
Shaving the head is not necessary to treat head lice!

Head lice and pubic lice may be treated with nonprescription and prescription *pediculicides*. OTC and Rx agents are both effective and, in the case of lindane lotion, OTC products are more effective and have a lower risk of toxicity. Drug resistance is a growing problem for OTC and prescription pediculicides, especially permethrins, due to the residue left after treatment. All treatments are more effective if a fine-tooth nit comb is used to remove eggs from the hair shaft and all family members are treated.

OVER-THE-COUNTER DRUGS

Two OTC pediculicides are available for the treatment of lice. They are pyrethrins and permethrin. They are formulated in various dosage forms including shampoo, creme rinse, lotion, and household spray.

PYRETHRINS AND PERMETHRINS

Pyrethrins are naturally derived from the chrysanthemum flower. Their effectiveness is boosted by the addition of piperonyl butoxide, a petroleum distillate. Pyrethrins are indicated for the treatment of head lice, pubic lice, and body lice. Permethrin is a mixture of synthetic isomers of pyrethrins. It is more effective for the treatment of head lice but less effective against pubic lice (as low as 57% efficacy). It is also effective against the scabies mite.

Pyrethrins are not ovicidal (kills the eggs), so retreatment is typically necessary in 7 to 10 days to kill newly hatched nymphs. Permethrin is ovicidal.

BOX 43-1 SYMPTOMS OF LICE AND SCABIES INFESTATION

HEAD AND PUBIC LICE
- Itching
- Feeling of something moving in hair or genital area
- Sores (from scratching)

BODY LOUSE
- Itching
- Rash
- Thickening and discoloration of skin

SCABIES
- Intense itching
- Pimple-like rash
- Sores (from scratching)

BOX 43-2 STRATEGIES TO PREVENT REINFESTATION

- Treat all household members.
- Use a nit comb to remove eggs.
- Wash clothing, linens, and bedding in hot water (130°F or 54°C).
- Dry clean clothing that is not washable.

- Place stuffed toys, clothing, and bedding that cannot be washed or dry cleaned in a large plastic bag and seal the bag for 2 weeks.

MECHANISM OF ACTION AND PHARMACOKINETICS

Pyrethrins and permethrin paralyze and kill lice by blocking repolarization of sodium channels. Their action is discontinued once the drug is washed off. Permethrins leave a residue on the hair that can destroy eggs and newly hatched nymphs.

ADVERSE REACTIONS

Adverse effects caused by topical application of pyrethrins are redness, itching and stinging, tingling, and minor swelling.

Pyrethins and Permethrin

Generic name	U.S. brand name(s) / Canadian brand(s)		Dosage forms and strengths
pyrethrins + piperonyl butoxide*	A-200 Lice treatment Solution, Clear Total Lice Elimination System, Pronto Plus Mousse Shampoo, Pronto Topical Spray, RID Mousse, RID pediculicide shampoo		**Lotion:** pyrethrins 0.3% + piperonyl butoxide 4% **Shampoo, mousse:** pyrethrins 0.33% + piperonyl butoxide 4% **Shampoo:** pyrethrins 0.3% + piperonyl butoxide 3%
	R&C Shampoo with Conditioner		**Solution:** pyrethrins 0.3% + piperonyl butoxide 3% **Spray:** pyrethrins 0.3% + piperonyl butoxide 3%
permethrin*	A-200 Topical Spray, Acticin, Nix, Elimite		**Lotion (creme rinse):** 1% **Cream:** 5%
	Nix		**Spray (A-200):** 0.5%

*Generic available.

TECH ALERT!
Pharmacy technicians must apply the warning label FOR EXTERNAL USE ONLY to prescription vials containing lindane lotion and shampoo.

PRESCRIPTION TREATMENTS

LINDANE

Lindane is an organochlorine pesticide known by the chemical name gamma benzene hexachloride. It is used in agriculture to control pests* and medically to kill lice. It is a scabicide and pediculicide, killing all type of lice, scabies, and their eggs.

Mechanism of Action and Pharmacokinetics

Lindane is absorbed through into the body of the scabies mite and lice, where it paralyzes and kills the parasite. Absorption of lindane through intact human skin increases with repeated applications and the half-life is long ($T\frac{1}{2}$ = 18 hours). Repeated use causes accumulation and increases the risk for neurotoxicity.

Adverse Reactions

Lindane is neurotoxic and can cause illness, vomiting, seizures, and death if accidentally swallowed. The Food and Drug Administration (FDA) has required manufacturers to place a Black Box warning in the package insert to alert health care providers that
- Lindane is not a first-line therapy and repeat applications should be avoided.
- Lindane should not be used by infants, young children, elders, adults weighing less than 110 lb [50 kg], or breastfeeding women.
- The drug should be dispensed in 1- to 2-ounce single-application vials (the maximum amount needed for a treatment).

*On January 1, 2005, Canada withdrew registration of lindane for agricultural pest control.

Lindane

Generic name	U.S. brand name(s) Canadian brand(s)	Dosage forms and strengths
lindane	Generics	Lotion: 1% Shampoo: 1%
	Hexit	

TECH ALERT!
Malathion is flammable, and individuals using the product should stay away from open flames, hair dryers and curling irons, and lit cigarettes, cigars, and pipes.

MALATHION

Malathion is an organophosphate pesticide that is used in agriculture to control pests and medically to kill head lice and their eggs. It was withdrawn from the U.S. market and then reintroduced in 1999 following labeling changes. It remains withdrawn from the market in Canada.

Mechanism of Action and Pharmacokinetics

Malathion paralyzes the central nervous system of parasites by causing an accumulation of acetylcholine (ACh). The lotion is applied to dry hair until the hair and scalp are saturated. The drug must dry naturally on the head and left on for 8 to 12 hours before being rinsed off. Retreatment is only recommended if crawling lice are found 7 to 10 days after initial treatment.

Adverse Reactions

The most common adverse reactions linked to malathion use are stinging, redness, minor swelling, itching, and tingling.

Malathion

Generic name	U.S. brand name(s) Canadian brand(s)	Dosage forms and strengths
malathion	Ovide	Lotion: 0.5%
	Not available	

CROTAMITON

Crotamiton is a scabicide. Its mechanism of action is not known. It is classified in FDA pregnancy category C and is an alternative to lindane.

Adverse Reactions

Crotamiton has few adverse reactions. Reactions are linked to drug allergy and include itchiness, minor swelling, and redness.

Crotamiton

Generic name	U.S. brand name(s) Canadian brand(s)	Dosage forms and strengths
crotamiton	Eurax	Cream: 10% Lotion: 10% (U.S. only)
	Eurax	

Summary of Drugs Used for the Treatment of Lice and Scabies

	Generic name	Brand name	Usual dose and dosing schedule	Warning labels
Over-the-Counter				
	pyrethrins + piperonyl butoxide	RID, R&C various	**Shampoo/creme rinse:** Saturate hair with product. Leave on for as long as instructed on product label. Rinse hair. Use nit comb to remove eggs. **Lotion/creme:** Apply after bathing to the skin over the entire body from the chin to the toes. Leave on overnight (or 8 hours). Wash off. Repeat treatment in 7 to 10 days if needed.	SHAKE WELL—lotion, creme rinse DO NOT RE-WASH HAIR FOR 1-2 DAYS AFTER TREATMENT TREAT ALL HOUSEHOLD MEMBERS RE-TREAT IN 7-10 DAYS IF CRAWLING BUGS ARE EVIDENT DO NOT OVERUSE PRODUCT
	permethrins	Nix, Elimite		
Rx only				
	crotamiton	Eurax	Apply after bathing to the skin over the entire body from the chin to the toes. Repeat in 24 hours. Bathe 48 hours AFTER second dose. Treatment may be repeated in 7 to 10 days if needed.	SHAKE WELL
	lindane	Generics	**Shampoo:** Saturate hair with product. Leave on for 4 minutes. Add a small amount of water a rub until a lather is formed, then rinse hair. Use nit comb to remove eggs. **Lotion/creme:** Apply 1 hour after bathing to the skin over the entire body from the chin to the toes. Leave on 8 to 12 hours. Wash off.	SHAKE WELL DO NOT RE-WASH HAIR FOR 1-2 DAYS AFTER TREATMENT TREAT ALL HOUSEHOLD MEMBERS RE-TREAT IN 7-10 DAYS IF CRAWLING BUGS ARE EVIDENT—malathion only DO NOT OVERUSE PRODUCT
	malathion	Ovide	Saturate hair with product. Leave on 8 to 12 hours then wash hair. Use nit comb to remove eggs.	

CHAPTER SUMMARY

- Lice and scabies infestations affect people around the globe without regard for social status or race.
- Head lice, body lice, pubic lice, and scabies are spread person-person through direct contact.
- Lice and scabies infestations are caused by parasites.
- A parasite is an organism that benefits by living in, with, or on another organism (host), usually to the detriment of the host.
- Head lice most commonly affects children aged 3 to 11 years and their families, but anyone can become infested.
- Infestation is caused by the parasite *Pediculus humanus capitis.*
- Head lice infestation is NOT caused by poor hygiene (lack of cleanliness).
- Adult head lice and pubic lice can live for only 2 days away from a human host.
- Adult body lice can survive away from a human host for 10 days.
- Body lice infestations are caused by the parasite *Pediculus humanus corporis.*
- Infestions are a serious public health concern because body lice may cause epidemics of typhus and louse-borne relapsing fever.
- Pubic lice, or "crabs," is sometimes classified as a sexually transmitted infection because it is most commonly spread through sexual contact.
- Individuals can NOT get pubic lice from sitting on public toilet seats.

- Lice infestation in the pubic region is caused by the parasite *Phthirus pubis.*
- Scabies infestations are common and are caused by a parasitic mite called *Saroptes scabei.*
- The mite flourishes and spreads person-person in environments where the population density is high, such as hospitals, nursing homes, child care facilities, and schools.
- Like lice, *S. scabei* feeds on blood and dies if away from a human host for greater than 48 to 72 hours.
- Strategies to prevent lice and scabies reinfestation include the following: (1) Treat all household members; (2) use a nit comb to remove eggs (lice); (3) wash clothing, linens, and bedding in hot water (130°F or 54°C); (4) dry clean clothing that is not washable; and (5) place stuffed toys, clothing, and bedding that cannot be washed or dry cleaned in a large plastic bag and seal the bag for 2 weeks.
- Head lice and pubic lice may be treated with nonprescription and prescription pediculicides.
- A pediculicide is a drug that kills lice.
- OTC and Rx agents are both effective and, in the case of lindane lotion, OTC products are more effective and have a lower risk of toxicity.
- Drug resistance is a growing problem for OTC and prescription pediculicides, especially permethrins, due to the residue left after treatment.
- Pyrethrins and permethrin are nonprescription treatments for lice infestation.
- Pyrethrins are naturally derived from the chrysanthemum flower.
- Permethrin is a mixture of synthetic isomers of pyrethrins.
- Pyrethrins are indicated for the treatment of head lice, body lice, and pubic lice, whereas permethrin is only approved for the treatment of head lice.
- Permethrin is ovicidal (kills eggs), whereas pyrethrins are not.
- Lindane and malathion are pesticides that are used in agriculture to control pests and medically to kill lice.
- Lindane, also known as gamma benzene hexachloride, is also a scabicide.
- Absorption of lindane through intact human skin increases with repeated applications. Repeated use causes accumulation and increases the risk for neurotoxicity.
- Lindane can cause illness, vomiting, seizures, and death if accidentally swallowed.
- Pharmacy technicians must apply the warning label FOR EXTERNAL USE ONLY to prescription vials containing lindane lotion and shampoo.
- Malathion paralyzes the central nervous system of parasites by causing an accumulation of acetylcholine.
- Malathion is flammable, and individuals using the product should stay away from open flames, hair dryers and curling irons, and lighted cigarettes, cigars, and pipes.
- Crotamiton is a scabicide that is classified in FDA pregnancy category C and is an alternative to lindane.

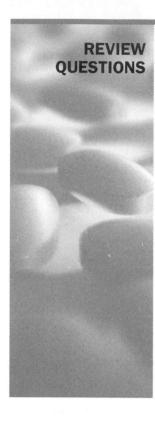

REVIEW QUESTIONS

Multiple Choice

1. A _____ is an organism that benefits by living in, with, or on another organism (host); usually to the detriment of the host.
   a. parasite
   b. protozoan
   c. proteus
   d. bacteria

2. The life cycle of a head louse is about _____.
   a. 1 to 2 weeks
   b. 2 to 3 weeks
   c. 3 to 5 weeks
   d. 4 to 6 weeks

3. Body lice infestations are a serious public health concern because body lice may cause epidemics of typhus and louse-borne relapsing fever.
   a. true
   b. false

4. _____, or "crabs," is sometimes classified as a sexually transmitted infection.
   a. Scabies
   b. Head lice
   c. Pubic lice
   d. Body lice

5. The scabies mite lives on the surface of the skin.
   a. true
   b. false

6. _____ may be treated with nonprescription and prescription pediculicides.
   a. Scabies
   b. Head lice
   c. Pubic lice
   d. b and c

7. Pyrethrins are naturally derived from the _____ flower.
   a. passion
   b. chrysanthemum
   c. periwinkle
   d. coneflower

8. Lindane _____.
   a. is neurotoxic
   b. should not be used by anyone weighing less than 100 lb (50 kg)
   c. in only dispensed in 1- to 2-oz applicator bottles
   d. all of the above

9. Malathion, an organophosphate pesticide that is used in agriculture to control pests and medically to kill head lice and their eggs, is sold both in the U.S. market and in Canada.
   a. true
   b. false

10. Crotamiton is a(n) _____. It is classified in FDA pregnancy category C and is an alternative to lindane.
    a. scabicide
    b. pediculocide
    c. insecticide
    d. pesticide

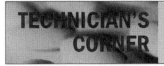

1. Crotamiton is a scabicide that is classified in FDA pregnancy category C. What kind of effects would it have on a developing fetus?
2. What is a "black box warning" put on some drugs like lindane?

BIBLIOGRAPHY

Center for Drug Evaluation and Research: *Lindane shampoo and lindane lotion: questions and answers,* U.S. Food and Drug Administration, updated April 15, 2003. Available at: http://www.fda.gov/cder/drug/infopage/lindane/lindaneQA.htm.

Gold Standard Inc., Clinical Pharmacology: Available at: http://www.clinicalpharmacology.com/apps/default.asp?entry=11&rNum=897

Health Canada Drug and Health Product Database. Available at: http://www.hc-sc.gc.ca/dhp-mps/prodpharma/databasdon/index_e.html.

Lance L, Lacy C, Armstrong L, Goldman M: *Drug information handbook for the allied health professional,* ed 12. Hudson, OH, 2005, APhA Lexi-Comp.

National Center for Infectious Diseases, Division of Parasitic Diseases: *Head lice infestation: fact sheet,* Centers for Disease Control and Prevention, reviewed August 18, 2005. Available at: http://www.cdc.gov/ncidod/dpd/parasites/lice/factsht_head_lice.htm.

National Center for Infectious Diseases Division of Parasitic Diseases: *Pubic lice infestation: fact sheet,* Centers for Disease Control and Prevention, reviewed October 19, 2004. Available at: http://www.cdc.gov/ncidod/dpd/parasites/lice/factsht_pubic_lice.htm.

National Center for Infectious Diseases, Division of Parasitic Diseases: *Scabies: fact sheet,* Centers for Disease Control and Prevention, reviewed February 10, 2005. Available at: http://www.cdc.gov/ncidod/dpd/parasites/scabies/factsht_scabies.htm.

National Center for Infectious Diseases Division of Parasitic Diseases: *Treating head lice: fact sheet,* Centers for Disease Control and Prevention, reviewed August 18, 2005. Available at: http://www.cdc.gov/ncidod/dpd/parasites/lice/factsht_head_lice_treating.htm.

National Center for Infectious Diseases Division of Parasitic Diseases: *Treating head lice: fact sheet,* Centers for Disease Control and Prevention, reviewed November 17, 2004. Available at: http://www.cdc.gov/ncidod/dpd/parasites/lice/factsht_body_lice.htm.

National Center for Infectious Diseases Division of Parasitic Diseases: *Treating head lice infestation with malathion: fact sheet,* Centers for Disease Control and Prevention, reviewed October 18, 2004. Available at: http://www.cdc.gov/ncidod/dpd/parasites/lice/factsht_malathion.htm.

Unintentional Topical Lindane Ingestions—United States, 1998- 2003, *MMWR Morbid Mort Wkly Rep.* Available at: http://www.cdc.gov/mmwr/preview/mmwrhtml/mm5421a2.htm.

USP Center for Advancement of Patient Safety: *Use caution–avoid confusion,* USP Quality Review No. 79, Rockville, MD, April 2004, USP Center for Advancement of Patient Safety.

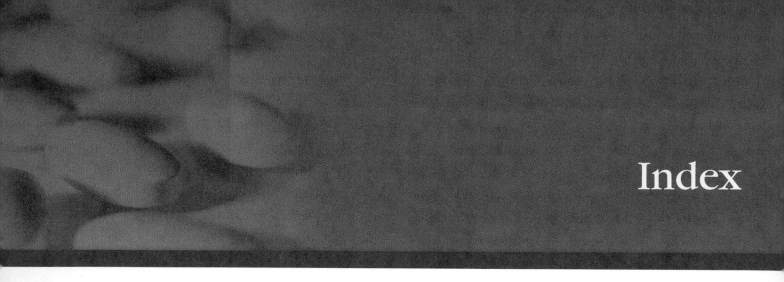

Index

A

Abacavir (ABC)
    dosage and warnings for, 617
    dosage forms and strengths of, 612
    overview of, 610-611
Abbreviation, inappropriate, 58, 60
Abciximab
    drug dosage and warnings, 385
    mechanism of action, 376
Absorption, **21**
    factors influencing, 25-26
    process of, 22
Abstinence, 546
Accuzyme, 690
ACE inhibitor
    drug dose strengths and schedule for, 366
    indications for, 366
Acetylcholine (ACh), 68, **196**
    cholinesterase and, 275
    mechanism of action, 200f
    Parkinson's disease and, 118, 118f, 119
    spasticity, role in, 212
    synthesis and release of, 198, 198f
Acetylcholinesterase, **116, 163**, 169
Acetylcholinesterase inhibitors, 171
Acinar cell, 406
Acini, 512
Acne, **700**
    in adult, 701f
    cause of, 703
    characteristics of, **700**
    factors exacerbating, 703
    medication triggering, 703b
    myths about, 703
    treatment of
        dosage and warnings for, 710-711
        hormonally influenced, 710
        mild, 704-705
        moderate to moderately severe, 706-708
        severe, 708-709
Acne vulgaris, **700**, 702
Acquired immune deficiency syndrome. *See*
    AIDS
Actinomycin D
    dosage and warnings for, 641-642
    overview of, 641-642
Action
    duration of, **21, 22**, 24f
    mechanism of, **40, 41**
    onset of, **22**, 24f
Action potential, 68, 76
Active transport, 25, 25f

Acupuncture, **144**
Acute lymphocytic leukemia, 640-641
Acute nonlymphocytic leukemia (ANLL), 47
Acute pain, **144**, 145
Acyclovir
    adverse reactions from, 606
    mechanism of action and
        pharmacokinetics of, 605
Adapalene, 706
Adaptive immunity, 576
Additive effect, **53**, 54
Adenohypophysis, 510
Adherence, **601**, 610
Adjunct, **86**
Adrenal cortex, 511
Adrenal gland
    hormones of, 512
    location of, 511
Adrenal medulla, 511
Adrenergic agonist
    aqueous humor, increasing drainage of,
        274-275
    glaucoma, as treatment for, 273
    types of, 278
Adrenergic antagonist, 273
Adrenergic antagonist, beta, 272
Adrenergic drug, alpha$_2$, 215
Adrenergic inhibitor, 355
Adrenergic receptor, types of, 71-72
Adverse drug reaction (ADR), 46-47
    from antidepressants, 80-81
    avoidance of, 57
    from benzodiazepines, 77-78
    from carbamazepine and oxcarbazepine,
        134
    as factor influencing adherence
        to therapy, 50
    in GI tract, 55f
    from MAOIs, 95
    from neuroleptics, 107
    from opioids, 149
    Parkinson's disease treatment, 121
    from phenytoin and fosphenytoin, 133
    reporting to FDA, 50
    from SSRIs, 93
    from succinimide, 136
    from tricyclic antidepressants, 91
    from valproates, 133
Aerosol inhaler, 14, 14f
Afferent neuron, 68
Affinity, **29, 40**, 41
Affordability, of drug therapy, 50

Age
    atrial fibrillation and, 392t
    cancer and, 626, 626b
    gastroesophageal reflux disease and, 408
    immunization schedule by, 654f
    metabolism, effect on, 33
    pharmacotherapeutics, effect on, 45
    stroke and myocardial infarction, 374
    yeast vaginitis and, 675
Agglutination, 310
Agonist, **40, 41**, 149
Agonist/antagonist, mixed, 149, 153t
Agonist binding, 42f
Agoraphobia, 75
Agranulocyte, 310
AIDS (acquired immune deficiency syndrome),
    601
    HAART therapy for, 603
    overview of, 609
    pharmacotherapy for, 610
Alcohol
    additive effects of, 54
    cancer and, 626b, 627
    gout, as risk factor for, 257-258
    Ménière's disease and, 284
    peptic ulcer disease and, 411
Aldosterone, **332**, 340
    role of, 476
    secretion of, 475
Aldosterone receptor blocker, 340, 366
Alimentary canal, 404
Alkylating agent, 630f, 634
Allergen, **461**, 462
    T lymphocyte response to, 462f
Allergic asthma, **443**
Allergic rhinitis, **461**, 463
Allergy, **461**
    antihistamine as treatment for, 465-466
    drugs used to treat, 464
    glucocorticosteroid as treatment for,
        466
    immunotherapy for, 468-469
    mast cell stabilizers as treatment for, 466
    overview of, 462
    symptoms of, 464, 464b
    triggers of, 462-463
Allylamine antifungal
    adverse reactions from, 679
    dosage and warnings for, 683
    dosage forms and strengths of, 679
    mechanism of action and
        pharmacokinetics of, 678

Alosetron
  IBS, as treatment for, 426
Alpha$_1$-adrenergic antagonist
  benign prostatic hyperplasia, as treatment
    for, 479
  types of, 480
Alpha$_1$-blocker, 348-349, 352
Alpha$_2$-adrenergic drug, 215
Alpha$_2$-agonist, 349-350
Alpha-adrenergic agonist
  glaucoma, as treatment for, 273
  types of, 277
Alpha blocker, **477**
Alpha bungarotoxin, 200f
Alpha cell, 512
Alpha-glucosidase inhibitor
  diabetes and, 535-536
  dosage and warnings for, 540
Alpha-lipoic acid, diabetes and, 539
Alpha receptor, 71-72
Alpha reductase inhibitor, **477**
Alprazolam, 81t
Alprostadil, 484
Alzheimer's disease, **163**
  acetylcholinesterase inhibitors, 171
  adverse reactions from treatment, 170
  drugs used to treat, 169-170, 171
  neurotransmitters, role in, 168-169
  N-Methyl-D-Aspartate receptor inhibitor,
    171
  pathophysiology of, 167
  prevalence and risk factors for, 165, 167
  symptoms of, 167
Amantadine, 603-604
Amenorrhea, **545**, 557
  pregnancy and, 546
  treatment of, 565
Amiloride, 340
Amine, 68
Aminoglycoside, **295**-296
  infections, treatment for, 300
  overview of, 583
Aminosalicylates
  mechanism of action, 428
  pharmacokinetics and adverse reactions of,
    429
  types of, 432-433
Amiodarone, 394
Amitriptyline, 54
Amphetamine
  adverse reactions and precautions for,
    184
  mechanism of action and pharmacokinetics
    of, 184
Amphiarthroses joint, 190
Amphotericin B
  dosage and warnings for, 683
  overview of, 679-680
Amprenavir (APV)
  dosage and warnings for, 618
  drug form and strengths, 615
  overview of, 614
Amputation, 690
Amylin analog, 539
Amyotrophic lateral sclerosis (ALS), **209**, 211
Anabolic agent, 250-251
Anakinra
  dosage and warnings for, 662
  as interleukin 1 (IL-1) receptor antagonist,
    660

Anal canal, 405
Analgesia, 148
Analgesic, **144**, 227
  for ear conditions, 285
  gout, as treatment for, 258
Anaphase, 635t
Anaphylactic shock, **196**, 202
Anaphylaxis, **461**
Anastrozole
  dosage and warnings for, 642
  dosage forms and strengths of, 633
Androgen, 512
Androgen agonist, 562-563, 568-569
Anemia, 311
Anesthetic, 158
Aneurysm, 315, **371**
Angina, 318
  drug dosage and warnings, 327-328
  drugs used to treat, 320, 320t
  nonpharmacological treatment for, 320
  types of, 319-320
  See also Heart disease; Nitrate
Angina pectoris, **317**
Angioedema, **461**, 463
Angiotension-converting enzyme (ACE),
  332, 353
  overview of, 341
  types of, 342-343
Angiotension-converting enzyme inhibitor
  (ACEI)
  mechanism of action, 397
  types of, 399
Angiotension II, **332**, 353-354
Angiotension II receptor antagonist
  drug dose strengths and schedule for, 366
  indications for, 366
  overview of, 344
  types of, 344-345
Angle, obstruction of, 271
Angle closure glaucoma, **270**, 271, 274
Anion, **490**, 491
Anorexia nervosa, 560
Anoxia, **129**, 130, **371**, 372
Antacid
  mechanism of action and adverse reactions
    for, 416
  types of, 417
Antagonism, **53**, **55**
Antagonist, 42, 149
Antagonist binding, 42f
Anterior pituitary gland, 510
Anthracenedione, 636-637
Anthracycline, 636-637, 643
Anthralin
  dosage and warnings for, 726
  overview of, 723
Antiarrhythmic drug
  adverse reactions and precautions for, 394
  classification of, 394, 395-396, 397-399
  digoxin and phenytoin as, 396
  drug dosage and warnings, 397
  mechanism of action, 394
  types of, 394t
  uses for, 393-394
Antibacterial drug, 691
Antibiotic, **578**
  acne, for treatment of, 706
  bacterial cell wall and, 579-581
  bacterial protein synthesis, inhibition of, 581f
  enzymes inactivating, 582

Antibiotic-modifying enzyme, production of,
  582
Antibody, 576
Anticholinergic, 123
  IBS, as treatment for, 427
  types of, 432
Anticoagulant, **371**
  heparin as, 377
  mechanism of action, 378
  types of, 380, 386
Antidepressant
  adverse reactions from, 80
  effectiveness of, 88-89, 89f
  indications for, 80
  migraine headache, treatment for, 164
  pain, treatment of, 158
  second- and third-generation, 95-96
  summary of use, 82t
Antidiarrheal, **423**
  drug form and strengths, 428
  types of, 432
Antidiuretic hormone (ADH)
  role of, 476
  secretion of, 475
Antiestrogen, 560
Antifolate, 581
Antifungal medication, **672**
  infections, treatment for, 301
  mechanism of action, 675
  polyene class of, 679-680
Antigen, 310
Antihistamine
  asthma and COPD, as treatment for, 467-468
  classification of, 464
  cyproheptadine as, 215
  overview of, 465
  types of, 465-466
Antiinfective, **578**
  classification of, 583
  corticosteroid and, 296-297
  Crohn's disease, as treatment for, 431
  indications for, 691
  infections, treatment for, 300-301
Antiinflammatory
  glucocorticosteroid as, 227
  glucocorticosteroids as, 449
  gout, as treatment for, 258
Antimalarial
  dosage and warnings for, 236-237
  indications and adverse effects of, 229
Antimetabolic, 630f
Antimetabolite
  dosage and warnings for, 644
  overview of, 640-641
Antimicrobial
  acne, for treatment of, 704-705
  drug dosage and warnings, 419
  factors influencing therapy with, 579f
  indications for, 417
  mechanism of action, 579
Antineoplastic agent, 629, 631
Antinuclear antibody (ANA), **221**
  actions of, 226f
  elevation of, 225
Antiplatelet agent, **371**
  adverse reactions and precautions for,
    377
  mechanism of action, 376, 376f
  pharmacokinetics of, 376
  types of, 377, 385-386

Antiresorptive agent, 247
Antiretroviral, **601**, 610
Antirheumatic drug, disease-modifying, 232–234
Antiseizure drug
  broad-spectrum, 137–138, 141
  migraine headache, treatment for, 164
  pain, treatment of, 158
Antiseptics
  burns, for treatment of, 696
  decubitus ulcer, for treatment of, 691
Antithrombotic, **371**
Antithrombotic drug, 375
Antithrombotin III, 378
Antithymocyte globulin (ATG)
  adverse reactions from, 658
  dosage and warnings for, 661
  dosage forms and strengths of, 658
  mechanism of action and
    pharmacokinetics of, 657
Antithyroid drug, **514**
Antiviral medication, **601**
  factors influencing outcome, 602–603
  infections, treatment for, 301
  mechanism of action, 603
  role of, 602
Antiviral resistance, **601**
Anvil (incus), 268, 268f
Anxiety, **74**
  benzodiazepines for, 78t, 81t–82t
  beta-adrenergic antagonist for, 81
  disorder, types of, 75
  neurochemistry of, 76
  treatment of, 76
Anxiety Disorders Association of America, 75
Anxiolytic, **74**
  benzodiazepine as, 77f
  hydroxyzine as, 82t
  mechanism of action, 76
Aorta, 312f, 316f
Aortic semilunar valve, 312, 313f
Aplastic anemia, 311
Apocrine sweat glands, 671
ApoE4 allele, **163**
Apoliprotein E, 165, 167
Appendicular skeleton, 190, 191f–192f
Appendix, 404, 405
Aqueous humor, 267, **270**
  abnormal collection of, 271
  drugs decreasing formation of, 272
  flow of, 272f
  increasing drainage of, 274–276
Aromatase inhibitors
  dosage and warnings for, 642
  overview of, 632–633
Arrhythmia
  formation of, 392
  prevention of, 397
  symptoms of, 392b
  treatment of, 393–394
  types of, 392–393
  See also Antiarrhythmic drug
Arteriosclerosis, 315, **317**
Artery, 313, 318f
Arthritis, **144**, 145–146
  gouty, 257f
  See also Rheumatoid arthritis, 223
Articulation, 190
Artificial immunity, 576
Aseptic technique, 47
Aspartame, 33

Aspirin
  drug dosage and warnings, 385–386
  mechanism of action, 376
  pain, treatment of, 150, 155
  peptic ulcer disease and, 410
  uses for, 228–229
  warfarin and, 54
Asthma, **443**
  airway challenges in, 445f
  antihistamine as treatment for, 467–468
  beta$_2$-adrenergic agonist
    long-acting, 448–449, 455
    short-acting, 447–448, 455
  classification of, 444b
  drugs used
    for acute symptoms of, 447
    to prevent flare-ups, 447
  gastroesophageal reflux disease and, 408
  glucocorticosteroid as treatment for, 449
  inhaled corticosteroid for, 449–450, 456
  leukotriene modifiers for, 450, 456
  management of, 446
  mast cell stabilizers for, 451, 456, 468
  medication, delivery devices for, 454, 454f
  monoclonal antibodies for, 453, 456
  pathophysiology of, 444
  prevalence and cause of, 444
  symptoms of, 444–455, 445b
  triggers of, 445b, 446b
  xanthine derivative for, 452, 453, 456
Ataxia, **221**
Atazanavir (ATV)
  dosage and warnings for, 618
  drug form and strengths, 615
  overview of, 614
Atheroma, **317**, 318
Atherosclerosis, **317**, **371**
  cause of, 373
  HDL and, 381
Atherothrombosis, **371**, 373
Athlete's foot
  prevention of, 674b
  symptoms of, 673
  view of, 674f
Atopic, **715**, 716
Atopic dermatitis, **715**
  irritants of, 716b
  prevalence of, 716
  symptoms of, 717
Atria, 312, 312f, 313f
Atrial fibrillation, **391**
  prevalence of, 392, 393
  risk factors for, 392t
  stroke, as risk factor for, 374
Atrial flutter, **391**, 392
Atrial natriuretic hormone (ANH), 476
Atrioventricular bundle (bundle of His), 315, 316f
Atrioventricular node (AV node), 315, 316f
Atrioventricular valve, 312, 313f
Atrophic vaginitis, **545**, 553
Attention-deficit/hyperactivity disorder
  amphetamine as treatment of, 184
  cause of, 182–183
  mechanism of action and
    pharmacokinetics of, 184
  pathophysiology of, 183
  signs of, 183f
  symptoms and subtypes of, 182
  treatment of, 183, 184–185

Auditory ossicles, 268, 268f
Auditory tube, 268
Aura, **129**
Auralgia, 285
Auricle, 268, 268f
Autoantibody, **221**
Autoimmune disease, **221**
  musculoskeletal system and, 222
  rheumatoid arthritis and, 234t–235t
  symptoms, control of, 234
  treatment of, 225
  types of, 222
Autoimmune hearing loss, 282
Autoimmunity, 222
Automaticity, **360**, **391**, 394
Autonomic nervous system (ANS)
  anxiety disorders and, 75
  divisions of, 68
  drugs used to affect, 73
  function of, 71
Axial skeleton, 190, 191f–192f
Azaperone, 79
Azapirone, 79t, 82t
Azathioprine, 230–231, 722–723
Azelaic acid, 707

B

Bacterial cell wall
  function, inhibition of, 580
  synthesis, inhibition of, 579, 580
Bacterial DNA/RNA, synthesis inhibition, 580
Bacterial infection
  athlete's foot and, 673
  cancer and, 626b, 627
  drugs used to treat, 594–597
  of eye, 293
  topical ophthalmics for, 295–297
  treatment for, 300–301
Bacterial protein, 581f
Bacterial transport mechanism, mutations
  changing, 582
Bactericidal, **578**
Bactericidal agent, 579
Bacteriostatic, **578**
Bacteriostatic agent, 579
B-adrenergic blocker, nonselective, 346–347
Balance, 268
  disorders affecting, 283
  physical therapy for, 284
Balsam Peru
  dosage forms and strengths of, 691
  drug dosage and warnings, 696
  indications for, 690
Barbiturates
  binding of, 42
  dose effects of, 178f
  mechanism of action, **177**, 177–178
  pharmacokinetics and adverse reactions of,
    178
  seizure, treatment of, 136, 137, 140
  types of, 179, 181
Barrier
  to drug distribution, 29
  types of, 30f
Basal ganglia, **116**
  composition of, 117
  Parkinson's disease and, 120f
Basal nuclei, 70
Basiliximab
  adverse reactions from, 659

Basiliximab *(Continued)*
  dosage and warnings for, 661
  dosage forms and strengths of, 659
  mechanism of action, 658
Basophil, 308f, 310
B cell, 577
Bed sore. *See* Decubitus ulcer
Benign, **624**
Benign paroxysmal positional vertigo (BPPV), 283
Benign prostatic hyperplasia (BPH), **477**
  diagnosis of, 478–479
  symptoms and risk of, 478
  symptoms of, 479, 479b
  treatment of
    5-alpha-reductase inhibitor, 481, 482
    alpha₁-adrenergic antagonist, 479–480, 482
    nonpharmacological options, 481
    summary of, 481f
Benzixazole, 109, 112
Benzodiazepine, 179
  adverse reactions from, 77–78
  half-life and peak effect of, 180
  half-life of, 77t
  indications for, 76
  mechanism of action, 76
  pharmacokinetics of, 77
  precautions for, 79
  seizure, treatment of, 136, 137, 141
  summary of use, 81t–82t
  tolerance and dependence of, 78
  types of, 78t, 179, 181
  withdrawals from, 78–79
Benzothiazolylpiperazine, 110, 112
Benzoyl peroxide, 705
Beta₂-adrenergic agonist
  long-acting, 448–449, 455
  short-acting, 447–448, 455
Beta-adrenergic antagonist, 81
  glaucoma, as treatment for, 272
  types of, 273, 277
Beta-adrenergic blocker
  drug dosage and warnings, 327
  overview of, 324
  types of, 325
Beta blocker, 81
  adverse reactions and precautions for, 346
  drug dose strengths and schedule for, 366
  mechanism of action, 344, 346, 365
  migraine headache, treatment for, 164
  types of, 352
  ventricular arrhythmia and, 394
Beta-carotene, 670
Beta cell, 406, 512
Beta-lactam antibiotic
  destruction of, 582
  structure of, 580f
Beta-lactamase, **578**, 582
Beta receptor, 71–72
Bicarbonate, **490**, 492
Bicuspid valve, 312
Biguanide antidiabetic agent
  dosage and warnings for, 540
  mechanism of action, 534
  pharmacokinetics and adverse reactions of, 535
  types of, 535

Bile acid sequestrant, 384, 387
Bioavailability, **2**, **15**, **21**, 36
Bioengineering, 3
Bioequivalence, 36
Bioequivalent drug, **21**, 36, 36f
Biofeedback, **144**
Biogenic amine theory, 87
Biologic amine hypothesis, 88f
Biologic response modifier, 235t
  dosage and warnings for, 237
  role of, 231
Biologic therapy, 629
Biopharmaceuticals, **2**
  bioengineering of, 3
  examples of, 5
Biopsy, **624**, 629
Biotransformation, **21**, 30–31
Biphosphonate, 247–248, 251
Bipolar affective disorder (BPAD), 87, 100
Bipolar disorder, **86**, 87, 96
  drugs used to treat, 98
Blackhead (open comedone), **700**, 702, 702f
Black widow spider, 198
Bleeding
  antiplatelet drugs and, 377
  warfarin causing, 55
Bleomycin
  dosage and warnings for, 644
  overview of, 641–642
Blepharitis, **292**, 293, 298f
Blepharoptosis, **196**, 202
Blindness
  fusarium keratitis causing, 298
  glaucoma and, 271
  uveitis causing, 295
Blister, **687**, 689
Blood
  clot formation
    drugs controlling rate of, 375
    process of, 375f
  clotting disorders, 311
  clotting pathways, 378f
  components of, 308
  disorders of, 311
  supply, imbalance of, 319f
Blood-brain barrier, 29–30, 30f
Blood flow
  drug absorption, effect on, 26
  pathway of, 313–314, 314f
Blood glucose
  diabetes mellitus and, 526–528
  hormone regulation of, 526
  monitoring of, 530
Blood glucose monitor, 531f
Blood groups, 310
Blood loss anemia, 311
Blood-placenta barrier, 29–30, 30f
Blood poisoning, 691
Blood pressure
  classification of, 335–336, 336t
  control, sites for, 333
  kidneys, role of, 337
  measurement of, 333
Blood-testicular barrier, 29–30, 30f
Blood types, 310
Blood vessel
  disorders of, 315
  types of, 313
  view of, 313f
Blood volume, 310

B-lymphocyte, 310
Body
  fluid compartments of, 493, 493t
  of stomach, 405
Body lice
  infestation of, 732
  symptoms of, 733b
Body mass index, **332**
Body surface area (BSA), 692
Bone
  Paget's disease of, 245
  See also Osteoporosis
Bone marrow disorder, 311
Bone mineral density (BMD), **242**, 243
Bone remodeling. *See* Remodeling
Bony labyrinth, 268
Booster shot, 653
Botox. *See* Botulinum toxin
Botulinum toxin, **196**
  acetylcholine, effect on, 198
  mechanism of action, 200f
  use of, 199
Bowman's capsule, 475
Bradykinesia, **116**, 119
Bradykinin
  pain, role in, 147
Brain
  divisions of, 68, 69f
  memory, parts controlling, 170f
  stroke and, 210
Brain stem, 70
Brand name drug, **8**
  generic drugs, comparisons between, 8
  See also Proprietary name
Breast cancer
  alkylating agents for, 634
  aromatase inhibitors, 632–633
  estrogen receptor downregulator, 632
  platinum compounds for, 639
  prevalence and mortality rate of, 627
  progestins for, 634
  screening test for, 629
  signs and symptoms of, 628b
  taxanes as treatment for, 634
  topoisomerase inhibitors for, 638–639, 638f
  vinca alkaloid as treatment for, 636
Bretylium, 394
Broad-spectrum antiseizure drug, 137–138, 141
Bronchial airway, 447
Bronchodilator, **443**
Buccal tablet, 11
Bulk-forming laxative
  IBS, as treatment for, 427
  polycarbophil as, 432
Bundle branch, 316f
Bungarotoxin, alpha, 200f
Bupropion, 96
Burn
  classification of, 692, 694f
  complications of, 692
  drug dosage and warnings for, 696
  estimating body surface area of, 692
  precautions for, 693
  treatment of
    drugs used to treat, 694
    rehabilitation, 695
Burns, 146
Butenafine
  adverse reactions from, 679
  dosage and warnings for, 683

Butenafine *(Continued)*
 dosage forms and strengths of, 679
 mechanism of action and
  pharmacokinetics of, 678
Butyrophenone, 106, 108, 111

C

Calcineurin inhibitor, 721, 725
Calcipotriene
 adverse reactions from, 722
 dosage forms and strengths of, 722
 mechanism of action and
  pharmacokinetics of, 721
Calcitonin, 248-249, 252
Calcium
 calculating in food, 246t
 dosage and warnings for, 502
 electrolyte replacement therapy for, 498
 levels of, 244f
 needs by age, 245t
 percent per calcium salt, 246t
 in serum, 243-244
Calcium channel blocker
 blood pressure, lowering, 349
 as class IV antiarrhythmic agent, 394
 drug dosage and warnings, 328
 gastroesophageal reflux disease and, 408
 mechanism of action, 365
 overview of, 325
 types of, 326, 354
Calcium ion, storage and release of, 212f
Calyx, 474
Canadian Community Health Survey (CCHS),
  318
Canadian Controlled Drug and Substances Act,
  78
Cancer, **624**
 cause of, 626
 risk factors for, 626, 626b
 screening tests for, 629
 staging of, 629
 treatment of, 629
 types of, 627-629
Candida, **672**, 673f
 location of, 673
 potassium hydroxide (KOH) stain, 673
Candidiasis
 oral, 676f
 sites for, 674
Capillary, 313
Capsule, 11, 11f
Carbamazepine, 97, 134
Carbapenems, 591
Carbidopa, 32
 levodopa and, 54-55
 Parkinson's disease, as treatment of, 121
Carbohydrate, 528b
Carbonic anhydrase inhibitor, 273, 277
Carcinogen, 626, 626b
Carcinogenicity, 47
Cardiac muscle
 function of, 195
 types of, 190
Cardiac output, **332**, 333
Cardioglycoside, **360**
 digoxin/digitalis as, 363-364
 drug dosage and warnings, 365
 drug dose strengths and schedule for, 366
 types of, 365-366
Cardiomyopathy, 315

Cardiotoxicity, 95-96
Cardiovascular disease
 prevalence of, 372
 See also Angina; Heart disease
Cardiovascular system, 311
Castor oil
 dosage forms and strengths of, 691
 drug dosage and warnings, 696
 indications for, 690
Catatonia, **103**, 104
Catecholamine, 68, 511
Catechol-O-methyl transferase (COMT), 72, 121
Cation, **490**, 491
CD4 count, **601**, 609
CD4 T lymphocyte, **601**
Cecum, 405
Ceiling effect, 44
Celecoxib (Celebrex), 229
Cell life cycle
 chemotherapeutic/antineoplastic agents
  interrupting, 629
 mitosis and, 630t, 635t
 summary of, 630t
Cell-mediated immunity, 576
Cell membrane
 drug movement across, 24-25
 weak acids and bases crossing, 26f
Center for Drug Evaluation and Research
  (CDER)
 drug naming, role in, 7
 Labeling and Nomenclature Committee, 8
Centers for Disease Control and Prevention
  (CDC)
 immunization schedule, 653f, 654f
 ocular toxoplasmosis, prevalence of, 298
Central acting alpha$_2$-agonist, 349-350, 354-355
Central acting muscle relaxant, **196**, 199
 for muscle strain, 215
 pharmacokinetics of, 201t
 spasticity, as treatment for, 214
Central nervous system
 blood pressure, drop in, 333-334
 skeletal muscle relaxants and, 215
Central nervous system (CNS)
 composition of, 68
Central vision, **270**
Cephalosporin, 303
 dosage and warnings for, 594-595
 drug form and strengths, 584-585
Cerebellum, 70
Cerebral cortex, 70
Cerebral hemisphere, 70
Cerebral palsy, **209**, 210
Cerebral tracts, 70
Cerebral vascular disease, seizures and, 130
Cerebrum, 70
Cerumen, 268, **281**, 671
 impaction of, 286
 removal of, 287
Ceruminous glands, 671
Cervical cancer
 prevalence and mortality rate of, 627-628
 screening test for, 629
Chancroid, 558
Chemical digestion, 404
Chemical name, **7**
Chemotherapeutic agent, 629, 630f
Chemotherapy, **624**, 629
Chewable tablet, 11
Chickenpox, treatment for, 605

Chief cell, 405
Children
 atopic dermatitis in, 716
 congenital glaucoma in, 271
 eczema in, 716, 717f
 gastroesophageal reflux disease in, 408
 immunization schedule for, 653f, 654f
 juvenile-onset diabetes mellitus, 527
 Lund-Browder chart, 692
 rheumatic heart disease and, 315
Chlamydia, 558
Chloramphenicol
 dosage forms and strengths of, 594
 indications for, 593
Chloride, **490**
 electrolyte replacement therapy for, 497
 role of, 492
Chloride ion (Cl$^-$), 76
Cholecystokinin (CCK), 105
Cholesterol, **371**
 heart disease and, 318
 stroke, as risk factor for, 374
Choline acetyltransferase, 125
Cholinergic agonist, 275, 278
Cholinergic receptor
 blockade of, 91
 types of, 72
Cholinesterase inhibitor, 275, 278
Choreiform movement, 125
Chronic obstructive pulmonary disease
  (COPD), **443**
 antihistamine as treatment for, 467-468
 mast cell stabilizers for, 468
 overview of, 446-447
Chronic pain, **144**, 145
Ciclopirox, 681, 683
Cidofovir
 adverse reactions from, 606
 indications for, 606
Ciliary body, 266, 266f
Cimetidine, 55-56
Circadian rhythm, **175**
Circular plicae, 405
Clindamycin
 acne, for treatment of, 707
 dosage and warnings for, 597
 dosage forms and strengths of, 594
 indications for, 593
Clinical depression, 87
Clomiphene, 560
Clomipramine, 80, 80-81, 80t
Clonazepam, 81t
Clonus, **209**, 210
Clopidogrel
 drug dosage and warnings, 385
 mechanism of action, 376
Clorazepate, 81t
Closed comedone. *See* Whitehead
Clostridium histolyticum, 690
Clotting
 formation of, 375, 375f
 pathways of, 378f
Clozapine, 112
Cluster headache, **163**, 164
Coagulation, 310
Cochlea, 268-269, 268f, 269, **281**
Codeine, 55
Cognitive function, **116**
 in Alzheimer's disease, 168
 in Parkinson's disease, 119

Cognitive symptoms, 104
Cold chain, **649**
    importance of, 651
    maintenance of, 651-652
    pharmacy technician's role in, 652, 652f
    for vaccines, 650
Colitis. *See* Inflammatory bowel syndrome
Collagenase
    debridement and, 690
    dosage forms and strengths of, 691
    drug dosage and warnings, 696
Collecting duct, 475
Colloid, **490**, 501
Colon, 404, 405
Colonoscopy, **423**
    performance of, 424
    view of, 424f
Colorectal cancer
    prevalence and mortality rate of, 628
    screening test for, 629
Combat Methamphetamine Epidemic Act
    (CMEA), 9
Comedolytics, 704
Comedone, **700**, 702
Commission error, 59
Communication, between nerve cells, 68
Complement, 577
Complementary and alternative medicine
    (CAM), **624**
Complex focal seizure, **129**, 130
Computed tomography (CT) scan, **624**, 629
Condom, **545**, 548
Conduction, 315
Conduction impairment, 269
Conductive hearing loss, **281**
Cone, 266
Congenital glaucoma, 271
Congestive heart failure
    compensatory mechanisms in, 361, 362f
    potassium-sparing diuretics and, 340
    See also Heart failure
Conjugate vaccine, **649**, 650
Conjunctiva, 267, **270**
Conjunctivitis, **292**
    cause and effects of, 293
    viral, view of, 294f
Constipation, **423**
Contraception
    emergency, 552, 566
    methods of, 547b, 548-552
Contractility, 195
Contraindication
    drug, **53**
    drug-disease, **53**
Controlled substance, **2**
    access in Canada, 10
    access to, 9
    schedules, classification, dispensing and
        examples of, 9t
Convergence, 267
Convulsion, **129**, 130
Cornea, 266, 266f, **270**
Coronary artery, 313f, 314
Coronary artery disease, **317**
Coronary heart disease, 257
Corpus callosum, 70
Corti, organ of, 269
Corticosteroid
    eczema and psoriasis, as treatment for,
        718

Corticosteroid *(Continued)*
    indications and adverse reactions for, 429
    inhaled
        for allergies, 467
        for asthma, 449-450, 456
        intranasal, 468
        types of, 430, 433
        See also Topical corticosteroid
COX-2 inhibitor, **144**
Crabs. *See* Pubic lice
Craniopharyngioma, **545**
Cream, 12
Crohn's disease, **423**
    diagnostic testing for, 424
    drugs used to treat, 431-433
    immunomodulators for, 431
    immunosuppressants for, 430
    lifestyle modifications for, 425, 426t
    symptoms of, 424t
Cross-resistance, **601**, 611
Crotamiton, 735
Crystalloid, **490**, 501, 501t
Curare (C), 200f
Cutaneous, **715**
Cutaneous immunosuppression, 722
Cuticle, 671
Cyclophosphamide, 230-231
Cyclopyrrolone derivative, 179
Cyclosporine, 230-231
    for atopic dermatitis and psoriasis,
        722-723
    dosage and warnings for, 661, 725
    dosage forms and strengths of, 657
    overview of, 656
Cyproheptadine, 215
Cyst, **700**, 702
Cysticercosis, 299
Cytochrome P-450 system, 31
Cytokine, 145, 575
Cytokine inhibitor
    dosage and warnings for, 661
    overview of, 660
Cytokinesis, 630t
Cytomegalovirus (CMV)
    drug dosage and warnings, 608-609
    drugs used to treat, 605-607
    exposure to, 297
Cytomegalovirus retinitis, **292**, 297

D

Daclizumab
    adverse reactions from, 659
    dosage and warnings for, 661
    dosage forms and strengths of, 659
    mechanism of action, 658
Dactinomycin
    dosage and warnings for, 644
    overview of, 641-642
Danazol, 563-564
Darunavir (TMC114)
    dosage and warnings for, 618
    drug form and strengths, 615
    overview of, 614
Data Standards Manual (DSM), 7
Debridement
    decubitus ulcers and, 690
    drug dosage and warnings for, 696
Decamethonium (D), 200f
Decimal point, misuse causing medication
    error, 58

Decubitus ulcer, **687**
    care, prevention and treatment of, 689-690
    characteristics of, 688
    drug dosage and warnings for, 696
    mechanism of formation, 688
    Norton Scale, 690t
    stages of, 688-689, 688f
    topical treatment of, 690b
    treatment for, 691
Deep vein thrombosis (DVT), 316
Deflection, 267
Deglutination, 405
Dehydration, **490**, 493
    burns and, 692
Delavirdine
    dosage and warnings for, 618
    overview of, 613
Delayed-action tablet, 10
Delta cell, 512
Delusion, **103**, 104
Dementia, **163**
Demyelination, **221**
    cause of, 223
Deoxyribonucleic acid. *See* DNA
Dependence, 47
    on Barbiturates, 178
    of benzodiazepines, 78
Depolarization, **391**, 392
Depolarizing neuromuscular blocker, **196**, 199
    mechanism of action, 200f
    pharmacokinetics of, 201t
    types, dosage forms and strengths of, 202
    See also Neuromuscular blocking agent
Depo-Provera, 550
Depressant, **175**
Depression
    drugs used to treat, 88, 98-99
    neurochemistry of, 87
    prevalence and types of, 87
Dermal-epidermal junction, 668, 668f
    role of, 669
Dermatitis, **715**
Dermatomyositis, **221**
Dermatophyte infection, 673
Dermatophytes, **672**
    location of, 673
Dermis, 668, 668f
    function of, 669
    layers of, 670
Desensitization, 46
Dexamethasone, 235
Diabetes
    cause of, 529
    complementary and alternative medicine
        for, 539
    complications of, 529-530, 530b
    drugs used to treat, 540-541
    hyperuricemia as risk factor for, 257
    nonpharmacological management of, 530
    thiazide diuretics and, 338
Diabetes mellitus, **525**
    diagnostic testing for, 529
    lifestyle modifications for, 530b
    overview of, 526
    risk factors for, 529t
    symptoms of, 529b
    treatment of, 530-531
    types of, 526-528
Diabetic neuropathy, **144**, 146, **525**
Diaphoresis, **196**

Diaphragm, 405, **545**
  contraception, as method of, 548
  types of, 549
  view of, 404
Diarrhea, **423**
Diarthroses joint, 190
Diastolic blood pressure (DBP), **332**, **333**
Diastolic heart failure (DHF), 361
Diazepam, 81t
Dibenzodiazepine, 112
Dibenzothiazepine, 110, 112
Dibenzoxazepine, 110, 112
Didanosine (ddI)
  dosage and warnings for, 617
  dosage forms and strengths of, 612
  overview of, 611
Diencephalon, 70
Diethylstilbestrol, 47
Diffusion, **21**, 26
Digestion, 404
Digestive system
  anatomy of, 404-405, 404f
  role of, 404
Digitalis, 363
Digitalization, **360**, 364
Digital rectal exam (DRE), **477**
Digoxin, 45
  arrhythmia, as treatment for, 396
  dosage strengths and schedule for, 365
  for heart failure, 363f
  overview of, 364
  potassium-sparing diuretics and, 340
Dipeptidyl peptidase-4 inhibitor
  diabetes and, 538
  dosage and warnings for, 540
Dipivefrin, 32, 275
Direct vasodilator, 350-351, 355
Disease
  drug-disease contraindication, **53**
  elimination, effect on, 34
  metabolism, effect on, 33
  pharmacotherapeutics, effect on, 46
Disease-modifying antirheumatic drug
  (DMARD)
  dosage and warnings for, 238
  rheumatoid arthritis, treatment of, 232-234
  uses for, 235t
Disinhibition, **175**, 178
Distal tubule, 475
Distribution, **21**
  factors influencing, 29-30
  process of, 27, 28f
Diuretic, **332**
  drug dose strengths and schedule for, 366
  indications for, 365
  role and classification of, 337
  types of, 351-352
DNA (deoxyribonucleic acid)
  anthracycline damaging, 637
  replication, 630t
    inhibition of, 605-606
    process of, 637f
Dopamine, 32
  depression, role in, 87, 88
  drugs affecting levels of, 124
  drugs enhancing activity of, 123
  drugs that deplete, 125
  Parkinson's disease, role in, 119
  Parkinson's disease and, 42, 118, 118f
  pathways of, 106f, 117f

Dopamine *(Continued)*
  schizophrenia, role in, 104-105
  secretion of, 70
Dopamine receptor, drugs blocking, 104
Dosage form, **2**, 5
  for oral (enteral) administration, 10-12
  for topical administration, 12
Dose, **2**, 5
Dose-response curve, 43, 43f
Dose-response relationship, 43
Dosing schedule, **2**, 5
  understanding, 50
Dosing unit, confusion causing medication
  error, 58, 60
Double-blind study, 46
Double-contrast barium enema, **624**, 629
Doxorubicin
  for breast cancer treatment, 636-637
  dosage and warnings for, 643
  dosage forms and strengths of, 637
Doxycycline, 706
Drug, **2**
  absorption of, 22, 24-26
  administration of, 14-17
  adverse reactions from, 46-47
  anxiety disorder, treatment of, 76
  bioavailability and bioequivalence of, 36
  chemical, generic and proprietary name, 8t
  classification and sources of, 5
  common endings of, 8t
  controlled substances, 9, 9t
  dependence and tolerance, 47
  development phases for, 7f
  distribution of, 27, 28f
  distribution phases of, 23f
  dopamine, blocking and depleting of, 125
  efficacy of, 43
  elimination of, 34-36
  enteral administration of, 10-12
  food and drug, interaction with, 54
  formulation of, 14
  GI interactions, 55f
  inhibitors and inducers of, 56t
  interactions, avoiding, 57
  interactions, effects of, 57t
  investigational processes of, 6f
  metabolism of, 30-34
  movement across cell membrane, 24-25
  multiple, effect on elimination, 35
  multiple, effect on metabolism, 33
  origin of, 5
  pharmacokinetic phases of, 22
  pharmacological class of, 7
  potency of, 43-44, 44f
  research and development of, 5-7
  safety categories for pregnancy, 30, 30t
  systemic effects of, 14-15
  topical administration of, 12
  transport mechanisms of, 25
  as weak acids or bases, 25-26
  See also Adverse drug reaction (ADR);
    Medication error
Drug contraindication, **53**
Drug delivery system, **2**
Drug dependence, **74**
Drug-disease contraindication, **53**, 57
Drug-drug interaction, **53**, 54
Drug Evaluation and Research. *See* Center for
  Drug Evaluation and Research (CDER)
Drug-food interaction, 54, 57-58

Drug Identification Number (DIN), 7
Drug legislation, 8-10
Drug nomenclature, 7-8
Drug Price Competition Act, 9
Drug Product Reference File (DPRF), 7
Drug property, 29
Drug-receptor binding, 42
  effects of, 42t
Drug-receptor interaction
  process of, 41f
  types of, 41-43
Drug-receptor theory, **40**
Drug Registration and Listing System
  (DRLS), 7
Drug resistance testing, **601**, 610
Drug therapy
  factors influencing adherence to, 48, 50
  improving adherence to, 48
  insufficient monitoring of, 61
Dry eyes, 267
Duodenal ulcer, **407**
Duodenum, 405
Duplication, therapeutic, **53**
Duration of action, **21**, **22**, 24f
Durham-Humphrey Amendment, 8
Dynorphin, **144**, 148
Dysfunctional uterine bleeding, **545**
Dysfunctional uterine bleeding (DUB),
  557-558
Dysmenorrhea, **545**
  NSAID as treatment for, 557, 565
  symptoms of, 555
Dysphoria, **144**
Dysthymia, 87

E

Ear
  anatomy of, 268f, 282f
  bacterial infections of, 302
  ceruminous glands of, 671
  disorders affecting, 285-287
  drug dosage and warnings, 287
  physiology of, 268
  water-clogged, 285-286
  See also Hearing
Ear canal, 268
Eardrum, 268
Earwax. *See* Cerumen
Eccrine sweat glands, 671
Echinocandins
  dosage and warnings for, 683
  overview of, 680-681
Echothiophate iodide
  acetylcholine and, 275
  preparation of, 276b
Ectopic, **391**
Ectopic heart beat, 394
Eczema, **715**
  drug dosage and warnings, 724-726
  nonpharmaceutical treatment of, 718
  pharmaceutical treatment of, 718
  phases of, 717f
  prevalence of, 716
  signs and symptoms of, 718b
  skin care for, 718b
  types of, 716b
Edema, **490**
  cause of, 494
  management and treatment of, 494b
Edrophonium (E), 200f

Efavirenz
    dosage and warnings for, 618
    overview of, 613-614
Effect
    additive, **53**, 54
    ceiling, 44
    first-pass, **21**, 32-33, 32f
    peak, **22**, 24f
    placebo, 46
    synergistic, **53**, 54
    therapeutic, 24f
Effector T cell, 577
Efferent neuron, 68
Efficacy, **40**
Efficacy, of drug, 43-44
Ejaculation, **477**
Ejection fraction, **360**
Electrical cardioversion, **391**, 393
Electrolyte, **490**
    depletion, management of, 497b
    homeostasis and, 491
    imbalance, treatment for, 497
    intravenous fluid, treatment with, 500
    in urine, 476
    values of, 492t
Electrolyte disorder
    disorders of, 491
    treatment of, 502-503
    types of, 493-497
Electrolyte replacement therapy
    calcium, potassium, phosphorus, 498
    for magnesium, 499
    sodium and chloride, 497
    types of, 502
Elimination, **21**
    factors influencing, 34-36
    process of, 34
    routes of, 34t
Elimination half-life (T½), 35-36
Elixir, 12
Embolic stroke, **371**, 372
Emergency contraceptive
    dosage and warnings for, 566
    indications for, 552
Emtricitabine (FTC)
    dosage and warnings for, 617
    dosage forms and strengths of, 612
    overview of, 611
Emulsion, 12
Endocarditis, 315
Endocardium, 312
Endocrine cell, 405
Endocrine system, 508
Endolymph, 269
Endometrial cancer
    medroxyprogesterone acetate as treatment
        for, 633-634
    prevalence and mortality rate of,
        627-628
    tamoxifen and, 631
Endometriosis, **545**, 563-564, 568
Endorphins, **144**
    pain, role in, 148, 148f
Endoscopy, **407**
Endotracheal intubation, **196**
    indications for, 199
Endplate, **196**, **197**
Enfuvirtide, 619
Enkephalins, **144**
    pain, role in, 148, 148f

Enteral, **2**
    advantages and disadvantages of, 15, 15t
    capsules as dosage form, 11, 11f
    oral liquid as dosage form, 11-12
    suspensions as dosage form, 11f
    tablets as dosage form, 10
Enteric-coated tablet, 10, 10f
Enuresis, **86**
Environment pollutant, 626, 626b
Enzyme, **21**
    induction and inhibition, 31f
    role of, 30-31
Eosinphil, 308f, 310
Epicardium, 311, 312, 312f
Epidermal cell, 669
Epidermal growth/repair, 669
Epidermis, 668, 668f, 669
Epilepsy, **129**, 130
Epinephrine, 55, 68, 71-72, 511
Epirubicin
    for breast cancer treatment, 636-637
    dosage and warnings for, 643
    dosage forms and strengths of, 638
Equilibrium, 268, **281**
    disorders affecting, 283
Erectile dysfunction (ED), **477**
    cause and treatment of, 482
    phosphodiesterase inhibitors for,
        483, 486
    prostaglandins for, 484-485, 486
Ergot alkaloid, 164
Error. *See* Medication error
Erysipelas, 692
Erythroblastosis fetalis, 310
Erythrocyte, 308, 308f
Erythromycin, 706
Erythropoiesis, 309
Erythropoietin, 3, 5
Eschar, **687**
Escharotomy, **687**
Esophagus, 404, 405
Estrogen
    deficiency of, 249
    dosage and warnings for, 566-567
    products, examples of, 553t, 554t
    types of, 555
Estrogen receptor downregulator
    dosage and warnings for, 642
    overview of, 631
Estrogen-receptor positive breast cancer,
    631
Etanercept
    dosage and warnings for, 662, 726
    dosage forms and strengths of, 723
    as tumor necrosis factor inhibitor, 660
Ethosuximide, 135
Etoposide
    dosage and warnings for, 644
    overview of, 638-639
Euphoria, **144**, 148
Eustachian tube, 268
Euvolemic hyponatremia, 494
Exacerbation, **715**
Excisional biopsy, **624**
Excitability, 195
Excitation, 197f
Exemestane
    dosage and warnings for, 642
    dosage forms and strengths of, 633
Exertional angina, 319

Extensibility, 195
External auditory meatus, 268, 268f
External ear
    divisions of, 268
    view of, 268f
External radiation, **624**
External urinary meatus, 475
Extracellular fluid, **490**
Extracellular fluid compartment, 493
Extrapyramidal symptoms, **103**, 107
Extrinsic eye muscles, 267
Eye
    anatomy and physiology of, 266f
    bacterial infections of, 293
    fungal and protozoal infections of, 298
    infections, treatment for, 300-301
    parasitic infection, treatment for, 299
    structure of
        accessory structures, 267
        cavities and humors, 267
        muscles, 267
        parts and layers, 266
    viral infections of
        drug dosage and strength, 298
        types of, 297
    See also Vision

F

Factor VIII, 308
Famciclovir, 606
Family history, cancer and, 626b, 627
Farsightedness, 267
Fasting blood glucose, **525**
Fatal hepatotoxicity, 613
Fatal liver toxicity, 613
Fatigue, 235t
Febrile seizure, **129**, 130
Fecal occult blood test (FOBT), **624**
Female condom, 548
Femidom, 548
Fentanyl, 5
Fetal circulation, 314
Fetal skull, 190
Fiber supplement, 427
Fibric acid derivative, 384, 387
Fibrinolytic agent, 375
    See also Thrombolytic
Fibrous layer, 266
Fibrous pericardium, 311, 312f
Film-coated tablet, 11
Filtration, 476
First-degree burn, **687**, 692, 694f
First messenger, 509
First-pass effect, **21**, 32-33, 32f
Fissures, 70
Fistula, **423**, 431-433
Five-alpha-reductase inhibitor, 480
Floater, **292**, 297
Fluid disorder, 491
    intravenous fluid, treatment with,
        500
    treatment of, 502-503
    types of, 493-497
Fluoropyrimidine
    dosage and warnings for, 643
    overview of, 640
Fluoroquinolone
    dosage and warnings for, 595
    dosage forms and strengths of, 586
    mechanism of action, 585

Fluoroquinolone *(Continued)*
  pharmacokinetics and adverse reactions of, 586
Fluoxetine, 80, 80t
Flu vaccine, 653
Focal (partial) seizure, 130
Folate deficiency anemia, 311
Folic acid
  bacterial synthesis of, 581
  deficiency of, 311
  UV radiation and, 670
Follitropin, 560
Fontanels, 190
Food
  drugs, interaction with, 54, 57–58
  griseofulvin, interaction with, 55
  purine content in, 260, 261b
Food and Drug Administration
  adverse drug reactions, reporting to, 50
  calcineurin inhibitors and, 721
  iPLEDGE program, 709
  selective COX-2 inhibitor, removal of, 229
  Voluntary Reporting Form 3500, 49f
Forced expiratory volume (FEV₁), **443**
Fosamprenavir (FPV)
  dosage and warnings for, 618
  drug form and strengths, 615
  overview of, 614
Foscarnet, 606
Fosphenytoin
  adverse reactions from, 133
  mechanism of action, 132
  pharmacokinetics of, 132–133
Fourth-degree burn, **687**, 692
Fracture, osteoporosis and, 243
Frequency, **477**
Frontal sinus, 190
Full-thickness burn, **687**, 692, 694f
Fulvestrant
  dosage and warnings for, 642
  dosage forms and strengths of, 632
Fundus, 405
Fungal infection
  imidazoles and triazoles for, 677–678
  treatment for, 300–301
  treatment of, 675
Fungus, **672**
  types of, 673
Furanocoumarin
  dosage and warnings for, 726
  overview of, 722
Fusarium keratitis, **292**, 298
Fusion inhibitor
  dosage and warnings for, 617
  overview of, 616

G

Gallbladder, 406
Gamma aminobutyric acid
  binding, drugs enhancing, 214–215
  Parkinson's disease, role in, 119
  seizure, role in, 130–131
  spasticity, role in, 212
Gamma aminobutyric acid (GABA)
  anxiety, role in, 76
  schizophrenia, role in, 105
Gamma aminobutyric acid analog, 135, 140
Ganciclovir, 606
Gangrene, 692
Garlic, diabetes and, 540

Gastric acid, 408, 414f
Gastric glands, 405
Gastric pit, 405
Gastric ulcer, **407**
Gastroenteritis, **423**, 425
Gastroesophageal junction, 409f
Gastroesophageal reflux disease (GERD), **407**
  antacids for, 416
  drugs used to treat, 411, 412
  factors contributing to, 408
  H₂-receptor antagonist drugs for, 412, 417
  lifestyle modifications for, 411b
  prevalence of, 408
  prokinetic drugs for, 415, 418
  proton pump inhibitor drugs for, 412–413, 418
  symptoms of, 411, 411t
Gastrointestinal (GI) tract, 404
  conditions relating to, 424
Gender
  atrial fibrillation and, 392t
  metabolism, effect on, 34
  pharmacotherapeutics, effect on, 45
  stroke, as risk factor for, 374
Generalized anxiety disorder, **74**
  prevalence and symptoms of, 75
Generalized seizure, **129**, 130
Generic name, **7**
  approval of, 9
  brand name, comparisons between, 8
Genetics
  metabolism, effect on, 33
  pharmacotherapeutics, effect on, 45
Gestational diabetes, **525**
  prevalence and cause of, 528
Gestational hypertension, 335
Gingival hyperplasia, **129**, 133
Glaucoma, 271
  angle closure, **270**
  congenital, 271
  laser surgery for, 278
  marijuana as treatment for, 276
  neovascular, 271
  normal vision versus, 271f
  open angle, **270**
  pathophysiology of, 271
  prevalence of, 271
  treatment of, 272, 277–278
Glial cell, 68
Glomerular capillary, 474
Glomerulus, 474, 475
Glucagon
  alpha cells secreting, 406, 512
  storage of, 526
Glucocorticosteroid, 227f
  adverse reactions and precautions for, 228
  allergies, as treatment for, 466
  asthma, as treatment for, 449
  disease treated with, 228
  gout, as treatment for, 259
  indications and pharmacokinetics of, 227
  suppressive effects of, 227f
Glutamate
  Alzheimer's disease, role in, 168
  pain, role in, 147
  Parkinson's disease, role in, 119
  schizophrenia, role in, 105
  spasticity, role in, 213
Glutamic acid decarboxylase, 125
Glycine, 213

Glycophospholipid, 669
Gold, 233
Gonad, 512
Gonadotropin-releasing hormone agonist (GnRH)
  dosage and warnings for, 643
  overview of, 633
Gonadotropin-releasing hormone analog, 564, 568
Gonadotropins, 560, 561
Gonorrhea, 559
Gosrelin
  dosage and warnings for, 643
  dosage forms and strengths of, 633
Gout, **256**
  drug dosage and warnings, 260
  drugs used to treat, 258
  hyperuricemia and, 257
  nonpharmacological treatment for, 260
  pathophysiology of, 257–258
  thiazide diuretics and, 338
Gouty arthritis, 257f
Granular leukocyte, 308f
Granulated eyelids, 293
Granulocyte, 310
Grapefruit juice, 33–34, 56
Graves' disease, **514**
Gray matter, 70
Griseofulvin
  dosage and warnings for, 683
  fatty food, interaction with, 55
  overview of, 681
Gynecomastia, **332**
  symptoms of, 412

H

Haemophilus influenzae type B (Hib), 650
Hair, 671
Hair cell, 268
Half-life (T½), **21**
  elimination, 35–36
Hallucination, **103**, 104
Haloperidol, 126
Hammer (malleus), 268, 268f
Hard palate, 405
Hashimoto's disease, **514**
Hazardous chemicals, cancer and, 626–627, 626b
HDL. *See* High-density lipoprotein (HDL)
Headache, 146
Head lice
  adult, 731f
  infestation of, 731–732, 731f
  symptoms of, 733b
Hearing, 268
  disorders affecting, 282
  impairment of, 269
Heart, 311
  blood supply, 314
  conduction system of, 315
  disorders of, 315
  drug dose strengths and schedule for, 366
  structure of, 312, 313f
  See also Arrhythmia; Blood flow
Heart attack
  prevalence of, 372
  seizure, as cause of, 130
Heart disease
  hyperuricemia and, 257
  lifestyle change, 320t

Heart disease *(Continued)*
  See also Angina; Coronary heart disease;
    Ischemic heart disease
Heart failure, **360**
  classification and management of, 362t
  digoxin therapy for, 363f
  doxorubicin and, 637
  drugs used to treat, 361
  lifestyle modifications for, 364b, 374b
  pathophysiology and stages of, 361
Heart murmur, 315
Heart rate, 333
Heart valve, 312
Helicobacter pylori (H. pylori)
  antimicrobials for, 419
  peptic ulcer disease and, 410
Helminthes, **292**
Helminthic infection, 299
Helper T cell, 577
Hemoglobin, 309
Hemoglobin A1c, **525**
Hemolytic anemia, 311
Hemophilia, 311
Hemorrhagic stroke, **371**, 373
Hemorrhoid, 316
Hemostasis, 310, **371**, 375
Heparin
  indications for, 377
  mechanism of action, 378
  overdose of, 379
  pharmacokinetics and adverse reactions of,
    379
Hepatic portal, 314
Hepatitis virus, 608-609
Hepatotoxicity, **40**, **47**
Herceptin, 642
Herpes simplex keratitis, **292**, 297
Herpes simplex virus (HSV), 297
  drug dosage and warnings, 608
  drugs used to treat, 605-607
Herpes zoster ophthalmicus, **292**, 297
Herpetic blepharitis, 298f
Herpetic eye disease, 297
Hiatal hernia, **407**
  effects of, 408
  view of, 409f
High blood pressure. *See* Hypertension
High cholesterol, stroke and, 374
High-density lipoprotein (HDL), **371**, 381
Highly active antiretroviral therapy (HHART),
  601
  for HIV treatment, 603, 610
Hilum, 474, 474f
Hirsutism, **129**, 133, **332**
Histamine, 310
  pain, role in, 147
Histamine₁-receptor antagonist
  allergies, as treatment for, 464
  types of, 465-466
Histamine₂-receptor antagonist
  overview of, 412
  types of, 413, 417
Histamine receptor, blockade of, 91
HIV (human immunodeficiency virus)
  fungal infection and, 675
  fusion inhibitors and, 616
  HAART therapy for, 603
  life cycle of, 609-610
  non-nucleoside reverse transcriptase
    inhibitor (NNRTI), 613-614, 618

HIV *(Continued)*
  nucleoside/nucleotide reverse
    transcriptase inhibitor (NRTI), 610-612
  overview of, 609
  pharmacotherapy for, 610
  protease inhibitors, 614-616, 618-619
Homeopathic medicine, **2**
Homeostasis, **490**, 491
Hormone, 68
  classification of, 509
  secretion, regulation of, 510
  in urine, 476
Hormone replacement therapy (HRT),
  249-250, 252
  adverse reactions from, 554
  benefits versus risks of, 553
  regimens, examples of, 554b
  treatment protocols for, 554
  See also Estrogen; Progestin
Host, **601**
  virus invasion of, 602f
Human immunodeficiency virus. *See* HIV
Human insulin, 3, 5
Humoral immunity, 576
Huntington's disease, **116**
  drugs used to treat, 125, 126
  neurochemistry of, 125
  prevalence and symptoms of, 124-125
Hydantoins
  adverse reactions from, 133
  dosing and warnings for, 139
  mechanism of action, 132
  pharmacokinetics of, 132-133
Hydration, 689
Hydrocortisone, 235
Hydrophilic, **21**
Hydrophobic, **21**
Hydroxychloroquine, side effects of, 229
Hydroxymethylglutaryl (HMG) CoA reductase
  inhibitor, 381, 387
Hydroxyurea
  dosage and warnings for, 644
  overview of, 641-642
Hydroxyzine, 79-80, 80t, 82t
Hyperchloremia, **490**, **491**, 496
Hyperglycemia, 338, **525**
  symptoms of, 532b
Hyperhydrosis, **196**
Hyperkalemia, 332, **491**, 495-496
  management of, 496b
  potassium-sparing diuretics and, 340
Hyperlipidemia, **317**, **372**
  drugs used to treat, 381, 387
Hypernatremia, **332**, **490**
  cause of, 495
  management of, 495b
Hyperplasia, **477**
Hyperpolarization, 76
Hypersomnia, rebound, **175**
Hypertension, **332**
  cause of, 334-335
  complications of, 336
  drugs causing, 335b
  drugs used to treat, 351-355
  hyperuricemia and, 257
  prevalence of, 334
  risk factors for, 335b
  stage 1-3, 335
  stroke, as risk factor for, 374
  treatment of, 336

Hypertensive crisis, 95
Hyperthyroidism, **514**
  drugs used to treat, 521
  prevalence of, 515
  symptoms of, 517, 517b
  treatment of, 517-518
  TSH and T₄, comparison of, 516f
Hypertonic, **491**
Hypertonic fluid, 500f, 501
Hyperuricemia, **256**, **332**, 338
  medical conditions associated with, 257
  prevalence of, 257
Hypervolemic hyponatremia, 494
Hypnotic, **175**
Hypocalcemia, **491**, 496
Hypochloremia, 338, 496
Hypodermis, 668, 668f
  composition of, 670
Hypoglycemia, **525**, 532b
Hypogonadism, **545**, 568
  prevalence and cause of, 559-560
  treatment of, 561-562
Hypokalemia, **332**, **491**, 495
  thiazide diuretics and, 338
  ventricular arrhythmia and, 365
Hypomagnesemia, **491**, 496
Hypomagnesia, 338
Hyponatremia, **332**, 338, **491**
  management of, 495b
  types of, 494
Hypophosphatemia, **491**, 496
Hypophysis, 510
Hypothalamus, 70, 510
Hypothyroidism, **514**
  drugs used to treat, 521
  overview of, 519-520
  prevalence of, 515
  symptoms of, 519b
  TSH and T₄, comparison of, 516f
Hypotonic, **491**
Hypotonic fluid, 500-501, 500f
Hypovolemic hyponatremia, 494
Hypoxia, **372**
Hysterectomy, **545**, 553

I

Idarubicin, 636-637
Idiosyncratic reaction, **40**, 46
Ileum, 404, 405
Imidazoles
  dosage and warnings for, 682-683
  dosage forms and strengths of, 677-678
  fungal infection, as treatment for, 677
Imidazopyridines, 179
Imionstilbenes, 134, 139
Immune response, treatment for, 234t
Immune system, 575
Immunization, **649**, 654f
  indication and effects of, 650
  schedules for, 653f
Immunoglobin (Ig), 576
Immunoglobin IV, 659
Immunomodulator, 431
  calcineurin inhibitors as, 721
  types of, 433
Immunosuppressant, 430, **649**
  atopic dermatitis and, 722
  dosage and warnings for, 661-662
  dosage forms and strengths of, 723
  fungal infection and, 675

Immunosuppressant *(Continued)*
    role of, 656
    types of, 433
Immunosuppressive
    dosage and warnings for, 237, 725
    types of, 230-231
Immunotherapy, 468-469
Impaired fasting glucose (IFG), 526
Impaired glucose tolerance (IGT), 526
Implant radiation, **625**
Inactivated, killed vaccine, **649**, 650
Incontinence, 476, **477**
Incretin mimetic, 538
Incus (anvil), 268, 268f
Indinavir (IDV)
    dosage and warnings for, 618
    drug form and strengths, 615
    overview of, 614
Induction
    of cytochromes P450, 56t
    enzyme, 31f
Infant
    eczema in, 716, 717f
    gastroesophageal reflux disease in, 408
    HIV transmission to, 611-612, 611t
    milia in, 703
Infarction, **372**
Infection
    from burns, 692
    stroke, as risk factor for, 374
Infertility, **545**
    dosage and warnings for, 567-568
    prevalence and cause of, 559
    treatment of, 560, 561
Inflammation, **145**
    glucocorticosteroid
        indications for, 227
        suppressive effects of, 227f
    treatment for, 234t
Inflammatory bowel syndrome (IBS), **423**
    cause of, 425
    diagnosis of, 424
    drugs used to treat, 426
    lifestyle modifications for, 425, 426t
    serotonin levels and, 425
    symptoms of, 424t
Infliximab, 431
Influenza, 607-608
Influenza A, 603
Influenza B, 603
Infundibulum, 510
Inhalation administration, 16
Inhaled corticosteroid
    allergies, as treatment for, 467
    asthma, as treatment for, 449-450, 456
Inhaler, aerosol, 14, 14f
Inhibition
    of cytochromes P450, 56t
    enzyme, 31f
Injection, forms of, 16f
Innate defense, mechanism of, 575-576
Innate immunity, 575
Inner ear, 268, 268f
Inner layer, 266
Insomnia, **175**
    medication for, 179-180, 181
    medication half-life and peak effect of, 180
    natural remedies for, 180
    nonpharmacological treatment for, 181
    prevalence and categorization of, 177

Insulin
    action of, 528f
    administration of, 531
    adverse reactions from, 531
    beta cell secreting, 406, 512
    dosage and warnings for, 540
    human, 3, 5
    mechanism of action and
        pharmacokinetics of, 531
    onset and duration of action of, 532t
    physiological effects of, 526, 528b
    role of, 528f
    types of, 533
    vials and cartridges, storage of, 532t
Insulin-dependent diabetes mellitus (IDDM),
    526-527
Insulin resistance, **525**
Integument, 668
Integumentary system, 668
Interaction
    avoidance of, 57
    drug-drug, 54
    drug-food, 54, 57-58
    effects of, 57t
    See also Adverse drug reaction (ADR)
Interaction, drug-drug, **53**
Interferon, **221**, 604-605
    types of, 231
Interleukin 1 (IL-1) receptor antagonist, 660
Interleukin antagonist, 232
Interneuron, 68
Interphase, 630t
Intestinal villi, 28f
Intestine
    biotransformation in, 30-31
    drug absorption and, 26
    wall with villi, 27f
Intraarticular solution, 13
Intracellular fluid, **491**
Intracellular fluid compartment, 493
Intradermal injection, 16f
Intradermal solution, 13
Intramuscular (IM) injection, 16, 16f
Intramuscular (IM) solution, 12
Intranasal corticosteroid, 468
Intraocular hypertension, 275
Intraocular pressure (IOP), **270**
    excessive, cause of, 271
    measuring of, 272
Intrathecal solution, 13
Intraurethral pellet, administration of,
    485
Intrauterine device (IUD), **545**
    adverse reactions from, 550
    mechanism of action, 549
    types of, 549
    use and warnings of, 566
Intravascular administration, 15t
Intravenous (IV) solution, 12, 57-58
Intrinsic eye muscles, 267
Inverse agonist, **40**, **41**
Investigational New Drug (IND), 6-7
Invisible condom, 548
Ion, **491**
Ion channel
    regulation of, 131
    seizure, role in, 132f
Ionization, **21**, 26
    elimination, effect on, 34
Ionizing radiation, **625**

iPLEDGE program, 709
Irinotecan
    dosage and warnings for, 644
    overview of, 638-639
Iris, 266f, **270**
Iritis, **292**
    cause and effects of, 294
    with Rosacea Keratitis, 294f
Iron deficiency anemia, 311
Irritable bowel syndrome (IBS), **423**,
    431-433
Ischemia, 315, **317**, **372**
Ischemic heart disease, **317**
    angina and, 318
Ischemic stroke, **372**
Islets of Langerhans, 512
Isoniazid
    dosage and warnings for, 597
    dosage forms and strengths of, 594
    indications for, 593
Isosorbide dinitrate
    dosage forms and strengths of, 323
    indications for, 322
Isosorbide mononitrate
    dosage forms and strengths of, 323
    indications for, 322
Isotonic fluid, **491**, 500, 500f
Isotretinoin, 708-709
IUD (intrauterine device), **545**
    adverse reactions from, 550
    mechanism of action, 549
    types of, 549
    use and warnings of, 566

J

Jejunum, 405
Joint
    categories of, 190
    gout affecting, 257f
    rheumatoid arthritis and, 224
The Joint Commission
    "Do Not Use" list, 60t
    error avoidance, 60
Juvenile-onset diabetes mellitus, 526-527
Juxtaglomerular apparatus, 475

K

Kallman's syndrome, **545**, 559
Kefauver-Harris Amendment, 8-9
Keratin, 669
Keratinocyte, 669
Keratitis, **292**
    iritis and, 294f
    prevalence and cause of, 294
Keratoconjunctivitis, treatment for, 606
Keratolytic, **700**, 704
Keratotomy, **270**
Ketoconazole, 54
Ketolide, 596
Kidney
    anatomy of, 474f
    biotransformation in, 30-31
    blood vessels of, 474
    characteristics of, 474
    diuretics and, 337
    function, effect on elimination, 34
    function of, 475-476
    renal blood supply, drop in, 333
Killed vaccine, **649**, 650
Klinefelter's syndrome, **545**, 559

L

Labeling, improper causing medication error, 62
Labyrinth, 268, **281**
Lacrimal apparatus, 267, **270**
Lambskin condom, 548
Lamivudine (3TC)
    dosage and warnings for, 617
    dosage forms and strengths of, 612
    overview of, 611
Lamotrigine, 97
Langerhans cell, 669, 716
Large intestine
    divisions of, 405
Laryngopharyngeal reflux (LPR), **407**
    drugs used to treat, 411, 412
    H₂-receptor antagonist drugs for, 412, 417
    overview of, 408–409
    prevalence of, 408
    prokinetic drugs for, 415, 418
    proton pump inhibitor drugs for, 412–413, 418
    symptoms of, 411, 411t
Larynx
    view of, 404
Laser cyclophotocoagulation, 278
Laser peripheral iridotomy, 278
Laser surgery, 278
Laser trabeculoplasty, 278
Latex, products containing, 464b
Latex condom, **548**
Laxative, **423**
    IBS, as treatment for, 427
    polycarbophil as, 432
LDL. *See* Low-density lipoprotein (LDL)
Lea's contraceptive, 549
Lea's shield, 549
Leflunomide, 233
Left bundle branch, 315, 316f
Legend drug, **2**
    over-the-counter versus, 8–9
Letrozole, 633, 642
Leukemia, 311, **625**
Leukocyte, 308, 308f
Leukocytosis, 311
Leukopenia, 311
Leukotriene modifier
    mechanism of action, 450
    pharmacokinetics of, 450–451
    types of, 451, 456
Leukotriene pathway, 450f
Levodopa, 32
    carbidopa and, 54–55
    Parkinson's disease, as treatment of, 120–121
Levonorgestrel, 552
Levothyroxine, 519t
Lice, **730**
    infestation of, 731–732
    prevention of reinfestation, 733b
    symptoms of, 733b
    treatment of
        over-the-counter medication, 733–734, 736
        prescription medication, 734–735, 736
Lifestyle modification
    for diabetes mellitus, 530b
    gastroesophageal reflux disease and, 411b
    for gastrointestinal disorders, 425, 426t
    heart disease and, 320t
    for hypertension management, 336, 337t

Lifestyle modification *(Continued)*
    peptic ulcer disease and, 411, 411b
    stroke and myocardial infarction, 374
Lindane, 734–735
Liothyronine
    levothyroxine, comparison to, 519t
Lipid, **22**
    metabolism, insulin and, 528b
Lipid-lowering drug, 381
Lipid metabolism pathway, 381, 382
Lipophilic, **22**
Lipoprotein, **372**
Lithium, 96–97
Live, attenuated vaccine, **649**, 650
Liver
    biotransformation in, 30
    function, effect on metabolism, 33
    function of, 406
    role of, 314
    view of, 404
Loop diuretic, 339
    drug dose strengths and schedule for, 366
    for fluid and electrolyte disorders, 499, 502
Loop of Henle, 475
Loperamide, 55
Lorazepam, 81t
Lou Gehrig's disease, 209
Louse-borne relapsing fever, 732
Low back pain, 146
Low-density lipoprotein (LDL), **372**, 381
Lower esophageal sphincter
    view of, 409f
Lower esophageal sphincter (LES), 405, **407**
Lower motor neuron, **209**
    spasticity and, 210
Low-molecular-weight heparin
    indications for, 377
    mechanism of action, 378
    pharmacokinetics and adverse reactions of, 379
Loxapine, 110
Lozenges, 11
Lund-Browder chart, 692
Lung
    biotransformation in, 30–31
Lunula, 671
Luteinizing hormone-releasing hormone agonist, 633
Lymph, 574
Lymphatics, 574
Lymphatic system
    overview of, 574
Lymph node, 574
    cancer and, 629
    role of, 575
Lymphocyte, 308f, 310
Lymphoma, **625**
Lymph vessels, 574

M

Macrolides, 296
    dosage and warnings for, 595, 661
    dosage forms and strengths of, 587–588, 657
    infections, treatment for, 300
    overview of, 586–587, 657
Mafenide
    drug dosage and warnings, 696
    overview of, 695

Magnesium, **491**
    acetylcholine, effect on, 198
    for diabetes, 539
    dosage and warnings for, 503
    electrolyte replacement therapy for, 499
    role of, 492
Major depression, **86**, 87
Malathion, 735
Malignant, **625**
Malleus (hammer), 268, 268f
Mammogram, **625**
Mania, 87
Manic-depressive disorder, 87
Marijuana
    glaucoma and, 276
Mast cell, **461**
Mast cell stabilizer
    allergies, as treatment for, 466, 467
    asthma and COPD, as treatment for, 468
    pharmacokinetics and adverse reactions of, 451
    types of, 452, 456
Mastication, 405
Mastoid sinus, 190
Materia medica, **2**, 3
Mechanical barrier, 546
Mechanical digestion
    process of, 404
Mechanism of action (MOA), **40**, **41**
Medication error, **53**
    administration error, 60–62
    avoidance of, 63
    cause of, 58
    decimal point error, 59f
    dispensing error, 60–62
    improper preparation of drug, 61
    by patient, 62–63
    by prescribers, 58–59
Medicine
    history of, 3
    peptic ulcer disease and, 410
Medroxyprogesterone acetate, 633–634
Medulla oblongata
    composition of, 70
Megestrol acetate, 633, 643
Meglitinide
    diabetes and, 536
    dosage and warnings for, 541
Meiosis, 630t
Melanin, 670
Melanocyte, 669
Melanoma, **625**
Melatonin, 70, **175**
Melphalan, 47
Membranous labyrinth, 268
Memory
    brain controlling, 170f
    See also Alzheimer's disease
Memory T cell, 577
Ménière's disease, **281**
    drug dosage and warnings, 285
    treatment of, 284
    vertigo, as cause of, 283–284
Menopause, **546**, 552–553
Menorrhagia, **546**, 549
Menotropins, 560
6-mercaptopurne
    dosage and warnings for, 644
    overview of, 640–641

Metabolic enzyme
  induction and inhibition, 31t
  location of, 32
Metabolic syndrome, **332**, 334
Metabolism, **22**
  biotransformation and, 30–31
  factors influencing, 33–34
  products of, 32t
Metabolite, **22**, **30**
Metaphase, 635t
Metastasis, **625**
Metered-dose inhaler, 447
Metformin
  drug form and strengths, 535
  mechanism of action, 534
  pharmacokinetics and adverse reactions of, 535
Methicillin-resistant *Staphylococcus aureus* (MRSA), 581
Methotrexate, 232–233
  dosage and warnings for, 644, 725
  overview of, 640–641
Methoxsalen
  for atopic dermatitis and psoriasis, 722–723
  dosage and warnings for, 726
Methylprednisone, 236
Metoclopramide, 55, 418
Metric system, confusion causing medication error, 59, 60
Metronidazole
  dosage and warnings for, 597
  dosage forms and strengths of, 594
  indications for, 593
Microbial keratitis, 294
Microbial resistance, **578**
  cause of, 581
  mechanisms of, 582
Microtubule inhibitor, 630f
Micturition, 476
Midbrain, 70
Middle ear, 268, 268f
Migraine headache, **163**
  drugs used to treat, 164, 166
  pathophysiology of, 164
  prevalence and characteristics of, 164
  See also Triptans
Milia, **700**
  characteristics of, 703
Millequivalent (mEq), **491**
Minocycline, 706
Miotic, 274
Miscommunication, medication errors from, 58
Misinformation, errors from, 59
Misoprostol
  adverse reactions and precautions for, 415
  drug dosage and warnings, 418
  drug form and strengths, 416
  mechanism of action, 414
Mitomycin
  dosage and warnings for, 644
  overview of, 641–642
Mitosis, 630t
  major events of, 635t
Mitoxantrone, 230–231, 636–637
  dosage forms and strengths of, 638
Mitral valve prolapse, 315
Mitral valve stenosis, **372**
Mixed agonist/antagonist, 149, 153t

Modafinil, 182
Moniliasis
  risk factors for, 675
Monoamine neurotransmitter
  antidepressants and, 88–89
  depression and, 87
Monoamine oxidase, **86**
Monoamine oxidase inhibitor (MAOI)
  adverse reactions from, 95
  anxiety disorders and, 80
  for depression treatment, 99
  dosage forms and strengths of, 96
  food and beverages to avoid, 96t
  mechanism of action, 94, 95f
  migraine headache, treatment for, 164
  for Parkinson's disease treatment, 121
  pharmacokinetics of, 94
  precautions for, 95
Monoamine theory of depression, 87
Monoclonal antibody, 453, 456, 630f
  adverse reactions from, 659
  for breast cancer treatment, 642
  dosage and warnings for, 661
  dosage forms and strengths of, 659
  mechanism of action, 658
Monocyte, 308f, 310
Mononucleosis, 311
Montelukast, 450–451
Mood disorder, **86**
Mood stabilizer, 96
Morphine
  as natural drug, 5
Mother-to-child transmission, **601**
M phase, 630t
MRI, 629
Mucosal protectant
  mechanism of action, 413
  types of, 416, 418
Mucosal villi, 27f
Multidrug-resistant tuberculosis (MDR-TB), 581
Multiple sclerosis, **209**, **221**
  antiinflammatories and analgesics, 227
  drug dosage and warnings, 235–238
  effects of, 224f
  glucocorticosteroid as treatment for, 228
  NSAID as treatment for, 229
  overview of, 223
  spasticity, as cause of, 211
  symptoms, control of, 234t–235t
Mupirocin
  dosage and warnings for, 597
  dosage forms and strengths of, 594
  indications for, 593
Muromonab
  adverse reactions from, 659
  dosage and warnings for, 661
  dosage forms and strengths of, 659
  mechanism of action, 658
Muscarinic (M) receptor, 72, 169f
Muscle
  calcium ion, storage and release of, 212f
  of the eye, 267
  function of, 192
  types of, 190, 193f–194f
Muscle relaxant
  categorization of, 199
  indications for, 199
  mechanism of action, 199–200
Muscle spasm, 210

Muscle strain
  muscle spasm and, 212
  treatment of
    adverse effects from, 216
    central acting drugs, 215, 216–217
Muscular system, 190
Musculoskeletal system
  autoimmune diseases affecting, 222
Myasthenia gravis, **221**
  drug dosage and warnings, 235–238
  glucocorticosteroid as treatment for, 228
  neuromuscular junction and, 223f
  NSAID as treatment for, 229
  prevalence and effects of, 222
  symptoms, control of, 234t–235t
Mycophenolate mofetil, 658
  dosage and warnings for, 661
Mycoses, **672**
  See also Fungal infection
Myelin, **221**
Myelin basic protein, **221**
Myocardial infarction
  drugs used to treat, 375
  ischemia and, 318
  nonprescription drug used for, 385–387
  pathophysiology and risk factors for, 373
  prevalence of, 372
  risk factors for, 374
  stroke versus, 373t
  symptoms of, 373
Myocardial ischemia, 318
  symptoms of, 319
Myocardium, 312
Myoclonic, 130
Myoclonic seizure, **129**
Myopia, 267
Myositis, **222**
  prevalence and effects of, 222–223
Myosititis, 382

N

Naftifine
  adverse reactions from, 679
  dosage and warnings for, 683
  dosage forms and strengths of, 679
  mechanism of action and pharmacokinetics of, 678
Nail
  composition of, 671
  fungal infection of, 673
Nail bed, 671
Nail body, 671
Naloxone, 55
Narcolepsy
  characteristics of, 177
  treatment of, 182
Nasopharynx, 268, 405
Natamycin
  dosage and warnings for, 683
  overview of, 679–680
National Coordinating Council for Medication Error Reporting and Prevention
  dangerous errors, 61t
  error avoidance, 60
Natriuretic peptide, **360**
  cardiac physiology and, 361
Natural drug, 5
Natural immunity, 576
Nearsightedness, 267
Nebulizer, **443**, 447, 454, 454f

Necrosis, **317**, **372**
    ischemia and, 318
Negative feedback loop, 510
Negative symptoms, **103**, 104, **209**
    spasticity and, 210
Negative-symptom schizophrenia, 88
Nelfinavir (NFV)
    dosage and warnings for, 618
    drug form and strengths, 616
    overview of, 614-615
Neoplasm, **625**
Neovascular glaucoma, 271
Nephron, 35t, 338f, 475
Nephrotoxicity, **40**, **47**
Nerve impairment, 269
Nerve impulse, 68
Nerve root, 71
Nervous system, divisions of, 68, 69f
Neuraminidase inhibitor, 604
Neurochemistry
    of anxiety, 76
    of depression, 87-88
    of Huntington's disease, 125
    of pain, 147-148
    of Parkinson's disease, 119
    of schizophrenia, 104
    of seizures, 130-131
Neurodegeneration, **163**
    cause of, 168
Neurodegenerative, **116**
Neurohypophysis, 510
Neuroleptic, **103**
    adverse reactions from, 107
    atypical types of, 108-110
    classification of, 105-106
    mechanism of action, 106
    pharmacokinetics of, 106-107
    precautions for, 107-108
    side effects of, 107t
    typical types of, 108
Neuroleptic malignant syndrome, **103**
Neuromuscular blocking agent
    adverse reactions from, 202
    mechanism of action, 200f
    pharmacokinetics of, 201
    reversal of, 203
    safe management of, 205
    safe use of, 204, 205
    types of, 203-204, 234
Neuromuscular junction, **196**
    excitation at, 197f
    function of, **197**
    myasthenia gravis, 223f
Neuron
    disintegration of, 169f
    types of, 68
Neuropathic pain, **144**, 145
    drugs used to treat, 158, 159
    types of, 146
Neuroprotective, **163**
Neuroprotective agent, 169
Neurotensin
    schizophrenia, role in, 105
Neurotransmitter, 68, 71
    Alzheimer's disease, role in, 168-169
    depression and, 87
    gamma aminobutyric acid as, 76
    painful stimuli triggering, 146-147
    seizure, role in, 130
    serotonin as, 76

Neutrophil, 308f, 310
Nevirapine
    dosage and warnings for, 618
    overview of, 613
Nicotinic (N) receptor, 72, 169f
Nicotinic acid derivative, 385
Nigrostriatal pathways, **116**, 117
Nitrate
    adverse reactions and precautions for, 322
    angina and, 320t
    dosage forms and strengths of, 323-324
    drug dosage and warnings, 327
    mechanism of action, 321f
    pharmacokinetics of, 321-322, 323t
Nitrogenous waste, 475, 476
Nitroglycerin, 32-33
    dosage forms and strengths of, 324
    indications for, 321
    potency of, 322
Nits, **730**
    hair shaft, attached to, 731f
N-Methyl-D-Aspartate receptor inhibitor, 171
Nociceptor, **144**, 145
Nocturia, **333**
    diuretics and, 338
Nodule, **700**, 702
Noncompetitive antagonist, **40**
Nondepolarizing competitive blocker, **196**, 199
    mechanism of action, 200f
    pharmacokinetics of, 201t
    See also Neuromuscular blocking agent
Nongranular leukocyte, 308f
Non-nucleoside reverse transcriptase inhibitor (NNRTI)
    overview of, 613-614
Nonopioid analgesic, 155
    NSAIDs and aspirin, 150
    types of, 156t-158t
Non-REM sleep, **175**
Nonsteroidal antiinflammatory drug (NSAID), **145**, 150, 155
    dosage and warnings for, 236, 565
    dysmenorrhea, treatment of, 557
    gastroesophageal reflux disease and, 408
    gout, as treatment for, 258-259
    peptic ulcer disease and, 410
    thiazide diuretics and, 338
    uses for, 228-229
Nonsteroid hormone
    categories of, 509
    mechanism of action, 509
Noradrenaline-dopamine reuptake inhibitor (NA/DRI), 95, 99
Norepinephrine, 68, 511
    anxiety, role in, 76
    binding of, 71-72
    depression, role in, 88
    depression and, 87
Norton Scale, 690t
Notice of Compliance (NOC), 7
Nucleoside/nucleotide reverse transcriptase inhibitor (NRTI)
    adverse reactions from, 612
    dosage and warnings for, 617-618
    dosage forms and strengths of, 612
    role of, 610
    types of, 610-611
NutraSweet, 33
Nutrition, 33-34
Nymph, **730**, 732

Nystatin
    dosage and warnings for, 683
    overview of, 679-680

O

Obesity
    atrial fibrillation and, 392t
    cancer and, 626b, 627
    gastroesophageal reflux disease and, 408
    hyperuricemia and, 257
Obsessive-compulsive disorder (OCD), **74**, 75
Occupational allergen, 463-464
Ocular toxoplasmosis, 298
Ointment, 12
Omega-3 fatty acid, diabetes and, 540
Omission, medication errors from, 59
Onchonoceriasis, 299
Onset of action, **22**, 24f
Onychomycosis, **672**, 674
Open angle glaucoma, **270**, 271
    beta-adrenergic antagonist as treatment for, 272
    carbonic anhydrase inhibitor as treatment for, 274
Open comedone. *See* Blackhead
Ophthalmic antifungals, 299
Opiate naïve, **145**
Opioid, **145**
    classification of, 149
    comparison of, 150t
    indications for, 148
    mechanism of action, 148-149
    pharmacokinetics and adverse reactions of, 149
    reversing dependence and effects of, 153t
    side effects of, 151t
Opioid agonist, 151t-153t
Opioid analgesics, 153t-155t
Opioid antagonist, 153t
    indications for, 149
Opioid antidiarrheal
    drug form and strengths, 428
    IBS, as treatment for, 427
Opsonization, 577
Optic chiasma, 70
Optic disc, 266, 266f, **270**
Optic nerve, **270**
Oral administration. *See* Enteral
Oral candidiasis, 676f
Oral cavity, 405
Oral contraceptive
    acne, for treatment of, 710
    dosage and warnings for, 565-566
    drug form and strengths, 551-552
    mechanism of action and pharmacokinetics of, 550
    types of, 550t
Oral hypoglycemic agent (OHA), 533
Oral liquid, 11
Oral suspension, 11f
Organ of Corti, 269
Ortho-Evra, 551
Orthostatic hypotension, **333**
Oseltamivir, 604
Osmolarity, **491**
Osteoblast, 242, 243
Osteoclast, 242, 243
Osteolysis, **242**
Osteopenia, **242**, 243

Osteoporosis, **242, 546**
  antiresorptive agent as treatment for, 247
  conditions producing, 244
  drug dosage and warnings, 251-252
  drugs producing, 244b
  pathophysiology of, 243-244
  prevalence and effects of, 243
  prevention of, 245
  treatment of, 246
Otalgia, 285
Otic drops, 285, 286
Otic suspension, 11f
Otitis, **281**
Otitis externa, **292**, 302
Otitis media, **281, 292**
  antiinfectives for, 303
  prevalence and cause of, 302
  treatment for, 303
Otolith, **281**
Otorrhea, **292**
Otosclerosis, **281**, 282
Ototoxicity, **281**
Outer ear, 268
Oval window, 268, 268f
Ovary, cancer of, 627-628
Over-the-counter (OTC) drug, **2**
  legend drug versus, 8-9
  for lice and scabies treatment, 733
  for mild acne, 704-705
Ovicidal, **730**
Ovicidal drug, 733
Oxazolidinone, 588
Oxcarbazepine, 134
Oxidative stress, 392
Oxygen
  heart and, 314
  imbalance of, 319f
  P. acne destroying, 705

P

Packaging error, 62, 62f
Paget's disease
  antiresorptive agent as treatment for, 247
  drug dosage and warnings, 251-252
  pathophysiology of, 245
  prevalence of, 245
  treatment of, 246
Pain
  low back, 146
  neurochemistry of, 147-148
  neurotransmitters, triggering of, 146-147
  nondrug treatment of, 158
  opioids for treatment of, 148
  perception of, 147f
  treatment for, 234t
  types of, 145
Palpitation, 81
Pancreas, 406, 512
Pancreatic hormone, 512
Pancreatic polypeptide, 512
Panic disorder, **74**, 75
Papain
  dosage forms and strengths of, 691
  drug dosage and warnings, 696
  indications for, 690
Papillae, 405
Papillary region, 668, 670
Pap smear, **625**, 629
Pap test, **625**
Papule, **700**, 702

Paranasal sinus, 190
Paranoid schizophrenia, 104
Parasite, **730**, 731
Parasympathetic nervous system, 68
  anxiety disorders and, 75
  function of, 71, 72f
Parasympathetic system, 68
Parathyroid gland, 510-511
Parathyroid hormone analogue, 250-251, 252
Parenteral, **3**
  advantages and disadvantages of, 15-16,
    15-16
  dosage forms for, 12-13
  typical containers for, 14f
Parietal cell, 405
Parietal layer, 311, 312f
Parkinson's disease, **116, 117**
  acetylcholine and dopamine levels in, 118,
    118f
  adverse reactions from treatment, 121
  carpidopa and levodopa, 54-55
  cholinergic activity, drugs reducing, 123
  comparison of drugs for, 122t
  dopamine, drugs affecting level of, 124
  dopamine and, 42
  drugs used to treat, 120
  mechanism of action, 120
  neurochemistry of, 119
  pharmacokinetics of, 120-121
  prevalence and cause of, 118
  signs of, 117f, 119
Parotid gland, 404, 405
Paroxetine, 80t
Partial agonist, **40**, 42
Partial-thickness burn, 692, 694f
Partial thromboplastin time (PTT), **372**
Passive transport, 25
Patch, transdermal, 12, 13f
Patent Restoration Act, 9
Pathophysiology, **14, 22, 41**
Patient-controlled analgesia (PCA), **145**
PCA (patient-controlled analgesia), **145**
Peak effect, **22**, 24f
Peak flowmeter, **443**
Pediculicide, **730**, 733
Pediculus humanus capitis, 731
Pediculus humanus corporis, 732
Pelvic inflammatory disease (PID), **546**, 558
Pemetrexed, 640-641, 644
Penciclovir, 606
Penicillamine, 233
Penicillin, 54
  dosage and warnings for, 596
  dosage forms and strengths of, 589-591
  overview of, 588-589
  resistance to, 581
  types of, 303
Penis
  intracavernosal injection, administration of,
    486
  intraurethral pellets, administration of, 485
  relaxing muscle of, 483b
  structure of, 485f
  See also Erectile dysfunction
Pentostatin, 640-641
Pepsin, 408
Peptic ulcer disease (PUD), **407**
  antacids for, 416
  antimicrobials for, 417, 419
  drugs used to treat, 411, 412

Peptic ulcer disease *(Continued)*
  H_2-receptor antagonist drugs for, 412, 417
  lifestyle modifications for, 411b
  mucosal protectants for, 413, 415, 418
  prevalence of, 408
  proton pump inhibitor drugs for, 412-413,
    418
  risk factors for, 409-410
  symptoms of, 411, 411t
Pericardial fluid, 311
Pericarditis, 315
Pericardium, 311, 312f
Perilymph, 269
Perinatal mother-to-child transmission
  (PMTCT)
  guidelines for, 611t
  of HIV, 611-612
Perinatal transmission, **601**
Periodic leg movements, 177
Peripheral acting muscle relaxant, **196**
  classification of, 199
  spasticity, as treatment for, 213
Peripheral nervous system (PNS), 68, 71
Peripheral vascular disease, 315
Peripheral vascular resistance, **333**, 334
Peripheral vision, **270**, 271
Peristalsis, **407**, 408
  cause of, 195
  drugs impairing, 408
Permethrins
  dosage forms and strengths of, 734
  indications for, 733
  mechanism of action and adverse reactions
    from, 734
Pernicious anemia, 311
Petit mal seizure, **129**, 130
PET scan. *See* Positron emission tomography
  (PET) scan, 629
pH
  drug absorption, effect on, 25-26
Phantom limb, 146
Pharmaceutical alternative, **22**, 37
Pharmaceutical equivalent, **22**, 37
Pharmaceutical phase, 23f
Pharmacodynamic phase, 23f
Pharmacodynamics, **40, 41**
Pharmacognosy, **3**, 5
Pharmacokinetic phase, 22, 23f, 24-26
Pharmacokinetics, **22**
Pharmacological class, 7
Pharmacology, 5
  definition of, **3**
  importance of study, 54
  timeline of, 4
Pharmacotherapeutics, **40**, 45-47
Pharmacotherapy, **3**
Pharmacy technician
  cold chain, role in, 652, 652f
  pharmacology knowledge of, 3
Pharynx, 404, 405
Phenobarbital, 31, 136
Phenothiazine, 106, 107, 108, 111
Phenylalanine, 33
Phenylketonuria (PKU), 33, **209**
Phenytoin, 33
  adverse reactions from, 133
  arrhythmia, as treatment for, 396
  mechanism of action, 132
  pharmacokinetics of, 132-133
Phlebitis, 316

Phobia, 74, 75
Phosphodiesterase inhibitors
 adverse reactions and precautions for, 484
 mechanism of action and pharmacokinetics of, 483
 types of, 484
Phosphorus
 content of, 499t
 electrolyte replacement therapy for, 498
 role of, 492
Photopsia, 292, 297
Photosensitivity, 333, 338
Phototherapy, 715
Phthirus pubis, 732
Physostigmine (P)
 mechanism of action, 200f
Pigment, in urine, 476
Pilosebaceous unit (PSU), 700
 normal, 701f
 open comedone, 702f
Pimecrolimus
 drug dosage and warnings, 725
 indications for, 721
Pimple. *See* Pustule
Pineal gland, 70
Pink eye. *See* Conjunctivitis
Pinna, 268, 268f
Piperonyl butoxide, 733
Pituitary gland
 hormones of, 511
 parts of, 510
Placebo effect, 46
Plant
 medicinal use of, 3
Plaque, 163, 222, 317, 372
 build-up of, 318f
 embolic stroke and, 372
 multiple sclerosis and, 223
Plasma, 308
Plasma membrane, 24f
Plasma protein, 29
Plasticity, 145, 146
Platelet, 308, 308f, 310
Platelets, 372
Platinum compounds
 dosage and warnings for, 644
 overview of, 639
Pneumonia, 692
Polycystic ovary disease, 546, 559
Polycythemia, 311
Polyene
 dosage and warnings for, 683
 overview of, 679–680
Polymyositis, 222
Polyp, 625, 629
Polypeptide cell, 512
Polyurethane condom, 548
Pons, 70
Positive inotropic effect, 360, 364
Positive symptoms, 103, 104, 209
 spasticity and, 210
Positron emission tomography (PET) scan, 625, 629
Posterior pituitary gland, 510
Postprandial, 525
Postsynaptic adrenergic blockade, 91
Postsynaptic neuron, 68
Post-traumatic stress disorder (PTSD), 74, 76
Postural hypotension, 103

Potassium, 491
 content of, 499t
 dosage and warnings for, 502, 503
 electrolyte replacement therapy for, 498
 role of, 492
Potassium hydroxide (KOH) stain, 673, 673f
Potassium-sparing diuretic, 339–340
Potency, 40, 43–44, 44f
Potentiation, 53, 54–55
Povidone-iodine
 adverse effects from, 695
 drug dosage and warnings, 696
 fungal infection, as treatment for, 681–682
Prediabetes, 525, 526
Prednisone, 236
Preeclampsia, 333, 335
Pregnancy, 546
 drug safety categories for, 30, 30t
 gastroesophageal reflux disease and, 408
 multiple births, prevalence of, 561
 pharmacotherapeutics, effect on, 46
 physiological changes during, 547t
 prevention methods, 546
 symptoms of, 546
 teratogenic effects on, 47
 warfarin and, 379
Prehypertension, 333, 335
Premenstrual dysphoric disorder, 546
 SSRI as treatment for, 555, 565
 symptoms of, 555
Premenstrual syndrome (PMS), 546
 symptoms of, 555
Presbycusis, 269, 281
Presbyopia, 267
Prescription Drug Users Fees Act, 7
Pressure sore. *See* Decubitus ulcer
Presynaptic neuron, 68
Primary amenorrhea, 557
Primary dysmenorrhea, 555
Primary tumor, 625
Probenecid, 259
Procainamide, 394
Prodrug, 22, 32
Progesterone-receptor positive breast cancer, 631
Progestin
 for breast cancer treatment, 633
 dosage and warnings for, 643
 products, examples of, 554t
Prokinetic drug, 55
 indications and adverse effects of, 415
 metoclopramide as, 418
Prolactinoma, 546, 559
Prophase, 635t
Propionibacterium acnes (P. acnes), 701–702
Proprietary name drug, 8
 See also Brand name
Prostaglandin, 228–229
 adverse reactions from, 485
 alprostadil as, 486
 mechanism of action and pharmacokinetics of, 484
 as tissue hormone, 510
Prostaglandin analog, 276
 types of, 278
Prostate cancer, 629
Prostate gland, 477
 normal versus enlarged, 478f
 role of, 478
Prostate-specific antigen (PSA), 477

Prostate-specific antigen (PSA) test, 477–478, 625
 indications for, 479
Prostatitis, 478
 symptoms of, 478
Protease inhibitor
 adverse reactions from, 615
 dosage and warnings for, 618–619
 drug form and strengths, 615–616
 role of, 614
 types of, 614–615
Protein
 metabolism, insulin and, 528b
 neurotransmitters as, 68
Protein binding
 distribution, effect on, 29
 drug interactions and, 56
 free faction of drugs, 29f
Protein synthesis, 630t
Prothrombin time (PT), 372
Pro-Time, INR, 372
Proton pump inhibitor drug
 mechanism of action, 412
 pharmacokinetics and adverse reactions of, 413
 types of, 414–415, 418
Proximal tubule, 475
Pseudonatremia, 494
Pseudoparkinsonism, 103, 116, 119
Psoriasis, 715
 characteristics of, 716
 factors exacerbating, 717
 nonpharmaceutical treatment of, 718
 pharmaceutical treatment of, 718
Psoriatic blepharitis, 293
Psychogenic polydipsia, 494
Psychomotor seizure, 130
Psychosis, 103
 drugs used to treat, 105–106, 111–112
 neuroleptics as treatment for, 105–106
Psychotherapy
 anxiety, as treatment for, 76
Pubic lice
 infestation of, 732
 view of, 732f
Pulmonary semilunar valve, 312
Pupil, 266, 266f
 constriction of, 267
Pure Food and Drug Act, 5
 role of, 8
Purine
 beer, levels in, 258
 food, content in, 260, 261b
 metabolism of, 257
Purine antimetabolite
 overview of, 640–641
Pustule (pimple), 700, 702
Pyloric sphincter, 405
Pylorus, 405
Pyrethrins
 dosage forms and strengths of, 734
 indications for, 733
 mechanism of action and adverse reactions from, 734

Q

Quetiapine, 110
Quinidine
 mechanism of action and precautions of, 394

Quinolones, 296
  infections, treatment for, 300

R

Radiation therapy, **625**
Radioactive iodine, 517–518
Radioactive iodine uptake (RAIU), **514**, 516
Radionuclide scan, **625**, 629
Radon, **625**
Raloxifene, 248
Range-of-motion exercise, 689
Rapid eye movement (REM), 176
Rapid-onset formulation, 16
Rasagiline, 121
Raynaud disease, 316
Reaction, idiosyncratic, **40**
Rebound hypersomnia, **175**, 177
Receptor site, **40**, 41
Rectal suspension, 11f
Rectum, 404, 405
Red blood cell, 308, 308f
  disorders of, 311
  formation of, 309
Referred pain, 145
Reflux, **407**, 408
Refraction, 267
Refractory period, **391**, 392
Rehabilitation, 695
Remission, **715**
Remodeling, **242**
  process of, 243–244, 243f
REM sleep, **175**
  necessity of, 176
Renal cortex, 474, 474f
Renal medulla, 474, 474f
Renal pelvis, 474, 474f
Renal pyramid, 474, 474f
Renin-aldosterone-angiotensin system (RAAS), **333**, 334f
  activation of, 361
Repeat-action tablet, 10
Repolarization, **391**, 392
Reproductive system
  drugs that affect, 565
  infection/inflammation, disorders caused by, 558
Resorption, **242**
Respiratory syncytial virus (RSV)
  treatment of, 606
Respiratory tract administration
  dosage forms for, 14
  inhaler, proper use of, 14f
Restless leg syndrome, 177
Reticular formation, 70
Reticular region, 668, 670
Retina, 266, 266f
Retinoid
  acne, for treatment of, 706
Rh$_0$ immune globulin
  adverse reactions from, 660
  dosage and warnings for, 662
  dosage forms and strengths of, 660
  mechanism of action and pharmacokinetics of, 659
Rhabdomyolysis, **372**
Rheumatic heart disease, 315
Rheumatoid arthritis, **222**
  drug dosage and warnings, 235–238
  glucocorticosteroid as treatment for, 228
  methotrexate as treatment for, 640–641

Rheumatoid arthritis *(Continued)*
  NSAID as treatment for, 229
  pathogenesis of
    cytokine network in, 226f
  phases of, 224
  prevalence of, 223–224
  symptoms, control of, 234t–235t
Rheumatoid factor, **222**, 224
Rh factor, 310
Ribavirin
  indications for, 606
Ribonucleic acid. *See* RNA
Ribosomal target, modification of, 582
Ribs, 190
Right bundle branch, 315, 316f
Rimantadine, 603–604
Ringworm, **672**, 673
Risperidone, 109, 112
Ritonavir (RTV)
  dosage and warnings for, 619
  drug form and strengths, 616
  overview of, 615
RNA (ribonucleic acid)
  replication, inhibition of
    mechanism of action and
      pharmacokinetics of, 605–606
Rod, 266
Rosacea keratitis, 294f
Rugae, 405, 475
Rules of nines, **687**, 692
Rules of palms, **687**, 692

S

Saccule, 268, **281**
Salicylate, 410
Salicylic acid, 704
Salivary glands, 405
Salpingitis, **546**, 558
Saquinavir (SQV)
  dosage and warnings for, 619
  drug form and strengths, 616
  overview of, 615
Sarcomere, **209**, **210**
Sarcoptes scabei, 732
Sassafras tea, 47
Scabicide, **730**
Scabies, **730**
  prevalence of, 732
  prevention of reinfestation, 733b
  sites of infestation, 733
  symptoms of, 733b
  treatment of
    over-the-counter medication, 733–734, 736
    prescription medication, 734–735, 736
Scar
  from acne, 701
  from burns, 692
  prevention of, 695
Schizophrenia, 88, **103**
  drugs used to treat, 105–106
  neurochemistry of, 104
  prevalence and cause of, 104
Sclera, 266, 266f
Seasonal allergic rhinitis (SAR), 462
Sebaceous glands, 671
Sebum, 671
Secondary amenorrhea, 557
Secondary dysmenorrhea, 556
Second-degree burn, **687**, 692, 694f

Second-generation antidepressant, 95–96
Second messenger, 41, 509
Secretory gland
  types of, 510–512
Sedation, Barbiturates and, 178
Sedative, **175**
Sedative-hypnotic, 177–178
Seizure
  classification of, 130, 131f
  drugs used to treat, 131–132, 138–141
  ion channel regulation, 131
  neurochemistry of, 130–131
Seizure threshold, **129**, 130
Selective estrogen receptor modulator (SERM), 248, 251
  for breast cancer, 631
  dosage and warnings for, 642
Selective serotonin reuptake inhibitor (SSRI)
  anxiety disorders and, 80
  comparison of, 93
  depression and, 93, 99
  dosage and warnings for, 565
  dosage forms and strengths of, 94
  PMDD, treatment of, 555
Selegiline, 121, 122f
Semen, **478**
Semicircular canal, 268–269, 268f
Semilunar valve, 312
Serotonin (5-HT)
  anxiety, role in, 76
  depression and, 87, 88
  inflammatory bowel syndrome, 425
  pain, role in, 147
  schizophrenia, role in, 105
Serotonin-noradrenaline reuptake inhibitor (SNRI), 95, 99
  migraine headache, treatment for, 164
Serotonin receptor antagonist
  IBS, as treatment for, 426
  types of, 431
Serotonin syndrome, 80t, **86**
Serous pericardium, 311
Sertraline, 80, 80t
Serum calcium, 243–244
Serum urate
  levels of, 257
Sexually transmitted infection (STI)
  cause of, 558
  pubic lice as, 732
  treatment of, 558–559
Shingles, **145**, 146
Shingles, treatment for, 605
Sigmoidoscopy
  view of, 424f
Sildenafil, 483, 483f
Silver nitrate
  drug dosage and warnings, 696
  overview of, 695
Silver sulfadiazine
  dosage forms and strengths of, 695
  drug dosage and warnings, 696
  overview of, 694
Simple focal seizure, **129**
Sinoatrial node (SA node), 315, 316f
Sinus cavity, 190
Skeletal muscle
  contraction of, 197
  function of, 195
  relaxant, categorization of, 199, 215
  types of, 190

Skeleton, 190, 191f-192f
Skin
    appendages of, 671
    classification of, 668
    color of, 670
    function of, 670
    fungal infection of, 673
    structure of, 668f
    See also Burn; Decubitus ulcer
Skin cancer
    prevalence and mortality rate of, 628
    signs of, 628b
Skin care
    eczema and, 718b
Skin glands, 671
Skin infection, 692
Skull, fetal, 190
Sleep
    cycle of, 176f
    overview of, 176-177
Sleep apnea, 177
Sleep deprivation, 177
Sleep disorder
    prevalence and types of, 177
    treatment of, 177
Slow-onset formulation, 16
Small intestine
    divisions of, 405
    drug absorption and, 26
Small-molecule transmitter
    chemical classes of, 68
Smoking
    cancer and, 626, 626b
    metabolic enzymes, effect on, 33
    peptic ulcer disease and, 411
Smooth muscle
    function of, 195
    types of, 190
Social phobia, 75
Sodium, **491**
    content of, 499t
    dosage and warnings for, 502
    electrolyte replacement therapy for, 497
    role of, 492
Sodium sulfacetamide, 704-705
Soft palate, 405
Soft spot, 190
Soleplate, **197**
    composition of, 198
Somatic nervous system (SNS), 68
    composition of, 71
    drugs used to affect, 73
Somatostatin, 512
Sonogram, **625**, 629
Sotalol, 394
Sound, 283
Spacer, **443**, 454, 454f
Spasticity, **209**
    conditions producing, 210-212
    neurotransmitters involved in, 212
    overview of, 210
    pathophysiology of, 210
    treatment of, 235t
        central acting drugs, 214
        central acting muscle relaxants,
            216-217
        direct acting muscle relaxants, 217
        peripheral acting drugs, 213
Specific immunity, 576
Spermicide, 546

Sphygmomanometer, 333
Spider, black widow, 198
Spinal cord, 71
    injury causing spasticity, 210
    stroke and, 210
Spinal nerve, 71
Spirometry, **443**
Spironolactone, 340-341
Spleen
    function of, 575
    view of, 404
Stable angina, 319
Stage, **625**
Stapes (stirrup), 268, 268f
Statin
    adverse reactions from, 382
    mechanism of action, 381
    types of, 382-383
Status epilepticus, **129**, 130
Stavudine (d4T)
    dosage and warnings for, 617
    dosage forms and strengths of, 612
    overview of, 611
Stem cell, **625**
Stem cell transplantation, **625**
Stenosis, **372**
Sternum, 190
Steroid hormone
    classification of, 509
    mechanism of action, 509
Stimulant, **175**
Stirrup (stapes), 268, 268f
Stoke volume, **360**
Stomach, 404, 405
Stomach cancer, 408
Strata, 669
Stratum basale, 668, 669
Stratum corneum, 669
Stratum granulosum, 668, 669
Stratum lucidum, 668, 669
Stratum spinosum, 668, 669
Streptococcal infection, 315
Stress, angina and, 318
Stroke
    atrial fibrillation and, 374, 392
    drugs used to treat, 375
    ischemia and, 318
    myocardial infarction versus, 373t
    nonprescription drug used for, 385-387
    pathophysiology and risk factors for, 373
    prevalence of, 372
    risk factors for, 374
    seizure, as cause of, 130
    spasticity, as cause of, 210
    symptoms of, 373, 373t
    types of, 372-373
Stye, **292**
    cause of, 294
    treatment of, 295
    view of, 295f
Subcutaneous (SC) injection, 16, 16f
Subcutaneous (SC) solution/suspension, 13
Subcutaneous layer, 670
Sublingual gland, 405
    view of, 404
Sublingual tablet, 11
Submandibular gland, 404, 405
Substance P, **145**, 147
Substantia nigra, **116**
Succinimide, 135-136, 140

Succinylcholine (S), 200f
Sucralfate
    drug dosage and warnings, 418
    drug form and strengths, 416
    indications and adverse effects of, 415
Sudden sensory hearing loss (SSHL), 282
Sudoriferous glands, 671
Sugar-coated tablet, 11
Sulfasalazine, 233
Sulfonamide, 56
    for bacterial infections, 296, 581
    dosage and warnings for, 596
    dosage forms and strengths of, 592
    infections, treatment for, 300
    overview of, 591
    types of, 303
Sulfonylureas
    dosage and warnings for, 540
    mechanism of action and
        pharmacokinetics of, 533-534
    types of, 534
Sulfur-resorcinol, 704
Sunburn, 692
Superficial fascia, 670
Superior vena cava, 313f
Suppository, 12, 12f
Suppressor T cell, 577
Supraovulation, **546**, 560
Supraventricular tachycardia, **391**, 393
Suspension, 11, 11f
Sustained-release tablet, 11
Sweat glands, 671
Swimmer's ear, 285-286
Sympathetic nervous system, 68
    anxiety disorders and, 75
    function of, 71, 72f
Sympathetic system, 68
Sympathomimetic, **175**
Sympathomimetics, 182
Synapse, 68
Synarthroses joint, 190
Synergistic effect, **53**, 54
Synovial joint, 225f
Synovium, **222**, 224
Synthetic drug, 5
Syrup, 12
Systemic circulation, 314
Systemic lupus erythematosus, **222**
    antimalarials as treatment for, 230
    drug dosage and warnings, 235-238
    effects of, 225
    glucocorticosteroid as treatment for, 228
    NSAID as treatment for, 229
    prevalence and triggers of, 224
    symptoms, control of, 234t-235t
Systolic blood pressure, 333
Systolic heart failure (SHF), 361

T

T_4 test, **514**, 516
Tablet, types of, 10-11, 10f
Tacrolimus
    drug dosage and warnings, 725
    indications for, 721
Tamoxifen
    dosage and warnings for, 642
    dosage forms and strengths of, 631
Tangles, **163**, 169f
Tardive dyskinesia, **103**, 107
Target cell, 510

Taste bud, 405
Taxane
    adverse reactions from, 635
    dosage and warnings for, 643
    dosage forms and strengths of, 636
    mechanism of action, 634
Tazarotene, 707
T cell, 577
Tear deficiency, 267
Tegaserod, 426-427
Telophase, 635t
Temporal lobe seizure, 130
Teniposide
    dosage and warnings for, 644
    overview of, 638-639
Tenofovir (TDF)
    dosage and warnings for, 617
    dosage forms and strengths of, 612
    overview of, 611
Tension headache, 146
Teratogenicity, 47
Terbinafine
    adverse reactions from, 679
    dosage and warnings for, 683
    dosage forms and strengths of, 679
    mechanism of action and
        pharmacokinetics of, 678
Tetanus, **197**
    indications for, 199
Tetrabenazine, 125, 126
Tetracycline, 54
    acne, for treatment of, 706
    dosage and warnings for, 597
    indications for, 593
    overview of, 592
Tetraiodothyronine (T_4), **514**, 515
Thalamus, 70
Theophratus, 3
Theophylline, 33
    pharmacokinetics of, 452
    serum blood levels, modification of, 452b
Therapeutic alternative, **22**, 37
Therapeutic duplication, **53**, 59
Therapeutic effect, 24f
Therapeutic index (TI), **40**, 44-45
    of benzodiazepines, 78
Thiazide diuretic
    adverse reactions and precautions for,
        338
    dosage forms and strengths of, 339
    drug dose strengths and schedule for, 366
    pharmacokinetics of, 337
Thiazolidinedione
    diabetes and, 536-537
    dosage and warnings for, 541
Thienobenzodiazepine, 109, 112
Thioamide, 518
Thiocarbamates
    dosage and warnings for, 683
    overview of, 680
6-thioguanine
    dosage and warnings for, 644
    overview of, 640-641
Thioxanthene, 106, 108, 111
Third-degree burn, **687**, 692, 694f
Third-generation antidepressant, 95-96
Thrombocyte, 308, 308f
Thrombocytopenia, 311
Thrombolytic, **372**
    mechanism of action, 379-380

Thrombolytic *(Continued)*
    pharmacokinetics and adverse reactions of,
        380-381
    sources of, 380t
    types of, 381, 386
Thrombophlebitis, 316
Thrombopoiesis, 310
Thrombosis, **372**
    formation of, 318
Thrombotic stroke, **372**, 372
Thrombus, **317**, 372
Thrush, 675, 676f
Thymus gland, 575
Thyroid antibody test, **514**, 516
Thyroid disorder
    diagnosis of, 515-517
    drugs used to treat, 521
    prevalence and risk factors for, 515
    types of, 517
Thyroid gland, 510
    TSH and T_4, comparison of, 516f
Thyroid hormone
    control and synthesis of, 515
    medication interacting with, 520, 520b
    physiological actions of, 515b
    structural formula for, 516f
Thyroid-releasing factor (TRF), **514**, 515
Thyroid replacement therapy, 520
Thyroid-stimulating hormone (TSH), **514**, 515
Ticlopidine
    drug dosage and warnings, 386
    mechanism of action, 376
Time-release tablet, 11
Tincture, 12
Tinea capitis, 674, 675f
Tinea corporis, 674, 675f
Tinea manus, 674
Tinea pedis. *See* Athlete's foot
Tinea unguium, 674
Tinnitus, **281**, 283
    quinidine toxicity, as sign of, 394
Tipranavir
    dosage and warnings for, 619
    drug form and strengths, 616
    overview of, 615
Tissue plasminogen activator (t-PA), **372**
T-lymphocyte, 310
    allergen, response to, 462, 462f
Tolcapone, 121
Tolerance, 47, **74**
    of Barbiturates, 178
    of benzodiazepines, 78
    of nitrates, 322
Tolnaftate
    dosage and warnings for, 683
    overview of, 680
Tonic-clonic (grand mal) seizure, **129**, 130
Tonometer, 272
Tonometry, **270**, 272
Topical administration
    ointments and transdermal patches, 12
    side effects of, 17
    suppository shapes, 12f
Topical antibacterials
    burns, for treatment of, 696
    decubitus ulcer, for treatment of, 691
Topical antiinfective, 302
Topical corticosteroid
    dosage forms and strengths of, 719-721
    drug dosage and warnings, 724-725

Topical corticosteroid *(Continued)*
    eczema and psoriasis, as treatment for, 718
    potency classification of, 719b
Topical ophthalmics, 295-297
Topoisomerase inhibitor
    adverse reactions from, 639
    dosage and warnings for, 644
    dosage forms and strengths of, 639
    mechanism of action and
        pharmacokinetics of, 638
    site of action, 638f
Topotecan
    dosage and warnings for, 644
    overview of, 638-639
Torimefene
    dosage and warnings for, 642
    dosage forms and strengths of, 631
Toxicity, Barbiturates and, 178
Toxic megacolon, **423**
Toxicology, **3**
Toxic shock syndrome (TSS), **546**
    diaphragms causing, 548
Toxin, in urine, 476
Toxocariasis, 299
Toxoid vaccine, **649**, 650
Toxoplasmosis, 298
Trabecular meshwork, **270**, 271
Trachea, 404
Transcription
    inaccuracy of, 61
    inhibitors of, 604-605
Transcutaneous nerve stimulation unit, 160f
Transdermal administration, 16
Transdermal drug delivery system (patch),
    12, 13f
Transdermal patch, 13f, 322
Transfusion reaction, 310
Transient ischemic attack (TIA), **372**, 373
Transverse colon, 404
Trastuzumab, 642
Trauma, 146
Trazodone, 96
Tretinoin, 706-707
Triamterene, 340
Triazolam, 54
Triazoles
    dosage and warnings for, 682-683
    dosage forms and strengths of, 677-678
    fungal infection, as treatment for, 677
Tricuspid valve, 312, 313f
Tricyclic antidepressant (TCA)
    adverse reactions of, 91f
    anxiety disorders and, 80
    comparison of, 91-92
    for depression treatment, 89, 98
    dosage forms and strengths of, 92
    mechanism of action, 89-90, 91f
    pharmacokinetics of, 90-91
    precautions for, 92
    three-ring structure of, 90f
Trifluridine, 606
Trigeminal neuralgia, **145**, 146
Trigger, **222**
    for acne flareups, 703b
    for allergic response, 462-463
    for asthmatic episode, 445b, 446b
    for hearing and balance, 268
    types of, 222
Triglyceride, **372**, **525**
Triiodothyronine (T_3), **514**, 515

Triptans
    comparison of, 166
    drugs used to treat, 167
    mechanism of action, 165f
    migraine headache, treatment for, 164-165
Troches, 11
Trypsin
    dosage forms and strengths of, 691
    drug dosage and warnings, 696
    indications for, 690
TSH test, **514**, 515
Tubal ligation, 546
Tubular reabsorption, 476
Tubular secretion, 476
Tumor, **625**
Tumor marker, **625**
Tumor necrosis factor, **222**, 232, **478**
Tumor necrosis factor inhibitor
    dosage and warnings for, 726
    etanercept and, 660, 723
    psoriasis, as treatment for, 723
Turner's syndrome, **546**, 559
Tympanic cavity, 268
Tympanic membrane, 268, 268f, **281**
Type 1 diabetes, **525**, 526
Type 2 diabetes, **525**, 527-528
Typhus, 732

U

Ulcer, **407**, **423**
Ulcerative colitis, **423**
    aminosalicylates for, 428-429
    cause of, 425
    diagnostic testing for, 424
    drugs used to treat, 431-433
    lifestyle modifications for, 425, 426t
    symptoms of, 424t
Undecylenic acid, 681, 682
United States Phamacopoeia, 7
Unstable angina, 319
Upper esophageal sphincter (UES), 405, **407**
Upper motor neuron, **209**, 212
Urates, **256**, **257**
Urea
    dosage forms and strengths of, 691
    drug dosage and warnings, 696
    indications for, 690
Ureter, 474, 475
Urethra, 474, 475
Urgency, **478**
Uric acid
    clearance of, 259
    synthesis, inhibitors of, 259-260
Uricosuric, **256**, 259
Urinalysis, **478**
Urinary bladder, 474, 475
Urinary system, 474
Urinary tract infection, 548
Urine
    composition of, 476
    volume, regulation of, 476
Urticaria, **461**, 463
Utricle, 268, **281**
Uveitis, **292**, 295
UV radiation, 670
Uvula, 405

V

Vaccine, **649**
    dosage forms and strengths of, 654-656
    refrigeration of, 650b
    types of, 650
Vaginitis, **546**, 558
Valacyclovir
    adverse reactions from, 606
    mechanism of action and
        pharmacokinetics of, 605-606
Valproate, 133-134, 139
Valproic acid, 97
Vancomycin-resistant enterococci (VRE), 581
Variant angina, 320
Varicella zoster virus (VZV), 605
Varicose vein, 316
Vascular headache. *See* Migraine headache
Vascular layer, 266
Vasectomy, 546
Vasodilator
    drug dose strengths and schedule for, 366
    indications for, 366
Vasodilator, direct, 350-351, 355
Vasospasm, **317**
Vasospastic angina, 320
Vein, 313
Venlafaxine, 96
Ventricle, 312, 312f
Ventricular arrhythmia, 365
Ventricular fibrillation, **391**, 393
Ventricular tachycardia, **391**, 393
Vertebral column, 190
Vertigo, **281**
    cause of, 283
    drug dosage and warnings, 285
    treatment of, 284
Very-low-density lipoprotein (VLDL), 384
Vestibule, 268, 268f
Villi, 27f, 405
Vinblastine
    dosage and warnings for, 644
    dosage forms and strengths of, 636
Vinca alkaloid
    for breast cancer, 636
    dosage and warnings for, 644
Vincristine
    dosage and warnings for, 644
    dosage forms and strengths of, 636
Vinorelbine
    dosage and warnings for, 644
    dosage forms and strengths of, 636
Viral conjunctivitis, 294f
Viral infection
    cancer and, 626b, 627
    drug dosage and warnings, 298
    of the eye, 297
    treatment for, 300-301
Viral load, **601**
    in HIV/AIDS, 609
Viral replication
    antiviral role in, 603
    in host cell, 602f
Viral resistance, 603
Viral undercoating, inhibitors of, 603-604
Virion, **602**, 602f
Virostatic, **602**

Virus, **602**
Visceral layer, 311, 312f
Vision
    process of, 267
    role of, 266
    See also Glaucoma
Vitamin A, 670, 706
Vitamin D analog
    adverse reactions from, 722
    dosage and warnings for, 725
    dosage forms and strengths of, 722
    mechanism of action and
        pharmacokinetics of, 721
Vitamin K, 55, 378
Vitreous humor, 267
Voluntary Reporting Form 3500, 49f
Vulvovaginal candidiasis, **672**
    risk factors for, 675, 676b
    signs of, 676b

W

Warfarin, 33
    aspirin and, 54
    indications for, 378
    overdose of, 379
    as protein bound, 56
    vitamin K and, 55, 378
Water-clogged ear, 285-286
Water intoxication, 494-495
Weak acid, 25-26, 26f, 55
Weak base, 25-26, 26f, 55
Weight, 45
Wheal, **461**
White blood cell, 308, 308f
    disorders of, 311
    types of, 310
White coat hypertension, 336
Whitehead (closed comedone), **700**, 702
White matter, 70
Wound
    debridement of, 690
    stages of, 688-689

X

Xanthine derivative, 452, 453
    types of, 456

Y

Yeast, 673
Yeast infection, 675
Yeast vaginitis, 675

Z

Zafirlukast, 450-451
Zanamivir, 604
Zero, misuse causing medication error, 58
Zidovudine (AZT)
    dosage and warnings for, 617
    dosage forms and strengths of, 612
    overview of, 611
Zileuton, 451
Ziprasidone, 110